Tabbner's Nursing Care:

Theory and Practice

Jacqueline Ormsby Chandler RN RM DNE FRCNA has almost 30 years nursing experience in Victoria, England, and Canada. Her particular area of interest is in nurse education, and she has spent 18 years involved in teaching enrolled nurse students. She was a member of the Panel of Examiners for Enrolled Nurse Examinations conducted by the Victorian Nursing Council from 1974–1987.

Tabbner's Nursing Care:
Theory and Practice

Jackie Chandler RN RM DNE FRCNA

Foreword by

Michael Drake MBBS FRCPA FRCPath FRACP FIAC
Consultant Pathologist, Prince Henry's Hospital and Victorian
Cytology (Gynaecological) Service
Chairman, Committee of Management, Melbourne School for Enrolled
Nurses

SECOND EDITION

CHURCHILL LIVINGSTONE
MELBOURNE MADRID EDINBURGH LONDON NEW YORK AND TOKYO 1991

CHURCHILL LIVINGSTONE
Medical Division of Longman Group UK Limited

Distributed in Australia by Longman Cheshire Pty Limited,
Longman House, Kings Gardens, 95 Coventry Street, South
Melbourne 3205, and by associated companies, branches and
representatives throughout the world.

First edition 1981
Second edition 1991
  Reprinted 1992

ISBN 0-443-04030-3

British Library Cataloguing in Publication Data. A catalogue record for
this book is available form the British Library.

Produced by Longman Singapore Publishers (Pte) Ltd.
Printed in Singapore

Foreword

The Melbourne School for Enrolled Nurses is justifiably proud of its record in the publication of books designed specifically to meet the needs of the State Enrolled Nurse. As early as 1961 a *Handbook for Nursing Aides* was published, this book being revised on a number of occasions, the thirteenth and last edition being published in 1978. At that time it had become apparent that, valuable though this book was, it was inadequate to meet the needs of the State Enrolled Nurse. Accordingly it was decided to produce an entirely new book. The task was undertaken by Miss A. R. Tabbner, a former Principal Teacher of the School, who worked in collaboration with the School's editorial committee. These efforts led to the publication, in 1981, of the first edition of *Nursing Care: Theory and Practice*. The book was an immediate success and is now used throughout the world by many thousands of nurses, both state enrolled and general.

In the decade that has elapsed since the publication of the first edition there have been further major advances in medical technology and nursing care. To assist the nurse in meeting these new challenges this second edition of *Tabbner's Nursing Care: Theory and Practice* has been produced. In producing this second edition much of the original text has been completely re-written. The author, Ms J. O. Chandler, has worked closely with the current members of the School's editorial committee to produce a book that reflects most comprehensively recent advances in medical knowledge and nursing care. The book has been expanded greatly and a considerable quantity of new material has been introduced. There is no doubt that this second edition will provide the nurse, both state enrolled and general, with the knowledge necessary to meet their expanded roles in the health care team. All those connected with the Melbourne School for Enrolled Nurses are proud to be associated with this new edition, which is commended to all members of the nursing profession, and indeed to everyone concerned with the care of the sick.

Melbourne 1991   Michael Drake

Preface

Tabbner's Nursing Care: Theory and Practice is an Australian textbook for students who are undertaking an enrolled nurse programme. The textbook introduces students to the basic concepts, process, skills and techniques of nursing practice, and provides them with a foundation for further nursing studies. This second edition is based upon the curricula of the nursing councils or registration boards in the various Australian states. It has been revised and updated extensively to reflect the changes which have occurred in, and to meet the needs of, enrolled nurse education programmes.

The book is presented in 5 parts. Part 1 introduces the students to various theories and models of nursing; normal growth and development throughout the lifespan; behavioural, legal, and ethical aspects of nursing; and to the nursing process. Part 2 introduces the students to aspects of physics and chemistry which are relevant to nursing practice, and provides information on structure and functions of the human body. Part 3 discusses basic human needs and how, when necessary, nursing care may be planned and implemented to assist an individual to meet these needs. Part 4 addresses the care of an individual with a body system disorder. Each body system is presented in a separate chapter which includes a brief review of anatomy and physiology, pathophysiological influences and effects of dysfunction, major manifestations of disorders of that system, diagnostic tests which may be performed, and nursing care guidelines. Part 5 introduces the students to care of an individual with a specific need, or special circumstance.

Learning objectives appear at the beginning of each chapter. These provide a general overview of the chapter content, and may assist students to evaluate their understanding.

Some information has been placed in tabular form or displayed prominently in boxes for easier access and learning. Suggested methods of performing nursing activities have been presented in a format consisting of nursing actions and their rationale, so that students have an understanding of why specific actions are taken. A large number of illustrations has been included to provide clear and meaningful visual aids.

At the end of each chapter is a list of references and further reading which can be used as a guide for students who wish to explore topics in greater depth.

It should be noted that no sexism or gender-specific incidence of occupation or disease is implied by the use of pronouns relating to nurses, patients, or others in the text.

The terms patient, person, and individual are used interchangeably in this text. The term 'client' has been avoided. Despite the trend towards its use by some authors, it seems inappropriate in an Australian text while the current illness-care system prevails.

Melbourne 1991   J.O.C.

Acknowledgements

The author would like to thank those people who provided encouragement, advice, information, criticism, and support during the preparation of this book. In particular I thank: Lyn Bradley, Robyn Gordon, Beverley Anne Knight and Geoffrey Parsons, members of the editorial committee, who gave generously of their time, and whose recommendations helped to develop this text to meet the needs of enrolled nurse students; Ita Kearney (Director of the Melbourne School for Enrolled Nurses) who gave me the opportunity to become involved in this exciting and challenging project; Kate Taylor (Director of Nursing) and the Board of Management at Warrnambool and District Base Hospital, who granted me secondment leave to undertake the writing of this book; Shelley Blair, Kwei Cheung, Judy Duffy, Bernadette Keane, Barbara Piesse, John Ravenhall, Christine Thompson, and Deborah Tsorbaris, each of whom provided invaluable advice in their area of special expertise; colleagues in the Nursing Division, NSW Department of TAFE who provided encouragement and support; the Anti-Cancer Council of Victoria, Association for the Blind, Australian Bureau of Statistics, Better Hearing Australia, Blood Bank (Red Cross Society), Diabetes Foundation (Victoria), Dietetics Department at the Warrnambool and District Base Hospital, and The Family Planning Association of Victoria, who supplied current information, statistics, and ready assistance; John Ward, whose careful and clear artwork complements that of the first edition and serves to clarify the text; Judy Waters (Publisher at the Melbourne Office of Churchill Livingstone), whose experience in developing textbooks has been invaluable, and whose support and encouragement helped to make this a less daunting task than it might have been.

Contents

An introduction to nursing

1. An outline of the history and theories of nursing

INTRODUCTION

A study of the historical background of nursing can help the nursing student to understand and appreciate the influence of the past on modern nursing.

This chapter addresses a brief historical perspective of nursing, various nursing theories and models, and the nursing student.

A BRIEF HISTORY OF NURSING

The word 'nurse' is derived from a Latin word meaning to nourish or cherish and as birth, illness, injury and death are common to all human beings there has always been a need for someone to take on the task of caring for others.

In earlier times superstition and witchcraft formed the basis of the treatment of illness, and for many centuries it was believed that sickness was a punishment for wrong-doing and that the signs of illness were evidence of the presence of evil spirits. Treatment was prescribed by witch doctors and priests and, although much of it was barbaric and caused more suffering than the illness, many old herbal remedies are still used in a modified form today. Until well into the eighteenth century those who suffered a mental illness were considered to be possessed by the devil, and were treated with extreme cruelty.

Some of the earliest organized nursing was performed by men who staffed the hospitals founded by military religious orders during the crusades, e.g. the Knights of St John of Jerusalem, the Teutonic Knights, and the Knights of St Lazarus.

During the twelfth and thirteenth centuries several secular orders were active in caring for the sick, and their members included men and women. Some of the orders were the Ursulines, the Poor Clares, the Beguines, and the Benedictines. Also at this time a religious order called the Augustinian sisters of the Hotel Dieu was founded in Paris, and it is the oldest order in the world of nuns who are devoted purely to nursing.

During the sixteenth century, Henry VIII ordered the dissolution of the English monasteries and the confiscation of their property and enormous wealth. This meant that large numbers of sick and destitute people were left to die. Workhouses were built to house the poor, many of whom were sick. They lived in appalling conditions and were required to work in return for the accommodation provided.

Finally conditions in the city of London became so dreadful that Henry VIII was forced to allow hospitals such as St Bartholomews, St Thomas's and St Mary's to be re-founded, and others to be established, following many petitions from the people of London. The hospitals were badly staffed with untrained workers, many of whom were of very poor character. Patients were housed in grossly overcrowded, dreary wards.

The period from the beginning of the eighteenth century to the middle of the nineteenth century has been termed the 'Dark Ages' of nursing, during which the care of the sick and the status of the nurse reached the lowest level imaginable.

The squalid conditions in hospitals and the undesirable character of those attending the sick were publicised by people such as the prison reformers John Howard and Elizabeth Fry, and the writer Charles Dickens, who created the unsavoury characters Sairey Gamp and Betsy Prig to typify the nurses of the time.

In 1836, a Lutheran clergyman named Theodor Fliedner established, with the help of his wife, an institution called Kaiserwerth situated near Dusseldorf in Germany. There they trained carefully selected women as deaconesses, and Kaiserwerth became famous for the high standard of training given and for the quality of care given to the sick. It became the centre of nurse training and received many trainees from overseas countries, some of whom set up similar institutions in their own countries.

Modern nursing has evolved as a result of the influence that Kaiserwerth had on people like Elizabeth Fry, who founded the Protestant Sisters of Charity as an attempt to ensure that the sick were cared for by women of good reputation; Agnes Jones, who revolutionized conditions in the workhouses and established a school of nursing to train nurses in the care of sick people in the workhouses; and Florence Nightingale—the founder of modern nursing.

Florence Nightingale was born in 1820 during a trip made by her English parents to the Italian city of Florence after which she was named. Her parents were wealthy and cultured, and Florence received an extensive education which was far beyond the standard usually received by the young women of her time. She travelled widely and led the full social life common to one in her place in society but, in spite of this, felt unhappy and dissatisfied. She was interested in nursing but this met with strong opposition from her family, and it was not until she was over 30 years of age that Florence Nightingale was able to realize her ambition. In 1850 she spent two weeks at Kaiserwerth and visited again in 1851 when she was appointed as Superintendent of the 'Establishment for Gentlewomen During Illness'. Florence Nightingale first achieved fame when, in 1854, she was asked to take a party of 38 nurses to Scutari in the Crimea. On arrival the nurses met with fierce opposition from the medical officers who would not allow them to care for the sick and injured soldiers. Miss Nightingale devoted her energies to improving the filthy conditions, obtaining supplies, organizing a good food supply, and establishing sanitary conditions generally. Within 2–3 weeks opposition had been overcome and the nurses were invited to take over the care of the sick. To the soldiers Miss Nightingale became an idol and, as she brought ease and comfort to the very sick by the light of the lamp she carried at night, she became known as the 'Lady of the Lamp'.

After the Crimean war the English public raised almost fifty thousand pounds as a mark of appreciation of Miss Nightingale's work and, with the money, she established a School of Nursing at St Thomas's Hospital in London. The first probationer nurses were admitted to the Nightingale School in June, 1860, and they were given one year of training followed by two years of experience in the hospital. Many of these nurses became Matrons of the large hospitals in London and elsewhere, and by the time Florence Nightingale died in 1910 at the age of 90 years remarkable progress had been made in nursing service and education of the nurse.

In 1868 Lucy Osburn, who was a graduate of the Nightingale School of Nursing and a personal friend of Miss Nightingale, arrived in Sydney to take up the appointment as Matron of Sydney Hospital. The hospital was in a filthy, dilapidated state, and it took many years of fighting against hostility and obstruction by the hospital staff before Miss Osburn was able to change the old order and establish a satisfactory level of patient care.

Changes in nursing education

It was not until late in the nineteenth century that any thought was given to the desirability of placing the care of the sick into the hands of those who could read and write, and it took until the early twentieth century for nursing to be accepted as a suitable occupation for young women who had received a good upbringing. By this time the training courses had been extended to three years but the hours of work were from 60–80 hours a week and, in some hospitals, nurses worked without pay and were required to pay a premium.

Conditions gradually improved and Preliminary Training Schools came into being. These allowed the nurse to attain a level of proficiency and learn basic principles before being required to attend to sick patients.

With the advances made in medical knowledge and the treatment of illness, it became necessary for nurses to acquire a greater depth of knowledge, and, therefore, study days and block systems were introduced to free nurses from their service commitments for days or weeks at a time in order to concentrate on study. More recent changes have been the establishment of alternative schemes of nursing education such as college-based courses and university degree courses.

Changes in the function of nurses

Dramatic changes have taken place since the early days when the nurse was an illiterate person required only to give custodial care of a very indifferent nature to the sick person.

The modern nurse is an intelligent and well educated person who assumes responsibility for a large portion of total patient care. The nurse must understand the nature of illness and the treatment given, and is required to make major decisions which influence patient care. Nursing today is very involved in the inescapable need for change, since nursing must reflect the health needs of the individual and the community, and these needs have changed dramatically during the past decades.

There are many avenues now open to the nurse who may work in general or specialized hospitals, community health areas, industrial areas, the armed forces, and other fields.

The enrolled nurse

Since training programmes were first established for the preparation of enrolled nurses in Australia, the role and function of enrolled nurses have undergone many changes.

Consequently the nature and content of educational programmes have changed in order to prepare the enrolled nurse for her expanded role in the nursing team.

The nature, requirements for entry into, the curriculum, and the conduct of enrolled nurse courses vary from state to state. Debate continues as to the role and function, the length of course, and the most appropriate setting for the education of enrolled nurses.

Despite the lack of consensus there appears to be general agreement that an enrolled nurse educational programme should prepare the individual to practice in co-operation with and under the direction and supervision of a registered nurse. Enrolled nurses work with registered nurses in the delivery of nursing care which includes health promotion and illness prevention, patient education, and the provision of care to individuals in hospital and community health care agencies.

Each level of nurse participates in the delivery of nursing care which has the individual's health needs as the central focus, using the nursing process as a tool to facilitate and improve nursing care.

THEORIES AND MODELS OF NURSING

Nursing, as a profession, is in the midst of change. Society is changing and nursing is affected by social forces which require that a community receives a system of health care delivery that will make quality care available for all people. The demand for quality care is reflected in the philosophical belief in the dignity and value of the individual. In order to provide quality care, nursing must focus on the needs of both the individual and the community.

Over recent decades the growth of nursing as a scientific health care profession has led to the development of various philosophies of nursing and theoretical models on which nursing practice can be based. A nursing model provides the basis for the framework of nursing practice, and the direction for nursing research.

In earlier times the responsibilities of nurses were centred around sanitation measures, nutrition, hygiene and comfort, prevention of cross infection, and relief of the prime symptoms of infection. Nurses functioned not only as nurses, but as housekeepers, dietitians, and cleaners.

Nursing has changed, and continues to change, as society changes and as the emphasis on health care changes. Nursing is shifting from being primarily illness-oriented to being a profession that is health-oriented. Nurses practice in a growing variety of settings, and nursing roles continue to expand as the focus of nursing care expands.

Current nursing philosophies and theoretical models reflect the trend to address the *total* person, in all dimensions, as an individual in interaction with the family and the community.

A *theory* is an abstract statement formulated to explain or describe the relationships among concepts or events.

A *model* is a conceptual framework developed from a set of concepts and assumptions; it is a conceptual representation of reality. A model provides the outline for which theory provides the functions.

Thus, a model represents *structure* while a theory suggests *function*. Numerous conceptual models of nursing practice have been devised, most of which:

- are based on sound theory
- contain implied or explicit assumptions, values and goals
- are implemented by the nursing process.

Peplau's theory

Hildegard Peplau made an attempt to analyze nursing action using an interpersonal theoretical framework (1952). Her theory focuses on the relationships formed by people as they progress through each developmental stage. She viewed the goal of nursing as developing a relationship between the nurse and patient whereby the nurse acts as resource person, counselor, teacher, and surrogate.

Abdellah's theory

Fay Abdellah, with her colleagues, devised a theory which emphasized the delivery of nursing care to the whole person (1960). Using a problem solving approach the nurse formulates a plan to help the patient meet his physical, emotional, intellectual, social, and spiritual needs. Abdellah identified 21 basic nursing problems. These are to:

1. maintain good hygiene and physical comfort.
2. achieve optimal activity, exercise, rest, and sleep.
3. prevent accident, injury, or other trauma and prevent the spread of infection.
4. maintain good body mechanics and prevent and correct deformities.
5. facilitate the supply of oxygen to all body cells.
6. facilitate the maintenance of nutrition to all body cells.
7. facilitate the maintenance of elimination.
8. facilitate the maintenance of fluid and electrolyte balance.
9. recognize the physiological responses of the body to disease conditions—pathological, physiological, and compensatory.
10. facilitate the maintenance of regulatory mechanisms and functions.
11. facilitate the maintenance of sensory function.
12. identify and accept positive and negative expressions, feelings and reactions.

13. identify and accept the interrelatedness of emotions and organic illness.
14. facilitate the maintenance of effective verbal and nonverbal communication.
15. facilitate the development of productive interpersonal relationships.
16. facilitate progress toward achievement of personal spiritual goals.
17. create and/or maintain a therapeutic environment.
18. facilitate awareness of self as an individual with varying physical, emotional, and developmental needs.
19. accept the optimum possible goals in light of limitations-physical and emotional.
20. use community resources as an aid in resolving problems arising from illness.
21. understand the role of social problems as influencing factors in the cause of illness.

Henderson's theory

Virginia Henderson saw the goal of nursing (1964) as helping the patient to gain independence as rapidly as possible, and she defined nursing as 'assisting the individual (sick or well) in the performance of those activities contributing to health or its recovery (or to a peaceful death) that he would perform unaided if he had the necessary strength, will or knowledge, and doing it in such a way as to help him gain independence as rapidly as possible'.

Virginia Henderson identified 14 basic needs which provide a framework for nursing care. These are to:

1. breathe normally
2. eat and drink adequately
3. eliminate by all avenues of elimination
4. move and maintain a desirable position
5. sleep and rest
6. select suitable clothing; dress and undress
7. maintain body temperature within normal range
8. keep the body clean and well groomed
9. avoid dangers in the environment
10. communicate with others
11. worship according to faith
12. work at something that provides a sense of accomplishment
13. play or participate in various forms of recreation
14. learn, discover, or satisfy the curiosity that leads to normal development and health.

Johnson's theory

Dorothy Johnson viewed the goal of nursing (1968) as reducing stress so that the patient can recover as quickly as possible. Johnson viewed man as a collection of behavioural subsystems which interrelate to form a whole person, and her theory focuses on man's needs in terms of his behaviour:

- security-seeking behaviour
- nurturance-seeking behaviour
- mastery of oneself and one's environment according to internalized standards of excellence
- taking in nourishment in socially and culturally acceptable ways
- ridding the body of waste in socially and culturally acceptable ways
- sexual and role identity behaviour
- self-protective behaviour.

Johnson saw the nurse's role as identifying the patient's inability to adapt to stress, and as providing the nursing care necessary to assist him resolve problems in meeting his needs.

King's theory

Imogene King viewed the goal of nursing (1971) as helping individuals and groups to attain, maintain and restore health, or to die with dignity. King saw nursing as a process of interaction between nurse and patient whereby, through communication, goals are set and agreement reached on ways to achieve goals.

Orem's theory

Dorothea Orem viewed the goal of nursing (1973) as helping the patient to achieve health through self-care. Orem saw nursing as a service required when individuals, or their significant others, are unable to care for themselves, i.e. when demands exceed their self-care abilities. The nurse identifies why an individual is unable to care for himself, and implements measures which assist him to meet his needs. The overall goal of nursing care is to assist the patient to achieve self-care whenever possible.

Roy's theory

Callister Roy viewed the goal of nursing (1981) as assisting man towards health by promoting and supporting his ability to adapt to various demands:

- meeting basic physiological needs
- developing a positive self-concept
- performing social roles
- achieving a balance between dependence and independence.

Roy saw nursing as being concerned with man as a total being, and intervening when necessary to assist him to adapt to one or more of these demands.

Roper, Logan and Tierney's theory

Roper, Logan and Tierney viewed the goal of nursing (1985) as helping people to prevent, alleviate, solve, or cope with problems related to activities of living. Their model of nursing is based on their model for living and includes five main concepts:

1. activities of living
2. lifespan
3. dependence–independence
4. factors affecting activities of living
5. the nursing process.

The activities of living, which are the focus of the model, are:

- maintaining a safe environment
- communicating
- breathing
- eating and drinking
- eliminating
- personal cleansing and dressing
- controlling body temperature
- mobilizing
- working and playing
- expressing sexuality
- sleeping
- dying.

The lifespan, in this model, serves as a reminder that nursing is concerned with people of all ages, and that an individual may require nursing assistance at any stage of the lifespan from conception to death.

The dependence/independence continuum is included in this model to acknowledge that there are certain stages in a person's life when he is unable to perform various activities of living independently. The continuum ranges from total dependence at one end to total independence at the other, and the concept of the dependence/independence is widely utilized in nursing practice. At certain times nurses help patients towards independence in the activities of living, and at other times help them to accept dependence.

Factors affecting the activities of living, or individuality in the activities of living, include those that are physical, psychological, sociocultural, environmental, and politico-economic. Therefore, the nurse needs to acknowledge that there are many differences in the way individuals perform the activities of living.

The nursing process is seen by Roper, Logan and Tierney as the means by which individualized nursing can be achieved. Information on the nursing process is provided in Chapter 12.

It becomes apparent, when comparing various models, that most include similar concepts of what constitutes nursing. Selection of a particular model of nursing practice depends on numerous factors, and health care agencies may consider several before deciding on the one they consider to be most appropriate. As nursing continues to grow as a health care profession, new philosophies of nursing and theoretical models will undoubtably be developed.

THE STUDENT OF NURSING

The nurse undertakes an educational programme which prepares her to fulfil her role, as a member of the health care team, in the delivery of safe nursing care.

The functions and responsibilities of enrolled nurses vary from state to state, therefore each nurse needs to understand her *specified role and function*. Each state has its own requirements for registration. The nurses' registration body in each state prescribes the curriculum and formulates policies which control the standard of nursing practice. Each nurse must, therefore, familiarize herself with the specified functions, degree of responsibility and accountability, and the legal responsibilities and limitations pertaining to enrolled nursing practice. **It is essential that the enrolled nurse performs only those functions that are within her specified role**.

Throughout the educational programme, the nurse is prepared to fulfil her nursing role as care-giver, decision-maker, patient-advocate, communicator, and teacher. To fulfil these roles the nurse is required to develop skills in three domains:

1. The cognitive domain deals with knowledge and understanding, involving the recall of concepts and principles and their application to problem solving situations. Cognitive function involves all aspects of perception, thinking, reasoning, and remembering.

2. The affective domain is concerned with attitudes, values, interests, and feelings.

3. The psychomotor domain deals with a variety of motor skills that depend on physical ability, e.g. learning to perform a specific skill such as changing a wound dressing.

All three skills must be developed in order for the student nurse to become a thinking, responsive, and feeling person who is capable of performing specific motor skills.

The student nurse learns to develop the skills through a variety of learning techniques. Learning experiences and activities may be described as the events which a student participates *actively* in to achieve specific objectives and goals. Learning involves receiving knowledge, comprehension and responding, and the integration of knowledge and practice. The student is involved in learning activities such as large group sessions, lectures, films, audiovisual tapes, reading, independent study, small group sessions, individual tutorials, discussions, role play, observation of others, simulated patient situations, and clinical application.

Practice laboratories are used for the development of particular nursing skills, whereby the student is able to practice until she is competent with a skill. Sufficient time and facilities must be available to enable the student to increase her technical proficiency and confidence in interpersonal skills. Clinical practice forms part of the curriculum, and focuses around actual patient care. Supervised clinical practice situations enable the student to apply knowledge, perfect expertise in skills, and to develop confidence in problem solving and interpersonal skills.

Nurses are encouraged to join a nursing organization which is concerned with professional and industrial issues of the nursing profession. The Australian Nursing Federation (ANF) is the national professional and industrial organization for nurses in Australia, and is affiliated to the International Council of Nurses (ICN). The Hospital Employees Federation (HEF) is another organization to which nurses can belong.

This text contains information which should prove helpful to the student as she learns the theory and practice of nursing necessary to fulfil her role as a member of the nursing team within the health care team.

CONCLUSION

The aim of this chapter is to introduce the student to a brief history of nursing, and to some of the theories and models of nursing which have been developed.

A study of the historical background of nursing can help the student to understand and appreciate the influence of the past on modern nursing.

An overview of the nursing models which have been developed by various nursing theorists helps to demonstrate how nursing has changed since the days of Florence Nightingale.

REFERENCES AND FURTHER READING

Abdellah F G, Martin A 1973 New directions in patient-centered nursing. Macmillan, New York
Knepfer G 1989 Nursing for life. Pan Books, Sydney, ch 1, 14–24
Potter P A, Perry A G 1985 Fundamentals of nursing. C V Mosby, St Louis Riehl J P, Roy C 1974 Conceptual models for nursing practice. Appleton-Century-Crofts, New York
Trembath R, Hellier D 1987 All care and responsibility. Florence Nightingale Committee, Australia

2. Theories of growth and development

OBJECTIVES

1. Compare and discuss the various theories of development.

INTRODUCTION

A nurse cares for people who are in different stages of development. Therefore, a basic understanding of growth and development enables her to recognize the needs of each individual and, thus, to provide appropriate care.

Human growth and development are orderly processes that begin at conception and continue until death. Every person progresses through definite phases of growth and development, but the rate and behaviours of this progression vary with each individual.

Every person is a unique individual and, while growth and development are generally categorized into age stages or in terms that describe the features of an age group, categorization does not take into account individual differences. The categorization does, however, provide a means of describing the characteristics associated with the majority of individuals at stages when comparative developmental changes appear.

Growth and development affect the whole person and, although defined separately, overlap and are dependent on each other.

Physical growth results when cells divide and synthesize new proteins, causing an increase in the number and size of cells and, consequently, an increase in the size and weight of the body or any of its parts. Growth can be measured in height and mass, and in the changes in physical appearance and body functions that occur as a person grows older.

Development refers to the behavioural aspects of a person's progressive adaptation to his environment, and is related to changes in psychological and social functioning.

Maturation is the process of attaining complete development; and is the unfolding of full physical, emotional, and intellectual capabilities. The term maturation is generally used to describe an increase in complexity that enables a person to function at a higher level.

An individual's development encompasses motor, emotional, personality, intellectual, moral, and spiritual growth. There are several theories, or approaches, regarding growth and development. This chapter addresses those approaches, while Chapter 3 describes each stage of development.

THEORIES OF DEVELOPMENT

The various developmental theories differ in how the human being is viewed. Some theories view development as a continuous process that moves from the simple to the complex, while other theories view development as a process characterized by alternating periods of equilibrium and disequilibrium. The major theories, or approaches, are maturational, psychoanalytic, cognitive-developmental, social learning, and moral.

The maturational approach

This approach emphasizes that development occurs regardless of practice or training. Physical development and the sequences involved—which are the same for every person—are part of specific hereditary information. This approach recognizes that while maturational patterns are controlled by heredity, they may be altered by factors such as nutrition or illness.

The psychoanalytic approach

This approach to, or theory of, development was founded by Sigmund Freud, who lived from 1856 to 1939. Freud's theory stresses the formative years of childhood as the basis for later psychoneurotic disorders, primarily through the unconscious repression of instinctual drives and sexual desires. His theory emphasizes the drives of sex and aggression which he sees as motivating much human behaviour. According to Freud, an individual's personality is composed of the id, the ego, and the superego.

1. *The id* is that part of the psyche that is the source of instinctive energy, impulses, and drives. Based on the pleasure principle, it directs behaviour towards self gratification.

2. *The ego* represents the conscious self and is that part of the psyche which maintains conscious contact with reality, and tempers the primitive drives of the id and the demands of the superego with the physical and social needs of society.

3. *The superego* is the individual's conscience, which is formed as the result of internalization of societal demands and restrictions.

Freud's theory of development is based on a series of psychosexual stages through which an individual must pass. Successful completion of each stage is necessary before the next stage can be entered without detrimental effects on future development. According to Freud specific body areas are the primary sites for expression and achievement of needs, and these sites change from stage to stage. Table 2.1 outlines the stages of development according to Freud's theory.

Table 2.1   Developmental stages according to Freud

Stage	Age	Behaviours
Oral	0–18 months	Uses mouth as source of satisfaction
Anal	1½–3 years	Focuses on pleasurable sensations arising from the anal region. Learns muscular control of urination and defaecation Exhibits increasing independence: learns to walk, talk, dress and undress Learns to say 'no'
Phallic	3–6 years	Focuses on pleasurable sensations arising from the genital region Learns sexual identity Perceives parent of same sex as a rival Identifies with parent of same sex Emergence of superego Develops refinement of motor and intellectual activities
Latency	6–12 years	Enters quiet stage; sexual development lies dormant, emotional tension eases Experiences normal homosexual phase Identifies with peers and teachers Increases intellectual capacity
Genital	12 years-adult	Experiences reawakened sex drives Develops secondary sex characteristics Exhibits concern over appearance Strives towards independence Matures intellectually Experiences identity crisis

Erikson's theory

Using the psychoanalytic framework, Erik Erikson based his (1963) theory of development on the process of socialization. He describes another series of stages of personal and social development as the 'Eight ages of man', and views development as a continuous struggle for an emotional—social balance.

According to Erikson, a person spends his whole life constructing, shaping, and reshaping his personality—which is influenced by psychological, biological, social, and environmental factors. Erikson identifies core problems that the individual tries to master during each stage of personality development. Progression to the next stage depends on resolution of the problem; however, no core problem is ever entirely resolved, as each new situation will present a conflict in a new form. Table 2.2 outlines the stages of development according to Erikson.

Table 2.2   Erikson's stages of development

Stage	Age	Conflict	Behaviours
I	0–1 year	Trust versus mistrust	Develops basic trust in someone who consistently responds to his needs. When his needs are not met, he may develop basic mistrust of others.
II	2–4 years	Autonomy versus shame and doubt	Develops a sense of self control and independence. Feelings of shame and doubt may arise if he is made to feel self conscious, or when he is expected to be dependent in areas where he is not capable.
III	4–8 years	Initiative versus guilt	Plans and undertakes tasks, and initiates a fantasy life whereby he can work out fears and conflicts. A sense of guilt may arise if a child is made to feel that his activities or imaginings are bad.
IV	8–12 years	Industry versus inferiority	Engages in tasks and activities that can be carried through to completion. Needs and wants real achievement. Feelings of inferiority or inadequacy may arise if a child believes that he cannot measure up to the standards set for him by others.
V	13–20 years	Identity versus role confusion	Establishes own identity and intimate relationships. Role confusion may result if the individual is unable to solve conflicts about his role in society.

Table 2.2 (cont'd) Erikson's stages of development

Stage	Age	Conflict	Behaviours
VI	20–30 years	Intimacy and solidarity versus isolation	Enters into intimate relationships, by allowing others to share the psychosocial and physical aspects of his personality. The individual may experience a sense of isolation if he is unable to become close to others.
VII	30–60 years	Generativity versus self-absorption and stagnation	Establishes and guides the next generation, and strives to ensure the continuation of his work and life-style. If the individual is unable to assume responsibility for promoting the future, he may experience a sense of stagnation. As a result he becomes self-absorbed, and experiences difficulty in relating to the world.
VIII	60 years-death	Integrity versus despair	Strives to feel a sense of worth. A sense of integrity develops when an individual feels satisfied with his past achievements. Despair arises when an individual is unable to recognize or accept his worth, or when he feels remorse for that which might have been.

Table 2.3 Piaget's stages of cognitive development

Stage	Age	Intellectual development
Sensorimotor	Birth–2 years	This stage of intellectual development is governed by sensations in which simple learning takes place. Problem solving is primarily trial and error, as the child progresses from reflex activity—through repetitive behaviours—to imitative behaviour. The child gradually acquires a sense that external objects have a separate and independent existence, and that they exist even when they are not visible to him.
Preoperational	2–7 years	During this stage the predominant characteristic is *egocentricity*, whereby the child considers his viewpoint as the only one possible. Thinking is concrete and tangible, and the child lacks the ability to make deductions or generalizations. Problem solving does not usually follow logical thought processes.
Concrete operational	7–11 years	Thought becomes increasingly logical, and problems are solved in a systematic fashion. The child is able to consider points of view other than his own. Towards the end of this stage, the child demonstrates a greater reasoning ability.
Formal operational	11 years–	Thinking is characterized by logical reasoning. The adolescent is able to think in abstract terms, draw logical conclusions and solve problems.

Cognitive-developmental approach

The theory of cognitive development focuses on the gradual development of cognitive processes, such as problem solving, and on the gradual development of intellectual growth. Cognitive development is the process by which a child becomes an intelligent person, acquiring knowledge and the ability to think, learn, reason, and abstract.

Jean Piaget's (1952) theory of cognitive development, which deals only with cognition and does not take into account all psychosocial aspects of the personality, views development as gradual, progressive, and related to age. Piaget's views are that, in order for learning to occur, a variety of new experiences or stimuli must exist. He believed that there are four major stages in the development of logical thinking, and that each stage builds on the accomplishments of the previous stage. Table 2.3 outlines Piaget's stages of cognitive development.

Social learning approach

Theorists who adopt the social learning approach, view development as a process of learning and changing behaviour whereby specific behaviours are learned through a process of *reinforcement*. Reinforcement may be positive or negative; and reinforcements may be tangible, e.g. toys or food, or they may be abstract, e.g. a smile, frown, verbal praise or admonishment. Positive reinforcement generally increases a behaviour, whereas negative reinforcement generally causes the specific behaviour to cease. Social learning theorists also view *imitation* as a major source of learned behaviour, whereby an individual imitates the behaviours of a person he views as worthy.

Theory of moral development

Moral development involves the establishment of a moral code that is consistent with society, and it depends on the individual's ability to accept his social responsibility.

Kohlberg's (1973) theory states that moral development follows the development of the ability to reason, and that it occurs in three levels. His theory of development focuses only on the development of morality, and does not consider other psychosocial issues. The three levels of moral development, according to Kohlberg's theory, are:

1. Pre-conventional (pre-moral) level. The child's behaviour is motivated by the desire to receive reward

or to avoid punishment. During this phase, the child begins to conform to rules for his own interest and social acceptance.

2. Conventional level. The child conforms to rules to please others, in order to avoid negative reinforcement of his behaviours. He begins to realize that he can earn approval by being 'nice'. Internal standards begin to develop, and behaviour is group oriented.

3. Post conventional (principled) level. The individual, from adolescence onwards, experiences conflict between social standards. During the later stage of this level, the individual internalizes moral standards and feels a need to do what is morally right regardless of the consequences. The most advanced level of moral development is one in which the individual's chosen ethical principles guide his decisions of conscience.

CONCLUSION

Growth and development are interrelated processes which are influenced by a variety of factors.

The theoretical approaches outlined in this chapter, together with various other approaches provide a framework for understanding the complexities of growth and development.

Each approach emphasizes different aspects of development, e.g. cognitive-developmentalists concentrate primarily on intellectual development, psychoanalytical theorists emphasize social and personality development, while maturational theorists focus primarily on physical growth and development.

Chapter 3 provides information on growth and development throughout the life cycle, and on the special needs at each stage.

REFERENCES AND FURTHER READING

Hilgard E R, Atkinson R C, Atkinson R L 1975 Introduction to psychology, 6th edn. Harcourt Brace Jovanovich, New York
Schuster C S, Ashburn S S 1986 The process of human development, 2nd edn. Little, Brown and Company, Boston

3. Stages of growth and development

OBJECTIVES

1. State the factors which influence growth and development.
2. Describe the major physical and psychosocial changes which occur during each stage of development.

INTRODUCTION

Growth and development are processes which begin at conception and continue through each stage of the life cycle. Human development involves both biological and psychosocial components. Biological science is concerned mainly with structure and function, while the psychosocial sciences focus on the behavioural aspects of development. Growth may be defined as the *physical* changes that occur in a steady and orderly manner, while development relates to changes in *psychological* and *social* functioning.

Adult behaviour and personality characteristics are shaped by events occurring during the early years of life. In order to understand the psychological processes of the adult, it is necessary to know how these processes originate and how they change with time. Developmental psychologists are concerned with how certain behaviours develop, and why they appear when they do. Chapter 2 addressed various *theories* of development, while this chapter focuses on the major physical and psychosocial changes which accompany each stage of development.

Factors influencing growth and development

An individual's development is influenced both by genetic factors and by the environment. Genetic factors are often referred to as the natural forces which influence development, while environmental factors are referred to as the nurturing forces. It is difficult to separate the effects of 'nature' and 'nuture', as an individual's development is affected by the interaction between these two forces.

Another factor which influences development is *maturation*: an innately governed sequence of physical changes that does not depend on particular environmental events. Many behavioural changes that occur in the early months of life are related to maturation of the nervous system, muscles, and glands. These changes represent a continuation of the growth processes that guided the development of the fetus within the uterus. Maturation can be accelerated or impeded by the *quality* of the environment, and by life experiences.

Genetic factors

Genetic factors influence many aspects of an individual's physical and psychosocial being. Research indicates that as well as determining physical characteristics, genetic factors also influence parts of a person's psychological make-up, e.g. his temperament.

The central structure of a living cell is its complement of *genes*, which are located on the chromosomes within the cell nucleus. Genes, the basic units of heredity, are molecules of DNA. Many thousands of genes are carried by the chromosomes.

In the human, each cell normally contains 46 chromosomes arranged in 23 pairs. When conception occurs the sperm and the ovum unite, each contributing 23 chromosomes to the zygote. These 46 chromosomes form 23 pairs, which are duplicated in every cell of the body as the embryo develops. Because of the high number of *genes* in each chromosome it is very unlikely that two human beings would have the same heredity—even with the same parents. One exception is identical (monozygotic) twins who, having developed from the same ovum, have the same chromosomes and genes.

During fertilization, a spermatozoa and an ovum unite to form one new cell. This one cell is capable of multiplying and developing into a fetus, with its sex and characteristics e.g. hair and eye colour, race, physical stature predetermined. Each individual's genetic structure is unique and life-lasting, therefore heredity affects all stages of development. While each person's capacities are inherited, the extent to which they are used in development is influenced by the environment.

Environmental factors

The hereditary potential with which an individual is born is greatly influenced by the environment he encounters. Therefore, the environmental conditions to which an infant is exposed are a major influence on development. Environment refers to the people with whom the individual has contact, the experiences he has throughout life, and the physical surroundings.

Attachment (bonding) is the process by which the parents and infant establish a relationship. Both parents and the infant have a role to play in the attachment process, whereby each establishes emotional ties with the other. As the parent responds to the infant, the infant must respond to the parent, e.g. by cooing or eye contact. Creating a situation in which the parent's and the infant's eyes meet in visual contact is significant in the formation of emotional ties. Research has suggested that this early social attachment provides the security necessary for the child to explore his environment, and that it forms the basis for interpersonal relationships in later years.

Failure to form an attachment to one or a few primary persons in the early years, has been related to an inability to develop close personal relationships in adulthood.

Early stimulation is important in providing the background necessary to cope with the environment at a later stage. Stimulation is provided by handling the infant, allowing him to move about freely and assume different positions, and by providing conditions whereby the infant receives visual and auditory stimuli, e.g. coloured objects, mobiles, the sound of voices and music. Many studies have been performed which indicate that a stimulating early environment is important for later intellectual development. Conversely, too much stimulation too soon could be upsetting for an infant, who may exhibit distress at being unable to respond to multiple stimuli.

The *family* and *peer group* are the most influential forces on an individual's psychosocial growth and development, as it is through these groups that an individual learns about himself, others and society.

The family, through its functions, exerts a major influence on development. It is through the family environment that the individual first learns about self, the world, and his place within a society. Initially, the individual adopts the family's values and belief systems. Family functions include providing love and security; meeting the basic needs such as food and warmth; facilitating emotional and social development; and helping the individual to learn about society, roles, and behaviours.

An individual's *peer group* exerts a major influence on

development, as it is through the peer group that an individual learns skills of socialization, and different ways of interacting with others. The peer groups also places demands and expectations on the individual to adapt his behaviour to achieve group purposes. It is often through the peer group that an individual learns about success and/or failure, receives support or rejection, and learns to question his thoughts and feelings.

Experiences, which may promote learning, enable an individual to progress developmentally through the lifespan. At each developmental stage the individual must learn to master a task or skill before progressing to the next stage. Gradually, an individual uses his accumulated skills and experiences to develop a range of effective behaviour.

Factors within the everyday *environment* such as nutrition, housing, and socioeconomic status, have been found to influence development. For example, the adequacy of nutrients in the diet influences how physiological needs are met, and subsequent growth and development. When a diet is lacking in adequate nutrients, deficits in height, mass, and developmental progression occur.

STAGES OF DEVELOPMENT

As described in Chapter 2, some theorists and psychologists perceive development as proceeding in definite stages rather than as a continuous process. As a developmental concept, a *stage* usually defines a set of behaviours that occur together. Stages follow in an orderly sequence, and the transition from one stage to another usually involves a process of integration, whereby the behaviour from the earlier stage is transformed into the next—along with some new elements. While environmental factors may accelerate or impede development, they do not change its sequence.

The stages of development are the stages of the lifespan, from conception to death:

- prenatal
- infancy
- early childhood
- late childhood
- adolescence
- early adulthood
- middle adulthood
- late adulthood.

The aspects of development during each stage are physical, intellectual, emotional, personality and social.

Prenatal development

The prenatal period is the stage of development from conception to birth, normally lasting 40 weeks.

Life begins as a single cell. Within a few days of conception the fertilized ovum implants in the wall of the uterus. Once implantation has occurred the lining of the uterus undergoes changes, so that by approximately the thirteenth day after conception the *embryo* is almost entirely embedded in the uterine lining. Embryonic blood vessels grow outward and come into intimate contact with the maternal blood. This enables the embryo, and later the fetus, to receive nutrient substances from, and to transfer wastes into, the maternal blood. As the embryo grows, differentiation of cells and tissues gives rise to specific tissues, and the shape of the embryo changes to gradually assume a human appearance.

By the 7th or 8th week, the developing organism is called a *fetus*, and the principal external features of the body are visible. Growth and development occur first in a cephalocaudal direction (head to tail), then in a proximo-distal direction (from the centre of the body outwards). Thus, the head of the fetus is more developed than the legs, and arm buds appear before leg buds. Development in the limbs proceeds from the shoulders and hips, to the hands and the feet.

Prenatal development occurs in three main stages, each lasting 3 months:

- The first trimester is the first 3 months
- The second trimester is the period from the third to the sixth month
- The third trimester is the last 3 months of intrauterine life.

Different tissues and regions of the body mature at different rates, while growth in length and mass proceeds at a predeterminal rate. Growth in length and mass depends on factors inherent in the fetus, placenta, and mother. Growth and development of the fetus may be impeded by factors such as infectious agents, e.g. the rubella virus, chemical agents, e.g. ionizing radiation or certain drugs, immunologic factors, e.g. the Rh factor, and by nutritional factors, e.g. maternal mineral deficiency.

The first trimester of intrauterine life is the most crucial for the developing fetus, as it is during this period that the fetal cells differentiate and develop into essential organ systems. Any factors which causes interference with growth, can result in extensive structural or functional alteration or congenital absence of an organ or system.

By the end of the *second trimester*, most organ systems are complete and capable of function, and the fetus is considered viable: capable of life outside the uterus. If a fetus is born at this stage, extensive environmental support is necessary to promote survival.

During the *third trimester*, the fetus grows in length and mass. When born, the infant is able to make the transition from intrauterine to extrauterine life. The cardiovascular system adapts so that blood circulation no longer bypasses the lungs, and the lungs are able to inflate—thereby enabling gaseous exchange.

Infancy

Infancy is the stage of development from birth to 12 months. The first 28 days of extrauterine life are referred to as the *neonatal* period.

Physical development

At birth the spinal cord and lower brain centres are well developed and, while not capable of co-ordinated movement, the infant exhibits a number of reflexes:

- *Eye reflexes*: when a bright light is directed towards the eyes, the pupils contract; blinking is elicited when objects are brought towards the eyes.
- *Oral reflexes*: the rooting reflex is elicited when the infant's cheek contacts the mother's breast and in response to peri-oral touch. This reflex enables him to find a nipple in order to feed.
- *Startle reflex*: elicited by a sudden loud noise. On hearing this, the infant startles and flexes the elbows.
- *Moro reflex*: consists of abduction and extension of the arms with the hands open, followed by adduction of the arms. This reflex is accompanied by extension of the trunk and head, movement of the legs, and crying. It is elicited by holding the infant's hands and raising him gently, then releasing the hands rapidly.
- *Grasp reflex*: elicited when the palm is stimulated so that the fingers flex and grip the object.
- *Walking reflex*: elicited when the infant is held upright with the sole of his foot pressing on a firm surface. This initiates flexion and extension of the legs, thus simultating walking.
- *Tonic neck reflex*: when an infant is in the supine position, he generally lies with the head turned to one side and with the arm of that side extended toward the head.

After several months, these basic reflexes disappear and are gradually replaced by conditioned reflexes.

Locomotion proceeds in stages. First, the infant learns to position the head in space, then crawl on hands and knees, later to move about while sitting upright; and finally to stand, balance, and walk. Thus, motor development occurs in the cephalocaudal direction.

At birth an infant is approximately 50–55 cm long, and weighs about 2.8–4.5 kg. During the first 12 months the infant increases in length by over a third, and his mass almost triples.

As the infant grows in height and mass, his internal organs also grow and develop in order to cope with the increasing demands made on them. Growth is influenced by hormones, especially thyroxine and growth hormone.

At birth the infant will follow a moving person with his eyes, binocular vision begins at 6 weeks and is established by 4 months. At approximately 6 months the infant moves his head and eyes in every direction. By 12 months he recognizes familiar people and objects at a distance.

At birth the infant can hear, and by 1 month he is able to move his eyes towards a sound. The brain is not sufficiently developed initially for any meaning to be attached to sounds, but by 5–6 months he turns immediately to his mother's voice—even when she is quite a distance away.

Speech develops from 'vocalizing' at birth and crying as a means of communication, until at 12 months the infant is able to say one or two recognizable words. With time the number of words spoken increase and become clearer. The rate of vocabulary gain varies, and is related to factors such as the amount and type of speech the infant hears.

Intellectual development

The process of acquiring intellectual skills is often referred to as 'cognitive' development. Cognitive activities, e.g. reasoning, thinking, and problem solving, involve two main processes—perception and conceptualization.

Perception is the sensory process by which an individual obtains information about himself and his environment. Through the senses, an infant perceives many stimuli, e.g. pressure, pain, warmth, cold, sound, taste, and visual images.

Conceptualization is the process of concept formation, and is an intellectual activity which facilitates reasoning, thinking, and problem solving. Concepts allow sense to be made of the information received through the senses.

The best known theory regarding cognitive development is the one postulated by Jean Piaget, a Swiss psychologist. Information on Piaget's theory is provided in Chapter 2. More recent research about cognitive development indicates that infants have the ability to think, deduce, and reason.

Emotional development

Emotion is the term used to describe a 'feeling'. Anger, fear, joy, and sorrow are typical emotions. Emotional development depends on a number of factors, e.g. maturation, heredity, socialization, and the environment. Most emotional expressions appear to be learned, and emotional development is related to age. Some forms of emotional expression appear to be inborn or to develop through maturation, but learning is important in modifying emotional expression to conform to the patterns approved by a specific culture.

At birth the infant is able to exhibit distress and pleasure; by 3–6 months he can express anger, distrust, and fear; and by about 8–10 months he can exhibit anxiety, surprise, dissatisfaction, obstinacy, anticipation, and frustration.

Personality development

Personality may be defined as the characteristic patterns of behaviour, and modes of thinking, that determine a person's adjustment to his environment. An individual's personality encompasses many factors: intellectual abilities, motives, emotional reactivity, attitudes, beliefs, and moral values.

An infant is born with certain potentialities, the development of which depend upon maturation and experiences encountered in growing up. Therefore, personality is the product of heredity and environment; and personality development is a complicated process involving all aspects of the individual and his environment.

Sigmund Freud's and Erik Erikson's theories of personality development are outlined in Chapter 2. According to Freud, personality develops as a result of a variety of processes, stresses, and experiences. Erikson's theory emphasizes the social rather than the psychosexual dimension of development.

Hans Eysenck developed a (1963) theory of personality based on the concepts of introversion–extraversion, and stability–instability. He claims that personality is the product of learning, especially as a result of early conditioning in infancy.

Although various theories provide a simple way of looking at personality, in actuality development of personality is far more complex. Broadly, personality development can be viewed as a process that begins in infancy, continues into adulthood, and is the way in which a person relates to his environment and circumstances. Personality is shaped by *inborn potential* as modified by experiences that affect the person as an individual.

Social development

Social development refers to how an individual learns to interact with others, and it begins early in an infant's life, e.g. smiling can be considered a social response. Initially, a smile can be elicited in response to strangers, but after about 6 months the infant's smile becomes more selective. As the infant begins to vocalize and later to speak, social interaction is increased.

The family is the first, and most important, social institution for the infant. Later on, other people become significant in a child's social network, e.g. kindergarten and school.

Social roles, e.g. those of brother or sister, playmate, are gradually acquired during social development in infancy. Play provides the opportunity for social development, whereby the infant learns the social expectations that accompany relationships.

Childhood

Childhood may be divided into two stages of development:

early childhood (which is the period from 12 months to approximately 5 years), and late childhood extending from 6 years to adolescence.

Physical development

During early childhood there is a steady increase in growth, so that by approximately 30 months the birth mass is quadrupled. Physical growth slows and stabilizes during the preschool years, so that at 5 years the child is approximately 18.6 kg in mass and 109 cm tall.

During the 'toddler' years, 12–24 months, chest circumference continues to increase in size and exceeds head circumference. After the second year the chest circumference exceeds the abdominal measurement, the lower extremeties grow, and the child assumes a taller, leaner appearance.

By the end of 'toddlerhood' most of the body systems are relatively mature. The internal structures of the ear and throat continue to be short and straight, and the lymphoid tissue of the tonsils and adenoids remains large. (These circumstances account for a high incidence of ear, throat, and upper respiratory tract infections during this stage of development). In later childhood most systems are mature and can adjust to moderate stress and change.

Motor development continues rapidly during early childhood so that the toddler is able to walk up and down stairs, kick a ball, and jump. By the end of the third year, most children can run well, and ride a tricycle. Drawing progresses from spontaneous scribbling to drawing stick-people, circles, and other recognizable objects. Improving motor skills allow more intricate manipulations during later childhood.

Towards the end of childhood, a child grows on an average of 2.5–5 cm per year and increases in mass by approximately 1.5–3 kg per year. The 'average' 12 year old is approximately 150 cm tall, and weighs approximately 38 kg. Body proportions take on a slimmer appearance, as fat gradually diminishes and its distribution patterns change. Cardiovascular functioning is refined and stabilized so that the heart rate averages 70–90 beats per minute, the ventilations average 16–18 breaths per minute, and blood pressure normalizes at approximately 110/70 mm Hg. Development of all body systems continues during middle childhood to become more efficient and adult-like in function.

Bones continue to ossify, but small and long bone ossification is not complete during this stage of development.

By about 10 years of age all temporary teeth have been shed, and the majority of permanent teeth have erupted.

The school age child gains increasing control over his muscular co-ordination and fine motor co-ordination.

Intellectual development

The major cognitive achievement of early childhood is the acquisition of language, and verbal language skills are further developed with an increased vocabulary and fluency of speech.

By the beginning of the second year, the child is able to think and reason; and the concepts of time, space, and causality (cause and effect) begin to have meaning.

By approximately 5 years, egocentric thinking is replaced partially by intuitive thought. The child begins to acquire the ability to use his thought processes to make sense of experiences, events and actions. Piaget describes this stage of development as 'concrete operational' (see Table 2.3).

The ability to read becomes a valuable means of increasing knowledge.

During the ages of 6–12 years, the ability to think abstractly and to solve problems develops or improves.

Emotional and personality development

As a child learns to be more specific in the expression of emotions, he begins to learn the effects of his own behaviour on others. New motives appear, that are learned by interacting with other people. While an infant's early behaviour is largely determined by basic biological needs, e.g. crying when hungry, much of his later behaviour is involved with meeting psychological needs, e.g. security, acceptance, approval, and feelings of self worth. *Emotions* can activate and direct behaviour in the same way as biological drives.

Relationships with others play an important role in emotional and personality development. As the child interacts with other people he learns to cope more effectively with them, and an ability to co-operate or compete with others involves a sense of accomplishment. The more positive a child feels about himself, the more confident he will feel about trying for success. Every small success increases the child's self image and a positive self image makes him feel likable and worthwhile. If a child is incapable of, or unprepared for, assuming the responsibilities associated with a sense of accomplishment, he may develop a sense of inadequacy or inferiority.

Freud and Erikson created their own milestones of emotional development, as outlined in Chapter 2. Freud based his theories on the fact that children have various physiological needs which must be met, while Erikson believed that adequate 'mothering' provided an infant with basic trust in himself and his environment. Piaget viewed emotional development in a more biological sense, with a child learning to adapt what is seen to what is known.

It is generally recognized that if a child's need for love and security is not met, he may become insecure and unable to relate effectively to others in later life. Therefore, throughout childhood, emotional and personality development depend largely on having psychological needs met. Emotional *deprivation* results in developmental retardation.

Young children especially do not thrive if their main caregiver is hostile or indifferent to them and their needs.

Social development

With increasing age, social development becomes less family-dominated than in infancy. Not only do the quality and quantity of contacts with other people exert an influence on the growing child, but a widening range of contacts is essential to learning and to the development of a healthy personality.

Each group the child becomes involved with, e.g. school friends, provides a social relationship of varying strength and type. One of the most important socializing agents in a child's life is the peer group with whom he explores ideas and his physical environment. Through peer relationships, children learn ways in which to relate and deal with others, e.g. those in positions of authority.

As a child interacts with his peers he becomes aware that there are views other than his own. As a result he learns to persuade, bargain, and co-operate in order to maintain friendships. The child becomes increasingly sensitive to the social norms and pressures of the peer group, and the need for peer approval becomes a powerful influence toward conformity. Peer relationships, in which a child experiences love and closeness for a friend, seem to be important as a foundation for close relationships in adulthood.

Although increased independence is the goal of middle to late childhood, children still feel secure knowing that there is someone, e.g. the parents, to implement controls and restrictions. With a secure base in a loving family, a child is able to develop self confidence and independence.

Adolescence

Adolescence is the period of development between 12–13 years and 18–20 years, and is the stage that marks the transition from childhood to adulthood.

Physical development

The physical changes of early adolescence (puberty) are primarily the result of hormonal activity. Physical changes occur rapidly in both males and females. Sexual maturation occurs with the development of primary and secondary sex characteristics.

The main physical changes are:

- increased growth rate of the skeleton and muscles
- alteration in the distribution of muscle and fat
- gender-specific changes, such as changes in shoulder and hip width
- development of the reproductive system and secondary sex characteristics.

Growth in length of limbs and neck precedes growth in other areas, increases in hip and chest width take place in a few months, followed by an increase in shoulder width several months later.

Fat becomes redistributed into adult proportions as height and mass increase, and the adolescent gradually assumes an adult appearance.

All physical changes are the result of hormonal influences when the hypothalamus begins to produce 'releasing' factors. The gonadotropic releasing hormones signal the pituitary gland to secrete gonadotropic hormones, which stimulate testicular cells to produce testosterone and ovarian cells to produce oestrogen. These hormones contribute to the development of secondary sex characteristics, and play an essential role in reproduction. The changing concentration of these hormones is also linked to problems of adolescence, such as body odour and acne:

- Sebaceous glands become very active
- Eccrine sweat glands become fully functional
- Apocrine sweat glands reach secretory capacity
- Body hair assumes characteristic distribution patterns and texture changes: pubic and ancillary hair appears, and facial and body hair appears on males
- Blood pressure increases, heart rate decreases, and respiratory efficiency improves
- In females, the initial appearance of menstruation (menarche) occurs, and ovulation usually occurs 12–24 months after menarche. Breasts begin to develop from about 10 years of age, and development continues until approximately 17 years of age
- In males, nocturnal emissions of seminal fluid generally indicates the onset of puberty. The testicles and penis enlarge, and the voice deepens.

The physical changes that occur during adolescence are rapid and dramatic, and play a significant role in psychosocial development.

Intellectual development

Adolescents are capable of using deductive reasoning and abstract thinking, and can consider the logic of a problem. Being able to think logically about role behaviours, enables an adolescent to develop his own thoughts and means of expressing his identity. Intellectual development continues, through formal education and the pursuit of personal interests. Language development is relatively complete by adolescence, although vocabulary continues to expand. The main focus becomes the development of communication skills that can be employed effectively in various situations.

Emotional and personality development

Adolescence is often a period of emotional turmoil and insecurity, caused by the conflict between the need and desire for independence and the need to retain dependence on others. It is a time when identity is consolidated, and a time when choices about vocation and lifestyle must be made. Relationships with parents undergo change, and the adolescent begins to assert his individuality and desire for independence—often by resisting adult authority and advice.

The adolescent usually displays mood swings, and experiences confused emotions. In later adolescence, emotions are better controlled and more mature. However, an older adolescent is still subject to heightened emotion and his expressive behaviour reflects feelings of insecurity and indecision.

The adolescent's search for *identity* involves the quest for individual, sex-role, and group identity. A sense of identity is the individual's concept of who he is and where he is going in life. To find out who he is, the adolescent must formulate standards of conduct for himself; he must know what he values as important and worth doing, and he needs a sense of his own worth and importance. As the adolescent moves away from the family, the values of his peer group and their appraisal of him become increasingly important. When parental views and values differ greatly from those of his peers and other important figures, the possibility for conflict is great. As a result the adolescent may experience *role diffusion*, as he tries out one role after another, and has difficulty in synthesizing the different roles into a single identity. A positive identity eventually emerges following periods of confusion and adjustment, as the adolescent makes choices about his future.

Social development

Social development involves an expansion of the network of social relationships and social activities. The peer group remains the most important social group, serving as a strong support for the adolescent and providing him with a sense of belonging.

Relationships with members of the opposite sex assume a new importance, and attachments can be intense. Sexual experimentation is common among adolescents, as a result of peer pressures, physiological and emotional changes, and societal expectations. Many adolescents experience homosexual attractions, which may result in feelings of guilt and confusion.

Adulthood

Early adulthood is the period of development from 19–20 years to approximately 45 years of age. From 46–65 years is classed as middle adulthood, while late adulthood is the period from 65 years on. Adult development involves orderly and sequential changes in characteristics and attitudes.

Early adulthood

Physical development. Physical changes are minimal during this stage of development, with the exception of the major physical changes that accompany a pregnancy.

Intellectual development. Formal and informal educational, and life, experiences together with occupational opportunities increase the young adult's conceptual and problem-solving skills. Decision making processes need to be flexible as the young adult is constantly adjusting to changes; in the home, workplace, and in personal life.

Emotional and personality development. Emotional development concerns adjustment to independent adult life, and centres on the formation of adult relationships. Erik Erikson describes this stage of development as that between 'intimacy and solidarity' and 'isolation' (see Table 2.2). The young adult chooses to adopt one of various lifestyles whereby emotional relationships are established. Some of the choices which may need to be made include whether to marry, whether to become a parent, or whether to pursue a career.

Social development. During this stage the young adult generally gives more attention to occupational and social pursuits, and attempts to improve his socioeconomic status. His network of relationships provide opportunities for the fulfillment of a variety of social roles, and to enter a number of different social systems. The young adult can choose to remain within the prescribed expectations of his society, or to relate to the society in his own way.

Middle adulthood

Physical development. Major physiological changes occur between the ages of 45 and 65 years. Physical growth is replaced by physical degeneration, bringing about changes including:

- slow decrease in skin turgor
- greying and loss of hair
- decreased muscle mass
- decreased range of joint motion
- changes in menstrual cycle precede menopause, due to declining production of oestrogen and progesterone
- decreased level of androgen leads to male andropause
- diminished acuity of the senses may occur.

Intellectual development. Changes are relatively uncommon, except in the presence of disease or trauma, and the middle aged adult is able to continue learning. Some individuals may experience difficulty with concentration and retention of information.

Emotional and personality development. Erik Erikson describes middle adulthood as the stage characterized by 'generativity' versus self-absorption. Some individuals achieve a sense of generativity by rearing a family, and others by developing careers. This is regarded as the stage when an individual is interested in establishing and guiding the next generation, and one in which the individual strives to ensure continuation of his work and life-style. If an adult is unable to assume responsibility for promoting the future he may experience a sense of stagnation, become self-absorbed, and be unable to relate effectively to his world.

Social development. This is a stage where there are likely to be many changes in the individual's life, e.g. children moving away from home, change in career, and assuming responsibility for the care of ageing parents. Loss of a spouse or partner by divorce or death is not uncommon. Retirement will be a reality for most adults towards the end of this stage, therefore it is necessary to plan for the future well before the event. Individuals generally build up a framework of leisure pursuits, hobbies, relationships, and financial security in preparation for retirement.

Late adulthood

The last developmental stage begins when an individual reaches approximately 65 years of age. Older adults undergo a number of changes and in order to understand the reasons for these changes, it is necessary to have some knowledge of the various theories of ageing. There are a number of theories regarding the process of ageing, but there are no certain conclusions as to the cause. *Pathological* changes due to disease should not be confused with normal ageing, and it is necessary to make distinctions between what are the *degenerative* changes of ageing and the pathological changes superimposed on the ageing process.

Ageing is a complex process which begins at conception and ends with death. Theories of ageing include:

- *Genetic theory.* There is little doubt that heredity is a factor in the ageing process, and the genetic theory states that an individual's life span is programmed within the genes. This means that an individual inherits the family's tendencies for long or short life.
- *Stress theory.* This theory proposes that natural changes occur in the body throughout the individual's life time, and that the ability to replace worn out cells is decreased by the stresses experienced throughout life.
- *Cell ageing.* The chemical structure of the cell and its nucleus have been studied in relation to ageing. One suggestion is that chemical errors could be incorporated in the cells of ageing tissues which would adversely affect overall cell function. There are two main theories about what is thought to take place in cells as they age and eventually die. The first suggests that the cell itself is the main cause of the ageing process; while the other theory suggests that ageing affects the organization of cells, and implies a failure of communication between cells and the environment around them.
- *Immunological theory.* Some theorists suggest that there

are several cellular mechanisms capable of attacking various body tissues, and that these mechanisms act more frequently in ageing.
- *Psychological theories.* Various theories state that factors other than heredity, e.g. life style, personality, and the environment, also influence an individual's life span. These theories attempt to explain the psychosocial changes which occur with advancing age. For example, the 'disengagement theory' suggests that even under optimal personal and social circumstances, decreased physical and psychic energy characterize the later years of the life cycle. This theory states that decreasing social involvement and activity are inevitable, and necessary for successful ageing.

Therefore, while the process of ageing is complex and inevitable, there is no one theory to explain why it occurs.

Physical changes. There are certain physical changes associated with ageing, which are not pathological processes. They occur in all individuals, but take place at different rates and depend on accompanying circumstances:

- loss of subcutaneous fat and collagen, leading to inelastic and wrinkled skin
- atrophy of sweat glands, leading to skin dryness
- osteoporosis (thinning of bone) is common
- shortening of the trunk as a result of intervertebral space narrowing
- decreased joint mobility and range of joint motion
- decreased muscle mass and strength
- decreased rate of voluntary or automatic reflexes
- decreased ability to respond to multiple stimuli
- decreased visual acuity and accommodation
- diminished hearing acuity and pitch discrimination
- decreased senses of smell and taste
- increased chest rigidity, increased ventilatory rate with decreased lung expansion
- loss of blood vessel wall elasticity and change in cardiac function, e.g. diminished cardiac output
- decreased secretion of saliva, and digestive enzymes
- diminished intestinal motility
- decreased liver function
- decreased renal efficiency, reduced bladder capacity and control
- decreased breast tissue and uterine size, atrophy of vaginal epithelium
- decreased testicular size, and decreased sperm count.

While the general picture of ageing suggests a gradual diminution of system function, it should be remembered that many older adults show undiminished vigour, and organ function little different from that in earlier years.

Behavioural changes. There is a general misconception that all older adults experience decreasing intellectual function, and that learning becomes impossible. It is important to understand that structural and physiological changes occurring in the brain during the ageing process, do not necessarily affect the individual's intellect. Intellectual performance improves with environmental stimuli and, if an older adult receives sufficient stimuli, cognitive function is generally retained or improved.

Emotional and personality changes may occur, particularly in respect to how an older adult views himself. Many elderly people experience social isolation for many reasons, and an older person's self esteem partially depends on whether he is accepted into social relationships and interactions. An older person may choose to reject personal interactions, preferring his own company to that of others. Some elderly individuals may be isolated from society because of people's attitudes towards, and rejection of, the aged. When society emphasizes the negative aspects of ageing, and rejects the positive aspects, older individuals experience a loss of self respect and a sense of worthlessness. Erik Erikson describes this stage of development as that which is characterized by 'integrity versus despair' (see Table 2.2).

Many psychosocial changes occur with ageing, and how an individual copes with these changes depends on many factors, e.g. personality and network of friends. Changes may include:

- retirement
- loss of a life-long partner
- altered socioeconomic status
- decreased independence
- change in health status
- change in housing and/or environment.

These, and other, social changes which can occur during the later years of life may be seen as a threat by an elderly person who fears loss of control. A person's need to control his environment is not diminished simply because he is becoming older. When control over what is happening to and around him is decreased, an older person may experience loss of self esteem and worth. As a result, the individual may experience severe psychological distress, which can be reflected in physical ill health.

CONCLUSION

Growth and development are processes which begin at conception and continue throughout each stage of the life cycle.

Growth may be defined as the physical changes that occur in a steady and orderly manner, while development relates to changes in psychological and social functioning.

The stages of growth and development are generally described as being prenatal, infancy, childhood, adolescence, and adulthood. Characteristic changes occur at each stage, but the pace and behaviours of growth and development vary with each individual.

REFERENCES AND FURTHER READING

Clements A (ed) 1986 Infant and family health in Australia. Churchill Livingstone, Melbourne
Turner J S, Helms D B 1987 Lifespan development, 3rd edn. Holt, Rinehart and Winston, New York

4. Introduction to the behavioural sciences

OBJECTIVES

1. Discuss the basic psychological and sociological concepts introduced in this chapter.
2. State the broad functions of the major departments within a hospital.

INTRODUCTION

The terms 'behavioural sciences' and 'social sciences' are both used to describe the fields of study such as anthropology, political science, psychology, and sociology. *Behavioural science* is a term which is frequently used to describe those fields which focus more particularly on individual behaviour; anthropology, psychology, and sociology.

This chapter aims to introduce the nurse to basic psychological and sociological concepts relevant to understanding human development and behaviour. An introduction to basic concepts should help the nurse to understand why people behave as they do, provide an insight into her own attitudes and reactions, and enhance her interpersonal skills. In the latter part of the chapter the structure of a hospital, as an organization, is described.

A beginning knowledge of psychology is relevant to nursing because its subject matter is that of *human behaviour*. Knowledge of sociological concepts should assist the nurse towards a better understanding of the differing social needs of people, and their different reactions, e.g. to illness and health care.

Psychology can be broadly defined as the science that studies behaviour and mental processes. *Sociology* can be broadly defined as the study of how individuals interact with one another in society. There is a close relationship between the two, as psychology is concerned with the behaviour and mental processes of the individual, and the individual is the basic unit of society. Both are, therefore, concerned with individuals; psychology mainly with human beings as individuals and sociology with the individual as part of a social system. *Social psychology* is concerned with those aspects of individual behaviour which stem from group membership.

Approaches to psychology

In addition to the study of human behaviour, psychologists are also concerned with human experience, language and other forms of communication. Because the range of psychology is so vast, the work of a psychologist is often restricted to one section of the science. For example, some psychologists are concerned with the study of learning, others are interested in the phenomena of perception, while others are concerned with the study of child behaviour or development. Because psychologists differ in their interests, and in the ways by which they approach the subject, there have emerged various 'schools' of psychology which are different approaches to the psychological study of the individual. Each approach, or viewpoint, offers a somewhat different explanation of why a person acts as he does, and each makes a contribution to an understanding of the total person. The major approaches are outlined below.

1. Neurobiological approach. This approach to the study of the human being attempts to relate his actions to events taking place within his body, particularly within the brain and nervous system. It attempts to reduce observable behaviour and mental events, e.g. emotions, to neurobiological processes. It is generally accepted that there is an intimate relationship between brain activity and behaviour and experience; and emotional reactions, e.g. fear, have been produced in humans by mild electrical stimulation of specific areas in the brain.

2. Cognitive approach. This approach is concerned with the way the brain actively processes incoming information, by transforming it internally in various ways so that it is converted into the individual's version of comprehension and understanding. *Cognition* refers to the mental processes that transform sensory input, store it in memory, and retrieve it for later use. Therefore, people can think, plan, and make decisions on remembered information.

23

3. Behavioural approach. This approach studies an individual by looking at his behaviour, and focuses on activities that can be observed and measured. This approach considers that both conscious and unconscious experiences are too subjective for scientific study, and concentrates on patterns of behaviour as conditioned responses. Stimulus-response psychology studies the stimuli that elicit behavioural responses, the rewards and punishments that maintain these responses, and the modifications in behaviour obtained by changing the patterns of rewards and punishments. Behaviourists, then, believe that all behaviour occurs in response to a stimulus. This school of psychology studies and interprets behaviour by observing measurable responses to stimuli—without reference to consciousness, mental states, or subjective phenomena such as ideas and emotions.

4. Psychoanalytic approach. This approach emphasizes unconscious motives stemming from repressed sexual and aggressive impulses in childhood. This concept, which was developed by Sigmund Freud (1856–1939), is based on the assumption that much of the individual's behaviour is determined by innate instincts that are largely *unconscious*. Freud viewed unconscious processes as the thoughts, fears, and wishes of which an individual is unaware but which influence his behaviour. Freud believed that all of the individual's actions have a cause, but the cause is often some unconscious motive—rather than a rational reason the individual may give for his behaviour. Freud's view was that man is driven by the basic instincts of sex and aggression, and that he is continually struggling against a society that stresses control of these instincts.

5. Humanistic approach. This approach focuses on the individual's subjective experiences, freedom of choice, and motivation towards self-actualization. Psychologists who adopt this approach see the individual as capable of controlling his own destiny and changing the world around him. This approach rejects the concept of the individual as a mechanism controlled by external stimuli or by unconscious motives, and considers that an individual's main motivational force is a tendency towards self-actualization (developing his potential to the fullest).

In order to understand human behaviour and mental functioning it is first necessary to have some knowledge of the underlying biological processes involved. Behaviour depends on the integration of numerous processes within the body. For example, the nervous system, special sense organs, muscles and glands, enable an individual to be aware of and adjust to the environment. *Perception* of events depends on how the sense organs detect stimuli, and how the brain interprets information coming from the senses. Much of human behaviour is motivated by needs such as thirst, hunger, and the avoidance of pain or extremes of temperature. The ability to use language, to think, and to solve problems depends on a brain structure that is incredibly complex. Information on the structure and functions of the nervous system and special sense organs is provided in Chapters 20 and 27. The remainder of this chapter aims to provide the nurse with a beginning knowledge of the basic aspects of psychology and sociology.

Sensation and perception

An individual receives information about the environment through the sense organs: the eyes, ears, nose, tongue, and skin. Thus, he is able to experience the sensations of sight, sound, smell, taste, and touch.

A sense organ, sometimes referred to as a receptor, is a specialized part of the body which is *selectively* receptive to stimuli. For example, the eye is a receptor for sensations of light waves yet is impervious to sound stimuli. A sensory *stimulus* is any kind of mechanical, physical, or chemical change that acts upon a sense organ, e.g. the eye will respond to stimulation from light waves. The behavioural reaction brought forth by a stimulus is termed a *response* and, in effect, every human response is preceded by a stimulus. Information on the physiology of sensation is provided in Chapter 27, and summarized as follows:

- The eye responds to electromagnetic energy, i.e. light. Light waves from an object enter the eye through the pupil and pass through the lens. They focus on the retina which is the true receptor of visual stimuli. The optic nerve attaches to the retina, and serves as a medium for carrying the visual impulses to the nervous system.
- The ear is sensitive to mechanical energy, i.e. to pressure changes among the molecules in the atmosphere. *Hearing* occurs when sound acts as a stimulus to the auditory sense. The external ear collects sound waves, which strike the tympanic membrane (ear drum). Behind the tympanic membrane is the middle ear containing three small bones (ossicles), which interlock and serve to conduct the sound impulses to the inner ear. The inner ear connects with the middle ear by an oval-shaped window, into which is fitted one of the ossicles. The oval window conducts the sound waves to the cochlea the auditory portion of the inner ear. Within the cochlea is a section called the Organ of Corti, containing sensitive hair cells which are connected to the acoustic nerve. The acoustic nerve acts as a medium for carrying the sound waves to the nervous system.
- The sense of *smell* is activated when gaseous particles of a substance reach the epithelium of the nasal cavity. The receptors for smell are cells embedded high in the nose, and are connected to the olfactory nerve. The olfactory nerve serves as a medium for carrying the impulses of smell to the brain.
- The sense of *taste* is activated when a substance in solution reaches the taste buds on the surface of the tongue. There are four types of taste bud which respond to salty, sweet, sour, and bitter tastes. Within the taste

buds are the taste receptors which are receptive to chemicals. Taste impulses are carried to the brain via the glossopharyngeal and facial nerves.

• Receptors in the *skin* enable an individual to distinguish the sensations of touch, pressure, pain, warmth, and cold.

For each type of sensation there are specialized nerve endings which react to the specific type of stimuli. For example, the application of heat to the skin activates different nerve endings from those which respond to tactile pressure. The sensory tracts for impulses of pressure, pain, and temperature follow separate paths through the spinal cord to the brain.

Thus, *sensation* is the act of receiving a stimulus by a sense organ. *Perception* is the act of interpreting a stimulus registered in the brain by one or more sense mechanism. It is the way by which we experience and interpret reality. While the mechanics or physiology for receiving stimuli are similar from one individual to the next, the interpretation of these stimuli may differ. What an individual perceives at any given time depends on:

• the nature of the stimulus
• previous sensory experiences
• personal feelings, attitudes, drives, and goals.
• cultural, religious, and social experiences and responses.

Perceiving is a *learnt* activity as, to perceive, it is necessary to remember a previous experience and to recognize a sensory stimuli as identical or similar to stimuli previously experienced. For example, when an infant first experiences the sensory stimulus which an orange presents, a coloured round object appears on the retina. Similar images are produced by objects such as the sun or a ball. Later the infant learns to handle the orange, puts it into his mouth, smells it, bites it. Thus, he learns about its size, mass, texture, smell, and taste. Eventually he hears the word 'orange' used in connection with the object. He uses all his knowledge about the object to interpret the visual sensation, and *perceives* it as an orange—not the sun or a ball. Thus, in most situations, perception is largely a process of inference based on past experiences.

When there is a discrepancy between what an individual perceives and the actual facts, the experience is termed an *illusion*. An illusion is the fleeting misinterpretation of a sensory stimulus. The senses can be deceived in many ways, and illusions have long intrigued psychologists.

Perception is not a simple mechanical process of receiving specific stimuli which produce specific results, but it is the result of action and reaction. Just as the nature of a stimulus and previous sensory experiences affect perception, so does the nature of the individual. For example, any emotional state or attitude has an influence on a perceptual response. What a person perceives and how he perceives it may also be determined by his needs and personal values. For example, what is *seen* at a particular time depends on what the observer expects to see, on his attention, and on the meaningfulness of what is perceived.

To illustrate this concept of perception: a nurse is required to perceive details about an individual for whom she is caring. She is required to assess the individual's condition through observing his vital signs, facial expression, colour, posture, and many other indicators. An experienced nurse will have learned to perceive a situation accurately and to recognize the significance of a sign or symptom. Conversely, a beginning student of nursing will be unable to perceive such a sign or symptom accurately, because she does not yet know what to expect when she assesses the individual's condition. The beginning student has not learned to perceive, among a mass of details, those which are relevant or significant to the individual's condition.

Learning and thinking

Learning may be defined as a 'relatively permanent change in behaviour that occurs as the result of a prior experience'.

How learning occurs is not easy to explain, and a number of controversies exist about the process of learning. Many psychologists and teachers consider learning to be 'a relatively permanent change in behaviour that is a result of reinforced practice'. However, not everyone agrees that reinforcement (reward) plays a part in learning.

The process of learning can consist of one, two, or all, of three steps:

• thinking—inventing an original solution to a problem
• memorizing—committing to memory
• becoming efficient at applying a solution to a problem, or forming a habit.

Regardless of how it is explained, the kinds of tasks that psychologists use to study the phenomena of learning can be grouped into four categories: classical conditioning, operant conditioning, multiple—response learning, and cognitive learning.

1. Classical conditioning is a form of learning in which a previously neutral stimulus comes to elicit a response through associative training. The most precise examples of this form of learning were provided by the famous conditioned-response experiments of the Russian physiologist Ivan Pavlov (1849–1936). He noticed that just prior to being fed, dogs drooled saliva from their mouths. In his first experiments, Pavlov served the dogs food at the same time as a bell was rung. After many presentations of bell and food, the dogs salivated at the sound of the bell alone. The sound of the bell had come to substitute for the originally effective stimulus of food, so that the bell alone was able to make the dog's saliva flow. In psychological language, the salivation response had become conditioned to the new bell-ringing stimulus. Pavlov's experiments provided several principles useful in the understanding of *habit formation*.

Because classical conditioning represents a simple form of learning, it has been regarded by many psychologists as an appropriate starting point for investigation of the learning process.

2. Operant conditioning is a form of learning in which a person is rewarded for a correct response and not rewarded for an incorrect response. Operant behaviour acts on the environment to produce *reinforcement*, and becomes strengthened by reinforcement.

To demonstrate operant conditioning B.F. Skinner (1904–) devised an experiment involving a rat or pigeon, a box, and food. In a typical experiment a rat was placed in a closed box, one side of which was glass. Inside the box was a lever and a receptacle for food. Prior to the experiment, the rat was deprived of food so that it would be motivated by hunger. The lever was set up so that each time it was pressed by the rat a pellet of food would fall into the dish. The rat soon learned that a press on the lever would produce food. The food *reinforced* lever-pressing. In other words, the correct response (lever-pressing) was rewarded or reinforced. If the rat did not press the lever, food was not delivered.

Operant conditioning is a method used in a form of treatment called *behaviour modification*. For example, an intellectually disabled child can learn self-help skills such as the use of a toilet or dressing and undressing by reinforcing (rewarding) every success (correct response) immediately.

3. Multiple-response learning is a form of learning involving more than one action or response, unlike classical or operant conditioning. Much of our learning consists of acquiring patterns or sequences of behaviour, e.g. in learning how to play a guitar or ride a bicycle.

The skills involved in multiple-response learning can be classified as sensorimotor and verbal. A sensorimotor skill is one in which muscular movement is prominent but under sensory control, e.g. learning to type requires the typist to operate a keyboard, stay within specified boundaries, and follow a manuscript.

Memorizing the lines of a play or poem involves rote learning, which is largely a verbal skill. When rote memorization is used, the person may not *understand* what is learned.

4. Cognitive learning is a form of learning that is concerned with acquisition of problem-solving abilities, and with intelligence and conscious thought. The cognitive approach to learning attempts to go beyond specific stimuli and responses, and to being the whole person into an interpretation of learning. An underlying assumption of cognitive learning is that stimuli in the environment act on the individual in the sense that they cause change to occur

at the level of feelings, interests, attitudes, values, and perceptions. Changes in an individual's thoughts, feelings, and attitudes are believed to bring about changes in the way a person behaves—and changed behaviour is considered to be an indication that *learning has occurred*.

The cognitive approach to learning recognizes the importance of the use of cognitive processes, beyond simple recall.

Humans have the ability to *reason*, and reasoning is a form of *thinking* in which the possible solutions to a problem are tried out symbolically.

Trial-and-error thinking differs from reasoning in that an individual faced with a task of learning will start out in a 'hit-or miss' fashion, varying his responses until he strikes upon the successful sequence of acts. Most people are likely to engage in trial-and-error when faced with unfamiliar mechanical tasks, instead of using reasoning to find the solution. When trial-and-error thinking is used, it is quite likely that if a solution is arrived at it will be only by chance.

Learning by *insight* is solving a problem as the result of forming a rearrangement of previous experiences to new patterns of thought, i.e. of gaining insight into a new relationship between the elements of a problem. Insight is sometimes referred to as the 'Aha' experience, as an individual discovers the correct solution to a problem in a flash. Such abrupt insight into the structure of a problem usually moves an individual to some expression of satisfaction, e.g. 'Aha!'

An account of human reaction when such insight comes is told about Archimedes. When the great mathematician discovered the principle of specific gravity while in his bath, he jumped up shouting 'Eureka, I've found it!' and ran naked through the streets. He was so delighted with the solution to the problem which had been bothering him, that he forgot he had no clothes on.

Creativity, a stage of reasoning, is a process which generally consists of three steps:

- Preparation, in which facts are learned and observations made.
- Incubation, a period of seeming inactivity in which the thinker's mind seems to be 'hatching' something.
- Inspiration, in which an idea suddenly occurs and a concept emerges.

Problem solving is a way of finding answers to problems. In a problem-solving situation, one of the basic steps is not only to recognize the problem but also to define it. In the problem-solving technique, the problem must be identified, data must be collected and analyzed, a decision must be made, and the decision must be evaluated.

Information on problem-solving, which is a technique used extensively in the practice of nursing, is provided in Chapter 12.

Memory and forgetting

Memory is recollection, and remembering can be defined as the present knowledge of a past experience. Remembering can occur in several forms.

- Recognition: when an individual recognizes something, he acknowledges that it is familiar that he has met it before. For example, an individual may recognize a piece of music that he has heard before as it has previously registered on his sensory perceptors.
- Recall: an individual is said to recall something when, without it being present to the senses, he becomes aware of having experienced it in the past. For example, an individual may recall a poem in its entirety, without the written poem being available to him at that time.
- Performance: an individual may perform certain actions so well learned that they are highly automatic. For example, a nurse may be able to make several beds in a hour without really thinking about each step of the technique.

In order for an individual to *remember* something, he must have first acquired the material. Acquiring is the first step in the complete process that culminates in remembering. A specific type of acquiring is associated with each form of remembering. In order to recognize or to recall, the individual must be able to perceive. In order to perform a habit or action, the individual must first form the habit.

Memory can be viewed in three stages:

- Encoding, which refers to the transformation of sensory information into a form that can be processed by the memory system.
- Storage, which is the transfer of encoded information into memory.
- Retrieval, which refers to the process by which information is remembered when it is needed.

Some form of *forgetting* is inevitable, and the reasons why people forget things can be explained in three ways:

- Decay through disuse: which means that forgetting takes place simply through the passage of time. This explanation assumes that learning leaves a 'trace' in the brain, which involves some sort of physical change that was not present prior to learning. With the passage of time the normal metabolic processes of the brain cause a fading or decay of the memory, so that traces of material once learned gradually disappear. There is no direct evidence to support this theory, and some evidence suggests that it is an incomplete explanation as to why people forget.
- Interference effects: which means that the course of forgetting is determined by what an individual does in the interval between learning and recall, and that *new* learning may interfere with material previously learned.
- Motivated forgetting: which means that an individual's motives play an important part in remembering and forgetting. Forgetting is often associated with the individual's emotional state. Everybody tends to forget unpleasant or painful experiences, and this process is called *repression*. The theory of repression states that the memories are not recalled because their retrieval would in some way be unacceptable to the individual, e.g. because of the anxiety they would produce or the guilt they might activate.

Repressed material is not necessarily permanently forgotten, and it may be recalled into consciousness when current circumstances evoke a connection and when the individual's emotional state makes it possible to remember.

Motivation and emotion

The term *motivation* refers to those factors that energize and direct behaviour. Psychologists study not only *what* people do, but *why* they do it, i.e. they look behind an individual's actions to find their origin or motive. Motivation may be described as an impulse to act as the result of a motive.

The most fundamental motives are those which stem from the body's physiology and chemistry. These body forces which activate individuals to satisfy needs, such as the need for food and water, are called drives.

A *drive* is a stimulus, usually of physiological origin, which demands a response to meet a bodily or tissue *need*. A drive motivates the individual to initiate behaviour to remedy the need. Hunger is a typical example of a basic drive. The hunger stimulus results from a lack of food in the body, and this lack causes the stomach to contract rhythmically. In response to this drive, an individual will eat something to satisfy his body's *need* for food.

It is apparent, however, that biological needs alone do not account for the diversity and complexity of human behaviour. Abraham Maslow (1908–1970) proposed an interesting way of classifying human motives. He assumed a hierarchy of motives ascending from the basic biological needs present at birth, to more complex psychological motives that become important only after the more basic needs have been satisfied (refer to Fig. 28.1). Maslow's scheme provides an interesting way of looking at the relationships among motives, and the opportunities afforded by the environment.

Although many theories have been developed to explain human motivation, there is little consensus. Two of the theories that adopt very different views concerning human nature and motivation are the psychoanalytic theory, and the social learning theory.

Psychoanalytic theory of motivation was developed by Sigmund Freud (1856–1939) and it proposes that an individual's behaviour is determined by inner forces and impulses—often operating below the level of consciousness. Freud considered that the two basic human motives were sex and aggression. He stated that these two motives arise in infancy, but as their expression is forbidden by parents, *repression* occurs. The repressed tendency remains active as an *unconscious motive*, and finds expression in indirect or symbolic ways, e.g. through dreams.

Social learning theory of motivation was formulated by Albert Bandura (1925–), and it focuses on patterns of behaviour that are learned in coping with the environment. The emphasis is on the interaction between behaviour and environment. According to this theory, the type of behaviour an individual exhibits partly determines the reward or punishment he receives, and these in turn influence behaviour. Patterns of behaviour can be acquired through direct experience or by observing the behaviour of others. Some action may be successful while others may produce unfavourable results. Through a process of *reinforcement*, an individual eventually selects the successful behaviour patterns, and discards the others. Reinforcement may be either external or self-evaluative. That is, a specific behaviour produces an external outcome such as praise or approval, but it also produces a self-evaluative reaction. An individual sets his own standards of conduct or performance, and responds to his behaviour in a self-satisfied or self-critical way.

Motivation and *emotion* are closely related. Feelings determine an individual's reactions and, conversely, behaviour often determines how an individual feels. Emotions can activate and direct behaviour in the same way as biological or psychological motives. Emotions can be a goal, and they can also accompany motivated behaviour.

Emotion is a difficult term to define, but when a person experiences an emotion the most striking aspect is the *feeling* it produces. Most emotions can be divided into those that are pleasant, e.g. joy or love, and those that are unpleasant, e.g. anger or fear. In addition to the feelings produced, emotion is generally accompanied by changes in immediate behaviour, e.g. laughing or crying. There are also many *internal* changes that occur in response to stimuli which provoke an intense emotional state:

- Blood pressure and heart rate increase
- Ventilations become more rapid
- Pupils of the eyes dilate
- The hairs on the skin erect, causing 'goose pimples'
- Blood glucose level increases to provide more energy
- Motility of the gastrointestinal tract decreases.

Most of these physiological changes which occur during intense emotion, e.g. anger or fear, result from activation of the autonomic nervous system as it prepares the body for emergency action. Information on the nervous system is provided in Chapter 20.

The basic ways of *expressing* emotion are innate. Infants and children cry when they are sad or hurt, and laugh when they are happy. Many of the facial expressions, postures, and gestures that are associated with different emotions develop through maturation; they appear at the appropriate age even when there is no opportunity to observe them in others. Studies of children who are blind and deaf from birth indicate that appropriate facial expressions and gestures develop in response to a specific emotion, e.g. smiling when happy.

Certain facial expressions, e.g. of happiness, anger, or surprise, seem to have universal meaning regardless of the culture in which an individual is raised.

Although certain emotional expressions may be largely innate, many modifications occur through *learning*. For example, *anger* may be expressed by using abusive language, by fighting, or by removing oneself from the situation.

Sometimes emotions are not immediately expressed, but continue to remain unexpressed or unresolved. This state of suppression can affect an individual's ability to function efficiently, and continual emotional tension can impair physical and psychological health. A number of different conditions, e.g. high blood pressure, migraine headaches, peptic ulcers, are related to emotional stress. Even when emotion does not contribute to the cause of an illness it can interfere with the course of a disease, e.g. an individual who has undergone surgical intervention may be so afraid of experiencing pain that he tends to lie very still, and this restricted mobility may result in the formation of deep vein thrombosis.

Personality

Personality may be defined as the behaviour and characteristics that distinguish one individual from another, or as the characteristic patterns of behaviour and modes of thinking that determine a person's adjustment to the environment. Personality is shaped by inborn potential and by the unique experiences that affect the person as an individual.

Psychologists are interested in how personality develops and changes, and in attempting to measure certain personality characteristics. How personality develops, and how personality can be described, has been the subject of many theories. Most theories can be grouped into one of four classes: trait, psychoanalytic, social learning, and humanistic.

The trait approach. Trait theories assume that a personality can be described by its position on a number of continuous scales or dimensions. A *trait* refers to any characteristic in which an individual differs from another in a relatively permanent and consistent way. A trait may also be defined as a tendency to behave in a consistent manner in various situations.

In studies of personality to discover the basic traits of individuals, two dimensions which are found fairly consistently are introversion-extraversion, and stability-instability. *Introversion-extroversion* refers to the degree to which an individual's basic orientation is turned toward the self, or outward toward the external world. As defined by Carl Jung (1875–1961), the *extrovert* is a person who is most interested in the external world of objects and people, while the *introvert* is most interested in his own thoughts and feelings.

Stability–instability is a dimension of emotionality varying from calm, well-adjusted, reliable individuals at the stable end to those who are moody, anxious, temperamental, and unreliable at the other end of the scale.

Characteristics such as patience, honesty, perseverance, conscientiousness, and initiative are other examples of personality traits.

The psychoanalytic approach. Psychoanalytic theory assumes that much of human motivation is *unconscious* and must be inferred indirectly from behaviour. This approach does not deny that external experiences are important, but draws special attention to the importance of unconscious motivation. The theory, developed by Sigmund Freud, suggests that personality is composed of three major systems—each of which has its own functions but all interact to govern behaviour:

• The *id* is the original source of personality, present in the newborn infant. It consists of everything that is inherited; it is irrational and impulsive, seeking immediate gratification of pleasure-seeking impulses. The id endeavours to avoid pain and to obtain pleasure, regardless of any external considerations.

• The *ego* develops out of the id because of the necessity for dealing with the real world. It is realistic and logical, postponing gratification until it can be achieved in socially acceptable ways. The ego is that part of the personality which decides what actions are appropriate, which instincts will be satisfied, and in what manner.

• The *superego* judges whether an action is right or wrong according to the standards of society. It is composed of the *conscience* and the *ego-ideal*. Conscience is the moral, self-critical sense of what is right and wrong. Ego ideal is the image of the self to which an individual aspires, and against which an individual measures himself and his performance. The superego develops as the standards of society are incorporated into the ego.

The social learning approach. Social learning theory assumes that personality differences result from variations in learning experiences. Social learning theorists claim that *reinforcement* is not necessary for learning, although it may facilitate learning by focusing attention. This theory claims that much of human learning occurs as a result of watching the actions of others, and by noting the consequences of those actions.

Social learning theorists regard the *situation* as an important determinant of behaviour. Thus, a person's behaviour in a given situation depends on the specific characteristics of the situation, the individual's appraisal of the situation, and on observations of others in similar situations.

Social learning theory focuses on behaviour patterns and cognitive activities in relation to the specific conditions that evoke, maintain, or modify them. The emphasis is on what individuals *do* in relationship to the conditions in which they do it.

The humanistic approach. Humanistic theories of personality are concerned with the individual's personal view of the world, his self-concept, and his ability to reach his fullest potential despite the limitations of personality and circumstance. Most humanistic theories place their emphasis on the 'here and now' rather than on events in early childhood that may have shaped the individual's personality.

Personality is a complicated arrangement of internal forces that mould the way in which an individual goes about being the kind of person that he is. While the four theories outlined above focus on different aspects they do not fully explain the complexities of personality, and pay little attention to the role of cognitive processes and social interactions in personality.

Intelligence and aptitudes

Intelligence, one aspect of personality, is difficult to define but it has to do with the ability to learn. In the view of many researchers in psychology and education, intelligence is defined broadly as a general ability to learn, to reason, to grasp concepts, and to deal with abstractions. While heredity is involved, so too is the environment to which the individual is exposed. Few experts doubt that there is some genetic basis for intelligence, but opinions differ as to the relative contributions of heredity and environment. The question is whether people are born with varying amounts of a general ability for learning or whether the differences are a result of variations in environmental experiences; that is, the result of differences in *opportunities* to learn. This question has come to be known as the 'nature-nurture controversy', and it is an issue that has excercised the minds of many researchers.

Some psychologists put forth the theory that, as there are people who seem to be more intelligent in some fields than in others, intelligence is a mixture of particular abilities called *aptitudes*. Others put forth the idea that there are several kinds of general intelligence, while some psychologists suggest that a person's total ability is the sum of his special abilities and his general intelligence. Professor E. L. Thorndike (1874–1949) suggested that intelligent behaviour might be broadly classified into three kinds: mechanical, social, and abstract. According to Thorndike:

• Mechanical intelligence is skill in manipulating tools and managing the working of machines
• Social intelligence covers the understanding of people and the ability to interact appropriately in human relationships

- Abstract intelligence is the ability to handle symbols and ideas such as words, numbers, formulae, and scientific principles.

Psychologists who believe in the *aptitude* theory of intelligence suggest that Thorndike's classification is too broad. In general, the modern concept of intelligence can be represented by an arrangement of factors:

- many particular *aptitudes*
- several *kinds* of intelligence
- *general* intelligence.

According to this concept, aptitudes are abilities to form habits efficiently; the kinds of intelligence are the abilities to form concepts of different parts of the environment; and general intelligence can be thought of as a tendency to experience insight.

Many tests have been developed to *measure* intelligence, including:

- Binet's method. Alfred Binet (1857–1911) decided to scale intelligence as the kind of change that ordinarily comes with growing older. Accordingly, he devised a scale of units of *mental* age. The average mental age scores correspond to chronological age. Thus, a bright child's mental age is above his chronological age, while a dull child has a mental age below his chronological age.
- Intelligence quotient (IQ). Louis Terman (1877–1956) adopted a convenient index of brightness that was suggested by a German psychologist William Stern (1871–1938). This index is the intelligence quotient (IQ) which expresses intelligence as a ratio of mental age to chronological age. A modern IQ is merely a test score adjusted for the age of the person being tested. It is no longer a 'quotient' but the expression IQ persists because of its familiarity and convenience.
- The Wechsler Intelligence Scales. This is a widely used intelligence test which has both a verbal and a performance scale. Using this test, separate information can be obtained about each type of ability.

While most intelligence tests measure *convergent* thinking (solving a problem that has a well-defined correct answer), J. P. Guilford (1897–) devised tests that also measure divergent thinking (arriving at many possible solutions to a problem). There are other ability tests which measure *aptitude* and *achievement*:

- Aptitude tests measure the capacity to learn, and predict what an individual can accomplish with training.
- Achievement tests measure accomplished skills, and indicate what an individual can do at present.

While intelligence and aptitude tests can be valuable, they do not predict personality variables such as creativity, special talents, motivation, and perseverance.

Norms

Norms operate as guidelines for behaviour. A norm can be defined as a measure of a phenomenon generally accepted as the *ideal* standard of performance, against which other measures of the phenomenon can be assessed. Norms are also referred to as codes, models, or standards. In sociology the rules, standards, or expectations within a *group* are called norms. Norms may operate as folkways, mores, customs or laws; and norms are called *prescriptive* if they require the individual to do something and *proscriptive* if they required the individual to avoid something.

Folkways are the simplest and least strongly enforced norms, and are standard practices and customs which people in a particular society are generally expected to follow. They are usually followed as a matter of course, passed on from one generation to another, and easily adopted by most people. Many of the norms which existed in previous generations are now no longer observed, e.g. once it was the norm for a male to open a door for a female. Many folkways vary from one society to another, e.g. in Australia 'burping' throughout a meal is considered a breach of etiquette, while in other societies it is considered to indicate appreciation of the food.

Mores are those customs and practices which must be observed strictly, and are considered to be more important than folkways. Failure by an individual to observe a more generally results in strong disapproval. Mores are associated with moral ideas of what is right and wrong, and are seen as being important to the welfare of a community. Mores may be expressed as prohibitions, such as 'Thou shalt not steal', while many mores are expressed in the form of laws.

Customs may be defined as the established modes of thought and action which are characteristic of a culture. Customs are generally enduring, related to a total culture, and may be extremely resistant to change. Customary ways of behaving are usually taken for granted by the members of a society, until people come into contact with other cultures and become aware that not all societies adopt the same customs. It is only by reflecting on the value of established customs, that people begin to question their purpose and place in society.

Laws, in a sociological context, refer to 'enacted law' which means any rule or regulation made by authority. Many of the rules and regulations made by the nursing administration department of a hospital may be regarded as enacted laws.

Role and status

In a sociological context, *role* is closely related to the concept of *function*. Roles are behaviours prescribed for and expected of persons who perform certain functions. A role may be viewed as the culturally prescribed behaviour of any person in a given social situation. The term 'role' is used in several ways: sometimes it is used to refer to other people's expectations of a person, sometimes to the activities that a person engages in, and sometimes to the way a person himself thinks he is expected to behave. Any individual plays a number of roles at any given time. For example, a 40-year-old male may be a husband, father, brother, uncle, salesman, a member of a particular religion, a rate payer, and a voter.

Role conflict may arise when a person is required to play two different roles that are competing or antagonistic. For example, a nurse may experience conflict if she is involved in caring for a person who is a close friend. Role conflict may also occur when different people expect a role to be carried out in different ways. As a result the person carrying out that role may be confused as to what is expected of her—what her role actually is.

The concepts of role and *status* are closely related. Status refers to a socially identified *position*, and a role is the expected pattern of behaviour that goes with that position. Thus, in a sociological context, status is considered in terms of the particular expectations that society has of people in particular positions. Status may be considered in terms of its:

- *causes*, which are associated with social class, wealth, education, occupation
- *results* such as recognition, privileges, benefits
- *responsibilities*, which are the expectations that society has of those who hold particular status positions.

There are two kinds of status: those that are ascribed by society and cannot be chosen or avoided, and those which an individual achieves by his own personal efforts. *Ascribed status and role* is that which has been ascribed to an individual by members of a society on the basis of personal attributes, and over which the individual has no control. For example, the status of an individual usually changes as he grows old. *Achieved status and role* is that which an individual achieves through choice, effort, and performance. Achieved statuses are acquired during an individual's lifetime and generally reflect individual talents. For example, a person may choose to pursue a career in nursing and through her efforts and performance go on to become an expert clinical nurse or administrator.

Attitudes and values

Attitudes are not behaviours but are perceptions which usually affect behaviour in relation to people, objects, and situations. An attitude can be defined as a *feeling* that affects behaviour. An individual's attitudes involve his perception and evaluation of a situation and of the people in the situation. A person's attitudes influence his choice of friends, hobbies, career; and affect the development of his social conscience and political opinions. Not only do his attitudes determine how he behaves towards other people, but also how other people behave towards him. Attitudes play a vital role in the way in which people communicate with others.

Attitudes generally develop over a long period of time, and many are acquired almost subconsciously from other people. Unconscious attitudes can influence conscious thought or behaviours. Attitudes can also be habitual, as when a person consistently despises members of a particular race, religion, society, or economic class. An attitude may be based on false assumptions, e.g. an individual may 'stereotype' another person and behave towards him accordingly.

Changes of attitude and, subsequently of, behaviour often come about with increased knowledge, maturity, and new insights gained from experience. For example, people's attitudes towards and behaviour regarding smoking have changed in recent years. As a result of anti-smoking campaigns people have acquired more knowledge about the hazards associated with smoking, and as a result the attitudes of many people towards smoking have changed.

Values are beliefs about particular modes of conduct, and they act in important ways in guiding conduct. The term 'value' refers to that which a person feels to be extremely important, e.g. material items such as money, or abstract phenomena such as competition, or power. Thus, people may, for example, value freedom, security, family, or social status. Values motivate individuals towards attaining a desired standard, and they act as standards by helping individuals to evaluate themselves and others. For example, people tend to choose as friends those who share many similar values. Values tend to remain fairly constant, whereas attitudes tend to be more flexible.

Attitudes about abstract ideas such as freedom, democracy, justice, hatred for suffering are pervasive and create a *value system* which affects an individual's attitudes in his work, choice of friends, and his interest in world affairs. A person's values are one of the most influential factors in that person's behaviour.

Stereotypes and labels

Stereotypes are clusters of interrelated traits and attributes that people assume to be characteristic of individuals in certain categories or groups. Stereotypes often have no factual basis, and are sometimes formed to rationalize prejudices or to justify shabby treatment of individuals on the basis of some assumed group characteristics that neither the individuals nor the group actually possess.

Stereotypes are often over-simplifications and generalizations about racial, national, religious, social, or professional groups. When the stereotype consists of many unfavourable characteristics it is often associated with *prejudice*. For example, an individual may build an idea for himself of the 'typical Asian' or 'typical Jew' and then behave towards all Asians and Jews—not according to their real personality but according to his own ideas. An individual may be quite surprised when he finds that the people he meets are quite different from his preconceived ideas.

The danger of forming judgements about whole groups of people on the basis of stereotype lies in the difficulty this creates in communication and understanding. For example, an individual who dislikes all Roman Catholics and has a stereotyped view of Roman Catholics is unlikely to be friendly, sympathetic and sincerely interested when he makes the acquaintance of a person who is a Roman Catholic. Some individuals are much more inclined than others to stereotype people, and those who are given to stereotyping often find it difficult to change their opinions—being rigid or inflexible in many of their attitudes.

The concept of stereotyping is closely linked to that of labelling. A *label* attached to a person, because of a preconceived bias, tends to make others approach him in a predetermined way. A consequence of 'labelling' people is the implication that all people covered by the label are alike. Labelling may occur in a health care institution, e.g. an individual may be labelled as a 'diabetic' rather than as a person who happens to have a physical condition. As a consequence some health care workers may expect that individual to behave in the same way as all other 'diabetics'.

Labels not only prevent people from getting to know the facts about an individual, but they may also have the effect of making the individual fit the label. For example, to label a child 'dull' may cause people to behave towards him as if he were dull, and may result in the child accepting the label so that he feels and acts as if he were dull.

Morale

The term 'morale' is often used to describe the atmosphere that exists between people which affects their happiness, attitude to their place of employment, the quality of their work, and work satisfaction. When morale is high everything seems to go well, and when it is low there are many indications of disturbance, and many aspects of work are affected, e.g. low productivity, poor quality of work. Among the most common results of low morale are rapid turnover in personnel, absenteeism, and increased incidence of accidents.

Morale is usually high when there is job satisfaction. Job satisfaction depends on many factors including work that is stimulating but not so difficult that it cannot be accomplished, opportunities for self-fulfilment, good relationships with fellow workers, and effective leadership and management.

The influence of morale is experienced by all members of a group; each person is aware that his own attitude and behaviour are part of the group as a whole, and each is aware that some external factors are affecting him. Morale is influenced by the extent to which people in a group are able to solve their problems of status and role definition.

To promote high morale the management needs to create, among the people with whom he works, a sense of loyalty and a commitment to the goals of the organization. This means that each person must understand the purpose of the work to which they contribute. It also requires management to be aware of each person's attitudes, aspirations, and difficulties sufficiently to bring about mutual understanding. The extent to which a 'manager' succeeds in creating group cohesiveness may depend on the intrinsic value of the work, or on his own personal authority.

When there is high morale there tends to be high confidence in the leader of the group which may, in part, be due to the confidence the manager has in his own ability to lead.

Socialization

Socialization is the process by which a person learns to become a member of a group or culture. A *culture* is comprised of many things; it is the learning, thoughts, beliefs, behaviour patterns, traditions, institutions, rituals and wisdom of a people. Transmission of a culture from generation to generation is achieved by the process of socialization—whereby individuals acquire the attitudes, values, and practises of the groups in which they live and work.

Socialization prepares an individual for the roles he has to play by defining situations, providing beliefs and values, developing habits, skills and knowledge. These factors, together with cultivation of appropriate emotional responses, combine to make an individual a social being. Socialization is an ongoing process that begins in infancy and continues throughout life, and it takes place all the time in interactions with significant others.

George Herbert Mead (1934) defined those people who are significant to an individual in the process of socialization as 'significant others'. Significant others may include parents, teachers, friends, and spouses or lovers.

Socialization is seen more dramatically in early life, as it transforms the totally dependent infant into a thinking, talking, acting individual. Early socialization serves the child in many subsequent situations as he will have been taught the general belief system of his culture, the customary ways of doing things, the important mores, as well as the language of the culture.

The process of socialization does not prepare the child for all the roles he will have to play during his lifetime.

With each new change in status, e.g. becoming a secondary school student, there will be new norms to learn. Until he has mastered the prescribed role behaviour, the individual will not have been adequately socialized for any new position. Some new roles are learned incidently, some are learned informally, e.g. as an individual joins a new group such as a sports club, while others will be learned on joining the workforce.

When an individual becomes an adult he is the product of the socialization process that has been operating continuously since he was born. Thus, an individual becomes socialized first by his parents and later by many other people, all of whom consciously or unconsciously influence him towards conforming to *group values*, confidentiality, loyalty and integrity.

Groups

In a sociological context a group consists of members who interact with each other in certain ways, and who interact with people outside that group in other ways. Social groups may be classified in terms of size, group interest, quality of social interaction, and in their degree of organization. Groups are either primary or secondary:

• A primary group is one that is small enough for all the members to know each other and to develop a strong group identity, e.g. a family, cricket club, or a student nurse group.
• A secondary group is larger in nature and all members of the group may not be within close range of each other, e.g. a state or national nurses organization or a trade union. Relationships within a secondary group tend to be less personal and more formal.

For a person to become an accepted member of a group he must become like the other people in the group in ways which are important to them as a group. The new member is introduced to the way of life of the group by verbal or written communication of the rules, or by example. He will be expected to conform, and the group will let him know by words or actions whether he is seen as conforming to their expectations.

The more individual group members feel *identified* with the group, the more likely the group is to be successful in the pursuit of its common interests. Some groups impose specific rules and regulations on their members in an effort to promote a sense of group identity, e.g. the wearing of a uniform or particular standards of behaviour.

The influence of a group on the individual is strong, and most people are aware of group pressures. In a group, an individual is more likely to modify what might otherwise be a spontaneous reaction because he has other people's reactions in mind.

Of all the groups to which a person may belong the most significant ones are his 'reference' groups. These are groups with whom he identifies as a referral point for his standards, whose values he prefers, and which serve him as a model. Examples of reference groups are families, social clubs, and professional or industrial organizations.

Organizations

An organization is a formal structure, comprised of people, which is deliberately constructed to achieve specific goals. An organization is generally an open system which is sensitive to, and interacts with, its environment.

A hospital is a highly structured bureaucratic organization, and each member has a defined role and status. A hospital is organized into a series of hierarchies which are reputed to produce efficient management, and lines of communication are developed within those hierarchies.

A bureaucratic organization, e.g. a hospital, has certain characteristics:

• a hierarchy of positions, or a hierarchical structure of management
• a clear division of labour
• lines of authority
• rules and regulations
• promotion by merit (not by favour)
• an authoritarian character.

The sociologist Max Weber, in 1946, developed a theory of bureaucracy, and identified two main characteristics: a hierarchical structure of management, and division of labour. In his theory, bureaucracy plays a central role which, in his view, is the product of a search for rational efficiency. Weber was interested in the rational means employed to direct the activities of individuals doing various jobs in the organization towards given objectives.

While Weber's model attempts to explain the social structure of an organization by showing how each of its elements contributes to effective operation of the organization, it does not reveal the inconsistencies and conflicting tendencies in organizations.

ORGANIZATION OF A HOSPITAL

The main objective of any hospital is the provision of the highest standard of care for each patient. Such an objective may, for example, be expressed as, 'To provide health care to all members of the community whether as inpatients, outpatients or domiciliary patients, achieving the highest standards of patient care and community health'.

A hospital, like any other organization, develops an organizational chart which depicts the hierarchical structure of management and the lines of communication and authority between various departments. A typical organizational chart shows the structure of each major department within the organization.

A hospital may be said to consist of three administrative

areas: general, nursing, and medical. Therefore, an organizational chart depicts the structure of each of the three administrative areas.

Heading the organizational structure is the *Board of Management* comprised of members who participate in various committees such as finance, education, house and works, quality assurance, and medical appointments.

The chief Executive Officer, who is accountable to the Board of Management, has responsibility for overall general and financial administration of a hospital.

The Director of Administrative Services (general) is responsible for those services which include catering, linen, engineering, domestic, and supply.

The Director of Nursing is responsible for nursing services and nursing education. In the larger hospitals there are one or more deputies with specific areas of responsibility, e.g. in nursing administration.

Other personnel in the nursing department may include assistant directors of nursing, supervisors, charge nurses, nurse specialists, clinical resource nurses, nursing projects officers, nurse teachers, registered nurses, enrolled nurses, and students of nursing.

The Director of Medical Services is responsible for the administration of all medical services and medical ancillary departments such as pathology, physiotherapy, occupational and speech therapy, radiology, and pharmacy.

The health team

The health team is spoken of as being *multi disciplinary*, meaning that it is made up of people with education and expertise in a number of different aspects of patient care.

The most important members of the team are the patient and his significant others, e.g. his family. The rest of the team, which varies according to the needs of the individual, is made up of medical officers and nurses, physiotherapists, occupational therapists, social workers, speech therapists, dietitians, chaplains and other paramedical personnel. Teams may be formed within the team e.g. the nursing team or the medical team in order to ensure that complex care plans are adequately carried out.

The success of team work in any situation depends on a number of factors including:

● Every member of the team needs to have a true appreciation of the skills and qualities of every other member, and of the inter-relationships of all team members.
● There must be a common goal, and all team members should be involved in planning the methods to be used to achieve that goal.
● Good communications are essential, so that every individual is aware of his/her role and is aware of any changes that occur.
● The team leader is important, and is responsible for co-

ordinating the efforts of individual members of the team and for organizing regular reviews of progress.

Classification of hospitals

Health care delivery systems are either community or hospital based. This chapter focuses on the latter classification.

A hospital performs curative, preventive, and rehabilitation functions. In addition, a hospital is involved in the areas of research and education. Hospitals may be described according to their size, ownership, services, or the length of stay of the patients. Hospitals are generally classified according to the services they provide:

● *Public hospitals* are administered by the Health Commission (a state government authority) and provide free care for patients. A public hospital may also offer private accommodation for fee-paying patients.
● *Private hospitals* are owned by organizations, e.g. churches, companies or private individuals, and provide care for fee-paying patients.

Both public and private hospitals may be specialized in function, for example:

● Children's hospitals, which care for infants and children.
● Geriatric hospitals, which provide short- and/or long-term accommodation for elderly people. Many geriatric hospitals have a rehabilitation section where incapacitated elderly people are helped to regain as much independence and mobility as possible.
● Rehabilitation hospitals in which incapacitated people are restored to their maximum ability.
● Psychiatric hospitals, which provide short-and long-term treatment for people with psychiatric disorders.
● Infectious diseases hospitals, where people with infectious diseases are treated.
● Day-care hospitals, where people attend on a daily basis for one or more days each week and receive various forms of treatment. Overnight accommodation is not provided. Day-care hospitals are available for people requiring geriatric, psychiatric, or rehabilitation care. In addition, there are some hospitals which provide day care services for people requiring minor surgical intervention.
● Women's hospitals, which are concerned with disorders or conditions experienced only by women.
● Cancer hospitals, which provide care and treatment for people with malignant disorders.
● Eye and Ear hospitals, which provide care for people who have conditions affecting the eye, ear, nose, or throat.
● Maternity hospitals, which provide care for mothers and newborn infants.

Hospitals which are not specialized in nature are referred

to as general hospitals. They may contain specialized units which are staffed by specially trained personnel, e.g.:

- Renal unit, where individuals with disorders of the kidneys are treated.
- Intensive care unit, which provides intensive medical and nursing care for critically ill people.
- Coronary care unit, which provides medical and nursing care for people with cardiac disorders, e.g. suspected or confirmed heart attack.
- Plastic surgery unit, for individuals who require surgery for the purpose of restoring or rebuilding a part of the body.
- Burns unit, which provides medical and nursing care for people who have experienced burn injuries.

There may also be specialization at ward level. For example, a neurological ward is for individuals with disorders of the nervous system; a urological ward is for people with urinary tract disorders; individuals with bone or joint conditions may be cared for in an orthopedic ward; and midwifery wards provide facilities for prenatal care, birth, and post-natal care.

Medical wards are for individuals with disorders that do not usually require surgery, and *surgical wards* are for individuals who are treated by surgical intervention.

Departments within a hospital

The many services within a hospital can be broadly divided into three groups: patient care services, institutional services, and financial services. The following departments are commonly found in most major hospitals.

Operating rooms (theatre suite)

Depending on the size of the hospital, there may be one or a number of operating rooms. In addition to the rooms where surgery is performed, there are:

- sterilizing rooms
- anaesthetic rooms
- recovery rooms
- utility and storage rooms
- staff amenities such as offices, toilets and shower rooms.

Accident and emergency department

In most large hospitals, people who are classified as 'emergency' admission are received into this department. Such people are those for whom admission to hospital has not been pre-arranged, e.g:

- the victims of road, industrial, or domestic accidents

- people who have suddenly become very ill
- victims of assault.

The individual is assessed by a medical officer, any urgent treatment is given, and arrangements for admission to hospital are made if necessary.

Some accident and emergency departments have their own operating room where minor surgery can be performed, a plaster room where plaster casts are applied, and other services such as X-ray or pharmacy.

Out-patients department

In this department clinics are conducted by specialists, and the clinics are attended by individuals who have been referred by a general practitioner, or who have been in-patients of the hospital. Individuals may attend this department for the purpose of receiving treatment, or to enable a medical officer to assess their progress following discharge from hospital.

Radiology department

A radiology department generally provides services for both in-patients and out-patients. The work of this department may be both diagnostic and therapeutic. *Diagnostic* procedures include plain X-rays of hard structures such as bone, and other radiological procedures whereby soft structures such as internal organs may be visualized. *Therapeutic* procedures include various forms of radiotherapy to destroy malignant tissues.

Pathology department

A pathology department generally consists of a number of highly specialized areas, including those where specimens obtained from individuals are investigated for evidence of disease or abnormality. Other areas within the pathology department may include haematology which studies the blood and blood-forming organs, and biochemistry which studies the chemistry of living organisms and life processes. Small hospitals, which do not have a pathology department, send specimens to be investigated to a central pathology service or to a major hospital.

Pharmacy

The pharmacy department is responsible for supplying a wide range of products for use throughout the hospital, e.g:

- drugs prescribed for in-patients and out-patients
- intravenous fluids
- substances for topical application such as lotions, ointments, or pastes

- disinfectants and antiseptics
- some items of medical or surgical equipment.

Central sterilizing department

All sterile equipment is issued, as required, to the wards and departments. After use non-disposable equipment is returned to the central sterilizing department for cleaning and resterilization. The method of issuing sterile supplies varies slightly from one hospital to another.

Physiotherapy department

The personnel of this department are concerned with many forms of treatment including exercising of muscles for the purpose of restoring function, encouraging mobility, and assisting with breathing. Individuals are taught how to manage the activities of daily living, and in some instances they may be helped to retrain for some type of employment. The work of the physiotherapist is one part of the total patient care plan, and it is therefore co-ordinated with the medical treatment, nursing care, and occupational therapy.

Occupational therapy department

The function of this department is twofold.

First it works closely with the physiotherapy department and sets similar goals when designing activities, e.g. to encourage the use of certain muscles. Incapacitated individuals are taught how to use devices to help with the activities of daily living. Some individuals may be taught how to perform activities which will enable them to seek full or part time work, or work in a sheltered workshop.

Secondly it conducts diversional therapy aimed at providing long-term patients with mental and physical stimulation. Diversional therapy may be in the form of handwork and craft activities, film shows, music, concerts, etc.

Speech therapy department

The personnel in this department are responsible for assisting individuals with speech problems arising from causes such as deafness, surgery of the larynx, cerebro vascular accident, or head injuries.

Medical social worker's department

Medical social workers, as part of the health team, help individuals and their significant others who have social problems. They assist with financial problems, accommodation difficulties, home help, travel to and from hospital, sheltered employment, and they advise on the agencies through which help of various kinds can be arranged.

Catering department

The organization of food services differs from hospital to hospital, but there is usually a catering officer who is responsible for the ordering of supplies and the supervision of all staff engaged in the preparation and delivering of food.

Dietitians are responsible for the planning of menus particularly when special diets are prescribed. Dietitians also consult with individuals who request special types of food for religious or personal reasons, and they educate individuals on the subject of special diets to be followed before or during hospitalization, and after discharge from hospital.

Engineers department

This department is responsible for construction and maintenance work, and it is generally divided into sections which are staffed by plumbers, electricians, carpenters, painters, and gardeners. One of the main responsibilities of this department is the maintenance of all parts of the hospital in a safe and functional condition; and the supply of water, power, heat, oxygen and other gases.

Domestic services department

The domestic services department is responsible for cleaning throughout the hospital and, as such, plays an important role in hospital hygiene and infection control.

Laundry department

Laundry services may be provided by an individual hospital, or a Central Linen Service may be used.

In addition to the departments already mentioned, large hospitals may provide other services such as an Education department, Supply department, Sexual assault unit, Aboriginal health liaison unit, District nursing service, Blood bank, De-toxification unit, Medical library, Medical records, and specialist referral services such as audiology, ophthalmology, orthodontics, or podiatry.

Structure of a ward

The environment of a ward is made up of two basic components: the physical aspects of furniture, furnishings, lighting and fixtures; and the psychosocial aspects created by the customs, cultural values, norms, and interpersonal relationships of the health agency providing health care.

The design of hospital wards has changed considerably over the years. Currently there are old-style wards in very old hospitals, modernized wards in old hospitals, and wards of various designs in modern hospitals. Changes in the treatment of diseases have progressively reduced the length of time that patients are confined to bed, and it has been necessary to design wards for more ambulatory patients. This has entailed an increase in bathroom and toilet facilities, more sitting room areas with suitable chairs and recreationing facilities, and the provision of dining areas. A greater awareness of the dangers of cross infection, and increased respect for the dignity of the individual and the right of privacy have resulted in wards designed to accommodate small groups of patients. Wards are generally divided into single, two bed, or four-bed rooms.

A *patient's unit* is the small section of the ward inhabited and used by each patient, and it includes:

- a bed and bedding
- a signal device
- a bedside locker
- a bed table
- a bedside chair
- a cupboard or wardrobe
- screens around the bed (in a multi-bed room)
- a handbasin.

In addition to the patient's rooms, each ward is equipped with several annexes such as:

- *Offices*, which may include an office for the nurse in charge and other areas commonly, referred to as 'nurses stations', where the patient's documents, ward records, and order books are kept.
- *Pantry*, which contains a refrigerator for food storage, and tea and coffee making facilities.
- *Pan room*, where bedpans, urinals, wash bowls and items such as urine-testing equipment are stored. It usually contains a bedpan emptying machine and sanitizer, sinks, slop-hopper, and containers for waste and soiled linen.
- *Service room*, which contains equipment used in nursing procedures, e.g. sterile items and lotions.
- *Cleaner's room*, where the equipment needed for ward cleaning is stored.
- *Flower room*, containing a sink, cupboards, and a receptacle for rubbish. Flowers may be arranged, or placed in vases, in this area before being delivered to the patients.
- *Bathrooms and toilets*, and areas for the storage of clean linen.

The environment in which an individual is being cared for influences his reaction to illness and admission to hospital, and can play a role in his recovery. Therefore, the provision of a pleasant environment should be the aim of everyone concerned with the welfare of the patient.

- The ward should be light, decorated and furnished in appropriate colours.
- Furniture and fittings should be clean and in good condition. Modern hospital furniture is for less institutional in appearance than in the past, and this factor helps to create a warm and friendly environment.
- Adequate cupboard and wardrobe space should be provided for each patient.
- Every patient should be encouraged to have a number of personal items, e.g. photographs or flowers, in his unit.
- Ventilation should be adequate without causing draughts, and the ward should be kept free from unpleasant odours.
- An even, comfortable temperature should be maintained in the ward.
- Noise should be kept to a low level.
- All equipment used for nursing activities and cleaning should be removed from the ward immediately after use.
- Personnel should strive to maintain a pleasant and harmonious atmosphere at all times. People, when ill, become more sensitive to the atmosphere around them and can become very distressed by any signs of discord. Information on reactions to illness and hospitalization is provided in Chapter 6.

CONCLUSION

This chapter aims to introduce the nurse to basic psychological and sociological concepts relevant to understanding human behaviour and development. A beginning knowledge of the basic concepts should help the nurse towards understanding why people behave as they do, provide some insight into her own attitudes and reactions, and enhance her interpersonal skills.

The latter part of the chapter looks at the overall structure of a hospital as an organization.

REFERENCES AND FURTHER READING

Altschul A, Sinclair H C 1981 Psychology for nurses, 5th edn. Baillière Tindall, London

Hilgard E R, Atkinson R C, Atkinson R L 1975 Introduction to psychology, 6th edn. Harcourt Brace Jovanovich, New York

Lopez F 1982 Sociology and the nurse, 2nd edn. W B Saunders, Sydney

Sallis E, Sallis K 1988 People in organisations. Macmillan Education, Houndsmills

Smith J P 1976 Sociology and nursing. Churchill Livingstone, Edinburgh

5. Communication

INTRODUCTION

One of the most vital components of all nursing practice is communication. A great deal of nursing practice involves interpersonal communication and the establishment of relationships, e.g. between the nurse and patient, or between the nurse and other members of the health team.

The nurse performs a variety of functions, each of which calls for specific communication behaviours. Nurses act as 'patient advocates', by assisting the individual to communicate his requests and needs; nursing activities in all areas of practice call for judgement which relies on thought processes, interpersonal communication skills and interpersonal communication ability; and nurses' interpersonal communication skills are essential to successful functioning whether it is with patients, members of the health team, personnel in other resource agencies, or the public. Nurses' ability to communicate effectively with government agencies and legislative bodies is a critical factor in attempting to achieve quality health care for all people.

This chapter aims to introduce the nurse to various aspects of human communication, in order that she may be able to interact effectively with other people.

HUMAN COMMUNICATION

Communication is a two-way process in which information is conveyed by verbal and/or non-verbal means by one person, and received and understood by another. Communication has *not* occurred if the information is not understood by the recipient.

Human communication may also be defined as an ongoing dynamic series of events in which meaning is generated and transmitted. Communication occurs when a person responds to a *message* and assigns *meaning* to it. Messages can take many forms: spoken words, written words, facial expressions, gestures, thoughts, or feelings. Messages may be internal—those we send to ourselves, or external—those we react to from our environment and other people. *Meanings* are mental images we create to develop a sense of understanding. When communicating, people respond to messages and create meanings for those messages.

Levels of communication

Human communication occurs at various levels, the most basic of which is intrapersonal communication.

1. Intrapersonal communication occurs when a person communicates with himself. It is a process that occurs *within* the individual himself whereby meaning is generated. For example, if a person looks outside and sees that it is raining and thinks, 'I had better bring the washing in', he is communicating intrapersonally. Thus, intrapersonal communication involves an ongoing dialogue of *thoughts*.

2. Interpersonal communication is communication that occurs between two people (a dyad). It can occur face-to-face, or via means such as a telephone.

3. Small-group communication occurs between three or more people interacting with one another. Small-group communication usually occurs face-to-face, but it may also develop through the use of a communication media, e.g. when several people are able to hold a conference via a link-up of telephones.

4. Organizational communication refers to human communication between members of an organization, e.g. a

hospital, during the performance of their organizational tasks. This level of communication encompasses the other three levels of communication: intrapersonal, interpersonal, and small-group.

5. Public communication involves interaction with large groups of people, e.g. when a speaker addresses an audience.

6. Mass communication occurs when a small number of people send messages to a large, anonymous audience through the use of some specialized media, e.g. films, television, radio, newspapers, and books.

The communication process

Communication is a process whereby an individual shares something of himself, e.g. his ideas, thoughts, values, or feelings, with others. In order to understand the process, many models of communication have been developed which provide a framework for observing, understanding, and predicting what happens during communication.

Many of the early models of human communication were oversimplified, in that they assumed that one person (the sender) sent another person (the receiver) a message. These models were too simple because, in human communication, no one individual is merely a sender or receiver of information. In much of human communication each participant simultaneously sends and receives numerous messages at many different levels.

Figure 5.1 depicts the basic elements of communication, and shows that communication is an *active* process between sender and receiver. The elements of the communication process are the sender, receiver, message, channel, feedback, and the variables:

1. The sender is the individual who initiates the interpersonal communication. The role of sender may alternate between participants at any time when information is transmitted.

2. The receiver is the individual to whom the message is transmitted. The role of receiver may alternate between participants at any time when information is transmitted.

3. The message is the information that is transmitted by the sender, and it may be comprised of both verbal and non-verbal information.

4. The channel is the means by which the message is conveyed, e.g. through the visual, auditory and tactile senses. The sender's facial expressions and body gestures *visually* convey a message to the receiver; the spoken word is transmitted via *auditory* channels; touching an individual while communicating with him uses the *tactile* channel.

5. Feedback helps the sender to recognize whether the meaning of his message has been received. The receiver's verbal and non-verbal responses convey feedback to the sender to reveal the receiver's understanding of the message. Feedback helps to clarify communication as it guides people in adjusting the messages they send to one another. Effective communicators continuously seek feedback from the people with whom they are communicating, to determine whether the information they are transmitting is being received and understood.

6. Variables are the factors which influence the contents of a message and the manner in which it is shared. They include factors such as the setting in which communication takes place, the presence of distractors such as background noise; and the language, perceptions, values, knowledge, culture background, role, and emotions of each person taking part in the communication.

When communication is occurring and information is being transmitted from one person to another, two processes must take place: encoding and decoding:

• *Encoding* refers to the cognitive processes which occur in the mind of the person who is to send the message. These thoughts must be translated into a *code*, e.g. verbal language to be transmitted to the person who is to receive the message.

• *Decoding* refers to the cognitive processes used by the receiver of the message to 'make sense' of what he hears and/or sees.

The following scenario illustrates a basic communication process in action:

Mr Smith, who has been in hospital for several days is about to be discharged home. Before his discharge, the nurse in charge must make certain that Mr Smith understands he has to attend an appointment with his medical officer in two weeks time. The nurse in charge (the sender) thinks about the best way to pass on the information (the message), and decides (encodes) to write the time and date of the appointment on a card in addition to telling Mr Smith. Thus, both spoken and written words (channels) are used to

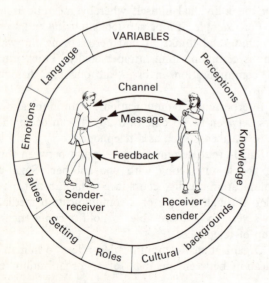

Fig. 5.1 The communication process.

transmit the message. Mr Smith (receiver) listens to the nurse in charge and looks at the appointment card. Because the words used are familiar to him, he is able to understand (decode) the information. He tells the nurse in charge that he realizes he is to attend the appointment at 11.00 hours on Tuesday 2nd October (feedback).

Even though the above scenario illustrates a simple act of communication between two people, many factors could have influenced the way in which the message was transmitted and/or received.

Factors that influence communication

There are a variety of factors that influence the effectiveness of communication, many of which are potential barriers to effective communication. These factors are frequently referred to as the *variables* in the communication process, and may be anything that will prevent the message which is being sent from being the message which is received. Barriers to effective communication may be problems associated with the sender of the message, the means of communication, or problems associated with the recipient.

Perceptions. Perception is a process by which individuals become aware of, and interpret, messages into meanings. Perceptions are closely related to past experiences, e.g. an individual may make a decision about another person's personality as a result of previous experiences in observing human behaviour. If an individual perceives another person as ignorant, uneducated, and naive, it may take a great deal of communication with that person before the individual's perception of him is altered.

Because people cannot possibly perceive everything there is in a given situation, e.g. all the external messages such as visual, auditory and tactile sensations, and the internal messages such as fatigue, nervousness, and decision-making, no two individuals will perceive a situation in exactly the same way. Each person needs to use the cognitive process of *selective perception*, in order to select the most important message from all the potentially perceivable messages in a situation. He must then use those selected messages to make sense out of the current situation. Thus, in order to give full attention to a message an individual must be able to 'block out' competing messages, such as his first impressions and initial judgement of another person's personality.

Values. The way an individual communicates with another person is influenced by the convictions he holds about certain ideas or behaviours. An individual's values, because they reflect what is important to him, have a significant influence on the way he communicates with other people. It is important to appreciate that no two people possess the same values, and that every individual considers his own values as right. Because people's values dif-

fer, effective communication may be prevented when one person judge's another person's values. For example, if a nurse held strong values about 'no sex before marriage' those values may affect the way she communicates with an unmarried pregnant woman.

Emotions. Emotions strongly influence how an individual relates to other people, and the power of emotion in communication should not be underestimated. In nursing practice, a nurse must be careful to prevent her personal feelings from affecting her interactions with those for whom she is caring. Effective communication can be disrupted if one person is experiencing personal emotional distress or is in an mood that is inappropriate for a specific situation. For example, if a nurse is experiencing anger and sadness resulting from the breakdown of a close relationship, she may find that those emotions hinder her communication in the workplace. It is possible that the nurse may transfer her anger and sadness to a patient for whom she is caring.

Nurses must also be aware that if they become too emotionally involved with the suffering experienced by a patient, they may be unable to effectively meet that patient's needs. This aspect is one of the most difficult situations faced by nurses, as on the one hand a nurse must become emotionally involved in order to assist a patient— while on the other hand she cannot allow emotions to adversely affect her care. All nurses need to be aware of their emotions, and many find it helpful to talk with other experienced nurses about what they are feeling and experiencing.

It is also important to realize that, if people cultivate 'emotional distance' in an interpersonal interaction, they prevent any deep sharing of meaning and may even arouse animosity. For example, if a patient feels that a nurse is treating him as an 'interesting case' or a 'problem' rather than as a *person*, he is likely to feel resentful and real communication between them is not likely to occur.

Another way by which emotions influence communication is when the receiver of a message becomes irritated or annoyed by any distracting mannerisms of the sender, e.g. irritating gestures, persistent coughing or throat clearing. Because the listener is annoyed by the mannerisms, he fails to concentrate on the *message* being conveyed.

Differences in knowledge. Where the levels of knowledge between two people are different, communication can be difficult. For example, an individual's level of knowledge may be so far above that of the person he is addressing, that the meaning of his message may be lost entirely. A nurse must always remember this possible barrier to communication when she is talking with patients, and she must be careful to express messages in words and phrases that will be understood. For example, a nurse who is familiar with nursing or medical language and jargon may forget that a patient may not be, and if she uses words or phrases that are not part of the patient's vocabulary he may not understand her message. The use of specific language that is familiar to members of a subculture or profession may confuse, frighten, or alienate people who are not part of that subculture or profession.

Ambiguity of language. Language itself may create barriers to mutual understanding, as words can confuse as easily as they can clarify. Individuals need to be aware of the ambiguity of words so that they can appreciate how easily some remarks can be misunderstood.

To illustrate how one word can have two meanings: A 6-year-old boy was being prepared for a surgical operation, and the nurse told him he would be going to the theatre in 2 hours time. Imagine his surprise and distress when he arrived in the operating room to have his tonsils removed, when he thought that he was being taken to see a film!

Sociocultural background. Communication difficulties can arise when there is a difference in education, social standing, or culture between individuals; and the greater the difference the less people are capable of understanding the intended meaning of a message.

Culture influences the way people behave and communicate as the language, gestures, and attitudes a person communicates reflects his cultural origins. It is important for individuals to acknowledge and accept other people's cultural socialization. For example, it is important that a nurse understands that 'wailing' is a normal and acceptable expression of grief or pain for people from certain cultures.

Relationships and roles. Individuals communicate with others in a way that is appropriate to their relationships and roles. Individuals communicate in different ways, depending on the roles they assume, with friends, colleagues, family members, employers, and casual acquaintances. A person generally feels more comfortable when communicating with another person with whom he has developed a positive and close relationship. Communicating with a person one is meeting for the first time is likely to be quite different in style.

Environmental setting. Effective communication is more likely to occur if it takes place within a setting which is conducive to listening and concentrating. An area which is free from noise and other distractions is suitable, whereas an area where there is noise or lack of privacy may create tension and confusion—thus making communication difficult. For example, background noise and the movements of other people in the environment may distract the listener, or cause him to miss a vital word in a sentence with resulting loss of meaning of a whole sentence.

Physical discomfort. Communication is likely to be poor if one or both participants are experiencing fatigue, pain, or other physical discomfort. Physical, like emotional, discomfort can distract an individual so that he is not really able to concentrate on communication.

Pressures of time. Because the majority of people have many pressures on their time, the urge to speed up communication must often be overcome. It takes time to explain, to listen, to reduce fears or anxieties, to assimilate facts; and an act of communication is rarely improved by speeding it up. This can cause conflict at times, e.g. when one individual needs someone to just sit and listen to him, while the listener is conscious that she has several other things she should be doing at that time.

Absence of feedback. Feedback is a communicated response to another person's communication, and it provides the communicator with information about how his message is being perceived. Feedback can be obtained by the person who is sending the message, e.g. by asking the receiver to express how he understood the message. Alternatively, the receiver of the message can provide the sender with feedback, e.g. by verbal or facial expressions to show that the message was received. If the receiver of a message is not providing any feedback, the sender has no way of knowing whether his message has been received or understood.

Inappropriate means of communication. The means of communication may be inappropriate and, in some instances, communication may be misconstrued:

• Oral communication may be face-to-face, or it may be by means of telephone, radio, tape-recording, or television. In all but the direct method (face-to-face), distortion of sound waves is possible leading to mishearing. When the speaker cannot be seen, there is no communication by means of facial expressions, gestures, or the use of written material and illustrations to reinforce the message.
• The message may be too involved or too lengthy to be effectively communicated via the medium chosen.
• The channel of communication may be inappropriate for a specific person or situation. In some situations a touch or facial expression can be more eloquent than the spoken or written word.

The factors that influence, and the potential barriers to, communication are innumerable and those just described are but a few of the most common ones that operate as people relate to others.

Barriers to effective listening

If an individual does not really listen to another person, effective communication can be blocked. Some of the ways by which an individual can block communication are by:

• Being defensive. When an individual becomes defensive, e.g. experiences a need to defend himself against criticism of his behaviour, he tends not to really listen to the person who is being critical. In addition, his defensive mood is conveyed through his words and non-verbal behaviour to the other person. Consequently, any further interactions between the two participants may be strained, and effective communication may be blocked.
• Changing the subject inappropriately. When one person

abruptly interrupts the flow of a conversation by changing to an unrelated subject, the other person's thoughts and ideas may become confused and he may experience resentment or anger. People sometimes change the subject when they are uncomfortable with, or unwilling to discuss, a specific topic. For example, a patient may ask a nurse 'Am I going to die?'. If the nurse feels unable to deal with that question she may abruptly switch the conversation to a more 'comfortable' subject, e.g. the weather. Thus, the patient feels that the nurse is not sensitive to his concerns, and effective communication between the two is blocked.

• Offering false reassurance or using cliches. For example, a nurse may try to alleviate a patient's anxiety by telling him that he is all right or by promising something that will not occur. Saying to an anxious patient, 'You will be fine, don't worry' does nothing to allay his anxiety. In fact, the patient may become more anxious as he may wonder if the nurse is trying to hide something about his condition.

• Offering advice or giving an opinion. Often an individual needs an opportunity to express his feelings, and giving an opinion or offering advice may reduce his independence and ability to make decisions. Frequently, when a person asks for advice what he really wants is an opportunity to discuss his options. If advice or an opinion is offered too readily, the individual may feel frustrated that he has been unable to discuss all possible solutions to a problem.

• Ignoring non-verbal cues. An individual's non-verbal communication may convey a totally different message from his spoken words. If another person fails to notice these cues, and concentrates only on the spoken words, the real message may be misinterpreted. For example, a patient may say to a nurse that he feels better when his facial expression, tone of voice, and body posture are conveying just the opposite. If the nurse ignores the non-verbal cures, the patient's real feelings will not be communicated to her. Further information on non-verbal communication is provided later in the chapter.

Facilitating communication

Communication is neither innately nor intuitively derived, but is an activity that must be learned. Effective communication cannot be learned except through interaction with others, and effective communication is perhaps the most important attribute of successful nursing.

Human communication requires knowledge of the concepts and theories of the communication process, as well as skill in applying them. Effective communication requires practice, time and effort, and a desire to improve. Communication can generally be improved if an individual:

• increases his understanding of the process itself
• improves his awareness of self
• becomes more sensitive to others.

Communication is the successful passing of a message from one person to another, and is a two-way process. For effective communication to occur, there must be:

• a message, sender, and recipient
• a clear, simple, and unambiguous message
• a message in a suitable form for the recipient
• a message which is received and understood.

The following guidelines can facilitate effective communication:

• Be clear about the message you wish to convey to someone else, how you will convey it, and why.
• Use the most appropriate medium (channel) for conveying a message.
• Use language which is appropriate for the recipient's level of intellectual understanding, his emotional status, and culture.
• Choose the right timing, and length of message, for each occasion.
• Use every means to receive and interpret feedback from the other person, e.g. *watch* his facial expressions and gestures, and *listen* to his words.
• Observe for clues and contradictions in what the other person is trying to get across.
• Wait for questions, and answer them clearly.
• Ask appropriate questions and listen to the response.
• Examine your own self-image because that determines how you present yourself to others, how others perceive you, and how they respond to your messages.
• Be aware of your own habits, attitudes and values, as these affect communication.
• Be sensitive to individual differences in communication behaviour, and adjust your methods of communication to accommodate these differences.
• Be aware of the barriers to effective communication, and try to minimize them.

Some of the skills that can be used to facilitate communication include:

• the art of listening
• conveying empathy, trust, honesty, respect, acceptance, and openness
• asking questions
• using silence
• paraphrasing, clarifying, and reflecting
• recognizing and understanding non-verbal communication.

The art of listening

Listening is an active process which requires skill, understanding, patience, and perseverance. Many people fail to appreciate that listening is not a passive act or that, in conversation, listening is required from both speakers. It could be said that the art of good conversation lies in the ability to listen with perception.

Listening is as important to the process of communication as speaking.

Listening requires attention and concentration in order to hear the *meaning* of words. To be an effective listener an individual must try to improve his listening ability in the areas of sensations, interpretation, and comprehension. Sensations can be a barrier to listening as sights, sounds, and smells in the vicinity of a conversation can distract both the speaker and the listener. Interpretation, such as prejudging, or criticizing a person rather than the message can impede the listening process. Comprehension must be adequate, and can be improved by concentrating on the spoken words and by being genuinely interested in what is being said. An individual's listening ability can be improved if he:

- keeps an open mind
- is self-perceptive
- stays mentally alert
- attempts to understand values, attitudes, and relationships
- focuses on the speaker's ideas
- listens with intuition and feeling
- pays attention to what is said
- shows reaction (feedback) to what is being said, e.g. by a nod or a smile
- does not interrupt the other person's speech or be anxious to 'butt in'
- encourages the speaker to continue by using expressions such as, 'go on', 'then what?'
- does not try to think too far ahead while listening
- remains alert for an unexpected remark
- uses silence appropriately
- concentrates on the content of a message, rather than on style or delivery
- concentrates on the speaker's main theme, rather than on isolated remarks
- takes time to summarize what he has heard.

An individual may have difficulty in actively listening to another person for a variety of reasons (barriers to hearing). An individual may have trouble hearing another person if:

- The speaker's values, ideas, culture, or level of knowledge are different from the listener's
- The vocabulary used is unfamiliar, or if the person speaks with an accent or dialect
- The views or feelings being expressed shock the listener or make him feel anxious
- The speaker is telling him something he does not want to hear
- Background noise or activity distracts the listener
- Hearing acuity is diminished

- He is pre-occupied, or is experiencing stress or discomfort
- He is self-centred
- He has preconceived ideas, e.g. the listener has already decided to dislike the speaker before he hears him speak
- The listener engages in an activity, e.g. watching television, while someone is speaking to him
- He is so concerned about having to answer a question that he does not hear the question being asked.

Conveying empathy

Empathy refers to the ability to develop an understanding of another person's situation and feelings, and to relate that understanding to the person. Empathic communication is associated with sincerity, genuine liking of the other person, sensitive understanding, and an ability to communicate those feelings to the other person.

Often, the best expression of empathy is non-verbal, e.g. by maintaining eye contact, by providing feedback to let the other person know that he has been understood, or by using touch as a means of communication. A nurse can often communicate caring and understanding through touch, e.g. by holding a patient's hand or by putting her arm around him.

A common misconception regarding empathy is that it is necessary to have actually undergone the same experience as someone in order to empathize. This is not true: it is a matter of understanding *how* a person feels rather than having a qualitative or quantative knowledge of the feeling itself. So when someone says, 'You don't know how I feel', it is reasonable and empathic to say, 'Not exactly, no. But I can understand why you feel the way you do'. (Hase & Douglas 1986)

Expressions of empathy usually results in mutual trust. If an individual is able to show that he understands how another person is feeling, rapport is established between the two which usually leads to mutual *trust*. Trust is a belief that a person will respect another's needs, and will behave towards him in a responsible and predictable manner. When people trust each other they feel more comfortable in their relationship, and communication is more effective.

Communication is further enhanced when an individual is able to show *acceptance*, i.e. when he is nonjudgmental of another person. Acceptance means respecting the other person, his values and ideas, as important and worthwhile. Acceptance does not necessarily mean agreement, but is a willingness to hear a person's message without conveying disagreement. To convey acceptance, an individual must avoid gestures or facial expressions, e.g. frowning, which suggest that he disagrees or disapproves of the other person's statements.

Openness, which requires self-awareness and the ability to give of one's self, facilitates communication. Self-disclosure, whereby an individual relates his own experiences and feelings to another person, helps to develop trust. For example, if a nurse enters a relationship with a patient as a person rather than by assuming the role of 'nurse', the patient is more inclined to feel free to express himself.

Honesty refers to the ability to communicate truthfully, frankly, and sincerely. Honest communication is intended to be a truthful representation of information as the individual knows it.

Asking questions

Questioning is a technique of communication, whereby one person attempts to elicit information from another. The type of question asked depends on the situation and the type of response required. Some questions call for simple and direct responses, while others are more probing in nature. A carefully constructed question can facilitate communication, while a question which is poorly constructed can inhibit communication.

Closed questions are those which elicit a simple 'yes' or 'no' or a short and factual answer. Closed questions often start with *who*, *where*, or *when*. For example, 'when did you begin your nursing career?' is a closed question, and the expected response to this question would be merely a date. Closed questions limit options, are restrictive by nature, and sometimes specify answers in the questions themselves. The answers to closed questions often fail to reveal feelings or attitudes.

Open-ended questions are those which generally evoke a long answer, or which enable a person to respond in any way he chooses. Open-ended questions often start with *why*, *what*, or *how*. Open-ended questions are more effective in encouraging an individual to elaborate, as such questions cannot be answered with a simple 'yes' or 'no'. This style of questioning invites the person to give his perceptions, views, thoughts, and feelings. Often, open-ended questions help in establishing rapport between the participants.

For example: 'What were the reasons for beginning your nursing career when you did?' is an open-ended question. This type of question affords the individual more scope to answer in as much detail, and in the style, he chooses.

Primary questions are those which introduce new topics or areas, while *secondary* questions attempt to elicit more information. Secondary questions are sometimes referred to as probing or follow-up questions which are used to get more complete or accurate data. Both primary and secondary questions may be closed or open-ended.

Summary questions reflect or summarize a series of questions and answers to make sure that an accurate understanding has taken place, for example, 'Let me see if I have understood what you have told me. You began nursing when you were 18 years old, and you always considered a nursing career as your first choice?'

Reflective questions are sometimes used to help correct real or suspected inaccuracies, for example 'Didn't you say that you had applied to undertake a physiotherapy course before you were accepted into a nursing course?'

Rhetorical questions are those to which a reply is not usually expected. An example of a rhetorical question is, when greeting a friend, a person may ask 'How are you?'. More often than not the questioner does not expect a response, and may be annoyed if the friend begins to tell him!

Using silence

It is necessary to be silent if an individual wishes to listen to another person, and many people are not good listeners for this reason. They feel uncomfortable when they are not speaking, and cannot wait for the other person to finish so they can talk again.

Silence, used correctly, can be as effective and as supportive as words. There are instances where words seem inadequate when an individual wishes to convey his thoughts and feelings to another person. In such instances it may be most helpful to sit quietly with the person and *share* the silence. Just to be with another person at moments when he is experiencing grief, sorrow, conflict, or joy, may be more helpful than trying to fill the silence with useless words or cliches.

In some situations, silence is not productive and can cause discomfort. Silence can be used to indicate approval or disapproval of a situation, or it may be used to punish or hurt another person. In such instances silence causes barriers to communication, and may cause a person to feel inferior or rejected.

Individuals should be aware of the ways in which they use silence in communicating, and they must be sensitive to situations in order to know when silence is appropriate.

Paraphrasing, clarifying and reflecting

Paraphrasing is a technique whereby one individual restates another's words, usually in order to make sure the message has been received correctly, for example—

First person: 'I can't stand it. The nurse in charge of the ward doesn't understand that I can't be everywhere at once.'

Second person: 'You're saying that you feel frustrated and angry with the nurse in charge?'

First person: 'Yes, she obviously can't remember what it's like to be a student nurse.'

Clarifying is a technique used whereby the conversation is stopped to clarify the meaning of a person's message. If the person who is receiving the message fails to understand its meaning, he can either attempt to repeat the message or ask the other person to restate the message, for example—

First person: '*I knew I might have difficulty in managing all the work. My mother has always told me I'd be like her. I didn't tell you about it last time.*'

Second person: '*I'm sorry you seem to have a problem. Could you tell me what the problem is ?*'

Reflecting is a skill which may be used when listening to another person. Paraphrasing and clarifying are sometimes described as reflective listening skills.

By 'reflecting' back the message received from the other person, e.g. by paraphrasing or clarifying, it lets the person know that he is being listened to. Reflecting also helps the listener to discover whether he has really understood the other person's message, and it encourages the speaker to provide more information.

Porrit (1990) provides the following example whereby the use of reflective listening would have enhanced communication.

There is nothing quite so deflating as when a person shares a feeling of wellbeing and joy, such as 'I had a marvelous day today and everything went right' only to receive a response of 'Lucky you; I wish I had!' stated in a gloomy and despairing tone. Instead of being able to share and talk about a satisfying day it becomes difficult to continue and more acceptable to commiserate with the other person about their gloom and doom. Some people would find themselves going so far as to feel guilty because they had a good day and the other person did not! A sad waste of a successful and happy day.

Non-verbal communication

During communication, people's actions are being transmitted as clearly as their spoken words. Approximately 60% of the information people pass on to others, in face-to-face conversation, is transmitted non-verbally.

When a person is communicating it is essential to *look* as you listen, for his non-verbal messages can tell you what he *really* means. If you just concentrate on what the person says *verbally*, you may miss much of what he is telling you.

Non-verbal communication involves:

- facial expressions
- body movements and gestures
- touch
- space
- tone of voice and other vocal aspects of speech
- eye behaviour
- time
- artifacts.

Facial expressions

The face is a strong communicator; it provides us with non-verbal feedback from others as we speak to them. For example, a frown or an eyebrow raised in disbelief, tell us how the other person is reacting to what we are saying. Facial expressions, used by the person who is speaking, can reinforce or contradict his words. If a listener pays attention to a speaker's facial cues, he is generally able to pick up any discrepancy between facial cues and the spoken words. For example, a person may be telling you that he is not angry, when his facial expression is giving you a different message.

Facial expressions convey emotional states, and much information can be obtained about a person's feelings by observing his facial expressions. Although some researches disagree, there seems to be specific universal facial expressions of emotion which convey surprise, fear, disgust, anger, happiness, and sadness:

- *Surprise* is expressed by raised eyebrows, wide open eyes, and dropped jaw.
- *Fear* is expressed by eyebrows which are raised and drawn together, wide open eyes, and lips stretched back.
- *Disgust* is expressed by wrinkled nose, lowered bottom lip, and lowered eyebrows.
- *Anger* is expressed by eyebrows which are lowered and drawn together, tensed eyelids, and lips pressed together.
- *Happiness* is expressed by the corners of the mouth drawn back and up, raised cheeks, lower eyelids raised but not tense, and 'crows' feet' wrinkles running outward from the outer corners of the eyes.
- *Sadness* is expressed by either loss of muscle tone of the face (expressionless); or the corners of the lips drawn down, trembling lips, and raised inner corners of the upper eyelids. The lower eyelid may appear raised.

Facial expressions can also mask true emotions, e.g. a person may smile to hide his feelings of sadness, anxiety, or boredom.

Body movements and gestures

Although body language can communicate much about how a person is feeling, it is a mistake to interpret a single movement or gesture in isolation. For example, touching or rubbing his nose while speaking may indicate that a person is not telling the truth or it could simply mean that his nose is itching! Therefore, all body movements and gestures should be considered in the context in which they occur.

Body language may sometimes take the place of speech, e.g. a shrug of the shoulders to say 'I don't know'. Body movements, and gestures such as pointing may also be used to emphasize the spoken word.

When a person's actions or gestures do not match his spoken words, the actions are described as being *incongruent*. This means that the body movements or gestures are conveying one message, while the verbal words are conveying a different message. When this situation occurs, other people tend to rely on the non-verbal message and the verbal content may be disregarded.

Some of the basic communication gestures are the same throughout the world, and convey the same message. For example, nodding the head is almost universally used to indicate 'yes' or affirmation. Conversely, just as verbal language differs from culture to culture, the non-verbal language may also differ. A specific gesture may be meaningless, or assume another meaning in different cultures. For example, the 'V' sign may mean victory, the number 2, or something rather rude! Interpretation of this gesture depends on whether it is made with the palm facing out or in, and the culture of the person either making or receiving the gesture.

Touch

Touch (tactile communication) is one of the most powerful means of expression, and it may be performed with or without words.

Touch is the most personal form of communication because it brings people into a close relationship. Touch is also the most basic of the senses: the newborn's first contact with extrauterine life is through touch, and the infant uses touch to explore his environment. An individual's first comfort in life comes from touch and, frequently, his last—since touch may communicate with a dying person when words cannot. A person who has no apparent verbal capacity can usually feel a touch, and understand its message of caring interest.

In nursing, touch may be the most important of all non-verbal behaviours. In fact, there is no way to practice nursing without touching. *How* a nurse uses touch in patient care conveys a great deal about the way she feels towards individuals and their illnesses.

In nursing practice touch is used to comfort, to evaluate some physical symptoms, e.g. determining the rate, rhythm, and volume of a pulse, and when performing activities such as bathing or administering medication. Touch can transmit positive feelings of understanding, compassion, or reassurance; or it can transmit negative feelings such as anger, hostility, and fear. To be effective, tactile communication must be used at the appropriate time and place. Individuals consider a certain amount of space

around them as private, and touch can be seen as an invasion of that privacy unless it is desired. Touch must be used at the right time and in the right way, otherwise misinterpretation of the message will occur.

Some people, including nurses, appreciate the significance of touch as a therapeutic act so much so that they perform the techniques of relaxation massage or the 'laying-on-of-hands'. Massage, performed skillfully and sensitively, can produce relaxation and can communicate caring. 'Laying-on-of-hands' involves placing the hands on or near the body of an ill person in an attempt to heal him.

Space

The concept of 'space' is important in communication, as it determines the distance an individual usually keeps between himself and other people. The individuals involved, and the context or situation, dictate acceptable distance zones.

Every individual surrounds himself by 'informal' space, which is invisible and mobile. There are four categories of space or zone (Fig. 5.2):

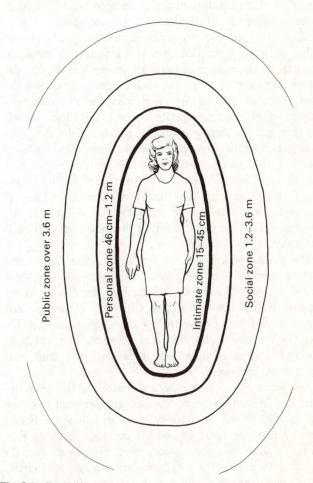

Fig. 5.2 Zone differences.

1. The intimate zone (between 15 and 45 cm from the body surface) is the most important to an individual, who guards it as if it were his own property. Only those who are emotionally close to the individual, e.g. spouse or lovers, parents, children, close friends, and relatives, are permitted to enter this zone.

2. The personal zone (between 46 cm and 1.2 m) is approximately the distance individuals keep between them at friendly gatherings and social functions.

3. The social zone (between 1.2 m and 3.6 m) is the distance individuals keep between themselves and strangers or people who are not well known to them.

4. The public zone (over 3.6 m) is a comfortable distance at which an individual generally chooses to stand when he is addressing a large group of people.

Each person has his own tolerance for closeness and distance, in addition to his cultural patterning. For example, it is generally more acceptable in most cultures for a male and female to touch and hold hands, but less acceptable for two people of the same sex to do so. Individuals desire less personal space in social situations with people with whom they are comfortable, and more personal space in social situations in which they feel uncomfortable.

When two people are communicating, each person makes personal space decisions and attempts to maintain 'acceptable' boundaries of personal space. Sometimes, the personal space expectations of each person conflict and the result is *spatial invasion*. Spatial invasion makes people very uncomfortable, and precipitates a communication reaction of either fight or flight—neither of which is helpful in promoting communication. Most people have experienced a situation when, during communication with one other person, that person moves in very close to make his point. The first person often sees this as an invasion of his personal space and responds by pulling his head back. If this first non-verbal cue is not received, he may even step back and away.

The nature of nursing practice means that nurses frequently invade a patient's intimate or personal space—often without first seeking his permission. Many patients will be uncomfortable with this closeness, and nurses should be sensitive to how each patient is responding. Conversely, such necessary closeness may promote rapport between a nurse and a patient, and emotional attachments can occur.

Territoriality is another aspect of space, and this term denotes the human tendency to mark out personal territory just as animals do. A territory is an area or space that a person claims as his own, which includes the area that exists around his possessions, e.g. his home that is bounded by fences, his own bedroom or a favourite chair. People will generally protect their territory vigorously, and will become quite angry if their territory is limited or thei possessions are taken from them.

The concept of territoriality is relevant to nursing practice. When an individual is admitted to a health care facility his new territory commonly consists of the bed, bedside locker, bed table, and chair. The individual tends to regard the new territory as his own, and becomes more possessive of it the longer he remains in the facility. Consequently, if he is required to move to another room or ward, he may be distressed by the loss of his familiar territory. Therefore, when a patient is to be transferred he must be given sufficient notice so that he has time to adjust and 'let go' of his territory.

Long-term patients often have special problems in initially relating to a health care facility environment. To remind himself of his 'old' territory, a patient may surround himself with many personal possessions and memorabilia. Nurses should be sensitive to an individual's need to retain these links with his previous territory.

Architectural design and environmental planning also have a major effect on human communication. Small rooms with low ceilings and no windows can cause people to feel trapped and depressed, whereas larger rooms with windows looking out on open spaces tend to evoke feelings of contentment.

The spatial arrangement of furniture in a room can also have an impact on communication. For example, it is easier to have a group discussion when people sit in a circle or around a table, than it is if they sit in rows. People will communicate more actively with one another if they are positioned face to face, than if they are positioned away from one another.

Vocal aspects of speech

In addition to the words used, speech involves non-verbal elements, e.g. tone of voice, pauses, volume, rate of speech, and inflection—all of which provide information about the speaker's message.

A person's tone of voice, the inflections of his voice, and his regard for the other person are factors that give *meaning* to his words. The tone and inflection of a voice can help to get a message across, e.g. they can give emphasis to words and can be instrumental in enabling another person to understand the meaning of a message. Tone of voice can cause people to listen, or it can cause people to be inattentive and unresponsive. An individual's personal warmth, credibility, and competence is often displayed by the tone he uses with others.

An individual can determine another person's level of sincerity and caring more from the *way* in which the words are spoken than from the actual words used. Loud, rapid, forcefully spoken words can intimidate and communicate aggression or contempt. Expressionless speech can communicate lack of interest.

Eye behaviour

The eyes may well provide the most revealing and accurate of all communication signals, because they are a focal point on the body. Eye behaviour, which includes eye contact and gaze, can convey an individual's emotional state and his level of interest in a situation or person. The eyes send out accurate cues, and therefore it is not surprising that *trust* is related to an individual's ability to look one straight in the eye. The eyes serve as a valuable message source, and something seems to be missing in an exchange when a person is wearing dark glasses or fails to use eye contact.

Like most body language and gestures, the length of time that eye contact is maintained is culturally determined. For example, the Japanese tend to gaze at the neck rather than at the face when conversing; Southern Europeans have a high frequency of gaze that may be offensive to others. Being raised in a specific culture teaches people the acceptable level of eye contact in that culture. In most cultures, people try to balance their eye contact somewhere between staring and avoiding all contact. Generally, during normal conversation between two people, direct eye contact is maintained one third of the time, with the listener initiating more eye contact than the speaker.

While some people can make others feel quite comfortable when they are conversing, others can make us feel ill-at-ease. This has to do primarily with the length of time that they look at us, or hold our gaze as they speak. Total lack of eye contact may signal low self-esteem, while too much eye contact (staring) is inappropriate.

Time

Time is, perhaps, the form of non-verbal communication that people are least aware of, yet time has a major impact on human interaction. The more time an individual spends communicating with others, the more he is telling them that he believes they are important people. Conversely, the less time spent with other people, the more you are implying that they are insignificant. The commitment of time becomes, in itself, communication.

In nursing practice time spent with a patient, particularly when no procedure is being performed, communicates interest and caring to the patient. It is sometimes difficult, in a busy health care facility, to spend enough time with each patient. A caring nurse will try to utilize her time to meet each patient's needs, and a nurse who spends time communicating with a patient demonstrates her interest in that person.

Artifacts

Artifacts, e.g. personal appearance, body shapes and sizes, smells, hair styles, clothing styles, jewellery, and the objects that people choose to decorate their environment, have a strong influence on the initial perceptions and first impressions people have about others. People tend to judge others by their appearance, a habit that can be detrimental as it can lead to incorrect assumptions. For example, the social or financial status of an individual may be incorrectly inferred from his clothes. Conversely, the physical dress and appearance of an individual *may* provide information about him, e.g. his personality and occupation. Traditionally, nurses and various other health care workers have identified themselves through the use of easily recognizable cues such as uniforms.

Communicating in special situations

The nurse is frequently expected to communicate with groups of people who require a special approach, e.g. individuals who are hearing, visually, or speech impaired. Information on communicating with hearing and visually impaired people is provided in Chapter 50, and information on communicating with speech impaired individuals is provided in Table 43.3. Other groups of people with whom the nurse will be required to communicate include children, relatives, and those whose first language is not English.

Communicating with children

Some important aspects of communicating with children include:

● Putting a child at ease, e.g. by asking his name or talking about his friends. A child who is relaxed generally communicates quite freely.
● Talking directly to a child, and asking him questions which he can answer on his own. If parents are present, the nurse should look to them for confirmation or reply only when necessary.
● Explaining, in terms a child can understand, any procedure or activity to be performed. Children are more likely to accept intervention if they know what to expect.
● Including the child in the discussion when a plan of care is being explained to the parents.
● Talking with a child as you would with an adult, e.g. being honest, and being careful not to disregard any information he volunteers.
● Answering a child's questions sensibly and truthfully whenever possible. For example, if a child asks if a procedure is going to hurt it is much better to be honest. If he

has been told that it will not hurt, and it does, his trust in the nurse will be reduced.

- Respecting a child's confidences.

Communicating with relatives

It is important for nurses to appreciate that the relatives or friends will often need assistance to cope with an individual's illness. A person's illness can be a very disruptive episode in the life of his loved ones, and they may need to discuss their concerns and to share the frustrations of the illness. Some important aspects of communicating with relatives include:

- Introducing yourself to the relatives and informing them that you are helping to look after their loved one.
- Providing them with opportunities to express their concerns and anxieties.
- Answering their questions, or referring questions to the nurse in charge.
- Including the relatives in discussions about the individual's care when appropriate, e.g. if the individual gives his approval.
- Demonstrating warmth, e.g. by touch, close proximity, body posture, and facial expressions. This is of particular relevance when relatives are confronted with a loved one who is seriously ill or dying.

Communicating when there are language differences

The nurse may be required to communicate with someone whose first language is different. Many health care facilities provide interpreters and/or other-language phrase books which can be most helpful. Some important aspects of communicating include:

- Developing a sensitivity to the significance of cultural factors in people's lives.
- Speaking slowly, clearly, and not shouting.
- Using gestures and/or pictures to illustrate what you mean.
- Keeping the information simple, e.g. by using short sentences and avoiding nursing or medical terminology and jargon.
- Repeating, and rephrasing, a sentence if it is not understood.
- Making sure, that when an interpreter is used, the patient trusts him and his ability to maintain confidentiality.

An interpreter provides a vital verbal communication link and whenever possible trained, skilled, and professional interpreters should be used. The nurse should remember that she is communicating with the *patient*, and is using the *services* of the interpreter. In other words, the nurse must not ignore or forget the patient, and she should speak directly to and maintain eye contact with him not the interpreter. The nurse should be aware of the Health Care Interpreter Services that are available.

Written communication

The art of conveying thoughts and information to paper is effectively accomplished as a result of logical thinking.

Nurses are required to compile notes, answer questions on examination papers, write reports about patients, maintain various types of charts, record treatments and nursing care, etc. In all of these situations, effective communication depends on certain principles:

- The words used should be chosen with care to avoid inaccuracy or ambiguity. Words which are open to misinterpretation should not be used.
- Meaning is conveyed not only by the words used in a written text, but also by the way in which they are used and by means of punctuation. Wrong use of words, omission of conjunctive words, and mistakes in punctuation can sometimes cause a sentence to convey a meaning which was not intended.
- The finished product should fulfil the purpose of the exercise, e.g. nursing care notes should present a clear picture of the condition of a patient as observed by the writer, plus accurate details of care given and the effects produced. An examination candidate should provide a clear, complete, and accurate answer to each question asked and refrain from including irrelevant material.
- Writing should be legible. Poor handwriting leads to misinterpretation, and it can cause mistakes to be made which adversely affect a patient.
- Correct spelling is very important incommunications containing people's names or technical words. Some medical products have names which contain only minor differences in spelling and are, therefore, easily confused.
- Plain simple English should be used, and jargon avoided. Users of jargon are often unsure of its precise meaning, and there may be a breakdown in communication caused by the reader's inability to grasp its meaning.

Further information on reporting and recording skills is provided in Chapter 14.

CONCLUSION

Communication is a process whereby people share their ideas, attitudes, values, and feelings; it is the generation and transmission of meaning.

Nursing practice involves the nursing process which is a process of assessment, planning, implementation, and evaluation of nursing care. All steps in the nursing process depend strongly on the communication skills of the nurse.

Therefore, the nurse requires an understanding of the communication process, the factors which facilitate or inhibit communication; and the significance of verbal, non-verbal, and written communication.

REFERENCES AND FURTHER READING

Argyle M 1978 The psychology of interpersonal behaviour. Penguin, Harmondsworth
Hase S, Douglas A J 1986 Human dynamics and nursing. Churchill Livingstone, Melbourne
Porrit L 1990 Interaction strategies: an introduction for health professionals. 2nd edn. Churchill Livingstone, Melbourne, p 84

6. Reactions and interactions

INTRODUCTION

To be effective in her role a nurse needs to think in terms of 'a person' instead of 'a patient' and to view each person as an individual member of a complex society with all the rights, privileges and responsibilities this bestows. No member of society can exist as a separate entity but all are interdependent, affecting and being affected by the behaviour of others.

People enter a health care agency as individuals with different personalities, sets of values, socio-economic and academic backgrounds, attitudes and reactions to illness, and different degrees of rehabilitation potential.

All human beings inherit certain physical and mental characteristics, but the way in which these are developed depends upon environment and life experiences. It is, therefore, helpful for a nurse to have some knowledge of an individual's background in order to be able to know him as a person. Through talking with a person and his family the nurse gains some insight into the factors that have influenced his growth and development, e.g. his place in the family, home background, beliefs and values, in- terests and hobbies. Detailed information on the factors that influence growth and development is provided in Chapters 2 and 3.

To develop helping relationships which promote the delivery of effective nursing care, a nurse requires knowledge about how the experience of illness affects people. Illness is a major stressor which affects not only the person who is ill but also those who are close to him.

This chapter aims to introduce the nurse to the concepts of stress and stressors, and it addresses the various ways by which people react to and deal with stress—particularly in relation to the experience of illness as a stressor. It also addresses the development of effective nurse-patient relationships, as a means of assisting individuals to cope with illness and/or hospitalization.

Stress

Stress may be described as a combination of physical and psychological responses to threat and conflict. Stress threatens an individual's physical and/or emotional homeostasis.

A *stressor* is any factor, e.g. emotional, physical, social or economic, that causes stress and which requires a response or change to avoid or reduce stress.

It is important to realize that, while people generally recognize traumatic events as being stressful, stress is also associated with events that are seen as being positive, e.g. promotion at work. Identifying sources of stress (stressors) helps to anticipate them, and most people are able to deal more effectively with stressful events when they are prepared for them. Every individual experiences stressful events throughout his life, e.g. death of a spouse or close family member, marriage, divorce or separation, personal injury or illness, change in financial status, change in living conditions, change to a different line of work, or change in social activities.

When a person becomes ill, and/or is admitted to hospital, he is faced with a number of new stressors, for example:

- loss of independence
- an unfamiliar environment

- being surrounded by strangers
- loss of income
- disruption of family life
- facing the unknown
- pain or discomfort
- loss of privacy
- unfamiliar sights, sounds, smells
- potential altered body image
- diagnosis and prognosis.

The body is able to respond to changing internal and external stimuli. *Homeostasis* is the body's tendency to maintain itself in a state of relative constancy, in which the body systems continually adapt to changes. Homeostasis is maintained by physiological mechanisms that control various body functions and monitor body organs. These mechanisms are generally controlled by the nervous system, e.g. the medulla oblongata controls heart beat, blood pressure, and respiration. Therefore, these mechanisms do not involve conscious behaviour. In a healthy person the mechanisms are effective in maintaining homeostasis so that the body's physiological needs are met. However, illness, injury, or prolonged stress can decrease the adaptive capacity of homeostatic functions. Further information on homeostasis is provided in Chapter 15.

When stress occurs, an individual uses both physical and emotional energy to respond and adapt:

- The body produces various kinds of *localized responses* to stress, e.g. the inflammatory response (see Chapter 59), blood clotting, and wound healing (see Chapter 59). These localized responses do not involve entire body systems, they require a stressor to stimulate a response, they are of short-term duration, and they assist in restoring homeostasis to the body area.
- The general adaptation syndrome (GAS), as described by Dr Hans Selye (1976) is a defense response of the whole body to stress. Selye called the three stages of the syndrome: the alarm reaction, the resistance stage, and the exhaustion stage. The three stages reflect the body's physiological response to stress over time. The *alarm reaction* involves a number of physiological changes, e.g. release of certain hormones into the blood, which prepare the individual to adapt to a stressor. During the *resistance stage* the body stabilizes and the individual attempts to adapt to the stressor. The *exhaustion stage* occurs if the body is unable to adapt to the stress, e.g. if the individual is experiencing a long-term severe illness. If the stress is not relieved, death may result.
- Exposure to a stressor also results in *psychological* adaptive responses. These behaviours, which are directed toward stress management, are also referred to as coping mechanisms and may be either constructive or destructive.

Physiological responses to stress

Physiological stress response is regulated by the hypo-thalamus, in the brain, which controls autonomic nervous activity. The majority of physical signs and symptoms that occur in acute stress are the result of sympathetic arousal and the release of hormones, and include:

- tachycardia
- raised blood pressure
- increased rate and depth of ventilation
- vomiting, diarrhoea or constipation
- frequency of micturition
- loss of appetite
- dry mouth
- sweating
- pallor
- dilated pupils
- muscle tension, tremor
- lack of co-ordination
- insomnia, restlessness.

This homeostatic mechanism, which is known as the 'fight or flight' response, is designed to release glucose in a usable form, to provide oxygen, and to direct both glucose and oxygen in large quantities to cardiac and skeletal muscle.

Psychological responses to stress

The psychological responses to stress involve mood changes and changes in behaviour including:

- anxiety
- depression
- withdrawal
- anger
- fear
- emotional lability, crying
- irritability
- hostile and aggressive behaviour
- poor memory
- inability to concentrate
- intolerance of disturbing stimuli, e.g. noise
- impulsive actions
- over-reaction to minor events
- inability to make decisions
- increased use of alcohol, drugs, nicotine
- changes in sleep patterns
- changes in eating patterns or appetite
- increase in the frequency of accidents.

Results of prolonged stress

Although short exposures to stress can be productive and can promote change, longer exposures can adversely affect an individual's health. Prolonged stress can contribute to physical illness, and can lead to changes in a person's emotional behaviour, in his intellectual processes, e.g. impaired decision making, to 'burnout', a chronic anxiety state, or a psychiatric disorder. Stress is associated with various disease states such as:

- cardiac arrhythmias
- hypertension
- coronary artery disease
- peptic ulcers
- colitis
- irritable bowel syndrome
- increased susceptibility to infection and neoplasia
- allergies
- psychotic and neurotic symptoms
- personality changes.

It is important for nurses to understand the relationship between stress and illness, and that the leading causes of death are diseases, e.g. heart diseases and malignant neoplasms, which are related to life-style stressors. The nurse is often in a position to consider the possible effects on an individual of a stressful life-style or stressful events. Illness and/or hospitalization are considered to be stressful events in themselves, and the nurse has a responsibility to help a patient to avoid, reduce, minimize, or deal with stressors.

Dealing with stress

How an individual reacts to, and deals with, stress depends on various factors, e.g. the intensity and duration of a stressor, his general health status, personality, mental state and abilities, knowledge, experience, social conditioning, and the type of support available. The presence of *several* stressors at the same time means that the individual needs more energy to adapt to any one of them, thus multiple stressors reduce a person's ability to adapt.

Individuals develop adaptive behaviours to cope with stressors. These adaptive behaviours are referred to as coping mechanisms, and they may be either:

- conscious techniques used to cope with the threats themselves
- unconscious ego-defence mechanisms, which serve to protect the individual from anxiety and stress.

Conscious mechanisms used by individuals to cope with an actual threat include problem-solving techniques, physical withdrawal from a threatening situation, and compromise. Information on *problem solving* is provided in Chapter 12.

An individual may *physically remove* himself from a stressor, e.g. if he has been unable to resolve a long-time conflict with his employer he may choose to resign. Depending on the effect such as action has on the individual, physical withdrawal may be a positive or negative means of coping with a stressor.

In a stressful situation an individual may choose *compromise* as a means of dealing with or avoiding stress. Compromise may involve substituting goals, changing a usual way of behaving, or delaying the satisfaction of certain needs. Increased anxiety or loss of self esteem may occur if an individual is required to continually compromise in order to cope with stressors.

Ego-defence mechanisms are unconscious mechanisms which protect an individual from anxiety and stress by reducing internal conflict and threatening feelings. These defense mechanisms do not alter the stressful situation, they simply change the way the person thinks about and responds to it. People use defense mechanisms in everyday behaviour and, used in moderation, they are helpful modes of adjustment. It is only when an individual becomes over-reliant on, or misuses, an inappropriate defence mechanism that difficulties arise. Ego defence mechanisms include:

1. *Repression*. The most common mechanism used, whereby an individual 'blocks out' unpleasant thought, memories, or feelings from his consciousness. Sometimes the repressed thoughts and feelings find indirect expression, e.g. in dreams.

2. *Denial*. A mechanism whereby emotions, thoughts, or external factors, which would cause distress, are ignored their existence is not acknowledged. Denial is quite normal in early childhood, e.g. a child who is so tired that he can't keep his eyes open will vehemently deny that he is tired! Adults may unconsciously use this mechanism in the face of serious threats such as the loss of a limb or a terminal illness. Initially, the adult may deny the situation has occurred.

3. *Sublimation*. A mechanism whereby unacceptable drives or urges are transformed into more socially acceptable activities. Sublimation is considered to be a healthy coping device. For example, many 'sporting' activities allow the expression of aggressive behaviour which would, in other situations, be unacceptable.

4. *Regression*. A mechanism whereby an individual avoids a threat or personal responsibility by reverting to behaviour which is characteristic of an earlier stage of development. A previously toilet trained child may revert to bedwetting in the face of a threat, or an adult may behave in an immature manner.

5. *Projection*. A mechanism whereby an individual's unacceptable thoughts, feelings, or urges are attributed to others. An individual may criticise another person's faults and weaknesses, unaware that these are aspects of his own personality. For instance, a person may protect himself from recognizing his own undesirable qualities, e.g. aggressiveness, by assigning them in exaggerated amount to other people.

6. *Rationalization* A mechanism whereby an individual attempts to preserve his self esteem by trying to justify his actions. The individual may present apparently logical reasons for an action or thought that is otherwise unacceptable to him. Rationalization serves two purposes; it eases an individual's disappointment when he fails to reach a goal, and it provides him with acceptable motives for his behaviour. For instance, an individual who failed to be accepted into a university course may state, 'I didn't want to do that course anyway', or 'The questions they asked me were ridiculous'.

7. *Displacement*. A mechanism whereby emotion is transferred from the provoking person or object, to another person or object. For instance, if an individual feels angry towards his employer he may express this anger by shouting at a friend or kicking the cat! The individual may regard this as more acceptable than expressing his anger towards his employer.

8. *Conversion*. A mechanism whereby a conflict or repressed feeling becomes manifested as a physical symptom. The body functions affected are those normally under voluntary control. For instance, a singer about to make her debut on stage may suddenly lose her voice, or a soldier about to face combat may develop paralysis of the legs. The physical symptom thus replaces the anxiety and saves the person from a stressful situation.

9. *Compensation*. A mechanism whereby an individual over-emphasizes a positive personal attribute to avoid the painful emotions which result from a sense of inferiority or inadequacy. For instance, an individual may substitute hard work and excellence in academic studies for a lack of ability in sporting activities.

10. *Reaction formation*. A mechanism whereby an individual displays an emotion which is opposite to the emotion he is actually experiencing. The individual avoids anxiety through behaviour and attitudes that are the opposite of his repressed feelings and impulses, and which serve to conceal those unacceptable feelings. For instance, an individual who is being admitted to hospital for surgery may be petrified but appears to be calm or indifferent, or he may laugh and joke about his situation.

11. *Withdrawal*. A mechanism whereby an individual responds to stress by becoming apathetic, lethargic, depressed, and retreating into himself. Withdrawal becomes pathological if it interferes with an individual's perception of reality and the ability to function in society.

12. *Dissociation*. A mechanism whereby an idea, thought, or emotion is separated from the consciousness and thereby loses emotional significance so that the individual does not experience an appropriate emotional response. For instance, grief at the loss of a loved one may not be felt at the time because it is too painful to bear; however it may be experienced later.

Defense mechanisms, therefore, help an individual to avoid or reduce anxiety in various ways: they give him *time* to solve a problem that may otherwise overwhelm him, they may assist him to learn new ways of adjusting to situations, and they may assist him to behave in a more rational manner in the future.

Defense mechanisms, while affording protection until the individual can reach a realistic solution to a problem, can fail to provide satisfactory adjustment. For instance, an individual who depends only on defence mech- anisms may never learn other ways of dealing with stress and anxiety.

Stress management

To reduce the undesirable impact of stress on physical and mental health, individuals can adopt certain preventive behaviours including:

- obtaining regular physical exercise
- consuming a balanced diet
- obtaining sufficient rest
- learning to manage time efficiently
- developing a support system of family and friends
- learning to think positively.

Stress can be relieved by either altering a situation itself so that it becomes less threatening, or by increasing the ability to cope with stressful situations. An individual can be assisted by:

- Providing him with adequate information before a stressful event occurs, so that he has time to plan a method of coping and so that he feels in control of a situation. For instance, prior to surgical intervention the nurse should ensure that a patient has received adequate explanation of what to expect post-operatively. Fear of the *unknown* generally results in greater anxiety and stress than would occur if a patient is adequately prepared.
- Attempting to alter his perception of a situation so that it is no longer seen as threatening. For instance, a patient who may be extremely anxious about experiencing severe post-operative pain should be informed that adequate pain relief is available and will be provided.
- Providing adequate psychological support so that he doesn't feel he has to cope with a threatening situation alone. For instance, a patient who is undergoing an invasive or uncomfortable examination may feel less anxious by the presence and comforting words of a supportive nurse.
- Teaching him various techniques which can help to reverse the effects of stress.

There are a variety of techniques an individual can use including:

1. Relaxation therapy, which involves the ability to relax specific muscles or the whole body. Relaxation may be achieved in a variety of ways including practising the systematic contraction and relaxation of muscles, and through meditation or massage.

2. Breathing exercises, which involve practising deep, slow and regular inhalations and exhalations in a quiet environment. The individual should be sitting comfortably, close his eyes, and concentrating on his breathing.

3. Visual imagery, which involves the individual closing his eyes and imagining a peaceful scene, e.g. a tropical beach. By imaging such a scene an individual is able to become relaxed, almost as if he were actually part of the peaceful scene.

4. Biofeedback, whereby an individual is instructed in techniques to gain control over physiological functions which are normally controlled by the autonomic system, e.g. heart rate and blood pressure. The process involves providing the individual with visual or auditory information about specific physiological functions, usually through the use of instruments. The individual gradually learns to *consciously* control these functions, e.g. he learns how to lower his blood pressure.

Assertiveness

As stress may result from an individual's inability to develop and maintain relationships with others, education in communication and social skills may be necessary. Information on communication skills is provided in Chapter 5.

Assertiveness can determine the effectiveness and satisfaction of interpersonal relationships, therefore an individual may need assistance to develop more assertive behaviour. Assertiveness should not be confused with aggression. Aggression generally involves behaving in a destructive manner, or engaging in activities that are forcefully expressed physically or verbally. Aggressive behaviour involves the expression of feelings at another person's expense.

Assertive behaviour means the honest, direct, and appropriate expression of feelings, beliefs and opinions—but not at the expense of others. Assertive behaviour involves *respect* for self and for others, and being able to stand up for yourself while taking other people's interests and feelings into account. Thus:

- Assertive behaviour involves the ability to stand up for yourself without infringing the rights of others
- Aggressive behaviour violates the rights of others
- Passive behaviour denies our own rights.

Assisting a person to become self-assertive focuses on helping him to express direct and honest statements of his feelings and beliefs. By practising assertive responses, the individual not only reduces anxiety but also develops more effective coping techniques. Some aspects in developing assertiveness include the ability to:

- make a distinction between assertiveness and aggressiveness or submissiveness
- state clearly what you want
- make requests politely and not apologizing for making requests
- refuse requests as politely as possible
- avoid criticism, threats and sulking as methods of exerting or resisting influence
- recognize that saying 'No' and meaning 'No' will reduce pressure from others in the future
- accept that everyone has the right to say 'No'
- express your opinions and attitudes.

Reactions to illness

The nurse who thinks in terms of 'people' rather than 'patients' will readily accept that people react as individuals to every situation they face in life, and that their reactions are influenced by a number of factors, e.g. their age, nationality, cultural background, intellectual level, temperament, and state of health.

There are usually three stages through which the 'average' person passes when illness occurs, but there are variations in the behaviour patterns exhibited at each stage. It is important to remember, however, that each individual responds uniquely to the experience of illness.

During the initial stage, when the manifestations of illness appear, the person's reaction may be one of refusal to acknowledge any health problems, aggression, extreme anxiety, apathy, or a concerned acceptance of his situation.

The middle stage is reached as the illness develops, and reactions vary considerably. Some people become very self-centred, dependent and demanding, others may be extremely anxious but outwardly appear to be philosophical. Not all reactions to illness are negative, and many people accept the reality of the situation and maintain an optimistic outlook.

Convalescence, or terminal illness, marks the final stage, where various reactions may be experienced. Adjustment to the convalescent stage of illness can be a difficult process for some individuals who may subconsciously fear the return to independence.

When illness occurs both the individual and his significant others experience:

- behavioural and emotional changes, e.g. anxiety, shock, denial, anger, or withdrawal
- changes in roles, e.g. a woman who is the main care-giver in the family may be unable to care for her children while she is ill
- changes in body image, e.g. an illness resulting in changes to an individual's physical appearance can affect both the individual and his significant others.
- changes in self-concept, e.g. an individual's self-concept may be altered when he loses some of his independence as a result of illness.

A nurse should try to understand why an individual reacts in a certain way, and she should appreciate that an individual's behaviour is not always a true expression of the way he is feeling. An individual may react to illness and/or hospitalization by becoming withdrawn or aggressive. He may regress, so that he becomes passive and dependent on others, and behave in an immature way. He may become totally introspective and self-absorbed, showing no interest in anything other than himself and his illness. He may constantly complain and criticize as a means of demonstrating his frustration at being ill or of feeling neglected. In order to help identify the reason for any type of behaviour, and to help a patient resolve his problems, the nurse must get to know him as a person and she must be able to establish a helpful relationship with him.

Nurse-patient communication

If a nurse is to help an individual cope with the implications of his illness and/or hospitalization, it is important that she implements measures which will reduce fears, stress, and anxiety. To do this the nurse must communicate with the individual, and establish a helpful relationship with him and his significant others.

Communication is the foundation on which all relationships are developed. Information on communication is provided in Chapter 5, while this chapter specifically addresses the importance of communication in establishing and maintaining relationships between nurse, patient, and his significant others.

Communication in a nurse-patient relationship is essential as it allows the two individuals to get to know each other, it provides the nurse with the information necessary to plan and deliver effective nursing care, and it provides the patient with information which is important to him.

The relationship between a nurse and a patient should be based on *mutual trust* and *respect*. The nurse should know the patient as a person, and she must respect his rights and privileges as an individual. The nurse's level of professional knowledge and proficiency should inspire in the patient a feeling of confidence and a willingness to share in the task of coping with illness in the best possible way. There must be adequate communication between nurse and patient and, in particular, a nurse needs to ensure that she has time to listen to and talk with the patient. Aspects of establishing and maintaining a therapeutic relationship include:

● Preserving the patient's identity by always addressing him by name, learning about his family, friends and interests; showing respect for him as an individual, involving him in decisions about his care, preserving his dignity, and promoting his continued contact with family and friends.
● Providing the patient with information, e.g. about events that are to occur, the reasons for any procedures or use of equipment, and the plans for his care. It is important that information is specifically tailored to meet the needs of the individual. When imparting information the nurse must consider the language used, the manner in which it is given, the nature and timing of information, and the possible need for repetition. The nurse must also ascertain whether the patient has understood the information he has been given.
● Being prepared to sit and listen to the patient, and encouraging him to verbally express any fears or anxieties.

The nurse should remain sensitive to the patient's verbal and non-verbal cues (as discussed in Chapter 5). She should recognize that the patient will be experiencing many changes which may result in stress and anxiety, e.g. altered eating, sleeping, and lifestyle habits.
● Encouraging the patient to retain as much independence as possible, by allowing him to participate actively in his care and treatment. It is also important to ask the patient for his permission and co-operation in treatments or procedures.
● Developing mutual trust. The degree of interpersonal trust is an important factor that influences people's communication and interaction. Trust facilitates effective communication as individuals become more free and open in expressing their true feelings and thoughts to others. In a climate of mutual trust, information sharing and better planning can be achieved. For trust to develop a person must be comfortable with an awareness of himself, his goals, motivations, and doubts and he must be able to share this awareness with others. A person must also be prepared to accept others who deviate from his own way of thinking, feeling, or acting without experiencing the desire to change them. In addition, a person must demonstrate a consistency between words and actions.

CONCLUSION

To develop a helping relationship which promotes the delivery of effective nursing care, a nurse requires knowledge about how the experience of illness affects people. Illness is a major stressor which affects not only the person who is ill, but also those who are close to him.

Stress is a phenomenon in which an individual perceives various stimuli as threatening to the physical, emotional, or social aspects of his being.

A stressor is any factor that causes stress and which requires a response or change to avoid or reduce stress.

When stress occurs, an individual used both physical and emotional energy to respond and adapt. Responses to stress include those which are localized, e.g. the inflammatory response, a general response known as the general adaptation syndrome, and psychological responses such as changes in mood and behaviour.

How individuals react to, and deal with, stress depends on various factors including age, general health status, mental state, and the intensity of the stressor.

Methods used by individuals to cope with stress include problem-solving techniques, withdrawal from a threatening situation, compromise, and unconscious ego-defence mechanisms.

To reduce the impact of stress on physical and mental health, individuals can adapt certain preventive behaviours such as obtaining adequate exercise, rest, and nutrition.

Stress can be relieved by either altering a situation so

that it becomes less threatening, or by increasing the ability to cope with stressful situations.

Illness and/or hospitalization are major stressors to which an individual is required to adapt. One of the most effective ways in which a nurse can assist the individual to adapt is by establishing and maintaining a therapeutic relationship with him.

REFERENCES AND FURTHER READING

Hase S, Douglas A J 1986 Human dynamics and nursing. Churchill Livingstone, Melbourne
Potter P A, Perry A G 1985 Fundamentals of nursing. C V Mosby, St Louis, ch 2, 51–61
Selye M 1976 The stress of life. McGraw-Hill, New York

7. Culture

INTRODUCTION

Australia is a multi-cultural society; therefore nurses, as members of that society, need to have an understanding of the many aspects that make up a culture, and an understanding of the diversity of cultures within Australia. As a member of the health care team the nurse needs to appreciate that a person's culture influences his health beliefs and practices and his perceptions of, and reaction to, illness. Because they are required to care for people from a variety of cultural backgrounds, nurses need to acknowledge the existence of various cultural and religious beliefs and practices. Part of the International Code of Nursing Ethics (1973) states that, 'The need for nursing is universal. Inherent in nursing is a respect for life, dignity and the rights of man. It is unrestricted by considerations of nationality, race, creed, colour, age, sex, politics, or social status'.

According to information from the office of Multicultural Affairs (1989) more than 3 000 000 Australians were born overseas, at least 2 000 000 regularly use a language other than English, and at least 4 000 000 have recent ancestors who came from areas other than the British Isles. Catholics are the largest religious denomination, and there are more than 300 000 non-christians, comprising mainly Muslims, Buddhists and Jews. Figures, from the same source (1988), show the ethnic composition of the Australian people as:

- Aboriginal   2%
- Anglo-Celt   74.6%
- Other European   19.3%
- Asian   4.5%
- Other   0.6%

From this information it is obvious that Australia is, indeed, a multi-cultural society. The National Agenda, unveiled by the Prime Minister in July 1989, contains the government's statement of the meaning of multiculturalism. It states, 'In a descriptive sense, multiculturalism is simply a term which describes the cultural and ethnic diversity of contemporary Australia. We are, and will remain, a multicultural society'.

Culture

The term 'culture' is difficult to define because it is used in a variety of contexts. Broadly, culture may be defined as a collection of behaviour patterns, language, values, beliefs, dietary practices, actions, rituals, attitudes, institutions, rules, ceremonies, and artifacts that a group accepts and by which members of the group live. Culture is the way of life which guides the thoughts, feelings, and actions of individuals who belong to a particular group.

Culture is learned through socialization, the process by which an individual learns to live in accordance with the expectations and standards of a group in society. It is through socialization that an individual acquires the beliefs, values, customs, and behaviour expected of a particular group. Such acquisition occurs primarily through imitation, family interaction, and educational systems.

Culture involves material aspects such as the objects with which people surround themselves, e.g. clothing, ornaments, eating utensils, and style of housing. Culture involves much more than its physical aspects as it includes rituals of social behaviour, methods of communication, ideologies, and attitudes, e.g. to religion, marriage, and death. Cultural values are also reflected in education systems, in art and literature, and in political institutions.

Within each culture there are many subcultures to which people belong. *A subculture* may be described as a group of people who, although members of a larger cultural group, share certain values and characteristics that distinguish them as a sub-group. Thus, a subculture is a group of people that exists within the geographical boundaries of a dominant culture. Subcultures may, for example, be based on religious definition, on the particular profession to which an individual belongs, or on the definition of a group which deviates by choice from the national norms or culture. Many subcultures consist of people who have some form of common identity, e.g. the nursing profession, and types of behaviour that are distinctive.

Within each culture or subculture there are individual differences and variations based on many variables including socio-economic background, age, religion, language gender identity and roles, geographical location, and the degree of contact with older group members who are the main sources of traditional values.

Stereotyping

Stereotyping occurs when people over-generalize about a particular cultural group. A stereotype is a cluster of inter-related traits and attributes *assumed* to be characteristic of certain kinds of people. Stereotyping can be misleading and harmful, and often has no basis in fact. Stereotypes are frequently formed to rationalize prejudices or to justify poor treatment of certain individuals on the basis of some assumed group characteristics. Some stereotypes are born out of racism, e.g. some are developed about status and role, while others are directed towards specific physical characteristics, e.g. 'all blondes are dumb'. Stereotyping, like ethnocentrism, is a major barrier to cultural understanding.

Ethnocentrism

Ethnocentrism is a belief in the inherent superiority of the race or group to which one belongs, or a tendency to consider other ethnic groups in terms of ones own racial origins. Ethnocentric people tend to judge all other groups according to the values of their own culture.

Ethnocentrism can be a significant problem in health care if a member of the health care team is not accepting of someone from a different culture. For example, a nurse who holds definite beliefs about a particular aspect of health care may become intolerant of a patient from a different cultural background who holds opposing values or beliefs. An ethocentric nurse would assume that the patient should adopt her values and beliefs which she considers to be more appropriate.

Thus, both stereotyping and ethnocentrism may have detrimental effects on patient care if a health worker fails to consider each patient as an individual.

Cultural similarities and differences

While there are differences between people of different cultures, there are also similarities. People do have the same basic needs and feelings which cut through cultural boundaries.

As effective communication is central to nursing practice, the nurse should have an understanding of what can be done to improve intercultural communication. Every individual needs to know more about the culture of others so that perceptions which differ from their own can be better understood. To facilitate effective intercultural communication, the nurse should:

- develop sensitivity to the significance of cultural factors to an individual .develop an open attitude to the behaviour of different cultural groups
- try to identify a person's cultural values
- be willing to learn from other cultures
- avoid stereotyping and ethnocentrism
- avoid judging a person's intellectual ability or emotional status on the basis of how he uses language
- appreciate that it may be necessary to vary communication techniques, e.g. reduce eye and body contact to a level which is appropriate and acceptable to an individual
- try to understand the person's non-verbal communication
- enunciate clearly and slowly, avoiding the use of slang and abstract terms, when talking to a person who speaks little English
- make use of the services of a health-care interpreter when a patient speaks little or no English
- admit when it is impossible to understand what the other person is saying, rather than run the risk of misunderstanding.

While it is beyond the scope of this text to provide detailed information about the similarities and differences of each cultural group, the following aspects must be considered when interacting with a person from a different culture:

- language differences
- personal space and territoriality
- gender role behaviours and attitudes
- emotional expression
- food and eating habits, dietary taboos
- attitudes towards the family structure
- susceptibility to specific diseases
- health-illness beliefs and practices
- religious beliefs and practices
- cultural sanctions and restrictions
- modesty and concept of the body
- reactions to pain and death.

This chapter does not attempt to identify or describe various cultural beliefs or attitudes towards illness and health care as, in doing so, there is the risk of reinforcing stereotypes or developing new ones. For detailed information on 'culture' the nurse is advised to refer to the texts listed at the end of this chapter.

It is important that nurses appreciate the influence that cultural factors have on the activities of daily living, for example:

- Each culture has its own concept of safety and what constitutes safe behaviour
- Cultural variations affect verbal and non-verbal communication
- Various cultural practices and constraints are associated with eating and drinking
- There are differences in words used in association with, and attitudes towards, elimination
- Not all cultures place the same emphasis on personal cleanliness
- Certain cultures prescribe the type of clothing worn and specify those areas of the body which may be exposed in public
- In some cultures the type of work or leisure activities an individual engages in are determined by sex
- Most cultures have their own code of acceptable sexual behaviour, and some cultures contain specific customs associated with sexuality, e.g. male and female circumcision
- Some cultures determine where a person sleeps and with whom, e.g. in a communal bed or room or in the open air
- There are various social customs which surround dying and death.

CONCLUSION

Australia is a multi-cultural society and, as members of that society, nurses need an understanding of the aspects that comprise a culture and of the diversity of cultures within Australia.

Nurses, as members of the health care team, need to develop an awareness of the significance of cultural factors to an individual. This chapter has introduced the concepts of culture, subcultures, stereotyping and ethnocentrism, and the aspects which must be considered when interacting with a person from a different culture.

REFERENCES AND FURTHER READING

Clements A 1986 Infant and family health in Australia. Churchill Livingstone, Melbourne, ch 21, 212–226
Gray G, Pratt R 1989 Issues in Australian nursing 2. Churchill Livingstone, Melbourne, ch 5, 53–70
International council of nurses 1973, ICN code for nurses: ethical concepts applied to nursing. Imprimeries populaires, Geneva
Knepfer G 1989 Nursing for life. Pan Books, Sydney, ch 2, 25–59
Leininger M 1981 Transcultural nursing: its progress and future. Nursing and health care II (7): 365–371

8. Health and illness

OBJECTIVES

1. Discuss the concepts of health and illness.
2. State the causes of disease.
3. Describe the body's response to injury.
4. State the factors which are either beneficial or detrimental to health.
5. Discuss the promotion of community health.
6. State the personal and environmental health services which are available.
7. Differentiate between primary, secondary, and tertiary health care.

INTRODUCTION

To assist in meeting the health care needs of individuals, the nurse requires an understanding of the concepts of health and illness, and its relevance to the individual, the family, and to society. This chapter addresses the concepts of health and illness, the factors which contribute to the promotion of health and prevention of illness, the meaning of disease, and the role of various health care systems.

Health

Although the term 'health' is used frequently there is little agreement as to its precise definition. Most people have their own idea of what constitutes health, and one individual's concept often varies greatly from the concepts of others.

Despite the difficulty in accurately defining 'health', there seems to be general agreement amongst health professionals that health is something more than simply the absence of disease. The World Health Organization (1974) has defined health as a 'state of complete physical, mental and social wellbeing, not merely the absence of disease or infirmity'. While this definition provides a broad statement about health, it fails to consider the variable and personal nature of health. It does, however, include two important concepts:

- that physical, mental, and social factors are linked in an interdependent relationship
- that an individual should *feel* well, not merely be free of illness.

These two important concepts can be incorporated into a definition which recognizes health as a *dynamic* (ever-changing) state. Thus, health should be viewed as a state of balance which is achieved when an individual succeeds in adapting to a constantly changing environment. An individual must constantly adapt to the environment in order to maintain health—or homeostasis. Homeostasis is a relative constancy in the body's internal environment, which is naturally maintained by adaptive responses that promote healthy survival. Information on homeostasis is provided in Chapter 15.

An individual is being constantly exposed to variations and changes in his physical and social environment. Physical variations include factors such as the climate, and exposure to environmental pollutants or pathogenic micro-organisms. Changes in an individual's social environment include events such as the breakdown of a relationship, altered financial status, and commencing a new job. In order to maintain or restore health, an individual is required to adapt to such variations and changes, through behaviour which seeks to restore balance. At times a combination of changes causes stress to such a degree that an individual is unable to adapt and, thus, the possibility of ill-health is increased. Health, therefore, should be viewed as a state of *dynamic balance* of many physical and environmental factors requiring constant adjustment and adaptation.

Because both health and illness are relative, and exist in varying degrees, it is helpful to consider both in terms of a scale or continuum. The health-illness continuum is a model (scale) which depicts high-level wellness at one end of the continuum and severe illness at the opposite end, with a range of states in between.

Community health

Community health refers to the health and welfare of individuals, families, and community groups. A community may be defined as a segment of a larger population. The basic social structural unit of the community is the family unit. The family unit has been an important unit of social structure from primitive times onwards, and its main functions are the reproduction and the economic and social development and support of family members. Many changes have occurred throughout the centuries which have influenced the family as an institution, so that in modern times the characteristics of families differ according to race, religion, and the social and economic structures of the country of residence. These differences are responsible for the wide variety of health care needs in the community, and thus affect the planning of health care services.

The individual in the community has certain needs which must be met to ensure the establishment and maintenance of physical, mental, and social wellbeing. These needs are described later in this chapter.

Ill-health

Ill-health or illness may be described as an abnormal event in which aspects of an individual's social, physical, emotional, or intellectual condition are impaired—compared to that individual's previous condition. Illness is not simply the presence of a disease process, as the concept of illness is strongly related to the *total* individual, his environment and culture. Illness is directly related to all the factors which affect an individual's life. It is, however, important that the nurse has an understanding of the classification of diseases and causes of illness.

Disease may be defined as a disturbance in structure and/or function of any part of an individual. Diseases may be classified according to their cause, the way in which they are acquired, or according to the body system that is affected.

Causes of disease

The causes of disease may be categorized broadly into those that are genetic or inherited, those due to environmental factors, and those that are due to degeneration.

1. Genetic or inherited diseases are those which are transmitted *genetically* from the parents to the embryo. Inherited disorders involve a single gene mutation, chromosomal aberrations, or multiple causative factors. Examples of disorders involving abnormalities of single genes include:

- phenylketonuria, a metabolic disorder
- achondroplasia, a skeletal condition
- Huntington's chorea, a disorder characterized by progressive chorea and mental deterioration

- cystic fibrosis, a disorder of the exocrine glands
- haemophilia, a blood disorder.

Examples of disorders involving chromosomal aberrations include:

- Down syndrome, caused by presence of an extra chromosome 21 in the G group
- Klinefelter's syndrome, characterized by an extra X chromosome in males
- Turner's syndrome, characterized by the absence of one X chromosome in females.

Examples of disorders involving more than one factor, e.g. genetic and environmental, include:

- spina bifida, a neural tube defect
- anencephaly, congenital absence of the brain
- cleft palate, congenital failure of fusion between the right and left palatal processes
- congenital heart disease.

2. Environment-caused disorders may be the result of physical injuries or trauma, nutritional abnormalities, micro-organisms, or harmful substances such as chemicals.

Traumatic disorders include those that result from physical injury, e.g. sprains, dislocations, or fractures; and those that are psychological, e.g. a psychiatric disorder resulting from stress.

Nutritional disorders include those that result from the effects of deficiency or excess of specific nutrients, e.g. scurvy resulting from insufficient intake of vitamin C, or cardiovascular disease resulting from an excessive intake of lipids.

Infective disorders result from invasion of the body by micro-organisms, and multiplication of micro-organisms within the body, e.g. influenza, rubella, varicella, or cystitis. Information on infection is provided in Chapters 9 and 38.

Chemically-induced disorders include those that result from exposure to chemicals, poisons, or toxins, e.g. some malignant neoplasms, alcoholism and drug dependence

3. Degenerative disorders are those which involve deterioration of structure or function of tissue, e.g. osteoarthritis, Alzheimer's disease, varicose veins, nephrosclerosis.

Causes of death

According to the latest information from the Australian Bureau of Statistics (1987) the leading causes of death in Australia were:

1. heart disease.
2. malignant neoplasms.
3. cerebrovascular diseases.
4. respiratory diseases.
5. accidents, poisoning, violence (external causes).

Of the 117 321 deaths registered in 1987, 40 000 were due to heart disease. Heart disease, malignant neoplasms, and cerebrovascular diseases accounted for 68.3% of *all* deaths.

In the 10 years from 1978–1987 the crude death rates for heart and cerebrovascular disease decreased by 9.5% and 21.6% respectively, while the death rate for malignant neoplasms increased by 14.2%. The most common primary sites of malignant neoplasms continued to be located in the digestive system and peritoneum, with the colon being the most frequently reported site. The leading cause of death, according to age groups, was:

- from 1–44 years of age: accidents, poisoning, violence (external causes)
- from 45–64 years of age: malignant neoplasms
- from 65 years and over: heart disease.

Response to trauma

Trauma is a term which denotes any type of injury to the body. Body tissues respond to damage by the processes of:

- inflammation
- metabolic response
- degeneration and necrosis
- repair and regeneration.

1. Inflammation is the local response to cell injury. When tissues are injured, e.g. by mechanical trauma, blood is lost from damaged vessels. Vasoconstriction occurs, followed soon after by vasodilation which increases the blood flow to the area—thereby delivering leucocytes and plasma proteins. As a consequence of increased localized blood volume, the area becomes red and warm. As the permeability of capillaries and venules increases, due to the release of histamine and other substances from damaged cells, protein, fluid, and leucocytes escape into the surrounding tissues producing oedema. Accumulation of fluid and cells at the site of injury is known as the inflammatory exudate. Pain in the inflamed area is due to pressure from the localized oedema.

This inflammatory response enables the process of phagocytosis, whereby the migrating leucocytes ingest foreign material, e.g. micro-organisms. In addition, antibodies in the exudate come into contact with micro-organisms or toxins, and the fluid in the exudate may dilute the substance which is causing the injury.

Acute inflammation exists when the inflammatory response is of short duration, and *chronic* inflammation exists when the response is prolonged.

Further information on the inflammatory process is provided in Chapter 59.

2. Metabolic response to trauma occurs in three phases:

- Ebb phase, which lasts approximately 24 hours. Metabolism is decreased to promote adequate perfusion of vital organs.

- Stress phase, which varies in duration according to the severity of the injury. Numerous metabolic changes occur in response to the stress of trauma, e.g. the release of glucocorticoids to help convert protein into carbohydrate which raises the metabolic rate, and increased secretion of aldosterone leading to sodium retention and potassium loss. As a result of these metabolic changes there is generally weight loss, possible fluid and electrolyte loss, and possible increase in heat production and body temperature.
- Recovery phase, which varies in duration depending on the severity of the injury and the extent of nutrient depletion. In this phase there is a release of hormones, e.g. insulin and growth hormone, to promote tissue repair and restoration of muscle mass.

3. Degeneration and necrosis. Some types of cell, e.g. nerve cells, respond to injury by degeneration, which may be reversible or which may result in death of cells and necrosis. Degeneration of cells, and cell death, may be caused by lack of vital substances such as oxygen or by the direct action of damaging agents such as toxins.

4. Repair and regeneration. Damaged tissues may be replaced either by fibrous connective tissue (repair), or by the proliferation of surrounding healthy cells (regeneration). Regeneration results in restoration of normal tissue function. Further information on healing is provided in Chapter 59.

Manifestations of disease

When there is a disturbance of normal function, the individual generally experiences some manifestations of disease, i.e. signs and symptoms. A *sign* is something that can be noted by an observer, while a *symptom* is a sensation experienced by the ill person.

An individual is likely to seek medical advice if he is experiencing manifestations of a disease which disrupt his normal lifestyle. However, not all individuals perceive signs or symptoms in the same way. For example, one person may seek medical advice immediately if he experiences a severe headache, while another individual may dismiss such an event as nothing more than a nuisance. Or, one woman may seek medical advice as soon as she detects a breast lump, while another woman may be so frightened of the possibility of cancer that she may defer seeking advice for months. Factors that influence an individual's reaction and response to the manifestations of disease include:

- the nature of the illness, e.g. whether it is acute or chronic
- whether the manifestations are perceived as serious or life-threatening
- how severely the manifestations affect the individual's usual life-style

- whether the significance of specific manifestations are understood
- how long a sign or symptom persists
- the availability of medical assistance, e.g. whether the individual has to travel a long distance to consult a medical officer
- financial status, e.g. an individual may not seek advice or treatment if he is unable to meet any costs incurred.

It is important for the nurse to understand how these and other factors may influence whether an individual seeks medical assistance. To help illustrate how various factors do influence an individual's behaviour in recognizing an illness and seeking assistance, the following example is provided.

An 80-year-old woman was admitted to hospital following a fall at home. Her daughter had visited her mother at home and had noticed several bruises on her face and arms. On asking her about the origin of the bruises, the daughter discovered that her mother had fallen over the previous day. She rang the local medical officer who suggested that it would be a good idea if he examined her mother. It was the first time that the woman had consulted a doctor in 30 years, as she had considered herself to be fit and healthy. On examining the woman, the doctor decided to admit her to hospital as he suspected she may have a fractured cheek bone.

Thus, the woman was admitted to hospital for facial X-rays and possible surgery. As a nurse was helping her to undress and get into bed, she noticed the woman was wearing several absorbent pads between her legs. When the nurse asked the reason for this, the woman told her that she had worn pads for the last 10 years—ever since she developed a prolapse. When the pads were removed, the nurse observed that the woman had a third degree uterine prolapse (the uterus was completely outside the vulva). On questioning, the woman told the nurse that she had never sought medical advice because she thought such a prolapse was a normal part of growing old! The nurse was further amazed when the woman said, 'Well, it's never really bothered me or stopped me doing the things I normally do.'

This example illustrates how the woman's perception and understanding of her condition differed greatly to that of the nurse, who understood that a prolapse is not a normal part of ageing and who viewed it as a significant health problem.

Many of the signs or symptoms, or manifestations, associated with specific diseases are described in Chapters 41–50. This chapter mentions some of the more common manifestations of disease which may prompt a person to seek medical advice.

The *significance* of signs and symptoms lies in the patho-physiology that results in their manifestation. Signs and symptoms may result from:

- a disturbed homeostatic mechanism, e.g. an elevated temperature due to an infection
- a direct manifestation of the disorder, e.g. pain in the joints with osteoarthritis
- a consequence of disturbed function, e.g. skin pallor due to anaemia
- a sign of some underlying disorder, e.g. spontaneous bruising due to a blood disease
- the body's attempt to adapt to disturbed function, e.g. sweating to increase heat loss when the body temperature is elevated
- a reaction or response to treatment, e.g. hair loss from the effects of chemotherapy.

Common signs associated with disease include:

- alterations in normal skin colour, e.g. pallor, cyanosis, jaundice
- skin rashes or lesions
- vomiting or diarrhoea
- abnormal vital signs, e.g. elevated temperature; rapid, slow, or irregular pulse, shallow ventilations, elevated or lowered blood pressure
- oedema, swelling, or distension of a body part
- abnormalities in the urine or faeces
- abnormal blood values
- abnormal discharge from a body orifice, e.g. purulent drainage from the ear
- bleeding.

Common symptoms associated with disease include:

- pain
- nausea
- cough
- difficult breathing
- fatigue
- loss of appetite
- constipation
- depression or anxiety.

Factors influencing health and illness

An individual's health status depends on many personal, social, and environmental factors which include:

- Lifestyle, e.g. whether the individual engages in behaviours which promote health or contribute to ill-health.
- Time and place. Disease patterns vary in relation to time, i.e. certain diseases are more prevalent during a specific season. For example, the incidence of the common cold and influenza increases during the winter months. The incidence of certain diseases, e.g. heart disease, is greater

in some countries than in others. The pattern of diseases can also vary within different geographical locations in the same country, e.g. the incidence of melanoma is greater in Queensland than in other Australian states.

- Age. The incidence of specific diseases and causes of death are related to age, e.g. the incidence of heart disease, cancer, and cerebrovascular disease increases with age. Infectious diseases such as rubella, measles and chickenpox are more common in the young.
- Sex. Certain diseases may more commonly affect individuals of one sex, e.g. the incidence of mesothelioma is higher in males.
- Race. Specific diseases, e.g. some genetic disorders are more common in particular ethnic or racial groups. For example, people of Mediterranean origin are more affected by thalassemia than others.
- Environmental elements. Exposure to harmful substances in the environment increases the risk of ill-health. For example, persons who are exposed to asbestos are at risk of developing mesothelioma.
- Availability and effectiveness of health promotion programmes.

Health promotion and disease prevention

Health care services recognize the need to focus on health rather than illness, therefore the emphasis is on health promotion and disease prevention at an individual and community level. Health promotion and illness prevention have become an important focus of health care for several reasons, e.g. there are still no cures for many diseases, health care costs are rising rapidly, and the community is more aware of the value of health maintenance.

The nurse has an important role to play in health promotion, therefore she needs an understanding of the factors that are beneficial or detrimental to health.

Factors which promote health

To promote physical, mental, emotional, and social health, individuals need to be aware of the importance of:

- A balanced diet, which contains all the essential nutrients in sufficient amounts. The Commonwealth Department of Health has developed guidelines to improve the health of all Australians, and the Australian Nutrition Foundation developed a Diet Pyramid (see Fig. 29.1) based on these guidelines.
Information on nutritional needs is provided in Chapter 29.
- Maintaining the ideal body weight for age, sex, height and build (see Table 29.2).
- Adequate movement and exercise which are necessary for maintaining normal body functions, e.g. muscle tone, circulation, and elimination.

Information on movement and exercise needs is provided in Chapter 37.
- Adequate sleep, rest, and relaxation which are necessary for an individual's physical and emotional health. Insufficient sleep and rest often results in inability to concentrate, increased irritability, and decreased ability to participate in the activities of daily living. The ability to relax physically promotes mental relaxation which relieves stress and anxiety.
Information on meeting the need for rest and sleep is provided in Chapter 35.
- Adequate elimination of wastes, e.g. faeces. Elimination of wastes from the bowel can be promoted by a diet high in fibre content, adequate intake of fluids, and sufficient exercise.
Information on elimination needs is provided in Chapter 30.
- Maintaining a high standard of personal hygiene which includes care of the skin, teeth, and eyes.
Information on hygiene needs is provided in Chapter 39.
- Preventing infection, e.g. through normal hygiene practices such as washing the hands after visiting the toilet, and by immunization against infectious diseases.
Information on prevention of infection is provided in Chapters 9 and 38.
- Avoiding accidental injury by promoting safe home and working environments, and by avoiding exposure to harmful elements in the environment.
Information on safety is provided in Chapter 38.
- Adopting measures which are directed at preventing, reducing, or dealing with stress.
Information on stress is provided in Chapter 6.

There are numerous health care programmes which are directed towards promoting healthy lifestyles, some of which encourage people to change 'unhealthy' behaviours or to adopt new habits which will promote health. Other programmes are directed towards a specific health problem, e.g. those that encourage and support people to give up smoking. The various health care programmes, which may be conducted by health-care or other agencies, are directed towards improving the health of individuals through education, preventive health services, and environmental protection.

Factors which are detrimental to health

People, for a variety of reasons such as lack of knowledge, may engage in behaviours that can have a negative effect on health. Detrimental practices include:

- smoking
- alcohol or drug abuse
- activities that involve a threat of accidental injury

- eating behaviours that lead to obesity or malnutrition
- insufficient rest or sleep
- insufficient exercise
- living a stressful lifestyle without practicing stress-management techniques
- engaging in unsafe sexual practices
- working or living in areas which are exposed to environmental pollutants
- living in overcrowded or unhygienic dwellings
- exposing the body to excessive amounts of sunlight.

Promoting community health

The health of a community is promoted when there is:

- safe water, food, and milk supplies
- safe disposal of sewerage and garbage
- adequate pest control
- control of environmental pollution
- control of communicable diseases
- safe and hygienic living and working environments, e.g. adequate ventilation, light, and heating
- equal opportunities for all people, e.g. to obtain employment and adequate housing
- provision of adequate health care services.

Community health care services

There are numerous services provided by Commonwealth and State Government departments, local government authorities, and voluntary agencies. The services may be classed as *personal* or those which directly serve individuals, and *environmental* which are concerned with the environment and therefore affect individuals indirectly.

Personal health care services

Personal health care services include:

- Health education in schools, encompassing subjects such as nutrition, hygiene, parenting, and sex. This is a responsibility shared between the Health Department and the Education Department.
- Fertility and family planning clinics conducted by some hospitals, community health centres and voluntary agencies.
- Antenatal clinics, conducted by maternity hospitals and community health centres, to educate prospective parents about pregnancy and childbirth.
- Maternal and child health centres which are run by local authorities under the auspices of the Health Department. Parents who attend these centres receive information and advice on all aspects of child care.
- Immunization programmes for children and adults, conducted by the Health Department and local authorities

as a means of reducing the incidence of communicable diseases.

- School health services which are the responsibility of branches of the Health Commission concerned with the general, dental, and mental health of children.
- Screening programmes conducted by Commonwealth and State Health Authorities for the purpose of detecting specific diseases, e.g. tuberculosis, in persons entering Australia.
- Occupational health and safety laws to promote safe and hygienic working conditions. Occupational health and safety acts set down standards to be maintained by employers, e.g. provision of safe and healthy work places, setting down safe and healthy work systems and procedures, provision of safe storage and use of plant, equipment, and substances.
- Rehabilitation services for children and adults with impairments, organized by hospitals, clinics, and voluntary agencies in conjunction with the Health Department. These services include sheltered workshops, where people with impairments may work at their own pace using specially adapted equipment.
- Mental health services supplied by agencies under the auspices of the Health Department, or voluntary organizations.
- Blood bank service, run by the Health Department and the Australian Red Cross Society, which is responsible for the collection of blood from donors and for much of the research into blood fractions.
- Visiting nurse services supplied to community members in their own homes, which include the Royal District Nursing Service and various domiciliary services run by hospitals and voluntary agencies.
- Occupational health nurses employed by many industries. An occupational health nurse provides emergency care, conducts health assessments, and provides information on matters relating to health promotion and safety.
- Services for the elderly are provided by numerous sources including public and private hospitals, various branches of the Health Department, local authorities, and voluntary agencies. Services available include meals on wheels, day-care facilities, elderly citizens clubs, hostel-type accommodation, and short-term and long-term accommodation in extended care hospitals and nursing homes.
- Educational literature provided by specialist agencies and voluntary organizations on subjects such as cancer, tuberculosis, sexually transmitted diseases, alcoholism, smoking, drug dependence, venomous bites and stings, safety, and nutrition.

Environmental health services

Services which focus on preventing community health hazards include:

• Environmental Protection Authorities and laws governing pollution, e.g. by noise, industrial waste, sewerage, and harmful chemicals.
• Control of the collection, storage, purification, and reticulation of a supply of clean water to all sections of a community.
• Safe disposal of waste such as garbage, excreta, industrial waste, and radioactive substances.
• Control of food standards to prevent infection of the community by food-borne diseases, via laws in respect of handling of livestock, processing and distribution of food.
• Control of building standards to ensure that the health of the community is not impaired as the result of poor conditions in residential buildings, restaurants, hospitals, entertainment areas, etc. There are standards set in respect of the height of ceilings, ventilation, heating, lighting, freedom from dampness, sanitary provisions, water supply, and the minimum size for a block of land used for any type of building.

Different parts of the responsibility for the provision and maintenance of community health is assumed by the four categories of health agency.

The Commonwealth Health Department is responsible for:

• quarantine procedures
• research laboratories
• institutes of anatomy and science
• diagnostic laboratories
• schools of public health and tropical medicine
• legislation in all matters relating to health.

The State Health Department is responsible for:

• control of the standards for the provision of clean water and food
• prevention and control of infectious diseases
• education of the public in the promotion and maintenance of health
• control of the standards of practice, e.g. nursing and medical
• registration of qualified health personnel
• maternal, infant, and child welfare services
• school medical services
• occupational health services
• administration of public hospitals
• registration and the control of the standard of private hospitals, nursing homes, and clinics.

Local authorities, e.g. shire or municipal councils working in conjunction with the State Health Department are responsible for:

• rubbish collection and disposal
• building regulations
• immunization programmes

• inspection of premises used for the production or selling of food
• pest control
• services for the elderly such as meals on wheels and home help.

Voluntary organizations, which provide various services including:

• blood bank
• disaster relief
• hospital visiting
• elderly citizens clubs
• accommodation and/or meals for homeless people
• counselling
• family planning and birth control
• promotion of breast feeding
• support and self-help groups, e.g. for people with cancer, visual or hearing impairment.

The influence of health services on community health

The services which are instrumental in promoting and maintaining the health of a community have developed gradually over many years, and when various statistics are consulted it can be seen that the standards of many aspects of community health has progressively risen:

• The infant mortality rate has been lowered considerably. It should be noted, however, that the infant mortality rate among the Aboriginal population remains at an unacceptably high level.
• There are fewer deaths among children of school age.
• Complications of pregnancy are less common, and maternal mortality has decreased significantly.
• Occupationally-induced diseases are less common and industrial accidents are fewer in number.
• There has been a considerable reduction in the incidence of infectious diseases and in the number of deaths or disabilities resulting from infectious diseases. It should be noted, however, that the increasing number of people with HIV infection poses a very real threat to community health. Information on HIV infection is provided in Chapter 44.
• A greater number of people can expect to reach old age, as a result of many factors such as better standards of nutrition and medical care. It is estimated that by the year 2000, approximately 12% of the population of Australia will be aged 65 years or over.

Delivery of health care

The health care industry involves a wide range of services which are provided by numerous systems and agencies. Health care services may be broadly classified as those that provide:

- primary care: health promotion and disease prevention
- secondary care: diagnosis and treatment
- tertiary care: rehabilitation.

While the traditional medical care system provides all 3 types of services, many people are looking towards alternative/complementary, systems of therapy, e.g. chiropractic, osteopathy, homeopathy, acupuncture, reflexology, or massage. There are increasing numbers of people who choose one or more of the less traditional approaches to health care. A person may choose an alternative/complementary system of health care for numerous reasons. One reason often given is the inability to obtain traditional health services in the way in which a person desires them, and at the time he needs them. For example a person may be dissatisfied because of:

- long waiting hours
- lack of availability of health professionals
- impersonality of care given
- increasing costs of medical care
- lack of comprehensiveness and continuity of care.

While it should be appreciated that every individual has the right to choose a particular system of health care, the nurse is more likely to work within a traditional setting.

The health care delivery system in Australia is varied and includes:

- health promotion programmes
- illness prevention programmes
- public and private hospitals
- specialty hospitals
- rehabilitation services
- community-based agencies
- clinics and outpatient services
- voluntary agencies
- hospices
- self-help groups.

Primary care

Primary care, which comprises health promotion and illness prevention activities, was described earlier in the chapter. Settings for primary care include community clinics, private homes, schools, industries, and physician's offices.

Secondary care

Secondary care, the diagnosis and treatment of illness, takes place in physician's offices, hospitals, clinics, outpatient services, home health agencies, and various community agencies such as drug rehabilitation centres.

Day-care centres and surgical centres offering one-day admissions offer people an alternative to hospitalization.

Home health care is increasing for many reasons, e.g. earlier discharge from hospital, and the development of support systems which enable persons with chronic illnesses, such as renal failure, to remain at home. In addition to home nursing care, people may utilize a range of other services such as meals on wheels or home help. Home care offers an alternative to hospitalization, a family-centred approach, and continuity of care.

Information on community-based care is provided in Chapter 62.

Tertiary care

Rehabilitation, or long-term care, is provided by rehabilitation centres, some hospitals, extended care facilities, hospices, and nursing homes. Rehabilitation also takes place in the individual's home through services provided by home nursing agencies, etc. Information on rehabilitation is provided in Chapter 60.

The health care team

The health care team is defined as a group of health professionals working together to provide health care. The health team is comprised of physicians, nurses, and allied health professionals, e.g. physiotherapists, occupational therapists, speech pathologists, dietitians, pharmacists, and social workers. Information on the role and function of health team members is provided in Chapter 4.

Changes in health care delivery

In the past the emphasis in health care was on the diagnosis and treatment of disease, however in recent decades the emphasis has shifted to health promotion and disease prevention. This shift in emphasis has occurred for a variety of reasons such as consumer influences, economic and political influences, and technological changes.

The health care delivery system has become more sensitive to the needs of the consumer and the community. Generally, individuals are now more knowledgeable about health and the importance of illness prevention, and are prepared to assume some responsibility for their own health. Consequently, health care services have responded by initiating and implementing a variety of health promotion programmes.

The rapidly escalating costs of health care, and the inability of large numbers of people to pay for health services, has led to many changes in the delivery of health care. People are discharged from hospitals much earlier and, consequently, there is a greater need for more home care agencies.

Health care services are required to match the economic resources available against the wants and needs of a community. There is much debate about the ethics of channelling vast sums of money into specific programmes which benefit a relatively small percentage of the population, e.g. organ transplant procedures, at the expense of the health needs of the majority.

People with lower economic status frequently defer seeking health services, or have to face long waiting periods before they can obtain a hospital bed. Conversely, people with adequate financial resources or private health insurance are generally able to obtain the health care they require.

Political decisions, e.g. health care legislation, also influences how health care is provided. Nurses are becoming increasingly aware of the role they can play in influencing the restructuring of the health care system, e.g. by advising local and state governments about specific health issues. Nurses, as a body, are able to exert political pressure to influence health policy reform so that the health care system responds to the needs of society as a whole.

Advances in medical technology have resulted in new and sophisticated equipment and procedures coming into use, and research has led to new treatments for life-threatening diseases. The development of sophisticated life-support equipment, and procedures such as implants and transplants, has undoubtedly saved the lives of many people. At the same time, however, technological advances have created numerous ethical dilemmas. Health care providers must consider the consequences of this scientific and technological 'explosion', e.g. the *quality* of life being saved.

Health care delivery is changing, and will continue to change, as health care services try to achieve the World Health Organization's (1978) aim of 'Health for All by the Year 2000'. The nurse has a responsibility to keep informed of change in order to deliver effective health care.

CONCLUSION

The nurse requires an understanding of the concepts of health and illness in order to deliver effective health care.

Health is a dynamic state in which the individual constantly adapts to changes to maintain a state of wellbeing.

Illness refers to a reduction in the individual's normal physical, mental, or social functioning.

Diseases—disturbances in structure or function—may be caused by genetic, environmental, or degenerative factors.

Body tissues respond to damage by the processes of inflammation, metabolic response, degeneration and necrosis, and repair and regeneration.

Signs and symptoms are manifestations of disease and may result from a disturbed homeostatic mechanism, be a direct manifestation of a disorder or a consequence of disturbed function, be a sign of some underlying disorder or the body's attempt to adapt to disturbed function, or be a reaction to treatment.

An individual's health status depends on many personal, social, and environmental factors such as lifestyle, time and place, age, sex, and race.

Health services recognize the need to focus on health promotion and disease prevention, therefore the nurse requires an understanding of the factors which are beneficial or detrimental to health.

Community health is promoted when there is safe water, food and milk supplies, safe disposal of sewerage and garbage, adequate pest control, control of environmental pollution, control of communicable diseases, safe and hygienic living and working conditions, and provision of adequate health care services.

Delivery of health care can be classified as primary, secondary, or tertiary. Primary care focuses on health promotion and disease prevention, secondary care involves the diagnosis and treatment of illness, while tertiary care involves rehabilitation and long-term care.

REFERENCES AND FURTHER READING

Potter P A, Perry A G 1985 Fundamentals of nursing. C V Mosby, St Louis, ch 2, 38–61
WHO UNICEF 1978 Primary health care. World Health Organization, Geneva

9. Microbiology, infection and immunity

OBJECTIVES

1. Name the major groups of microorganisms, and state the characteristics of each group.
2. Name the common diseases caused by each group of microorganisms.
3. Describe the process of infection (chain of infection).
4. Describe the body defences against infection.
5. Differentiate between innate and acquired, and passive and active immunity.
6. Practise recommended and approved infection control techniques when carrying out nursing activities.

INTRODUCTION

The nurse requires a knowledge of microorganisms, the infectious process, and the application of infection control principles to prevent the spread of infection. Control of infection is an essential component of every nursing activity.

Information on aspects of infection control, disinfection and sterilization, is provided in Chapter 38; and information on isolation nursing techniques is provided in Chapter 61. This chapter addresses a brief history of microbiology, micro-organisms, infection and immunity, prevention and control of infection.

A brief history of microbiology

Throughout history philosophers and scientists have debated the nature of disease, but it is within only a comparatively short space of time that accurate information has become available.

Microbiology is the study of living organisms of microscopic size. As early as 1546 the suggestion was made by *Fracastaro* that disease was spread by particles too small to be seen, but the microscopes which were made in the latter part of that century were primitive and capable of only very low magnification.

In 1676, a Dutchman, *Anton van Leeuwenloek* designed and made a microscope which he used to become the first person to see bacteria. He found many microorganisms in materials such as water, mud, saliva, and the intestinal contents of healthy subjects. He recognized these as living organisms because they moved actively, and he observed that very large numbers of bacteria appeared in solutions of animal or vegetable matter that were left to stand for several days at room temperature. He believed that these large populations of bacteria developed from a few organisms that were originally present in the animal or vegetable matter, or that they had entered the solution from the air.

Other scientists believed that microorganisms arose by *spontaneous generation*, i.e. by the spontaneous conversion of dead organic matter into living microbes. This suggestion began a controversy that lasted for approximately 200 years. An experiment which was to disprove this theory was first described by a Frenchman, *Louis Joblet* in 1718. Other scientists performed similar experiments, notably an Italian scientist, *Lazzaro Spallanzani*. The experiments demonstrated that bacteria multiplied by simple division, and so disproved the notion of spontaneous generation. (A considerable amount of progress was made in the field of microbiology in the nineteenth century, although the 'germ theory' of disease did not become firmly established until 1876.)

Edward Jenner (1749–1823), an English physician, was responsible for the discovery that a cowpox vaccine would produce immunity to smallpox. For many years immunization to smallpox was practised, and people were inoculated with infected material from smallpox sufferers—a dangerous practice which resulted in many deaths. Jenner noticed that farmworkers with cowpox showed no reactions to the smallpox inoculation, and so the idea of a cowpox vaccine was formulated.

Ignaz Semmelweiss, a Hungarian doctor, was appalled at the extremely high rate of death due to puerperal fever contracted by mothers following childbirth. He investigated and came to the conclusion that microorganisms were carried on the hands of doctors and nurses, on instruments, and on linen. Against a great deal of opposition he instituted a system of antiseptic procedures, which drastically reduced the mortality rate and paved the way for the development of antiseptic surgical techniques.

Louis Pasteur (1822–1895) was a French chemist whose work in solving the problems of wine makers and beet growers led to the discovery that bacteria cause fermentation, and enabled him to prove that dust particles carry bacteria. His efforts to prevent the spoiling of wine by bacteria led Pasteur to devise the system of preservation now known as pasteurization, which is used as a means of protecting perishable foods, notably milk. Other important contributions made to medical science by Pasteur were the development of vaccines against anthrax and rabies—two dreaded diseases prevalent at that time.

Robert Koch (1843–1910), a German scientist, is now regarded as the father of modern bacteriology. He introduced the technique of using solid media for bacterial culture, and he created the basic principles which are still applied in establishing the causative organism of a particular disease. Koch is also noted for his isolation of the bacilli which cause tuberculosis and anthrax.

Joseph Lister (1827–1912), an English surgeon, used the work carried out by Pasteur as a foundation for his own investigations into the prevention of bacterial invasion of wounds. As a result, he is acknowledged as the founder of modern antiseptic surgery. Lister's use of carbolic acid as a spray and as a wound dressing was not approved by his colleagues, who, in 1870, still thought that infection was an essential phase in the healing process and who refused to believe that infection could be airborne. Lister later applied the antiseptic procedures established by Semmelweiss and received a great deal of opposition, until it became obvious that these techniques dramatically reduced the number of postoperative infections.

Klebs, Loeffler, Roux, and *Behring* were medical scientists who, in the 1880s, succeeded in isolating the diphtheria bacillus—establishing that the damage to tissues was caused by a toxin produced by the organism, and that an antitoxin was produced by the sufferer of diphtheria. This led the team to the production of a serum to treat and prevent diphtheria, which was previously responsible for thousands of deaths.

Twentieth century progress includes the work carried out by *Ehrlich* that resulted in the discovery of a drug which, until the advent of penicillin many years later, was the most successful treatment of syphilis. Ehrlich's finding gave rise to the discovery of a wide range of antibiotics. Penicillin was discovered by *Alexander Fleming* in 1929, and developed in 1940 by *Florey* (an Australian) and *Chain*.

The production of a vaccine against poliomyelitis has been one of the most important developments in modern medical science, as it has resulted in almost complete eradication of the disease. In 1953 *Dr Jonas Salk* developed a vaccine which was given by injection, and in 1955 an oral vaccine was produced by *Dr Albert Sabin* which was found to be safer to use and more effective as an immunizing agent.

More recently, vaccines have been developed against measles, rubella, mumps, and other infectious diseases. Research continues, and modern technology makes it possible to adapt the principles and methods established hundreds of years ago in order to obtain results more speedily.

MICROORGANISMS

Microorganisms are forms of animal or plant life too small to be seen without the aid of a microscope.

Microscopes, which can magnify an object many thousands of times, are usually one of two main varieties:

- The light microscope, in which the specimen to be viewed is illuminated by ordinary light rays. It can magnify up to 2000 times.
- The electron microscope, which uses electrons instead of light rays. It is capable of much greater magnification than the light microscope, and can magnify several hundred thousand times.

Distribution of microorganisms

Microorganisms are found in millions, in every situation where it is possible for life to exist. Microorganisms are present:

- in the air
- in the water
- in the soil
- in dust
- in and on food
- on every surface
- in and on the bodies of other organisms, including the human being.

Microorganisms may be pathogenic or non-pathogenic. Only a small proportion of the microorganisms that abound in nature are *pathogenic*—capable of causing disease. *Non-pathogenic* microorganisms do not cause disease under normal circumstances and in their normal environment. Non-pathogenic microorganisms can become pathogenic if transferred to a different environment.

Most pathogenic microorganisms are free-living in soil, water and similar habitats, and are unable to invade the living body. Some free-living microorganisms obtain their energy from daylight or by the oxidation of inorganic matter, but the majority feed on dead organic matter and are termed *saprophytes*. In contrast, a *parasite* is defined as a microorganism or larger species (e.g. helminth) that lives in or on, and obtains its nourishment from, a living host.

Commensal microorganisms are also called *normal flora* because they live in or on the body without causing disease. They are, therefore, non-pathogenic. Under certain circumstances, e.g. when the body defences are impaired, they may invade the tissues and cause disease thus acting as *opportunistic pathogens*.

Normal flora perform a number of useful functions if they remain at their normal location, but are potentially pathogenic if they are introduced into an area which they do not normally inhabit. Normal flora are found:

* on the skin
* on the mucous membranes of the upper respiratory tract, intestines, and vagina.

The functions performed by non-pathogenic microorganisms include:

* decomposition, in the bowel, of the cellulose content in the diet which may then be excreted in the faeces.
* production of vitamins, i.e. by the activities of bacteria in the large intestine and in the soil.
* protection of the body, i.e. normal flora suppress invasion by pathogenic microorganisms.
* production of some antibiotic medications.

True pathogens are the organisms that are able to overcome the normal defences of the body and invade the tissues. Their growth in the tissues, or their production of poisonous substances such as toxins, damages the tissues and causes the manifestations of disease.

The process of microbial invasion of the body is called *infection,* and a microbial disease is often called an *infective disease.* Those infective diseases that are readily communicable from person to person are called infectious or contagious.

Virulence is a term used to describe the pathogenicity of an organism or, in other words, the extent to which it is capable of causing disease.

CLASSIFICATION OF MICROORGANISMS

The major groups are classified according to size, structure, and method of reproduction. They are generally classed as:

1. bacteria
2. viruses
3. fungi
4. parasites (metazoans and protozoans).

Bacteria

Bacteria (singular—bacterium) are single-celled microscopic organisms, varying in size from 0.3–14.0 micrometres.

Bacteria consist of a rigid cell wall enclosing cytoplasm which contains a nuclear body—but no nuclear membrane. When division occurs to form 2 similar daughter cells, a septum, which consists of new cell membrane and cell wall material, is formed across the cell—dividing it into 2 equal parts. The new cells usually separate but in some instances they remain adhered to each other and, in this way, chains or clusters of bacteria are formed.

Some bacteria develop a *capsule*, which is a thick protective covering—making the organism more resistant to adverse conditions and increasing its virulence by protecting it against *phagocytosis* (the process by which specialized cells in the body attempt to engulf and destroy harmful organisms).

Some bacteria have *flagella*, which are whip-like processes attached to the cell body and are used in a lashing movement for propulsion.

Some bacteria have *fimbriae*, which are hair-like processes that enable the bacteria to attach themselves to other cells, e.g. the host's tissue cells.

Mycoplasmas, classed as bacteria, lack rigid cell walls.

Chlamydiae and *rickettsiae*, classed as bacteria, multiply only in host cells.

Requirements of bacteria

Bacteria are able to grow and reproduce only if they are provided with favourable conditions: food and water, oxygen, carbon dioxide, suitable temperature and pH.

1. Food and water are required by all bacteria for growth and a supply of energy. Bacteria require the same basic nutrients as humans, but obtain them in a variety of ways. Bacteria contain enzymes which break down the nutrients obtained to supply energy, and food is stored in the cell.

2. Oxygen requirements vary with different groups of bacteria. Some can survive with or without oxygen (facultative anaerobes), some need oxygen (aerobes), while others flourish only in the absence of oxygen (anaerobes).

3. Carbon dioxide requirements. All bacteria require a small amount of carbon dioxide, and the concentration in air is sufficient for the needs of most bacteria. Some cannot be grown after removal from the host, unless they are provided with a concentration of carbon dioxide which is over 5%. Examples are the *Brucella abortus* and *Neisseria gonorrhoeae.*

4. Temperature requirements. Most bacteria grow best at body temperature (37°C), but they can multiply in a wide range of temperatures from 10°C to 60°C. Low temperatures inhibit the growth of most bacteria, and temperatures above 60°C can kill bacteria. As bacteria vary considerably in their reactions to temperature, other factors such as moisture and time of exposure have to be considered.

5. pH. Most bacteria require a neutral or slightly alkaline medium. Growth and reproduction usually cease in a highly acid or highly alkaline medium, but there are some exceptions. A few species will flourish in a highly acid environment, and a few prefer a highly alkaline environment.

Properties of bacteria

Bacteria, like other living cells, must be capable of three basic processes in order to survive. They must be able to:

1. reproduce exact replicas of themselves.
2. use materials available to them in their environment, to synthesize living matter.
3. produce energy by breaking down food, and to use the energy produced.

Spore formation. Some bacteria have the ability to develop round or oval structures, called spores, when exposed to adverse conditions. Spores contain condensed protoplasm which can exist in unfavourable conditions without nourishment for many years—then resume normal activity when conditions again become favourable. Spores are highly resistant to high temperatures, sunlight, freezing, and disinfectants—and therefore they are extremely difficult to destroy.

Production of toxins. Pathogenic bacteria produce two types of poisons called toxins:

1. exotoxins, which are produced by living bacteria and liberated into the surrounding tissues where they cause damage, e.g. tetanus and diphtheria toxins.
2. endotoxins, which remain inside the bacterial cell, and are released on the death and destruction of the bacterium.

Classification of bacteria

Bacteria may be classified by reactions to staining, and by shape.

1. Staining properties are the reactions of bacteria to a staining technique named after Gram, the scientist who invented it. A violet coloured stain is used to stain bacteria on a glass slide, then a solvent is used as a decolourizing agent. Counterstaining with a red dye follows, then the slide is rinsed with water:

- Gram-positive bacteria are those than retain the violet colour.
- Gram-negative bacteria are those that retain the red colour.

Acid-fast bacteria have a waxy envelope through which the stain is unable to penetrate, and a very strong hot stain is necessary. The organism holds this stain, and solvents are not able to decolourize it. This staining technique is called the Ziehl-Neelsen method. The tubercle bacillus (causing tuberculosis) is an example of an acid-fast bacillus.

Table 9.1 Bacterial diseases

Organism	Diseases caused
Bacilli (Singular–bacillus)	
Escherichia coli (E coli)	Gastroenteritis, urinary tract infections
Salmonella typhi	Typhoid fever
Chlostridium tetani	Tetanus
Chlostridium botulinum	Botulism
Myobacterium tuberculosis	Tuberculosis
Coryne bacterium diphtheriae	Diphtheria
Bacillus anthraces	Anthrax
Haemophilus pertussis	Pertussis
Proteus vulgaris	Urinary tract infections
Pseudomonas aeruginosa	Infected wounds and burns, bronchopneumonia
Cocci (Singular—Coccus)	
(A) Diplococci:	
Meningococci	Meningitis
Gonococci	Gonorrhoea
Pneumococci	Pneumonia, meningitis
(B) Streptococci:	
Strep. pyogenes	Pharyngitis, tonsillitis, cellulitis
Strep. agalactiae	Neonatal pneumonia and meningitis
Strep. faecalis	Urinary tract infection
Strep. viridans	Endocarditis
Strep. pneumoniae	Pneumonia, Meningitis, Otitis media
(C) Staphylococci:	
Staph. aureus	Boils, carbuncles, styes, wound infection, pneumonia, abscess formation, septicaemia
Staph. epidermidis	Colonisation of surgical prostheses
Staph. saprophyticus	Cystitis
Vibrio (singular-vibrium)	
Vibrio cholerae	Cholera
V. parahaemolyticus	Gastroenteritis (from seafood)
V. alginolyticus	Wound infection (following wounds sustained in sea water)
Spirilla (Singular–spirillum)	
Spirilla minus	Rat-bite fever
Spirochaetes	
Treponema pallidum	Syphilis
T. vincentii	Vincent's angina
Leptospira	Leptospirosis
Mycoplasmas	
Mycoplasma pneumoniaea	Pharyngitis, pneumonia
M. hominis	? Non-specific urethritis
M. urealyticum	? Salpingitis
Chlamydiae	
Chlamydia trachomatis	Trachoma, lymphogranuloma, cervicitis, salpingitis, non-specific urethritis
Rickettsieae	
Rickettsia prowazekii	Epidemic typhus
R. rickettsii	Rocky Mountain spotted fever
R. australis	Queensland tick typhus

2. Classification by shape. There are three basic types of bacteria:

- rod shaped, called bacilli
- spherical or round shaped, called cocci

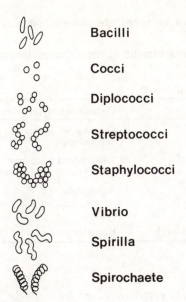

Bacilli

Cocci

Diplococci

Streptococci

Staphylococci

Vibrio

Spirilla

Spirochaete

Fig. 9.1 Bacterial shapes.

- spiral shaped, namely spirilla, vibrios, and spirochaetes.

Figure 9.1 illustrates the various bacterial shapes. Table 9.1 lists various diseases caused by bacteria

Culture of bacteria

When it is necessary to identify the causative organism of a disease, a sterile culture medium is used to promote growth and reproduction of the organism present in infected material.

A *culture medium* is a substance which contains all the nutrients needed by bacteria for growth and reproduction. It may be contained in a test tube, or in a flat dish called a Petri dish. There are several types of media which can be used, and certain bacteria will flourish on one medium while others prefer a medium with different ingredients. Examples of media are:

- nutrient broth, which is a liquid containing meat extracts.
- nutrient agar, which is made by adding agar to nutrient broth to solidify it.
- blood agar, which consists of nutrient agar to which blood has been added.
- heated blood agar, which contains blood that has been boiled.

Bacteria are cultured from infected material such as pus, blood, urine, faeces, sputum, and mucus.

A swab or a wire loop is used to spread some of the infected material over the medium in the culture plate. A cover is placed over the plate which is placed into an incubator at body temperature—a temperature which is ideal for promoting bacterial growth and reproduction. After 18–24 hours, the plate is removed from the incubator and the growth of bacteria is examined.

Each bacterium multiplies and forms a *colony*, containing up to 1000 million organisms. These colonies, which can be seen by the naked eye, are examined for size, shape, colour, and the effect they have had on the culture medium. For example, haemolytic organisms produce a *toxin* which destroys red blood cells. Haemolytic streptococci produce colonies which are surrounded by a clear halo, when grown on blood agar. *Pseudomonas aeruginosa* causes bluish-green discolouration of nutrient agar.

In addition to observation of colonies of bacteria, other investigative measures are used to help identify the organism:

1. Microscopic examination can be made after a smear of some of the growth is prepared on a glass slide, and stained.

2. Biochemical tests are used mainly to detect the presence of enzymes in bacteria. Some bacteria, which look alike under a microscope, are found to differ in their ability to ferment various types of sugars—so *fermentation reaction tests* (using specific sugars) are carried out to identify bacteria.

3. The ability to form *indole*, a substance produced during putrefaction of protein, is the basis of another test used to differentiate intestinal bacteria.

4. Serological tests are used to detect the presence of specific *antigens* on the bacteria.

5. Animal inoculation is used to identify organisms which cannot be grown on artificial media. The ability of an organism to produce characteristic disease in an animal, may be tested to establish or confirm the identity of the organism, e.g. guinea pigs are used for the isolation and identification of the tubercle bacillus.

Viruses

Viruses (singular-virus) are specialised microorganisms with a number of distinctive characteristics:

1. Most are ultramicroscopic, meaning that they are too small to be seen with a light microscope and can be viewed only with an electron microscope. Viruses vary in size from 10–350 nanometres (nm).

2. They will grow only within living cells, and cannot be cultured on dead or artificial media.

3. Viruses have no real cell structure: they lack a rigid cell wall; have no mitochondria or other organelles, no ribosomes, and are devoid of enzymes to generate high energy bonds. Their nucleic acid consists of either DNA or RNA, but not both.

4. Viruses may be referred to as *intracellular parasites* as they can reproduce only when they are within their host cells.

Viruses reproduce by invading living cells, and taking over the metabolic processes of those cells to reproduce themselves. The tissue cells usually degenerate and die, releasing viral particles, but in some instances cells survive and remain host to the virus, resulting in a latent infection, e.g. herpes simplex infections.

Culture of viruses

Viruses can be grown only in living tissue, and this is achieved by inoculating:

- tissue cells, which are grown under special conditions in a test tube
- a developing chick embryo in a fertile hen egg
- laboratory animals such as mice.

Serology tests are performed to detect specific antigens.

Table 9.2 lists various diseases caused by viruses.

Table 9.2   Viral Diseases

Organism	Diseases caused
DNA viruses	
Poxviruses	Variola, molluscum contagiosum
Herpesviruses	Herpes simplex, varicella, infectious mononucleosis, genital herpes, herpes zoster, encephalitis
Adenoviruses	Pharyngitis, pneumonia, conjunctivitis, upper respiratory tract infection
Papovaviruses	Warts, papillomata
RNA viruses	
Paramyxoviruses	Colds, croup, measles, mumps, acute respiratory infections, influenza
Orthomyxoviruses	Epidemic and endemic influenza, pneumonia, bronchitis.
Coronaviruses	Colds, acute respiratory infections
Arenaviruses	Meningitis, encephalitis
Reoviruses	Mild respiratory and enteric diseases
Picornaviruses	Meningitis, myocarditis, pericarditis, infectious hepatitis (hepatitis A), poliomyelitis, hepatitis B
Rhabdoviruses	Rabies
Togaviruses	Rubella, lympadenopathy, yellow fever
Retroviruses	
HTLV	Leukaemia, lymphoma
HTLV-III) Human	Acquired immunodeficiency syndrome
LAV) Immune	(AIDS)
ARV) Virus (HIV)	

Fungi

Fungi (singular-fungus) (moulds and yeasts) are present in the soil, air, and water.

Moulds reproduce by various kinds of spores, and form large filamentous colonies on artificial media.

Yeasts grow as single cells and reproduce by budding, and form creamy colonies on artificial media.

Most species of fungi are non-pathogenic, but a few cause disease.

Table 9.3 lists various diseases caused by fungi.

Table 9.3   Fungal diseases

Organism	Diseases caused
Candida species	Candidiasis—oral thrush, vaginitis, Skin infections
Dermatophytes	Tinea capitus (ringworm) Tinea pedis (athletes foot)
Aspergillus species	Aspergillosis, e.g. chronic infections of the ear canal, bronchopulmonary disease.
Histoplasma capsulatum	Histoplasmosis

Parasites

Metazoans and protozoans are collectively known as parasites.

1. Metazoans are multicellular animal organisms, which are classified initially according to external appearance:

- flatworms (platyhelminths)
- roundworms (nematodes)
- flukes (trematodes).

2. Protozoans are single-celled animal organisms, some of which are transmitted by insects (vectors) to man. All protozoa require large amounts of water, and they are abundant in soil and water, also in and on plants and animals.

Table 9.4 illustrates various diseases caused by metazoans and protozoans.

Table 9.4   Parasitic diseases

Organism	Diseases caused
Metazoans	
Enterobius vermicularis	Pinworm infestation
Trichinella spiralis	Trichinellosis
Platyhelminths (flat worms)	Tapeworm infestation
Nematodes (round worms)	Round worm infestation
Trematodes (flukes)	Infestation of liver, lungs, or intestines
Protozoans	
Toxoplasma gondii	Toxoplasmosis
Plasmodium	Malaria
Trichomonas vaginalis	Vaginitis
Entamoeba histolytica	Amoebic dysentery
Trypanosoma species	Sleeping sickness
Pneumocystis carinii	Pneumonia

INFECTION

Infection is a state which exists when pathogenic microorganisms have invaded and multiplied in the tissues, and there are manifestations of damage to the tissues.

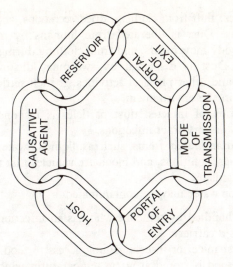

Fig. 9.2 Chain of infection.

Development of an infection (Fig. 9.2) occurs in a process (chain of infection) that depends on:

- pathogenic organisms in sufficient numbers
- reservoir for pathogen growth
- portal of exit from the reservoir
- means of transmission, or vehicle
- portal of entry to the host
- susceptible host.

If this 'chain' is uninterrupted, an infection will develop. *Infection control* is directed towards breaking the 'chain of infection'.

Reservoirs (sources) of infection

The reservoirs of pathogenic microorganisms are human, animal, or inanimate sources.

Human sources

The majority of organisms which infect humans are acquired from human sources. A variety of organisms reside on the surface of the skin and within body cavities, fluids, and discharges. Some areas of the body contain larger populations of *normal flora* than others, e.g. the skin, respiratory tract, colon, mouth, and vagina. Areas of the body which are usually considered sterile (without normal flora) include the bloodstream, urinary tract, peritoneal cavity, and spinal fluid. The entrance of a foreign object into a sterile site leads to a high risk of infection.

Normal flora can cause infection if they are transplanted. *Auto-infection* occurs when organisms from one part of the body, e.g. the colon, are transferred and cause infection in another part of the body, e.g. the urinary tract, of the same individual.

Cross-infection may occur when organisms from one person, e.g. the nurse's hands, are transferred to an abnormal environment, e.g. a patient's wound.

A person *incubating* a disease is another source of infection. During an incubation period the organisms multiply and can be transmitted to others. The host has no manifestations of disease at this stage, and is unaware of the infection.

A person with an infection usually liberates large numbers of pathogens into the environment. In some diseases this lasts only for a short time as the organisms are killed rapidly, but in other diseases pathogens continue to be released by the infected person over a long period. For example, in tuberculosis the organism may be present for years.

A carrier is someone who harbours pathogenic microorganisms in the tissues. A carrier state may exist during the incubation period of a disease, following an attack of the disease, or without the person ever experiencing the disease which the organism causes.

Animal sources

Animals, plants, and insects can also be reservoirs for infectious organisms. Diseases which can be acquired from animal sources include:

- tuberculosis, from cattle
- anthrax, from sheep, cattle, pigs
- ringworm, from dogs, cats, cattle
- toxoplasmosis, from cats
- brucellosis, from cattle, goats
- rabies, from dogs
- psittacosis, from birds
- plague, from rats
- intestinal infections, from mice, poultry, pigs
- cholera, from contaminated shellfish
- malaria, from the anopheles mosquito.

Inanimate sources

Soil, seawater, food, water, and milk are additional reservoirs for pathogens. Many organisms live in the soil and obtain their nourishment from decaying vegetable and animal matter. A few anaerobic, spore-forming bacteria cause disease if they gain entry to human tissue or produce a lethal toxin in canned food. Diseases caused by anaerobic spore-forming bacteria include:

- tetanus
- gas gangrene
- botulism.

Legionnaires' disease is caused by the bacterium *Legionella pneumophilia*, which lives in contaminated pooled water.

Portals of exit (from the reservoir)

If microorganisms are to enter another host and cause disease, they must find a portal of exit. When the human is the reservoir, microorganisms can exit through a variety of sites:

1. in mucus from the upper respiratory tract, and in saliva from the mouth.
2. in faeces excreted from the bowel.
3. in vomitus.
4. in discharges from infected wounds, or discharges from infected organs, e.g. eye, ear, nose, vagina, penis.
5. in infected blood.
6. in urine, when there is an infection of the genito-urinary tract.

Modes of transmission

There are a variety of vehicles for the transmission of microorganisms from the reservoir to a host:

1. Direct contact is direct physical transfer between an infected or colonized person and a host. Examples of diseases spread by direct contact are syphilis, gonorrhoea, skin infections, glandular fever, Hansen's disease, and AIDS.

2. Indirect contact is personal contact of the host with a contaminated inanimate object. Contaminated inanimate objects are sometimes referred to as *fomites*. Organisms can be transferred to items such as clothing and bedclothing, books, papers, crockery, cutlery, toys, toilet utensils, furniture and fittings, dressing materials, needles, tubing, instruments, stethoscopes.

Examples of diseases spread by indirect contact are measles, hepatitis B, and AIDS.

3. Droplet contact occurs when pathogens, carried in droplets of moisture exhaled from the nose and mouth, come into contact with the conjunctivae, nose, or mouth of a host. Large droplets of moisture may fall rapidly after being expelled, but smaller droplets remain suspended in the air for several hours before falling.

During normal breathing the number of microorganisms expelled is small, but when there is forcible exhalation vast numbers of organisms are expelled. During the acts of coughing, sneezing, shouting, or blowing the nose, the number of microorganisms liberated may be as high as from 500 000 to 1 000 000.

Droplets of moisture which contain organisms do not have to be inhaled in order to spread infection. They contaminate all surfaces on which they fall, therefore infection may be transmitted by indirect contact.

Examples of diseases spread by droplet contact are influenza, tuberculosis, pneumonia, and meningitis.

4. Dust consists of environmental dust particles, dead skin flakes, fluff from clothing, dried secretions, and microorganisms. Dust is liberated from humans by means of normal body movements, and from clothing during normal activity. Dust is dispersed by sweeping, dusting, bed-making, and other physical activities. It then settles on all surfaces in the environment.

Inhalation of infected dust particles is responsible for many respiratory tract infections.

5. Contaminated items such as liquids, water, milk, food, drugs, solutions, and blood are vehicles that transmit microorganisms.

Food or water may be contaminated:

- when handled by someone who has an infection or who is a carrier.
- by rats, mice, or insects gaining access to food.
- when food is stored at warm temperatures which encourage the growth of bacteria.
- by cooking methods which use temperatures low enough to promote bacterial growth, and not high enough to destroy bacteria.
- if there are unhygienic conditions where food is prepared or processed, e.g. dirty utensils, dirty kitchens, inadequate handwashing facilities, inadequate refrigeration, infestations of rats, mice, flies, ants, or cockroaches.

Examples of diseases spread by contaminated items are food poisoning, hepatitis A, hepatitis B, gastroenteritis, AIDS, cholera.

6. Flies are capable of transmitting many microorganisms. Flies feed on rotting animal and vegetable matter or excreta. They are equipped with hairy legs covered with a sticky substance, so that material adheres to the hairs. In this way, particles of contaminated material are carried by flies and deposited wherever a fly alights. Examples of diseases spread by flies are gastroenteritis and hepatitis A.

7. Vectors such as mosquitoes, lice, fleas, ticks and mites transmit infection by biting. The vector becomes infected when it bites a host whose blood contains microorganisms. Mosquitoes can transmit malaria; lice, ticks and mites can transmit typhus.

Hands are frequently the vehicles by which infection is transmitted, particularly in a health care setting.

Portals of entry

Microorganisms can enter the body through the same routes they use for exiting:

- inhalation into the respiratory tract.
- ingestion through the mouth into the alimentary canal.
- inoculation through the skin or mucous membrane, which can occur when those tissues become cracked

or when they are broken during injury, surgical procedures, invasive activities such as injections, bites, or stings.

Transplacental entry can also occur when organisms from a pregnant woman cross the *placenta* to enter the fetal circulation.

Susceptible host

Susceptibility is the degree of resistance an individual has to pathogens. Whether an individual acquires an infection depends on his susceptibility to an infectious agent. The more virulent an organism, the greater the likelihood of a person's susceptibility.

Resistance to infection may be decreased by many factors such as:

- poor nutritional status
- age (both the very young and the elderly are more susceptible)
- stress
- the nature of a disease process
- hereditary conditions
- type of medical therapy received
- psychosocial and lifestyle factors.

An individual's defence mechanisms may be altered by conditions such as:

- extensive trauma, burns
- diabetes mellitus
- leukaemia
- immunosuppressive therapy
- broad-spectrum antibiotics
- chronic heavy alcohol use
- heavy tobacco smoking
- glucocorticosteroids.

Nosocomial infections

Nosocomial infections are those which are acquired by an individual in a hospital or other health care setting. Such infections are sometimes referred to as 'hospital-acquired infections'.

Factors which increase a patient's susceptibility, and lead to nosocomial infections, include:

- the use of invasive techniques such as catheterization, insertion of intravenous lines or endotracheal tubes
- the presence of a condition that alters the body's ability to combat microorganisms
- an impaired immune system
- poor techniques and practices by personnel caring for the individual, e.g. inadequate handwashing.

Nosocomial infections may be exogenous or endogenous.

An *exogenous* infection arises from microorganisms external to the individual, and *endogenous* infections may occur when part of the individual's own normal flora becomes altered and an overgrowth occurs. Endogenous infections can also occur when normal flora from one body site are transferred to another body site, e.g. transmission of enterococci in faecal material transferred via the hands to the skin may cause a wound infection.

Major sites for nosocomial infections include the respiratory tract, bloodstream, urinary tract, and surgical or traumatic wounds.

Body defences against infection

The human body is surrounded by non-pathogenic and pathogenic microorganisms, but it possesses defence mechanisms against infection. Some defence mechanisms prevent the entry of microorganisms, and others destroy microorganisms that gain entry to the tissues.

There are three principal lines of defence: outer defences, which are mainly mechanical barriers; inflammatory responses; and immunity.

First-line defences

1. The skin forms an intact, waterproof barrier against microorganisms and its sweat and sebum are bactericidal for some organisms.

2. Mucous membranes trap organisms until they can be removed, e.g. through washing out of the body by tears or saliva, or by coughing or sneezing.

Ciliated mucous membrane, which lines the upper respiratory tract, contains cilia which sweep particles away from the lungs and into the oropharynx to be expectorated or swallowed.

3. Body secretions such as saliva, tears, gastric juice, and bile are anti-bacterial. Some secretions are anti-bacterial because they cause abrupt changes in the pH of an area, and others because they contain an anti-bacterial such as *lysozyme*.

4. Lymphoid tissue, which is found in many areas of the body, filters microorganisms from the circulation and destroys them.

5. Normal flora, which are microorganisms that normally live in and on the human body, protect the body by suppressing invasions by pathogenic microorganisms.

Second-line of defence

Although often associated with infection, inflammation is the body's response to any form of injury. Once microorganisms have gained entry to the tissues, they will start to proliferate and release substances which act as stimulators of the inflammatory process. The damaged tissue cells also release substances, known generally as vasoactive amines, which cause an increased blood flow through the tissue by inducing dilation of the blood vessels. This results in redness and increased temperature in inflamed tissues. These substances also increase the permeability of the blood vessels, resulting in fluid seeping from the blood into the tissues.

The result of this inflammatory response to the invasion of tissues by microorganisms, is that large numbers of polymorphonuclear leucocytes and antibacterial substances are concentrated at the site of infection.

Polymorphonuclear leucocytes are macrophages which means that they are able to engulf and ingest microorganisms by a process called phagocytosis (see Fig. 15.5). Phagocytosis of microorganisms usually results in their death, however the process also results in the death of tissue cells—due possibly to the leakage of hydrolytic enzymes into the cell cytoplasm. The large numbers of cells which die results in the formation of pus.

If microorganisms survive these defence mechanisms, proliferation of microorganisms may lead to local abscess formation and, perhaps, spread of infection via the lymphatics to other parts of the body.

Third line of defence

The immune response is initiated during the inflammatory response, and involves a group of cells called lymphocytes. Lymphocytes are found in the blood but are particularly abundant in lymphoid tissue, e.g. spleen, lymph nodes, tonsils, bone marrow, and thymus gland.

When macrophages (leucocytes) engulf and ingest some of the micro-organisms, they transfer antigens to their own surface.

An *antigen* is a foreign substance, usually a protein, which is not normally present in the body. Antigens stimulate the formation of protective substances which are referred to as *immunoglobulins* (antibodies).

Circulating in the bloodstream are T-lymphocytes which are programmed to recognize the antigen on the surfaces of the leucocytes. Once recognized, the T-lymphocytes bind to the leucocytes and become activated as 'helper T-lymphocytes'. The helper T-cells multiply and travel to the lymph nodes and/or spleen, where they stimulate the production of further cells and chemicals against the invading microorganisms.

'Killer T-cells' are produced which recognize and destroy the invading microorganisms.

B-lymphocytes are produced which bind their immunoglobulins (antibodies) to the antigens.

Immunoglobulins are *specific*, and react only with the antigen responsible for their formation.

Immunoglobulins act in a variety of ways:

- Some cause agglutination of microorganisms
- Some cause the breakdown of cells
- Some render microorganisms more susceptible to phagocytosis
- Some, referred to as *antitoxins*, neutralize toxins produced by microorganisms.

As infected body cells are destroyed, macrophages (leucocytes) phagocytoze and remove debris from the site of infection.

The result of the immune response is that two forms of immunity develop: antibody-mediated (humoral) immunity, and cell-mediated (cellular) immunity.

Some of both the T and B lymphocytes become 'memory cells' that remain in the body and retain a memory of the original foreign substance (antigen) to which they were formed. Such memory cells can then respond on subsequent contact with the specific antigen—and start the immune response again. It is largely B-cells which become re-activated against bacterial invasion (humoral immunity), and T-cells which respond to viral invasion (cellular immunity).

Immunoglobulins (antibodies) are classified into 5 identifiable groups: IgM, IgG, IgA, IgE and IgD. Table 9.5 describes the properties of the various immunoglobulin groups.

Table 9.5 Immunoglobulins

Group	Functions
1gM	Early antibody in the primary immune response. Triggers the increased production of 1gG, and the complement fixation required for effective antibody response.
1gG	Main immunoglobulin of secondary immune response. Neutralizes toxins. Crosses the placenta and provides passive immunity during the first few weeks of life.
1gA	Plays a role in protecting mucous membranes from pathogenic micro-organisms. Principal immunoglobulin of saliva, tears, respiratory and intestinal fluids.
1gE	Provides the primary defence against environmental antigens. Plays a role as mediator of allergic reactions.
1gD	Increases in quantity during allergic reactions to various toxins and other substances.

IMMUNITY

Immunity is the ability of the body to resist an infectious disease, and results from the presence of *specific* immunoglobulins (antibodies). Therefore, immunity to one disease does not influence an individual's resistance to another disease.

Immunization is a process by which resistance to an infectious disease is induced or augmented.

Immunity may be innate (inborn) or it may be acquired.

Innate immunity

Effective defences against potentially harmful micro-organisms are present from birth, and do not depend upon having previous experience with any particular micro-organism. This is known as the innate immune mechanism, which is effective against a range of potentially infective agents and is, therefore, non-specific. Factors influencing innate immunity include:

- heredity
- age
- nutritional status
- hormonal influences
- intact skin and mucous membrane
- phagocytosis.

Acquired immunity

Acquired immunity (Fig. 9.3), which is not present at birth but is developed during life, may be passively or actively acquired.

Passive immunity

Passive immunity is the transfer of the products of an immune response to an individual without any involvement by that individual's tissues. Immunoglobulins (antibodies) may be passively conferred in one of three ways:

1. Before birth, immunoglobulins in the mother's bloodstream are transferred across the placenta to the fetal bloodstream.
2. After birth, a breast fed baby receives small amounts of immunoglobulins in the breast milk.
3. A serum (antiserum) prepared from pooled blood plasma containing antibodies may be injected, for example:

- Tetanus immunoglobulin may be injected to treat tetanus, and may be used in the management of a tetanus-prone wound.
- Antitoxins may be injected to treat diphtheria and gas-gangrene.

- Antivenoms may be injected to treat bites or stings sustained from venomous creatures such as snakes, box jellyfish, red back spider, or stone fish.

Human immunoglobulins may be injected to confer passive immunity in a variety of situations, e.g. for prophylaxis in persons accidently exposed to hepatitis B, rabies, hepatitis A, rubella, and other infectious diseases. Injection of human immunoglobulin may also be indicated in poliomyelitis, herpes zoster, and overwhelming bacterial infections. Rh (D) immunoglobulin may be given to an Rh negative (Rh−) mother within 72 hours of delivery of an Rh positive (Rh+) infant to prevent subsequent formation of anti-D immunoglobulins.

Passive immunity is of a *temporary* nature only, providing protection for approximately 2–3 weeks. The immunoglobulins passed from mother to baby remain in circulation for longer—up to a few months.

Active immunity

Active immunity is acquired as a result of the stimulation of an individual's immune system—therefore there is active involvement of the body in the production of its own immunoglobulins.

Active immunity is of a more *permanent* nature, providing protection for years or, in some instances, for life.

Active immunity may be acquired by:

1. An attack of an infectious disease. The degree of immunity varies, and in some instances it is high (e.g. measles, mumps) and a second attack of that disease is rare. In other instances, the degree of immunity is low and repeated attacks of the disease, e.g. the common cold, can be expected.
2. Repeated sub-clinical attacks of a disease. When a specific disease is common in a community, pathogenic microorganisms may invade the tissues of individuals repeatedly, but there may be no recognizable manifestations of disease—or they may be only signs and symptoms of a mild attack. The body produces immunoglobulins each time it is invaded, so the individual acquires an immunity against a full clinical attack of the disease.

Vaccination

Vaccines are antigenic materials which induce a specific active artificial immunity to infection by a specific microorganism. Vaccines are suspensions of either live, dead, or attenuated (weakened) organisms, which are introduced into the body to stimulate the production of specific immunoglobulins. Specific vaccines provide protection against some infectious diseases for months or years. Examples of vaccines:

- Bacillus Calmette-Guerin (BCG) is given to individuals

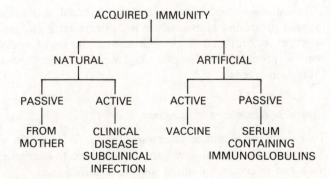

Fig. 9.3 Immunity.

Table 9.6 Recommended primary immunization schedule

Age	Disease	Vaccine	Route
2 months	Diphtheria-tetanus-pertussis	Triple antigen 'DTP'	Intramuscular
	Poliomyelitis	Sabin vaccine 'OPV'	Oral
4 months	Diphtheria-tetanus-pertussis	Triple antigen 'DTP'	Intramuscular
	Poliomyelitis	Sabin vaccine 'OPV'	Oral
6 months	Diphtheria-tetanus-pertussis	Triple antigen 'DTP'	Intramuscular
	Poliomyelitis	Sabin vaccine 'OPV'	Oral
Between 12–15 months	Measles/mumps/rubella	Measles/mumps/rubella 'MMR'	Subcutaneous
18 months	Diphtheria-tetanus-pertussis	Triple antigen 'DTP'	Intramuscular
5 years or prior to school entry	Diphtheria-tetanus	Childhood diphtheria and tetanus 'CDT'	Intramuscular
	Poliomyelitis	Sabin vaccine 'OPV'	Oral
15 years or prior to leaving school	Diphtheria-tetanus	Adult diphtheria and tetanus 'ADT'	Intramuscular

* Childhood immunization schedule recommended by the National Health and Medical Research Council

who are not immune to tuberculosis. A *Mantoux test* is performed first by injecting tuberculin into the skin on the forearm. Immunity to tuberculosis is demonstrated by a positive reaction at 72 hours, indicated by an area of oedema 5 mm or more in diameter. (A positive reaction may be due to a current infection, a previous infection, or previous vaccination with BCG vaccine). If the reaction to the Mantoux test is *negative*, BCG vaccine may be given by intradermal injection (inoculation).

• Sabin vaccine, which is ingested orally, provides protection against poliomyelitis.

• Other vaccines are given to provide immunity against cholera, diphtheria, pertussis, tetanus, typhoid fever, typhus, influenza, rabies, and hepatitis B.

Table 9.6 illustrates the recommended primary immunization schedule.

PREVENTION AND CONTROL OF INFECTION

The prevention and control of infection is a major aspect of the work of all members of the health team, whether working in the community or in hospitals. The basic principles employed in the prevention of spread of infection are the same in all situations, and are directed towards breaking the 'chain of infection' (see Fig. 9.2):

• control or elimination of reservoirs
• control of portals of exit
• control of transmission
• control portals of entry
• protection of a susceptible host.

The methods used to control infection at the *community* level, are described in Chapter 8, and listed here:

• provision of a pure water supply
• control of all aspects of food handling
• immunization against infectious diseases
• early diagnosis of infections
• provision of adequate drainage and sewerage
• collection and disposal of waste
• pest control facilities
• notification of infectious diseases
• isolation of individuals with specific infectious diseases
• quarantine and health requirements for travellers
• control of standards related to premises and staffing in the provision of goods and services to the public
• education of the public in the promotion and maintenance of good health.

Control of infection in health care settings

Wherever there are large numbers of people congregated together, there is an increased risk of infection being transmitted from one person to another. In a health care setting, e.g. a hospital, the risks are further increased and there is a need for constant enforcement of stringent measures to prevent the spread of infection.

As infection control measures are directed primarily towards protecting individuals in health care settings from infection, information on prevention and control of infection is provided in Chapter 38 (Meeting Safety And Protection Needs).

Control or elimination of reservoirs

To control or eliminate reservoir sites for infection in a health care setting, measures are implemented to eliminate *sources* of infection. Common sources of infection are:

- body excreta, e.g. faeces, vomitus, sputum, urine
- blood and other body fluids
- exudates from infected wounds or skin lesions
- secretions from the respiratory tract.

Other sources of infection are contaminated food, water, or milk; and items of equipment used in the care of an infected person.

Although patients form the largest reservoir of infection in a health care setting, hospital personnel and visitors can also be sources of infection.

To control or eliminate reservoirs, measures are implemented whereby all items contaminated with infective, or potentially infective, substances are handled and disposed of correctly: dressings, suction or drainage tubing and containers, intravenous therapy apparatus, needles and syringes; bedpans, urinals and other toilet utensils.

Control of portals of exit

Measures to control the exit of microorganisms include careful handling of all excreta and exudate, and soiled linen. Disposable gloves are worn when there is a likelihood of contact with a patient's blood or body fluids.

People are instructed to cover their nose or mouth when sneezing or coughing, and disposable tissues should be used to control the spread of micro-organisms. If a nurse has a respiratory tract infection, e.g. the common cold, she may be required to wear a mask—especially when performing a sterile technique.

Control of transmission

Correct handwashing is the most basic and important technique in preventing and controlling the transmission of pathogens. Information on handwashing technique is provided in Chapter 38.

Other measures to control transmission include using disposable equipment whenever possible; and cleaning, disinfecting, and sterilizing reuseable items. Information on these aspects of infection control is provided in Chapter 38.

Isolation precautions may be implemented to control the transmission of pathogens, and information on these precautions is provided in Chapter 61.

Control of portals of entry

Measures that control the entrance of microorganisms to the body include:

- maintaining skin and mucous membrane integrity
- cleansing the genital area in a direction away from the urinary meatus to the rectum

- implementing aseptic techniques, using sterile equipment, when invasive procedures are performed
- cleansing wounds outwards from the wound site, to prevent the entrance of microorganisms.

Protection of a susceptible host

Measures to improve an individual's resistance to infection include:

- promoting adequate nutritional intake
- promoting adequate rest
- maintaining skin and mucous membrane integrity
- immunization against infectious diseases.

Infection control personnel

Many health care facilities employ one or more persons who are responsible for the area of infection control. Infection control personnel are responsible for advising staff on safe aseptic practices, and for monitoring outbreaks of infection within the facility. They are also responsible for:

- educating staff and patents on infection control
- reviewing infection control policies and techniques
- researching laboratory reports and records for incidence of infections
- conferring with support services such as the 'housekeeping' department within the facility.

CONCLUSION

As control of infection is an essential component of every nursing activity the nurse requires a knowledge of microorganisms, the infectious process, and the application of infection control principles.

It is important for the nurse to understand the differences between pathogenic and non-pathogenic microorganisms, the distribution of microorganisms, and their classification.

As infection control is directed towards breaking the 'chain of infection' the nurse should know the components which make up the chain: pathogenic microorganisms in sufficient numbers, a reservoir for pathogen growth, a portal of exit from the reservoir, a means of transmission (vehicle), a portal of entry to the host, and a susceptible host.

It is important for the nurse to understand the factors which may contribute to nosocomial (hospital-acquired) infections, and she must understand the measures which should be implemented to reduce the incidence of nosocomial infection.

A knowledge of the mechanical barriers, inflammatory

responses, and immunity is important in understanding how the body defends itself against infection.

The importance of practising correct handwashing techniques to prevent the transmission of pathogens cannot be over-emphasized.

REFERENCES AND FURTHER READING

Burton G 1983 Microbiology for the health sciences, 2nd edn. Lippincott, Philadelphia

Duguid J P, Marmion B P, Swain R H A (eds) 1978 Mackie and McCartney medical microbiology, 13th edn. Churchill Livingstone, Edinburgh

Smith A L 1985 Principles of microbiology, 10th edn. Times Mirror/Mosby, St Louis

10. Legal aspects of nursing

OBJECTIVES

1. Discuss the distinctions between criminal law and civil law.
2. Discuss the legal responsibilities and obligations of nurses.
3. Discuss various legal issues that arise in nursing practice.

INTRODUCTION

In a democratic society the legal system provides a framework inside which all sections of the community interact. It establishes the rights and privileges of the individual, and makes provision for enforcement of rights and redress for wrongs suffered. All citizens should be aware of their legally defined rights and responsibilities, and should have an understanding of the laws which govern their personal and professional lives. Ignorance of a law is not accepted as an excuse for violation of that law.

Nurses have legal responsibilities common to all members of the community, and also the responsibilities imposed by the nature of their work which may be defined as responsibilities in respect of:

- the provision of safe, effective nursing care
- the health of the community
- the employing authority
- the nursing profession.

The aim of this chapter is to introduce the nurse to some legal concepts that are relevant to the practice of nursing. For further information on legal principles, the nurse is advised to refer to the texts listed at the end of this chapter.

Types of law

It is important to be aware of the distinctions between criminal and civil law.

1. Criminal laws are concerned with offences against people and their property. The government has the power to make rules as to what constitutes minimum levels of acceptable behaviour and then seeks to control behaviour, through the power of the police force, by ensuring that those rules are obeyed. A violation of a criminal law is called a *crime*, and it is sanctioned by some form of punishment, e.g. payment of a fine or imprisonment. Murder, robbery, rape, and kidnapping are examples of crimes which are regarded as offences against society as a whole.

2. Civil laws are concerned with the relationships between people. Such laws provide the means by which rights can be enforced and wrongs can be remedied. For example, an individual who is found to have broken the civil law will usually be required to pay a sum of money to the person alleging personal or property loss or damage. Areas of civil law include trespass, contracts, and negligence.

The employer

An employer, e.g. the Board of Management of a hospital, is legally responsible for the acts committed by all employees in the course of their duty. This principle of *vicarious liability* is relevant to all nurses, as it renders an employer liable for the actions of an employee committed in the course of employment. While the employer is held liable, he does have the right to seek a total financial indemnity from the offending employee, e.g. in the case of negligence. An employer must ensure that:

- Employees possess the required qualifications, registration, and level of competence.
- All legal requirements are met, including valid contracts of employment.
- Safety standards are observed in relation to standards of patient care, buildings and equipment.

The legal liability of the employer does not absolve a nurse from individual responsibility, and legal action can be taken against a hospital and a nurse or against a nurse as an individual.

The nurse's responsibilities

The nurse has a responsibility to be aware of certain legal principles, specifically in relation to:

- contracts
- standards of care, and negligence
- defamation
- false imprisonment
- assault and battery
- informed consent
- confidentiality
- documentation, e.g. of incident reports
- acts, e.g. Nurses Registration Acts
- witnessing wills
- coroner's court.

It is important for a nurse to realize that she is legally responsible for her own actions and that, although the enrolled nurse works under the supervision of a registered nurse, this does not relieve her of personal liability. A nurse has a responsibility, to herself and the patients, to refuse to perform an activity if:

- She is asked to do something that is beyond the legal and professional scope of her role
- She has not been prepared to perform a function safely
- Directions are unclear, unethical, illegal, or against the policies of the health care agency.

Nurses Registration Acts

Because the control and regulation of the nursing profession is determined on a state basis, each Australian state has its own Act and regulations. There is a Nurses Registration Board (in Victoria, called a Council) in each of the states, which is composed of members who are empowered to both register and de-register nurses. Nurses Registration Boards also have the power and authority to determine the character and conduct of examinations under the state Act, to appoint examiners in respect of the examinations, and, in most states, to approve of schools of nursing for nurse education purposes. Each state Act is divided into sections, each one of which deals with a specific aspect concerning registration. As each state has its own Act it is essential that nurses read a copy of the relevant state legislation so that they are aware of individual state requirements.

By defining the terms under which a nurse may practise in each of the categories of registration, the law protects the community by deeming the nurse who has qualified to be safe and competent to practise nursing. Nurses who do not fulfil the requirements of a Nurses Registration Act may not practise as nurses. A practising certificate must be obtained from the state Registration Board, or Council, annually by a person who is registered or enrolled and intends to practise in any branch of nursing. The responsibility for ensuring that registration or enrollment fees are paid each year rests with the individual nurse.

Each state registration body is empowered to de-register nurses in certain circumstances, e.g. a nurse's registration or enrolment may be cancelled if she unlawfully uses a registration number, or if she is found to be guilty of misconduct or negligence in a professional respect.

Contracts

A contract is an agreement between parties that is legally enforceable because of mutuality of agreement and obligation. A contract gives rise to rights and obligations which will be protected and enforced by the law.

A contract may be in writing, or it may arise by implication, e.g. the agreement that is reached between a patient and a health care agency to which he is admitted. While the patient is not required to sign a document, he will have entered into a contract as to the nature and extent of his proposed treatment. If the individual is a private patient he enters into a contract with his medical officer.

The nurse, as an employee, enters into a contract with the employer. Arising out of this contractual relationship are certain rights and obligations relevant to both the employee and employer, as defined in a written contract of employment. The creation of *industrial awards* has imposed specific provisions on employers relating to the health and safety of employees, the payment of wages and the provision of certain conditions. An industrial award is a document which sets out the wages and conditions of a particular group of employees, and it represents the contract of employment between the employer and employee. A copy of each award can be obtained from the Department of Industrial Relations, and employers are also required to have copies of the relevant awards available so that they are accessible to employees. Nurses have a responsibility to themselves to understand their contract of employment and their industrial award.

Standards of care

Standards of care are the guidelines by which a nurse should practice, and are determined by Nurses Registration Boards, professional organizations such as the Australian Nursing Federation, and the employing health care agency.

Each source defines standards of nursing care, e.g. a Nurses Registration Board (or Council) defines the scope of nursing practice; professional organizations develop standards for nursing service in policy statements, and the employing health care agency develops written policies and protocols which detail how a nurse is to perform her duties.

Nurses have a responsibility to know the standards of care they are expected to meet, and to understand the importance of not undertaking tasks which are outside their defined role and function.

Negligence

Negligence, in a legal sense, describes conduct which falls below the standard required by law. If a nurse gives care that does not meet accepted standards she may be held liable for negligence, e.g. if her actions result in harm to a patient.

Generally, negligence means failure by a nurse to take appropriate actions to protect the safety of a patient, and it may involve failing to do something which should be done or doing something that should not be done. Situations which have occurred involving negligent acts include incorrect administration of medications, e.g. the wrong medication being administered, failure to communicate important information about a patient's condition, and failing to take appropriate measures so that a patient has consequently sustained an injury, e.g. from falling out of bed.

There are three elements a plaintiff must prove to succeed in an action for negligence, namely:

1. That the defendant owed the plaintiff a duty of care.
2. That this duty of care was breached, by failure to conform to the appropriate standard of care.
3. That the plaintiff suffered injury as a result of the breach of duty. In this regard there must be a reasonably close causal connection between the defendant's conduct and the injury or damage to the plaintiff.

The likelihood of injury to a patient, and the risk of liability, is reduced when the nurse adheres to the principles of sound nursing practice and follows the established policies relating to standards of care.

Defamation

The term 'defamation of character' refers to any communication, spoken or written, about an individual that injures his reputation. The term 'libel' is used when the communication is written, whereas the term 'slander' is used when the communication is spoken. With regard to nursing practice, all patients have a right to expect their privacy and confidentiality to be respected, and colleagues have a right to expect that their personal and professional reputations will not be harmed.

Nurses should, therefore, exercise extreme caution when discussing or documenting information relating to patients, and when discussing members of staff, e.g. a nurse may not be openly critical of the standard of care provided by another nurse. While recognizing that, at times, such criticism may be valid, a nurse who is genuinely concerned about standards of nursing care should direct her concern through the proper channels, e.g. to the department of nursing administration. Nurses should refrain from gossiping about colleagues, as this practice may lead to irreparable damage of an individual's personal or professional reputation. Nurses should avoid making statements in writing in a patient's documents that may be interpreted as being of a defamatory nature. Nurses must ensure that all statements relating to a patient are written in an objective, rather than a subjective, manner.

False imprisonment

False imprisonment refers to the wrongful deprivation of an individual's freedom of movement, e.g. restraining or detaining a person against his will. With regard to nursing practice, there are specific instances where a patient may be restrained or detained under statutory or common law, e.g. there are specific provisions for the *detention* of people with particular infective conditions in the interests of public health or safety. There are also certain situations where a patient may need to be *restrained*, e.g. to protect him from injury. Nurses must be aware that the application of any restraint is only performed in consultation with the patient's medical officer, and then only after very careful consideration. Written authorization by a medical officer is generally required for the application of a restraint. Apart from very specific instances there are no powers to detain a person in a health care agency against his wishes. All health care agencies have a document which a patient is asked to sign if he decides to leave the agency against medical advice.

Assault and battery

Assault and battery are considered criminal offences as well as breaches of civil law. Although, the term 'assault' is used to describe both actions, there is a distinction between the two. *Assault* can be described as a 'threat' to carry out a physical action on another person, thereby causing that person to be in fear of his safety. *Battery* involves the direct, intentional, and uninvited application of physical contact to another individual's body.

With regard to nursing practice a nurse could, intentionally or unintentionally, commit an act of assault if she does anything which provokes fear in a patient resulting in the patient's belief that he will be harmed. As many nursing activities involve direct physical contact with a patient, there is a possibility of committing the offence of battery. The important factor in these situations, i.e. where physical contact is involved, is to make sure you have the patient's *consent*. Consent may be implied, verbal, or in writing. Implied consent is frequently given in the performance of nursing activities, e.g. if a nurse requested a patient to hold out his arm so that she could measure his blood pressure, and he did so, then he has implied his consent to that procedure. Patients frequently give consent verbally, e.g. by agreeing to have a procedure performed. Written consent provides documentary evidence that consent was given, e.g. before any invasive procedure or surgical intervention is performed a patient is requested to sign a consent form.

Informed consent

Any consent must be valid, and for consent to be valid it must be voluntarily and freely given. Also, consent is only valid when the person giving it has the legal capacity to do so, when it is specific, and when the consent given is informed. *Legal capacity* to given consent is determined by age, and the individual's mental and intellectual function, i.e. legally, consent can only be given by a competent adult. Consent must be *specific*, i.e. it must cover the precise nature of the procedure to be performed. *Informed* consent means that a patient should be given adequate information about, and understand, the procedure to which he is consenting. The patient giving consent should understand the risks and benefits involved, as well as understanding the actual procedure. It is the responsibility of the medical officer to provide the patient with an adequate explanation of any medical or surgical treatment which is proposed, and it is the responsibility of the nurse to provide adequate information to the patient about any nursing procedure to be performed.

It is important to note that a patient has the right to withhold or withdraw consent at any time. If either situation arises the event must be reported immediately to the nurse in charge, and documented.

In some instances it is difficult to obtain consent, e.g. if the patient is unconscious. If such a situation arises, and the patient requires immediate intervention, no consent is required. Piesse (1989) states that, 'In this situation the professionals involved act as agents of necessity for the patient, as they undertake procedures often in life-threatening situations and to avoid greater harm occurring to the patient'. Piesse (1989) also states that:

In some circumstances legislation dispenses with the need for consent and provides legal justification for conduct which would otherwise be actionable trespass. For example, legislation authorizing the taking of blood samples from persons admitted to hospital as a result of road accidents, vaccinations and isolation in specialist units for contagious or infectious diseases, and blood transfusions for children regardless of parental consent. In these instances overriding public interest outweighs the individual's rights and the interests of children, in relation to transfusion, are safeguarded.

Confidentiality

Nurses have an ethical obligation not to disclose confidential information which is acquired about patients in their care, except when such disclosure occurs during the course of their professional duties. Information which may be classified as confidential may be anything related to a patient's condition, treatment being given, the prognosis, or anything relevant to a patient's private life. Disclosure of such information may lead to legal action against the health care agency.

Information communicated in a patient's nursing and medical records must be kept confidential and, therefore, nurses are responsible for protecting records from unauthorized readers. A patient's right to privacy must be respected, and his affairs must not be discussed with other patients, with non-professional staff, or with members of the general public. Discretion should be used by nurses during their off-duty hours, and they should avoid careless chatter about the health care agency, any of the patients or staff members. If approached at any time by a representative of an organization, press, radio or television, a nurse should refrain from giving information but should refer the enquiry to the administrative section or other appropriate department of the health care agency.

Documentation

In the course of her work a nurse is required to document information about patients on nursing care plans, progress notes, flow charts etc. Information about recording is provided in Chapter 14, and it should be referred to a conjunction with this chapter. A patient's records may be required in legal proceedings, e.g. as evidence in a case where negligence has been alleged. Therefore, in addition to ensuring that any information is recorded accurately and concisely for the purpose of communication between members of the health team, accurate detailing of all relevant information is necessary to provide adequate explanation to a court of law. If a patient's records are required in legal proceedings they will be subject to very close scrutiny by lawyers.

Piesse (1989) states that, 'Documentation provides the evidence that the patient has received the appropriate quality of care; it also provides the means of defence in any potentially litigious situation. In this regard the interests of the patient and the nurse go hand in hand'. A nurse must remember that written records are representative of the level of care provided for a patient, and are legal documentations of that care. Piesse (1989) also states that:

The quality of documentation influences not only recall, but also the ability with which the lawyer can defend a hospital and its staff against an action. Gaps in the records, uncertainties, subjective comments, and equivocal statements can all be utilized to cast the competence and credibility of the staff in unfavourable light. Liability can often arise purely because a hospital cannot show in its documentation that it has not been negligent.

The nurse must ensure, therefore, that all written information pertaining to patient care is:

- accurate, brief, and complete
- legibly written
- objectively written
- made at the time a relevant incident occurs, e.g. immediately following nursing intervention and not several hours later
- made on the correct patient's records, therefore the patient's name and registration number on each sheet must be checked before any entry is made
- prefaced by the date and time and followed by the nurse's signature
- not made on behalf of another nurse who was responsible for implementing care or making an assessment.

Incident reports

Nurses have an ethical and legal responsibility to report any accidents or incidents which occur within a health care agency. A written report must be made immediately after an accident or incident occurs in which a patient, a visitor, or a member of the staff was involved even when no injuries appear to have been sustained or the incident seems trivial. Most health care agencies have special forms for this purpose. Incident reports provide a source of information to improve the quality of care and to evaluate the effectiveness of policies.

There is always a possibility that the 'victim' may take legal action, in which case the written report becomes a very important document. The information included in the report must be factual, clear, concise, and objective. Personal opinions must not be included, and care must be taken to avoid using terms which could be misinterpreted.

Acts

There are, in each Australian state, various Acts, which are laws created by a parliament. Acts are commonly referred to as legislation, and Acts are often accompanied by Regulations which give directions to be followed in order to comply with the intent of the Act.

As the Acts vary from state to state, nurses are advised to become familiar with the specific Acts which are relevant to the practise of nursing, e.g.:

- Drugs, Poisons and Controlled Substances Act
- Mental Health Act
- Child Protection Act
- Human Tissue Act, or Human Tissue and Transplant Act
- Nurses Registration Act
- Coroner's Act
- Worker's Compensation Act
- Freedom of Information Act.

Witnessing wills

A patient wishing to make a will should be given all the assistance required, but it is policy in most health care agencies that nurses may not act as witnesses.

Coroner's court

A coroner's court is presided over by a magistrate called a coroner, whose main function is to detect unlawful homicide. A coroner is required to investigate any death that was unexpected, or if the person died in unusual or violent circumstances. An inquest into a death may be conducted as long as several years after the event occurred and, in the case of an inquest arising out of a patient's death in a health care agency, a nurse may be called upon to give evidence. If this situation arises, nurses are advised to seek legal advice prior to giving a statement to the police or appearing in court. The health care agency, in which the nurse is employed, will generally ensure that she is represented by the agency's legal representatives. Alternatively, a nurse can be represented by the professional nursing organization of which she is a member.

CONCLUSION

This chapter introduced the nurse to some legal concepts that are relevant to the practise of nursing. Nurses, as members of the community and because of the nature of their work, have legal responsibilities which may be defined in respect of the provision of safe and effective nursing care, the health of the community, the employing authority, and the nursing profession.

The legal liability of the employer does not absolve a nurse from individual responsibility. Nurses are more likely to fulfil their legal responsibilities if:

- They acquire the knowledge, understanding and level of competence necessary to promote safe, effective nursing care
- They do not undertake tasks which are beyond their level of educational preparation and competence
- They remember that all patients have the rights and privileges accorded to every citizen
- They maintain a high ethical standard in their professional life.

REFERENCES AND FURTHER READING

Game C, Anderson R, Kidd J (eds) 1989 Medical-surgical nursing: A core text. Churchill Livingstone, Melbourne, ch 3, 21–32
Staunton P J, Whyburn B 1989 Nursing and the law, 2nd edn. W B Saunders/Ballière Tindall, Sydney

11. Ethics in nursing

INTRODUCTION

A nurse is a member of multi-disciplinary health team and, as such, she has responsibilities which will vary according to the composition of the team and the status of the individual nurse. The primary concern of the health team must be the provision of very best standard of patient care and, to achieve this, it is necessary for all team members to respect the abilities and functions of their co-workers and to observe *ethical standards*.

Professional groups each have a code of ethics, which consists of standards of conduct that members of the group are expected to follow. *Ethics* may be defined as a set of moral principles which imply a commitment unrelated to monetary reward or prestige, and are derived from a system of values and beliefs that are concerned with rights and obligations. Ethics is concerned with ascribing moral values to, or passing moral judgement on, such things as people, situations, or actions. Ethics is also concerned with the justification of such ascriptions.

In the course of practice nurses are frequently confronted by ethical issues and ethical dilemmas. Consequently, conflict may arise over philosophies, personal values, and professional responsibility. It is most important that nurses have an understanding of their own values, and some understanding of how ethical problems may be resolved without compromising personal values.

Values

A value is a belief about the worth of a particular idea or behaviour, or something an individual views as desirable or important. Values are acquired or learned, initially in childhood, from the family and other significant people and experience. Values become part of an individual during his socialization and reflect his personal needs, the society and culture in which he lives, and the people to whom he relates. Values influence the way an individual interacts with others and the decisions he makes.

Personal values motivate and guide an individual's behaviour, and it is important to recognize that each person's set of values is unique. No two individuals give equal importance to the same values. Some people have very few specific values while others have many. People may value such things as honesty, skill, justice, privacy, friendship, material goods, physical well-being, knowledge, talent, wealth, courage, and creativity.

A consideration of values becomes important when an individual has to take a stand for that which he values. Moral or ethical dilemmas occur in health care when choices have to be made which involve putting one set of values against another. Morals relate to specific values and principles to which an individual is committed, and a moral belief is a conviction that something is absolutely right or wrong. For example, some people believe that abortion is absolutely wrong in all circumstances.

Code of nursing ethics

The nursing profession has its own code of ethics which is a statement about expected standards of behaviour, and which is used to guide ethically sound professional nursing conduct and practice. The International Council of Nurses (I.C.N.) has formulated an International Code of Nursing Ethics (1973) outlining the nurse's responsibilities to individuals, to society, to nursing practice, to co-workers and to the nursing profession. It reads:

The fundamental responsibility of the nurse is fourfold: to promote health, to prevent illness, to restore health, and to alleviate suffering.

The need for nursing is universal. Inherent in nursing is a respect for life, dignity and the rights of man. It is

95

unrestricted by considerations of nationality, race, creed, colour, age, sex, politics, or social status.

Nurses render health services to the individual, the family and the community, and co-ordinate their services with those of related groups.

Nurses and people

The nurse's primary responsibility is to those people who require nursing care. The nurse, in providing care, promotes an environment in which the values, customs and spiritual beliefs of the individual are respected.

The nurse holds in confidence, personal information and uses judgement in sharing this information.

Nurses and practice

The nurse carries personal responsibility for nursing practice and for maintaining competence by continual learning.

The nurse maintains the highest standards of nursing care possible within the reality of a specific situation.

The nurse uses judgement in relation to individual competence when accepting and delegating responsibilities.

The nurse when acting in a professional capacity should at all times maintain standards of personal conduct which reflect credit upon the profession.

Nurses and society

The nurse shares with other citizens the responsibility for initiating and supporting action to meet the health and social needs of the public.

Nurses and co-workers

The nurse sustains a co-operative relationship with co-workers in nursing and other fields. The nurse takes appropriate action to safeguard the individual when his care is endangered by a co-worker or any other person.

Nurses and the Profession

The nurse plays the major role in determining and implementing desirable standards of nursing practice and nursing education.

The nurse is active in developing a core of professional knowledge.

The nurse, acting through the professional organization, participates in establishing and maintaining equitable social and economic working conditions in nursing.

Professional ethics

Nursing is practised within certain legal constraints that promote safe and effective care. Information on legal aspects of nursing is provided in Chapter 10. In addition to legal constraints there are also ethical considerations which provide standards that guide a nurse's actions and decisions. Society expects professional people, such as nurses, to behave with integrity, dignity, competence, and compassion. The International Code of Nursing Ethics provides the nurse with guidelines to assume personal responsibility for providing a standard of excellence in clinical practice. Every nurse is responsible for determining and implementing desirable standards of nursing practice, and for following ethical standards in her professional conduct and in the care she delivers. The nurse has a responsibility to participate actively in developing a body of professional knowledge and the skills necessary which promote safe and effective nursing care.

Individual nurses assume responsibility for performing specific activities related to the care of patients, i.e. a nurse is responsible for her own actions. It is, therefore, essential that all nurses understand the scope of functions and duties associated with their role.

Accountability means that the nurse is responsible, legally and professionally, to herself, to the patients, to the employing institution, and to the nursing profession. Whenever a nurse delivers nursing care to a patient she must be able to answer for her own actions, i.e. no one else is accountable for her actions. Accountability means that a nurse must assume responsibility to report any behaviour that endangers a patient's safety, that she provides patients with adequate information about their care, that she maintains high ethical standards in her own practice, and that she follows the policies and guidelines developed by her employing institution and the professional organization to promote the delivery of safe and effective nursing care.

Advocacy, in a nursing context, means that the nurse acts for and on behalf of the patient. To act as an advocate for a patient the nurse must ensure that the patient is provided with adequate and accurate information relating to his care, and she must support him in any informed decisions he makes about his care. In this way the nurse meets the ethical requirement of honouring a patient's right to self-determination. Nursing ethics involves respecting a patient's right to:

- be informed
- make decisions and choices
- confidentiality
- privacy and dignity
- hold his own ethical and religious beliefs.

All nurses have a responsibility to ensure that, in relation to nursing practice, the patient is assured of safe and competent care and that his rights will be protected.

Ethical issues

It is beyond the scope of this text to discuss at length the ethical issues and moral dilemmas that confront nurses.

For detailed information the nurse is advised to refer to the texts listed at the end of this chapter.

There are numerous areas of medical and nursing practice in which ethical questions arise, and which may require nurses to be involved in resolving ethical problems. The following list is by no means complete, but it provides an outline of the common ethical issues currently facing the health care team:

- genetic engineering
- artificial fertilization
- contraception
- therapeutic abortion
- child abuse
- artificially prolonging life
- voluntary euthanasia
- 'not for resuscitation' orders
- selective non-treatment
- informed consent
- withholding information
- refusal of treatment
- quality versus quantity of life
- organ transplantation
- dying with dignity
- non-therapeutic research
- conflict of values and beliefs between members of the health team.

Ethical decision-making

Often, solving an ethical dilemma may seem almost impossible but using the standards stated in a code of ethics helps the nurse to view such problems objectively. When an ethical decision is to be made, the following factors must be considered:

- the ethical dilemma must be recognized and defined
- all the facts relevant to the issue and to the individuals involved must be obtained
- the people involved in making a decision must be understand the relevant moral rules and principles involved, and be able to apply them in an appropriate manner
- proper evaluation must be made of possible solutions to the problem and of the strategies to be implemented.

Moral dilemmas will continue to occur in health care so long as choices have to be made which involve putting one set of values against another. It is important, therefore, that nurses keep informed and are involved in discussions and debates about ethical issues and dilemmas so that they are able to make ethical decisions in an informed way rather than on a purely emotional basis.

Professional conduct

When nurses are acting in their professional capacity, they are expected to maintain a high standard of conduct, sometimes also referred to as professional etiquette.

Opinions regarding what constitutes proper professional conduct in nursing vary with individual health care agencies, but all codes are based on the fundamentals of courtesy, dignity, loyalty, and consideration for others. Nurses are expected to behave with dignity and to show respect for the dignity of patients, co-workers, and others. Some aspects of professional conduct are:

- Information about patients should not be imparted to other patients, and discretion should be used when information is imparted to professional personnel.
- Matters relating to patients, the health care agency or personnel should not be discussed in public.
- All members of the health care team should show respect for, and give support to, each other.
- Nurses should show loyalty to their profession by behaving in an appropriate manner when acting in a professional capacity.
- Nurses should familiarize themselves with the standards of behaviour set within their employing agency, and they should learn the reason for each policy.
- Nurses, and other health care personnel, should develop a sense of responsibility towards health care agency property and should refrain from extravagance in the use of supplies or misappropriation of supplies for personal use.

Each nurse is responsible for her own standard of behaviour and should refuse to be influenced by others with lower standards.

The nurse must appreciate that, in any group situation, chaos is likely to develop unless a leader is appointed who has the authority to establish priorities and, after consultation with the group, to accept responsibility for decision making. When there is a very large and complex group, such as a hospital community, there must be delegation of responsibility and sharing of the decision making process among a number of people. This leads to a complex administration structure which can function efficiently only if respected and supported by the community it serves. Nurses should learn the correct channels of communication within this system, and should be prepared to abide by the set rules and regulations.

Applying for a position

A written application for employment is a very important communication as it creates in the mind of the prospective employer an impression of the applicant. An applicant for a nursing position must demonstrate in the letter of application an ability to express oneself accurately, concisely, and with clarity.

The two parts to a job application are the application form or introductory letter, and a job resumé or curriculum vitae. Important aspects relating to the written letter include:

• Observation of the rules which apply to the writing of a business letter, e.g. a letter is signed 'Yours faithfully' if the letter begins with 'Dear Sir or Madam' and signed with 'Yours sincerely' if the letter begins with 'Dear Miss Jones' etc. Paragraphs should be short and well spaced. Spelling and punctuation should be correct.
• Plain white stationery should be used, and the applicant should write on only one side of the paper.
• State why you are interested in the position and the contribution you feel you are able to make in that position.
• Request a detailed job description for the advertised position.
• Include the names, addresses, and occupations of two referees who can recommend your personal characteristics, professional experience, and expertise.
• Indicate the date on which you would be free to commence work if appointed.
• The letter should be concluded with an expression of your willingness to support your application at interview.

The curriculum vitae (CV) consists of a summary of information describing professional education, employment experience, and professional activities. It should be typed on a separate sheet of paper and include:

• name
• work and home address and telephone numbers
• date of birth
• educational and professional qualifications
• continuing education activities
• employment history
• professional memberships
• other professional activities.

The personal interview

Prior to appointment to a position, a personal interview with the protective employer is required. The employer will wish to discuss the job application, and she will be trying to ascertain the applicant's suitability for the position as well.

The interview also provides an opportunity for the applicant to find out more about the position and the employing agency. It is important that the applicant who is to have an interview:

• arrives on time
• is neatly dressed and well groomed

• is prepared, e.g. brings any relevant educational documents to the interview, and has thought about the questions she may wish to ask the employer
• is aware that non-verbal messages are transmitted to the interviewer as well as verbal information.
• answers the interviewer's questions honestly and clearly.

Most people who are interviewing prospective employees are aware that it can be a stressful situation and, therefore, try to create a friendly and comfortable environment.

Information on the communication process is provided in Chapter 5.

Resigning from a position

Notification of intention to resign from a position should always be given in writing. There are regulations, e.g. in the relevant Nurses Registration Act or Industrial award, which govern the length of notice to be given. The date on which the resignation becomes effective should be clearly stated.

Reasons for resignation do not have to be given, but many employers prefer that this is done as it enables them to investigate any areas of dissatisfaction. A letter of resignation may also contain comments which express the degree of job satisfaction experienced by the writer. A letter of resignation is acknowledged by the employer either in an exit interview or in writing.

CONCLUSION

As a member of a multi-disciplinary health team the nurse is required to observe ethical standards. Nurses, like other professional groups, have a code of ethics which consists of standards of conduct that they are expected to follow.

Ethics may be defined as a set of moral principles which are derived from a system of values and beliefs concerned with rights and obligations.

A value is a belief about the worth of something, and personal values guide and motivate an individual's behaviour. Some people have very few specific values while others have many, and no two individuals give equal importance to the same values.

Morals relate to specific values and principles to which an individual is committed, and a moral belief is a conviction that something is absolutely right or wrong.

A consideration of values becomes important when an individual has to take a stand for that which he values. Moral or ethical dilemmas occur in health care settings when choices have to be made which involve putting one set of values against another.

Nursing is practiced within certain legal constraints and

ethical considerations which promote safe and effective care. While the International Code of Nursing Ethics provides a framework of standards to promote excellence in clinical practice, every nurse is responsible for determining and implementing desirable standards of practice and for following ethical standards in her professional capacity.

All nurses have a responsibility to promote safe and competent patient care.

REFERENCES AND FURTHER READING

Campbell A V 1984 Moral dilemmas in medicine. Churchill Livingstone, Edinburgh
Johnstone M-J 1989 Bioethics: a nursing perspective. W B Saunders/ Baillière Tindall, Sydney
Potter P A, Perry A G 1985 Fundamentals of nursing. C V Mosby, St Louis, Ch 14, 253–267
International council of nurses 1973, ICN Code for nurses: ethical concepts applied to nursing. Imprimeries populaires, Geneva

12. The nursing process

OBJECTIVES

1. Discuss the various methods of problem solving.
2. Identify the components of the nursing process.
3. Demonstrate use of the nursing process in the delivery of patient care.

INTRODUCTION

Problem solving is a way of finding answers to problems, and is the foundation of the nursing process.

The nursing process is a series of planned steps and actions directed towards meeting the needs and solving the problems of patients, and it forms the basis for all nursing practice.

This chapter addresses several methods of problem solving, and provides information about the nursing process as a problem solving process.

Problem solving

Individuals, as members of a group or alone, are frequently placed in problem solving situations. A problem can be defined as any question proposed for solution or consideration.

A problem may be something as simple as considering what to wear, or as complex as proposing a solution for world peace. Some problems are solved quite readily, while others require much thought and deliberation. People frequently fail to solve a problem efficiently because they:

- don't define the problem
- fail to specify aims or goals
- jump to conclusions as to the cause of a problem
- fail to consider all possible alternatives or solutions to a problem
- fail to consider the possible consequences of their actions.

The use of a systematic scientific process of problem solv-

ing can help to overcome these difficulties, and can assist the solver to make *logical* decisions.

The choice of which methods of problem solving to use depends on several factors such as the seriousness of the problem, and on the experience and skills of the problem solver. Common methods of problem solving include:

1. *Unlearned* problem solving, which is largely instinctive and involves mechanical reflexive reactions to problems. Animals use this method to solve problems of obtaining food or shelter.

2. *Trial and error* problem solving, which involves trying out possible solutions without much forethought and without recording the outcome. This method involves guesswork, because the problem solver does not actually know *why* some of his actions fail while others seem to work.

3. *Intuitive* problem solving, which arises when an individual has had some experience with similar problems in the past. The risk associated with this method is that a person's instincts, or hunches, may be right or they may be wrong. Intuitive feelings, or instincts, can be a valuable asset, but they must be followed up and substantiated with *facts*.

4. *Scientific method* of problem solving, which is a logical and *systematic* process for solving problems. The method is broken down into a series of distinctive steps:

- recognition and definition of the problem
- collection of data
- formulation of a hypothesis (a hypothesis is an unproven theory or proposition which can be tested)
- selection of a plan for testing the hypothesis
- testing the hypothesis
- interpretation of the test results
- evaluation of the hypothesis.

5. *Systems approach* to problem solving, which uses concepts derived from both the scientific method and from systems theory.

A *system* is composed of separate but interrelated components that are linked by a communications network, and the activities of systems are directed towards certain goals. A *cybernetic* system, which can be utilized in problem solving, depends on *feedback* to monitor and control its activities. The major elements in a cybernetic model are:

- input: information entering the system
- throughput: goal-directed activities
- output: end product of the system
- feedback: reinserting, into the system, results of its past performance.

In problem solving the possibility of finding cause-effect relationships seems to be increased with the systems approach. Numerous questions, possible solutions, and new problems can be raised and tested by this method. The advantages of using a systems approach for problem solving include the following:

- It provides a complete overview of the whole process of scientific problem solving
- It helps the solver to think clearly and methodically about problems
- The format helps to ensure that steps will not be missed
- It emphasizes the role of feedback in evaluation and modification of plans.

Nurses commonly use a modified form of *scientific* problem solving (the nursing process) in the practice of nursing, which involves data gathering, formulation of nursing diagnoses, planning, nursing intervention, and evaluation. The main goals of the nursing process are to enable nurses to help patients solve their immediate and long-term problems, and to help prevent further problems from arising. Problem solving is accomplished in 5 steps:

1. A problem is perceived or stated.
2. The problem is defined.
3. Investigation is made by collecting data.
4. Possible solutions are suggested and evaluated.
5. One of the solutions is accepted, or all possible solutions are discarded.

The following example is provided to demonstrate how the problem solving process is implemented.

Ms Jane Smith has decided to host a dinner party for 6 of her colleagues from work. She has not been working with them for long, and does not know any of them very well. She wants the party to be a success but does not know what to cook. She has no idea of her colleagues' food preferences, or whether anyone has special needs or is unable to eat specific foods. Ms Smith has a problem!

To solve the problem, Ms Smith should follow the 5 steps:
1. *She has already perceived that there is a problem.*
2. *The problem must be defined, e.g. 'How can I provide a meal that is acceptable and will be enjoyed by every guest?'*

3. *Collection of data. Ms Smith needs to find out as much as she can about her guests' food preferences and any special needs. She does this by asking each of them, and discovers that 5 of her colleagues enjoy any type of food while the sixth person is a vegetarian.*
4. *She thinks of several possible solutions to her problem, of what to cook! Her possible solutions are:*

- *cancel the party*
- *cook an all-vegetarian meal*
- *take them to a restaurant*
- *provide a buffet-style meal which consists of non-vegetarian and vegetarian dishes.*

Each possible solution is evaluated:

- *to cancel the party would be taking the easy way out*
- *to provide an all-vegetarian meal may not be appreciated by the 5 non-vegetarians*
- *to take the guests to a restaurant would allow them to choose what they preferred, but it would be expensive*
- *to provide a choice of vegetarian and non-vegetarian dishes would require more effort but it could be done.*

5. *Ms Smith accepts one of the solutions, i.e. to provide a buffet-style meal consisting of a variety of dishes. The problem is solved!*

Not all problems are as easily resolved as the one in this example but, by dividing the problem solving process into 5 steps, often seemingly hopeless problems become potentially manageable.

THE NURSING PROCESS

Essentially, the nursing process is a series of planned steps that produce a particular end result. Specifically, the nursing process is a modified scientific method of systematic problem solving. In simple terms the nursing process is a method used to assess, plan, deliver, and evaluate nursing care. The process of nursing, or scientific method of problem solving, remains the same whether the nursing care provided is a simple measure or a sequence of complicated nursing activities.

Providing the framework for nursing care, the nursing process consists of 5 components, each of which follows logically one after the other:

- assessment
- nursing diagnosis
- planning
- implementation
- evaluation.

It is important for the nurse to recognize that the process is on-going, (Fig. 12.1) as it is essential to revise and up-

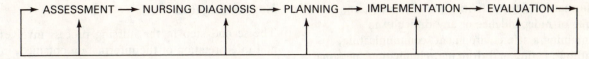

ASSESSMENT → NURSING DIAGNOSIS → PLANNING → IMPLEMENTATION → EVALUATION →

Fig. 12.1 The nursing process.

date any plan of care continually in order to meet a patient's changing needs.

By utilizing the nursing process each individual's *specific* needs are assessed, any problems are identified, and a care plan is developed and implemented in order to meet those needs. The effectiveness of any care given is continuously evaluated, in terms of the individual's needs.

Assessment

Nursing assessment is the process of obtaining and communicating information (data) about a patient, through a variety of methods. The purpose of obtaining information is to identify those areas in which nursing intervention is required.

Data may be obtained from the patient, from his significant others, from health team members, and from the patient's past or present medical and nursing records.

Data obtained may be either subjective or objective:

Subjective data is the patient's, or other significant person's, perceptions, ideas, and sensations about a health problem. For example, a patient may supply information about his sensations of a painful and itching skin, and state that he feels hot.

Objective data is the information observed or measured by the nurse. For example, the nurse may observe the presence of a rash on the patient's body, and she may measure his temperature and observe that it is elevated.

Methods of obtaining both subjective and objective data include:

- the nursing history
- physical examination and observation
- laboratory and diagnostic tests.

The nursing history

A nursing history is obtained by talking with the patient, and/or a significant other person, and is achieved by means of a structured interview. As it is essential that the information is recorded, the nurse uses a form that has been developed by the health care facility.

A nursing history, through the use of interviewing skills, elicits information from the patient about his current and past health problems, his life-style, activities of living, and his psychosocial history. A nursing history centres on the patient's description of his physical, psychological, and emotional reactions to his illness and on the resultant changes to his life-style. A nursing history:

- is the first stage of problem solving and planning for immediate and long-term patient care
- establishes an information base upon which the nursing diagnoses and plans for care can be built
- helps the nurse to initiate a positive relationship with the patient and enables the nurse to observe the patient's verbal and non-verbal communication
- provides the patient with an opportunity to discuss his feelings about himself and his health problems
- helps to reveal any past, present, and potential problems that may require nursing intervention
- helps the patient to remember certain aspects of his illness which he may have forgotten or elected not to tell the medical officer
- provides a written framework in which to record information about the patient's physical, functional, psychological, and emotional state
- creates a reference point from which the nurse can monitor a patient's progress throughout his illness.

A nursing history should be obtained as soon as possible after the patient's admission to the health care agency and it should be conducted, when feasible, by the nurse who has primary responsibility for planning the patient's care. Before beginning the interview the nurse must explain its purpose so the patient understands why certain questions will be asked. The interview setting should be quiet and private for the patient to feel comfortable about discussing personal details. If a patient is too ill, or unable to communicate effectively, a nursing history may be obtained by talking with a member of his family. It is important to record, on the nursing assessment form, from whom the information was obtained.

It is essential that any information obtained during the interview is documented accurately and concisely, as the nursing assessment form is retained for future reference together with other documentation.

The basic information which should be obtained in a nursing history includes:

- medical diagnosis
- previous illnesses and admissions to hospital
- any medications or known allergies
- patient's perception of his current state of health
- social data, e.g. type of accommodation and home conditions, interests and recreational activities, of kin and/or significant others in his life, life crises, employment status, religious practices, the name by which he prefe

- performance of the activities of daily living, e.g. degree of independence or any difficulty in maintaining a safe environment, communicating, breathing, eating and drinking, eliminating, personal cleansing and dressing, controlling body temperature, mobilizing, working and playing, expressing sexuality, sleeping, dying and grieving.
- use of any prosthesis, e.g. walking stick or artificial limb, and any impairments, e.g. visual, auditory, or speech
- habits, e.g. use of alcohol, nicotine or unprescribed drugs.

Physical examination and observation

The physical examination is conducted by a medical officer and his findings are recorded in the patient's notes. The medical officer uses the techniques of inspection, pal- pation, percussion, and auscultation to detect any abnormalities that may provide information about the patient's health problem. The nurse is able to refer to the medical officer's documentation for information about the patient which is relevant to the planning and implementation of nursing care.

Observation of the patient is made by the nurse during her interview with him and involves assessing factors such as his skin colour, general appearance, degree of mobility and independence, emotional status, and the presence of obvious abnormalities, e.g. a rash. Information about his general physical status is obtained by measuring his body temperature, pulse, ventilations, and blood pressure. The patient's weight (mass) and height are also measured and recorded.

Information obtained from physical examination and observation helps to provide baseline data on which to assess the patients present health status, and it may be useful in the identification of actual or potential nursing problems.

Laboratory and diagnostic tests

Laboratory and diagnostic tests, which are the most objective form of assessment data, provide another source of information about the patient.

Both subjective and objective data are required for comprehensive assessment of the patient as they provide more information than either could provide alone. For example, during the nursing interview a patient may reveal that he feels tired constantly, (subjective data) the nurse observes that he looks extremely pale and the laboratory test results indicate that his haemoglobin level is below normal (objective data). Thus, the laboratory test data provides verification of the alterations from normal (tiredness and pallor) identified during the interview.

Nursing diagnosis

The second step in the nursing process involves analysis and interpretation of the information obtained, in order to identify the *actual or potential problems* of the patient that the nurse can help to resolve or prevent through nursing intervention.

The term 'nursing diagnosis' is frequently used to describe a statement of an actual or potential problem that a patient is experiencing with the activities of living. Most health agencies have a listing of accepted nursing diagnoses but, in Australia, a complete classification of approved nursing diagnoses has not yet been compiled. Many health agencies use the diagnostic categories accepted by the North American Nursing Diagnosis Association (NANDA).

A nursing diagnosis is made once all the information has been obtained and compared with normal functioning for the patient. The nurse then makes judgments or inferences about the significance of the information, and identifies the patient's problems. When formulating a nursing diagnosis the nurse should ask herself, 'Is there a problem that nursing intervention can help to resolve?'.

Stating the problem (nursing diagnosis) can be a difficult task, as nurses sometimes become confused about problems versus needs. *A problem is a difficulty the patient is experiencing (actual) or may experience (potential)*. Another difficulty in stating a nursing diagnosis is that a nurse may state the problem as a *medical* diagnosis. The goal of a medical diagnosis is to identify the *disease*, whereas the goal of a nursing diagnosis is to identify the actual or potential health *problems* of the patient.

The following example is provided to help illustrate the difference between a medical and nursing diagnosis:

An elderly male has been admitted to hospital for investigation and treatment of his illness. Manifestations of his illness include joint pain and swelling, stiffness in the morning, 'grating' of some joints during motion, and limited movement. After a physical examination and X-rays of the affected joints, the medical officer makes a diagnosis of 'osteoarthritis'. The nurse, following her assessment of the patient makes a nursing diagnosis which is stated as, 'restricted mobility related to painful joints'.

A nursing diagnosis consists of 2 parts: the first part states the problem (restricted mobility), and the second part states the possible cause of the problem (painful joints). If the problem is a *potential* one, the words *potential for* or *at risk for* are written before the problem, e.g. 'potential for restricted mobility related to painful joints'.

Formulation of nursing diagnoses requires experience in nursing, and practise. Once the patient's problems are identified, each nursing diagnosis is placed in order of importance on the nursing care plan.

Planning

Once the patient's problems have been identified and the nursing diagnoses formulated, the nurse plans the care to be implemented. Planning involves setting goals, establishing priorities, and determining nursing interventions to achieve the goals.

1. Setting goals establishes the framework for a nursing care plan. Goals, or objectives, are the outcomes or results which are expected as a consequence of nursing or patient activities. Therefore, for each nursing diagnosis (problem) the nurse in conjunction with the patient sets the goals to be achieved.

A goal may be short-term, i.e. one that is expected to be achieved in a relatively short time, e.g. hours or days. A long-term goal is one that is to be achieved in the future, e.g. within several weeks or months.

Goals are expressed specifically and in behavioural terms. By expressing a goal *specifically*, everyone involved in the patient's care knows the expected outcome. Goals are written using a *verb* to express the expected behaviour, and as such are observable and measurable. Thus, the expected outcomes describe the behaviour the patient is expected to attain. For example, 'The patient will walk the length of the ward without assistance'. It is more helpful to all concerned if a time frame is included in the goal, e.g. 'The patient will walk the length of the ward without assistance by October 2nd.'

Any goals that are set must be realistic and attainable, in terms of the patient's limits and the ability of the nurse to assist him.

2. Priorities are established once the nursing diagnoses have been formulated and specific goals have been set, by grading them in order of importance. High-priority goals are those that require immediate attention, while low-priority goals are those which do not need to be attained as quickly. Basic physiological needs, e.g. the need for oxygen, nutrition, or water, are given priority over other needs. Information on Maslow's hierarchy of needs is provided in Chapter 28.

'Actual problems precede potential problems, and the problem seen as the most crucial would be stated first' (Game, et al 1989).

3. Determining nursing interventions involves selecting the activities which are expected to help the patient achieve the set goals (expected outcomes).

To select the most appropriate nursing activities (interventions) all possible alternatives are discussed, generally in consultation with the patient. Selection of appropriate nursing interventions must be based on sound nursing knowledge, using a scientific problem solving approach, with the patient's participation when possible. Once a decision has been made on the measures to be implemented, statements defining the selected actions are written in the nursing care plan. For example, one selected nursing activity may be expressed as, 'perform active leg and feet exercises every 2 hours whilst in bed'.

All proposed nursing interventions must be written specifically and in adequate detail to enable all nursing personnel to carry them out correctly.

Interventions may consist of activities which the nurse will perform, or actions to be taken by the patient with or without assistance from the nurse.

The nursing care plan is a document developed by the health care agency, which is organized in such a way that any nurse can readily identify:

- the nursing diagnoses
- the goals or expected outcomes
- the specific nursing interventions for each goal
- whether the goals are being achieved (evaluation).

While the structure of a nursing care plan may vary slightly from one health care setting to another the principles of formulating a care plan remain the same, i.e. the plan is structured so that the nursing diagnoses, goals, and nursing interventions are clearly stated. A correctly formulated nursing care plan facilitates the co-ordination and continuity of care.

An example of a fully documented nursing care plan is provided in Table 12.1.

Implementation

Implementation means putting the nursing plan into action, and is the actual performance of the activities which have been selected to help the patient achieve the set goals. Reassessment of the patient's needs is made continuously during the implementation stage, so that any new needs can be identified and so that the nursing care plan can be modified or adapted. During this stage of the nursing process the planned nursing interventions are implemented to achieve identified goals. If the nursing actions are not effective in helping the patient achieve the goals, the plan is reviewed and other appropriate measures are implemented. As problems are solved, the nursing diagnoses are revised, and deleted from the care plan if they are no longer relevant. As new nursing diagnoses are made they are added to the plan, together with specific goals and selected nursing actions to achieve those goals.

Evaluation

Once the planned nursing interventions have been implemented, the nurse must then evaluate the results to determine whether the interventions were effective. Evaluation is the process of determining the extent to which the set goals or objectives have been achieved, and it enables

Table 12.1 Nursing care plan

Nursing diagnoses	Goals/expected outcomes	Nursing interventions	Date commenced	Evaluation	Date ceased
1. Anxiety related to impaired eyesight	To understand the implications of surgery on her vision	Encourage her to express her fears	20.6.89	Is able to communicate her anxieties verbally	24.6.89
		Explain all pre- and post-operative procedures, their purpose and possible implications	20.6.89	States that she understands the nursing actions	
		Arrange for the surgeon to explain how her eye-sight should be improved after the operation	20.6.89	States that she has understood the surgeon's explanation and feels reassured	20.6.89
		Explain that new spectacles will be prescribed following surgery to aid her vision	20.6.89	Understands that the new spectacles will be provided soon after her discharge	21.6.89
2. Impaired ability to communicate due to impaired vision and hearing	To communicate effectively	Encourage her to wear her current spectacles	20.6.89	Occasionally needs reminding	25.6.89
		Face her when speaking and speak clearly	20.6.89	Is able to communicate effectively	25.6.89
		Attract her attention before starting to speak	20.6.89		
		Use gestures to enhance the spoken word	20.6.89		
		Ensure adequate lighting and reduced glare	20.6.89		
3. Potential for accidents due to impaired vision	To provide a safe environment	Assist when ambulating	20.6.89	Required assistance until the third day	24.6.89
		Remove obstacles from her path	20.6.89		25.6.89
		Place signal device within easy reach	20.6.89		25.6.89
		Place personal items within easy reach, in front of her	20.6.89		25.6.89
		Adjust the bed to a low level	20.6.89		25.6.89
		Elevate the bed-rails at night	20.6.89		25.6.89
		Assist with bathing and dressing	20.6.89		24.6.89
		Cut up food and pour fluids	20.6.89		24.6.89
4. Potential for pain and discomfort related to the operation	To be pain-free at all times	Assist her to assume a position of comfort	21.6.89		24.6.89
		Assess her continually for presence of pain	21.6.89		25.6.89
		Apply eye patch and shield correctly	21.6.89		25.6.89
		Administer prescribed analgesic medications	21.6.89		23.6.89
5. Potential inability to perform activities of living due to the effects of the operation	To achieve independence, within her limitations, before discharge from hospital	Allow her adequate time to perform the activities of daily living of which she is capable.	20.6.89	Manages well with some assistance	25.6.89
		Observe her ability to perform the activities independently.	20.6.89		
		Assist when she requests help or is unable to perform an activity independently.	20.6.89	Manages independently by third day	24.6.89
		Provide adequate support and preparation for her return home	20.6.89	States she understands what to expect when she is discharged.	25.6.89
		Contact the visiting nurse service to arrange for a nurse to instill the the prescribed eye drops at her home.	23.6.89	Community services will commence in the afternoon of 25.6.89	23.6.89
		Contact the community agencies to arrange Home help and Meals on Wheels on her return home.	23.6.89		23.6.89

the nurse to monitor the effectiveness of a nursing care plan. Whether the plan was a success or not is determined by comparing the patient's response to the nursing interventions, with the set goals. Evaluation also enables the nurse to identify any new health care problems experienced by the patient.

Evaluation is made by examining the results of the interventions, assessing the patient for possible side effects and adverse reactions to the nursing interventions, and by analyzing the results. Analysis involves determining whether the patient is better or worse or shows no change: in other words, have the set goals been achieved?. Based on the data obtained from the evaluation a nursing judgment is made.

Thus, evaluation allows the nurse to revise and, if necessary, to modify or change the plan at any stage of her delivery of patient care. If the set goals have been achieved the plan is deemed to be successful and the nursing interventions can usually be terminated. If the goals have not been achieved the patient's needs must be reassessed, new nursing diagnoses formulated if necessary, and the plan changed and reimplemented.

Evaluation is performed continuously throughout the nursing process, as it is the most important method of determining the effectiveness of a nursing care plan.

Effectiveness of a nursing care plan can also be determined by another method of evaluation, a nursing audit. *A nursing audit* is a thorough investigation made to evaluate the overall nursing care received by a patient. An audit is generally performed by an experienced nurse, or committee, who does not actually work in the ward where the audit is being carried out. Each health care agency develops its own nursing audit form, which is a checklist that includes specific criteria for each category of care. A nursing audit may be made during the patient's hospitalization or after his discharge from hospital. The purpose of an audit is to improve the quality of patient care.

A NURSING CARE STUDY

This nursing care study is provided to demonstrate how the nursing process is used to deliver care in a logical and systematic way.

Mrs Brown, a 77-year-old woman, was admitted to hospital at 1400 hours on 20th June 1989 for surgery the following day. After she had been admitted to the ward, introduced to the other patients in the 4 bed room, and given time to settle into her new environment, Nurse Charles came to obtain a nursing history.

Assessment

Nurse Charles introduced herself and explained that the purpose of the nursing history was to obtain the information necessary to develop a care plan for Mrs Brown.

Nurse Charles drew the screens around the bed, sat down, and began to talk with Mrs Brown. She asked the patient by what name she preferred to be known, and was informed that 'Mrs Brown' would be fine as she was not enamoured with her given name of Annie. During the 20 minute discussion with Mrs Brown, nurse Charles obtained and recorded the following information:

- Mrs Brown's husband had died of cancer two years previously. She had one daugher and one son, both of whom lived some distance away. Her daughter came to stay with her once or twice a month, while her son visited 2-3 times a year. Neither of her children had married.
- Mrs Brown lived alone in the house she had shared with her husband since their marriage. The house had all the facilities she required, but was located on a large block so that Mrs Brown was experiencing some difficulty in maintaining the garden without her husband's assistance. Mrs Brown had one cat which she enjoyed looking after and said, 'She is good company'.
- Mrs Brown had been an active member of several organizations, but had given up some of her social activities over the past 18 months when her eyesight began to fail. She still enjoyed reading, watching television, and working in the garden.
- The patient had been in hospital to have both her children, and was admitted for one day 5 years ago to have an operation on her wrist. She has also spent 3 days in hospital for treatment of a fractured ankle.
- Mrs Brown's past health problems included a deep vein thrombosis, a fractured wrist, and a urinary tract infection.
- Her current admission was so that she could have a cataract removed from her right eye. Mrs Brown told Nurse Charles that her vision had been deteriorating over the past 2 years, and that she had difficulty in seeing many things unless they were very close. She quite frequently bumped into, or tripped over, objects in her path. She understood that she would be in hospital for 2–3 days, and would be required to instil eye drops and wear an eye patch for several days after that. She expressed some anxiety over her eyesight, as her mother had become totally blind at about the same age. Mrs Brown was also concerned as to how she would manage at home after the operation during the time her right eye was covered.
- Mrs Brown had no difficulty in carrying out most of the activities of living, except that she was frightened of slipping during her evening bath or shower. She enjoyed porridge for breakfast and ate a lot of fruit during the day, and had experienced no problems with elimination. She usually went to bed at approximately 2200 hours, and slept well without the use of any medication.
- Recordings of Mrs Brown's vital signs showed that her temperature was 370°C, pulse 76 and regular, ventilations 18, and blood pressure 130/70. She weighed 64 kg, and her urine sample showed no evidence of any abnormalities.

During her conversation with the patient, Nurse Charles observed that Mrs Brown appeared to be generally in good condition, that she wore spectacles for reading and watching television, and that she appeared to be slightly hard of hearing. Following the interview with Mrs Brown, Nurse Charles looked at her medical history to see if there was any further information which would be relevant to the delivery of nursing care. She observed that the medical officer, who had examined Mrs Brown, had not detected any additional pathological abnormalities. The results of her chest X-ray, electrocardiogram, and full blood examination were within normal limits. The medical diagnosis was, 'Cataract in right eye for extraction and intro-ocular lens transplant'.

Nursing diagnosis

Nurse Charles examined all the information she had obtained, and determined that Mrs Brown's actual and potential problems were:

- impaired vision, which caused her to be more vulnerable to accidents, e.g. falls and burns
- anxiety about her vision and how she would manage after the operation
- some difficulty in maintaining her home garden
- some hearing impairment
- potential for pain and discomfort after operation
- potential inability to perform the activities of living independently after the operation, while her right eye was covered.

Nurse Charles then formulated the following nursing diagnoses:

- Anxiety related to impaired eyesight
- Impaired ability to communicate due to impaired vision and hearing
- Potential for accidents due to impaired vision
- Potential for pain and discomfort related to the operation
- Potential inability to perform the activities of living independently while her right eye was covered.

Planning

Once Nurse Charles had identified Mrs Brown's problems, and formulated the nursing diagnoses, she was able to plan the care to be implemented. For each nursing diagnosis Nurse Charles set objectives (expected outcomes), and decided on the nursing actions which would help Mrs Brown to achieve those objectives. This information, together with the nursing diagnoses, was recorded on a nursing care plan (Table 12.1).

Implementation and evaluation

During implementation of the nursing actions Nurse Charles continuously reassessed Mrs Brown in order to evaluate the effectiveness of the nursing care plan, and to detect any new problems should they arise.

Mrs Brown recovered well after the operation to remove the cataract, and was required to wear an eye pad during the day. At night the soft eye pad was covered by a rigid shield to provide added protection. During the day prescribed eye drops were instilled every 6 hours. Mrs Brown experienced some pain in the immediate post operative period, but the pain was relieved when prescribed analgesic medications were administered. She required some assistance with bathing, dressing, mobilising, and feeding herself for the first 2 days. By the third day she was able to perform the activities of daily living independently with supervision. Mrs Brown was unable to instill the eye drops or apply the eye pad correctly, so the visiting nurse service was contacted and twice daily home visits were arranged. As Mrs Brown did not feel confident in her ability to shop for or prepare food or attend to all the housework for a few days, home help and meals on wheels were arranged for her.

On the fourth day after operation, Mrs Brown was discharged. A discharge plan was completed, and the only remaining problem was 'potential inability to perform the activities of living independently due to the effects of the operation'. She was pleased to be going home and expressd the belief that she would be able to manage with the assistance of the support services which had been arranged. Nurse Charles ensured that Mrs Brown knew what times the visiting nurse would be coming to instill the drops and apply an eye pad. She was advised to wear the rigid shield over the eye pad when she retired for the night. An appointment was made to see the surgeon the following week.

Throughout the process of implementation and evaluation, Nurse Charles constantly assessed Mrs Brown. As a problem was solved, the nursing interventions were discontinued (Table 12.1). For example, Mrs Brown was not experiencing any pain or discomfort by the second postoperative day, therefore analgesic medications were no longer required.

SUMMARY

The nursing process forms the basis for all nursing practice, consisting of a series of planned steps and actions directed toward meeting patients needs and solving their problems.

The nursing process is based on a modified scientific method of problem solving which involves, assessment, formulation of nursing diagnoses, planning, implementation, and evaluation.

Apart from the scientific method, other problem solving methods include unlearned, trial and error, intuitive, and systems approach. People choose a method of solving problems based on factors such as their skills and experience, and on the seriousness of the problem.

Problem solving is accomplished in 5 steps: a problem is perceived or stated, the problem is defined, investigation is made through collection of data, possible solutions are suggested and evaluated, and one of the solutions is chosen.

The nursing process, then, is a problem solving approach to the delivery of nursing care. Using the nursing process, a nurse assesses, plans, delivers, and evaluates nursing care.

Assessment is the process of obtaining and communicating information about a patient. The information (data), which may be either subjective or objective, is obtained through a nursing history, physical examination and observation, and laboratory and diagnostic tests.

Nursing diagnosis is a term used to describe a statement of an actual or potential problem. An actual problem is a difficulty the patient is currently experiencing, whereas a potential problem is a difficulty that a patient may experience in the future.

Planning involves setting goals and determining which nursing interventions (actions) should be implemented to help the patient achieve those goals. A goal is the outcome or result which is expected as a consequence of nursing or patient activities. Short-term goals are those that are expected to be achieved in a relatively short time, and long-term goals are those which are set to be achieved within a longer period.

Once the most appropriate nursing interventions have been selected, a nursing care plan is developed. A nursing care plan is a document which is structured in such a way that any nurse can readily identify the nursing diagnoses, the expected outcomes, the specific nursing interventions for each goal, and evaluation of the effectiveness of each nursing action.

Implementation involves putting the plan into action, and is the actual performance of the activities which have been selected to help the patient achieve the set goals.

Evaluation is the process of determining whether the implemented actions were effective.

The nursing process is continuous, in that the nurse constantly assesses the patient, identifies his problems; plans, implements, and evaluates nursing care. At any stage, during delivery of care, the nursing care plan may be modified or changed in order to meet the patient's needs.

REFERENCES AND FURTHER READING

Game C, Anderson R E, Kidd J R (eds) 1989 Medical-Surgical nursing: a core text. Churchill Livingstone, Melbourne
McFarlane J K, Castledine G 1982 A guide to the practice of nursing. C V Mosby, London
Potter P A, Perry A G 1985 Fundamentals of nursing. C V Mosby, St Louis, ch 6, 128–136
Roper N, Logan W W, Tierney A J 1990 The elements of nursing, 3rd edn. Churchill Livingstone, Edinburgh

13. Observational skills

INTRODUCTION

Assessment is an essential part of the nursing process, as it enables the nurse to obtain information about the patient that will facilitate the identification of problems relating to his health status. Once his problems (actual or potential) are identified, steps can then be taken to plan appropriate care to meet his needs.

Continued assessment enables the nurse to determine:

- the progress being made by the patient
- any change in his condition
- the effectiveness of the nursing care plan in meeting the patient's needs.

Accurate assessments made, recorded, and reported by nurses also assist the medical officer in making a diagnosis, planning a programme of treatment, or altering a plan of treatment in the light of reported changes in a patient's condition. Information on the nursing process is provided in Chapter 12, and it should be referred to in conjunction with this chapter.

The nurse has an essential role to play in assessing patients and in recording and reporting her findings. In order to assess a patient effectively, the nurse requires knowledge of the normal so that she is able to identify any deviations or abnormalities.

Assessment skills

Assessment involves obtaining subjective and objective information about a patient, using various skills:

- interviewing
- observing and examining the patient by using the senses of sight, hearing, touch, and smell
- using equipment, e.g. to assess a patient's vital signs
- evaluating laboratory and diagnostic test results.

Subjective data (information) are the patient's perceptions of his health problems, while objective data are the observations or measurements obtained by the nurse or other personnel. Examples of subjective data are the presence of pain, nausea, fatigue, or anxiety. Examples of objective data are identifying the presence of a rash, abnormal skin colour, elevated temperature, or blood in the urine.

The ability to observe methodically and intelligently, and to report with accuracy what one has observed, is a fundamental element of nursing. While Chapter 12 addresses the interviewing component of assessment, this chapter focuses on use of the physical senses and equipment to assess a patient's physical and mental condition and the signs and symptoms which may be indicative of change.

Interpretation of specific observations depends on:

- comparison with the normal for a given group of people
- knowledge of the results of previous observations of a particular patient
- the sum total of all observations at the time of the present observation.

For example, to interpret the significance of a patient's pulse rate the nurse needs to know the normal pulse rate for people of that patient's age group, and the patient's previous pulse rate. Additional observations or assessment of that patient, e.g. his blood pressure, temperature, ventilations, colour, and degree of mental alertness, provide information which enables more accurate interpretation of his condition. Therefore, while a single observation provides some information about a patient, several observations enable a more accurate assessment of his condition.

Interpretation of any observation involves a *decision* as to its significance. The nurse has a responsibility to report her observations to the nurse in charge who makes a decision, e.g. to assess the patient more frequently, to take immediate action, or to notify the medical officer.

Assessment using the sense of sight

A nurse must learn how to really *see* things so that, even in passing or without conscious effort, she will be aware of patients and their general appearance, colour, expression, and body posture. During closer contact with the patient no significant external feature should escape the nurse's notice, and she must be able to recognize deviations from normal. In order to do this, the nurse must know what to look for, and what constitutes 'normal'.

Assessment of a patient is performed when he is first admitted to a health care institution or when community nursing care is commenced. Thereafter, assessment is performed continuously to evaluate his progress, and to identify new needs. Table 51.1 lists the observations to be made during the admission assessment, the normal findings, and various deviations from normal. In addition to the observations listed in this table, the nurse must assess:

- the patient's degree of independence
- his ability to perform the activities of daily living
- his ability to interact with others
- his reactions and responses to treatment, e.g. medications
- basic needs, e.g. for food, water, oxygen, safety, exercise, comfort.
- specific needs, e.g. for wound care or pain relief
- excretions and secretions, e.g. urine, faeces, vomitus, wound drainage.

Information on these topics is provided in the relevant chapters, e.g. Chapter 35 addresses comfort needs and Chapter 36 addresses the need for freedom from pain.

While observation of all the aspects mentioned is essential, one of the most important skills a nurse should develop is the ability to *look* at a patient and determine whether he appears comfortable. A person's comfort depends on many things, the most basic of which are that his needs for hygiene, posture, maintenance of body temperature, and freedom from pain are met. When looking at a patient, the nurse should ask herself various questions, for example:

- Is he positioned comfortably?
- Are all his limbs adequately supported?
- Does he have enough pillows?
- Are the pillows arranged to meet his needs?
- Does he have enough blankets?
- Can he reach his signal device and articles on the locker or bedside table?
- Does he require mouth care?
- Would he like his face washed or hair brushed?

- Is the light in the room too bright or inadequate?
- Is the room too hot or too cold?
- Does he appear to be experiencing any pain or discomfort?

As well as observing and assessing the patient and his needs, the nurse must also use her sense of sight to assess the functioning of equipment used in patient care. Nurses assess various items of equipment to determine whether they are functioning correctly when they are in use, for example:

- intravenous fluid apparatus
- oxygen apparatus
- urinary drainage systems
- wound drainage systems
- traction apparatus.

While the nurse may not be directly responsible for the management of specific items of equipment, she has a responsibility to *observe* their functioning and to *report* immediately to the nurse in charge if she suspects any malfunction.

Assessment using the sense of hearing

It is important that a nurse learns to *listen* effectively, so that not only what a patient says is registered, but also his tone of voice, which often conveys a great deal. A nurse must also learn how to recognize abnormal sounds. Information on the art of effective listening in communication is provided in Chapter 5, and it emphasizes the importance of recognizing that listening is an *active* process which involves much more than just hearing the spoken word. Recognition of *abnormal* sounds, in patient care, involves the ability to detect:

- abnormalities of breathing, e.g. ventilations that are wheezing, noisy, or distressed.
- abnormalities of heart sounds, blood pressure, bowel sounds, or fetal heart sounds when using a stethoscope.
- manifestations of a patient's distress, e.g. coughing, expectorating sputum, vomiting, crying or moaning.
- changes in the sound or rhythm of technical equipment such as suction or artificial ventilation apparatus.

Assessment using the sense of touch

The sense of *touch* should be developed so that a nurse is able to detect abnormalities, for example:

- abnormally hot, cool, moist, dry, inelastic, or roughened skin.
- an excessively hard, soft, or ropy arterial wall.
- a rapid, slow, weak, or irregular pulse.

- rigid or flaccid muscles.
- swelling of part of the body, e.g. a joint.

Touch is also used when examining a patient by palpation or percussion. Palpation, usually performed by a medical officer, is a technique whereby the examiner feels the texture, size, consistency, and location of certain parts of the body with the hands. For example, the examiner may palpate an abdomen to determine the size of the liver.

Percussion, usually performed by a medical officer, is a technique in which the examiner strikes the body surface with a finger producing vibration and sound. An abnormal sound suggests the presence of a mass or accumulation of fluid within an organ or cavity. For example, the examiner may percuss the posterior chest wall to determine the presence of fluid in the lungs.

Assessment using the sense of smell

A well developed sense of *smell* enables a nurse to detect odours which are characteristic of certain conditions, for example:

- the 'fishy' smell of infected urine
- the 'ammonia' odour associated with concentrated or decomposed urine
- the 'musty' or offensive odour of an infected wound
- the offensive 'rotting' odour associated with gangrene (tissue necrosis)
- the smell of 'ketones' on the breath in ketoacidosis (accumulation of ketones in the body)
- the smell of alcohol on the breath
- halitosis (offensive breath) accompanying mouth infections, e.g. gingivitis or certain disorders of the digestive system, e.g. appendicitis
- the foul odour associated with steatorrhoea (abnormal amount of fat in the faeces)
- the characteristic odour associated with melaena (abnormal black tarry stool containing blood)
- the 'faecal' odour of vomitus associated with a bowel obstruction
- bromhidrosis (offensisve smelling perspiration) caused by bacterial decomposition of perspiration on the skin.

Assessment using equipment

A nurse should acquire proficiency in the correct use of equipment which will provide information about a patient, for example:

- clinical thermometer
- sphygmomanometer
- stethoscope
- weighing scales
- urine testing equipment
- calibrated calipers to measure skinfold thickness
- tapemeasure, e.g. to measure head, limb, or abdominal circumference
- auriscope, to visualize the ear canal.

CONCLUSION

In order to assess a patient's condition, and to identify his health problems and needs, a nurse needs to develop skill in using her senses and various items of equipment to obtain information.

The ability to observe methodically and intelligently is a fundamental element of nursing, and in order to assess a patient effectively a nurse requires knowledge of the normal so that she can recognize deviations from normal.

Initial and continual assessment of a patient is performed to determine his progress, any change in his condition, and the effectiveness of nursing care in meeting his needs. Accurate assessments also assist the medical officer in making a diagnosis, planning a programme of treatment, or altering a plan of treatment.

REFERENCES AND FURTHER READING

Murray R B, Zentner J P 1985 Nursing assessment and health promotion through the life span, 3rd edn. Prentice Hall, Eaglewood Cliffs
Potter P A , Perry A G 1985 Fundamentals of nursing. C V Mosby, St Louis

14. Reporting and recording skills

OBJECTIVES

1. Develop and practise the skills of verbal and written reporting and recording in the delivery of patient care.

INTRODUCTION

Reporting and recording are two ways in which communication takes place among members of the health team, as both are an account of what has been assessed or observed about a patient and what care has been implemented. Health team members rely on reports and records to deliver care that is directed toward mutually agreed goals. Continuity of care and the pursuit of common objectives depends upon effective communication between members of the health team, which involves accurate and precise verbal and written reporting and recording of information. While Chapter 5 addresses the communication process in detail, this chapter focuses on the aspects of reporting and documenting information as part of the nursing process. Information on the nursing process is provided in Chapter 12.

REPORTING

Reporting involves the spoken or written exchange of information. A nurse has a responsibility to report verbally, to the nurse in charge, details of the observation she has made and the nursing care she has implemented. When reporting information verbally the nurse should provide prompt, accurate and concise information to the nurse in charge.

1. When reporting a patients' symptom, e.g. nausea or pain, the following details should be provided:

- description of the event
- severity, onset, and location of the symptom
- frequency and duration

- any precipitating or aggravating factors
- any associated symptoms.

For example, rather than just telling the nurse in charge that a patient has pain, it is more beneficial to provide detailed information, such as:

Mrs Brown was lying down with her legs drawn up to her abdomen. When I asked her how she was feeling she told me she had suddenly developed severe pain in the right side of her abdomen after eating lunch. She has had the pain intermittently for 20 minutes, she appears pale, and is feeling nauseated. Her temperature is 37°C, pulse 90, ventilations 24, and her blood pressure is 130/70.

Detailed information, such as provided in the example, enables the nurse in charge to make a better decision on what course of action to take.

2. When reporting about the nursing measures she has implemented, e.g. changing a wound dressing, the following details should be provided:

- the time the activity was performed
- what equipment was used, e.g. the type of lotion or dressing
- the observations made, e.g. type and amount of drainage from the wound
- the patient's response to the activity, e.g. appeared tired, pale, or in pain.

3. When reporting about a patient's behaviour, e.g. manifestations of anxiety or confusion, the following details should be provided:

- the behaviours exhibited, e.g. crying, restlessness, or inability to remember his name
- any precipitating or aggravating factors
- the nurse's response or actions taken
- the patient's response to nurse's actions.

When reporting a patient's behaviour the nurse must be objective and avoid interpreting her observations. Assumptions and interpretations can be both inaccurate and misleading. For example, an objective observation would be, 'Mr Smith is crying', whereas a subjective interpretation of his behaviour might be, 'Mr Smith seems depressed'. While that may very well be the cause of his crying, he may be crying for a variety of other reasons!

A more useful and accurate report would be:

When I went into his room I noticed that Mr Smith was crying. I went to him, put my arm around his shoulder, and asked him if I could help. He told me that he was very anxious about the results of his tests. I told him I would ask you to speak to him about them, and he said he would appreciate that.

4. When reporting about the effects of treatments, e.g. medications, the following details should be provided:

- the time the treatment was performed
- the patient's response, and whether the treatment produced the desired or any adverse reactions
- the patient's vital signs.

For example, following administration of intramuscular morphine 10 mg the nurse may report:

Since Mrs Jones was given intramuscular morphine 10 mg at 1300 hours she is not experiencing any pain, is resting quietly, and her vital signs are: temperature 36.8°C, pulse 82, ventilations 18, and blood pressure 120/70.

Alternatively, the report may be, 'Mrs Jones is still in pain since her injection of morphine 10 mg at 1300. She is feeling nauseated, is sweating and pale, and her pulse rate has dropped from 80 to 58.'

5. When reporting measurements or observations of body excreta or secretions, the nurse should provide adequate information. For example, little information is transmitted if a nurse uses expressions such as 'her pulse is normal', or 'her urine looks alright'. A more useful report would be, 'Mrs Jones' pulse is 80, regular, and strong', or 'Mr Black's urine is amber-coloured, clear, and has no offensive odour'.

In addition to verbal reports, written reports are made on all aspects of a patient's care and progress. To promote continuity of care, a verbal report, using written records, is given on each patient at each change of shift. The nurse who is giving the report should do so in a methodical manner, beginning with basic information on the reason for the patient's being in hospital followed by a detailed description of his progress.

Various methods of giving change-of-shift reports may be used, e.g. reading from the care plan and/or Kardex, and reports may be conducted in a nurse's office or while walking around and visiting each patient. If the latter method is used, nurses must be careful to report any information that may distress a patient out of his hearing.

A report on each patient generally includes the following information:

- the patient's name, age, and sex
- the medical diagnosis
- the name of the medical officer
- nursing diagnoses or problems, whether specific goals have been achieved, specific problems resolved, or whether any parts of the nursing care plan have been changed
- general description of the patient's physical and psychological status, and any recent changes in his condition
- the patient's degree of independence in performing the activities of daily living
- the patient's response to nursing intervention and treatments
- details of any diagnostic tests or surgical interventions which have been, or are to be, performed
- details of any new treatments, e.g. intravenous therapy, which have been prescribed
- significant medications, e.g. narcotic analgesics, and their effects
- any dietary or fluid restrictions or modifications, and whether the patient's fluid input and output are being measured and recorded
- details of the condition of any wound, e.g. degree of healing, amount and type of any discharge
- details of any deviations from normal, e.g. of the patient's vital signs or excreta
- pertinent information concerning the patient's family or other significant people.

As a verbal report is being given, the nurse who is receiving it should obtain an accurate assessment of each patient and his current condition. Use of the *nursing process* enables the nurse who is giving the report to systematically review the patient's identified problems and nursing diagnoses, and the nursing interventions and goals as stated on the care plan.

In addition to giving verbal reports at each change of shift, *team conferences* are held regularly to evaluate the progress of patients. The nursing team may hold a daily conference to review each patient and his nursing care plan, or a conference may be held whereby various members of the team, e.g. nurses, medical officer, and physiotherapist meet to discuss patient care and to exchange information. Team conferences are conducted in a variety of settings, e.g. hospitals, rehabilitation and psychiatric units, and community health agencies. The purpose of such a conference is the *evaluation* of:

- a patient's health problems
- the goals which have been set
- the interventions which have been planned and implemented
- a patient's progress
- plans for discharge.

RECORDING

Information about each patient is recorded in writing to communicate information about his health status and care. Various types of records are used for the purposes of:

- communication
- assessment
- auditing
- education and research
- legal documentation.

Records, which promote continuity of care, are the means by which various members of the health team *communicate* information about the patient's condition and the type of care which has been implemented.

Written records provide permanent and accurate *assessment* of the patient, his health status, and his progress: and they provide the data necessary to plan and implement care.

As part of quality assurance programmes conducted by health care agencies, *auditing* is performed whereby the information contained in patient records is reviewed on a regular basis. Audits are performed to determine the degree to which specified quality assurance standards have been met.

Written records provide a great deal of information, e.g. about nursing diagnoses, and evaluation of care which has been implemented, that may be used for *educational* purposes. The information contained in records may also serve as a source of data for *research*.

Records also become a *legal document*, e.g. if a patient takes legal action against a health care agency, patient records can be used as evidence in courts of law, where they are read and interpreted by lawyers. In addition, some records are now accessible by patients under the Freedom of Information Act.

The two most commonly used record formats are the traditional source records, and the problem-oriented records. In the *source method* information is grouped according to its source, i.e, the record is divided into the nurse's notes, the medical officer's record, laboratory reports, the physiotherapist's report, etc. Using this method, each member of the health team uses a separate section of the record to record data. While this method of recording enables each category of health team member to make detailed entries, it does lead to the fragmentation of data as the information is not written according to the patient's identified problems.

The *problem-oriented method* groups information from all members of the health team into sections according to a patient's specific health problems, whereby each member of the team contributes to a single list of identified patient problems. When this system is used, it is easy to recognize and locate, on a single record, the patient's health care problems. While each health care agency adopts its own record format, many use a problem-oriented system of total patient recording which includes all the information relevant to a patient's care.

The various types of records which may be used by a health care agency include:

- nursing and medical admission histories
- patient interview forms
- nursing care plans
- flow sheets
- progress notes/reports
- Kardex
- laboratory/diagnostic test reports
- consent forms
- incident reports
- pre-operative anaesthetic records, and post-operative surgical reports
- therapeutic order sheets
- medication records
- discharge summaries.

The nurse is most likely to be regularly involved in recording information on patient interview forms, nursing care plans, various flow sheets, progress notes, and the Kardex.

Information on patient interviews and nursing care plans is provided in Chapter 12, and a sample nursing care plan is shown in Table 12.1.

Flow sheets are used to record certain assessments or measurements, and provide an efficient method of recording such information. Types of flow sheets used include those to record:

- vital signs
- neurological assessments
- fluid input and output, e.g. fluid balance and intravenous therapy charts.

Sample flow sheets are provided in Figures 31.1, 33.2, and 43.3.

Progress notes involve recording information on the document which describes the patient's progress. Using the problem-oriented method, all members of the health team contribute to the progress notes by documenting information about a patient's identified problems. A specific format has been developed for writing these descriptive notes, which is referred to as the *SOAP* format.

The letters *SOAP* stand for *subjective* statement (made by the patient) that describe his perception of a problem, *objective* data which consists of information that can be measured, e.g. obtained via observations or tests, *assessment* of the subjective and objective data available, and the *plan* which is developed in response to assessment. Some health care agencies also extend the SOAP format to include *IER*, thus making the format SOAPIER. The letter *I* stands for implementation of the plan, *E* stands for evaluation, and *R* stands for reassessment of the patient's problems and needs.

The *Kardex* consists of flip-over cards, one for each patient, which contain pertinent information about a patient's ongoing plan of care. If Kardex is used, nurses are able to refer to it frequently throughout their shift and during the change-of-shift report. Each card provides a summary of information, e.g. medical diagnosis, medical officer's orders, nursing care plan, details related to the activities of daily living; and specific orders related to diet, current medications, scheduled tests or procedures etc. The Kardex provides a quick and easily accessible source of current information about each patient.

Principles of recording

When recording information on any chart or document is it essential that:

- Ink is used, as pencil does not provide a permanent record.
- Writing is neat and legible, as illegible entries can be misinterpreted.
- The patient's full name, U.R. number and other pertinent details are clearly stated on each sheet.
- The date and time are included for each entry.
- Only approved abbreviations are used, to avoid misinterpretations.
- Correct spelling is used, e.g. in relation to recording medications.
- Any errors made are not erased or scratched out. Instead, the nurse should draw a single line through the error, write the word 'error' and initial it or sign her name.
- No lines or spaces are left. A line should be drawn through the blank space in a partially completed line of writing to prevent others from recording in a space with someone else's signatures.
- The information is accurate, concise, and factual. The nurse should not record her own interpretations or speculations, but record only what she actually observed or measured. *Concise* communication enables better understanding of information. Be *specific* and avoid using ambiguous statements where the meaning is unclear.
- Nursing actions are not recorded before they have been performed. Once performed, they are recorded immediately to avoid errors or omissions.
- Recording is performed in a logical and sequential manner. An organized record, e.g. progress notes, addresses each topic thoroughly before a new topic is introduced.
- When recording subjective data the patient's own words are used whenever possible, using quotation marks to indicate that the statement is a direct quote.
- Each entry is signed by the person who records it. Most health care agencies require that a full signature and title is included, e.g. Jane Smith S.E.N.
- The nurse is aware of the health care agency's policies regarding charting and documentation.
- Confidentiality is respected, e.g. avoid leaving documentation in an area where it can be read by unauthorized persons. Nurses are legally and ethically required to maintain confidentiality about any information relating to a patient.

Computers are being used increasingly in major health care agencies, e.g. to record some patient information. It is possible that, in the future, manual recording of information will be replaced by computerized systems of recording. Instead of recording on a patient's chart, health team members will be able to enter the information directly into a computer. Information relating to the patient's care can then be retrieved when needed. It is, therefore, important for nurses to become familiar with any computerized information systems if they are being used.

CONCLUSION

Reporting and recording are the two major ways in which communication takes place among members of the health team.

Continuity of care and the pursuit of common objectives depends on effective communication, which involves accurate and precise verbal and written reporting and recording of information.

A nurse has a responsibility to report verbally, to the nurse in charge, details of the observations she has made and the nursing care she has implemented.

A verbal report, using written records, is given on each patient at each change of shift. The report must be delivered in such a way that the nurse who is receiving it obtains an accurate assessment of each patient and his current condition.

In addition to change-of-shift reports, team conferences are held regularly to evaluate the progress of patients.

All pertinent information is recorded in writing to provide a permanent form of communication about each patient. Written records, in whatever format, are used for the purposes of *communication*, assessment, auditing, education and research, and legal documentation.

REFERENCES AND FURTHER READING

Potter P A, Perry A G 1985 Fundamentals of nursing. C V Mosby, St Louis
Robinson J (ed) 1981 Documenting patient care responsibly: nursing skillbook, 2nd edn. Intermed communications, Pennsylvania

Structure and functions of the human body

15. Science in nursing

INTRODUCTION

A basic knowledge of two sciences, physics and chemistry, is helpful in many aspects of nursing. This chapter, therefore, addresses some of those aspects of physics and chemistry which help to:

- provide a framework which is of value in the study of physiology.
- provide the nurse with an understanding of the rationale behind many nursing practices.

Although the boundary between the two sciences is often indistinct:

- *Physics* may be defined as the study of the laws and properties of matter, particularly as related to motion and force.
- *Chemistry* may be defined as the science dealing with the elements, their compounds, and the chemical structure and interactions of matter.

The concepts of atoms, atomic structure, and bonding provide the link between physics and chemistry. Both physics and chemistry are interrelated and interdependent, and one action rarely happens in isolation. Therefore, this chapter does not divide the information into 'physics' or 'chemistry' as such, but outlines some of the physical and chemical principles which are commonly applied in nursing practice.

FORCES AND MECHANICS

One general area of physics is known as *mechanics*, which includes the concepts of motion, force, work, energy and power. A knowledge of some of the basic principles of mechanics will give an insight into many nursing activities, e.g. the most effective methods of assisting a patient into position, or an understanding of the traction systems that may be applied to part of a patient's body. Some aspect of mechanics is always being made use of in any nursing practice, e.g. in the way in which the nurse uses her body to assist a patient to move. The principles of body mechanics, which are based on the principles of mechanics, are described in detail in Chapter 37.

Velocity

Velocity refers to motion in a straight line. In physics, velocity denotes the speed of an object moving in a straight line at a given instant of time. Velocity involves *speed* and *direction*, i.e. velocity is a vector quantity. When something is said to have a constant velocity, this means that not only is its speed not changing—but also that the direction of motion remains the same.

Acceleration

Acceleration is the rate of change of velocity. Since velocity possesses both magnitude and direction, velocity is being changed if an object is speeding up or slowing down, or if the direction in which it is moving changes.

Force

A force is a push or a pull, and the unit of force is the newton (N). A force may act on an object in various ways. For example, if an object is at rest, a force acting on it may impart an acceleration to the object. Alternatively, if an object is moving a force may cause it to slow down, speed up, or change direction.

The force of gravity is a special example of a force. Any 2 objects in space exert an attraction, e.g. the sun and the earth. In the same way, a human being and the earth attract each other. Every object exerts a gravitational force on every other object, which is proportional to the product of the masses of the 2 objects and inversely proportional to the square of the distance between them.

The centre of gravity of an object may be defined as that point at which all the forces of gravity may be said to be concentrated. For a uniform, symmetrical object, the centre of gravity is at the geometric centre. In the human being, the centre of gravity is usually located in the pelvic region near the base of the spinal column.

Mass and weight

The *mass* of an object is the amount of matter of which it is made up, whereas the *weight* of an object is a measure of the force which gravity exerts on that object. Weight force is proportional to the product of the masses of 2 objects, and inversely proportional to the square of the distance between them. Mass is measured in kilograms (kg), and weight (being a force) is measured in newtons (N). When an individual is referring to his 'weight', he is usually referring to his mass.

Equilibrium

Equilibrium is a state of balance owing to the equal action of opposing forces. Any object which is balanced, and remains in a fixed position, is said to be in static equilibrium. The *sum* of the forces acting on the object is zero.

Homeostasis, discussed later in this chapter, is sometimes referred to as 'dynamic equilibrium', or a state of 'dynamic balance'.

Vectors

Vector quantities are those which possess both magnitude and direction. A vector is normally represented by a straight line with an arrowhead at one end (Fig. 15.1). The arrow shows the direction of the vector force, and its length may be used to represent its magnitude.

In the care of a patient who has an orthopaedic condition, traction is often used to exert a force on one of his extremities, e.g. a leg. When traction, or pull, is applied in one direction, an equal but opposite pull is also required to maintain stability. If a (traction) force is applied without countertraction to a leg, the patient's body tends to slide in the direction of the force, lessening magnitude of the force and the effect on the area being treated. By applying traction forces in 2 different but not opposite directions to the same body part, e.g. the leg, a resultant (vector) force is created.

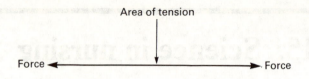
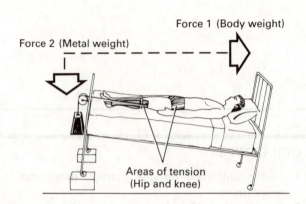

Fig. 15.1 Vectors.

Pulleys

A pulley serves to change the direction of a force. Fixed or moveable pulleys are used in traction setups, and allow a hanging weight to exert a force in almost any direction. Moveable pulleys are used to increase the effective force exerting traction (as in a "block and tackle" arrangement).

Levers

A lever (Fig. 15.2) consists of a rigid bar arranged in such a way that it can pivot about some definite point (the fulcrum) in order to overcome some resistance force. A force which is applied at one point on the bar is used to overcome another force at another point. Levers can be divided into three classes which are referred to as first, second, and third class levers.

A first class lever is one in which the pivot point (fulcrum) is somewhere between the effort and resistance forces (load), e.g. a pair of scissors.

A second class lever is one in which the resistance force is exerted between the pivot point and the effort force, e.g. a wheelbarrow, wheelchair.

A third class lever is one in which the effort force is exerted between the resistance force and the pivot, e.g. a fishing rod, scalpel.

Numerous examples of lever systems are found in the co-operative action of the muscles, ligaments, and bones of the body. For example, the action of the biceps muscle in lifting the forearm can be described as a third class lever—with the elbow being the pivot point or fulcrum.

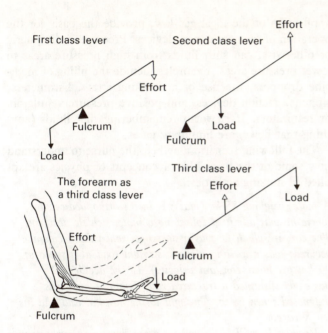

First class lever

Second class lever

Effort

Effort

Fulcrum

Load

Load

Fulcrum

Load

The forearm as
a third class lever

Third class lever

Effort

Effort

Load

Fulcrum

Effort

Load

Fulcrum

Fulcrum

Fig. 15.2 Levers.

Friction

When there is relative motion between 2 surfaces which are in contact, there will be a force which resists this motion. The degree of frictional force will depend on the nature of the surfaces, and upon the amount of force pressing the 2 surfaces together.

The force of friction is the force that enables an individual to walk, as friction normally exists between the soles of shoes and the surface on which an individual is walking. If this friction is reduced, e.g. because the floor surface is too smooth or wet, walking becomes difficult as the footwear cannot get a 'grip' on the floor.

Friction has some disadvantages, e.g. it can damage skin surfaces when the skin comes into contact with surfaces which are not smooth. The skin of a patient who is confined to bed may be damaged if care is not taken to maintain a smooth, wrinkle free surface under him.

Energy

Energy can be loosely defined as the ability or the capacity for doing work. Energy can take many forms such as heat, electrical, nuclear or mechanical energy.

Mechanical energy is divided into two classes; kinetic and potential energy. *Kinetic energy* is the energy associated with motion, whereas *potential* energy is the energy associated with position or configuration.

In physiology, kinetics is the study of the forces that produce, arrest, or modify the motions of the body.

Newton's laws of inertia are especially applicable to kinetics.

Newton's first law states that bodies at rest tend to stay at rest, and bodies in motion in a straight line tend to keep moving in the same direction.

Newton's third law states that action and reaction are equal in magnitude, but opposite in direction.

These laws are applicable to the forces produced by muscles of the body which act on joints. The reaction forces of the muscles contribute to the equilibrium and the motion of the body.

Potential energy of position refers to the energy an object possesses as a result of its height above a given reference point. For example, a weight in a traction apparatus has potential energy because it is higher than the floor.

Potential energy of configuration (state) is the energy possessed, e.g. by a stretched elastic band, a compressed coil spring—or other objects that have the ability to do work if released. Potential energy of state also refers to the storage of energy in a chemical form, in the chemical bonds of compounds.

Each form of energy (kinetic and potential) can be converted to the other form. For example, if a traction weight (which has no kinetic energy) is suddenly released, the potential energy possessed by the weight is changed to kinetic energy as the weight descends. Conversely if an object is thrown up into the air, the kinetic energy imparted by the object is changed into potential energy—as the object moves upwards.

Pressure

Pressure may be defined as force per unit area. Alternatively, pressure may be defined as a force (per unit area) or stress (per unit area) applied to a surface by a fluid or an object. The concept of pressure applies equally well to solids, liquids and gases, since the force involved may be applied equally well any a solid, liquid, or gas. Some of the principles and concepts relating to pressure that are relevant to nursing are described below.

Pascal's principle. A *law* stating that a confined liquid transmits pressure, applied to it from an external force, equally in all directions. Pascal's principle provides the basis for all hydraulic devices, e.g. a hydraulic lift used to move a patient from or into a bed. Another example where Pascal's principle is used is the water or air mattress. Nursing a patient on a water or air mattress tends to evenly distribute the pressure to all areas of his body thus reducing the possibility of skin and tissue damage.

Boyle's law. A law stating that the volume of a given mass of gas is inversely proportional to the pressure to which it is subjected, provided that the temperature remains constant.

Boyle's law provides the basis for the functioning of a

syringe. When the plunger is withdrawn while the needle end is immersed in a liquid, the volume of air below the plunger increases while the pressure decreases.

Boyle's law is able to be applied to the process of breathing. During inhalation the movements that occur serve to increase the volume of the thoracic cavity. By Boyle's law, this means that the pressure in the thoracic cavity is decreased below atmospheric pressure, so air, at a higher pressure outside the thoracic cavity, flows *into* the lungs. During exhalation the movements that occur serve to decrease the volume of the thoracic cavity. By Boyle's law, this means that the pressure in the thoracic cavity is increased above atmospheric pressure, so air flows out from the lungs.

Charles' law. A law stating that the volume of a given mass of gas is directly proportional to its absolute temperature, provided the pressure remains constant. For example, as the temperature of a gas is increased, at constant pressure, the gas expands.

The general gas law (or ideal gas law). Both Boyle's law and Charles' law deal with special cases of the ideal gas law. A gas which is composed of hard spherical molecules which move randomly at high speeds, and interact with each other only by collision, is referred to as an *ideal gas*. The state of an ideal gas can be specified by measuring the pressure, volume, and temperature of the gas. The *ideal gas law* considers those 3 variables at once.

An example of one application of the ideal gas law under *constant volume* conditions, is the safety precaution of keeping pressure packs away from direct heat. In this instance, the volume in the pack is *constant*, and the variables involved are pressure and temperature. If the temperature of the pack is increased, the pressure inside it is increased proportionally—and the risk of explosion is increased.

The concepts of *negative and positive pressure*. These terms are used when a pressure is being compared to normal atmospheric pressure:

- Any pressure *above* normal atmospheric pressure is regarded as a positive pressure.
- Any pressure *below* normal atmospheric pressure is regarded as a negative pressure.

One application of these concepts is in the use of 'suction' equipment. In practice, 'suction' amounts to a decrease in pressure compared to atmospheric pressure. Any fluid between a suction device and the atmosphere will be forced into the device.

Atmospheric pressure. The total pressure exerted by the atmosphere is called atmospheric pressure. Atmospheric pressure arises by virtue of the weight of the air above the earth's surface. It is for this reason that atmospheric pressure decreases as altitude increases. Even at a particular altitude, atmospheric pressure is not constant—but varies according to atmospheric conditions.

The combined effects of atmospheric pressure and the application of the ideal gas law, provide the basis for the operation of many common devices. Pressure, atmospheric or otherwise, can shift fluids from high pressure areas to lower pressure areas. Examples include the filling of medicine droppers, the use of a drinking straw, barometers, siphons, suction devices, and positive pressure ventilators or respirators. It is worth remembering that fluids (anything that flows) are liquids *or* gases.

The following scenario may help the nurse to understand how some of the principles or concepts of physics are applied in nursing activities:

A male weighing 85 kg (mass) is in the orthopaedic ward, where he was admitted following a motor vehicle accident. The car, in which he was a passenger when the accident occured, was travelling along a straight road at a speed of 90 km per hour (constant velocity). In the accident the passenger sustained a fractured right femur, which was diagnosed when he was brought to the hospital and had his leg X-rayed.

Because he will be in bed for some time, a sheepskin rug has been positioned under him to prevent friction between the bottom sheets and his skin. As part of his treatment, traction has been applied to his right leg. The traction apparatus applied to his leg exerts a pull (force) on the leg, by a system of weights, ropes and pulleys. The traction force consists of the weight, and countertraction is provided by the weight of his body—as the foot of the bed has been elevated. The pulleys in the traction system act to establish the direction in which the force (vectors) acts.

After several days in hospital, the medical officer requests an X-ray of his leg to assess the effectiveness of the treatment. Two people were required to wheel the bed, as their combined efforts meant that a greater force was applied—and thus a greater acceleration—to move the bed from its stationary position.

There was maximum friction between the rubber of the wheels and the floor, therefore the bed did not 'skid' as it was being moved. There was minimum friction in the wheel bearings, thus they were able to roll easily as the bed was being moved down the corridor. As the two people were wheeling the bed, their lower legs were acting as second class levers during the act of walking. The ball of the foot acted as the fulcrum, the force was applied by a muscle at the back of the leg to overcome another force of the body mass acting through the ankle bones.

MATTER

To assist in understanding normal body function, and body dysfunction, a knowledge of certain chemical principles is important. An understanding of chemistry is the basis for the study of homeostasis, which is described later in the chapter.

All living and non-living materials are generally classified as matter. *Matter* can be defined as that which occupies space and has mass. All matter can be broken down into about a hundred different elements, and the smallest 'working' unit of any element is the atom. Atoms, in turn, are composed of particles—electrons, protons, and neutrons, and even much smaller 'particles' which hold atoms together. The human body, like all other matter, is composed of atoms (which are the fundamental units of matter).

Atoms

An atom is composed of a positively charged nucleus of protons and neutrons, surrounded by negatively charged electrons in orbit around the nucleus. Protons carry a positive electrical charge, electrons carry a negative charge, and neutrons are neutral with no charge. Since atoms do not exhibit any nett or overall electrical charge under normal conditions, the number of positively charged protons in each neutral atom equals the number of negatively charged electrons. The number of neutrons may vary, but they do not affect the charge of the atom.

Isotopes are atoms of the same element having the same number of protons but different mass numbers, due to having different numbers of *neutrons* in the nucleus. Thus, isotopes differ in the number of their neutrons and atomic weights. For example, one isotope of carbon has 6 neutrons in the nucleus, another has 7, and another has 8. All have 6 protons, so all are carbon atoms. Many radioactive isotopes are used in diagnostic and therapeutic procedures.

Atoms differ from each other in the number of particles they contain; and to aid in the identification of atoms, each one is assigned an atomic number. The *atomic number* of an atom is the number of protons in its nucleus. For example, the carbon atom has 6 protons—therefore its atomic number is 6.

Elements

Matter which is composed entirely of the same kind of atoms, i.e. each with the same number of protons, is an *element*. Over one hundred chemical elements are known to exist, each with its own atomic number and its own particular chemical properties. Each element (and thus each kind of atom) is named, and has been given a unique symbol which is used as a 'shorthand' for that element. Table 15.1 lists some naturally occuring elements, their chemical symbol, and their atomic number. Elements can combine with each other to form new substances—thus one atom of sodium (Na) combines with one atom of chlorine (Cl) to form a salt—sodium chloride (NaCl); similarly one atom of Carbon (C) combines with *two* atoms of oxygen (O_2) to form carbon *di*oxide (CO_2).

Table 15.2 lists the common elements that make up the human body. Over 95% of the body is made up from the

Table 15.1 Some naturally occurring elements

Name	Symbol	Atomic Number
Aluminium	Al	13
Antimony	Sb	51
Argon	Ar	18
Arsenic	As	33
Barium	Ba	56
Beryllium	Be	4
Bismuth	Bi	83
Boron	B	5
Bromine	Br	35
Cadmium	Cd	48
Caesium	Cs	55
Calcium	Ca	20
Carbon	C	6
Cerium	Ce	58
Chlorine	Cl	17
Chromium	Cr	24
Cobalt	Co	27
Copper	Cu	29
Dysprosium	Dy	66
Erbium	Er	99
Europium	Eu	63
Fluorine	F	9
Gadolinium	Gd	64
Gallium	Ga	31
Germanium	Ge	32
Gold	Au	79
Hafnium	Hf	72
Helium	He	2
Holmium	Ho	67
Hydrogen	H	1
Indium	In	49
Iodine	I	53
Iridium	Ir	77
Iron	Fe	26
Krypton	Kr	36
Lanthanum	La	57
Lead	Pb	82
Lithium	Li	3
Lutetium	Lu	71
Magnesium	Mg	12
Manganese	Mn	25
Mercury	Hg	80
Molybdenum	Mo	42
Neodymium	Nd	60
Neon	Ne	10
Nickel	Ni	28
Niobium	Nb	41
Nitrogen	N	7
Osmium	Os	76
Oxygen	O	8
Palladium	Pd	46
Phosphorus	P	15
Platinum	Pt	78
Potassium	K	19
Praseodymium	Pr	59
Radium	Ra	88
Radon	Rn	86
Rhenium	Re	75
Rhodium	Rh	45
Rubidium	Rb	37
Ruthenium	Ru	44
Samarium	Sm	62
Scandium	Sc	21
Selenium	Se	34
Silicon	Si	14
Silver	Ag	47
Sodium	Na	11
Strontium	Sr	38
Sulfur	S	16

Table 15.1 (cont'd)   Some naturally occurring elements

Name	Symbol	Atomic Number
Tantalum	Ta	73
Tellurium	Te	52
Terbium	Tb	65
Thallium	Tl	81
Thorium	Th	90
Thulium	Tm	69
Tin	Sn	50
Titanium	Ti	22
Tungsten	W	74
Uranium	U	92
Vanadium	V	23
Xenon	Xe	54
Ytterbium	Yb	70
Yttrium	Y	39
Zinc	Zn	30
Zirconium	Zr	40

Table 15.2   Elements in the body

Element	Chemical symbol	Percentage (approximate)
Oxygen	O	65
Carbon	C	18
Hydrogen	H	10
Nitrogen	N	3
Calcium	Ca	1.5
Phosphorous	P	1
Potassium	K	0.4
Sulphur	S	0.3
Sodium	Na	0.2
Magnesium	Mg	0.1
Chlorine	Cl	0.1
Iron	Fe	Trace
Iodine	I	Trace
Copper	Cu	Trace
Zinc	Zn	Trace
Cobalt	Co	Trace
Fluorine	F	Trace

elements oxygen, carbon, hydrogen, and nitrogen; while the remaining 5% is comprised mainly of calcium and phosphorous with other elements in very small quantities.

Molecules

A molecule is the smallest unit of matter that can exist alone and exhibit the characteristic chemical properties of an element or a combination of elements. A molecule is composed of two or more atoms held together by electrical forces (chemical bonds). A molecule can consist of atoms of the same kind, or of two or more atoms of different kinds. A change in the structural position of any atom in the molecule will alter its chemical characteristics.

Molecules may be classified into two basic types; organic and inorganic:

- *Organic molecules* contain the element carbon, and are the principle materials from which the structures of living things are formed.
- *Inorganic molecules* may or may not contain carbon,

and are smaller and more simple than organic molecules.

Mixtures

A mixture is made up of two or more elements or compounds that have been mixed, without forming a new compound. Therefore, the elements present in the mixture retain their individual properties, and the components of a mixture can be separated by physical means.

Compounds

A compound is a substance composed of two or more different elements, chemically combined in definite proportions, that cannot be separated by physical means. A compound has different properties from those of its individual elements.

Ions and electrolytes

Elements or compounds that dissolve in water, or other solvents, to form separate ions are called electrolytes.

An ion is an atom or molecule that has gained or lost one or more electrons, and is therefore electrically charged. Movement of ions constitutes an electric current. Positively charged ions are called *cations*, and negatively charged ions are called *anions*.

Electrolytes are chemical substances which, when dissolved or melted, dissociate into ions and can conduct an electric current. Electrolytes are a major constituent of all body fluids, and they affect the functioning of many physiological processes. Electrolytes are, for example:

- essential to the normal function of all cells
- involved in metabolic activities
- involved in fluid homeostasis
- involved in creating charge differences on which the functioning of nerves and muscles depend.

The maintenance of electrolyte balance in the body depends on homeostatic mechanisms which regulate the absorption, distribution and excretion of water and the solutes dissolved in it. Many disease processes can cause an electrolyte imbalance, e.g. prolonged diarrhoea may cause a loss of many electrolytes.

Acids and bases

An acid is any substance which releases protons (hydrogen ions) when dissolved in water. Acids have chemical properties essentially opposite to those of bases.

A base is any substance which accepts protons in chemical reactions. *Alkalis* are bases which are soluble in water.

Acids react with bases to form a salt and water: bases react with acids to form a salt and water. *A salt* is a compound formed when an acid and a base react together. Salts are usually composed of a metal ion and a non-metal ion.

If a strong acid and a strong base react, the salt formed is *neutral* in solution.

If a weak acid and a weak base react, the salt formed is *neutral* in solution.

If a strong acid and a weak base react, the salt formed is *basic* in solution.

If a weak acid and a strong base react, the salt formed is *acidic* in solution.

Acid-base balance is a condition existing when the rate at which the body produces acids or bases, equals the rate at which acids or bases are excreted. The result of acid-base balance is a stable concentration of *hydrogen ions* in body fluids.

The meaning of pH

The pH scale is used to express the concentration of hydrogen ions in acids or bases. The 'p' stands for potential or power, and the 'H' stands for hydrogen. Therefore, pH represents the potential or power of hydrogen.

The pH of a solution is determined by measuring the number of hydrogen ions present. The pH scale is numbered from 0–14; and the lower the number on the scale, the more hydrogen ions are present—and the more acid the solution. At pH 7, the solution is neutral, if the pH is above 7 the solution is basic or alkaline; and a solution is acid if the pH is between 0 and 7.

The acid—base balance is critical in the human body, e.g. the pH of the blood needs to be kept within the range of 7.35–7.45 if problems are not to arise.

Acidosis is a condition where there is an abnormal increase in hydrogen ion concentration—owing to an accumulation of an acid, or the loss of a base.

Alkalosis is a condition characterized by an increased pH, above 7.45.

Buffer systems

A buffer is a chemical substance which resists changes in the pH of solutions. Buffers maintain the normal pH range of a solution by reacting with a relatively strong acid or base, and thereby decreasing the acidic or basic strength of the solution. Buffer systems provide the body fluids, especially the blood, with protection against drastic changes in acidity or alkalinity.

Some of the most important buffer systems in the body fluids are the bicarbonate system, proteins, and the phosphate system. Buffer systems compensate for any situation that tends to alter the normal pH of body fluids, and thus maintain *homeostasis*. Homeostasis is achieved by all the buffer systems working together.

Chemical energy

Chemical reactions, whereby one substance is changed into another substance or substances, are accomplished by a transfer of energy. Chemical reactions that take place in the body cells result in the release of energy. The major source of energy for the body is the food that is consumed. The energy which the cell extracts from the metabolic breakdown of food can be stored in ATP molecules until needed.

Adenosine triphosphate (ATP) is an organic compound produced in all cells, which can readily liberate its energy. When energy is required for cellular activity, a bond of ATP molecule is broken and its energy is released. ATP provides the energy necessary for most physiological processes to take place efficiently. Energy is required by all the cells to:

- synthesize large molecules from smaller ones (anabolism)
- act together to cause muscles to contract
- support the electrical energy of nerves
- effect active transport
- supply heat.

The energy for such activities is supplied by energy-releasing reactions; cellular respiration being the significant energy-releasing reaction in the human body. Cellular respiration is the process by which fuels such as glucose are utilized by means of a series of chemical reactions to produce energy. Oxygen is required, and water and carbon dioxide are released as by-products. Therefore:

$$Glucose + oxygen \rightarrow \begin{array}{c} Carbon \\ dioxide \end{array} + Water + ENERGY$$
$$(C_6H_{12}O_6) \quad (6O_2) \quad (6CO_2) \quad (6H_2O)$$

Most of the chemical reactions in the body require the assistance of catalysts to influence the rates at which chemical reactions proceed. The body's catalysts are a group of proteins known as enzymes.

Transport mechanisms

It is important to understand the mechanisms by which substances move in and out of the body cells. The transport mechanisms that move substances in and out of cells are diffusion, osmosis, active transport, phagocytosis, pinocytosis, and filtration.

Diffusion

Diffusion (Fig. 15.3) is the movement of molecules or ions

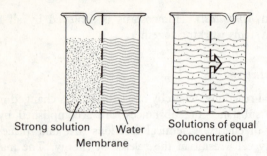

Fig. 15.3   Diffusion.

from one region to another, due to random molecular motion, until a dynamic equilibrium is reached. Normally, molecules will tend to move from a region of higher concentration to a region of lower concentration, until the concentration is the same in both regions. Sometimes, diffusion of fluids occurs through a membrane, e.g. the movement of oxygen from alveoli in the lungs through the fine capillary membrane into the blood stream. Many substances in the body diffuse, e.g. electrolytes, amino acids, and glucose. The rate at which diffusion occurs depends upon a number of factors which include:

- the size of the molecules, as larger molecules move less rapidly.
- concentration, as the greater the difference in concentration between the two regions the faster the rate of diffusion.
- temperature, as the higher the temperature the faster the rate of diffusion.

Osmosis

Osmosis (Fig. 15.4) is a term used to describe the *diffusion* of a solvent across a membrane. Osmosis is the movement of a solvent, e.g. water, through a semipermeable membrane from a solution that has a lower solute concentration—to one that has a higher solute concentration. Movement across the membrane continues until the concentrations of the solutions equalize. The rate at which osmosis occurs depends upon a number of factors which include:

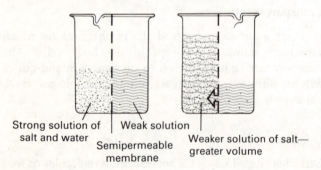

Fig. 15.4   Osmosis.

- the concentration of solute
- the temperature of the solution
- the electrical charge of the solute
- the difference between the osmotic pressures exerted by the solutions.

Osmotic pressure is the pressure exerted on a semipermeable membrane separating a solution from a solvent. The osmotic pressure of a solution is the pressure required to prevent the diffusion from a pure solvent into that solution.

Active transport

Active transport is the transfer of materials across a membrane, by means of chemical activity (using energy from ATP) that allows the cell to admit larger molecules than would otherwise be able to enter. Ions which are transported by this mechanism include sodium, potassium, hydrogen, calcium, iron, and chloride ions. Substances also transported in this way include sugars and amino acids.

Phagocytosis

Phagocytosis (Fig. 15.5) is the process by which certain cells engulf and dispose of micro-organisms and cell debris. One example of this is the ingestion of bacteria by leukocytes (white blood cells). The leukocytes ingest foreign substances by flowing around them in amoeboid fashion, and engulfing them. That part of the cell membrane around the foreign matter is pinched off, forming a vesicle (small sac).

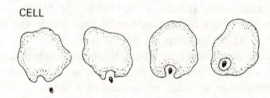

Fig. 15.5   Phagocytosis.

Pinocytosis

Pinocytosis (Fig. 15.6) is a similar process to phagocytosis, and is the process by which extracellular fluid is taken into a cell. The cell membrane develops an indentation filled with extracellular fluid, then closes around it—forming a

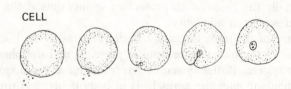

Fig. 15.6   Pinocytosis.

vaccule of fluid within the cell. Pinocytosis is the only mechanism by which large molecules, such as protein, can be transported into a cell.

Filtration

Filtration involves the removal of particles from a solution by allowing the liquid portion to pass through a membrane. In the body, filtration involves *hydrostatic pressure* which forces liquid with ions and small molecules dissolved in it, through a membrane—leaving behind larger molecules. Filtration, like diffusion, is a passive process and substances move from a higher pressure area to the lower pressure area. Filtration which occurs in the capillaries, and in the glomerulus of the kidneys, is a one way process—as distinct from diffusion.

Radiation

Radiation is the emission of energy, rays, or waves. Nuclear radiation refers to those particles or waves which emanate from the nucleus of the atom.

Radioactivity is the result of nuclear instability; if there are too many or too few neutrons in a nucleus, it is unstable (radioactive) and breaks up. Therefore, radioactive means giving off radiation as the result of the disintegration of the nucleus of an atom. Natural radioactivity is a property exhibited by all chemical elements with an atomic number greater than 83 (refer to Table 15.1). Artificial radioactivity is achieved through the bombardment of naturally occurring isotopes with subatomic particles or with high levels of gamma or X-radiation (see below).

Isotopes are the various forms of an element. All isotopes of a particular element have the same number of protons and electrons, but each has a different number of neutrons. Many isotopes are radioactive and are called *radioisotopes*. Radioisotopes are used in medicine for therapeutic and diagnostic purposes including:

- as radiotracers to locate abnormalities such as tumours, e.g. within the lungs, brain, or bones
- as a therapeutic measure to destroy tumours
- as a palliative measure to relieve pain in advanced cancer.

Radiation therapy can be administered externally through the use of X-ray machines or radioisotopic sources, or internally through the implantation of radioisotopes into the body. Internal radioisotope therapy can be:

- intracavity, where radioactive isotopes are placed in a body cavity or body organ
- interstitial, where radioactive isotopes are implanted directly into the malignant tumour tissue
- systemic, where radioisotopes are injected intravenously.

Half-life

All radioactive material decays, and the half-life of any radioactive material is the time required for half of the mass of material to decay. Not all the nuclei of a radioactive element breakup or decay simultaneously; individual nuclei decay at different times. Half-lives of radioisotopes range from seconds to many years, e.g. the half-life of fluorine (^{18}F) is 110 minutes, whereas the half-life of carbon-14 ($^{14}_6C$) is 5570 years. In the case of medical radioisotopes, the half-life must be known for accurate dose calculations.

Types of radioactivity

The 3 basic types of radiation are alpha particles, beta particles, and gamma rays.

Alpha radiation has poor penetration ability and is rarely used in therapeutic radiation therapy. Alpha particles are identical to helium nuclei (2 protons and 2 neutrons held together).

Beta radiation is generally emitted from radioactive isotopes and is used for internal source radiation. Beta particles are electrons, emitted after the breakup of par-ticles in the nucleus of atoms.

Gamma radiation penetrates deep areas of the body. Therapeutically, gamma sources are used more than any other form of radioactive emission.

X-rays (or Roentgen rays) are produced, for medical applications, by machines.

X-rays are produced when electrons, travelling at high speed, strike certain materials—particularly heavy metals. They can penetrate most substances and are used to investigate the integrity of body structures, to therapeutically destroy diseased tissues, and to make photographic images for diagnostic purposes, e.g. as in fluoroscopy.

Laser is an acronym for 'Light Amplification by Stimulated Emission of Radiation'. By exposing a large number of electrons to a high energy level in a gaseous, solid, or liquid medium, the electrons emit very narrow beams of light. The beams are all of one wavelength and parallel to each other, and it is possible to focus the beam to an almost microscopic point. The laser is sometimes used during surgery, e.g for certain operations on the eye.

Homeostasis

Homeostasis is the term that refers to the processes by which the internal environment of the body is maintained within narrow physiological parameters. Homeostasis can also be defined as the tendency of the body to maintain the stability of the internal environment. Homeostasis is dynamic and active, as the body constantly and actively pursues the maintenance of a stable internal environment.

Homeostatic regulation of the body is achieved by the

co-operative action of most organs and tissues, e.g. the lungs, the kidneys, the cardiovascular system, the pituitary gland, the suprarenal glands, and the parathyroid glands. Much of nursing practice is aimed at maintaining or restoring the individual's homeostasis. Many of the topics discussed in this, and other chapters, relate to the state of homeostasis. For example:

- acid-base balance in body fluids
- energy production
- fluid and electrolyte balance
- body temperature regulation.

Homeostatic mechanisms are the mechanisms by which the body is able to control the state of the internal environments. They are the processes and means by which the body is able to adapt to stresses (anything which threatens or upsets homeostasis), and yet maintain its inner balance.

Any stress situation which arises, activates protective homeostatic mechanisms which endeavour to compensate for that stress. Without homeostatic mechanisms to maintain the internal environment, the body cannot survive. When the ability of the body to maintain homeostasis is overwhelmed illness, and sometimes death, occurs.

For the mechanisms to maintain homeostasis, the body must be able to detect changes and to react appropriately to those changes. The ability of the body to detect changes is through the process of feedback. Two types of feedback exist:

Negative feedback brings the body's internal environment back to its optimum state. Negative feedback is a decrease in function in response to a stimulus, e.g. if the blood glucose level rises above normal, action is instituted by several control systems (such as the islets of Langerhans in the pancreas) to restore the blood glucose level to normal.

Positive feedback directs the body's internal environment away from its optimum state. Positive feedback is an increase in function in response to a stimulus, e.g. during childbirth one uterine contraction induces further contractions which keep increasing (in intensity and frequency) until the baby is born. Many positive feedback situations are undesirable, and can for example, result in the over production of a normal body chemical—thus compounding the problem.

CONCLUSION

Nursing practice encompasses the use of physical and chemical principles and concepts. This chapter has outlined some of those principles and concepts, in an effort to provide the nurse with information that will help in the study of physiology, and which will assist in understanding the rationale behind many nursing actions.

16. The human body: an orientation

OBJECTIVES

1. Describe the position of the body cavities, and list the structures contained in each cavity.
2. State the nine regions of the abdominopelvic area.
3. State the basic functions of each body system.

INTRODUCTION

The study of anatomy and physiology explores the structure and functions of the body:

- *Anatomy* is the study of the structure of the body and the relationship of one part to another.
- *Physiology* is the study of the function of all parts of the body.

Anatomy and physiology are interdependent because the structure determines the functions which can take place. The study of anatomy and physiology is important to the nurse so that she is familiar with the human body's normal structure and function. An understanding of the normal is essential before the nurse can recognize any deviations from normal. Knowledge of anatomy and physiology also helps the nurse to understand the patient's needs, and the rationale behind specific nursing or medical intervention when there is a disturbance of body structure or function.

BODY POSITION AND DIRECTION

In order to study anatomy it is necessary to understand the common terms used to describe areas of the body. Parts of the body are described in relation to other parts and, therefore, to avoid confusion it is assumed that the body is in the anatomical position. *The anatomical position*, as illustrated in Figure 16.1, is when the body is erect, the arms at the sides with the palms facing forward, and the feet together. The neck is straight with the face looking for-

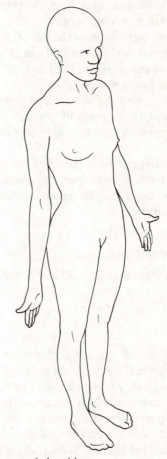

Fig. 16.1 The anatomical position.

ward. Terms that are used to describe the position of one body part in relation to another include:

- *Superior*: means upper or above, thus a superior structure is above other structures, e.g. the lungs are superior to the diaphragm.
- *Inferior*: means lower or below, thus an inferior structure is below other structures, e.g. the diaphragm is inferior to the lungs.

131

- *Anterior*: (ventral): means at or towards the front of the body or body part, e.g. the anterior surface of the body includes the face, chest, and abdomen.
- *Posterior*: (dorsal): means at or towards the back of the body or body part, e.g. the posterior surface of the body includes the back and buttocks.
- *Medial*: means towards the mid-line of the body or body part. An imaginary line drawn down the centre of the body is referred to as the median sagittal plane.
- *Lateral*: means relating to, or located at, the side of the body or body part, e.g. the arms are lateral to the trunk.
- *Superficial*: means on or near the body surface, e.g. the skin is superficial to the body's internal organs.
- *Deep*: means inward or away from the body surface, e.g. the stomach is a 'deep' organ.
- *External*: means pertaining to the outside or outer, e.g. the epidermis is the external layer of the skin.
- *Internal*: means pertaining to the inside or inner, e.g. the heart is an internal organ.
- *Proximal*: means near the centre or midline of the body, or nearest to the point of origin, e.g. the proximal interphalangeal joints are those closest to the hand.
- *Distal*: means farthest from the centre or midline of the body, or farthest away from any point of reference, e.g. the distal phalanges are those at the ends of the fingers.

Anatomical divisions

As illustrated in Figure 16.2, the body is divided into:

- the head and neck
- the trunk
- the limbs.

The head consists of the bony framework—the skull, which contains several cavities, these being the cranial, nasal, oral and orbital. *The neck* consists of the upper section of the spinal column, which contains part of the spinal cavity and the upper parts of the trachea and oesophagus, the thyroid gland, and the parathyroid glands.

The trunk is divided into the thorax, the abdomen, and the pelvis.

The limbs which are attached to the trunk consist of the upper limbs (or arms) and the lower limbs (or legs).

Body cavities

The cranial cavity (see Fig. 16.3) is the space inside the bones of the cranium. The cranium consists of eight bones joined together to form the boundaries of the cranial cavity. The cranial cavity contains the brain, the pituitary gland, blood vessels and lymphatic vessels.

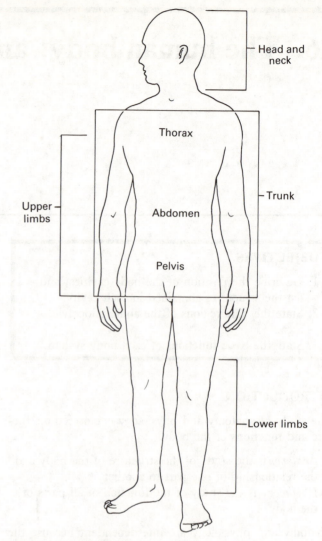

Fig. 16.2 Anatomical divisions.

The other cavities in the skull include the *nasal* cavities which are two passages inside the nose and are separated from each other by the nasal septum. The *oral* cavity is the area bordered by the teeth, and contains the tongue. The *orbital* cavities are the bony depressions in the skull which contain the eyes.

The spinal cavity, or neural canal, (Fig. 16.3) is the space inside the bones forming the vertebral column, and extends from the skull to the first or second lumbar vertebra. The spinal cavity contains the spinal cord which is surrounded by meninges, and the origins of the spinal nerves which exit from the vertebral column. Blood and lymphatic vessels are also contained in the spinal cavity.

The thoracic cavity (Fig. 16.3) is the space in the upper trunk. The boundaries of the thoracic cavity are the neck, the sternum and ribs, the thoracic vertebrae, and the diaphragm. The thoracic cavity contains the heart, lungs,

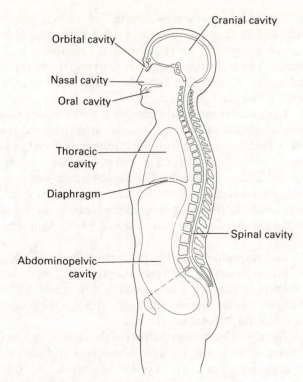

Cranial cavity

Orbital cavity

Nasal cavity

Oral cavity

Thoracic cavity

Diaphragm

Spinal cavity

Abdominopelvic cavity

Fig. 16.3 Body cavities.

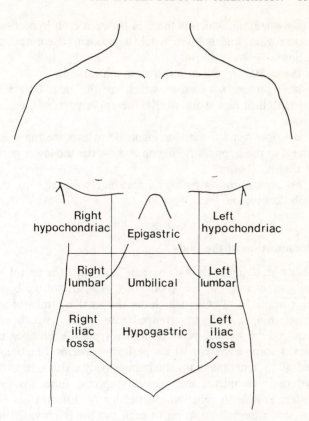

Right hypochondriac

Epigastric

Left hypochondriac

Right lumbar

Umbilical

Left lumbar

Right iliac fossa

Hypogastric

Left iliac fossa

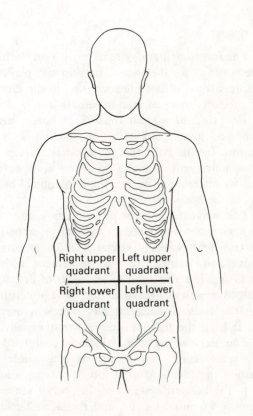

Right upper quadrant

Left upper quadrant

Right lower quadrant

Left lower quadrant

Fig. 16.4 Quadrants and regions of the abdominopelvic area.

lower trachea, the bronchi, the oesophagus, the thymus gland, blood and lymphatic vessels, and nerves.

The abdominopelvic cavity (Fig. 16.3) is the cavity inferior to the diaphragm and, although there is no physical structure dividing them, it is usual to consider the abdominal and pelvic cavities separately.

The *abdominal* cavity is the space in the middle trunk. The boundaries of the abdominal cavity are the abdominal muscle wall, the lumbar vertebrae, the diaphragm, and the pelvic girdle. The abdominal cavity contains the stomach, small and large intestine, liver, gall bladder, spleen, pancreas, kidneys, upper part of the ureters, suprarenal glands, blood and lymphatic vessels, and nerves.

The *pelvic* cavity is the lower portion of the abdominal cavity and is enclosed by the pelvic girdle. The floor of the pelvis is formed by muscles. The pelvic cavity contains the urinary bladder and urethra, the lower parts of the ureters and the intestine, and the reproductive organs. The female pelvic cavity contains the ovaries, uterus, uterine tubes and the vagina; while the male pelvic cavity contains the prostate gland, vas deferens, and seminal vesicles.

The abdominopelvic area can be studied more easily if it is divided into 4 equal regions or quadrants, or by further dividing it into 9 regions. Figure 16.4 illustrates the quadrants and regions of the abdominopelvic area. The regions are:

• *the right and left hypochondriac*, which are the regions lateral to the epigastric region, and overlie the lower ribs.

- *the epigastric*, which is the area between each hypochondriac region, and is immediately superior to the umbilical region.
- *the umbilical*, which is the most central area.
- *the right and left lumbar*, which are the areas lateral to the umbilical region and overlie the upper parts of the iliac bones.
- *the right and left iliac* (or inguinal), which are the areas lateral to the hypogastric region and overlie the lower parts of the iliac bones.
- *the hypogastric*, which is immediately inferior to the umbilical region.

Organization of the body

Before studying each body system in detail, it is useful to have an overview of the whole body. All parts of the body are comprised of cells, which are the smallest units of all living things. Cells are grouped into tissues, which are arranged in specific ways to form organs. A number of organs form a system which performs specific functions, and all systems make up the human body. Although each system is complete, and performs specific functions, no system is able to function independently. Information on the structure and function of each system is provided in Chapters 18–27.

Body systems

1. **The integumentary system** (or the skin) forms a protective covering for the body. The skin also plays a major role in regulation of body temperature, in the excretion of waste products in sweat, and in sensation.

2. **The skeletal system** consists of bones, cartilages, tendons and joints, and its major function is to form a framework for the body that the skeletal muscles can use to cause movement. Some of the bones also provide protection for internal organs, and the formation of blood cells occurs in the bone marrow.

3. **The muscular system** provides movement. Muscle tissue is classified as skeletal (or voluntary), smooth (or involuntary), and cardiac. Skeletal muscles are attached to the bones, and contract to cause movement of the body. Smooth muscle forms most of the walls of hollow organs and blood vessels, and enables the passage of substances within the body. Cardiac muscle is present only in the heart, and has the ability to contract rhythmically.

4. **The nervous system**, which is comprised of the brain, spinal cord, and nerves, is responsible for coordinating the functions of all other systems. Closely related to the nervous system are the special sense organs: the ears, eyes, nose, tongue, and the skin. These organs receive sensations from the environment and relay them to the brain for interpretation.

5. **The endocrine system** consists of various glands which produce chemical substances called hormones. Hormones are responsible for stimulating and regulating body activities. The endocrine glands are the pituitary, thyroid, parathyroids, suprarenals, islets of Langerhans, ovaries, testes, thymus, and the pineal gland.

6. **The circulatory system** consists of the cardiovascular system comprised of the heart, the blood vessels, and the blood. Closely associated with the cardiovascular system is the *lymphatic system* consisting of lymph, lymphatic vessels, lymphatic nodes and glands. The cardiovascular and lymphatic systems together form the circulatory system which is responsible for the transport of various substances to and from the cells, and which plays a major role in combating infection.

7. **The respiratory system** consists of the nasal passages, pharynx, larynx, the bronchial tree, the lungs, and the ventilatory muscles. The respiratory system enables the exchange of carbon dioxide and oxygen through the actions of external and internal respiration.

8. **The digestive system** consists of the alimentary canal (or digestive tract) and the accessary organs of digestion. The alimentary canal is comprised of the mouth, oropharynx, oesophagus, stomach, and the small and large intestine. The accessary organs, comprised of the salivary glands, the pancreas, and the liver, secrete substances into the alimentary canal which assist in the process of digestion. The digestive system is responsible for the digestion of food, the absorption of nutrients, and the elimination of wastes as faeces.

9. **The urinary system** consists of the kidneys, ureters, urinary bladder, and the urethra. The urinary system is responsible for the excretion of waste products in urine, and plays a major role in the maintenance of the body's fluid balance and acid-base balance.

10. **The reproductive systems**. The female reproductive system consists of the internal reproductive organs (the ovaries, uterine tubes, uterus, and vagina), and the external genitalia (the vulva). The male reproductive system consists of the internal reproductive organs (testes, epididymis, deferent duct, seminal vesicles, ejaculatory ducts, bulbo-urethral glands, the prostate gland), and the external genitalia (penis and scrotum). The reproductive systems are responsible for the continuation of the species.

SUMMARY

Anatomy is the study of the structure of the body, and physiology is the study of how a structure functions.

To plan and implement nursing care, the nurse should first have an understanding of the normal human body. The nurse should understand the terminology used to describe parts of the body in relation to other parts, and she should be aware that the descriptions are used on the assumption that the body is in the anatomical position.

Anatomically, the human body is divided into the head and neck, the trunk, and the limbs. The body contains the cranial, spinal, thoracic, and abdominopelvic cavities.

The cell is the fundamental unit of all living things, and cells are grouped to form tissues. In turn, tissues are arranged to form organs, and a number of organs form a system. Each system performs specific functions, but no system is capable of independent function. The body is comprised of ten systems: the integumentary, skeletal, muscular, nervous, endocrine, circulatory, respiratory, digestive, urinary, and the reproductive system.

17. Cells and tissues

INTRODUCTION

The human body develops from one microscopic cell which is formed by the fusion of a male reproductive cell or spermatozoon, with a female reproductive cell or ovum. The fertilized ovum grows, and then reproduces by dividing to form two cells which will also divide to form four cells. This process of division continues until millions of microscopic cells have been formed.

The cells formed in this way vary in shape, size and characteristics, and eventually group together to form tissues.

Tissues are groups of cells which are all similar in size, shape and characteristics, and they are the materials from which all parts of the body are made.

Organs are individual structures in the body formed by tissues.

A system is a group of organs which are all concerned with the same function.

Therefore, cells massed together form tissues, tissues form organs, and organs are grouped into systems.

CELLS

The cell is the fundamental unit of all living tissue, and cells vary in size from approximately 500 nm in diameter (bacteria) to as much as 1 m in length (some nerve cells). Cells also vary in shape, e.g. some are disc shaped, some have many threadlike extensions, while others are cubelike.

The human body contains approximately 75 trillion cells. Each type of cell is specially adapted to form one particular function, but all human cells have certain basic characteristics that are alike.

Cell anatomy

All cells (Fig. 17.1) consist of two major parts; the nucleus and cytoplasm. The nucleus is separated from the cytoplasm by a nuclear membrane, and the cytoplasm is enclosed by the cell membrane. The different substances that make up the cell are collectively called protoplasm. Protoplasm is comprised mainly of water, electrolytes, proteins, lipids, and carbohydrates.

Cytoplasm, which is colourless and jelly-like in consistency, consists of the material inside the cell membrane and outside the nucleus.

The nucleus is a dense area in the cytoplasm and is the central controlling body within the cell. Within the nucleus

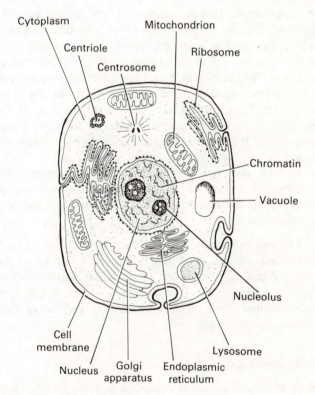

Fig. 17.1 Structure of a cell.

137

are the nucleolus containing RNA, and chromatin granules containing DNA that develops into chromosomes.

Ribonucleic acid (RNA) transmits genetic instructions from the nucleus to the cytoplasm.

Deoxyribonucleic acid (DNA) is the carrier of genetic information in the cell.

Chromosomes are the threadlike structures in the nucleus which carry genes that determine hereditary factors. A gene is the biological unit of genetic material and inheritance.

Organelles, which are structures contained in the cytoplasm, are the:

• Mitochondria. These small rodlike, threadlike, or granular structures function in cellular metabolism and respiration. Enzymes in the mitochondria carry out the reactions of cellular oxidation in which oxygen is used to break down foods. As the food is broken down energy is released, most of which escapes as heat, but some is retained and used to form adenosine triphosphate (ATP) molecules. ATP is used to provide the energy for the cell's activities. As the mitochondria provide most of the ATP, they are commonly referred to as the 'powerhouses' of the cell.
• Golgi apparatus. The golgi apparatus consists of a number of tiny sacs which are concerned with secretory activities of a cell, e.g. secretion of mucus.
• Vacuoles. These small cavities, or spaces, within the cell are used for storage of secretions or waste products (cellular debris).
• Centrosome. This structure, which is located near the nucleus, consists of the centrosphere and the centrioles. The centrosome is involved in *mitosis* (cell division).
• Lysosomes. These membrane-bound particles contain enzymes that function in the intracellular digestive process. The enzymes are capable of digesting worn out cell structures and foreign substances that enter the cell. If the enzymes are released into the cytoplasm they cause self-digestion of the cell, and for this reason they are commonly called the 'suicide sacs' of the cell.
• Endoplasmic reticulum. This extensive network of membrane-enclosed tubules functions in the synthesis of proteins and lipids, and in the transport of these substances within the cell.

The cell membrane (or cell wall) encloses the contents of the cell. As well as forming a protective barrier for the cell, the cell membrane determines which substances can enter or leave the cell. The membrane is believed to have many minute pores through which only very small molecules, e.g. water can pass.

Cell physiology

Each of the cell's internal structures perform specific func-

tions, and all cells possess the characteristics of living matter, i.e. they are capable of the following functions.

Functions of the cell

1. Respiration. All cells require oxygen for the combustion of food, and carbon dioxide is one of the waste products of combustion.

2. Ingestion and assimilation. From the fluid surrounding them, cells are able to select the chemical substances required for their structure.

3. Growth and repair. Substances supplied in food are used by the cells to synthesize new cytoplasm so that growth can occur, and to repair worn out parts of cells.

4. Excretion. Waste products are eliminated from the cells into the surrounding tissue fluid, and from there into the blood to be transported to various organs for excretion.

5. Irritability and activity. Cells are able to respond to a stimulus, which may be physical, chemical, or nervous. Response to a stimulus varies with individual types of cells, e.g. a stimulus will cause muscle cells to contract or relax, the cells in some glands will be stimulated to produce a secretion, and a nerve cell responds to a stimulus by conducting an impulse.

6. Metabolism. Activity requires a supply of energy, and cells are able to break down and use substances in food as fuel to supply energy.

7. Reproduction. Cells reproduce by simple division, and some cells reproduce more readily than others. Other cells, e.g. cells of the central nervous system, can never be replaced if they are destroyed.

Cell division

In all cells—except bacteria and some cells of the reproductive system—cell division consists of two events. Division of the nucleus (mitosis) occurs first, followed by division of the cytoplasm. Division of the cytoplasm takes place during the last stage of mitosis.

Mitosis

Mitosis (Fig. 17.2) is cell division that results in the formation of two genetically identical daughter cells which contain the diploid number of chromosomes characteristic of the species. (In humans, the normal diploid number is 46.) Mitosis consists of the division of the nucleus, during which the two chromatids of the chromosomes separate and migrate to opposite ends of the cell, followed immediately by division of the cytoplasm.

Mitosis, which is the process by which the body produces new cells for growth (and repair of injured tissue), consists of several stages. Prior to cell division, an event called *interphase* takes place. Interphase is the period in the

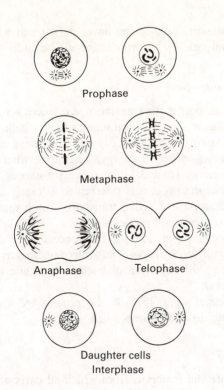

Fig. 17.2 Mitosis.

cell cycle during which no cell division is occurring. This period lasts from the completion of one mitosis until the beginning of the next. During interphase, the DNA molecules (or genetic material) that form part of the chromatin are duplicated exactly.

The stages of mitosis are described below.

1. Prophase. As a cell begins to divide, the chromatin threads coil and shorten so that chromosomes appear. Each chromosome consists of two strands, called chromatids, held together. The centrioles (in the centrosome) separate from each other and begin to move to opposite ends of the cell. A spindle of thin tubules forms to provide a scaffolding for the attachment and movement of the chromosomes. By the end of prophase, the nuclear membrane disappears and the chromosomes have become attached to the spindle fibres.

2. Metaphase. The centriole pairs are pushed far apart by the growing spindle, and the chromosomes become aligned at the centre of the spindle. The chromosomes form a straight line in the centre of the cell.

3. Anaphase. Each pair of chromosomes is pulled apart and the chromosomes begin to move slowly towards opposite ends of the cell. Therefore, 46 'daughter' chromosomes move towards one end of the cell, and 46 duplicate chromosomes move towards the other end.

4. Telophase. The chromosomes at each end of the cell uncoil to become threadlike chromatin again. The spindle breaks down and disappears, a new nuclear membrane

forms around each set of chromatin threads, and nucleoli appear in each of the daughter nuclei. The division of cytoplasm occurs during this stage, so that the original mass of cytoplasm is split into 2 parts. At the completion of cell division, 2 daughter cells exist. Each of the daughter cells is smaller than the original cell, but is genetically identical to it. The daughter cells grow and carry out normal cell activities until it is their turn to divide.

Meiosis

Meiosis (Fig. 17.3) is the type of cell division that occurs in the maturation of sperm and ova, and results in 4 daughter cells containing half the diploid number of chromosomes (23). Meiosis consists of 2 rapid divisions of the nucleus that result in 4 daughter cells. When the sperm containing 23 chromosomes, and the ovum also containing 23, unite to form a zygote, the normal number of 46 chromosomes is re-established. Thus, the child inherits some of the characteristics of both parents.

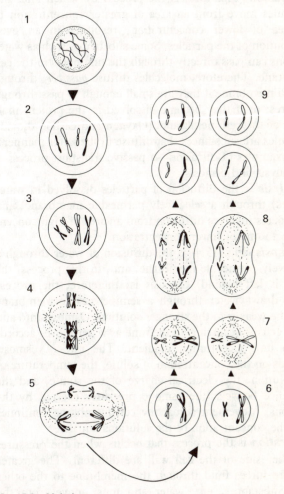

Fig. 17.3 Meiosis.

Membrane transport

The contents of each cell are enclosed by a semipermeable membrane that permits the passage of some molecules and ions, and prohibits the passage of others. The means by which substances pass in and out of cells depends on selective permeability. Selective permeability means that the cell membrane is selective about which substances pass through it.

Tissue fluid surrounds the cells, and there is a constant exchange between the fluid in the tissues (extracellular) and the fluid in the cell (intracellular). Movement of substances through the cell membrane, e.g. nutrients into the cell; and movement of substances out of the cell, e.g. carbon dioxide, takes place through passive and active transport.

Passive transport

Passive transport is the movement of small molecules across the cell membrane by diffusion. In passive transport, substances are moved across the membrane without any activity on the part of the cell.

Diffusion (Fig. 15.4) is the process by which ions and molecules move from an area of greater concentration to an area of lower concentration, resulting in an even distribution of the particles. Some substances such as water and ions can pass directly through the tiny pores in the cell membrane. Therefore, molecules diffuse *passively* through the cell membrane if they are small enough to pass through its pores; or if they become dissolved in the protein molecules of the cell membrane. (Oxygen and carbon dioxide molecules are substances that diffuse in the latter manner). Two examples of diffusion—a passive transport process—are dialysis and osmosis.

Dialysis is the diffusion of particles dissolved in water (solutes) through a selectively permeable membrane, and the process involves diffusion from an area of high concentration to one of lower concentration.

Osmosis (Fig. 15.4) is the diffusion of water through a selectively permeable membrane, and, in this process, the solute is left behind. Osmosis is, therefore, the process which draws water through a semipermeable membrane from the weaker to the stronger solution. Osmosis into and out of cells is occurring all the time as water moves according to its concentration gradient. The rate of osmosis depends on the concentration of solute, the temperature of the solution, the electrical charge of the solute, and the difference between the osmotic pressures exerted by the solutions. Movement across the cell membrane continues until the concentration of the solutions equalize.

Filtration is the process that occurs when the pressures on either side of the cell wall are different. The greater pressure forces fluid through the membrane to the other side. Substances, e.g. water and ions, move from the higher pressure area to the lower pressure area, while the larger molecules, e.g. protein are left behind.

Active transport

Active transport is the transfer of substances across a membrane against a concentration gradient. Such a process requires energy, and will only occur in living membranes which have a source of energy. Therefore, whenever a cell uses its energy from ATP to move substances across the membrane, the process is referred to as being active.

Two examples of active transport, which require ATP, are phagocytosis and pinocytosis.

Phagocytosis (Fig. 15.5) is the process by which certain cells engulf and dispose of micro-organisms and cell debris, e.g. the ingestion of bacteria by white blood cells (leucocytes).

Pinocytosis (Fig. 15.6) is the process by which extracellular fluid is taken into a cell.

TISSUES

Tissues are the materials from which all parts of the body are made, and they are formed by masses of cells connected by an intercellular substance. Following fertilization, a ball of cells is formed by repeated cell division, then cell differentiation occurs so that cells assume the shape, size, and characteristics which will enable them to perform a specific function.

Cells of similar characteristics are massed together to form each type of tissue. There are 4 types of tissue, each with subdivisions, and each type has a recognizable structure, pattern, and functions. The 4 types of tissue are:

1. epithelial tissue or epithelium
2. connective tissue
3. muscular tissue
4. nervous tissue.

Epithelial tissue

Epithelial tissue forms the covering of the body and the lining of various organs, and it is classified according to the number of layers of cells.

- *Simple epithelium* consists of a single layer of cells.
- *Compound epithelium* has many layers of cells.

Simple epithelium

Simple epithelium consists of one layer of cells lying on a basement membrane. It is a fragile type of tissue, and is therefore found where there is a need for a smooth surface, and where there is little wear and tear. There are 4 main varieties:

1. *Squamous or pavement epithelium* where the cells are fitted together rather like crazy paving. It is found lining blood vessels and forming air sacs in the lungs.

2. *Cuboidal epithelium* with cube shaped cells. It is found covering the ovary, and in the thyroid gland where it has a secretory function.

3. *Columnar epithelium* which has tall cells, like columns. It is found lining the stomach, intestines, urinary bladder, parts of the respiratory tract and other structures where it has a secretory function.

4. *Ciliated epithelium* is modified columnar epithelium. It has microscopic hair-like processes called cilia, projecting from its free surface. The cilia move together in a wave-like motion to sweep particles or mucus in one direction.

Ciliated epithelium is found lining most of the lower respiratory passage where it prevents the entry of particles into the lungs, and lining the uterine tubes where it aids in the passage of the ovum into the uterus.

Compound epithelium

Compound epithelium consists of many layers of cells with the deepest layer lying on a basement membrane. It may be stratified epithelium or transitional epithelium.

Stratified epithelium consists of layers of cells of differing shapes. It is found where there is a lot of wear and tear and, as superficial cells are rubbed off they are replaced by cells pushed up from deeper layers. Examples of stratified epithelium are:

- the skin
- the lining of the mouth, pharynx and oesophagus.

Transitional epithelium has pear-shaped cells arranged so that they form a waterproof lining in an organ which expands, e.g. the urinary bladder.

Glands

Glands are structures consisting of secreting epithelial cells, some of which have ducts through which they pour secretions while others are ductless.

Exocrine glands are glands with ducts to carry the secretion to the site of action, e.g. sweat glands, sebaceous glands and salivary glands.

Endocrine glands do not have ducts, but pour their secretions (called hormones) directly into the bloodstream, e.g. thyroid gland, pituitary gland and suprarenal glands.

Connective tissue

Connective tissue is the supporting, connecting and transport tissue and is widely distributed in the body. It consists of cells, fibres, and an intercellular substance called a matrix. The matrix may be soft, semi-solid or rigid. The types of connective tissue are:

1. white fibrous tissue
2. yellow fibrous tissue
3. areolar tissue
4. adipose tissue
5. haemopoietic tissue
6. lymphoid tissue
7. cartilage
8. bone.

White fibrous tissue is a tough tissue with many bundles of white fibres, but very little matrix. The fibres are wavy to allow for a certain degree of movement without stretching. White fibrous tissue forms the *ligaments* which bind bones together, and the *tendons* which attach muscles to bone.

Yellow fibrous tissue is similar to white fibrous tissue, but the fibres are more elastic and are yellow in colour. Yellow fibrous tissue is found in the walls of structures and organs that must be able to stretch and recoil, e.g. arteries, stomach and the lungs.

Areolar tissue consists of a soft matrix containing a network of white and yellow fibres. Areolar tissue is found under the skin, supporting and covering muscles, blood vessels and in the nerves.

Adipose tissue is similar to areolar tissue but contains an abundance of fat cells. Adipose tissue insulates the body against excessive heat loss, protects and supports some organs, and is a reserve store of fuel. Adipose tissue is found under the skin, surrounding the kidneys, behind the eyes, and as 'deposits' in areas of the body such as the breasts.

Haemopoietic tissue is blood forming tissue present in the cavities of bone where it continually replenishes the supply of red blood cells. Blood is also a connective tissue with a fluid matrix, and is described in detail in Chapter 21.

Lymphoid tissue is similar to areolar tissue, but is packed with specialised cells called lymphocytes. It produces white blood cells and antibodies, and filters harmful substances from circulation. Lymphoid tissue is found forming the tonsils, adenoids, spleen, lymph glands and nodes.

Cartilage is a firm yet pliant tissue with a firm elastic matrix. There are 3 varieties:

- White fibro-cartilage, which forms pads in some joints, e.g. the intervertebral discs.
- Yellow fibro-cartilage, which is elastic, is present in the external ear and the epiglottis.
- Hyaline cartilage, which is bluish-white in colour and has a smooth matrix, covers the ends of bones

involved in joint movement. Hyaline cartilage is also present in the nose, trachea, larynx, and forms the costal cartilage which joins the ribs to the sternum.

Bone (osseous tissue) is composed of bone cells surrounded by a hard matrix. The structure and functions of bone is described in detail in Chapter 19.

Muscular tissue

Muscular tissue (Fig. 17.4) is comprised of muscle cells, usually called muscle fibres, that contract or shorten to produce movement. The 3 types of muscle tissue are:

1. voluntary
2. involuntary
3. cardiac.

Voluntary muscle is also called skeletal or striated muscle. This tissue forms the muscles which are responsible for movement of the skeleton. It is under conscious control (voluntary), and when viewed under a microscope its fibres have a striped appearance. Further information on the structure and functions of voluntary muscle tissue is provided in Chapter 19.

Involuntary muscle is also called visceral or smooth muscle. This tissue forms the walls of internal organs which are not under conscious control, and its fibres contain no stripes.

Cardiac muscle is present only in the walls of the heart.

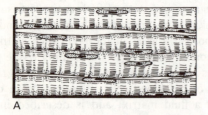

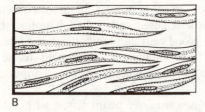

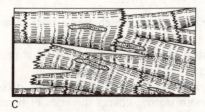

Fig. 17.4 Types of muscle tissue: (A) Voluntary (skeletal) muscle; (B) Involuntary (smooth) muscle; and (C) Cardiac muscle.

The cells are elongated, striated and branched, contain only one nucleus, and are not under the control of the will.

Nervous tissue

Nervous tissue forms the brain, spinal cord and the nerves, and is composed of cells called neurones bound together by neuroglia. Neurones receive and conduct electrochemical impulses from one part of the body to another. Further information on the structure and functions of nervous tissue is provided in Chapter 20.

Membranes

A membrane is a thin layer of tissue which covers an organ, lines an organ or cavity, or forms a partition in an organ or cavity. The 3 types of membranes are:

1. mucous
2. serous
3. synovial.

Mucous membrane is composed of a layer of epithelial cells resting on a deeper layer of connective tissue. It lines cavities or canals of the body that open to the exterior, i.e. the respiratory, and genitourinary tracts. Mucous membranes secrete mucus, which is a sticky fluid containing mucin, white blood cells, and inorganic salts. Mucus helps to protect against the entry of micro-organisms, and helps to filter and moisten inhaled air.

Serous membrane is composed of a layer of simple squamous epithelium on a basement membrane. Serous membranes consist of a *parietal* layer that usually lines a body cavity, and a *visceral* layer that covers the outside of the organs in that cavity. Examples of serous membrane are:

- pericardium, two layers around the outside of the heart.
- pleura, which lines the thoracic cavity and covers the lungs.
- peritoneum, which lines the abdominal cavity, and covers some abdominal organs.

Serous membranes secrete serous fluid, a thin fluid, which lubricates the organs and reduces friction as they slide across one another and the cavity walls.

Synovial membrane is composed of connective tissue, and lines the capsules of freely movable joints, and tendon sheaths. Synovial membrane secretes a lubricating fluid, synovial fluid, which allows bones to move without friction.

SUMMARY

Cells are massed together to form tissues, tissues form organs, and organs are grouped into systems.

The cell is the fundamental unit of all living tissue, and human cells range in size and vary in shape. While each type of cell performs a specific function, all cells have the same basic characteristics.

Human cells generally divide by mitosis. Mitosis is cell division that passes through four stages, and results in the formation of two genetically identical daughter cells. The daughter cells grow and carry out normal cell activities until it is their turn to divide. Meiosis is the type of cell division that occurs in the maturation of sperm and ova, and results in four daughter cells.

Substances pass in and out of cells by passive or active transport. The semipermeability of the cell membrane permits the passage of some substances, and not of others. The passive processes by which substances move in and out of cells are diffusion, dialysis, osmosis, filtration. Substances also move in and out by active transport involving chemical activity.

Tissues are formed from masses of cells connected by an intercellular substance. Each of the four main types of tissue (epithelial, connective, muscular, and nervous) has a different structure and different functions.

Glands are structures consisting of secreting epithelial cells, and are either exocrine or endocrine in nature.

Membranes, which consist of a thin layer of tissue, are mucous, serous, or synovial.

18. The integumentary system

OBJECTIVES

1. Describe the structure of the skin.
2. Describe the functions of the skin.

INTRODUCTION

The integumentary system consists of the skin and its appendages; the hair, nails, sweat and sebaceous glands. The skin (or integument) is the largest organ of the body, covering approximately 7500 cm² of surface area in an average adult. It is a protective barrier to the outside world, plays a vital role in homeostasis, and also provides a major means of communication through touch and sensation. The appendages of the skin—hair, nails and glands—arise from the epidermis but are present in the dermis.

STRUCTURE OF THE SKIN

The skin is comprised of two basic layers: the epidermis and dermis (Fig. 18.1). Under the dermis is a layer of adipose tissue called subcutaneous tissue. While this layer is not considered to be part of the skin, subcutaneous tissue does protect and insulate the deeper tissues.

The epidermis

The epidermis is the thin outermost layer, and is composed of epithelial cells which are arranged in layers of stratified epithelium. The number of layers vary according to the amount of wear and tear experienced, e.g. there are many more layers on the soles of the feet and the palms of the hands, than there are between the toes and the fingers.

The epidermis is divided into two layers described below.

1. The horny layer (stratum corneum) is the uppermost layer, and consists of keratinized cells. The keratinocytes contain a waterproof hard protein substance called *keratin*. Keratin, due to its waterproofing properties, protects the

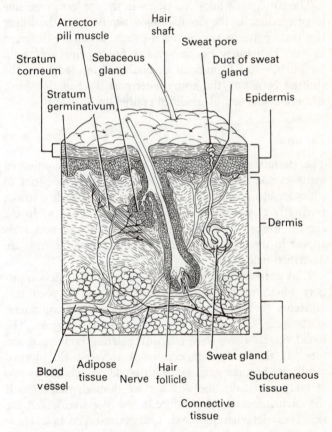

Fig. 18.1 Structure of the skin.

body and prevents escape of fluid from the deeper tissues. Keratin is also responsible for the formation of hair and nails.

2. The germinative layer (Stratum germinativum) is the deeper layer of the epidermis. It is here that new cells are constantly being formed, and pushed upward to replace cells that die and are rubbed off. Millions of new cells are produced daily, and are pushed up away from the source of nutrition, to become part of the outermost layer.

Melanocytes are present in the germinative layer, and their function is to produce a brown pigment called *mel-*

anin. Melanin gives colour to the skin, and protects the body against the damaging effects of ultra-violet rays in sunlight. Brown-toned skin results when large amounts of melanin are produced, whereas light-toned skin results when the body produces less melanin.

The epidermis does not contain any blood vessels, but receives its essential substances from fluid which comes from the blood supply to the dermis. As cells are pushed towards the surface, away from the source of nutrition, they die and are eventually rubbed off. Dead epithelial cells are flaked off in thousands every day, which means that they are deposited on clothing and on every surface touched. They become part of the dust in a room, serve as food for mites, and harbour microorganisms.

The patterns of lines and ridges in the epidermis are due to projections in the dermis called *papillae*. On the finger tips these patterns are the finger prints, which are different in every individual. For this reason, finger prints are useful for purposes of identification. Nails are formed from the stratum corneum (the horny outermost layer of the skin), and are composed of modified epithelium.

The dermis

The dermis consists of white fibrous tissue containing many elastic fibres. Elasticity of the skin is essential to allow for changes in the size of a part of the body without tearing, e.g. the abdominal area during pregnancy. In old age the fibres become less elastic, and wrinkles and folds appear in the skin. Structures contained in the dermis are described below.

1. A network of blood vessels. The blood vessels transport blood containing substances such as oxygen and nutrients to the dermis; and transport blood containing wastes, e.g. carbon dioxide, away from the dermis. The blood vessels also play a role in regulating body temperature. If the body temperature is elevated the dermal capillaries become engorged with blood, which allows loss of body heat from the skin surface through radiation. If the environmental temperature is low blood vessels in the skin constrict, therefore body heat is conserved as less heat is radiated from the body.

2. Nerve endings. The dermis has a rich nerve supply consisting of several types of nerve endings. Each type of nerve ending reacts to a different stimulus, e.g. pain, touch, pressure, temperature. Via the nerve endings, impulses are transmitted to the brain for interpretation.

3. Hair follicles and hairs. Hairs grow from hair follicles, which are deep pouch like cavities in the skin. Although hair follicles are present in most areas of the skin, they are not found on the palms of the hands or the soles of the feet. Hair is composed of modified epithelium, and grows from roots deep in the follicles. The part of a hair projecting above the epidermis is called the shaft. Hair colour reflects the amount of pigment, generally melanin, in the epidermis. Hair is a protection from the elements and from trauma, e.g. the scalp hair and eyebrows are barriers against sunlight, and the nasal hairs filter inhaled air.

4. Arrector pili muscles. These are minute involuntary muscles with one end attached to a hair follicle, and the other end to the dermis. When these muscles contract, e.g. during fear or exposure to cold, the follicles and hairs become erect. Contraction of the muscles also causes some elevation of the skin around the hairs, giving rise to the 'goose pimple' appearance.

5. Sebaceous glands. Sebaceous glands are small glands, most of which open into hair follicles. The glands produce *sebum*, which is an oily substance and a lubricant that keeps the skin soft and moist and prevents the hair from becoming brittle. Combined with sweat, sebum forms a moist, oily, acidic film that is mildly antibacterial. During periods of increased hormonal activity, e.g. adolescence, sebaceous glands become very active and the skin becomes more oily.

6. Sweat glands. Sweat glands, which are widely distributed, are either eccrine or apocrine. *Eccrine* glands are present all over the body and produce a clear perspiration. *Apocrine* glands are found mainly in the axillary and genital areas, and secrete sweat that has a strong characteristic odour. Sweat glands are coiled in appearance, with a straight duct which releases sweat on to the surface of the skin through an opening called the pore.

Sweat glands play a part in regulating body temperature. They excrete large amounts of sweat when the external, or body, temperature is high. When sweat evaporates off the skin's surface it carries large amounts of body heat with it. *Sweat* consists of water which contains sodium chloride, phosphates, urea, ammonia, and other waste products. Under normal circumstances, the amount of sweat secreted by an individual is approximately 700 ml per hour. Under some conditions, e.g. strenuous physical exertion or pyrexia, the amount can be increased to as much as 1500 ml per hour. Much of the water lost through the skin evaporates immediately, so it is not noticeable and is called *insensible perspiration*. Sweat that makes the skin damp is noticeable and is called *sensible perspiration*.

FUNCTIONS OF THE SKIN

The major functions in which the skin and its appendages play a role are protection, thermoregulation, metabolism, and sensory perception.

Protection

The skin is the first line of defence against the external environment. It provides a barrier to a variety of harmful agents, e.g. micro-organisms, radiant energy, and chemical substances. The skin acts as a barrier to harmful agents only as long as it remains intact.

The waterproof quality of the outer layer prevents excess water absorption, and abnormal loss of body fluids.

The skin contains nerve endings which are sensitive to painful stimuli. The nerve endings transmit impulses to the brain which alert the individual that damage is occurring.

Thermoregulation

The skin plays a major role in the maintenance of constant body temperature. Blood conducts heat from internal structures to the skin for dissipation. The skin dissipates excess body heat by radiation and evaporative cooling.

Body temperature is controlled by the hypothalamus—the heat regulating centre in the brain. This centre is sensitive to the temperature of the blood passing through it, and it also receives sensory stimuli from nerve endings in the skin (thermorecptors) that react to heat and cold. The hypothalamus, in turn, relays impulses requiring vasodilation and activation of the sweat glands (for cooling), or vasoconstriction (for heat retention). Thus, the hypothalamus acts like a thermostat which initiates heat—losing activities should the body temperature begin to rise, and heat—retaining activities should the body temperature start to fall:

• When the body temperature begins to rise impulses are generated which bring about vasodilation in the skin, the blood flow is increased; and heat from the skin is disipated by radiation, condition, and convection. The sweat glands are stimulated to secrete fluid on to the skin's surface, and it is the evaporation of this fluid which carries heat away.
• When the body temperature begins to fall impulses are generated which bring about vasoconstriction in the skin, the blood flow is decreased—which reduces loss of heat from the skin. In addition, sweating is inhibited and evaporation from the skin is reduced.

Regulation of body temperature is also described in Chapter 33.

Metabolism

The skin assists in the regulation of fluid and electrolyte balance by eliminating water and small amounts of sodium chloride through the sweat glands. Sweat consists of 99.4% water, 0.2% salts, 0.4% urea and other wastes.

In the presence of sunlight or ultra-violet radiation, the skin begins the process of forming vitamin D (calciferol), a substance required for absorbing calcium and phosphates from food.

Sensory perception

In addition to playing a role in the protective function of the skin through perception of a painful stimuli which causes an avoidance reaction—other receptors perceive sensations of pressure and touch. The skin is, therefore, an agent of communication between the outside environment and the body, as the activity of sensory nerve endings informs the individual of what is happening outside the body.

SUMMARY

The integumentary system consists of the skin and its appendages; the hair, nails, sweat and sebaceous glands.

The skin is the largest organ of the body, and is composed of two layers. The epidermis is the thin outermost layer composed of epithelial cells, many of which are keratinocytes. Keratin has waterproofing qualities, and is also responsible for the formation of hair and nails.

Melanin, which is produced by cells in the deeper layer of the epidermis, gives colour to the skin and protects the body against the damaging effects of ultra-violet rays in sunlight.

The dermis, or deeper layer of the skin, contains blood vessels, nerve endings, hair follicles and hairs, arrector pili muscles, sebaceous glands, and sweat glands.

Nails and hair protect certain areas of the body, e.g. nails protect the tips of toes and fingers, while hair protects areas such as the scalp.

The major functions of the skin are protection, thermoregulation, metabolism, and sensory perception.

19. The musculoskeletal system

OBJECTIVES

1. State the functions of the musculoskeletal system.
2. Describe the structures of bone, joints, and muscle.
3. Describe the position of the bones and joints.

INTRODUCTION

The musculoskeletal system is composed of many structures that function together to produce movement, support, and to provide protection of the body. These structures include the bones and joints of the skeletal system, the skeletal muscles, and the tendons and ligaments that connect muscle to bone or bone to bone.

SKELETAL SYSTEM

The skeleton is the framework which gives the body shape, and the skeletal system consists of approximately 200 bones and the ligaments that bind them together. Bones are composed of different tissues and have different shapes.

Formation of bone

By the 8th week of pregnancy the skeleton of the developing embryo is complete, but instead of bone the fetal skeleton is made of flexible cartilage and fibrous membrane. The cartilage and fibrous membrane is gradually hardened by the laying down of calcium, which has been absorbed from food and transported in the bloodstream to the foetus. This process of hardening is called *ossification*, and commences soon after the 8th week of pregnancy. The process is not completed in all bones until the individual reaches the early twenties, when all growth finally stops. Cartilage remains in isolated areas of the body, e.g. the joints, parts of the ribs, and the bridge of the nose.

Ossification is the conversion of cartilage and fibrous membrane into bone. Osteoblasts (bone building cells) remove calcium and phosphorous from the blood stream and lay them down as small plates in the cartilage. The process starts in the middle of the shaft of a strip of cartilage at the primary centre of ossification. From this centre, calcium and phosphorous are laid down in both directions forming the shaft of the bone. Secondary centres of ossification appear, one at each end of the cartilage, and these become the extremities of the bone.

At birth, there is a strip of cartilage (epiphyseal) remaining between the shaft and each extremity to allow for further growth. Cartilage (hyaline) remains as a covering over the upper and lower extremities of long bones.

Growth of bones

All bones are covered (except where there is hyaline cartilage) by a fibrous tissue called periosteum, from which bone cells arise which are responsible for growth in the circumference of a bone. Growth in the length of a bone can only take place while some epiphyseal cartilage remains. Bone is a dynamic structure that is continuously remodelled by bone cell activity. Old bone is removed, and new bone is formed.

Factors which influence the growth of bone

Dietary factors. There are several dietary factors:

- Protein is required to maintain the matrix or framework of bone.
- Calcium and phosphorus are essential to maintain the hardness of bone.
- Vitamin D is important for the absorption and use of calcium and phosphorus.
- Vitamin C influences the production of the intercellular substance.

Hormonal factors. Hormones produced by some endocrine glands play a very important role in promoting or inhibiting growth in bone.

These are discussed fully in Chapter 25 but some examples are:

- the growth hormone produced by the pituitary gland.
- a hormone (calcitonin) secreted by the thyroid gland.
- a hormone (parathormone) secreted by the parathyroid gland.

Physical factors. The normal growth and development of bone is affected by exercise and rest. Exercise stimulates the flow of blood to all structures, including bones, and this means an increased supply of the substances carried by blood, which are essential for growth. The attachment of skeletal muscles to bones, means that the shape of developing bones in children is influenced by posture and by the muscular activity during exercise. Rest enables the bones of the child to recover from the effects of a day of strenuous activity.

Tissue of the skeleton

Bone tissue

There are two types of bone tissue, an inner spongy tissue and a hard outer tissue.

1. Cancellous bone is latticelike—resembling honeycomb—porous and spongy. It is hard and strong but light in weight. The spaces in cancellous bone are usually filled with red bone marrow. Cancellous bone is present in the extremities of long bones, in the centre of short bones, and between the two surfaces of flat bones.

2. Compact bone is dense and hard, and forms a shell which gives the bone strength. Compact bone is present in the shafts of long bones, and forms the outer layer of short and flat bones.

Fibrous tissue

A sheet of fibrous tissue, called *periosteum*, adheres to all surfaces of bone except for the smooth areas where joints are formed. It provides a protective covering, and is permeated with the nerves and blood vessels that innervate and nourish underlying bone.

Hyaline cartilage

Hyaline (articular) cartilage is a smooth connective tissue with a bluish-white translucent appearance. It is present over the articulating ends of bones, and wherever there is a movable joint, and it allows the bones to glide freely on each other.

Adipose tissue

Bone marrow (red and yellow) is a fatty tissue filling the spaces in cancellous bone. Red bone marrow is present in many bones of infants and children, and in the cancellous bone tissue of adults. Yellow bone marrow is present in the medullary cavity of the long bones of adults.

Classifications of bones

Each bone belongs to one of four categories:

1. *Long bones*. All the bones of the limbs, except at the wrist and ankle, are long bones.
2. *Short bones*. Short bones are present in groups at the wrists and ankles.
3. *Flat bones*. These thin bones form the bony walls of the major body cavities, e.g. the skull, thorax , and pelvis.
4. *Irregular bones*. These are bones of varying shapes which cannot be classified as long, short, or flat. The bones of the face and the vertebrae are irregular in shape, and are classed as irregular bones.

Terms relating to bone markings

The surfaces of bones are marked with ridges, projections, processes and depressions. Bone markings indicate where muscles, tendons, and ligaments attach; where blood vessels and nerves pass, or where joints are formed:

- Crest—a narrow ridge of bone
- Condyle—a rounded projection
- Epicondyle—a raised area on a condyle
- Head—an extension supported by a narrow neck
- Fissure—a narrow opening
- Foramen—a round or oval opening
- Fossa—a shallow depression
- Spine—a sharp thin projection
- Trochanter—a large, irregularly shaped process
- Tubercle—a small rounded projection
- Tuberosity—a large rounded projection or elevation.

Structure of bones

Long bones

Long bones (Fig. 19.1) differ in size and shape according to their position and function, but all possess certain basic characteristics. A typical long bone has the following features:

- A shaft or central portion (diaphysis)
- Two extremities (epiphyses)
- Compact bone forming a complete outer shell. It is thin at the extremities and very thick in the shaft of the bone for greater strength
- Medullary cavity which is a central canal running the length of the shaft to lighten the weight of the bone
- Cancellous bone forming the two extremities
- Yellow bone marrow found filling the medullary cavity
- Red bone marrow which occupies the spaces in

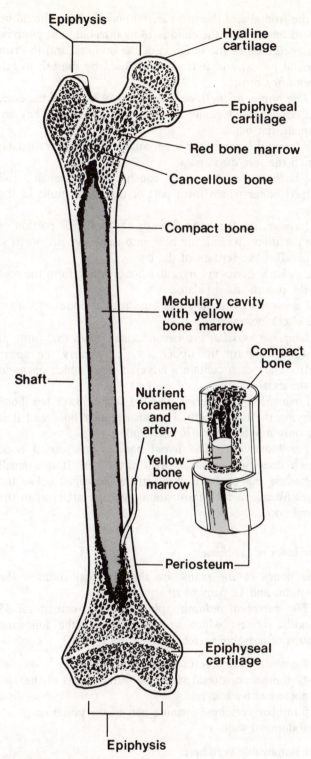

Fig. 19.1 A long bone.

cancellous bone at the extremities. It produces the cells of blood
- Periosteum, a tough fibrous tissue which covers the bone except at the extremities. It protects the bone and contains numerous blood vessels which help to

nourish the bone. It has a layer of bone forming cells on its under surface to allow for growth in the circumference of the bone
- Hyaline cartilage covering the extremities to allow for movement of bones without friction
- A nutrient artery which enters through an opening in the shaft of the bone, and divides into branches that carry blood to all parts of the medullary cavity.

Short and irregular bones

Short and irregular bones need to be light in weight and so they consist mainly of cancellous bone enclosed in a shell of compact bone, covered by periosteum.

Flat bones

Flat bones consist of a layer of cancellous bone sandwiched between two layers of compact bone, covered by periosteum.

THE BONES OF THE SKELETON

The skeleton (Fig. 19.2) may be divided for descriptive purposes into two parts:

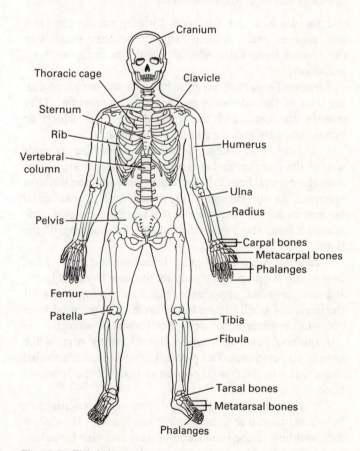

Fig. 19.2 The skeleton.

- 1. The *axial skeleton* forming the axis or upright, central part of the body and it is made up of the bones of the skull and the trunk.
- 2. The *appendicular skeleton* consisting of the bones of the appendages, i.e. the upper and lower extremities.

The axial skeleton

The bones of the skull

These comprise 8 bones of the cranium, and 14 bones of the face.

The cranial bones. The cranium is a box-like cavity formed by 8 bones which encloses the brain. The floor of the cranium is referred to as the base of the skull or cranium. The cranial bones are:

1 frontal bone, a flat bone forming the forehead and the roof of each orbit or eye socket. It contains 2 cavities, one above each eye, lined by ciliated mucous membrane and filled with air. They are called the frontal sinuses, and the functions of all air sinuses are:

- to lighten the weight of, and help to balance, the head.
- to give resonance to the voice.

They communicate with the nasal cavities by means of openings through which air passes.

2 parietal bones are flat bones forming part of the sides and roof of the cranium. They articulate (join) with the frontal bone anteriorly, and with the occipital bone posteriorly.

2 temporal bones are irregular bones at the temples forming part of the side walls and base of the cranium. They contain the ears, and the mastoid processes which lie behind the ears and contain many air cells.

1 occipital bone, a large, flat bone forming the posterior wall of the cranium and also part of the base. It articulates with the parietal bones. It has a large opening, the foramen magnum, for the passage of the spinal cord. The occipital bone rests on the first bone in the vertebral column, (the atlas) to form the joint which allows for nodding of the head.

1 ethmoid bone, an irregular bone forming part of the base of the cranium and separating the nose from the brain. It has a sieve-like appearance, due to many openings for the nerves of smell to pass to the brain. The ethmoid bone contains air sinuses that open into the nasal passages.

1 sphenoid bone, an rregular bone forming part of the base of the cranium. The pituitary gland of the endocrine system, lies in the central portion or body of the sphenoid bone.

The fontanelles. Fontanelles are areas of fibrous ssue in a baby's cranium due to incomplete ossification. They allow for moulding of the head during birth, and also for subsequent growth. The *anterior* fontanelle lies at the junction of the frontal and the two parietal bones, and it should be closed by the time the child is 18 months old. The *posterior* fontanelle lies at the junction of the occipital and the two parietal bones, and it is usually closed by the 6th to 8th week after birth.

The bones of the face. There are 14 bones of the face:

2 nasal bones forming the bridge of the nose. They are 2 small, flat bones.

2 lacrimal bones in the inner angle of the orbits through which the tear ducts pass.

2 turbinate bones or nasal conchae are the small scroll shaped bones which form part of the lateral walls of the nose.

1 vomer is a flat bone forming the posterior portion of the partition dividing the nose into right and left nostrils. It is called the septum of the nose.

2 palatine bones are irregular bones which form the roof of the mouth (hard palate).

2 zygomatic or malar bones are irregular bones which are the cheek bones.

2 superior maxillae are two irregular bones that unite at mid-line to form the upper jaw. They carry the upper teeth. They each contain a large air sinus which opens in to the nasal cavity.

1 mandible (or inferior maxilla) is the lower jaw bone carrying the lower teeth. It is an irregular bone and it is the only movable bone in the skull.

The hyoid bone. The hyoid bone is an isolated bone which does not articulate with any other. It is a small horseshoe shaped bone, lying in the neck just below the chin. Muscles which move the tongue are attached to the hyoid bone.

The bones of the trunk

The bones of the trunk are the vertebral column, the sternum, and 12 pairs of ribs:

The vertebral column (spinal column), consists of 33 irregular bones, which are divided into the following groups of movable vertebrae:

- 7 cervical vertebrae in the neck
- 12 thoracic or dorsal vertebrae forming part of the posterior thoracic wall
- 5 lumbar vertebrae forming part of the posterior abdominal wall.

and immovable vertebrae:

- 5 sacral vertebrae fused together to form a bone called the sacrum which is part of the pelvic girdle
- 4 coccygeal vertebrae fused together to form a bone called the coccyx or tail remnant, which is part of the pelvic girdle.

Intervertebral discs are pads of white fibro-cartilage situated between the bodies of the movable vertebrae.

Their functions are:

- to join the body of each movable vertebra with the one above and the one below
- to protect the brain and spinal cord from injury by acting as shock absorbers
- to allow a limited amount of movement of the vertebral column.

Curves of the vertebral column. The position of the fetus in the uterus gives rise to a convex backwards curve in the thoracic and sacral regions. After birth a forwards curve develops in the cervical region, as the baby lifts its head. The forward curve is developed in the lumbar region, as the child begins to stand and walk. The curves of the vertebral column are important as a means of maintaining good posture, and they provide some of the resilience needed in walking, running or jumping. Exaggeration of any of the curves can place a strain on ligaments and muscles, and can impair the functioning of internal organ, e.g. a hunckback deformity (kyphosis) interferes with the respiratory process as there is poor chest expansion.

Structure of typical vertebrae. Vertebrae vary in size, shape and general characteristics, but on the whole, each group comprises vertebrae which are similar to each other. Most movable vertebrae have certain characteristics in common. A typical vertebra (Fig. 19.3) consists of:

- A body or drum shaped block of bone located anteriorly as the weight-bearing part of the spinal column. The size of the body varies according to the position, with the bodies of the cervical vertebrae being small, those in the thoracic region larger, and the lumbar vertebrae having the largest bodies
- A neural arch or canal formed by bony processes projecting backwards from the body. When the vertebrae are in position one on top of another, a canal is formed which surrounds and protects the spinal cord as it passes through
- Two transverse processes, one projecting from either side of the arch of bone forming the neural canal, to provide attachments for spinal ligaments, and the tendons of muscles
- One spinous process projects backwards in the middle from the arch of bone and forms the bony prominence which can be felt under the skin of the back

It provides attachment for spinal ligaments, and the tendons of muscles

- Articular processes on the superior and inferior surfaces of the arch of bone, allow each vertebra to articulate (join) with the vertebra above and below.

Atypical (non-typical) vertebrae are those which do not possess all of the characteristics of the typical vertebrae. The atypical vertebrae (see Fig. 19.4) are:

- the atlas
- the axis
- the 5 sacral vertebrae
- the 4 coccygeal vertebrae.

1. The atlas is the first cervical vertebra and it supports the head, hence its name which refers to the mythical Greek god named Atlas, who carried the world on his shoulders. It consists mainly of a ring of bone, with no body and no spinous process. The occipital bone of the skull, has two rounded processes of bone called condyles, which rest on the atlas and allow for a nodding movement of the head.

2. The axis is the second cervical vertebra, and named the axis because it provides a pivot to enable the head to be turned from side to side. The atlas fits around a tooth-like projection of bone from the body of the axis, called the odontoid peg or dens which forms the pivot around which the atlas turns, to turn the head.

3. The sacral vertebrae in adults are fused to form a triangular shaped bone called the sacrum. The lines are clearly visible which show where the bodies of the five vertebrae have joined together, and there are rudimentary spinous processes present. The neural canal continues through most of the sacrum. The coccygeal vertebrae in an adult have become fused to form the bone called the coccyx, the last segment of the vertebral column.

The sternum or breast bone is a flat bone shaped like a dagger, lying in the centre of the anterior wall of the thorax. It is divided into 3 sections:

1. Manubrium, the upper part.

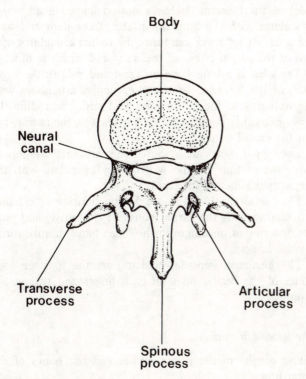

Fig. 19.3 Typical vertebra.

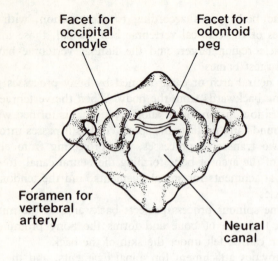

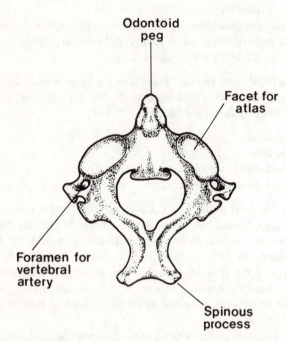

Fig. 19.4 Atypical vertebrae—the atlas (top) and the axis (bottom).

2. Body, the central portion.
3. The ensiform or xiphoid process forms the tip of the sternum and it usually consists of cartilage which has not become ossified. The sternum articulates with the two clavicles (collar bones) and most of the ribs.

The ribs are flat bones, and there are 12 pairs, all articulating posteriorly with the thoracic vertebrae. The ribs are divided into 3 groups:

1. pairs of true ribs which are joined directly to the sternum by means of strips of hyaline cartilage called costal cartilage.
2. pairs of false ribs, so called because they are attached only indirectly to the sternum, as the costal cartilage

of each is attached to the costal cartilage of the rib above.

3. 2 pairs of floating ribs which do not have any anterior attachment.

The appendicular skeleton (upper and lower extremities)

The upper extremities

These consist of the shoulder girdle, and the bones of the upper limbs:

The shoulder girdle. The shoulder girdle is formed by 2 scapulae or shoulder blades, and 2 clavicles or collar bones.

The scapula is a flat, shield-shaped bone lying over the ribs on the posterior wall of the thorax. A depression called the glenoid cavity situated on its lateral border receives the rounded head of the humerus (the bone of the upper arm) to form the shoulder joint. The clavicle is a long, S-shaped bone which articulates with the sternum, and with the scapula.

The bones of the upper limbs consist of the humerus (upper arm), the radius and the ulna (forearm), 8 carpal bones (wrist), 5 metacarpal bones (hand), and 14 phalanges (fingers and thumb).

The *humerus* is a long bone in the upper arm. Its rounded head fits into the glenoid cavity of the scapula to form the shoulder joint. The lower extremity of the humerus articulates with the radius and ulna at the elbow joint.

The *radius* is a long bone lying on the outer side (thumb side) of the forearm. It has a button-shaped head which articulates with the humerus at the elbow joint and with the ulna. At its lower extremity the radius articulates with two of the carpal bones of the wrist and with the ulna.

The *ulna* is a long bone on the inner side (little finger side) of the forearm. Its upper extremity articulates with the humerus at the elbow joint and with the radius. Its lower extremity is small and articulates with the radius, but not the carpal bones.

The *carpal* bones are 8 short bones arranged roughly in two rows of four, in the wrist. They articulate with the metacarpal bones of the hand.

The *metacarpal* bones are 5 long bones in the hand, articulating with the carpal bones of the wrist, and with the first row of phalanges in the fingers and thumb, forming the knuckles.

The *phalanges* (singular-phalanx) are the fourteen long bones of the digits, three in each finger and two in the thumb.

The lower extremities

These consist of the pelvic girdle, and the bones of the lower limbs.

The pelvic girdle is a basin-shaped bony ring formed by 2 innominate or hip bones (also called os coxae), 1 sacrum, and 1 coccyx.

The innominate bone or os coxae is a large, irregular bone formed by the fusion of 3 bones:

1. The *ilium* which constitutes the flat, upper portion of the innominate bone, and articulates posteriorly with the sacrum. The rim of the ilium is called the crest and can easily be felt through the skin.
2. The *pubis* which is the anterior portion of the innominate bone, articulating with the pubis of the other innomimate bone.
3. The *ischium* which is the posterior lower portion of the innominate bone. It has two protuberances called the ischial tuberosities which support the weight of the body when one sits down.

At birth these three bones are separated from each other by cartilage. During childhood, fusion of the three bones takes place and one solid bone is formed. A large cup-shaped socket is formed at the lateral junction of the three bones. It is called the acetabulum and it receives the head of the femur (thigh bone) to form the hip joint.

The sacrum and coccyx are the last portions of the vertebral column and they help to form the pelvic girdle. The sacrum articulates with the two innominate bones posteriorly.

Differences between the female and male pelvis. The pelvis of the female is shaped to allow for pregnancy and childbirth which means:

- The bones are lighter and smaller than in the male pelvis.
- The basin-shaped cavity in the female is shallow and round whereas the male pelvis is deep and funnel-shaped.
- The sacrum of the female is more concave to increase the size of the inlet and outlet of the pelvic cavity. The male is less concave, making the outlet narrower.
- The coccyx is more movable in the female than in the male, and this is an important factor during childbirth.

The bones of the lower limbs consist of:
the femur (thigh), the patella (kneecap), the tibia and the fibula (lower leg), 7 tarsal bones (the ankle), 5 metatarsal bones (the feet), and 14 phalanges (the toes).

The *femur* is the longest and strongest bone in the skeleton. It has a rounded head which fits in to the acetabulum of the innominate bone to form the hip joint. A neck of bone joins the head at an angle to the shaft. At its lower end the femur is broad and it articulates with the tibia to form the knee joint.

The *patella* is a flat, triangular-shaped bone, that is developed in the fibrous tissue forming the tendon of the thigh muscle. It lies over the anterior lower surface of the femur, in fron of the knee joint.

The *tibia* is the larger of the 2 bones in the lower leg. It is a long bone lying on the inner (medial) aspect of the leg, and is known as the shin bone. The upper extremity is broad, and articulates with the lower extremity of the femur to form the knee joint. It also articulates with the fibula just below the knee joint. At its lower extremity, the tibia articulates with the fibula and one of the tarsal bones to form the ankle joint.

The *fibula* is a long, slender bone, lying lateral to the tibia, on the outer aspect of the lower leg. Its upper extremity articulates with the tibia but does not enter into the formation of the knee joint. At its lower extremity the fibula articulates with the tibia and one of the tarsal bones to form the ankle joint.

The *tarsal* bones are 7 short bones in the ankle. Only one of these articulates with the tibia and fibula to form the ankle joint. The largest and strongest of the tarsal bones is the calcaneus (or os calcis), which is the heel bone. It transmits the weight of the body to the ground and gives attachment to the calf muscle by means of the tendon of Achilles.

The *metatarsal* bones are the 5 long bones of the foot articulating with some of the tarsal bones at the ankle and the phalanges of the toes.

The *phalanges* are the 14 long bones of the toes. There are 2 phalanges in the big toe, and 3 in each of the other toes.

Functions of the skeletal system

The skeletal system has several functions that are reflected in the structure of the bones:

1. The skeleton provides a rigid framework to give shape to the body.
2. It provides support and protection for softer structures in the body.
3. Individual bones serve as levers on which muscles can act to provide movement.
4. Bones serve as storage sites for minerals such as calcium and phosphorous. Lipids are stored in yellow bone marrow.
5. Bones are responsible for the production of blood cells, which are produced in the red bone marrow.

Joints, or articulations

A *joint* is an area where two or more bones are in close contact with each other. The bones forming the joint are held together by bands of white fibrous tissue called *ligaments*. Each joint is classified according to its structure and mobility.

Classification of joints

A joint is one of three types:

- fibrous or immovable
- cartilaginous or slightly movable
- synovial or freely movable.

Fibrous or immovable joints consist of bones held together by fibrous tissue in such a way that no movement is possible. The suture joints between bones of the skull are examples of this type of joint.

Cartilagenous or slightly movable joints are those where bones are separated by cartilage. This cartilage can be compressed to allow slight movement. The joints between the bodies of the vertebrae and the symphysis pubis, are two examples of this type of joint.

Synovial or freely movable joints are numerous and varied. They are classified according to their structure and/or the type of movement they allow but all synovial joints possess certain structural characteristics (Fig. 19.5):

- Two or more bones form the joint, held together by ligaments.
- Hyaline cartilage covers the articulating surfaces to prevent friction.
- A fibrous capsule encloses the joint, and helps to hold the bones in place.
- Synovial membrane lines the capsule, and secretes synovial fluid to lubricate joint structures.

Other structures are present in some joints, where they serve a specific purpose, for example:

- Extra ligaments are present for added strength or stability, e.g. cruciate ligaments are present in the knee joint to stabilize the joint by limiting the amount of movement.
- Extra cartilage is present to deepen a socket, e.g. semilunar cartilages (menisci) lie on top of the tibia to cushion it, and to deepen its rather flat surface to receive the articulating surfaces of the femur.
- *Bursae*, which are small sacs of synovial fluid, form cushions between ligaments and bones—or over bony prominences.

Types of synovial joints are ball and socket, hinge, gliding, pivot, and condylar.

1. Ball and socket joints are those where the rounded head of one bone fits into a cavity in another bone. Examples of ball and socket joints are the shoulder, where the head of the humerus fits into the glenoid cavity of the scapula: and the hip, where the head of the femur fits into the acetabulum of the innominate bone.

2. Hinge joints are those where the articulating surfaces are shaped to permit only a forward and backward movement, like the hinge of a door. Examples of hinge joints are the knee, where the femur articulates with the tibia:

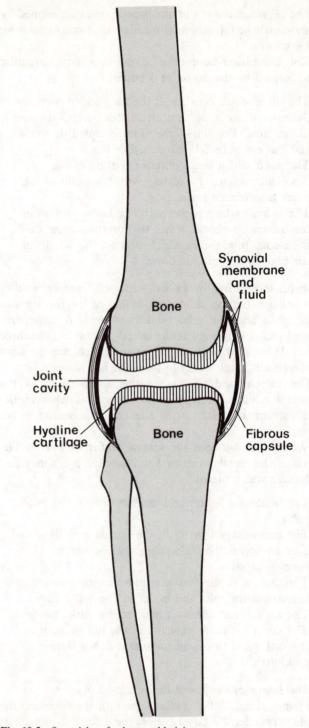

Fig. 19.5 Synovial or freely movable joint.

and the elbow, where the humerus articulates with the radius and ulnar.

3. Gliding joints are those where one articulating surface glides against another. Examples of gliding joints are the joints between the carpal bones of the wrist, and the joints between the tarsal bones of the ankle.

4. Pivot joints are those where one bone rotates on another. Examples of pivot joints are the joint between the radius and ulna, and the joint between the atlas and axis.

5. Condylar joints are those in which a condyle (rounded projection at the end of a bone) of one bone fits into an elliptical cavity of another bone. An example of this type of joint is the temporomandibular joint, which is a combined hinge and gliding joint, formed by the condyles of the mandible and the temporal bone.

Joints hold the bones together, and allow the rigid skeleton to become somewhat flexible.

Function of joints

Together with the muscles, ligaments, and tendons, movable joints provide stabilization and permit movement of the skeleton. The many joints of the body allow for a variety of movements. Terms associated with joint movements include:

- Abduction—movement away from the mid-line of the body
- Adduction—movement toward the mid-line of the body
- Flexion—bending
- Extension—straightening
- Hyperextension—a position of maximum extension
- Rotation—turning around a fixed axis
- Inversion—turning a part in toward the body
- Eversion—turning a part outward away from the body
- Circumduction—a circular movement which includes flexion, abduction, extension, adduction, and rotation.

Table 19.1 lists the joints where each type of movement is possible. Refer also to Figure 37.1 which illustrates the full range of motion joint exercises.

Table 19.1   Joint Movements

Type of movement	Joints where movement occurs
Flexion Extension	Shoulder, hip, knee, elbow wrist, interphalangeal joints
Abduction Adduction	Shoulder, hip, joints between metacarpals, wrist and phalanges, or metatarsals and phalanges
Rotation	Shoulder, radius and ulna joints, hip, the joint between the atlas and axis
Circumduction	Shoulder
Pronation or turning the palm downwards. Supination or turning the palm upwards	Radius and ulna joints

MUSCULAR SYSTEM

Skeletal muscles form the flesh of the body and, although there are two other types of muscle tissue: involuntary and cardiac, the term muscular system applies specifically to voluntary skeletal muscle.

Structure of muscle tissue

Skeletal, or voluntary, muscle is composed of large, elongated cells commonly called muscle fibres. Skeletal muscle fibres are multinucleated, and each fibre has horizontal light and dark stripes which gives the muscle a striped appearance. Muscle fibres are bound together by connective tissue into small bundles called *fasciculi*, which are bound into larger bundles which collectively form the muscle. Each muscle consists of many bundles of fasciculi enveloped in a sheet of fibrous tissue (fascia) which is continuous with the tendon.

Tendons are bands of white fibrous tissue attaching muscles to bones. Except at points of attachment, tendons are sheathed in a delicate fibrous connective tissue. Tendons are extremely strong and flexible, and occur in various lengths and thicknesses.

Aponeuroses are sheets of fibrous connective tissue that attach muscles to each other.

A muscle is usually attached to two or more bones, and either the muscle or its tendon crosses the joint moved by the muscle. The *origin* of a muscle is the point of attachment where movement does not occur. The *insertion* of a muscle is the point of attachment where movement does occur.

Muscle activity

Muscle tissue is capable of contraction and relaxation, and skeletal muscles must be stimulated by nerve impulses to contract. Skeletal muscle contraction begins with the stimulus of a muscle fibre by a motor neurone. Every motor neurone ends in many fine branches, each branch connecting with an individual muscle fibre. A group of muscle fibres activated by a single motor neuron is called a motor unit.

One motor neurone may stimulate a single muscle cell or hundreds of muscle cells, depending on the particular muscle.

Contraction (Fig. 19.6) occurs as a result of nervous, chemical, electrical, or thermal stimulation of muscle fibres, causing them to shorten and pull on the tendons attaching muscles to bones. Muscular contraction involves the expenditure of a great deal of energy. When a nerve impulse reaches the end of a motor neurone, a series of chemical changes involving glucose and oxygen occur, releasing the energy which makes the muscles contract.

Relaxation follows contraction as the muscle fibres resume their former length.

Muscle contraction can be classified as either isotonic or

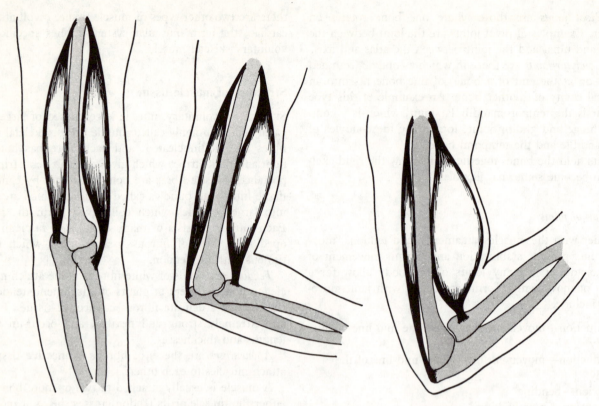

Fig. 19.6   The action or voluntary muscle showing contraction and relaxation.

isometric. In *isotonic* contractions, the muscle shortens and movement occurs. In *isometric* contractions the muscles do not shorten.

Muscle co-ordination

Most skeletal muscles work in pairs or groups, with one pair or group antagonizing the action of another pair or group to achieve controlled movement. For example, during elbow flexion, the triceps must relax to allow the forearm to be pulled up when the biceps contracts. Extension of the arm is made possible by the relaxation of the biceps, as the triceps contracts and pulls on the arm.

The erect position of the trunk is maintained as a result of co-ordination of groups of muscles.

Muscle tone is a state of steady, partial contraction of muscle fibres. It is present at all times in a healthy muscle, so that the muscle responds quickly when stimulated. Posture is influenced by the degree of muscle tone present.

Muscle fatigue can be caused by prolonged or repeated stimulation of a muscle which results in an accumulation of waste products. This interferes with the muscle's ability to contract and relax normally.

Skeletal muscles

The skeletal muscles are named according to one or more of the following:

- their shape and/or size.
- the direction in which their fibres run.
- the position of a muscle.
- the type of movement produced by the muscle.
- the number of points of attachment.
- the name of the bones to which the muscle is attached.

Muscles which move the arm

The pectoralis major lies on the anterior thoracic wall, and it pulls the arm forward and towards the body—flexion and adduction.

The deltoid is a triangular muscle lying over the point of the shoulder. Its action is to abduct (raise) the arm.

The latissimus dorsi is a large muscle, triangular in shape, which lies across the back of the lower thorax, and its action is extension and adduction of the arm at the shoulder joint.

The biceps lies on the anterior aspect of the upper arm. Its action is flexion of the elbow joint, and supination of the forearm.

The triceps lies on the posterior aspect of the upper arm. Its action is extension of the elbow joint.

The brachialis lies below the biceps on the anterior aspect of the upper arm. It helps with flexion of the elbow.

Muscles of the abdominal wall

There are 4 layers of muscle forming the anterior abdominal wall. They are:

- the rectus abdominis muscle is the most superficial, and is a broad flat muscle. It forms the anterior abdominal wall.
- the external oblique, the internal oblique, the internal oblique, and the transversus abdominis, which form the side walls of the abdomen.

These 4 muscles form a strong protective abdominal wall, and when they contract they compress the abdominal organs, thus aiding their emptying, and flex the vertebral column.

The posterior abdominal wall is formed by the quadratus lumborum, and the sacro spinalis.

Muscles of the pelvic floor

These are important muscles as they suppoprt the weight of the abdominal and pelvic organs. The muscles are the levator ani, and the coccygeus muscles.

In the female these muscles are pierced by 3 openings for the passage of the urethra, the vagina, and the rectum.

In the male the structures which pass through are the urethra, and the rectum.

Muscles which move the hip

The psoas, iliacus, gluteal muscles move the hip.

The psoas and iliacus lie in the region of the groin, and they flex the hip joint.

The gluteal muscles and form the buttocks, and they extend the hip joint.

Muscles which move the leg

The sartorius is the longest muscle in the body extending from the pelvic girdle to the upper part of the tibia. Its action is flexion and abduction at the hip, and flexion at the knee.

The quadriceps femoris is a large muscle of the front of the thigh. Its action is extension of the knee and flexion of the hip.

The hamstrings are the muscles at the back of the thigh and they flex the knee and extend the hip.

The tibialis anterior lies in front of the lower leg and its action is dorsiflexion of the foot. Injury to the nerve supply to this muscle results in footdrop.

The gastrocnemius is the calf muscle which is inserted into the os calcis (heel bone) by the tendon of Achilles. The muscle contracts to plantar-flex the foot.

The soleus is also a calf muscle lying deep to the

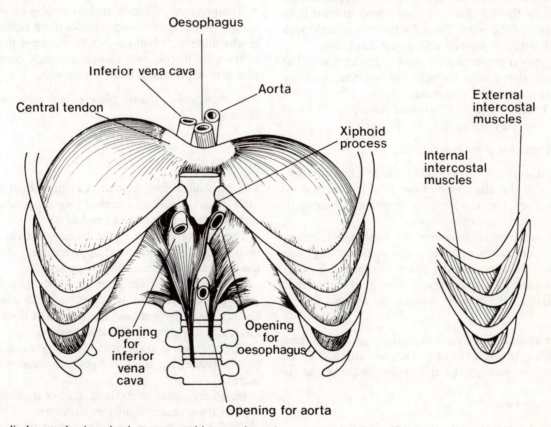

Fig. 19.7 The diaphragm, showing related structures and intercostal muscles.

gastrocnemius and it acts in conjunction with the gastrocnemius.

The muscles of respiration

A number of muscles in the neck, thorax and abdomen play a minor role in respiration under normal circumstances, but can become very important when breathing is laboured or forced in any way. They are called the accessory muscles of respiration.

The chief muscles of respiration are the diaphragm, and the intercostal muscles.

The diaphragm. The diaphragm (Fig. 19.7) is a dome-shaped muscular partition, forming the floor of the thorax and the roof of the abdomen. The diaphragm is formed by an outer section of striped muscle originating from the circumference of the trunk. Its origins are:

- Anteriorly—the xiphoid process of the sternum.
- Laterally—the lower 6 ribs.
- Posteriorly—the first 3 lumbar vertebrae.

Its insertion is a central sheet of white fibrous tissue called the central tendon and all the muscle fibres radiate to this central point of insertion.

There are 3 openings in the diaphragm to allow for the passage of important structures. The openings are for:

1. The aorta which is conveying blood to all parts of the body, and the thoracic duct bringing lymph drained from the lower part of the body. These 2 structures pass through an opening which is actually behind the diaphragm

2. The oesophagus conveying food to the stomach. The vagus nerve also passes through this opening, carrying impulses to most of the abdominal organs

3. The inferior vena cava, carrying deoxygenated blood from the lower part of the body to the heart.

The diaphragm has 3 main functions:

1. The diaphragm is the chief muscle of respiration. Contraction of the diaphragm causes it to flatten, and inspiration occurs. On relaxation the diaphragm resumes its dome shape, and expiration occurs

2. Contraction and flattening of the diaphragm increases the pressure on abdominal organs, and so aids in emptying of the bowel, bladder, and the uterus during childbirth

3. Movements of the diaphragm have a pumping effect on the inferior vena cava, so helping the upward flow of blood.

The intercostal muscles. There are 2 groups of these muscles, lying between the ribs. They are attached to the lower border of one rib and the upper border of the rib below.

The 2 groups are:

- 11 pairs of external intercostals with fibres running down and forwards.

- 11 pairs of internal intercostals with fibres running down and backwards.

The external intercostal muscles contract to move the rib cage upwards, and outwards to increase the size of the thorax on inhalation. The internal intercostals contract to pull the rib cage down and inwards to decrease the size of the thorax during exhalation.

Posture

The muscular system plays a vital role in maintaining correct body posture, by means of good muscle tone and co-ordinated activity. Factors which influence contraction of muscle and therefore muscle tone are:

- Satisfactory metabolic conditions, meaning that there is an adequate supply of food and oxygen, oxidation is complete, and waste products are removed, and not accumulated.
- Strength of the stimulus, so disorders of the nervous system can affect muscle contraction.
- Exercise, which increases the flow of blood and therefore increases the supply of oxygen and nutrients to muscle tissue, and enables waste products to be removed, thus reducing fatigue.
- Prolonged immobility, which can cause reduced muscle tone.
- Temperature. Warmth enables muscle fibres to react to stimuli more rapidly, and contract more efficiently, which is why athletes 'warm up' before a competition. Exposure of the skin to cold will stimulate muscle contraction as a means of maintaining body temperature.

The importance of good posture, and exercise, is outlined in Chapter 37.

SUMMARY

The musculoskeletal system is composed of many structures that function together to produce movement, support, and protection of the body.

The skeletal system is the framework which gives the body shape, and consists of approximately 200 bones and the ligaments that bind them together.

Bone is formed from cartilage by the process of ossification, and formation is complete when the individual reaches the early twenties. The growth of bone depends on dietary, hormonal, and physical factors.

The skeleton is comprised of two types of bone tissue, fibrous tissue, hyaline cartilage, and adipose tissue (bone marrow).

Bones are either long, short, flat, or irregular; and each type of bone varies slightly in structure.

The skeletal system provides a rigid framework for the body, provides protection and support for softer structures, provides levers for muscles, serves as a storage site for minerals, and produces blood cells in the bone marrow.

A joint, which is an area where two or more bones are in close contact with each other, may be fibrous, cartilaginous, or synovial. Each type of joint varies in structure. Synovial joints, which permit a wide range of movements, are ball and socket, hinge, gliding, pivot, or condylar joints.

The muscular system consists of the skeletal muscles that form the flesh of the body. Skeletal, or voluntary, muscles consist of bundles of muscle fibres bound together enveloped in a sheet of fibrous tissue. Voluntary muscles are attached to bones by tendons.

Muscle tissue is capable of contraction and relaxation. When muscle fibres are stimulated they contract; contraction pulls on a bone or bones producing movement at a joint.

20. The nervous system

INTRODUCTION

The nervous system is the most complex system in the body and it is responsible for the co-ordination of all other systems. It provides a network for communication within the body, and between the body and its environment. The brain is informed of events occurring both within and outside the body by nerve impulses which originate at a large number of sensory receptors. The receptors, which may be nerve endings, single specialized cells, or a group of cells forming a sense organ, convert the energy of a stimulus into impulses which pass to specific areas of the brain.

The nervous system develops in the embryo from a simple tube of ectoderm, called the neural tube. Ectoderm is the outermost layer of the 3 primary cell layers of an embryo. The cells lining the neural tube become the nervous tissue of the brain and spinal cord.

The nervous system can be divided into 2 primary divisions; the central nervous system consisting of the brain and spinal cord, and the peripheral nervous system consisting of nerves that connect the central nervous system with the body tissues.

CENTRAL NERVOUS SYSTEM

The central nervous system is composed of nervous tissue, which is commonly described as grey and white matter. Examination of a section of the brain reveals that it is grey on the outside and white on the inside. Microscopic examination reveals that the grey matter is composed of cells, and the white matter is made up of fibres. A cell and its fibres is called a neurone, and there are billions of neurones making up the nervous system.

Neurones

Neurones are the primary components of the nervous system. Functioning alone, or as units, neurones detect internal and external changes and initiate body responses needed to maintain homeostasis.

Each neurone is composed of a cell body with projections forming *dendrites* and one long *axon* (Fig. 20.1).

The dendrites are short branched fibres which receive impulses and conduct them towards the cell body of a neurone.

The axon, which may vary in length from miniscule to over a metre, conducts impulses away from the cell body of a neurone.

Generally, a neurone has only one axon but many dendrites. Axons leave the grey matter and become the fibres of the white matter. Each axon has a covering called a neurilemma, and most have a fatty sheath, the *myelin sheath*, which acts as an insulating material.

Neurones are bound together by a special type of connective tissue called neuroglia.

Neuroglia

The neuroglia include many types of cells that support and protect the neurones. They play a role in regulating neurone activity, and in providing the neurones with nutrients.

Neuroglia differ from neurones, in that they are not capable of transmitting nerve impulses, and they never lose their ability to divide.

The neuroglia are comprised mainly of 2 types of cells:

• *Astrocytes* are cells with small cell bodies and processes like dendrites. Astrocytes protect the neurones from harmful substances that may be in the blood, by forming a living

163

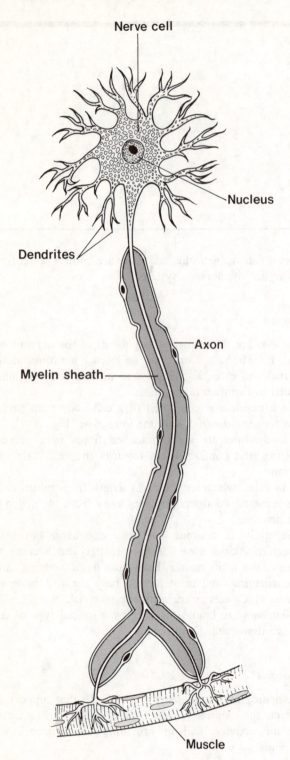

Fig. 20.1   A typical neurone.

barrier between the capillary blood supply and the neurones.

- *Oligodendrocytes* have few processes. They produce the myelin sheath around the processes of the neurones.

Functions of neurones

Neurones have 2 major functional properties; irritability and conductivty. *Irritability* is the ability to respond to a stimulus and convert it into a nerve impulse. *Conductivity* is the ability to transmit the impulse to other neurones, muscles, or glands.

An impulse is a complex electrical and chemical signal, transmitted along a nerve pathway in response to a stimulus. The speed of transmission varies with the size of the nerve fibre, and may be as much as 120 metres per second.

A synapse is the space between the axon of one neurone, and the dendrites of another neurone. By means of a chemical substance (neurotransmitter) which is released by the axons, impulses are transmitted through this space from one neurone to another. Many different types of stimuli can excite neurones so that they become active and generate an impulse. Most neurones are excited by the neurotransmitters released by other neurones, however other stimuli can excite neurones. For example, sound excites some of the ear receptors, and pressure excites some cutaneous receptors of the skin.

Receptors, or sensory nerve terminals, act as transducers converting the energy of a stimulus into impulses which pass to the brain.

The brain

The brain is a large organ weighing approximately 1.4 kg in the adult, held in position within the skull by membranes called the *meninges*.

In most parts of the brain the outer portion consists of grey matter, while white matter forms the inner portion. The grey matter is convoluted to provide a greater surface area. The brain is divided into:

- the forebrain—the cerebrum
- the midbrain
- the hindbrain—the pons varolii, medulla oblongata
- cerebellum.

The term 'brain stem' is also used to describe the stalk-like section which connects the brain to the spinal cord.

The cerebrum

The cerebrum is the largest part of the brain, filling the vault of the cranium from front to back. It is divided by fissures into the left and right *hemispheres*, and each hemisphere is further divided (Fig. 20.2) by fissues into 4 lobes:

- frontal
- parietal
- temporal
- occipital.

Within each hemisphere is a cavity called the *lateral*

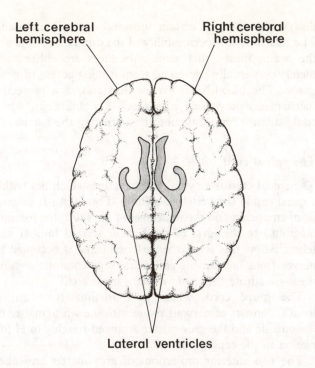

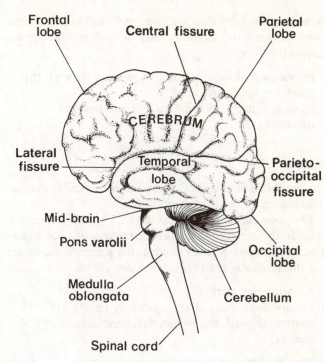

Fig. 20.2 The brain—cerebral hemispheres (left) and major structures (right).

ventricle, which is concerned with the formation of *cerebrospinal fluid*.

The left hemisphere is usually associated with language, mathematical skills and reasoning. The right hemisphere is generally associated with skills such as artistic awareness and imagination.

The cerebrum is divided into a number of areas, some of which are sensory and some of which are motor areas (Fig. 20.3). The sensory areas of each hemisphere receive and interpret sensations from the opposite side of the body

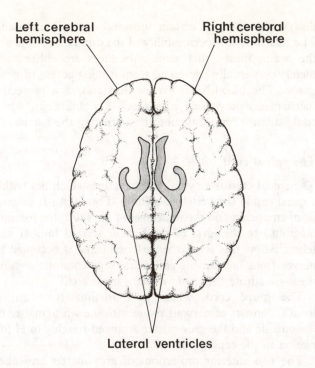

Fig. 20.3 The sensory and motor areas of the cerebrum.

including touch, temperature, pain, pressure, and an awareness of the position of the body in its environment. The motor areas of each hemisphere control all voluntary movement on the opposite side of the body. The centres of special sense are located in the various lobes, including the centres for hearing, speech, smell, taste, and sight.

The functions of the cerebrum are therefore:

1. to receive and interpret impulses from the sensory organs.
2. to initiate and control the movements of skeletal muscles.
3. to perform the higher levels of mental activity such as thinking, reasoning, intelligence, learning, and memory.

The thalami and the hypothalamus. The thalami are two oval masses of grey matter which form the lateral walls of the third ventricle. Each thalamus is subdivided into a number of nuclei. All sensory pathways (except smell) synapse in the thalamus, and the thalamus also plays a role in the control of somatic motor activity.

The hypothalamus lies beneath the thalamus, and the pituitary gland is closely connected to it. The hypothalamus controls all the activities of the autonomic nervous system, which is described later in this chapter.

The midbrain

The midbrain is a short, narrow segment (see Fig. 20.2)

connecting the cerebrum with the pons varolii. It is composed primarily of ascending and decending fibre tracts. Its functions are to:

- provide a pathway for impulses passing between the cerebrum and spinal cord.
- receive stimuli which initiate eye and postural movements.

The hindbrain

The hindbrain consists of 3 parts: the pons varolii, the medulla oblongata, and the cerebellum.

The pons varolii is approximately 2.5 cm long, lying anterior to the cerebellum and above the medulla oblongata. It contains two respiratory centres, the pneumotaxic centre and the apneustic centre. Its functions are to:

- act as a relay station
- modify the activity of the medullary respiratory centres, through the pneumotaxic and apneustic centres.

The medulla oblongata is approximately 2.5–3.0 cm long, lying between the pons and the spinal cord. It provides the link between the brain and the spinal cord, and it contains the cardiac, respiratory, vasomotor, and reflex centres. Its functions are:

1. to provide a pathway where nerve fibres to and from the brain cross over to the apposite side.
2. through the cardiac centre, to control heart beat.
3. through the respiratory centre, to control ventilation.
4. through the vasomotor centre, to control constriction and dilatation of blood vessels.
5. through the reflex centres, to initiate the reflex actions of swallowing, vomiting, coughing, and sneezing.

The cerebellum lies behind the pons and medulla, and below the occipital lobes of the cerebrum. Like the cerebrum, the cerebellum is divided into two hemispheres which have shallow convolutions in their surface of grey matter. Its functions are:

- Co-ordination of muscular activity and regulation of muscle tone.
- Maintenance of balance and posture.

Blood supply to the brain

The carotid and the vertebral arteries supply blood to the brain. These arteries branch and join up again, forming a circle of arteries at the base of the brain called the *Circle of Willis*. From here smaller cerebral arteries branch off to supply each region of the brain.

Blood returns from the brain via the jugular veins, to the superior vena cava.

The blood-brain barrier is a barrier which prevents, or delays, the entry of certain substances into brain tissue. The relatively low permeability of the capillaries supplying the brain, means that some substances are either completely or partially prevented from gaining access to brain tissue. The blood-brain barrier thus acts as a protective mechanism, preventing substances, e.g. bilirubin, which could disrupt brain function from crossing the barrier.

The spinal cord

The spinal cord is a cylindrical structure which lies within a canal inside the vertebral column (Fig. 20.4). It extends from an opening on the underside of the skull (the foramen magnum) to the level of the first or second lumbar vertebra. Below this level, the vertebral canal is occupied by nerves from the lumbar and sacral segments of the cord; these constitute the *cauda equina* ('horse's tail').

The spinal cord, which is approximately 46 cm in length, consists of nervous tissue with the white matter on the outside and the grey matter arranged roughly in H formation in the centre (Fig. 20.5).

The two anterior projections of grey matter are called the anterior horns, and the posterior projections are called the posterior horns. Sensory nerve fibres enter the posterior horns, and motor nerve fibres leave the anterior horns.

Leaving the spinal cord at intervals throughout its length are 31 pairs of spinal nerves.

The functions of the spinal cord are:

1. to receive sensory impulses from the tissues and convey them to the sensory areas of the brain, via ascending pathways
2. to convey motor impulses from the brain to various parts of the body, via descending pathways
3. to provide a pathway through which reflex actions take place.

A reflex action is an automatic motor response to a sensory stimulus—without conscious involvement. Most reflex actions are protective in nature, and take place more quickly than voluntary actions. The structures involved in a reflex action are:

- a sensory organ, e.g. the skin, to receive the stimulus
- a sensory (afferent) nerve fibre to carry the impulse to the spinal cord
- the spinal cord, where the posterior horn receives the impulse and transmits it directly to motor (efferent) neurones in the anterior horn
- a motor organ, e.g. a muscle, to receive and respond to the stimulus.

An example of a reflex action is when the hand comes into contact with a very hot object. The skin on the hand receives the stimulus of heat, an impulse travels from the sensory nerve endings in the skin to the posterior horn of

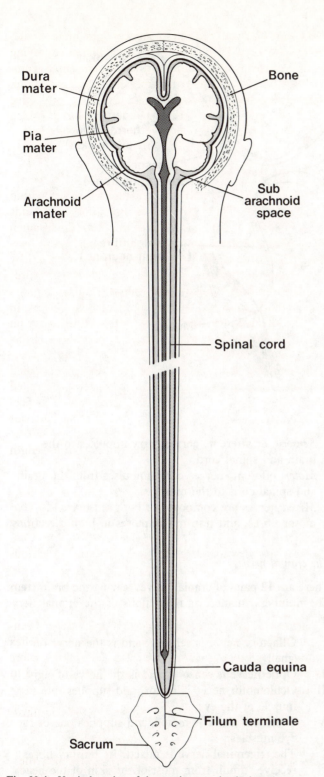

Fig. 20.4 Vertical section of the meninges and spinal cord.

Labels for Fig. 20.4:
Dura mater, Pia mater, Arachnoid mater, Bone, Sub arachnoid space, Spinal cord, Cauda equina, Filum terminale, Sacrum

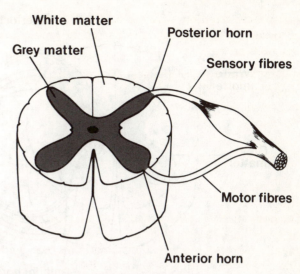

Fig. 20.5 Cross-section of the spinal cord.

Labels for Fig. 20.5:
White matter, Grey matter, Posterior horn, Sensory fibres, Motor fibres, Anterior horn

The meninges

The meninges (Fig. 20.4) are the three membranes which cover the brain and the spinal cord.

1. The dura mater (meaning 'hard mother') is the tough outermost layer. It consists of 2 layers of fibrous connective tissue, with one layer forming the periosteum covering the inner surface of the skull bones, and the other layer covering the brain and spinal cord. The dura mater extends further than the spinal cord, and ends as a blind sac at the level of the sacrum.

2. The arachnoid mater (meaning 'mother like a spider's web') is the middle layer. The name refers to the fact that it is so thin that, when viewed under a microscope, it resembles a spider's web. The arachnoid mater terminates with the dura mater at sacral level.

3. The pia mater (meaning 'gentle mother') is the delicate innermost layer. It adheres closely to the surface of the brain and spinal cord, dipping down into all the convolutions and fissures. The pia mater is richly supplied with blood vessels which carry blood to the brain and spinal cord, and ends as a thin cord attached to the sacrum.

The sub-arachnoid space is the space between the arachnoid mater and pia mater, filled with cerebrospinal fluid in circulation.

The functions of the meninges are:

1. to form a protective covering around the brain and spinal cord against physical injury
2. to help secure the brain to the cranial vault.

Cerebrospinal fluid

Cerebrospinal fluid (CSF) is a clear watery fluid with a composition similar to plasma. It contains substances in-

the spinal cord. From there, the impulse is transmitted to the anterior horn; then is passed along the motor nerves to the muscles of the shoulder, arm and hand. As a result, the hand is pulled rapidly away from the source of heat (Fig. 20.6).

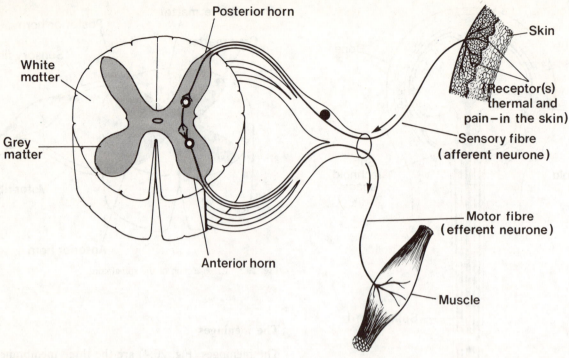

Fig. 20.6 A reflex arc.

cluding water, glucose, sodium, chloride, potassium, protein, and waste products such as urea.

Cerebrospinal fluid is formed from the blood, and is produced by a combination of filtration and active secretory processes by the choroid plexus in the ventricles of the brain. CSF circulates in the subarachoid space surrounding the brain and spinal cord.

The total volume of CSF is approximately 150 ml. The fluid is formed continuously in the ventricles at a rate of approximately 600–700 ml per day, and is reabsorbed into the blood at about the same rate.

The normal cerebrospinal fluid pressure, when the body is horizontal, is from 5–10 mmHg.

The functions of cerebrospinal fluid are:

1. to form a protective cushion around the brain and spinal cord

2. to maintain normal pressure around the brain and spinal cord

3. to provide a medium for the exchange of nutrients and waste products between the bloodstream and the nervous tissue.

THE PERIPHERAL NERVOUS SYSTEM

The peripheral nervous system consists of the 12 pairs of cranial nerves which leave the brain stem, 31 pairs of spinal nerves which leave the spinal cord, and the autonomic nervous system. The peripheral nerves may be sensory, motor, or mixed:

- *Sensory*, or afferent, nerves carry impulses to the brain and spinal cord.
- *Motor*, efferent, nerves carry impulses from the brain and spinal cord to the muscles.
- *Mixed* nerves are composed of both sensory and motor fibres, and transmit impulses in both directions.

The cranial nerves

There are 12 pairs of cranial nerves leaving the brain stem. The numbers, names, and functions of the cranial nerve are:

I. Olfactory nerve is sensory, and is the nerve of smell.

II. Optic nerve is sensory, and is the nerve of sight.

III. Oculomotor nerve is motor, and supplies the muscle of the eye.

IV. Trochlear nerve is motor, and supplies one of the eye muscles.

V. The trigeminal nerve is mixed. Its sensory fibres receive stimuli from most of the skin of the head and face, the membranes of the nose and mouth, the orbits, the upper and lower jaws and teeth. The motor fibres supply the muscles of mastication.

VI. Abducent nerve is motor, and supplies one of the eye muscles.

VII. Facial nerve is mixed. The sensory fibres convey the sensation of taste from the anterior portion of the tongue. The motor fibres supply the muscles of facial expressions.

VIII. Auditory nerve is sensory, and is the nerve of hearing and balance.

IX. Glossopharyngeal nerve is mixed. Its sensory fibres convey taste sensations from the posterior part of the tongue. Its motor fibres supply the pharynx.

X. Vagus nerve is mixed. It controls secretion and movement of the internal organs, e.g. oesophagus, larynx, trachea, heart, stomach, intestines, pancreas, spleen, kidneys and blood vessels.

XI. Accessory nerve is motor, and supplies the muscles of the neck, and also the pharynx and larynx.

XII. Hypoglossal nerve is motor, and supplies the tongue muscles.

The spinal nerves

The spinal nerves project out of the vertebral canal, one pair emerging below each vertebra, and one pair emerging between the cranium and the first cervical vertebra.

The spinal nerves are mixed nerves, containing both sensory and motor fibres. They allow for sensation and movement in peripheral parts of the body not supplied by the cranial nerves, e.g. skin, muscles, bones and joints of the trunk and limbs.

The spinal nerves are arranged in groups according to their region of origin in the cord. There are:

- 8 pairs of cervical nerves.
- 12 pairs of thoracic nerves.
- 5 pairs of lumbar nerves.
- 5 pairs of sacral nerves.
- 1 pair of coccygeal nerves.

In some regions the nerves divide immediately after leaving the cord, and these branch, then unite with each other to form what is called a plexus. Some of the plexuses are:

- *The cervical plexus* which supplies the muscles of the neck and shoulders, and also gives rise to the phrenic nerves which supply the diaphragm.
- *The brachial plexus* which gives rise to the radial, median and ulna nerves which supply the arm.
- *The lumbar plexus* which gives rise to the femoral nerve to supply the thigh muscles.
- *The sacral plexus* from which the sciatic nerve arises. It is the largest nerve in the body, running over the hip posteriorly down the back of the thigh to the knee where it divides into the peroneal nerve and tibial nerve.

The autonomic nervous system

The autonomic nervous system is that section of the peripheral nervous system which is concerned with the involuntary activity of the body.

It supplies nerves to all the structures in the body that are not under conscious control. The autonomic nervous system consists of two sections:

- the sympathetic nervous system.
- the parasympathetic nervous system.

The sympathetic nervous system consists of two chains of ganglia in front of the vertebral column, from the cervical region to the lumbar region. *A ganglion* (plural ganglia) is a knot-like mass of cell bodies.

The ganglia are connected to each other and to the spinal cord by nerves, and they give rise to nerves which supply internal organs and blood vessels.

Plexuses are formed by fibres from these ganglia, for example:

- the solar plexus lying behind the stomach and supplying the abdominal organs.
- the cardiac plexus supplying the heart and lungs.

The parasympathetic nervous system consists of cranial nerves numbers III, VII, IX, and X; and nerves that emerge from the sacral legion of the spinal cord. The vagus nerve (cranial nerve X) is the largest autonomic nerve.

Functions of the autonomic nervous system

The functions of the autonomic nervous system are to control the movements of internal organs and the secretions of glands.

The system provides dual control: the activity of an organ is stimulated by one set of nerves, and is inhibited by the other set of nerves. This dual control achieves smooth, rhythmic action of involuntary muscles and internal organs, maintaining a balance between activity and rest.

The sympathetic nerves can be affectd by strong emotions such as anger, fear, or excitement, and have a stimulating effect on most organs. The effect resembles that produced by by adrenalin, a hormone which is secreted by the suprarenal glands. This effect is called the 'fright, fight, and flight' effect, whereby the body is prepared to respond to fright—either by fighting or running away:

- The pupils of the eyes are dilated
- The force and rate of the heart beat is increased, so circulation improves
- Blood pressure rises and arterioles in the skin and internal organs are constricted to divert blood to all skeletal muscles, heart, lungs and brain
- Bronchi dilate to allow more oxygen to enter
- Digestion is slowed so that the digestive organs can receive a reduced blood supply, enabling blood to be diverted to vital structures

Table 20.1 Effects of sympathetic and parasympathetic stimulation

Organ	Sympathetic stimulation	Parasympathetic stimulation
Heart	Increases rate/strength of heart beat. Dilates coronary arteries to increase blood supply to the heart muscle.	Decreases rate/strength of heart beat. Constricts coronary arteries to decrease supply of blood to the heart muscle.
Bronchi	Dilates bronchi allowing more air to enter the lungs.	Constricts bronchi and so limits the air intake.
Digestive system	Decreases activity of the system and constricts digestive system sphincters. Inhibits production of saliva.	Increases peristalsis and relaxes sphincters. Stimulates production of saliva.
Urinary bladder	Relaxes bladder wall. Contracts internal sphincter muscle.	Contracts bladder wall. Relaxes internal sphincter muscle.
Eye	Dilates the pupil. Retracts the eyelids.	Constricts the pupil. Closes the eyelids.
Skin	Stimulates perspiration. Stimulates smooth muscles attached to hair follicles, producing 'goose bumps'.	No effect on sweat glands. No effect on muscles/hair follicles.

- Sweat glands secrete more sweat
- Blood sugar level rises, as the liver is stimulated to release more glucose for increased energy needs.

The parasympathetic nerves tend to slow down body processes, and so the end result of the antagonistic action of each division of the autonomic nervous system, is a balance between acceleration and retardation. After the 'fright' or stressful situation is over, the parasympathetic nervous system returns things to normal. The digestive organs receive more blood, the glands increase their secretions, the heart beat is decreased, and the blood pressure falls.

Information comparing some of the effects of sympathetic and parasympathetic stimulation on various body organs, is provided in Table 20.1.

SUMMARY

The nervous system is a complex system, responsible for communication within the body and between the body and its environment. It is divided into two primary divisions, the central nervous system and the peripheral nervous system.

The nervous system is composed of nervous tissue, which is commonly described as grey and white matter. The grey matter is composed of cells and the white matter is made up of fibres. Neurones are the primary components of nervous tissue, which are bound together by neuroglia.

Neurones have 2 functional properties, irritability and conductivity. This means that neurones are able to respond to a stimulus, convert it into an impulse, and transmit the impulse to other neurones, muscles, or glands. Impulses are transmitted through spaces, called synapses, between the neurones.

The central nervous system consists of the brain and the spinal cord. The brain is a large organ composed of the cerebrum, the midbrain, the pons varolii, the medulla oblongata, and the cerebellum. Each part of the brain has specific functions.

The spinal cord lies within a canal inside the vertebral column, extending from the base of the skull to the first or second lumbar vertebra. The spinal cord receives sensory impulses, conveys motor impulses, and is the centre through which reflex actions take place.

The meninges are three membranes which cover the brain and spinal cord to protect them against physical injury.

Cerebrospinal fluid is a clear watery fluid produced in the ventricles of the brain, which circulates in the subarachnoid space surrounding the brain and spinal cord. It protects the brain and spinal cord, and provides a medium for the exchange of nutrients and waste products.

The peripheral nervous system consists of 12 pairs of cranial nerves, 31 pairs of spinal nerves, and the autonomic nervous system. The nerves of the peripheral nervous system may be sensory, and carry impulses to the brain and spinal cord; motor, and carry impulses away from the brain and spinal cord; or mixed.

The autonomic nervous system is composed of the sympathetic nervous system and the parasympathetic nervous system. It is the section of the peripheral nervous system which is concerned with the involuntary activity of the body. Sympathetic nerves have a stimulating effect on most organs, while parasympathetic nerves tend to slow down body processes.

21. The circulatory system

INTRODUCTION

Every cell in the body requires a constant supply of nutrients and oxygen, and every cell must rid itself of waste products. The circulatory system is the means by which both these activities are achieved.

The circulatory system has 2 major subdivisions: the cardiovascular system, and the lymphatic system. The overall function of the circulatory system is transportation of substances to and from the cells. The circulatory system consists of:

- the heart, which acts as a pump to circulate the blood through the body.
- the blood, which carries essential substances to the cells and carries wastes from the cells.
- the blood vessels, which contain and transport the blood through the body.
- the lymphatic system, which filters and destroys harmful substances before they reach the bloodstream.

THE CARDIOVASCULAR SYSTEM

The structures which make up the cardiovascular system are the blood, the blood vessels, and the heart.

The blood

Blood, which is classed as a connective tissue, constitutes approximately 1/12th of the weight of the body. Depending on the weight of the individual, the total volume of blood is approximately 5 to 6 litres.

Blood varies in colour from bright red when it has a high oxygen content, to dark red when the oxygen content is low. The blood normally has a pH of approximately 7.4.

Blood is a viscous substance composed of a fluid portion (plasma) and solid components (cells).

Plasma

Plasma, the fluid part of blood, is a straw coloured watery fluid in which the blood cells are suspended. Plasma forms approximately 55% of the blood volume, and contains water, plasma proteins, mineral salts, nutrients, waste products, gases, hormones, antibodies and antitoxins, and enzymes.

1. Water. Approximately 90–92% of the plasma is composed of water, which is important in the maintenance of all body fluids and in the production of secretions.

2. Plasma proteins: Albumin, globulin, fibrinogen, prothrombin, and heparin are the proteins found in plasma.

Plasma proteins are produced by the liver, with the exception of serum globulin which is derived from lymphocytes. Plasma proteins have several important functions:

- They help to maintain the viscosity of blood, which is necessary to control the amount of fluid passing from blood into the tissues. The viscosity of blood is also a factor in the control of blood pressure.
- Prothrombin and fibrinogen are necessary for the normal clotting of blood.
- Heparin prevents blood clotting in the blood vessels.

3. Mineral salts. The mineral salts found in blood plasma are sodium chloride, iodine, potassium, phosphorus, calcium, iron, magnesium, and copper. Mineral salts are necessary for:

- regulation of tissue activity
- formation of protoplasm
- maintenance of the pH of blood.

4. Nutrients found in blood plasma are amino acids,

glucose, fatty acids and glycerol, and vitamins. Nutrients have been reduced to their simplest form by the digestive processes, and absorbed from the alimentary tract into the bloodstream for circulation to the cells.

5. Waste products found in blood plasma are urea, uric acid, and creatinine.

The waste products result from protein metabolism, formed by the liver and carried by the blood to the excretory organs.

6. Gases found in blood plasma are oxygen, nitrogen, and carbon dioxide. Oxygen and nitrogen enter the bloodstream following the inhalation of air, and carbon dioxide is an end product of oxidation in the tissues.

7. Hormones are chemical substances secreted directly into the bloodstream by endocrine glands, and are carried to the areas of the body where they are required to stimulate activity.

8. Antibodies and antitoxins are complex protein substances produced by the body in response to an invasion by a foreign protein (an antigen). They are part of the body's defence mechanism.

9. Enzymes produced by the body initiate or accelerate chemical reactions.

Blood cells

The blood cells float in the plasma, and form the solid part of blood. The 3 types of blood cell are erythrocytes, leucocytes, and thrombocytes.

1. Erythrocytes (red cells) are microscopic, biconcave, non-nucleated discs measuring approximately 7 microns in diameter. Erythrocytes are produced in the red bone marrow present in cancellous bone tissue, where they pass through several stages of development. They begin as large nucleated cells but, when mature and ready to be liberated into circulation and have been reduced in size, lose the nucleus and gain haemoglobin.

Haemoglobin is a complex protein containing a pigment and iron. It has a strong affinity for oxygen, and gives the blood its colour. The normal haemoglobin level is approximately 14–16 g per 100 ml of blood.

The number of erythrocytes is approximately 5 000 000 per cubic millimetre of blood, and the average life-span of an erythrocyte is 100–120 days. They become worn out in circulation, and are then destroyed in the spleen and liver. The haemoglobin is split, its iron is stored by the liver for future use, and the pigment is used by the liver in the production of bile.

The function of erythrocytes is to carry oxygen. In the lungs, oxygen combines with haemoglobin to form oxyhaemoglobin making the blood bright red in colour. As blood circulates through the tissues, the oxygen is released for use and the blood becomes dark red in colour.

2. Leucocytes (white cells) are microscopic blood cells measuring approximately 10 microns in diameter. They differ from erythrocytes in that they are larger, possess a nucleus and are less numerous. They also have the power of independent movement, which erythrocytes do not possess. There are 2 main types of leucocytes: granulocytes and granular leucocytes.

Granulocytes consist of neutrophils, basophils and eosinophils.

Neutrophils make up the largest number of the leucocytes, and are important to the body in defence against bacteria, as they have the ability to engulf and digest bacteria (phagocytosis). Neutrophils also play an important part in the inflammatory response. Injured tissues, and other leucocytes, are believed to secrete substances that stimulate the bone marow to release increased numbers of neutrophils.

Basophils are thought to prevent clotting in the microcirculation, to release substances in infected tissue that are toxic to many micro-organisms, and also play a part in the allergic response.

Eosinophils are also involved in phagocytosis because the ingest antigen-antibody complexes and parasites. They also play a role in clot retraction.

Agranular leucocytes consist of monocytes and lymphocytes.

Monocytes have the ability to move into the tissues where they become macrophages, capable of phagocytosis. They also secrete a number of substances involved in the body's defence, and play a role in the immune response.

Lymphocytes are either T-lymphocytes, or B-lymphocytes, both of which divide when stimulated by antigens. T-lymphocytes are responsible for cellular immunity, and adhere to cells identified as foreign to the body. They secrete cytotoxic substances which kill the foreign cells. B-lymphocytes are involved in humoral immunity, as they produce antibodies and are also responsible for immunoglobulin production.

The number of leucocytes is approximately 8000–10000 per cubic millimetre of blood, but this number increases considerably (leucocytosis) when there is any infection in the body. The life-span of a leucocyte is variable and depends to some extent on the degree of activity.

Lymphocytes may survive up to 100 days, but the span of life for granular leucocytes is only about 21 days.

3. Thrombocytes (platelets) are colourless microscopic cells measuring approximately 3 microns in diameter, and they do not possess a nucleus. Thrombocytes are produced in the red bone marrow which is present in cancellous bone tissue.

The number of thrombocytes is approximately 250 000–300 000 per cubic millimetre of blood, and the average life-span of a thrombocyte is from 5–9 days. The function of thrombocytes is to play a major role in the clotting of blood when an injury occurs.

The *clotting mechanism* occurs in order to reduce blood loss, when a blood vessel wall is injured. The process involves many substances that are normally present in the plasma (clotting factors), as well as some substances released by the platelets and injured tissues. Normally, a blood clot will form within two to six minutes after a blood vessel wall has been damaged.

The mechanism of clotting (haemostasis) involves 3 phases: vascoconstriction, formation of a temporary platelet plug, and formation of a clot. When a small vessel becomes damaged:

• Local vasoconstriction occurs, which reduces blood flow and, therefore, blood loss.
• Thrombocytes adhere to the damaged area.
• The thrombocytes release *serotonin* and adenosine diphosphate (ADP), which attracts other thrombocytes leading to the formation of a temporary platelet plug.
• The temporary platelet plug is converted into a clot, by the deposition of fibrin which is formed from fibrinogen. The conversion of fibrinogen to fibrin involves a 'cascade' of reactions which require a number of plasma factors (numbered I to XIII). A series of reactions culminate in the conversion of *prothrombin* to thrombin. This conversion requires the presence of platelets, factor V, factor X, and calcium ions. Vitamin K is necessary for the formation of factors VII, IX, and X.
• The fibrin forms a mesh-work of threads that traps the erythrocytes and forms the basis of a clot.
• The clot plugs the injured blood vessel, drawing the edges together. As the clot shrinks, a clean yellow liquid called *serum* appears.

The clotting mechanism is a complex one that will not occur if any of the necessary elements are missing.

Functions of blood

Blood has the following functions:

1. to transport oxygen, nutrients, and waters to all tissue cells, waste materials to the excretory organs, and hormones from endrocrine glands to the appropriate tissues.
2. to supply the materials from which glands make their secretions.
3. to protect the body against infection by means of the leucocytes and antibodies.
4. to regulate body temperature by distributing heat evenly throughout the body.
5. to prevent a loss of body fluid and blood cells by means of its clotting mechanism.

Blood groups

Human blood can be classified into 4 basic groups, depending on the substances present in the blood which are capable of inducing the production of antibodies. They are, therefore, types of antigens, although they are also known as agglutinogens.

There are a great number of antigens present in blood, but the two most important systems are the ABO and Rh (rhesus) systems. The antigens of these systems are present on erythrocyte (red cell) membranes.

ABO system refers to the group to which the blood belongs. An individual's blood may be one of 4 types: A; B; O; or AB.

If an individual's blood belongs to group A, his antigen is A but his antibody is Anti-B.

Individuals whose blood belongs to group B, have B antigens, and Anti-A antibodies.

Blood group O individuals have both Anti-A and Anti-B antibodies but no antigens.

Blood group AB individuals have neither Anti-A or Anti-B antibodies.

Because of potential transfusion hazards steps must be taken to ensure that the donor's blood is compatible with the blood of the recipient.

Incompatibility is due to the presence of agglutinins in the plasma of some blood groups, which will cause agglutination (clumping together) of erthrocytes in certain other blood groups. Clumps of cells block vital small blood vessels, and death may result.

Before a transfusion is given, erythrocytes from the donor's blood are mixed with plasma from the recipient's blood to test for agglutination. If no agglutination occurs, the donor's blood is considered safe to transfuse. Table 21.1 illustrates which blood groups are compatible or incompatible with other blood groups.

Table 21.1 Blood group compatibility

Blood type	Blood that can be received
Group A	A and O
Group B	B and O
Group AB (Universal recipient)	A, B, AB, and O
Group O (Universal donor)	O

Individuals who belong to Group AB can *receive* blood from all groups, and are therefore known as universal recipients. Individuals who belong to Group O can *donate* blood to all groups, and are therefore known as universal donors.

If an individual receives blood from an incompatible group (e.g. if a Group A person is given Group B blood) his plasma antibodies will vigorously attack the foreign erythrocytes, leading to a *transfusion reaction*. Information about blood transfusion and reactions is provided in Chapter 44.

Rh system refers to whether an individual does or does not possess the Rh factor in his blood. In the blood of approximately 80% of the world population, there is a substance called the Rhesus factor. The factor is named after the rhesus monkey in which the system was first studied. Individuals who possess the factor are said to be Rhesus positive (Rh+ve). Individuals who do not possess the factor are said to be Rhesus negative (Rh−ve).

Whether an individual is Rh positive or Rh negative, is very significant in two instances. The first is when receiving a blood transfusion, and the second instance is during pregnancy.

If an Rh negative person is transfused with Rh+ve blood, anti-Rh positive agglutinins will be formed slowly in the recipient's blood, usually without causing any immediate ill effects. A further transfusion of Rh+ve blood will cause an increase in the production of agglutinins—which will destroy the erythrocytes in the transfused blood.

A pregnant woman who is Rh−ve may be carrying a fetus who has inherited Rh+ve blood from its father. Erythrocytes containing this factor may escape from the fetal circulation into the mother's circulation. This causes her to develop anti-Rh positive agglutinins in her blood. There may not be any ill effects during the first pregnancy, but in subsequent pregnancies destruction of the baby's erythrocytes will occur due to the increase in the level of agglutinins in the mother's blood.

The blood vessels

In health, blood in circulation remains in the vessels responsible for its transport through the tissues (Fig. 21.1). The major blood vessel types are arteries, veins, and capillaries. Blood is pumped by the heart into the major arteries, which branch to form increasingly smaller arteries and eventually arterioles. Arterioles are continuous with a network of minute vessels, the capillaries. Blood then passes into venules which join with one another to form veins. Veins unite to form the largest veins which transport the blood back into the heart.

Arteries

Arteries are the vessels which always carry blood in a direction away from the heart. All arteries carry oxygenated (bright red) blood, with the exception of the two *pulmonary arteries* which carry deoxygenated (dark red) blood from the heart to the lungs.

Arteries vary in size, and large arteries divide to form smaller arteries. Further division, or branching, occurs until the smallest arteries are formed.

These smallest arteries are called *arterioles* which divide into capillaries. Arteries and arterioles have the same structure. The walls of arteries have 3 coats (Fig. 21.2):

- an outer coat of fibrous tissue
- a thick middle coat of involuntary muscle with elastic fibrous tissue
- a lining of endothelium to form a smooth surface for contact with blood.

The walls of arteries are structured to allow them to stretch and recoil as the blood is pumped into them by the heart.

Veins

Veins are the vessels which always carry blood in a direction towards the heart. All veins carry deoxygenated (dark red) blood, with the exception of the four *pulmonary veins* which carry oxygenated blood from the lungs to the heart.

Veins vary in size, and large veins divide to form smaller veins. Further division, or branching, occurs until the smallest veins are formed. These smallest veins are called *venules* which divide into capillaries (Fig. 21.1). The walls of veins are composed of the same 3 layers as those of arteries, but the walls are thinner. They are less rigid and contain less muscle and elastic tissue than arterial vessels. As a consequence, veins offer little resistance to blood flow back to the heart.

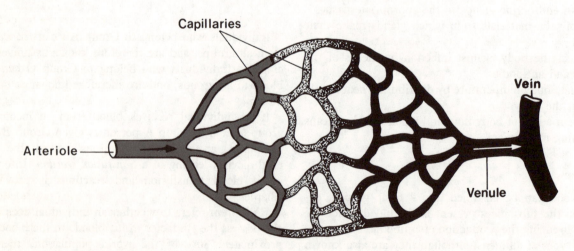

Fig. 21.1 Circulation of blood through the tissues.

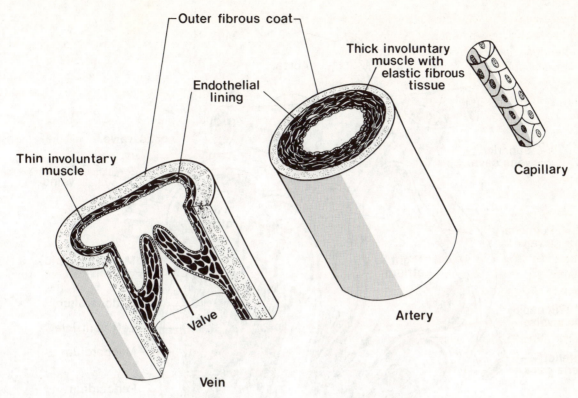

Fig. 21.2 Structure of blood vessels.

The larger veins possess pocket-like valves on their inner surfaces (Fig. 21.2). These valves aid the unidirectional flow of blood towards the heart, and prevent a backward flow of blood. Skeletal muscle activity also helps venous return; as the muscles surrounding the veins contract and relax, the blood is 'milked' through the veins towards the heart.

Table 21.2 illustrates the structural and functional differences between arteries and veins.

Table 21.2 The differences between arteries and veins

Arteries	Veins
Carry blood away from the heart	Carry blood toward the heart
Carry oxygenated blood (except for the two pulmonary arteries)	Carry deoxygenated blood (except for the four pulmonary veins)
Have thick muscular walls	Have thin muscular walls
Have elastic tissue in their walls	Have little or no elastic tissue in their walls
Do not possess valves	The larger veins possess valves

Capillaries

Capillaries are microscopic vessels, approximately 5–7 microns in diameter, and are composed of a single layer of endothelium with a little surrounding connective tissue. They form close networks through all tissues, and are structurally adapted for their role in the rapid exchange of substances between plasma and interstitial fluid.

The semipermeable membrane, formed by the single layer of endothelial cells, allows water, oxygen, nutrients, and other essential substances to pass from the blood to the tissue cells. Waste products from the tissue cells pass through the capillary walls to the blood.

The heart

The heart is a hollow, conical, muscular organ, situated obliquely in the thoracic cavity between the lungs and behind the sternum. One third of the heart lies to the right, and two thirds lie to the left of the median plane. Its base is uppermost and points towards the right shoulder, and its apex is below, pointing to the left. In size, the adult heart is approximately 12 cm × 8–9 cm × 6 cm, and weighs about 300 g.

Structure of the heart

The heart (Fig. 21.3) is divided into a right, and a left side by a muscular partition called the *septum*. Each side is further divided into an upper receiving chamber—the *atrium*—and a lower distributing chamber—the *ventricle*.

The walls of the heart consist of the pericardium, the myocardium, and the endocardium.

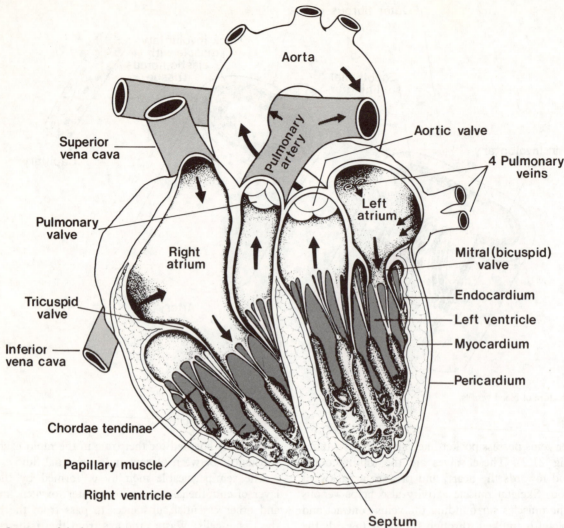

Fig. 21.3 Structure of the heart.

The *pericardium* is the outer coat consisting of two layers of serous membrane. Pericardium secretes a small amount of serous fluid to moisten the surfaces in contact with each other, so that the heart can beat without friction.

The *myocardium* is the middle muscular layer consisting of cardiac muscle, which is a highly specialized type of muscle tissue present only in the heart. It is of varying thickness, being thicker in both ventricles than in the atria, and thicker in the left ventricle than in the right.

The *endocardium* is the lining of the heart, and consists of endothelium which provides a smooth surface for the flow of blood. Folds of endocardium help to form the valves of the heart.

The *valves of the heart* consist of flaps of fibrous tissue covered by endocardium, which allow blood to flow in one direction only, thus preventing a backward flow.

The valves are:

● the *bicuspid* (or mitral) valve between the left atrium and left ventricle.

● the *tricuspid* valve between the right atrium and right ventricle.
● the *aortic* valve between the left ventricle and the aorta.
● the *pulmonary* valve between the right ventricle and the pulmonary artery.

Chordae tendinae (tendinous cords) are fine cords which are attached from the mitral and tricuspid valves to small projections from the muscle walls of the ventricles called *papillary muscles*. Contraction of the *papillary muscles* exerts a pull on the cords, to prevent the valve flaps from being carried up into the atria when the valves close.

Blood vessels. There are several blood vessels which either enter or leave the heart. The blood vessels which *enter* the heart (see Fig. 21.3) are:

1. The *inferior vena cava*, which enters the right atrium. It carries deoxygenated blood collected from the lower part of the body.

2. The *superior vena cava*, which enters the right atrium. It carries deoxygenated blood collected from the upper part of the body.

3. The *four pulmonary veins*, which enter the left atrium. Two pulmonary veins leave each lung and carry oxygenated blood into the heart.

The blood vessels which *leave* the heart are:

1. The *aorta*, which leaves the left ventricle. It carries oxygenated blood from the heart for distribution to all parts of the body.

2. The *pulmonary artery*, which leaves the right ventricle then divides into two branches. One branch carries deoxygenated blood from the heart to each lung.

Thus, the right side of the heart deals only with deoxygenated blood, and the left side deals only with oxygenated blood. The atria are the receiving chambers of the heart, and the ventricles are the distributing chambers.

Blood supply to the heart

As the aorta leaves the heart, it gives off two branches called the *coronary arteries*. These arteries pass into the heart wall to supply it with blood. The coronary arteries divide into smaller and smaller branches, until networks of capillaries are formed in the heart wall. Veins carry the deoxygenated blood from the tissues in the heart wall, and unite to form a vein which opens directly into the right atrium.

The conducting system of the heart

The conducting system of the heart (Fig. 21.4) consists of specially differentiated muscle tissue—nodal fibres and Purkinje tissue. This system is responsible for the initiation and maintenance of normal cardiac activity.

The *sinoatrial node* (pacemaker) is a narrow structure

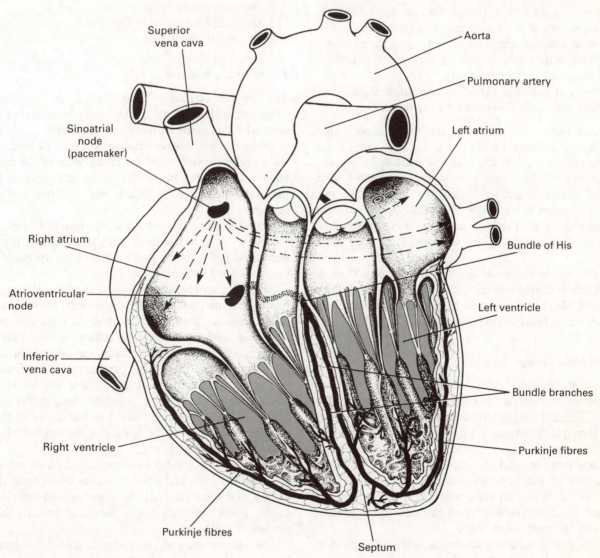

Fig. 21.4 The conducting system of the heart.

situated in the upper part of the right atrium. The *atrio-ventricular node* is smaller, and lies in the lower part of the interatrial septum of the heart.

The Purkinje fibres form a network in the tissue of the ventricles, and branch off from main bundles to supply the myocardium.

Functions of the heart

The function of the heart is to act as a pump:

1. It pumps deoxygenated blood to the lungs to get rid of carbon dioxide, and pick up oxygen.
2. It pumps oxygenated blood to all parts of the body.

The *cardiac cycle* is the series of pressure changes, valve actions and electrical potentials that bring about the movement of blood through the heart during one complete heart beat. The cardiac cycle takes about 0.8 of a second and consists of two phases:

1. *Systole*, or contracting, period. During this time both atria contract at the same time, emptying their contents into the ventricles. The two ventricles then contract simultaneously, forcing their contents into the aorta and pulmonary artery.
2. *Diastole*, or relaxing, period. A relaxation phase follows after each contraction of the heart.

The *heart beat* is controlled by the vagus nerve, which slows it and reduces the force of the beat, while sympathetic nerves quicken the beat and increase its force.

Individual cardiac muscle cells are capable of spontaneous, rhythmic, self-excitation. To be effective as a pump, the action of the whole heart must be co-ordinated. Co-ordination of the rhythmic movements is brought about by the specialized cells of the sinoatrial (SA) node (pacemaker).

Cardiac output is the volume of blood pumped out by each ventricle during one minute. It is dependent upon the volume of blood pumped at each beat (stroke volume) and the number of beats during one minute (heart rate).

Flow of blood through the heart

Deoxygenated blood is collected from all over the body by the superior and inferior vena cavae, which enter the right atrium. When the right atrium is full it contracts, forcing blood through the tricuspid valve into the right ventricle.

As the blood fills the ventricle, it carries the valve flaps back into position; and the chordae tendinae, pulled by contraction of the papillary muscles, prevent the flaps going too far. When the right ventricle is full, it contracts to force the deoxygenated blood through the pulmonary valve into the pulmonary artery.

The deoxygenated blood leaves the heart in the pulmonary artery which divides to send one branch to each lung.

In the lung the blood gives up its carbon dioxide, and picks up oxygen. It is now oxygenated blood and is carried from each lung by two pulmonary veins. The four pulmonary veins enter the left atrium of the heart. When full the atrium contracts to force blood through the mitral valve and into the left ventricle.

When the left ventricle is full the mitral valve closes, the ventricle contracts, and the oxygenated blood is forced through the aortic valve into the aorta. As the aorta leaves the heart it arches towards the left, then passes down behind the heart, pierces the diaphragm, and runs down the abdomen to divide into two branches in the pelvic region. Branches from the aorta supply every part of the body with oxygenated blood.

Circulation of blood

Blood is in constant circulation around the body, and the system of circulation can be divided into 3 parts:

1. the systemic circulation
2. the pulmonary circulation
3. the portal circulation.

The systemic circulation

The systemic circulation (Fig. 21.5) is the distribution of oxygenated blood to all tissues, and the return of deoxygenated blood from all tissues to the heart.

When the left ventricle contracts it forces blood into the aorta under pressure, and the elastic walls of the aorta distend to receive the blood. When the left ventricle relaxes the walls of the aorta recoil, and the blood is driven onwards.

Branches from the aorta also distend and recoil as the blood travels through them, and this wave of distension and recoil is felt as the pulse wherever a superficial artery crosses a hard structure, e.g. bone.

Arterioles supply networks of capillaries with oxygenated blood, and the pressure behind the blood causes water and other essential substances to pass through the capillary walls and wash over the tissue cells to become part of the tissue fluid. Tissue cells pick out the substances they require and excrete their waste products into the tissue fluid.

The pressure within the capillaries, will allow only a small amount of the fluid to return through the capillary wall, and back into the blood. The remainder of the fluid reaches the blood via the lymphatic system, which is discussed later in this chapter.

Venules carry the now deoxygenated blood away from the capillary beds and unite to forms veins, until the two largest veins are formed; the superior and inferior vena cavae. These two veins empty their contents into the right atrium of the heart.

The main vessels in the systemic circulation consist of arteries and veins.

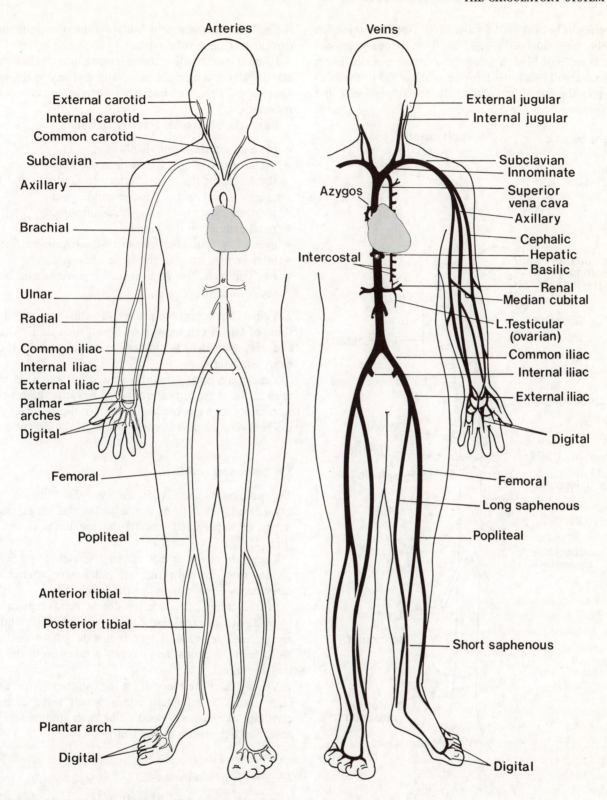

Arteries

External carotid
Internal carotid
Common carotid
Subclavian
Axillary
Brachial
Ulnar
Radial
Common iliac
Internal iliac
External iliac
Palmar arches
Digital
Femoral
Popliteal
Anterior tibial
Posterior tibial
Plantar arch
Digital

Veins

External jugular
Internal jugular
Subclavian
Innominate
Superior vena cava
Azygos
Axillary
Cephalic
Hepatic
Intercostal
Basilic
Renal
Median cubital
L.Testicular (ovarian)
Common iliac
Internal iliac
External iliac
Digital
Femoral
Long saphenous
Popliteal
Short saphenous
Digital

Fig. 21.5 Major arteries and veins of the systemic circulation.

Arteries. The aorta has four sections, each of which has a number of branches (Fig. 21.6). Two coronary arteries to the heart wall branch from the ascending aorta. From the aortic arch branch the left common carotid to the head and neck; the left subclavian to the left upper limb; and the right innominate, which divides into the right common carotid and right subclavian.

From the descending thoracic aorta branch the bronchial arteries to the lungs; the oesophageal artery to the oesophagus; and 10 pairs of intercostal arteries to the intercostal muscles.

From the abdominal aorta branch the:

- phrenic arteris to the diaphragm.
- coelic trunk which divides into the gastric artery to the stomach; the hepatic artery to the liver; and the splenic artery to the pancreas and spleen.
- superior mesentric to the small intestine.
- renal arteries to the kidneys.
- ovarian or testicular arteries to the ovaries or testes.
- inferior mesentric to the large intestine.
- two common iliac arteries to the pelvic organs and the lower limbs.

Veins. There are two groups of veins: superficial veins, some of which can be seen as bluish lines under the skin; and deep veins which run beside, and often have the same name as, arteries.

Veins rely greatly on the squeezing action of skeletal muscles to assist in pushing blood towards the heart. The respiratory movements also have a milking effect on the inferior vena cava as it passes through the diaphragm.

The pulmonary circulation

The pulmonary circulation involves the transport of deoxygenated blood from the heart to the lungs, and the return of oxygenated blood from the lungs to the heart (Fig. 21.7).

The pulmonary artery leaves the right ventricle and divides into the right and left pulmonary arteries which carry deoxygenated blood to the lungs.

In the lungs, the arteries divide until capillaries are formed, and an exchange of gases takes place through their semipermeable walls. Carbon dioxide passes out of the blood into the alveoli and oxygen is taken from the alveoli into the blood.

Veins collect the blood from the capillaries, and unite to form the two pulmonary veins which leave each lung, carrying oxygenated blood. The four pulmonary veins enter the left atrium of the heart.

The portal circulation

The portal circulation (Fig. 21.8) is responsible for carrying blood which is deoxygenated, but rich in digested nutrients, from some of the abdominal organs to the liver.

The *veins* which make up the portal system are:

- the splenic vein from the pancreas and spleen.
- the gastric vein from the stomach.

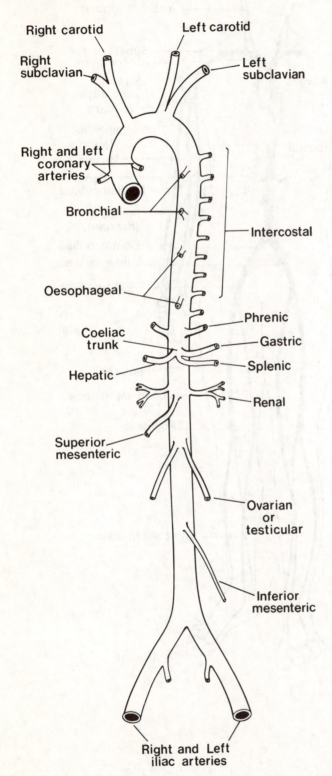

Fig. 21.6 The aorta and its branches.

Right carotid
Left carotid
Right subclavian
Left subclavian
Right and left coronary arteries
Bronchial
Intercostal
Oesophageal
Phrenic
Coeliac trunk
Gastric
Hepatic
Splenic
Renal
Superior mesenteric
Ovarian or testicular
Inferior mesenteric
Right and Left iliac arteries

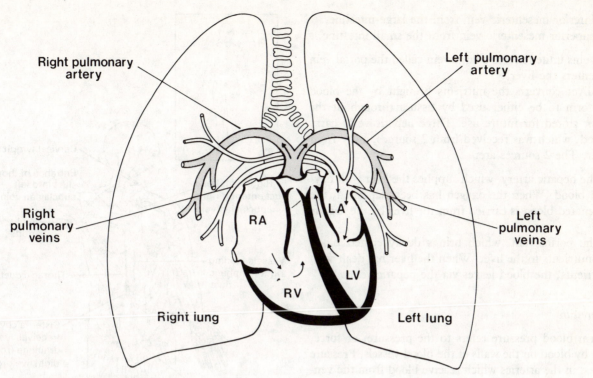

Fig. 21.7 The pulmonary circulation.

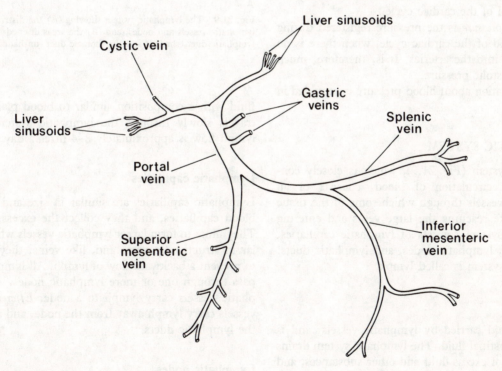

Fig. 21.8 The portal circulation.

- the inferior mesenteric vein from the large intestine.
- the superior mesenteric vein from the small intestine.

These veins unite to form a large vein called the portal vein which enters the liver.

The liver converts the nutrients brought by the blood into a form to be either used by tissues throughout the body, or stored for future use. Three hepatic veins carry the blood, which was received from 2 sources, away from the liver. The 2 sources are:

1. The hepatic artery, which supplies the liver with oxygenated blood. When the oxygen has been deposited, the deoxygenated blood is carried from the liver by the *hepatic veins*.

2. The portal vein, which brings deoxygenated blood rich in nutrients to the liver. When the liver has dealt with the nutrients, the blood leaves via the hepatic veins.

Blood pressure

The term blood pressure refers to the pressure, or force, exerted by blood on the walls of the blood vessels. Pressure is highest in the arteries which receive blood from the ventricles of the heart, then the pressure progressively lessens, so that there is only very slight pressure in the capillaries.

Systolic blood pressure is the pressure registered in a large artery as blood is forced out of the ventricle during the contracting period of the cardiac cycle.

Diastolic blood pressure is the pressure registered during the relaxing period of the cardiac cycle, when there is no ejection of blood into the arteries. It is, therefore, much lower than the systolic pressure.

Further information about blood pressure is provided in Chapter 34.

THE LYMPHATIC SYSTEM

The lymphatic system (Fig. 21.9), which is closely connected with the circulation of blood, consists of an additional set of vessels through which some of the tissue fluid passes before reaching the large veins and entering the blood. This system consists of lymphatic capillaries, lymphatic vessels, lymphatic nodes, and lymphatic ducts. The fluid in the system is called lymph.

Lymph

Lymph is the fluid carried by lymphatic vessels, and is formed from interstitial fluid. The lymphatic system drains the tissue spaces of excess fluid and other substances, and returns them to the blood.

When fluid leaks out of the capillaries of the cardiovascular system it accumulates in the tissue spaces. When this fluid is drained from the tissues and collected by the lymphatic system, it is called lymph. Lymph is a colourless

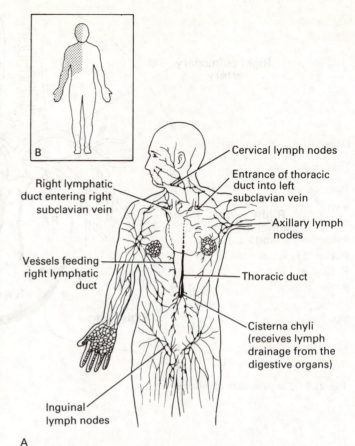

Fig. 21.9   The lymphatic system showing (A) the distribution of lymphatic vessels and nodes, and (B) the areas drained by the right lymphatic duct (shaded) and the thoracic duct (unshaded).

fluid with a composition similar to blood plasma. Lymph travels slowly through the lymphatic system, and total lymph flow is approximately 2–4 litres a day.

Lymphatic capillaries

Lymphatic capillaries are similar in size and structure to blood capillaries, and they collect the excess tissue fluid. They unite to form larger lymphatic vessels which are similar in structure to veins and, like veins, they have valves to prevent a backward flow of lymph. All lymphatic vessels pass through one or more lymphatic nodes. *Afferent* lymphatic vessels carry lymph to a node. *Efferent* lymphatic vessels carry lymph away from the node, and empty it into the lymphatic ducts.

Lymphatic nodes

Lymphatic nodes are found mainly in groups in many parts of the body, e.g. the neck, the thorax, the abdomen, the groin and the limbs. Lymphatic nodes consist of lymphatic tissue and they vary in size, the smallest being about the size of the head of a pin, and the largest the size of an almond. The functions of lymphatic nodes are to

1. filter bacteria from the lymph passing through the node, and destroy them.
2. produce lymphocytes which are added to the lymph.
3. produce antibodies and antitoxins.

Other areas of lymphatic tissue

Lymphatic tissue is found in a number of structures in addition to the nodes already described:

- the tonsils in the oropharynx
- the adenoids in the nasopharynx
- the appendix attached to the intestines
- the thymus gland in the thorax
- peyers patches—large groups in the small intestine
- the spleen in the abdomen.

The tonsils

The tonsils form part of a protective ring of tissue at the entrance to the respiratory and digestive tracts. Lymphatic vessels leave the tonsils and enter the cervical nodes.

The thymus gland

The thymus gland is a soft, grey-pink gland present in the thorax behind the sternum. It is large in infants and children, reaching its maximum size at puberty. After puberty this gland gradually shrinks, until in adulthood there is only a small piece of tissue left. The thymus gland functions in the production of lymphocytes.

The spleen

The spleen is a purplish, half-moon shaped organ in the left hypochondriac region of the abdomen. It lies below the diaphragm and behind the lower ribs, and is mainly composed of lymphoid tissue enclosed in a fibrous capsule. The functions of the spleen are to:

1. produce lymphocytes, some of which enter the bloodstream to carry out their phagocytic action.
2. destroy worn out erythrocytes, producing bile pigments and iron.
3. produce antibodies and antitoxins.
4. provide extra erythrocytes in emergency situations.

If haemorrhage occurs, the spleen contracts and empties its blood into the circulation in an attempt to restore normal blood volume.

Lymphatic ducts

Lymphatic ducts receive the lymph from lymphatic vessels and empty it into the bloodstream. They are:

- the thoracic duct.
- the right lymphatic duct.

The thoracic duct

The thoracic duct is the larger of the two lymphatic ducts, and commences in the abdominal cavity at lumbar level, as a dilated sac called the cisterna chyli. The duct passes upwards, through the aortic opening behind the diaphragm into the thorax, where it empties its contents into the left subclavian vein, so that lymph rejoins the bloodstream.

Lymphatic vessels from all parts of the body below the diaphragm, and the left side of the body above the diaphragm, empty their contents into the thoracic duct.

The right lymphatic duct

The right lymphatic duct is very small (about 1 cm long) and lies in the root of the neck. It receives lymph from the right side of the head and neck, the right side of the thorax and the right upper limb. The right lymphatic duct empties its contents into the right subclavian vein.

The lymphatics begin in the tissue spaces as tiny vessels a little larger than capillaries, empty into progressively larger branches of lymphatic vessels, pass through the lymph nodes, and ultimately empty their fluid (lymph) into the venous circulation.

The lymphatics serve an important function in preventing *oedema*, as the tiny vessels collect fluid and proteins from the interstitial spaces and promote their return to the blood circulation. They also collect the larger digested fat particles from the digestive system and empty them into the circulation. In addition, the lymphatics play a key role in the body's defence against microorganisms. They collect microorganisms in the interstitial spaces, and carry them to the lymph nodes where the lymphocytes (and macrophages) remove these foreign substances from the lymph.

SUMMARY

The circulatory system is the means by which every cell in the body is supplied with oxygen and nutrients, and the means by which the cells waste products are transported to various organs for excretion.

The circulatory system consists of the cardiovascular and the lymphatic systems.

The cardiovascular system is composed of the blood, the blood vessels, and the heart. The lymphatic system consists of lymph, lymphatic capillaries, vessels, nodes, and ducts.

Blood is a viscous substance composed of a fluid (plasma) in which 3 types of blood cells are suspended. Erythrocytes, leucocytes, and platelets are the types of blood cells; and each has specific functions to perform. The overall functions of blood are to transport oxygen, nutrients and other substances to the cells, to transport wastes away from the cells, to protect the body against infection, to distribute heat evenly throughout the body, and to prevent a loss of blood by means of a clotting mechanism. Blood belongs to one of four groups (A, B, AB, O) and may or may not possess the Rh factor.

The blood vessels are the means by which blood is transported through the tissues. Blood is pumped by the heart into the major arteries which then form increasing smaller arteries and eventually arterioles. Arterioles are continuous with a network of minute vessels, capillaries. Blood then enters small veins or venules, which join to form veins. The veins unite to form the major veins which transport the blood back to the heart.

The heart is a hollow muscular organ situated in the thoracic cavity, and acts as a pump. It pumps deoxygenated blood to the lungs, and it pumps oxygenated blood to all parts of the body.

Blood is in constant circulation around the body, either in the systemic, pulmonary, or portal circulation.

The lymphatic system drains the tissue spaces of excess fluid and other substances, and returns them to the blood. The lymphatic vessels pass through one or more nodes, the functions of which are to filter and destroy micro-organisms, and to produce lymphocytes, antibodies, and antitoxins.

22. The respiratory system

INTRODUCTION

Every cell in the body requires oxygen to carry out its metabolic functions, and every cell must rid itself of carbon dioxide—a waste product of cellular metabolism. The respiratory system is the means by which oxygen from the atmosphere is delivered to the bloodstream, and the means by which carbon dioxide from the blood is delivered to the atmosphere. The cardiovascular system, which is described in Chapter 21, transports oxygen to, and carbon dioxide from, the body tissues.

The function of the respiratory system is to bring about gaseous exchange, allowing the uptake of oxygen and the elimination of carbon dioxide. Respiration is the term used for the interchange of gases, and it includes external and internal respiration.

External respiration is the exchange of oxygen and carbon dioxide between the body and the surrounding air.

Internal respiration is the exchange of oxygen and carbon dioxide between the bloodstream and the tissues.

STRUCTURE OF THE RESPIRATORY SYSTEM

The structures which make up the respiratory tract, (Fig. 22.1) are the nasal cavities, pharynx, larynx, trachea, the bronchial tree, and the lungs. The muscles of ventilation are the diaphragm and the intercostals.

Nasal cavities

The nose is a bony cartilagenous structure, divided into a right and left nasal cavity by a septum. The anterior portion of the septum is cartilage, and the posterior portion is bone—formed by the vomer and part of the ethmoid bone.

Inside each nostril (nares) is a vestibule lined by skin containing sebaceous and sweat glands, and coarse hairs which act as filters. Apart from the vestibules, all other areas of the nasal cavities are lined by mucous membrane. In most of the cavity the membrane is covered by *ciliated* epithelium with many goblet cells. Mucous glands are also present in the underlying connective tissue. The inside of the nasal cavity is therefore covered by a thin layer of *mucus* which traps dust from the air.

Functions of the nose (nasal cavities)

1. Hairs in the nose filter foreign particles from the air breathed in.
2. Mucus, secreted by the lining, traps dust in inhaled air, and the cilia move particles of mucus towards the pharynx to be swallowed or expectorated.
3. Inhaled air is warmed and moistened as it passes over the mucous membrane which lines the nasal cavities.
4. The nose is an organ of sensation, as it contains the nerve endings for the sense of smell (olfactory receptors).

The pharynx

The pharynx is a muscular tube approximately 12 cm long, lying in front of the cervical vertebrae and behind the nose, mouth and larynx. It is lined with mucous membrane and has 3 sections:

*1. **The nasopharynx** is continuous with the nasal cavity above and with the oropharynx below. The *pharyngotympanic (Eustachian) tubes* which carry air to the middle ear, have openings into the nasopharynx. The *adenoids* are patches of lymphoid tissue which lie on the posterior wall of the nasopharynx.

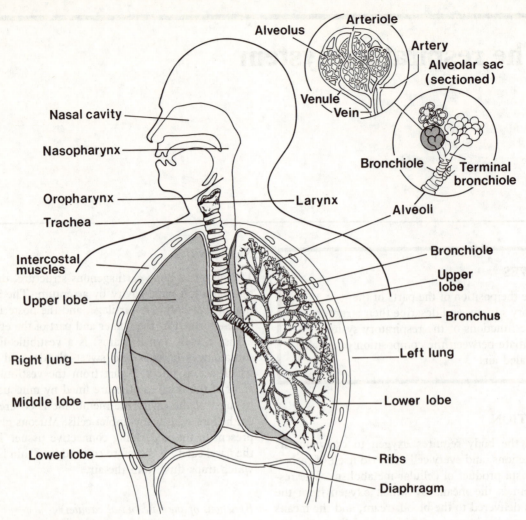

Fig. 22.1 The respiratory tract.

2. The oropharynx is the section which lies behind the mouth, and is separated from the cavity of the mouth by two folds of mucous membrane (the fauces). Between these folds lie the oral *tonsils*, which are patches of lymphoid tissue.

The *uvula* is a muscular projection of the soft palate in the middle of the arch formed by the fauces.

3. The laryngopharynx is the section which opens into both the larynx and the oesophagus. The *epiglottis* is a small flap of cartilage that covers the larynx during swallowing to prevent food or fluid from being aspirated. As a result, food or fluid is directed down into the oesophagus.

Functions of the pharynx

1. The nasopharynx warms and moistens inhaled air.
2. It allows for air to travel along the pharyngotympanic tubes to the middle ear, to equalize the pressure in the middle ear with the atmospheric pressure.

3. The oropharynx provides a common passage for air, food and fluids.

The larynx

The larynx is situated in the upper region of the neck, and extends from the pharynx above to the trachea below. It is composed of pieces of cartilage connected by membranes, and it is lined mainly by ciliated mucous membrane. Stratified epithelium lines the upper part of the larynx containing the vocal cords. The main cartilages forming the larynx are:

1. The thyroid cartilage is the largest, and forms a prominence known as the 'Adam's apple'.
2. The epiglottis is a leaf-shaped cartilage attached to the upper part of the thyroid cartilage. During swallowing, the larynx rises and the epiglottis covers its opening.
3. The cricoid cartilage lies below the thyroid cartilage, and is shaped like a signet ring.

The larynx is lined with mucous membrane which becomes ciliated in the lower part. In the upper part, two folds of membrane containing embedded fibrous and elastic tissue, form the *vocal cords*. The vocal cords extend from the anterior wall to the posterior wall of the larynx to form the *glottis* or voice box.

Voice production. The vocal cords are apart during normal breathing. Contraction of muscles attached to the cords brings them close together, and expired air is used to cause vibration of the cords. The brain, tongue, lips, and the facial muscles, all help to covert the resultant sounds into speech. The pitch of the voice depends on the length and tightness of the cords, and air sinuses in the skull bones influence the resonance of the voice. The vowels and consonants that make up speech are formed by various positions of the lips and tongue. Speaking requires coordination of the larynx, mouth, lips, tongue, throat, lungs, and abdomen.

The nerve supply to the larynx is from the laryngeal and recurrent laryngeal nerves, which are branches from the vagus nerve.

Functions of the larynx

1. It provides a passageway for air between the pharynx and trachea. As air passes through, it is further moistened, warmed, and filtered.

2. The vocal cords produce sounds.

3. The epiglottis prevents the entry of food or fluid into the trachea.

The trachea

The trachea is approximately 12 cm long extending from the larynx to the mid-thorax, where it divides into a right and a left bronchus. It lies in front of the oesophagus, in the mid-line.

The trachea consists of 15–20 C-shaped rings of cartilage joined by involuntary muscle and fibrous tissue. The deficiency in the rings of cartilage posteriorly is filled in by connective tissue and involuntary muscle. This ensures that the oesophagus can expand when food is swallowed, and the cartilage rings of the trachea maintain patency of the airway.

The trachea is lined with ciliated epithelium containing goblet cells and mucous glands. The cilia sweep mucus and any foreign particles which enter the trachea, up into the pharynx to be swallowed or expectorated.

Functions of the trachea

1. It provides a permanently open passageway for air travelling to and from the lungs.

2. Air is warmed and moistened as it passes through trachea.

The bronchi

At about the middle of the thorax, the trachea divides to form the right and left bronchus. The bronchi enter the lungs; the right bronchus dividing into three, and the left bronchus dividing into 2 branches. There are 3 lobes in the right lung and 2 lobes in the left lung, therefore one branch of each bronchus enters a lobe. The left bronchus is longer than the right, because of the position of the heart.

The bronchi are similar in structure to the trachea, but as the division of the bronchi continues the cartilage is gradually replaced with involuntary muscle.

The bronchioles

Bronchioles are the smallest branches from the bronchi, and their walls consist of involuntary muscle with elastic fibrous tissue allowing for expansion. They divide to form microscopic *alveolar* ducts which terminate in clusters of air sacs called alveoli.

Alveoli

Alveoli are microscopic air sacs in the lungs. Their walls are composed of one layer of epithelium, forming a semipermeable membrane. Alveoli are surrounded by networks of capillaries.

Functions of alveoli

The interchange of oxygen and carbon dioxide takes place between the air in the alveoli and the blood in the capillaries (Fig. 22.2).

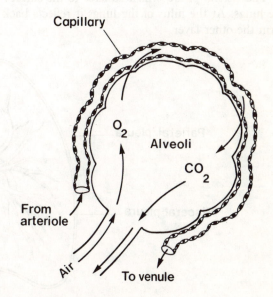

Fig. 22.2 Exchange of gases in the alveoli.

The lungs

The lungs are two structures that lie in the thoracic cavity on either side of the *mediastinum*. The mediastinum contains the heart, major blood vessels and the oesophagus. The lungs are light and spongy, and consist of the bronchioles, alveoli and blood vessels, supported by areolar tissue. There is also a great deal of elastic tissue to enable the lungs to expand and recoil freely during respiration.

The base of each lung rests on the diaphragm and the apex of each extends to just above each clavicle.

The right lung has 3 lobes and is shorter and wider than the left lung which has 2 lobes (Fig. 22.1). Each lobe is made up of lobules. On the medial side of each lung there is a depression called the *hilus* through which the bronchi and blood vessels enter and exit. The structures entering or exiting each hilus include:

- the bronchus, providing a passageway for air into and out from the lung.
- the pulmonary artery, carrying deoxygenated blood to the lungs for removal of carbon dioxide.
- the bronchial artery, supplying the lung tissue with blood rich in oxygen and other essential substances.
- the bronchial vein carrying deoxygenated blood from the lung tissue to the superior vena cava.
- two pulmonary veins, carrying oxygenated blood to the left atrium of the heart.
- lymphatic vessels, draining lymph from the heart into the lymphatic circulation.

The pleura

The pleura (Fig. 22.3) is a double layers of serous membrane, consisting of:

- 1. The *visceral pleura* which adheres to the surface of the lungs. At the hilus of the lungs it reflects back to form the other layer.

- 2. The *parietal pleura* which lines the thoracic cavity, and covers the superior surface of the diaphragm.

The pleura secretes a thin film of serous fluid which lies between the 2 layers, and prevents friction between them during breathing.

The muscles of ventilation

The main muscles responsible for ventilation are the diaphragm and the intercostal muscles. Information on these muscles is provided in Chapter 19. During difficult or forced breathing, accessory muscles are used, e.g. the muscles of the neck, thorax and abdomen.

PHYSIOLOGY OF RESPIRATION

As a result of forces exerted by respiratory muscles on the thorax, the intrathoracic pressure alters. Consequently air is drawn into and expelled from the lungs, which play an essentially *passive* role in these processes.

Respiration is the term used to describe an interchange of gases. The main purpose of respiration is to supply the body with oxygen and dispose of carbon dioxide. Three processes are involved:

1. *Ventilation* (breathing) is the passage of air into and out of the lungs.
2. *External respiration* is the exchange of oxygen and carbon dioxide between the blood and the alveoli.
3. *Internal respiration* is the exchange of oxygen and carbon dioxide between the bloodstream and the tissues.

Gas exchange is the term used to describe the movement of oxygen from the alveoli to the pulmonary blood, and the simultaneous movement of carbon dioxide from the

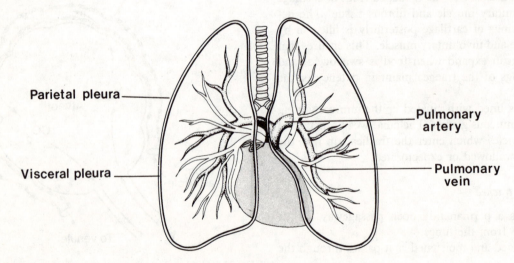

Fig. 22.3 The lungs and pleura.

pulmonary blood to the alveoli (Fig. 22.2). Gas exchange takes place by *diffusion* of molecules of dissolved gas.

Certain physical laws, in relation to gases, apply to both external and internal respiration:

- A gas will always move from an area of higher pressure to an area of lower pressure, or from a greater concentration to a lower concentration.
- The molecules forming a gas are in constant motion.
- Gases always exert pressure on the walls of containers in which they are held.
- Gases *diffuse* through semipermeable membranes.

The mechanisms of ventilation (breathing)

Ventilation has 2 phases; inhalation (breathing in) and exhalation (breathing out).

Inhalation

During inhalation the diaphragm contracts and flattens, enlarging the thoracic cavity lengthwise (Fig. 22.4). At the same time the external intercostal muscles contract, raising

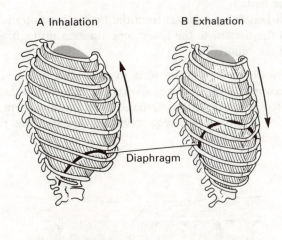

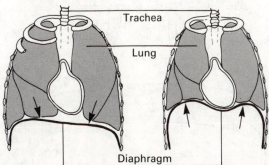

Fig. 22.4 Rib cage and diaphragm positions during breathing. (A) At the end of the normal inhalation: chest expanded (top left) and diaphragm depressed (bottom left).
(B) At the end of a normal exhalation: chest depressed (top right) and diaphragm elevated (bottom right).

the ribs and sternum thus increasing the size of the thoracic cavity from side to side and front to back.

As the chest wall moves up and outward the parietal pleura moves with it, and due to the negative pressure between the layers of the pleura the visceral pleura follows the parietal pleura. This causes stretching of the lungs which expand to fill the enlarged thorax, and air is sucked into the respiratory passages. The air is warmed, moistened, and filtered in the respiratory passages before it enters the lungs.

Exhalation

Exhalation is a more passive process than inhalation. During exhalation the diaphragm relaxes thus decreasing the size of the thoracic cavity. The intercostal muscles also relax, allowing the ribs and sternum to return to their former position—further decreasing the size of the thoracic cavity. The elastic lungs recoil, forcing air out of the respiratory passages.

Capacity of the lungs refers to the volume of gas breathed in and out of the lungs, and this volume can be measured using a spirometer:

- *Tidal volume* is the volume of air that enters or leaves the lungs at each breath. In normal breathing the resting tidal volume is approximately 500 ml of air.
- *Vital capacity* is the volume of air that can be expelled by the deepest possible exhalation following the deepest possible inhalation. The average vital capacity is between 4000 ml and 5000 ml.
- *Residual volume* is the amount of air left in the lungs following the deepest possible exhalation. There is always approximately 1000–1200 ml of air remaining in the lungs at the end of exhalation.

External respiration

External respiration is the exchange of gases between air in the alveoli, and the blood in the surrouning capillaries (Fig. 22.2). During this exchange, gases diffuse through the semipermeable walls of the alveoli and capillaries, until the pressure is equal on both sides:

- Oxygen moves from the higher concentration in the alveolar air to the lower concentration in the capillary blood.
- Carbon dioxide moves from the higher concentration in capillary blood to the lower concentration in the alveolar air.

Branches of the pulmonary artery bring deoxygenated blood to the capillary networks. Veins collect the blood rich in oxygen from the capillaries, and unite to form the two pulmonary veins which leave each lung to enter the left atrium of the heart.

Table 22.1 illustrates the concentration and movement of gases in the alveoli and capillary blood.

Table 22.1 External respiration

Gas	Concentration in alevoli	Movement	Concentration in blood
Oxygen	100 mmHg	→	40 mmHg
Carbon dioxide	40 mmHg	←	46 mmHg

Table 22.2 illustrates the approximate composition of inspired and expired air.

Table 22.2 Composition of air (approximate)

Substance	Inhaled air	Exhaled air
Nitrogen	78.62%	74.5%
Oxygen	20.84%	15.7%
Carbon dioxide	0.04%	3.6%
Water vapour	0.50%	6.2%
Total	100.0%	100.0%

Mechanisms of respiratory control

The rate and depth of inhalation and exhalation are regulated by nerve pathways that respond to various stimuli which signal increased or diminished oxygen requirements or carbon dioxide levels.

The respiratory centres that control the rhythm and depth of ventilation, are located in the medulla oblongata and pons varolii of the brain. Impulses are transmitted to these centres, and back from these respiratory centres to:

- the phrenic nerves which stimulate the diaphragm
- the intercostal nerves which stimulate the intercostal muscles.

The cerebral centres receive impulses from a wide array of nerve endings, some of which are sensitive to chemical stimuli and some of which are sensitive to mechanical stimuli.

Chemoreceptors are located centrally in the medulla. Ventilation is stimulated by an increase in arterial carbon dioxide pressure (PCO^2), a fall in arterial pH, and to a lesser extent a fall in arterial oxygen pressure (PO^2). The resultant increased ventilation will tend to reduce the changes back towards normal.

Mechanoreceptors are present in lung tissue and within the thoracic wall. The bronchioles and alveoli have stretch receptors that respond to extreme overinflation as well as extreme deflation. When overinflation occurs impulses are transmitted from the stretch receptors to the medulla by the vagus nerves, the *expiratory* centre is activated, and exhalation occurs. When extreme deflation occurs impulses

from the lungs activate the *inspiratory* centres, and inhalation occurs.

Any abnormal mechanical disturbance, e.g. the presence of chemical substances such as cigarette smoke, causes excitement of the lung irritant receptors. Excitement of the true lung irritant receptors induces hyperventilation and a reflex broncho constriction.

Information from other parts of the body may also be received by the respiratory centres, e.g. a rise in body temperature initiates an increase in the rate of ventilation. Conversely, a sudden cooling of the skin induces a sudden inhalation—followed by hyperventilation.

Other factors can modify the rate and depth of ventilation, e.g. exercise, conscious control, and emotional states.

Internal respiration

Internal respiration is the exchange of gases between the bloodstream and the tissues (Fig. 22.5). During this exchange, the gases diffuse through the semipermeable walls of the capillaries until the pressure is equal on both sides:

- Oxygen moves from the higher concentration in the blood in the capillaries to the lower concentration in the tissues.
- Carbon dioxide moves from the higher concentration in the tissues, to the lower concentration in the blood in the capillaries.

Arteries branch from the aorta to carry oxygenated blood to networks of capillaries in all tissues. Veins collect deoxygenated blood from the capillaries, and unite to form the inferior and superior vena cava which enter the right atrium of the heart.

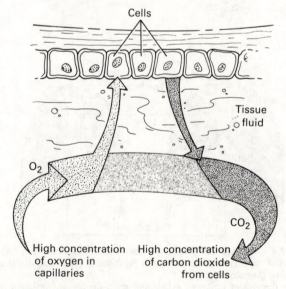

Fig. 22.5 Internal respiration.

Table 22.3 illustrates the concentration and movement of gases in the tissues and capillary blood.

Table 22.3 Internal respiration

Gas	Concentration in tissues	Movement	Concentration in blood
Oxygen	Low	←	High
Carbon dioxide	High	→	Low

SUMMARY

The function of the respiratory system is to bring about gaseous exchange, allowing the uptake of oxygen and the elimination of carbon dioxide.

The structures which make up the respiratory tract are the nasal cavities, pharynx, larynx, trachea, bronchial tree, and the lungs. The main muscles of ventilation are the diaphragm and the intercostals.

The nasal cavities are lined by ciliated mucous membrane, which secretes mucus to trap dust in inhaled air. The cilia sweep particles of mucus towards the pharynx to be swallowed or expectorated.

The pharynx has 3 sections; the naso-pharynx, oropharynx, and laryngopharynx. As inhaled air passes through the pharynx, it is warmed and moistened.

The larynx is composed of 3 cartilages, one of which is the epiglottis which covers the larynx during swallowing.

The larynx contains the vocal cords which form the glottis or voice box.

The trachea extends from the larynx to mid-thorax, where it divides into a right and a left bronchus. The trachea provides a permanently open airway for air travelling to and from the lungs.

The bronchi enter the lungs and divide into smaller branches which divide further to form the bronchioles. At the ends of bronchioles are alveolar ducts which terminate in clusters of air sacs called alveoli. The interchange of oxygen and carbon dioxide takes place between the air in the alveoli, and the blood in the surrounding capillaries.

The lungs lie in the thoracic cavity, one on either side of the mediastinum. Each lung is made up of spongy elastic tissue and contain the branches of the bronchi, the bronchioles, and the alveoli; together with important large blood vessels, nerves and lymphatic vessels that enter or leave the hilus of the lung.

The pleura is a double layer of serous membrane that covers the lungs and lines the thoracic wall. It secretes a serous fluid which prevents friction between the two layers.

Respiration supplies the body with oxygen and disposes of carbon dioxide. For this to occur, ventilation, and external and internal respiration must take place.

Ventilation (breathing) consists of inhalation and exhalation. External respiration is the exchange of oxygen and carbon dioxide between the air in the alveoli, and the blood in the capillaries which surround them. Internal respiration is the exchange of oxygen and carbon dioxide between the bloodstream and the tissues.

The rate and depth of ventilations are regulated by nerve pathways that transmit information to the respiratory centres in the brain. Impulses from the respiratory centres travel back to the diaphragm via the phrenic nerves, and to the intercostal muscles via the intercostal nerves. Thus the rate and depth of ventilations are adjusted to meet the body's respiratory demands.

23. The digestive system

INTRODUCTION

Every cell in the body requires energy in order to carry out its normal functions. Cellular energy is produced when nutrients in food are broken down and absorbed. Solid wastes that accumulate during the digestive process must be eliminated. The digestive, or gastro-intestinal, system is the means by which food is ingested and digested. In the digestive tract, food is digested (broken down) to its elemental components—nutrients, fluid, and electrolytes. The digested elements are absorbed into the bloodstream for transport to all the cells, and the solid wastes that accumulate during digestion are excreted from the body.

The digestive system consists of the alimentary canal and the accessory digestive organs.

THE ALIMENTARY CANAL

The alimentary canal is a muscular tube approximately 9–10 metres in length which extends from the mouth to the anus. The structure of the canal (Fig. 23.1) is similar for most of its length, and consists of an outer covering, layers of involuntary muscle and connective tissue, and a mucous membrane lining.

1. The outer covering consists of fibrous tissue (the serosa) or, in the abdomen, peritoneum which is a serous membrane.
Peritoneum is a double layer of serous membrane that secretes serous fluid which prevents friction between the abdominal organs. The two layers of the peritoneum are in contact with each other, but there is a potential space between them which is called the peritoneal cavity. The

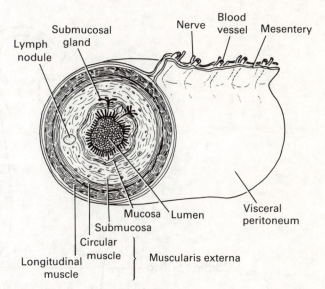

Fig. 23.1 Structure of the alimentary canal.

peritoneum forms a lining for the abdominal cavity (parietal layer) and a covering for most of the abdominal organs (visceral layer). The *mesentery* which is formed by the peritoneum, covers the intestines and attaches them to the posterior abdominal wall. Ligaments are formed by folds of peritoneum to attach some organs to each other, or to the abdominal wall, e.g.:

- the greater omentum, which is attached to the lower border of the stomach, hangs down like an apron and loops up to be attached to the transverse colon.
- the lesser omentum, which extends from the lower border of the liver to the lesser curvature of the stomach.

2. The second layer of smooth involuntary muscle (muscularis externa) has both circular and longitudinal fibres.

3. The third layer of connective tissue (the submucosa) contains many large blood and lymph vessels.

4. The inner lining of mucous membrane (the mucosa) secretes mucus. The mucosa also contains a small amount

193

of loose connective tissue and a thin layer of smooth muscle.

The parts which make up the alimentary canal (Fig. 23.2) are the mouth, the oropharynx, the oesophagus, the small intestine, and the large intestine.

The mouth

The mouth, or oral cavity, has boundaries of muscle and bone and is lined by mucous membrane. The lips protect its anterior opening, the cheeks form the lateral walls, the hard palate forms its anterior roof, and the soft palate forms its posterior roof (Fig. 23.3).

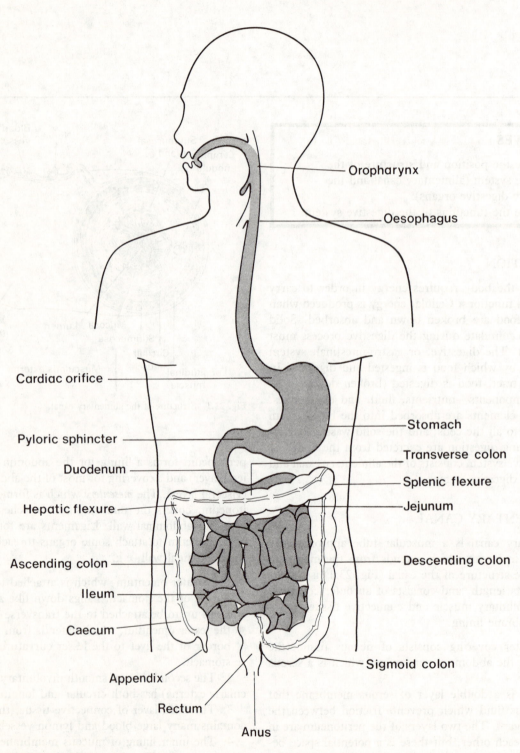

Fig. 23.2 The parts of the alimentary canal.

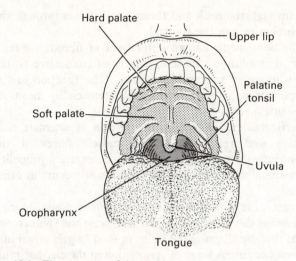

Fig. 23.3 The structures of the mouth.

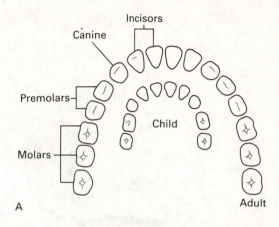

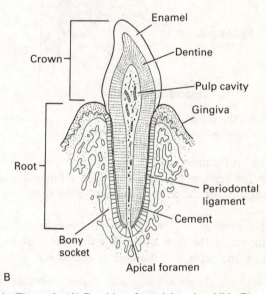

Fig. 23.4 The teeth. (A) Dentition of an adult and a child. (B) Structure of a tooth.

The uvula is a finger-like muscular projection hanging down from the midline of the soft palate. It helps to prevent the entry of food and fluids into the nasal cavities.

Contents of the mouth

The mouth contains the tongue and the teeth.

The tongue is a muscular organ which occupies the floor of the mouth. It is attached to the hyoid bone; and also to the floor of the mouth by folds of mucous membrane called the frenulum. The tongue consists of a mass of voluntary muscle and is covered by squamous epithelium. On the upper surface of the tongue there are many little projections called *papillae* which contain taste buds which are the endings of the nerve of taste. The tongue is a very mobile organ which:

- is the organ of taste
- is important in the chewing (mastication) of food
- assists in swallowing
- is essential for speech.

The teeth are embedded in the maxillae and the mandible. All teeth have the same basic structural organization (Fig. 23.4), but differ in shape and size. Each tooth has:

- one or more roots embedded in the maxilla or mandible
- a portion (the crown) above the gum
- a neck, which joins the root and the crown and which is surrounded by the gum.

Each tooth is made up of an ivory-like substance called dentine; a central pulp cavity containing blood and lymphatic vessels, nerves and connective tissue; and a thin layer of enamel covering the crown.

In children the deciduous (milk) teeth are 20 in number, consisting of 10 each in jaw. In adults there are 16 perma-

nent teeth in each jaw, and the teeth are named according to their shape and function. In each jaw (Fig. 23.4) there are:

- 4 incisors, used for biting
- 2 canines, used for tearing
- 4 premolars, used for crushing
- 6 molars, used for grinding.

A wisdom tooth is the third molar tooth and it is the last tooth to erupt. Wisdom teeth usually erupt between the ages of 18–25 years.

The salivary glands, of which there are three pairs, pour their secretions into the mouth (Fig. 23.5). The salivary glands are:

- The parotid glands, each of which lies below the ear and between the mandible and the sternocleidomastoid muscle. Each parotid duct opens through a papilla on the cheek opposite the crown of the second upper molar.

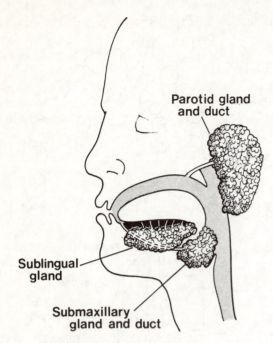

Fig. 23.5   The salivary glands.

• The submandibular (submaxillary) glands, each of which lies beneath the mandible. Each submandibular duct opens on either the left or right side of the frenulum of the tongue.
• The sublingual glands, situated beneath the mucous membrane of the floor of the mouth contain ducts which open on the surface of the floor of the mouth.

The salivary glands are accessory digestive organs, and as such, their function is discussed later in this chapter.

The oropharynx

The oropharynx is the muscular canal forming the passage between the oral cavity and the major parts of the alimentary canal. Lined by mucous membrane, it is a tube approximately 13 cm long and is continuous with the nasopharynx above and the oesophagus below.

Functions of the oropharynx

1. Through the act of swallowing, masticated food formed into a *bolus* is pushed into the oesophagus by the muscles of the pharynx.
2. Together with the other 2 sections of the pharynx, it forms part of the respiratory tract.

The oesophagus

The oesophagus is a muscular tube approximately 20–25 cm long, extending from the pharynx above to the stomach below. It lies behind the larynx and trachea, in the mid-line through the neck and thorax, and passes through the diaphragm to join the stomach.

The oesophagus has an outer layer of fibrous tissue, a layer of involuntary muscle, a layer of connective tissue, and a lining of mucous membrane. The function of the oesophagus is to carry food to the stomach by means of peristaltic action.

Peristalsis is a wave-like progression of alternate contraction and relaxation of the muscle fibres of the oesophagus or intestines, by which contents are propelled along the alimentary canal (peristalsis also occurs in other systems).

At rest, the opening to the oesophagus is closed. During swallowing the muscles contract and cause the sphincter to open, thereby allowing the bolus of food to pass down into the oesophagus. A wave of contraction in the circular muscle layer then propels the bolus down to the stomach. This peristaltic wave travels at a rate of approximately 4 cm per second.

The bottom end of the oesophagus acts as a functional sphincter which is normally in a state of tonic contraction. As the peristaltic wave approaches the sphincter, the muscle relaxes and allows food to enter the stomach. The sphincter then closes again and prevents regurgitation of gastric contents back into the oesophagus.

The stomach

The stomach (Fig. 23.6) is a hollow muscular organ that lies primarily in the upper left quadrant of the abdomen, beneath the diaphragm. It is commonly described as being 'J shaped', but the size and shape of the stomach varies according to its contents. The stomach is divided into 4 areas:

• the fundus, which is the upper portion
• the cardia, where the oesophagus joins the stomach
• the body, or main part of the stomach
• the pylorus, which is the narrowed lower portion.

The opening of the oesophagus into the stomach is called the cardiac orifice, and is surrounded by a functional sphincter called the *cardiac sphincter*. The pyloric orifice is the opening between the stomach and the small intestine, and it is surrounded by the *pyloric sphincter*. The pyloric sphincter, which consists of a thickened layer of circular muscle, is normally partly open. The peristaltic wave pushes some of the gastric contents through the orifice and into the duodenum. The orifice then closes.

The *curvatures* (Fig. 23.6) of the stomach are:

• the lesser curvature, which is the medial border
• the greater curvature, which is the lateral border.

The *stomach wall* consists of 4 layers:

• the serosa, an outer covering of peritoneum

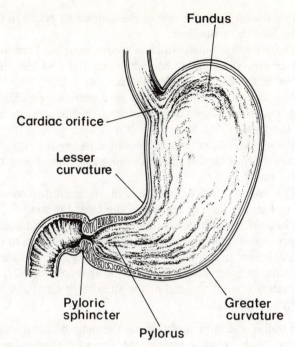

Fundus

Cardiac orifice

Lesser
curvature

Pyloric
sphincter

Pylorus

Greater
curvature

Fig. 23.6 The stomach.

- the muscular layer consisting of longitudinal and circular muscles and an additional oblique layer of muscle on the inside
- the submucosa
- the mucosa, which is a lining of mucous membrane arranged in folds which flatten out as the stomach distends.

The lining consists of a single layer of epithelial cells which continually secrete neutral mucus onto the surface. The mucosa is covered by small depressions which contain the openings of the gastric glands that secrete gastric juice.

Functions of the stomach

1. The stomach acts as a temporary reservoir for food allowing the digestive enzymes time to act.
2. Breaks up the food into a liquid state by muscular contraction of the stomach walls.
3. Produces gastric juice which contains hydrochloric acid, intrinsic factor, mucus, gastric enzymes (pepsinogens), and water.

Hydrochloric acid, which has several functions, is released in response to a hormone, gastrin. Hydrochloric acid:

- activates pepsins and provides an optimal pH for pepsin activity
- converts ferric iron to ferrous iron
- destroys bacteria.

Intrinsic factor is vital for the absorption of vitamin B_{12} from the diet, and therefore for the development of erythrocytes.

Mucus, secreted by the surface cells of the stomach mucosa, forms a protective lining layer about 1 mm thick. The mucus protects the mucosal cells from the gastric contents.

Pepsinogens are inactive until exposed to hydrochloric acid, when the active pepsins are released. Pepsins act as a catalyst in the chemical breakdown of protein, forming polypeptides and free amino acids.

The small intestine

The small intestine is a coiled muscular tube approximately 5–6 metres in length, extending from the pyloric end of the stomach to the large intestine. The small intestine is divided into a number of anatomically recognizable areas:

- The *duodenum*, which is the widest section, is approximately 20 cm long and is curved.
- The *jejunum*, which is the middle section, is approximately 2.5 metres long.
- The *ileum*, which is the last section, is approximately 4 metres in length.

At the junction of the ileum and the caecum of the large intestine, is the *ileo-caecal valve* which prevents a backward flow of countents from the large to the small intestine.

The wall of the small intestine consists of:

- the serosa, or outer covering of peritoneum
- the muscular layer consisting of longitudinal and circular fibres
- the submucosa
- the mucosa, which is a lining of mucous membrane arranged in folds.

Covering the mucosa are very fine projections called villi (Fig. 23.7).

Intestinal glands in the mucous membrane secrete a digestive juice, called intestinal juice, containing enzymes which complete the digestion of food.

Solitary and aggregated patches of lymphatic tissue, (Peyer's patches) are also found in the mucosa of the intestinal wall, especially in the lower ileum.

An opening in the duodenum (ampulla of Vater) (see Fig. 23.9) allows for the entry of the common bile duct carrying bile from the liver, and the pancreatic duct carrying pancreatic juice.

The functions of the small intestine

These are as follows:

1. secretion of intestinal juice
2. completion of chemical digestion of food
3. absorption of digested food through the villi.

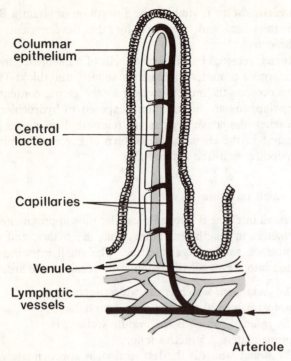

Columnar epithelium

Central lacteal

Capillaries

Venule

Lymphatic vessels

Arteriole

Fig. 23.7 A villus.

The large intestine

The large intestine (Fig. 23.8) is a muscular tube approximately 1.5 metres in length and 6 cm in diameter, and extends from the end of the ileum to the anus. Lying in the abdominal and pelvic cavities, the large intestine may be divided into regions which are distinguished by their anatomical structure and their position:

● The *caecum*, which is a blind-ended sac, approximately 6 cm long and 7.5 cm in diameter. The caecum, which leads into the ascending colon, has the appendix attached.
● The *ascending colon*, which is approximately 15 cm long

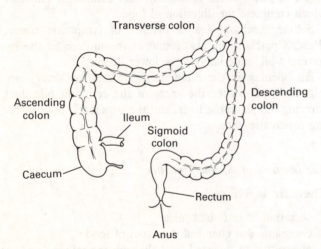

Transverse colon

Ascending colon

Ileum

Sigmoid colon

Descending colon

Caecum

Rectum

Anus

Fig. 23.8 The large intestine.

and passes up the right side of the abdominal cavity to the lower surface of the liver.
● The *transverse colon*, which is approximately 50 cm long and crosses the upper abdomen from right to left then curves in the vicinity of the spleen.
● The *descending colon*, which is approximately 25 cm long, and passes down the left side of the abdomen to the left iliac region.
● The *sigmoid colon*, which is variable in length, is the S-shaped continuation of the descending colon and lies in the pelvic cavity.
● The *rectum*, which is a straight tube approximately 12 cm long, is the last section of the large intestine.
● The *anal canal*, which is the terminal part of the rectum, is approximately 4 cm in length. The canal opens on to the external skin at an orifice called the *anus*. The anal canal contains the internal and the external anal sphincters. The sphincters seal off the end of the alimentary canal and are normally constricted.

The wall of the large intestine has the same basic structure as that of the small intestine (the serosa, muscular layer, submucosa, and the mucosa).

Functions of the large intestine

These are as follows:

1. The absorption of large amounts of water, and some mineral salts
2. Presence of microorganisms (mainly bacteria) which are necessary for the normal development of lymphatic tissue in the large intestine and thus, resistance to infection. The bacteria also synthesize vitamins B and K.
3. Transformation of the intestinal contents into semi-solid faeces, and storage of them until they are excreted.
4. Secretion of mucus to lubricate faeces.

THE ACCESSORY DIGESTIVE ORGANS

The accessory organs are those that pour into the alimentary canal, secretions (enzymes) which are actively involved in the process of digestion. *An enzyme* is a substance, usually protein in nature, that initiates and accelerates a chemical reaction. The accessary organs the salivary glands, the pancreas, and the liver and the biliary tract.

The salivary glands

There are 3 pairs of salivary glands which secrete saliva into the mouth, and the anatomical position of each pair was described earlier in this chapter.

Saliva

Saliva is a watery fluid containing ions, mucin, and the

digestive enzyme salivary beta-amylase (previously known as ptyalin). *Salivation* is largely initiated by sensory stimulation including the presence of food in the mouth, taste and smell. Salivation may also be induced by the presence of irritating substances in the stomach or small intestine. *Saliva* has several functions:

1. It moistens and softens food
2. The mucin acts as a lubricant to aid swallowing
3. It moistens the mouth
4. It has an antibacterial action
5. It enables molecules to dissolve on the surface of the tongue and stimulate the taste buds
6. The enzyme salivary beta-amylase commences the chemical digestion of starch.

The pancreas

The pancreas (Fig. 23.9) is a soft gland, lying across the abdominal cavity behind the stomach. It is divided into:

- a head, which fits into the curve of the duodenum
- a central portion, or body
- a tail, which extends out to the spleen.

The pancreatic duct runs centrally through the length of the pancreas, while smaller ducts carry the pancreatic juice secreted by the pancreas into the central duct. The pancreatic duct joins the common bile duct, from the liver, to enter the duodenum.

The bulk of the tissue in the pancreas is composed of *exocrine* cells which produce pancreatic juice. Scattered among the exocrine tissue are groups of hormone-secreting cells, the islets of Langerhans. The function of the islets of Langerhans is described in Chapter 25, as these cells belong to the endocrine system.

Digestive function of the pancreas

The exocrine tissues of the pancreas are responsible for the production of pancreatic juice, which contains major digestive enzymes. The pancreas secretes approximately 1200 ml of pancreatic juice daily.

Pancreatic juice is a watery alkaline fluid rich in digestive enzymes. The enzymes and their actions are summarized in Table 23.1. The overall function of pancreatic juice is the digestion of nutrients.

The liver

The liver is a large organ, weighing up to 1.8 kg in the adult male, and 1.4 kg in the adult female. It is situated in the upper part of the abdominal cavity, immediately beneath the diaphragm. The greater part of the liver lies in the right upper abdomen, but the organ extends across to the left upper abdomen. The liver is divided into two parts, a large right lobe and a much smaller left lobe (Fig. 23.10).

Like the alimentary canal, the liver is almost entirely covered by a layer of peritoneum. Beneath this is a fibrous capsule which is continuous with areolar connective tissue situated within the liver. The areolar tissue forms a tree-like structure which carries branches of the hepatic artery, hepatic portal vein, bile ducts, lymphatic vessels. These vessels enter and leave the liver through the *porta hepatis*, a short transverse fissure on the inferior surface of the liver.

The hepatic artery carries oxygenated blood to the liver.

The portal vein carries deoxygenated blood, rich in nutrients, to the liver.

Three hepatic veins carry deoxygenated blood from the liver to the inferior vena cava.

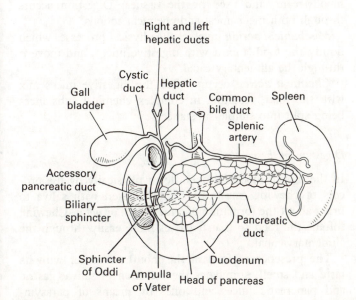

Fig. 23.9 The pancreas and neighbouring structures.

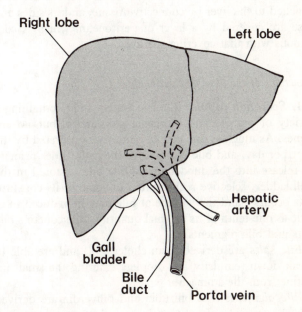

Fig. 23.10 The liver.

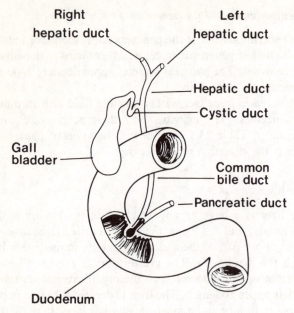

Right hepatic duct

Left hepatic duct

Hepatic duct

Cystic duct

Gall bladder

Common bile duct

Pancreatic duct

Duodenum

Fig. 23.11 The biliary tract.

The right and left hepatic ducts carry bile, secreted by the liver, to the common hepatic duct. The latter combines with the cystic duct from the gallbladder to form the *common bile duct* which drains into the duodenum.

The bilary tract (Fig. 23.11), which transports bile from the liver to the duodenum consists of the left and right hepatic ducts, the common hepatic duct, the cystic duct, the gall bladder, and the common bile duct.

The gallbladder

The gallbladder is a small muscular sac, which lies on the inferior surface beneath the right lobe of the liver. It is attached to the liver by connective tissue, and its sides and base are covered by a layer of peritoneum which is continuous with that covering the liver.

Functions of the liver and gallbladder

1. Secretion of bile. Bile is a watery fluid containing a variety of organic and inorganic substances, but no enzymes. As much as one litre of bile may be secreted by the liver per day, and bile is stored in the gallbladder prior to its release into the duodenum. While bile is stored in the gallbladder, selective reabsorption of some of its constituents occurs—and the volume of bile may be reduced to as little as one-tenth of its original quantity. Bile contains bile salts and bile pigments.

Bile salts are derived from cholesterol, and are able to break down (emulsify) fat droplets entering the small intestine from the stomach.

Bile pigments, i.e. bilirubin and biliverdin are derived from haemoglobin from worn out erythrocytes.

Bile has several functions:

- to provide the alkaline medium required by the enzymes in the small intestine
- to emulsify fats in preparation for the action of enzymes
- to stimulate peristalsis in the intestine
- to colour and deodorize faeces
- to help in the absorption of fats and vitamin K from the small intestine.

Bile not needed immediately travels from the common hepatic duct into the cystic duct, and passes into the gallbladder for storage. When bile is required in the duodenum, the gallbladder contracts and forces bile through the cystic duct into the common bile duct to enter the duodenum.

2. Preparation of nutrients. The liver converts any glucose, not needed immediately, into glycogen for storage. It converts excess protein to glucose to be used as an energy source, and changes the nitrogenous part of excess protein to urea which is excreted. The liver also converts fats into a form which can be used by the tissues.

3. Production of plasma proteins (albumin, globulin, fibrinogen, prothrombin, heparin), and production of vitamin A from carotene in the diet.

4. Storage of glycogen, iron, vitamin A, B. and D.

5. Destruction of worn out erythrocytes, and toxic substances such as alcohol, poisons, and drugs.

6. Production of a considerable amount of heat, as a result of the many activities of the liver.

Digestion of food

During the process of digestion, food is reduced to its simplest chemical form so that it can be absorbed into the bloodstream, and used by the tissues. Digestion occurs through both mechanical and chemical actions.

Mechanical action involves the physical processes which liquify the food, mix it with digestive juices, and move it through the alimentary canal.

Chemical action occurs when the digestive juices mix with the food, resulting in complex chemical substances being split into simple substances.

Digestion in the mouth

In the mouth food is broken down physically by the process of chewing (mastication), and mixed with saliva to bring about the formation of a moist ball or *bolus*. Chewing softens the food so that it passes more easily through the alimentary canal.

The presence of food in the mouth, together with its taste and smell, stimulates the secretion of saliva, gastric and pancreatic juices and bile (by means of parasympathetic pathways). The enzyme salivary beta-amylase in saliva begins to digest starches. Once the food has been formed into a bolus it is passed through the pharynx and down the oesophagus into the stomach. This is achieved by the act of swallowing.

Swallowing is a complex reflex which is regulated by a 'swallowing centre' in the medulla oblongata of the brain. Swallowing is initiated when the tongue muscles push the bolus upwards and backwards into the oropharynx. The soft palate is elevated and comes into contact with the posterior wall of the pharynx, thereby closing off the nasopharynx. The larynx is pulled upwards and forwards, and the bolus pushes the epiglottis back over the glottis to prevent food from entering the respiratory tract.

Peristaltic waves carry the bolus through the oesophagus, and the cardiac sphincter relaxes to allow food and fluids to enter the stomach. The cardiac sphincter contracts to close the cardiac orifice at the end of each wave of contraction of the oesophagus, then relaxes to open the orifice when the next wave of contraction begins.

Digestion in the stomach

The stomach stores the food and later releases it at a rate which is optimal for digestion. Food is mixed with *gastric juice*, thereby changing its consistency so that it will be more easily transported along the alimentary canal. The food is exposed to enzymes (pepsins) which begin the digestion of proteins, and the gastric juice converts ferric iron to ferrous iron.

When the stomach muscles are stretched by swallowed food, peristaltic contractions are stimulated which results in a *churning* movement. When the food is mixed with gastric juice it develops a pasty consistency and becomes known as *chyme*.

The rate of emptying of the stomach depends on:

- the consistency of the chyme
- the degree of opening of the pyloric orifice
- the force of the peristaltic contractions
- the type of food in the stomach. Fats tend to delay emptying, but carbohydrates are usually emptied quickly.

The average time for the stomach to empty after a meal is 4–6 hours. Once the food has been well mixed in the stomach, peristalsis begins in the lower half of the stomach and forces the chyme through the pyloric sphincter. Because this sphincter is only partially opened, only small amounts of chyme enter it at one time. When the duodenum is filled with chyme a nervous reflex (the enterogastric reflex) occurs. This reflex inhibits the *vagus nerves* from stimulating the stomach muscles, and slows the emptying of the stomach. This mechanism ensures that food does not enter the small intestine too fast to ensure its digestion.

Digestion in the small intestine

After it leaves the stomach, chyme is mixed with intestinal secretions as well as with bile and pancreatic juice. Digestion is completed and the products are absorbed through the villi of the intestinal wall. The wall of the small intestine is capable of several different types of movement (Fig. 23.12):

1. Peristalsis ensures an onward movement of the contents of the intestine.

2. Segmentation ensures mixing of the intestinal contents. Segmentation contractions occur regularly, causing the chyme to be broken up into segments.

3. Pendulum movements are small contractions that sweep forwards and then backwards, to cause more effective mixing of the intestinal contents.

Table 23.1 summarizes the process of chemical digestion in the mouth, stomach, and small intestine.

Absorption of digested food

Absorption is the passage of the end products of digestion, through the villi, into the bloodstream. Although absorption mainly occurs in the villi in the small intestine, some absorption takes place in the stomach and large intestine.

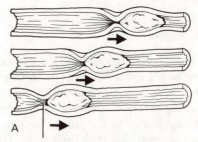

A

Site of muscular contraction

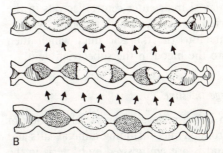

B

Neighbouring segments of the intestine alternately contract and relax, moving food along the tract.

Fig. 23.12 Movements of the small intestine. (A) Peristalsis: food moves along the digestive tract as neighbouring segments of the intestine contract and relax in turn. (B) Segmentation: single segments contract and relax alternately. Since there are inactive segments between the active ones, the food mixes but does not move along the tract.

Table 23.1   Summary of chemical digestion

Secretion	Approximate daily volume (ml)	Enzyme	Acts on	Result
Saliva	1000–1500	Salivary beta amylase	Starch	Dextrins Maltose
Gastric Juice	2000	Pepsin	Protein	Polypeptides and a few free amino acids
Bile	700	—	Fat	Facilitates action of lipase to emulsify fats
Pancreatic Juice	1200	Lipase Amylase Maltase Trypsin	Triglycerides Starch Maltose Proteins	Fatty acids and monoglycerides Maltose Glucose Peptides and Amino acids
Intestinal Juice	2000	Peptidases Amylase Maltase Lactase, Sucrose Lipase	Peptides Starch Maltose Disaccharides Glycerides	Amino acids Maltose Glucose Monosaccharides Fatty acids Glycerol Trypsin
		Enterokinase	Activates Pancreatic trypsinogen	

Absorption in the stomach

Substances which can be absorbed in the stomach are small and lipid-soluble and therefore able to diffuse through cell membranes, e.g. alcohol, water, glucose, and drugs such as salicylic acid (aspirin).

Absorption in the small intestine

Absorption of water and of digested nutrients occurs all along the length of the small intestine. Most substances, e.g. amino acids and monosaccharides, are absorbed through the villi walls (Fig. 23.7) by the process of *active transport*, and enter the capillaries in the villi to be transported in the blood to the liver—via the portal vein. The exception is lipids (fats), which are absorbed passively by the process of *diffusion*. Lipids enter central lacteals in the villi to be transported in the lymph. Lymphatic vessels empty their contents into the thoracic duct which then pours the lymph into the blood in the subclavian vein.

Absorption in the large intestine

The proximal colon is the main site for the absorption of certain substances from chyme, including mineral salts and water. Vitamins B and K are synthesized by bacteria in the colon, and absorbed into the bloodstream.

Excretion

Chyme enters the caecum through the ileo-caecal valve, which is normally closed but opens briefly to allow a small amount of chyme through with each peristaltic wave. Movement of chyme through the large intestine is a slow process. Various types of movement occur in the colon, including peristalsis, segmentation, and mass movements. Mass movements are brought about as a result of distension of the stomach or duodenum by ingested food. This sudden movement of colonic contents can push large amounts of faeces into the rectum and initiate the desire to defaecate.

Defaecation

Most of the time the rectum is empty of faeces, however when a mass movement forces faeces into the rectum the desire to defaecate is initiated.

Faeces are formed as the breaking down of cellulose continues, water is absorbed so that the contents of the colon become semi-solid, and the faecal matter is held together and lubricated by mucus. The faeces are composed of the indigestible remains of food, e.g. dietary fibre, fat, ions, water, digestive enzymes, mucus, cells from the alimentary canal lining, bile pigments, and bacteria.

Defaecation is the term used for emptying of the rectum. Faeces collect in the sigmoid colon prior to entering the rectum. As the faecal mass enters the rectum the defaecation reflex and the desire to defaecate are initiated. Impulses from sensory neurons in the rectal wall travel to the spinal cord, and peristalsis is stimulated in the descending colon, rectum, and the anal canal.

When the peristaltic wave reaches the internal anal sphincter it relaxes. Voluntary relaxation of the external anal sphincter enables the faeces to be excreted. Voluntary contraction of the abdominal muscles, and deep inhalation, raise the intra-abdominal pressure and assist evacuation. If it is not convenient, defaecation can be delayed temporarily, as within a few seconds the reflex contractions cease and the rectal walls relax.

Further information on defaecation and faeces is provided in Chapter 30.

SUMMARY

The digestive system is the means by which food is ingested and digested, so that nutrients can be absorbed into the bloodstream and transported to all the body cells. Solid wastes that accumulate during digestion are then excreted from the body.

The digestive system consists of the alimentary canal and the accessory digestive organs.

The alimentary canal is a muscular tube approximately 9–10 metres in length, extending from the mouth to the anus. It comprises the mouth, the oropharynx, the oesophagus, the stomach, the small intestine, and the large intestine. The structure of the alimentary canal is similar for most of its length, consisting of an outer fibrous covering, a layer of involuntary muscle, a layer of connective tissue, and a lining of mucous membrane.

The accessory organs of digestion are the salivary glands, the pancreas, and the liver. Each accessory organ secretes substances, which are actively involved in the process of digestion, into the alimentary canal. The salivary glands secrete saliva, the pancreas secretes pancreatic juice, and the liver secretes bile.

Food is taken into the mouth (ingested), mixed with saliva and mucus, and swallowed. The formed bolus passes down the oesophagus into the stomach by peristaltic action.

In the stomach, the food is churned and mixed with gastric juice which changes its consistency to chyme, and which begins the digestion of protein. Peristaltic action moves small quantities of chyme into the small intestine. In the duodenum, where bile and pancreatic juice mix with the chyme, most of the chemical digestion takes place.

Digestion is completed when intestinal juice is mixed with the chyme. The contents of the small intestine are moved along its length by waves of peristalsis.

Although absorption of some substances, e.g. alcohol and small amounts of water, takes place in the stomach, absorption mainly occurs in the villi of the small intestine. The digested nutrients and water are absorbed through the walls of the villi into capillaries or lymphatic lacteals, then into the bloodstream to be transported to all body cells. Mineral salts and large amounts of water are absorbed in the proximal section of the large intestine, and vitamins B and K are synthesized by bacteria in the colon and absorbed into the bloodstream.

Faeces which are composed of the indigestible remains of food and other substances, are formed and collect in the sigmoid colon. As the faecal mass enters the rectum, the defaecation reflex and the desire to defaecate is initiated. Voluntary relaxation of the external anal sphincter enables the faeces to be excreted.

24. The urinary system

INTRODUCTION

As a result of cellular metabolism, various wastes are produced. The urinary system plays a major role in the elimination of metabolic waste products and toxic substances, and in regulating the rates of elimination of water and electrolytes from the body. In addition, the kidneys conserve fluid and electrolytes as needed to maintain homeostasis.

By regulating the volume of the body fluid, the urinary system helps to maintain blood pressure, and the electrolyte content and the pH of the blood. Because of this role, the kidneys are considered to perform one of the major homeostatic functions of the body.

The urinary system (Fig. 24.1) consists of the kidneys which filter blood; the ureters which transport urine to the bladder, and the bladder which stores the urine until it is excreted through the urethra.

THE KIDNEYS

The kidneys are two bean-shaped organs situated behind the peritoneum on the posterior wall of the abdominal cavity, on either side of the vertebral column. The kidneys extend from approximately the 12th thoracic vertebra to the third lumbar vertebra. The right kidney is situated a little lower than the left, because of the space occupied by the liver.

Gross structure of the kidney

A kidney (Fig. 24.2) weighs between 120–170 g, is from

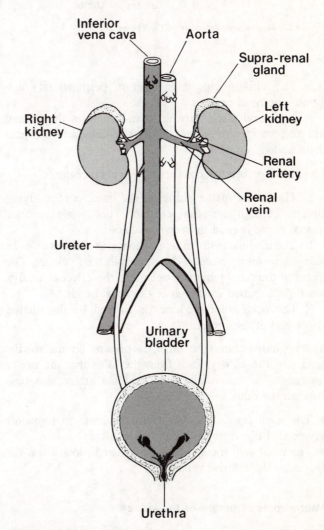

Fig. 24.1 The urinary system.

10–13 cm in length, 5–6 cm wide, and 3–4 cm in thickness. The kidneys are protected and supported by renal fascia, and by layers of perirenal fat. Each kidney is surrounded by 3 layers of tissue:

1. The fibrous renal capsule covers the surface of the kidney.

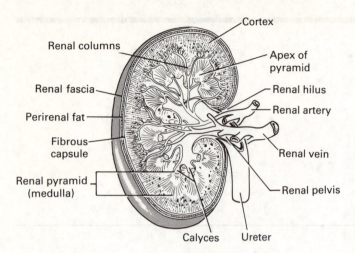

Fig. 24.2   Macroscopic structure of the kidney.

2. The adipose capsule (a layer of perirenal fat) surrounds the renal capsule.

3. The renal fascia surrounds and encloses the kidney and adipose capsule, and anchors the kidney to the posterior abdominal wall.

The kidney substance consists of 3 general regions:

1. The cortex of the kidney is the outer portion, lying directly beneath the renal capsule. This highly vascular area of tissue is reddish-brown in colour.

2. The medulla is the inner portion, and consists of 8–18 triangular *renal pyramids*. It is purplish in colour. The apices of the renal pyramids open into the calyces. A calyx is a funnel-shaped extension of the renal pelvis.

3. The pelvis of the kidney is formed by the dilated upper end of the ureter.

A deep indentation, the hilus, is present on the medial border of the kidney. It is from the hilus that the ureter emerges. The renal vein and the renal artery also pass through the hilus:

● The *renal artery* branches from the aorta to transport oxygenated blood to the kidney.

● The *renal vein* transports deoxygenated blood from the kidney to the inferior vena cava.

Microscopic structure of the kidney

Each kidney contains at least 1 000 000 nephrons, together with their collecting tubules or ducts. The nephron is the functional unit of the kidney and has the structure necessary for urine formation.

The nephron

Each nephron (Fig. 24.3) is composed of a vascular and tubular system that allows for the formation of urine. The nephrons are located in the renal tissue, with most in the cortex and with some extending deep into the medulla of the kidney. A nephron consists of a number of anatomically distinct regions:

● Malpighian bodies, or renal corpuscles, are located in the cortex. Each malpighian body is composed of a tuft of capillaries called the *glomerulus*, which is inserted into the horseshoe-shaped commencement of a renal tube—the Bowman's capsule. The outer wall of the Bowman's capsule is composed of flattened squamous epithelium. The inner layer of the Bowman's capsule is made up of very specialized cells which form a porous membrane surrounding the glomerulus.

● The proximal convoluted tubule is the first part of the renal tubule, and is situated in the cortex.

● The loop of Henle consists of the straight portion of the proximal tubule and the straight part of the distal tubule.

● The distal convoluted tubule is the last portion of the renal tubule. It empties into a straight collecting tubule in the cortex which joins other collecting tubules.

● The collecting tubules fuse in the inner medulla of the kidney to eventually open into the calyces. A second set of capillaries is formed by division of the *efferent vessels* (the arterioles which carry blood away from the capillaries). The veins that collect blood from these capillaries unite to eventually form the renal vein.

Function of the kidneys

The function of the kidneys is to filter the blood to maintain its normal composition, volume, and pH. In carrying out this function, the kidneys secrete urine.

The formation of urine

The formation of urine occurs in 3 phases: simple filtration, selective reabsorption, and secretion.

1. Filtration occurs through the semipermeable walls of the glomerulus and glomerular capsule. Blood enters the glomerular capillaries under relatively high pressure, and is forced into the lumen of the Bowman's capsule.

Water and small molecules pass through the semipermeable walls; while blood cells, plasma proteins, and other large molecules are unable to pass through healthy capillary walls. The resultant glomerular filtrate is, therefore, plasma minus the plasma proteins.

The major factor assisting filtration is the difference between the blood pressure in the glomerulus, and the pressure of filtrate in the glomerular capsule. A capillary hydrostatic pressure of approximately 70 mmHg builds up in the glomerulus—because the calibre of the efferent arteriole is less than that of the afferent arteriole. The capillary pressure is opposed by the lower osmotic pressure of the blood, and the lower filtrate hydrostatic pressure in the glomerular capsule.

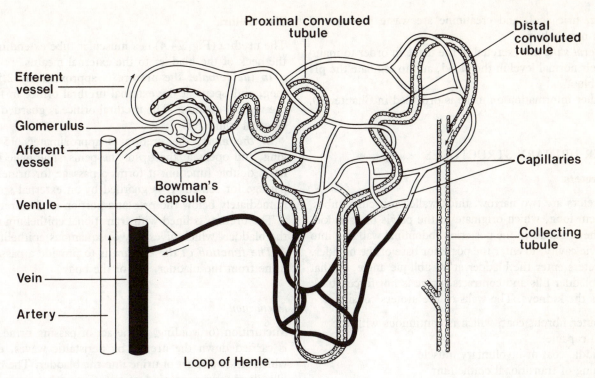

Fig. 24.3   The nephron showing (A) the parts of the nephron.

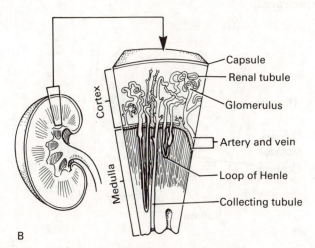

Fig. 24.3   (B) The position of a nephron in the kidney.

The amount of dilute filtrate which is formed in 24 hours is approximately 100–150 litres. The amount actually excreted as urine, in 24 hours, is approximately 1–1.5 litres.

2. Selective reabsorption occurs as the filtered fluid flows through the renal tubules. During this phase, substances such as glucose, amino acids, hormones, mineral salts, vitamins, and most of the water are reabsorbed into the blood. Not reabsorbed are some of the water, substances in excess of body needs, and wastes. Selective reabsorption, therefore, helps to maintain fluid and electrolyte balance and blood pH.

3. Secretion is the process by which substances such as hydrogen and potassium ions move from the blood of the peritubular capillaries through or from the tubule cells into the filtrate to be eliminated in urine. The fluid (urine) which flows from the collecting tubules contains substances not needed by the body.

Urine is poured into the pelvis of the kidneys for transport, via the ureters, to the urinary bladder.

Control of urine formation

The control of kidney function is both nervous and hormonal.

1. Nervous control maintains the level of blood pressure required for filtration to occur.

2. Hormonal control consists of:

• adrenaline secreted by the suprarenal glands, which helps to maintain the high level of blood pressure in the glomerulus.
• anti-diuretic hormone (A.D.H.) secreted by the pituitary gland, which controls the amount of water reabsorbed from the tubules.
• aldosterone secreted by the suprarenal glands, which controls the tubule's reabsorption of mineral salts.

Composition of urine

Urine is a clear, amber coloured fluid which is slightly acidic, and is composed of 96% water, 2% urea, and 2% mineral salts, uric acid and creatinine.

Urea, uric acid, and creatinine are waste products of protein metabolism.

Mineral salts are excreted in the urine in order to maintain their normal level in the blood, and to regulate the pH of the blood.

Further information on urine is provided in Chapter 30.

OTHER URINARY STRUCTURES

The ureters

The ureters are two narrow, thick-walled muscular tubes, 25–30 cm long, which originate in the pelvis of each kidney. They pass down the posterior abdominal wall and into the pelvic cavity, to enter the posterior base of the bladder. The ureters enter the bladder at an oblique angle, so that as the bladder fills and contracts, urine is not forced back towards the kidneys. The walls of the ureters consist of:

- an outer fibrous coat, which is continuous with the renal capsule.
- a middle coat of involuntary muscle
- a lining of transitional epithelium.

The function of the ureters is to carry urine from the kidneys to the bladder, by means of peristaltic action. The involuntary muscle layer, in the walls of the ureters, contract from 1–5 times per minute to force urine into the bladder.

The urinary bladder

The urinary bladder is a hollow muscular organ lying in the pelvic cavity behind the symphysis pubis. In the female, the bladder lies in front of the uterus; in the male it lies in front of the rectum. The walls of the bladder consist of:

- a covering of peritoneum over the upper portion (the fundus)
- a layer of involuntary muscle
- a layer of connective tissue
- a lining of mucous membrane composed of transitional epithelium.

The trigone of the bladder is a triangle formed by the three orifices:

- 2 ureteric orifices where the ureters enter
- 1 urethral orifice where the urethra leaves.

Below the neck of the bladder lies the striated muscle which constitutes an external *sphincter*.

The function of the urinary bladder is to act as a reservoir for urine.

The urethra

The urethra (Fig. 24.4) is a muscular tube extending from the neck of the bladder to the external meatus.

In the female, the urethra is approximately 2.5–4 cm long, and opens at the external urethral orifice in front of the vaginal opening. The urethral orifice is guarded by the external sphincter.

In the male, the urethra is approximately 15–20 cm long, and opens at the tip of the penis. The male urethra has a double function: it forms a passage for urine, and a passage for semen. It is guarded by an external sphincter immediately below the prostatic portion of the urethra.

The urethra is lined with transitional epithelium near to the bladder, which gives way to squamous epithelium.

The function of the urethra is to provide a passage for urine from the bladder, out of the body.

Micturition

Micturition (or voiding) is the act of passing urine. Urine is carried down the ureters by peristaltic waves, each of which sends a spurt of urine into the bladder. The bladder fills slowly over a period of time, and when it holds approximately 300 ml a desire to empty the bladder is experienced.

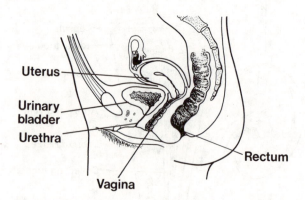

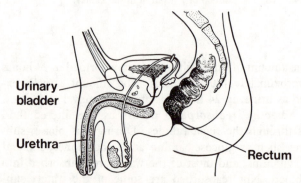

Fig. 24.4 Position of the female and male urethra.

The process of micturition is regulated by a reflex which is initiated by impulses from stretch receptors in the bladder wall. The sensory neurons transmit the impulses to the spinal cord, where they are relayed to parasympathetic neurons which innervate the bladder wall and cause it to contract. Simultaneously, the external sphincter relaxes and urine can be voided.

Further information on micturition is provided in Chapter 30.

SUMMARY

The urinary system is essential for homeostasis. It is the means by which the body rids itself of a variety of metabolic wastes, and the means by which fluid and electrolytes are conserved or excreted.

The urinary system consists of the kidneys, the ureters, the urinary bladder, and the urethra.

The kidneys filter the blood to maintain its normal composition, volume, and pH. In carrying out this function, the kidneys secrete urine.

Urine is formed by the processes of filtration, selective reabsorption, and secretion. Urine is composed of water, urea, mineral salts, uric acid and creatinine.

When urine is formed by the kidneys it passes down the ureters by peristaltic action, to the urinary bladder. Urine is stored in the bladder until it is excreted from the body through the urethra.

Micturition is initiated when the bladder walls are stretched. Normally when the bladder holds about 300 ml of urine the micturition reflex is initiated.

25. The endocrine system

INTRODUCTION

The endocrine organs do not make up an anatomical system, but are a number of small glands (Fig. 25.1). Some of the glands are located within other organs, while others are structurally independent.

The endocrine glands function as an inter-related system together with the nervous system, to maintain homeostasis. Endocrine glands are ductless glands that secrete hormones directly into the bloodstream. The glands that make up the endocrine system are the:

- pituitary gland
- thyroid gland
- 4 parathyroid glands
- 2 suprarenal (adrenal) glands
- islets of Langerhans (in the pancreas)
- gonads (ovaries and testes)
- thymus gland
- pineal gland.

ENDOCRINE GLANDS AND HORMONES

A hormone is a chemical substance secreted into the blood by an endocrine gland. The hormone is transported via the blood to areas of the body where it is needed to stimulate a specific cellular activity. Organs that respond to a particular hormone are the *target organs* of that hormone.

Some hormones have a controlling effect on other hormones by influencing their action, metabolism, synthesis or transport. Table 25.1 summarizes the major hormones, their sites of origin, their target organs, and their effects.

Hormones

A hormone can be described as a 'chemical regulator', which integrates and co-ordinates cellular activities. Hormones are either *steroids* or *proteins*, and only target cells have the ability to respond to a specific hormone. After entering the blood, some hormones become bound to plasma proteins while others are transported in an unbound state. Most hormones are continuously secreted. The rates of secretion are modified as a result of stimuli to the glands from which they are released.

The pituitary gland

The pituitary gland (hypophysis) weighs approximately 500 mg, and is positioned the base of the brain in a depression in the sphenoid bone. It lies just beneath the hypothalamus, to which it is connected by a stalk containing blood vessels and nervous tissue. The pituitary gland is composed of an anterior lobe (adenohypophysis) and a posterior lobe (neurohypophysis). Each lobe performs specific functions.

The anterior lobe of the pituitary gland

The anterior lobe produces:

1. The growth hormone, concerned with body growth, particularly of bones and muscles.
2. The thyrotrophic hormone responsible for controlling the growth and activity of the thyroid gland.
3. The adrenocorticotrophic hormone (ACTH) which stimulates the cortex of the suprarenal glands to produce hormones.
4. The gonadotrophic hormones which control the development and functions of the ovaries and testes.
   In the female, the hormones are
   (a) the follicle stimulating hormone (FSH) which stimulates the developing ovarian follicle to secrete oestrogen, and

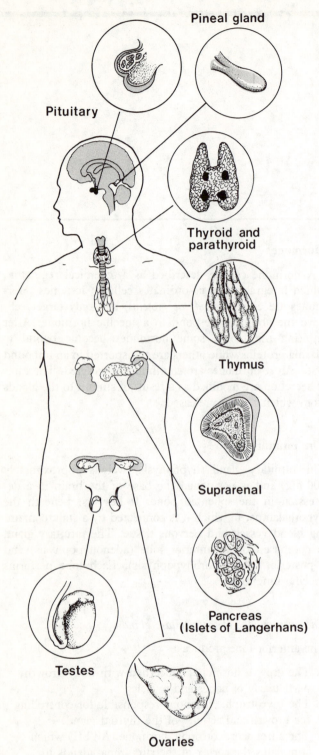

Pineal gland

Pituitary

Thyroid and parathyroid

Thymus

Suprarenal

Pancreas (Islets of Langerhans)

Testes

Ovaries

Fig. 25.1 The endocrine system.

(b) the luteinizing hormone (LH) which is secreted after ovulation has occurred and stimulates the development of the corpus luteum in the ruptured follicle. The corpus luteum secretes progesterone.

In the male, the hormones are
(a) the follicle stimulating hormone (FSH) which stimulates the seminiferous tubules to produce spermatozoa, and
(b) the interstitial cell stimulating hormone (ICSH) which stimulates the testes to secrete testosterone.
5. The lactogenic hormone, also called prolactin, which stimulates the mammary glands to secrete milk after the birth of a baby.

The posterior lobe of the pituitary gland

The posterior lobe produces:

1. Oxytocin which has two functions: (a) it causes contraction of the muscle walls of a pregnant uterus, and (b) it causes the ducts of the mammary glands to contract, expelling milk.
2. Anti-diuretic hormone (ADH) which stimulates the kidney tubules to re-absorb water, and so causes decreased excretion of water in the urine.

The thyroid gland

The thyroid gland usually weighs less than 30 g, and lies in the neck just below the larynx. It is composed of two lateral lobes, one lying on either side of the trachea, and a narrow strip called the isthmus which lies anteriorly across the trachea and joins the two lobes.

The thyroid gland is covered by a connective tissue capsule and, from this, trabeculae pass inwards to divide the gland into lobules. The thyroid gland produces:

1. *Thyroxine*, containing large quantities of iodine which is derived from the diet and stored in the thyroid gland. The function of thyroxine is to control the metabolic rate, and it therefore influences:
- physical and mental development
- body temperature
- the health of skin and hair.
2. *Calcitonin*, which decreases blood calcium levels by causing calcium to be deposited in the bones. In the kidneys, the hormone promotes the excretion of phosphate and calcium. Calcium, therefore, contributes to the regulation of blood calcium levels.

The parathyroid glands

The parathyroids are four small glands, with a combined weight of between 20 and 40 mg. Two glands are embedded in the posterior surface of each lobe of the thyroid gland. The parathyroid glands produce *Parathormone* (PTH), which is primarily responsible for the regulation of blood calcium and phosphate levels. Parathormone promotes the reabsorption of calcium and inhibits the reabsorption of phosphate in the renal tubules.

Table 25.1 The major hormones

Endocrine gland	Hormone	Target	Effects
Pituitary —Anterior lobe	Growth (GH)	Bones, muscles, organs.	Promotion of growth and metabolism.
	Thyroid—stimulating (TSH)	Thyroid gland	Regulates thyroid hormone.
	Adrenocorticotrophic (ACTH)	Adrenal Cortex	Secretion of cortisone, aldosterone, and sex hormones.
	Follicle—stimulating (FSH)	Ovaries	Secretion of oestrogen.
		Seminiferous tubules	Production of sperm.
	Luteinizing (LH)	Ovarian follicle	Formation of corpus luteum.
	Interstitial cell—stimulating (ICSH)	Testes	Production of testosterone.
	Prolactin (LTH)	Corpus luteum	Secretion of progesterone.
		Breasts	Stimulates milk secretion.
—Posterior lobe	Oxytocin	Uterus	Stimulates uterine contractions.
		Breasts	Stimulates milk production.
	Anti-diuretic (ADH)	Tubules of kidneys	Reabsorption of water.
Thyroid	Thyroxine	Widespread	Energy metabolism.
			Increases metabolic rate.
			Regulation of growth.
	Calcitonin	Skeleton	Decrease in plasma calcium levels.
Parathyroids	Parathormone (PTH)	Bones	Increase in plasma calcium levels.
		Kidneys	Regulates phosphorous excretion.
Adrenals —Cortex	Glucocorticoids, e.g. cortisone.	Widespread	Metabolism of protein, fat and carbohydrate.
			Promotes gluconeogenesis.
			Mobilization of amino acids.
			Suppression of inflammation.
			Effect on plasma glucose levels.
			Lipolysis.
	Mineralocorticoids, e.g. aldosterone.	Renal tubules	Reabsorption of sodium.
			Excretion of potassium.
			Maintenance of fluid balance.
	Sex, e.g. androgens, oestrogens.	Gonads	Influence on development of secondary sex characteristics and growth.
—Medulla	Epinephrine and norepinephrine	Widespread	Vasoconstriction.
			Increase in blood pressure.
			Gluconeogenesis.
			Response to stress.
			Stimulation of metabolism.
			Secretion of ACTH.
Islets of Langerhans	Insulin	Widespread	Decrease in plasma glucose.
			Aids glucose transport into cells.
			Decrease in protein catabolism.
	Glucagon	Liver	Increase in plasma glucose.
		Muscles	
		Adipose cells	
Gonads —Ovaries	Oestrogen	Reproductive tissues	Development of secondary sex characteristics.
			Maturation of sexual organs.
			Sexual functioning.
	Progesterone	Uterus	Development of mammary tissue.
		Breasts	Maintenance of pregnancy.
			Preparation of endometrium.
—Testes	Testosterone	Widespread	Development of secondary sex characteristics.
			Maturation of sexual organs.
			Sexual functioning.
Thymus	Thymosin	Immune system	Lymphocyte development.
Pineal	Melatonin	Hypothalamus	Regulating the gonads.
		Midbrain	
		Gonads	

The suprarenal (adrenal) glands

There are two suprarenal glands, each weighing approximately 10 g, one lying on top of each kidney. Each gland is bounded by a capsule and contains two areas; an outer cortex and an inner medulla.

The adrenal cortex

The cortex, or outer portion, produces 3 major groups of steroid hormones collectively called corticosteroids.

1. The glucocorticoids, which include cortisone, hydrocortisone, and cortisol. These hormones are concerned with:

- metabolism of protein, fat, and carbohydrate
- conversion of protein to glucose
- storage of glycogen and its conversion to glucose
- release of fat, stored in a depose tissue, for use as a fuel.

2. The mineralocorticoids, mainly aldosterone which is concerned with: The reabsorption of sodium ions and the elimination of potassium ions, in the kidneys.

3. The sex hormones. The male sex hormones are the androgens, and the female sex hormones are the oestrogens. Both hormones are concerned with: the development of secondary sexual characteristics, and The functioning of the reproductive organs.

The adrenal medulla

The medulla, or inner portion, produces two similar hormones, the catecholamines:

1. epinephrine (adrenaline)
2. norepinephrine (noradrenaline).

When the medulla is stimulated by sympathetic nervous system neurons, the two hormones are released into the bloodstream. The physiological activities of the medullary hormones are similar to those of the sympathetic nervous system, and are:

- dilation of the coronary arteries, and arteries to skeletal muscle.
- constriction of blood vessels in the skin and internal organs.
- increase in the rate and strength of the heart beat.
- increase in blood pressure.
- dilation of the bronchial tubes.
- reduction of peristalsis in the alimentary canal.
- stimulation of the liver to release more glucose into the bloodstream.
- dilation of the pupils of the eyes.
- increase in the metabolic rate.

Adrenaline prepares the body for fight or flight, and its secretion is increased as a result of strong emotions such as fear, anger, or excitement.

Islets of Langerhans

The islets of Langerhans are small groups of cells scattered throughout the pancreas. They produce two hormones, insulin and glucagon, both of which help to regulate the amount of glucose in the blood.

1. Insulin is released in the presence of high blood glucose levels. Some amino acids and fatty acids also increase insulin release.

Insulin increases the uptake of glucose into cells and reduces the release of glucose from the liver, thereby decreasing the levels of glucose in the blood. Insulin also promotes the conversion of glucose to fatty acids, within the liver. Insulin acts generally to stimulate protein synthesis. Insulin is essential for the use of glucose by the body cells, as it increases their ability to transport glucose across the cell membranes.

2. Glucagon is released by the islets of Langerhans in response to a reduced blood glucose level. Its output is reduced in the presence of raised blood glucose and insulin.

Glucagon raises blood glucose levels by stimulating the breakdown of glycogen in the liver and inhibiting glycogen synthesis.

The gonads

The female gonads are the ovaries, and the male gonads are the testes.

The ovaries

The ovaries are two small almond-shaped organs of the female reproductive system lying in the pelvic cavity, one either side of the uterus. The hormones produced by the ovaries are:

- Oestrogens, which influence development of the reproductive organs and the secondary sexual characteristics. Oestrogen also stimulates the lining of the uterus to thicken in preparation for reception of a fertilized ovum.
- Progesterone, which promotes the final stages in the development of a thick, engorged uterine lining. Progesterone inhibits the contraction of uterine muscles to prevent expulsion of a fertilized ovum, inhibits ovulation during pregnancy, and stimulates the mammary glands to produce milk.

The testes

The testes are two small organs of the male reproductive system, lying in a loose pouch of skin called the scrotum. The hormone produced by the testes (*testosterone*) is responsible for the development of male characteristics and the growth and function of the reproductive organs.

The thymus gland

The thymus gland is situated in the upper thorax behind the sternum. It consists mainly of lymphoid tissue, and its functions are those performed by all lymphoid tissue. The thymus gland is large in childhood, reaching its maximum size at puberty, then it gradually decreases in size during adulthood.

It is believed that the thymus gland produces a hormone, thymosin, which is thought to promote the growth of lymphoid tissue in the body.

The pineal gland

The pineal gland is a small cone-shaped structure situated in the brain. It begins to atrophy early in life, and is replaced by fibrous tissue.

The endocrine function of the pineal gland is unknown, but it is believed that it produces two hormones:

1. melatonin, which is concerned with regulating the gonads.
2. adrenoglomerulotropin, which is involved in stimulating the adrenal cortex to release aldosterone.

The placenta, which is a temporary organ formed during pregnancy, produces hormones from approximately the third month of pregnancy. Further information on the structure and function of the placenta is provided in Chapter 52.

SUMMARY

The endocrine system is made up of a number of glands, some of which are structurally independent while others are located within other organs.

Endocrine glands secrete hormones directly into the bloodstream. A hormone is a chemical substance which is transported in the blood to areas of the body where it is needed to stimulate a specific cellular activity.

Each of the endocrine glands secrete specific hormones, which have specific functions. The endocrine glands are the pituitary gland, the thyroid gland, the four parathyroid glands, the two suprarenal glands, the islets of Langerhans, the gonads (ovaries and testes), the thymus gland, and the pineal gland.

Each of the glands of the endocrine system has one or more specific functions, but they are all dependent upon the other glands in the system for maintenance of normal hormonal balance in the body.

26. The reproductive systems

OBJECTIVES

1. Describe the position, structure, and functions of the components of the male reproductive system.
2. Describe the position, structure, and functions of the components of the female reproductive system.
3. State the actions of the reproductive hormones.
4. Outline the stages of the menstrual cycle.

INTRODUCTION

The purpose of both the human male and female reproductive systems is propagation of the species. In addition, the reproductive organs are a means of obtaining sexual pleasure.

The reproductive role of the male is to manufacture and deliver sperm to the female reproductive tract, while the role of the female in reproduction is more complex. The female produces ova and her uterus houses the developing fetus during the 9 months of pregnancy.

THE MALE REPRODUCTIVE SYSTEM

The male reproductive system consists of external and internal structures (Fig. 26.1).

External genitalia

The external male genitalia consists of the penis and the scrotum.

The penis

The penis is a pendulous soft tissue structure attached to the anterior and lateral walls of the pubic arch by muscles and suspensory ligaments. It is composed of three columns of spongy erectile tissue: a central column containing the

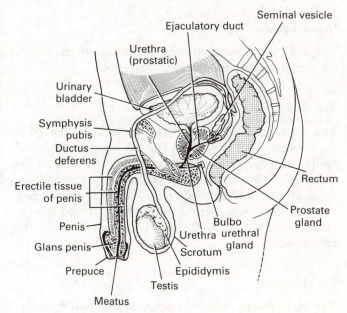

Fig. 26.1 The male reproductive system.

urethra, and two encompassing columns that provide the organ's main structural support. The erectile tissue is overlayed with subcutaneous tissue and a fibrous sheath. The skin covering the penis is continuous from the base of the penis to the glans penis, or tip, where it folds inward and backward on itself and is called the prepuce or foreskin.

Blood supply to the penis is via the pudendal arteries that form a network within the erectile tissue. When the erectile tissue becomes filled with blood during sexual excitement, the penis becomes enlarged, firm and erect.

The penis contains the urethra to transport urine to its external orifice, the meatus. It is also the organ which deposits sperm in the female vagina.

The scrotum

The scrotum is a thin-walled pouch of skin that is suspended from the perineal region posterior to the penis. The interior of the scrotum is divided into two compartments, each of which contains a testis, an epididymus, and a ductal system. Under normal conditions, the scrotum hangs loosely which keeps the testes at a temperature suitable for sperm viability. When the external temperature is cold, or during tactile stimulation, the scrotum draws up and pulls the testes closer to the body.

The breasts

While the male breasts do not serve any reproductive purpose, they are a site of sexual pleasure for some men. The male breasts are structurally the same as the female breasts, consisting of glandular tissue and a nipple.

Internal genitalia

The male internal reproductive structures are the testes, the ductal system, and the accessory glands.

The testes

The testes, or gonads, are two glands that lie suspended in the scrotum. They are first formed in the upper abdominal cavity, then they gradually descend into the scrotum before birth. Each testis is surrounded by a connective tissue capsule, and the body of each testis is divided into wedge-shaped lobes. Within each lobe are coiled tubules called the *seminiferous tubules*, which unite to form the epididymis.

The ductal system

The ductal system, which transports sperm from the body, is composed of the epididymis, the vas deferens, and the urethra.

The epididymis is the first part of an efferent ductal system leading from each testes, through the inguinal canal, and finally opening· into the prostatic portion of the urethra. The epididymis provides a temporary storage site for immature sperm which enter it from the testes. While in the epididymis, the sperm become mature and fully functional.

The vas deferens, or deferent duct, is a continuation of the epididymis and passes into the pelvic cavity and arches over the top of the bladder. The vas deferens is suspended and contained within the *spermatic cord* through most of its length. The end of the vas deferens empties into the *ejaculatory duct*, that carries the sperm through the prostate gland into the urethra.

The urethra passes through the penis and is a passage for the expulsion of both urine and semen.

The accessory glands

The male accessory glands are the seminal vesicles, urethral and bulbo-urethral glands, and the prostate gland.

The seminal vesicles lie posterior to the bladder at the base of the prostate gland. They secrete a thick, nutritive, alkaline fluid which forms part of the semen.

Semen is the fluid ejaculated by the male, and consists of spermatozoa and secretions from the seminal vesicles, the bulbo-urethral glands, and the prostate gland.

The bulbo-urethral (Cowper's) glands are two pea-sized glands located on either side of the urethra and opening into it. They produce a lubricating alkaline mucus that drains into the urethra during ejaculation.

The prostate gland is a spherical gland that encircles the upper part of the urethra just below the bladder. It secretes a thin, milky, fluid that forms part of the semen.

Functions of the male reproductive system

Spermatogenesis

The production of sperm, or spermatogenesis, begins at sexual maturation (puberty). Sperm is produced, under the influence of gonadotrophic hormones, in all the seminiferous tubules in the testes. The sperm originate from a primordial cell that appears in the embryo early in gestation. As these cells multiply by *mitotic division*, they form spermatogonia. At sexual maturity, spermatogenesis begins. The process of sperm production includes mitosis (proliferation), growth, and meiosis (division). At the end of the process sperm, or *spermatozoa*, are formed.

The mature sperm consists of a head, neck, body, and tail (Fig. 26.2). The head contains the genetic material (DNA), the neck contains the centrioles, and the body contains mitochondria. The tail contains adenosine triphosphate (ATP), which is necessary to sustain the continued movement of the tail as it propels the sperm through the female reproductive tract.

Sperm are transported through the male reproductive system in semen. The average sperm density in semen is approximately 40 000 000–100 000 000 sperm per ml of semen. Viable sperm may be stored in the male reproductive tract for up to six weeks, but will survive usually no more than 48 hours in an inhospitable external environment.

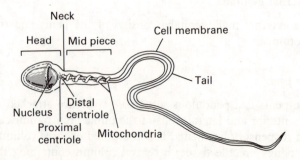

Fig. 26.2 The structure of a sperm.

Testosterone production

The interstitial cells that lie between the seminiferous tubules produce the hormone, testosterone. During puberty, the interstitial cells are activated by follicle-stimulating hormone (FSH) and interstitial cell-stimulating hormone (ICSH) which are released by the anterior lobe of the pituitary gland. From puberty onwards, testosterone is produced for the remainder of the male's life span.

The chief function of testosterone is to stimulate the development of the male reproductive organs, and the secondary sex characteristics:

- deepening of the voice due to lengthening and thickening of the vocal cords.
- appearance of pubic, axillary, and facial hair.
- increased activity of the sebaceous glands.
- broadening of the shoulders due to increased bone density, and a general increase in muscle mass.
- increase in the length and width of the penis, and genital pigmentation.

Testosterone is also necessary for the secretion of fructose by the seminal vesicles—for the nourishment of sperm.

THE FEMALE REPRODUCTIVE SYSTEM

The female reproductive system consists of external and internal structures (Fig. 26.3).

External genitalia (Vulva)

The external genitalia consists of the mons pubis, the labia majora, the labia minora, the clitoris, the perineum, the urethral and vaginal orifices, and the Bartholin's glands.

The mons pubis

The mons pubis (mons veneris) is a rounded pad of fatty tissue over the symphysis pubis, and it is covered by hair after puberty. The mons pubis protects the pelvic bones, and enhances sexual arousal.

The labia majora

The labia majora are two rounded mounds of tissue that form the lateral boundaries of the vulva. They originate in the mons pubis and end in the perineum, and are covered by hair after puberty.

The labia majora serve as a protective covering for the genitals, and serve as a source of sexual pleasure.

The labia minora

The labia minora are two thin longitudinal folds of tissue, enclosed by the labia majora. Their surface is smooth and does not contain hair follicles. They divide anteriorly to

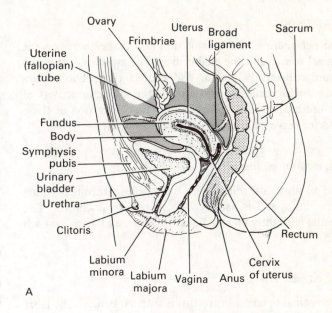

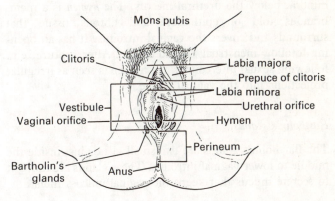

Fig. 26.3 The female reproductive system. (A) Sagittal section of the female reproductive system. (B) External genitalia of the female.

form the prepuce of the clitoris, and posteriorly they unite to form a fold called the *fourchette*. The urethral and vaginal orifices are enclosed by the labia minora.

The tissue of the labia minora is erectile, and becomes engorged during sexual excitement.

The clitoris

The clitoris is an area of erectile tissue, visible between the folds of the labia minora at the anterior junction. The clitoris is approximately 5–6 mm in length, and 6–8 mm in diameter.

The external portions are the body and the glans, and there is a prepuce (hood) overlying the glans. The glans consists of mucous membrane with a large number of free nerve endings, which makes the clitoris an area very sensitive to stimulation. The prepuce also contains an abundance of free nerve endings.

The perineum

The perineum is the area of skin and tissues between the vaginal orifice and the anal orifice. The muscles of the perineum collectively anchor and protect the pelvic viscera and external genitalia, and provide the sphincter activity of the urethra, vagina, and rectum. The contraction of these muscles serve as a major stimulus of orgasm.

The urethral meatus

The urethral meatus forms the opening through which urine flows, and is usually 2–3 cm below the clitoris. The meatus is slightly elevated and has depressed areas on each side.

The vaginal orifice

The vaginal opening (introitus) is situated beneath the labia minora, below the urethral meatus. The *hymen* is a membranous fold of epithelium and fibrous tissue that surrounds and covers the vaginal introitus. It has an opening to allow menstrual flow to escape. After rupture, e.g. following sexual intercourse, the hymen is seen as irregular projections into the vaginal orifice.

Bartholin's glands

The Bartholin's glands are two small glands just inside the middle to lower vaginal introitus. These glands are thought to secrete mucus that keeps the vaginal mucosa moist.

The internal genitalia

The internal genitalia consists of the vagina, the uterus, the uterine (fallopian) tubes, and the ovaries.

The vagina

The vagina is a musculo-membranous passageway, approximately 9 cm long. It extends from the uterus to the vulva where it opens to form the vaginal opening. The lining of the vagina is stratified epithelium, which is arranged in folds (rugae) to allow for stretching.

The upper part of the vagina is called the vaginal vault. The cervix of the uterus projects into the upper part of the anterior vaginal wall. The four arches that result from the projection of the cervix into the vaginal vault are called the vaginal *fornices*. The anterior fornix is short, the lateral ones are deeper, and the posterior fornix is deepest.

About one-third to one-half way into the vagina, on the anterior surface of the vaginal wall, is a small area called the Gräfenberg spot (G-spot). It has been reported, that when this spot is stimulated, small amounts of fluid are expelled and sexual sensation is enhanced. The vagina is acidic from menarche to menopause, and its surface is moist from fluid secreted by the vaginal epithelium.

Functions of the vagina are to:

- receive the penis during sexual intercourse
- provide a passageway for menstrual flow to leave the body
- provide a passageway through which the fetus is expelled from the uterus.

The uterus

The uterus is a hollow pear-shaped muscular organ, located at the centre of the pelvic cavity behind the bladder and in front of the rectum. The uterus is suspended in the pelvis by a peritoneal fold (the broad ligament). Normally the uterus is in an anteverted position, which means that it is leaning forward so that the upper portion rests on the bladder. The walls of the uterus consist of:

- an outer covering of peritoneum (perimetrium).
- a middle layer of thick involuntary muscle (myometrium).
- a lining of mucous membrane (endometrium).

The uterus consists of two parts, the uterine body and the cervix.

The uterine body forms the upper two-thirds of the uterus, and the *fundus* is the portion above the point where the fallopian tubes enter.

The cervix is the lower one-third of the uterus which protrudes into the vagina. The openings of the cervix are the internal os at the uterine end, and the external os at the vaginal end.

Squamous stratified epithelium covers the vaginal portion of the cervix, and columnar ciliated cells with mucus-secreting glands line the upper portion of the cervix. The mucus-secreting glands produce mucus, which provides lubrication and acts as a bacteriostatic agent.

The functions of the uterus are to:

- receive the fertilized ovum which embeds itself in the endometrium.
- provide 'housing' and nourishment for the fetus.
- expel the fully developed fetus at the end of pregnancy.
- shed the superficial layer of the endometrium if fertilization of the ovum does not occur.

The uterine (Fallopian) tubes

From each side of the upper part of the uterus arise the uterine (Fallopian) tubes. Each tube is muscular, approximately 10 cm long, and extends from the uterus into the peritoneal cavity. The distal end of each tube curves over an ovary, where the tube fans out to a trumpet-like shape.

Around the small orifice at the distal end of the uterine tube are folds of tissue called *fimbriae*. The largest fimbria attaches to the ovary, keeping the tube close to the ovarian surface. The fimbriae are mobile, moving the ovum into the tube.

The walls of the uterine tubes consist of:

- an outer covering of peritoneum
- a middle layer of involuntary muscle
- a lining of ciliated mucous membrane.

The function of the uterine tubes is to transport the ovum from the ovary to the uterus, by means of peristaltic action. The ciliated cells in the lining move to help the ovum towards the uterus.

Fertilization of the ovum occurs in the distal $\frac{1}{3}$ of the uterine tube, which provides a favourable nourishing environment.

The ovaries

The ovaries, or gonads, are two almond-shaped organs, one on either side of the uterus. Each ovary is attached to the broad ligament, the ovarian ligament, and the suspensory ligament. An ovary is composed of an inner portion which contains nerves and lymph vessels, and an outer portion which contains follicles and ova.

Graafian follicles are microscopic sacs, each containing an immature ovum (female sex cell).

Functions of the ovaries are oogenesis and hormone production.

1. Oogenesis is the development of mature ova. Immature ova are present in the graafian follicles at birth, but they are not discharged from the ovary until maturation begins at puberty. The cells of the developing ovarian follicle are stimulated by the follicle stimulating hormone (FSH) to secrete oestrogen. The oestrogen enhances the growth and maturation of the maturing follicle. Eventually, Luteinizing hormone (LH), from the pituitary gland, acts on the follicle—and ovulation occurs.

Ovulation is the rupturing of a mature follicle to release an ovum. The ovary usually releases one mature ovum each month. When a follicle matures, it becomes distended with fluid and bulges on to the surface of the ovary. When the follicle ruptures, the ovum is liberated into the peritoneal cavity near the distal end of a uterine tube which it will enter.

The corpus luteum is a mass of specialized tissue, which develops in a ruptured follicle after the ovum has been discharged.

2. Hormone production by the ovaries begins at puberty. The follicle cells of the growing and mature follicles produce oestrogen. *Oestrogen* causes the development of the secondary sex characteristics:

- enlargement of the uterine tubes, uterus, vagina and external genitals

- development of the breasts
- increased deposits of fat, particularly in the hips and breasts
- widening of the pelvis
- onset of the menstrual cycle
- appearance of pubic and axillary hair.

Oestrogen also stimulates the lining of the uterus to prepare for the reception of a fertilized ovum.

The second ovarian hormone, *progesterone*, is produced by the *corpus luteum* (which also produces some oestrogen). Progesterone:

- promotes the final preparation of the uterine lining to receive the fertilized ovum
- inhibits contraction of the walls of the uterus
- suppresses further ovulation
- stimulates the mammary glands to produce milk
- blocks the effect of aldosterone, and has an indirect effect on fluid and electrolyte balance.

The mammary glands

The female breast (Fig. 26.4) is a cutaneous gland that is an accessory organ of the reproductive system. The reproductive function of the breasts is to produce milk for breast feeding.

The breast is a complex structure composed of a glandular and ductal network, fat, connective tissue, fascia, blood vessels, nerves, and lymphatic vessels. In the centre of the breast is a pigmented area, the *areola*, which surrounds the nipple. The areola contains Montgomery's tubercles, which secrete a fluid that protects the nipples during breast feeding. Internally, each breast contains 15–20 lobes which radiate around the nipple, and which are separated from each other by adipose tissue. The lobes consist of lobules which contain clusters of alveolar glands that produce milk during lactation. The alveolar glands pass the milk into the *lactiferous* ducts, which open at the nipple.

The hormones *oestrogen* and *progesterone*, secreted by the ovaries, are responsible for the development of the breasts at puberty. *Prolactin*, secreted by the anterior lobe of the pituitary gland after the birth of a baby stimulates the production of milk.

Oxytocin secreted by the posterior lobe of the pituitary gland, stimulates the release of milk during breast feeding.

The menstrual cycle

The menstrual cycle consists of a series of changes, which occur at regular intervals, involving the reproductive organs. The events of the menstrual cycle (Fig. 26.5) are the changes that the *endometrium* goes through, as it responds to changes in the levels of ovarian hormones in the blood.

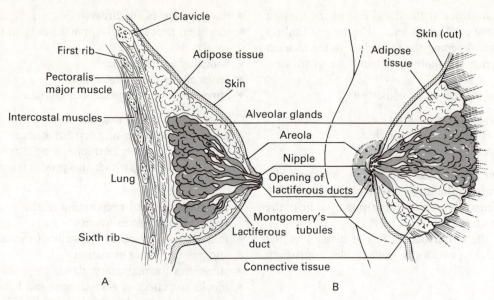

Fig. 26.4 The breast. (A) Sagittal section. (B) Anterior section.

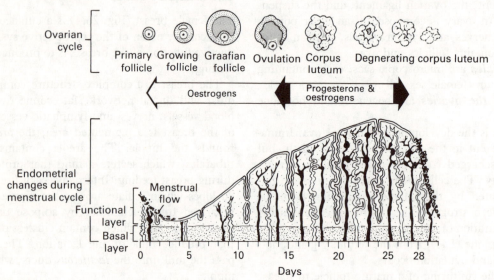

Fig. 26.5 The menstrual cycle.

The average menstrual cycle is of 28 days duration, and the stages of the cycle are:

1. Days 1–5: Menstruation (menses) Menstruation occurs if the ovum released during ovulation is not fertilized, and therefore the specially prepared endometrium is not required. The superficial layer of cells, together with extra secretions and blood, is discharged from the uterus.

2. Days 6–14: Follicular stage and ovulation. Under the influence of oestrogens produced by the growing follicles of the ovaries, the endometrium is repaired. The graafian follicle in the ovary ripens, and the ovum begins to mature. The mature ovum ruptures the surface of the ovary at about the 14th day (ovulation), and the ovum is discharged into the pelvic cavity. Ovulation occurs in response to a release of LH from the anterior lobe of the pituitary galnd.

3. Days 15–28: Premenstrual (secretory) stage. The endometrium is once again prepared to receive a fertilized ovum. Rising levels of progesterone, and oestrogen produced by the corpus luteum, increase the blood supply to the endometrium. Progesterone also causes the endometrial glands to increase in size and to begin secreting nutrients into the uterine cavity.

Unless pregnancy occurs, the corpus luteum begins to

regress and the secretion of oestrogen and progesterone decreases. Lack of ovarian hormones in the blood, causes the blood vessels supplying the endometrium to go into spasm. When deprived of oxygen and nutrients, the endometrial cells begin to die. The endometrium is sloughed off, and the menstrual cycle begins again.

Fertilization

Fertilization is the fusion of a spermatozoon and an ovum, and it occurs in the uterine tube. Millions of spermatozoa are deposited in the vagina during sexual intercourse, and they have a life span of between 24–48 hours. The spermatozoa move through the cervix and up towards the uterine tube, but only a small percentage of the total number reach the tube. The ovum enters the fimbriated end of the uterine tube, and is moved towards the uterus by means of the peristaltic action of the tube walls, and the sweeping action of the cilia lining the tube.

Fertilization occurs in the distal one-third of the tube, when a spermatozoon and an ovum fuse to form one cell. After penetration by the spermatozoon, the ovum develops a tough outer coat to prevent penetration by other spermatozoa. The resulting zygote embeds itself in the uterine wall and becomes an *embryo*. Further information on the development of the embryo is provided in Chapter 52.

HUMAN SEXUAL RESPONSE

Both male and female sexual responses are determined by psychological and tactile stimuli. Sympathetic and parasympathetic autonomic nerves carry the motor impulses that result in the responses to stimulation. Sexual response can be initiated by many different types of stimuli, including sight, sound, touch, smell, or thought. Although the phases of sexual response are the same for both males and females, the duration of each phase varies.

Male sexual response

As a physiological event, the male sexual response is designed to prepare the male for reproductive union with the female. The response consists of two components:

1. Genital vasocongestive reaction, which produces penile erection.
2. Reflex muscular contractions, which result in orgasm.

The four phases of male sexual response are; excitement, plateau, orgasm, and resolution.

In the excitement phase, the penis becomes erect, and the testes begin to elevate and engorge.

During the plateau phase, the bulbourethral glands secrete a lubricating mucus, the penis remains erect, and there is complete engorgement and elevation of the testicles.

Male orgasm consists of emission, where sperm is expelled into the urethra, and ejaculation where spurts of semen are forced out from the urethra.

During the resolution phase, there is a refractory period where erection begins to subside, the testes descend, and the scrotum returns to its pre-excitement state.

Female sexual response

As a physiological event, the female sexual response is designed to prepare the female for reproductive union with the male. The four phases of female sexual response are excitement, plateau, orgasm, resolution.

During the excitement phase, vasocongestion in and around the vagina causes a lubricating transudate to pass through the tissue of the vaginal walls. Vagocongestion of the labia majora and minora occurs, the glans of the clitoris increases in size, there is an upward and backward movement of the cervix and uterus, erection of the nipples, and a breast flush may occur.

In the plateau phase, the lower one-third of the vagina becomes engorged, the labia minora's colour deepens, and the clitoris retracts.

The orgasm phase is characterized by rhythmic contractions of the muscles of the clitoris, vagina and uterus.

During resolution, the clitoris descends and returns to its unaroused state, the labia majora and minora return to their unaroused position and colour, and the vagina loses its distention.

SUMMARY

The biological purpose of both the male and female reproductive systems is propagation of the species.

The reproductive role of the male is to manufacture and deliver sperm to the female reproductive tract, while the female role is to produce ova and to house the developing fetus during pregnancy.

The male reproductive system consists of external and internal structures.

The testes, or male gonads, are concerned with the production of sperm and the hormone, testosterone. Testosterone's chief function is to stimulate the development of the male reproductive organs, and the secondary sex characteristics.

The female reproductive system also consists of external and internal structures.

The functions of the uterus are to receive the fertilized ovum, to provide 'housing' for the developing fetus, to expel the fetus at the end of pregnancy, and to shed its superficial layer of endometrium if fertilization of the ovum does not occur.

The ovaries, or female gonads, are concerned with the production of mature ova and the hormones, oestrogen and progesterone. Oestrogen's chief function is to stimulate the development of the female reproductive organs, and the secondary sex characteristics. Progesterone plays a major role in the menstrual cycle by promoting the final preparation of the uterine lining.

The menstrual cycle consists of a series of changes in the endometrium, as it responds to changes in the levels of ovarian hormones in the blood.

Fertilization which occurs in the uterine tube, is the fusion of a spermatozoon and an ovum to form one cell.

Male and female sexual responses can be initiated by many different types of stimuli. As a physiological event, the human sexual response is designed to prepare the male and female for reproductive union.

27. The special senses

OBJECTIVES

1. Describe the position of each special sense organ.
2. Describe the structure of each special sense organ.
3. Describe the physiology of taste, smell, sight, and hearing.

INTRODUCTION

The sensory abilities of taste, smell, touch, sight and hearing enable the individual to pick up signals that provide information about the environment. Perception of sensory stimuli has its origin in the five special sense organs; the tongue, nose, skin, eyes, and ears. Receptors in the sense organs pick up stimuli from the environment, and transmit this information to the brain via pathways in the nervous system. In the brain, the information is processed and interpreted.

The special sense organs are those which are specially adapted for the reception of specific stimuli:

- the tongue—taste
- the nose—smell
- the skin—touch
- the eyes—sight
- the ears—hearing, and maintenance of balance.

SPECIAL SENSE ORGANS

The tongue (taste buds)

The specific receptors for the sense of taste are the taste buds. They are chemoreceptors which respond to substances present in food, and generate nerve impulses which are transmitted to the brain for interpretation. Taste buds are widely scattered throughout the oral cavity, and are most numerous on the upper and lateral surfaces of the tongue (Fig. 27.1).

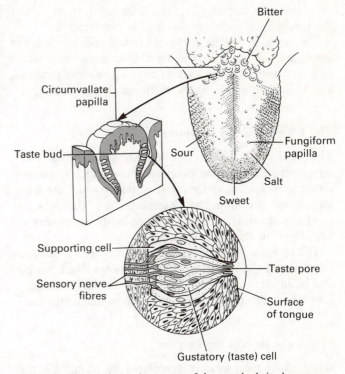

Fig. 27.1 The location and structure of the taste buds in the tongue.

The upper surface of the tongue is covered with small projections, *papillae*, some of which contain the taste buds. Each taste bud consists of sensory and supporting cells situated in the epithelium, and opening onto the surface through a small *gustatory* pore. Between the cells of the taste bud lie the endings of afferent nerve fibres derived from a number of cranial nerves.

Taste buds on the anterior two-thirds of the tongue connect with fibres of the *facial* (7th cranial) nerve. Taste buds on the posterior one-third of the tongue are associated with the fibres of the glosso-pharyngeal (9th cranial) nerve, while pharyngeal taste buds send impulses to the brain via the vagus (10th cranial) nerve.

Function of taste buds

The four basic tastes are sweet, sour, salty and bitter. The tip of the tongue is most sensitive to sweet and salty substances, the edges of the tongue are most sensitive to sour substances, and the back of the tongue is most sensitive to bitter substances.

Substances must be in solution (in saliva) so that they can enter the opening in a taste bud, and stimulate the nerve ending. Molecules pass into solution on the surface of the tongue, and then combine with the surface membranes of the receptor cells. Transmitter substances are released which evoke action potentials in the sensory nerve fibres.

Fibres from the seventh, ninth and tenth cranial nerves carry the taste impulses, via the brain stem, to an area of the cerebral cortex where the taste is experienced.

The sense of taste is intricately linked with the sense of smell, and the sense of taste depends on stimulation of the olfactory receptors. Both senses have a protective function, e.g. in detecting substances which may be harmful.

The nose (olfactory receptors)

The specific receptors for the sense of smell are the olfactory receptors. They are chemoreceptors which respond to airborne chemicals, and generate impulses which are transmitted to the brain for interpretation. The olfactory receptors are situated in the mucous membrane lining the upper part of the nose (Fig. 27.2).

The receptor cells are sensory neurones with a cell body lying within the epithelium, and a process which terminates in an olfactory vesicle. From the vesicle, a number of long cilia—olfactory hairs—project above the epithelium.

Function of the olfactory receptors

When these receptors are stimulated by chemicals, they transmit impulses along the olfactory (1st cranial) nerve to the brain.

The receptor cells respond to the presence of molecules. Generator potentials from a number of different receptor cells promote the formation of action potentials, which pass from the receptor cells to the olfactory bulb (Fig. 27.2). From the olfactory bulb, nerve fibres pass through the olfactory striae to the olfactory areas of the brain, where the sense of smell is experienced.

There is a close relationship between the sense of smell and the sense of taste, and therefore they are not always easily distinguishable. Smell receptors are very sensitive, and can adapt readily. This adaptation means that an individual can become accustomed to an odour when constantly exposed to the same stimulus. The sensations of smell and taste play an important part in stimulating the secretion of digestive juices.

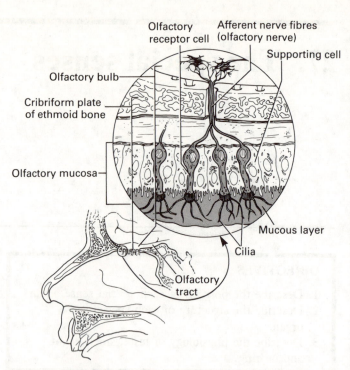

Fig. 27.2 The location and structure of the olfactory receptors in the nose.

The skin (as an organ of sensation)

In addition to the functions described in Chapter 18, the skin is an organ of sensation. Distributed widely in the skin are many nerve endings or receptors, that allow reception of external stimuli. There are four basic sensations that are perceived by specific receptors in the skin: pain, temperature, pressure and touch.

Touch, as a sense, is detected by the general cutaneous receptors of the skin. Afferent, or sensory, neurons carry impulses from these receptors to the brain where the sensation of touch is interpreted. The skin is, therefore, a sense organ that reacts to external stimuli as well as reacting to stimuli occuring within the body.

The eyes

Sight, or vision, is the result of light rays being received by the eyes and transmitted by the optic (2nd cranial) nerve to the brain where they are interpreted.

The eyes are located within the orbits of the skull, one on either side of the nose. The eyeball is protected by the bony socket within which it is located, and by the eyebrow ridge. The frontal surface of the eyeball is protected by the eyelids, and tears prevent friction between the eyelids and surface of the eye.

Structure of the eye

The eye is a spherical structure (Fig. 27.3) approximately

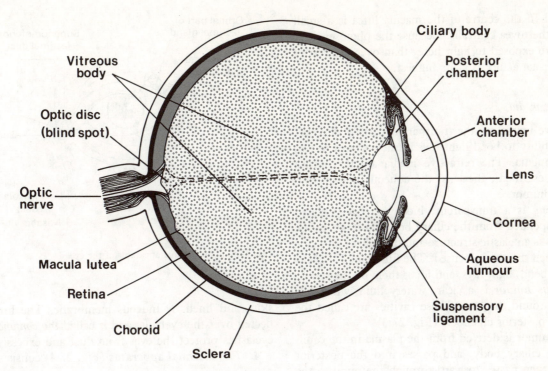

Fig. 27.3 The eye.

2.5 cm in diameter, consisting of three principal layers: an outer fibrous layer, a middle pigmented, vascular layer, and a thin innermost layer (retina).

1. The outer fibrous layer consists of the *sclera* and the *cornea*, which is a transparent structure that is continuous with the sclera. About five-sixths of the outer surface is made up of a tough white opaque fibrous layer (sclera), while the cornea comprises the anterior one-sixth. Both the sclera and the cornea consist of layers of collagen fibres. In the cornea, the fibres are regular in size and arrangement and this leads to the transparency of the cornea. The cornea functions as a refracting and protective layer through which light rays pass en route to brain.

2. The middle pigmented vascular layer is composed of three structures: the choroid, the iris, and the ciliary body.

The choroid is a layer of tissue that lies between the sclera and the retina. It is composed largely of blood vessels, and contains highly pigmented cells that absorb light and prevent it from being reflected within the eyeball.

The iris is the pigmented circular membrane behind the cornea, in front of the lens, that gives the eye its colour. Sphincter and dilator muscles within the iris regulate the central aperture, the pupil. By either dilation or constriction of the pupil, the amount of light entering the eye is regulated. The pupil appears black because light rays entering the eye are absorbed by the choroid, and are not reflected.

The ciliary body is a thickened area of the choroid, and is anterior to the choroid extending to the root of the iris.

A circular array of tiny fibres stretches from the ciliary body to the *lens* to hold it in place. The ciliary body controls focusing of the lens, and it contains glands which secrete aqueous humor.

3. The innermost layer is a thin structure called the *retina*. The retina lines the inner wall of the posterior portion of the eyeball, and is comprised of a number of layers. The two main layers are:

- *the pigmented layer* which is the outermost layer of the retina, lying next to the choroid. The cells in this layer contain melanin.
- *the rod and cone layer* lies next to the pigmented layer.

Rods and cones (specialized nerve endings) are distributed as a tightly packed mass throughout the retina, except at the point where the ganglionic fibres coverage to form the *optic nerve*. This area, which is approximately 1.5 mm in diameter, is termed the 'optic disc'. Since it possesses no photosensitive cells it is also known as the 'blind spot'.

The prime function of rods and cones is to absorb light. *Rods* can be stimulated by dim light, and they also allow perception of shapes and movement in dim light. Rods also provide far peripheral vision. *Cones* are specialized for fine visual discrimination and colour perception. There are three types of cones: one type responds most to blue light, another to red light, and the third type responds to green light.

In the centre of the retina is an oval, yellowish area, the

macula lutea. In the centre of the macula lutea is a small depression, the fovea centralis. Because the photosensitive cells are more exposed to light here, than over the rest of the retina, visual acuity is at its highest.

The refractive media

The refractive media are the transparent parts of the eye, having the ability to bend light rays at the surfaces of two transparent media. The refractive media are the cornea (previously described), the lens, the aqueous humor, and the vitreous humor.

1. The lens is a transparent, biconvex, encapsulated structure suspended from the ciliary body posterior to the iris. The lens is an elastic structure and this allows its shape to change when the eye is focused. The function of the lens is to refract (bend) light rays, and focus them on the retina.

2. Aqueous humor is a clear, watery fluid which fills the cavities around the lens. These cavities are called the anterior and posterior chambers (Fig. 27.3).

Aqueous humor is derived from the plasma in the capillaries of the ciliary body, and passes into the posterior chamber. It then passes forward through the pupil to the anterior chamber, where it is absorbed into the ciliary veins. The rate of secretion and reabsorption is balanced, so that intra-ocular pressure is regulated. Aqueous humor serves as a refractory medium and provides nutrients to the lens and cornea.

3. Vitreous humor is a clear jelly-like substance which fills the intra-ocular space from the posterior lens to the retina. Because it does not regenerate, any significant loss of vitreous humor, e.g. as a result of injury to the eye, may distort other ocular structures. Vitreous humor helps to maintain the shape of the eyeball, helps to keep the retina in position, and helps with the refraction of light rays.

Accessory apparatus

The eyeball is anchored into position by a number of structures including the extra-ocular muscles, the conjunctiva, and the eyelids. The eyeball is further protected by the bony socket, the eyebrow ridge, and some fatty tissue. It is lubricated by the lacrimal glands.

1. The extra-ocular muscles are the muscles which bring about rotational movements of the eyeball. The muscles arise from the orbit, and consist of four *rectus* muscles which are attached to the sclera, and two *oblique* muscles. The oblique muscles are arranged so that, for part of their length, they lie around the circumference of the eyeball. The nerves which supply the extra-ocular muscles are the oculomotor (3rd cranial), trochlear (4th cranial) and the abducens (6th cranial).

2. The eyebrows protect the eyes from dust, sweat, and excessive light.

3. The eyelids consist of connective tissue covered by

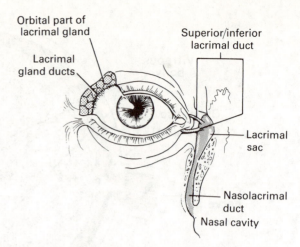

Fig. 27.4 The lacrimal apparatus of the eye.

skin, and lined by mucous membrane. The lining is reflected over the eyeballs, and is called the *conjunctiva*. The eyelashes protect the eyes from dust and excessive light.

4. The lacrimal apparatus (Fig. 27.4) consists of:

- the lacrimal gland, which is situated over the eye at the upper outer corner, secretes tears which constantly wash over the conjunctiva.
- the lacrimal ducts, which carry tears from the lacrimal gland.
- the lacrimal canal, which leads from the inner angle of the lids to the lacrimal sac.
- the lacrimal sac, which lies on the lacrimal bone at the inner angle of the eye.
- the nasolacrimal duct, which runs from the lacrimal sac to open into the nasal cavity.

Tears are secreted on to the anterior surface of the eyeball, and are spread over it by the blinking movements of the eyelids. An antimicrobial substance in tears protects the eyes against micro-organisms. Excess tears drain down into the nasal cavity.

The lacrimal glands are stimulated in response to chemical and mechanical irritants , thus producing tears to wash away the irritants. Tears may also be produced as a result of emotion, e.g. sadness, or happiness.

The physiology of sight

Light travels to various objects where it undergoes reflection. This reflected light can then travel towards the eye, where it passes through the cornea, aqueous humor, the lens and the vitreous humor, before forming an image on the retina. Nerve endings in the retina transmit electrical impulses along the optic nerve to the brain.

A co-ordinated process of refraction, accommodation, regulation of pupil size, and convergence makes normal binocular vision possible.

1. Refraction. Refraction, or bending of light rays, occurs as the light waves pass through the cornea, aqueous humor, the lens and the vitreous humor, so that they are focused on the retina of each eye.

2. Accommodation. Accommodation is the process whereby the curvature of the lens in altered so that the eye is able to focus light from objects at different distances. As an object moves closer to the eye the curvature of the lens increases, so that the image remains in focus on the retina.

3. Regulation of pupil size. The diameter of the pupil influences image formation, and the muscles of the iris respond reflexly to changes in light intensity. An increase in light intensity initiates constriction of the pupil, whereas a decrease in light intensity causes dilation of the pupil. Adjustment of pupil size, therefore, regulates the amount of light entering the eyes. Too much light may damage the retina, and too little light fails to stimulate the retina.

4. Convergence. Convergence is the medial movements of the two eyeballs so that they are both directed towards the object being viewed. Convergence allows light rays to fall on and stimulate two identical spots on the retinas, resulting in the perception of a single image.

After an image has been formed on the retina by the processes of refraction, accommodation, regulation of pupil size and convergence, light impulses are coverted into nerve impulses by the rods and cones. The light breaks down the photosensitive chemicals in either rods or cones, which stimulates electrical impulses to the brain for interpretation.

Nerve impulses travel from the retina along the optic nerve. The optic nerve emerges from the back of the eyeball and passes to the *optic chiasma*, an area at the base of the brain. At the optic chiasma the left and the right optic nerves come together, and one half of the fibres then cross to opposite sides of the brain. The fibres then form the left and right optic tracts, which continue to the visual area of the brain in the occipital lobes. Here, further processing occurs so that the image is given meaning.

The ears

The ear is specially adapted as the organ of hearing, but it is also concerned with sense of position, balance and equilibrium. Hearing is a complex mechanism in which the ears receive sound waves and convert them into nerve impulses. The nerve impulses are transmitted by the acoustic (8th cranial) nerve to the brain where they are interpreted.

The externally visible portion of each ear is located on the lateral surface of the head on each side. The remaining parts of each ear are embedded in the bone of the skull beneath.

Structure of the ear

Each ear (Fig. 27.5) can be divided into three areas; the external, middle, and inner ear.

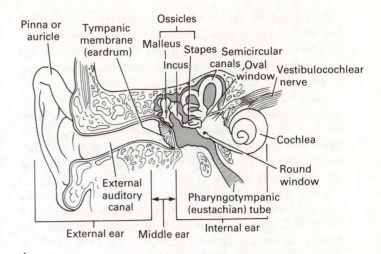

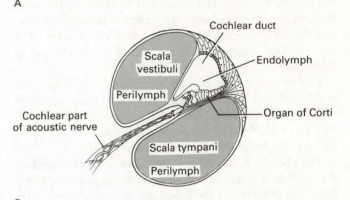

Fig. 27.5 The ear. (A) The parts of the ear, and (B) a section of membranous cochlea showing the organ of Corti.

1. The external ear consists of the auricle (pinna), together with the external acoustic meatus.

The auricle (pinna) consists of a piece of elastic cartilage with a number of associated ligaments and muscles, and it is covered by skin.

The **ear lobe** does not contain cartilage, but is composed of fibrous and adipose tissue.

The skin of the auricle is covered with fine hairs, and it is continuous with the skin lining the external acoustic meatus.

The external acoustic (auditory) meatus is an S-shaped canal approximately 2.5 cm long. It extends from the auricle to the tympanic membrane (ear drum). The skin lining the meatus contains glands which produce cerumen (wax), that protects the lining from damage and keeps dust particles away from the ear drum.

The tympanic membrane at the end of the external acoustic meatus, is a semi-transparent sheet of membrane consisting of three layers. The outermost layer consists of hairless skin, the middle layer is connective tissue, and the innermost layer is continuous with the mucous membrane lining the middle ear.

2. The middle ear, or tympanic cavity, is a small chamber within the temporal bone. It is lined by mucous membrane and filled with air, so that the pressure on the inner surface of the ear drum equals the atmospheric pressure—and the drum is kept taut.

The pharyngotympanic tube (also known as the auditory or Eustachian tube) connects the middle ear with air from the nasopharynx. It is approximately 36 cm long and is lined with mucous membrane. Normally, the tube is flattened and closed at the pharyngeal orifice, but swallowing or yawning will open it briefly.

There are three small bones, or *ossicles*, lying in the middle ear which transmit sound from the tympanic membrane to the oval window. Because of their shapes, the bones are named the malleus (mallet), the incus (the anvil), and the stapes (the stirrup). The malleus is attached to the tympanic membrane, the stapes is attached to the oval window, and the incus articulates with the other two ossicles. The three ossicles are attached to the wall of the middle ear by ligaments.

3. The internal ear consists of a bony cavity within the temporal bone, known as the *osseous labyrinth*. It is lined with periosteum, and is filled with a fluid called *perilymph*. The three divisions of the osseous labyrinth are the cochlea, the vestibule, and the semicircular canals.

The cochlea is a spiralling bony cavity, which resembles the shell of a snail. It contains the nerve endings which carry sound waves to the acoustic (8th cranial) nerve, for transmission to the brain.

The vestibule lies between the cochlea and the semicircular canals. It contains nerve endings which enable the individual to know the position of his head in space.

The semicircular canals consists of three canals (in each ear) that are arranged at right angles to each other. They are filled with *endolymph*, and contain specialized nerve endings which are stimulated by the movement of the endolymph.

The membranous labyrinth is a membrane consisting of three layers, and lies within the osseous labyrinth. In the areas where it is not attached to the osseous labyrinth it is surrounded by perilymph. The fluid contained within the membranous labyrinth is known as endolymph. Part of the membranous labyrinth is concerned with hearing, and part is concerned with the position of the head in space. The ear is responsible for hearing and for maintenance of equilibrium.

Physiology of hearing

Sound waves are collected and directed by the auricle into the external acoustic meatus, where they pass through and cause the tympanic membrane to vibrate. They then pass through the middle ear by vibration of the ossicles and into the internal ear. From the internal ear sound waves are transmitted to the brain, via the acoustic nerve, for interpretation. Perception of sound involves interpretation of pitch and intensity. The entire process of hearing involves the following steps:

- The movement of air molecules cause a sound wave to form.
- The sound wave travels through the air to the auricle, which directs it into the external acoustic meatus.
- The sound wave enters the acoustic meatus and comes in contact with the tympanic membrane, causing it to vibrate.
- The vibrations are transferred to the ossicles which begin to vibrate, and the sound wave is transmitted across the middle ear cavity to the oval window and into the fluid-filled internal ear.
- Sound waves set the cochlear fluids into motion. The receptor cells are stimulated, and the sound waves are transmitted along the acoustic nerve to the temporal lobe of the brain for interpretation.

Two qualities of sound, pitch and intensity, are important in the interpretation of sound.

Pitch is related to the frequency of the sound wave. A high frequency sound stimulates the neurones supplying the cells near the base of the cochlea. Low frequency sounds stimulate neurones nearer to the apex of the cochlea. An individual is normally able to distinguish pitch over a frequency range of about 30 to about 20 000 cycles per second.

Intensity is related to the loudness of sound, and is measured in decibels. A loud sound causes the nerve endings to be stimulated at a greater rate, than does a softer sound. The intensity of normal conversational speech is approximately 60 decibels (db), and a decibel level of 160 can cause bursting of the tympanic membrane.

Maintenance of equilibrium (balance)

Two structures within the internal ear—the semicircular canals and the vestibule—work together to help an individual maintain his balance, or equilibrium. Components of the semicircular canals alert the brain to rotational movement, and components of the vestibule alert the brain to gravitational movement. Movement of fluid in the canals gives a constant flow of information about body position, and the speed and direction of any body movement. This information is used to co-ordinate movements and to main balance.

SUMMARY

The special sense organs are those which contain receptors that pick up stimuli from the environment, and transmit impulses to the brain for interpretation. The special sense organs that allow the individual to obtain information about the environment are the tongue, the nose, the skin, the eyes, and the ears. Through these organs, the individual is able to experience taste, smell, touch, sight and sound.

The tongue contains taste buds which respond to substances in the food, and generate nerve impulses which are transmitted to the brain for interpretation. Taste buds are capable of detecting sweet, sour, salty and bitter tastes when substances are in solution.

Olfactory receptors in the mucous membrane lining the upper part of the nose are stimulated by chemicals, and transmit impulses to the brain where smell is interpreted.

The sensations of taste and smell are closely related, and both play and important part in stimulating the secretion of digestive juices.

The skin, as one of its several functions, allows the perception of touch. It is, therefore, an organ of sensation as it contains receptors that transmit impulses to the brain where the sense of touch is perceived.

Sight is the result of light rays being received by the eyes and transmitted to the brain for intepretation. Each eye receives light from the environment and forms images on the retina, which converts them into nerve impulses which are transmitted to the visual centres of the brain.

A co-ordinated process of refraction, accommodation, regulation of pupil size, and convergence makes normal binocular vision possible.

The eyeballs are anchored into position by extra-ocular muscles and the conjunctiva; and are further protected by the bony socket, the eyebrow ridge and the eyelids. The lacrimal apparatus secretes tears and directs them onto the anterior surface of the eye, where they are spread over it by the blinking movements of the eyelids.

Hearing is a complex mechanism in which the ears receive sound waves, and convert them into nerve impulses. The nerve impulses are transmitted to the brain for interpretation. Perception of sound involves interpretation of both pitch and intensity.

The ears also, through structures contained in the internal ear, help the individual to maintain balance.

REFERENCES AND FURTHER READING

Hinwood B G 1981 Integrated science applied for nurses. Cassell, Australia
Marieb E N 1984 Essentials of human anatomy and physiology. Addison-Wesley, California
Nave C R, Nave B C 1975 Physics for the health sciences. W B Saunders, Philadelphia
Wilson K J W 1987 Ross and Wilson Anatomy and physiology in health and illness, 6th edn. Churchill Livingstone, Edinburgh

PART 3

Nursing care and basic needs

28. An introduction to human needs

INTRODUCTION

Fundamental to the practice of nursing is the understanding that all people have needs. A 'need' may be described as a requirement that is necessary or desirable for maintaining physical or psychosocial well being. In psychological terms, 'motivation' is any inducement or force that directs behaviour towards satisfying needs or achieving goals. According to theories of motivation based on the concept of need gratification, stimuli called 'drives' occur within the individual. If a need is not fulfilled, drives cause responses directed towards meeting this need. For example, an unsatisfied need for food will motivate the individual to take certain actions which will result in taking food into the body. The intake of food will satisfy the need, and as a result the drive stimuli are reduced.

Abraham Maslow, a psychologist, devised a theory of need gratification and identified basic human needs which he arranged into a hierarchy. He believed that some needs are basic to others, and that certain basic needs must be satisfied before individuals will be motivated to satisfy higher needs. Maslow's hierarchy of needs is illustrated in Figure 28.1. According to Maslow, physiological needs are the strongest and once these needs have been satisfied, needs at the next level emerge; the process continues until all categories of needs in the hierarchy have been fulfilled. Another theorist, Richard Kalish, suggested modification to Maslow's hierarchy. He believed that the order of importance in which Maslow had placed the needs should be altered. For example, Kalish placed more importance on the need for knowledge than Maslow who placed it in the 'self actualization' category.

It is generally agreed that these needs are common to all people, and that they apply throughout the life span. However, the nature of needs and their relative importance to an individual's well being, vary with his age and stage of development. Some needs require particular attention at each stage of development, for example:

● During pregnancy, the need for food is of great importance to supply the mother and developing fetus with the nutrients necessary for growth of new tissue.

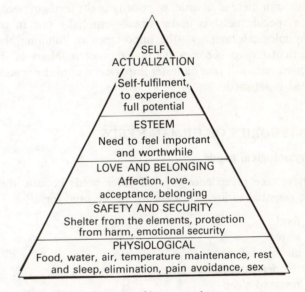

Fig. 28.1 Maslow's hierarchy of human needs.

● During early childhood, the need for safety and protection becomes considerable. The child aged between eighteen months and three years, has little concept of danger but is at the stage where he is developing independence and insatiable curiosity about his environment. To tivities and surroundings in order to ensure his protection and safety.

● Adolescence is a stage of many physical changes and, as the appearance of adolescents begins to alter from that of children to that of adults, their need for love and belonging becomes very important. Relationships with peers play a vital role in adolescents' sense of acceptance, and are an important influence in the development of a sense of belonging.

● During the later years many of the changes associated with the ageing process tend to result in the elderly person becoming more vulnerable to accidents and injury, therefore protection and safety needs become of vital importance.

In normal circumstances people are usually capable of meeting their own needs, but during illness or periods of dependence they may require assistance. The foundation of nursing practice is based on the principle of assisting individuals to meet their needs when they are unable to do so independently. Nursing actions that may be required to assist the patient meet his basic needs are described in Chapters 29–40.

Maslow suggested five basic categories of human needs arranged in order of priority for satisfaction. They are:

- physiological needs
- safety and security needs
- need for love and belonging
- esteem needs
- need for self actualization.

Although there is an order of priority in the levels of needs, if a specific need is under stress—especially one in the physiological category—the importance of fulfilling that particular need becomes the major concern. Many of the other needs will take on lesser importance until the specific need is satisfied.

CATEGORIES OF HUMAN NEEDS

Physiological needs

These take precedence over all other needs because they are essential to life. They consist of the need for:

- food
- water
- air
- temperature maintenance
- rest and sleep
- elimination
- pain avoidance.

If a person is deprived of food or water he will begin to feel ill and weak, and will be stimulated to take actions satisfy his hunger and relieve his thirst. A patient who is unable to eat or drink normally, will require nursing assistance to ensure that his nutritional and fluid needs are met.

Oxygen is essential to life and if cells are deprived of oxygen for more than a few minutes they will die. A patient who is experiencing difficulty in meeting his oxygen needs through normal breathing, will require nursing intervention to ensure an adequate oxygen supply.

The maintenance of a constant body temperature is essential for normal function. During illness deviations from the normal range of body temperature may occur. A patient with an abnormally high or low body temperature will often require nursing actions to restore the temperature to normal.

Rest and sleep are two closely related needs that both depend on and contribute to a person's comfort. Periods of reduced physical activity are considered to be necessary for the restoration and growth of body cells. Because of illness

and the many disruptions to his usual routine, a patient may require assistance to ensure that adequate rest and sleep are attained.

Elimination of wastes from the body is essential for normal function. Due to a variety of factors, a patient may experience difficulty with normal elimination, and nursing actions may be indicated to prevent the accumulation of waste and to assist elimination.

Pain is a response to a number of stressors, e.g. infection, and is a protective mechanism because it is commonly a warning that something harmful is occuring to the body. Pain is a common symptom of illness, and nursing intervention is required to reduce or relieve the patient's pain.

Safety and security needs

This category includes the need for adequate shelter from the elements, appropriate clothing, and protection from harmful factors in the environment. People also have a need to feel emotionally secure and protected, and are more likely to feel secure when they are in familiar surroundings with people they know and trust. It is not uncommon for people to feel threatened and insecure in an unfamiliar environment, or when their usual pattern of living is disrupted, or when they are among people who are not known to them.

An important function of the nurse is the promotion of patient safety, and therefore the nurse must be aware of the factors that make a patient more at risk of being harmed. Patients who are more vulnerable to accidents include those at each end of the life span and those with impaired mobility, senses, or consciousness. In addition to the factors that may result in physical injury, a patient must also be protected against infection. The importance of preventing the spread of infection in health care institutions, is emphasized throughout this text.

It is also important for the nurse to realize the significance of emotional security. When people are admitted to hospital their usual way of living is disrupted. A patient often experiences anxiety about his illness, and about being away from his normal environment and associates. Being ill and in hospital often results in increased dependence on others, and this may result in feelings of insecurity. A patient will usually feel less anxious if he is given adequate explanations about what is happening, and why nursing actions are being implemented. The patient's need for knowledge about his illness and treatment, will be partially fulfilled if the nurse provides him with sufficient information.

The high priority that Richard Kalish considered the need for knowledge should be given in a hierarchy of human needs, is further highlighted in a number of studies which have shown that a patient's recovery is hastened by the provision of knowledge about his illness and its treatment. The nurse's manner towards patients should be warm and friendly, and the explanations given should take into account each patient's individuality.

Need for love and belonging

Every person needs to feel that he is accepted and loved, and to experience warmth and closeness in his relationships with other people. Regardless of age, a person's emotional and social development is enhanced when he feels loved and needed. Failure to thrive of well fed and physically well cared for infants, has been attributed to deprivation of affection. It is also possible that some elderly people experience the same fate. The nurse must be careful not to neglect the emotional needs of a patient and should develop communication skills that promote effective nurse-patient interaction.

It is important to understand that all individuals have a right to their views and beliefs, and to follow their preferred life style. Acceptance of a person requires that his thoughts, feelings, beliefs, strengths and weaknesses are respected. The interaction between a nurse and a patient is enhanced when the nurse is able to communicate her acceptance of him as an individual. The patient's family and loved ones should be encouraged to keep close contact with him during his illness, and to participate in his care when appropriate.

The need for sexual activity, although not vital to the survival of the individual, is vital to the survival of the human race. The sex drive is fundamental and strong, but the expression of sexuality is much more than the physical act of sex. Human sexuality is expressed in attitudes, feelings, and behaviour, and is part of an individual's need to give and receive love.

Esteem needs

Every person has a need to feel important and worthwhile as a human being. A person with low self esteem will feel inadequate and alienated from others. Illness may lower a person's self esteem due to his increased dependence on others. This dependence may be on assistance from other people, or on special aids and equipment. A person who has been independent all his life may find it difficult to accept assistance, and the nurse must ensure that it is offered in a manner that enables him to maintain self respect and dignity.

Part of a person's self esteem is related to how his physical being, or body image is perceived. Nurses should be aware that a person's self esteem can be reduced when the body image is altered. For example, if a woman has to have a breast removed she may feel that the changes in her body image will affect her relationships with other people. A patient with a bowel tumour, may require an artificial opening in the abdomen through which wastes are elimin-ated. These alterations to normal body function and, consequently, to the person's body image can seriously affect self esteem. It is important for the nurse to implement actions that will help a patient to develop or maintain a positive self image, and as a consequence to retain his self esteem. It is important that a patient does not feel that he is any less a person because of his health problem.

Need for self actualization

People have a need to achieve self fulfilment and to experience their full potential. Maslow has included in this category the need for knowledge, and the need to appreciate the beautiful things in life. Illness or temporary dependence may prevent a person from achieving his full potential. The nurse has a role to play in assisting the patient to reach his full potential, particularly in rehabilitation settings, or when considering the needs of people who are physically, emotionally, or mentally disabled. Assistance should be provided that will enable such people to develop to the full extent of their capabilities. The nurse should be aware that any potential or actual disruption to the achievement of self actualization may be a cause of great anxiety for people who are ill. Illness can interfere with a person's career, or with his need to reach his full potential. For example, the loss or threatened loss of the ability to use an arm, would be overwhelming for a person who relies on his hands for work or leisure.

Basic human needs can be categorized into the physiological or survival needs, and the secondary or psychosocial needs. All needs are closely related, and the deprivation of physiological needs will have psychosocial effects. For example, if a person is experiencing prolonged or chronic severe pain, obtaining relief from the pain becomes the major focus in his life. Not only will other physiological needs, such as the need for food, be neglected, but so may his self esteem; and he would have little interest in achieving self fulfilment. Conversely, if a psychosocial need is not fulfilled, the individual's motivation or ability to meet his physiological needs is affected. For example, a person with low self esteem may either neglect his diet or engage in overeating; or he may experience altered sleep patterns.

It is important for the nurse to be aware that people who are unable to fulfil their basic needs may react to the associated frustration in different ways. Reaction to any frustration in a person's attempt to fulfil his basic needs varies with each individual and is influenced by factors such as age, state of health, temperament, and environment. Some patients who are dependent on others to assist them meet their needs may regress. Regression is a return to a type of behaviour more appropriate to a younger age group. An adult who is experiencing frustration in fulfilling certain basic needs may instinctively use a form of behaviour which met with success during childhood or adolescence, or a child may revert to infantile behaviour. For example, a child who was previously toilet trained may revert to bed wetting, or if able to feed himself independently, may demand to be fed.

A patient may react to his loss of independence by behaving in an aggressive manner. Aggressive behaviour is a common way of expressing and partially relieving anxiety. In a health care setting, aggressiveness may take the form of complaints about the care, the food, or the staff. Aggression may be directed towards the person perceived by the patient to be the one who is preventing fulfillment of a need, e.g. the nurse or the medical officer.

Further information on people's reactions to illness and loss of independence is provided in Chapter 6.

Nursing care is thus concerned with assisting patients to meet those needs they are unable to achieve independently. Care plans are developed from this model of nursing and are structured around one of the various theories of nursing, some of which are introduced in Chapter 1. Although they are expressed in different terms, the activities of living as described in the Roper/Logan/Tierney model for nursing, relate to the categories of needs as identified by Maslow. This chapter will thus briefly address their model for nursing which is based on a model of living, and focuses on activities of living. The activities of living identified by Roper, Logan and Tierney in their book *The Elements of Nursing*, are:

- maintaining a safe environment
- communicating
- breathing
- eating and drinking
- eliminating
- personal cleansing and dressing
- controlling body temperature
- mobilizing
- working and playing
- expressing sexuality
- sleeping
- dying.

The activities of living are the main focus of the model, and Roper, Logan and Tierney view nursing as, 'helping

patients to prevent, solve, alleviate or cope with problems with the activities of living'.

The model consists of five components:

- activities of living (AL)
- lifespan
- dependence/independence continuum
- factors influencing the activities of living
- individuality in living.

The activities of living and the level of dependence or independence, are influenced by the stages of development during a person's life span from conception to death. Individuals carry out the activities of living differently because of a variety of factors that are:

- physical
- psychological
- sociocultural
- environmental
- politico-economic.

Although deciding that there should be no fixed priority among the activities of living, Roper, Logan and Tierney agree that those activities which are vital to survival and safety, should take precedence over the others. They state that when the nurse is making decisions about the relevance and relative priorities of the activities of living, she should keep in mind that different circumstances create different priorities. They cite the example that although 'working and playing' takes up much time in ordinary life, this activity of living will assume a low priority during a period of critical illness.

Whether a nursing care plan is based on the human needs theory or on a specific theory of nursing, the nursing process is commonly used as a means of ensuring that appropriate care is planned for each patient. Information on the nursing process is provided in Chapter 12.

The remaining chapters in this section examine the human needs in detail, and their significance to well being. Information is provided about various nursing actions that may be required to assist the patient meet his needs when he is unable to do so independently.

29. Meeting nutritional needs

INTRODUCTION

The intake of food has psychosocial and cultural significance in life; but the major roles of food are the provision of nutrients necessary for the development and growth of cells, and the replacement of substances required by cells to maintain efficient body function.

Information about the ingestion and digestion of food, and the absorption of nutrients, is provided in Chapter 23. After the digested nutrients have been absorbed into the blood and lymph, they are distributed to the cells for further chemical processing which releases the energy necessary for body function. The process of *metabolism* converts the nutrients into chemical forms that produce energy and rebuild body tissue. The two phases of metabolism are:

- *Anabolism* (or constructive phase), when simple substances derived from the nutrients are converted into complex substances that can be used by the cells.
- *Catabolism* (or destructive phase), when these complex substances are reconverted into more simple forms in order to release the energy necessary for cell function.

The term *nutrition*, is used to describe all the processes by which the body uses food for energy, maintenance, and growth. Nutritional requirements vary in response to changes throughout the life span. Factors that increase the body's metabolic demand include the periods of rapid growth during infancy and adolescence, and periods of stress related to disease or trauma. Metabolic requirements diminish with reduced energy demands, decreased physical activity, and age.

Adequate nutrition is partially dependent on the ability of the body to ingest and digest food, to absorb nutrients from the small intestine, and to excrete waste products. In addition, the quality and quantity of food consumed has an important influence on an individual's current and future health status. A diet containing the essential nutrients is vital throughout each stage of the life span.

Many factors influence the individual with regard to his pattern of eating, and include:

- the availability of food
- economic status
- influences such as the family, or advertising
- food fads and fallacies
- beliefs, values, and cultural heritage
- the social and emotional aspects of food
- the physical or psychological status of the individual such as an allergy or intolerance to specific foods; difficulty in chewing or swallowing; level of independence; disorders that interfere with nutrition and result in maldigestion, malabsorption, or loss of

nutrients; and emotional states such as depression or anxiety.

NORMAL NUTRITION

Assessment of an individual's nutritional status is achieved by obtaining information about his appetite, his food preferences, his height and weight, his level of activity, and from observing his general appearance. Observation of an individual's general appearance provides information about his nutritional status, and the characteristics of nutritional status are presented in Table 29.1.

Table 29.1 Characteristics of nutritional status

Body area	Normal appearance	Signs of poor nutrition
Hair	Smooth and glossy	Dull, dry, or brittle
Nails	Firm, healthy colour of nail bed	Brittle, ridged, or spoon shaped. Pale nail bed
Skin	Healthy colour, good turgor	Unhealthy colour. Poor turgor. Dry or scaly. Bruising unrelated to trauma
Mouth	Firm gums. Reddish-pink mucous membranes and tongue	Spongy or bleeding gums. Pale mucous membrane. Swollen or smooth tongue
Eyes	Bright and clear Reddish-pink mucous membrane No discharge	Dull Pale mucous membrane Purulent discharge
Muscles	Firm, good tone	Wasted, lack of tone
Limbs	Straight	Bowed arms or legs

From the assessment made of an individual's eating pattern and his nutritional status, any problems or risk factors can be identified.

In addition to the physical characteristics associated with poor nutritional status, psychological symptoms may be evident. An individual with a poor nutritional status may experience irritability, lethargy, apathy, or inability to concentrate. It is possible, however, that these symptoms plus the physical signs presented in Table 29.1, may be related to conditions other than the individual's nutritional status.

Certain groups of people may be more at risk of a poor nutritional status, including those who are:

- physically inactive
- alcohol, drug, or nicotine dependent
- pregnant or breastfeeding
- elderly
- unaware of nutritional values
- strict vegetarians
- following 'fad' diets
- experiencing certain physical or emotional disorders.

In order to maintain or promote an appropriate intake of food, and therefore a good nutritional status, people should be encouraged to follow the principles of a well balanced diet that provides the body with essential nutrients.

Balanced diet

A balanced diet is one that consists of foods taken regularly, in sufficient quantities, from each of the basic food groups. In order to achieve a diet that is balanced and contains sufficient essential nutrients, a diet composed of 60% carbohydrate, 20% protein, and 20% fat is recommended.

The recommended number of daily servings from each of the five food groups varies slightly according to the individual's stage of development. The five food groups, and the recommended daily allowances are given below.

1. Milk and dairy products. The major nutrients provided by foods from this group are protein, fat, and calcium. 300–600 ml of milk, or equivalent substitutes such as cheese and yoghurt, should be consumed daily. During pregnancy or lactation this amount should be increased to 900 ml of milk, or equivalent substitutes, daily.

2. Meat, fish, and eggs. The major nutrients provided by foods from this group are protein, fat, and iron. 1–2 servings from this group is the recommended daily allowance.

3. Fruits and vegetables. The major nutrients provided by foods from this group are carbohydrate, fibre, water soluble vitamins, and water. The recommended daily allowance is at least 4 servings of either fruits or vegetables, or a combination of both.

4. Breads and cereals. The major nutrients provided by foods from this group are carbohydrate, protein, vitamins, iron, and fibre. Depending on energy requirements, at least 4 servings daily are recommended.

5. Fats (butter, margarine, oils). The major function of foods in this group is to provide a vehicle for the fat soluble vitamins: A, D, E, and K. The recommended daily allowance of fats is 15–30 g.

Energy requirements

In addition to the consumption of foods from the 5 food groups that provide essential nutrients, dietary requirements are also considered in terms of energy requirements. Energy is needed for all the chemical and physical activities of the body, e.g. muscular activity, production of gland secretions, and the synthesis of substances in the cells. The amount of energy required by an individual is the amount necessary to maintain physiological processes, and is dependent on factors such as:

- age
- sex
- climate
- body build, height, and weight

- level of physical activity
- normal function or dysfunction.

Energy requirements are increased during periods of rapid growth, e.g. during pregnancy, infancy, and adolescence; and when the individual engages in a high level of physical activity. Certain body dysfunction, e.g. a disorder of the thyroid gland, also increases the amount of energy required. Energy requirements are decreased when an individual's level of physical activity is low, and during stages of development when there is little growth, e.g. old age.

The two units of measurement that specify the energy value of food, are calories and joules. A calorie is defined as the amount of heat required to raise 1 gram of water through 1 degree Celsius. One calorie is equal to 4.184 joules. A joule, which is the SI unit of energy and heat, is equivalent to the amount of work performed when a 1 kilogram mass is moved 1 metre by the force of 1 newton. As joules are very small units, it is more convenient to measure food energy in terms of kilojoules. One kilojoule is 1000 joules.

The energy value of the three major nutrients are:

- 1 gram of protein produces approximately 17 kJ
- 1 gram of carbohydrate produces approximately 17 kJ
- 1 gram of fat produces approximately 38 kJ.

Energy expenditure varies with the level of physical activity an individual engages in, and ranges from approximately 5 kJ per minute during sleep, to approximately 120 kJ per minute during hard physical labour. When the intake of kilojoules is increased, or energy expenditure is decreased, weight gain occurs. Conversely, loss of weight occurs when the intake of kilojoules is decreased, or energy expenditure is increased.

Basal metabolism is the term used to describe the minimal maintenance of essential body functions, e.g. circulation and respiration. The amount of energy required to support basal metabolism is measured when an individual is awake but at complete rest and has not eaten for at least 12 hours. The measurement is expressed as basal metabolic rate (BMR), according to the number of kilojoules consumed per hour per square metre of body surface area (or per kilogram of body weight). Variations in BMR occur during certain disease states, and estimation of the BMR is one diagnostic test that is commonly used.

A table of acceptable weight for height for Australians, Table 29.2, was adopted by the National Health and Medical Research Council in 1984. This table is based on body mass index (BMI) which is calculated using the following formula:

$$BMI = \frac{Weight\ in\ kilograms}{Height\ in\ metres^2}$$

The value obtained when this formula is used should be

Table 29.2 Acceptable weights-for-height*

Height (cm) (without shoes)	Body weight (kg) (in light clothing without shoes)
140	39–49
142	40–50
144	41–52
146	43–53
148	44–55
150	45–56
152	46–58
154	47–59
156	49–61
158	50–62
160	51–64
162	52–66
164	54–67
166	55–69
168	56–71
170	58–72
172	59–74
174	61–76
176	62–77
178	63–79
180	65–81
182	66–83
184	68–85
186	69–86
188	71–88
190	72–90
192	74–92
194	75–94
196	77–96
198	78–98
200	80–100

After an adaptation by the Commonwealth Department of Health from Garrow 1981 Treat obesity seriously: a clinical manual. A classification of obesity p3. Churchill Livingstone.
Consistent with minimal mortality and least risk for morbidity, based on data from a number of studies.
*Based on Body Mass Index (BMI) in range of 20–25 and suitable for use with both men and women from the age of 18 years onwards.

rounded to the nearest whole number. A value below 20 denotes underweight, from 20–25 is within the healthy weight range, from 25–30 indicates overweight, over 30 is defined as obesity, and a value above 40 signifies morbid obesity.

Nutrients

Nutrients are chemical substances in food that provide energy, build and maintain cells, or regulate body processes. The essential nutrients are:

- carbohydrates
- proteins
- lipids (fats)
- water
- fibre
- vitamins
- mineral salts.

Carbohydrates. Carbohydrates are a group of organic compounds comprised of sugar, starch, and cellulose, and are composed of one or more units of monosaccharide. Sugars can be classified as either simple or complex, and are divided into groups according to the complexity of their molecular structure.

Simple sugars or monosaccharides, include glucose, fructose, and galactose. Sucrose, lactose, and maltose, are classified as disaccharides—which are a combination of two sugars. For example, glucose and fructose combine to form sucrose. Complex sugars, or polysaccharides, include starch, glycogen, and cellulose. Before carbohydrates can be utilized by the body cells, they must be converted by chemical digestion into glucose.

Carbohydrates provide energy, assist in the metabolism of fat, and act as a protein sparer. (If there is insufficient carbohydrate in the diet, protein is converted to glucose and used for energy). Carbohydrate foods also supply indigestible cellulose which adds bulk to the intestinal contents, resulting in stimulation of peristalsis. The major food sources of carbohydrate are:

- Sugars; present in fruits, honey, cane sugar, milk, and cereals
- Starches; present in vegetables, cereals and foods made from cereals, e.g. bread and pasta
- Cellulose; present in vegetables, fruits and cereals (complex carbohydrate).

Proteins. Proteins are a group of nitrogenous compounds composed of amino acids. Amino acids are the individual units from which all proteins are constructed, and 22 different amino acids have been identified. The 8 essential amino acids are those which the body is unable to make, and must be obtained from dietary sources. The remaining 14 non-essential amino acids can be synthesized by the body. Before proteins can be utilized by the cells, they must be converted by chemical digestion into amino acids. According to the number and type of amino acids present, proteins are classed either as complete or incomplete.

Proteins build and repair tissue, or supply energy. (Protein that is not needed for growth and repair of tissues is converted into glucose and stored in the liver and muscles as a reserve store of energy). The major food sources of protein are:

- complete (or first class) protein; present in meat, fish, eggs, cheese, milk, poultry, and soya beans.
- incomplete (or second class) protein; present in cereals, lentils, legumes, and nuts.

Lipids (fats). Lipids, or fats, are a group of substances that are insoluble in water and are composed of fatty acids. Fatty acids are classed as saturated or unsaturated. Saturated, or solid, fats are chiefly of animal origin, e.g. butter, and contain a full complement of hydrogen. Unsaturated, or soft/liquid, fats are chiefly of vegetable origin, e.g. margarine, and are capable of adding more hydrogen to their molecular structure.

Before fats can be utilized by the body cells they must be converted by chemical digestion into fatty acids and glycerol. These substances may either be used in the tissues or stored. Fat supplies energy, and forms adipose tissue which supports and protects some organs. Adipose tissue also insulates the body to prevent excessive heat loss, and is a reserve store of fuel. Fats also supply the fat-soluble vitamins A, D, E, and K. The major food sources of fat are:

- animal fats; present in meat, butter, cream, egg yolk, cheese, and fish oils.
- vegetable fats; present in margarine, cocoa, and oils such as olive, safflower, corn and peanut.

Water. Water is a chemical compound which is obtained by the body from food and fluid; and as a result of the metabolism of protein, fat, and carbohydrate in the tissues. Water constitutes approximately 66% of the total body weight and is present as intracellular fluid and extracellular fluid. Water is also the basis of all body secretions and excretions.

Water is necessary for the digestion, absorption, and metabolism of food; for the production of secretions; and for the maintenance of body fluids. Water is also necessary for the regulation of body temperature by means of evaporation of sweat, and for the elimination of waste products through the kidneys, bowel, skin and lungs.

Water is present in all fluids and as part of the cellular structure of solid foods. Foods vary in water content, e.g. fruit and vegetables contain approximately 80–90%, meat contains approximately 70%, and bread contains approximately 35% water.

Fibre. Dietary fibre, often referred to as cellulose, is the fibrous parts of food that are not digested or absorbed. Fibre creates bulky stools which are easily excreted, and is also thought to help in the prevention of certain disorders, e.g. haemorrhoids, diverticular disease, the formation of gallstones, simple constipation, and intestinal cancer. Foods that have a high fibre content are fruits, vegetables, and wholegrain products.

Vitamins. Vitamins are a group of organic compounds which, with few exceptions, must be obtained from dietary sources. Although they have no nutrient value, vitamins are essential for metabolic and physiologic function. The word 'vitamin' was first used in 1912 and letters of the alphabet were given to the substances it described. Now that more is known about their composition, the chemical name for a vitamin is frequently used.

Vitamins are classed as either water or fat soluble. The water soluble vitamins are easily destroyed during the preparation and cooking of food. If they are consumed in excess of the body's need, water soluble vitamins are excreted in the urine. Fat soluble vitamins can be oxidized by exposure to air, light, and high temperatures. As fat soluble vitamins are not soluble in water, any excess is stored in the body and a condition known as hypervitaminosis may occur.

Information about the functions and the effects of a deficiency of vitamins is provided in Table 29.3.

Excessive intake of Vitamin A over long periods can result in Hypervitaminosis A, a condition which is characterized by yellow discoloration of the skin, loss of appetite, and dry itchy skin. Excessive intake of Vitamin B may result in allergic type reactions. Hypervitaminosis D is a condition that may occur if excessive amounts of Vitamin D are taken, and is characterized by nausea, vomiting, diarrhoea, general irritability, and impairment of kidney function. In normal circumstances, a well balanced diet will provide the body with sufficient quantities of all vitamins.

Mineral salts. Mineral salts are a group of compounds which play an important role in metabolism, maintenance of blood pressure, cardiac function, acid-base balance, and the regulation of other body processes. Storage and processing of food does not alter its mineral content, although mineral salts may be lost when food is soaked or cooked in water. Mineral salts are classed as either major or trace elements, with the trace elements being those minerals that are present in only minute quantities in the body. A mineral salt that has the property of being a conductor of electrical currents, is referred to as an electrolyte. Information about functions and the effects of a deficiency of mineral salts is provided in Table 29.4.

Diets to meet individual needs

An individual's pattern of eating, and the food he chooses, depends on the factors mentioned previously (see p. 239). An individual's dietary practice may change during illness, e.g. he may avoid eating foods that cause adverse reactions such as indigestion, nausea, or diarrhoea. His diet may also need to be adapted as part of his therapy during certain disease states, and a therapeutic diet may be prescribed.

While acknowledging the factors that influence an individual's choice of foods, and observing any restrictions to diet in the management of disease, nurses should encourage the consumption of well balanced meals following the principles of good nutrition. The principles of good nutrition are that:

- A variety of foods from each of the basic food groups should be eaten each day.
- The intake of fat, sodium, sucrose, and alcohol should be limited.
- The intake of complex carbohydrate and dietary fibre should be high.
- Adequate amounts of water should be consumed.

Food should be prepared and cooked in such a way that the nutrient value is not lost.

- Dietary intake and energy expenditure should be adjusted in order to achieve and maintain the appropriate weight for height.
- Breast feeding for babies is recommended.
- People should become aware of the information contained on the labels of prepared and packaged foods. Notice should be taken of the expiry date, the presence of preservatives and other additives. The listing of ingredients in the container denotes the relative quantities of each, with the major ingredient listed first. The remainder are listed in order of decreasing quantities.

The Commonwealth Department of Health has developed guidelines to improve the health of all Australians, and the Australian Nutrition Foundation developed a Diet Pyramid based on these guidelines (Fig. 29.1).

The various diets that an individual may choose, or which may be prescribed for therapeutic purposes include:

Regular diet

A regular diet is one without dietary restrictions or modifications, and, in hospital an individual may select the foods he prefers within the principles of good nutrition.

Diets based on health, cultural, or religious beliefs.

Some individuals choose to follow a diet in which specific foods or nutrients are restricted or increased, as part of a commitment to a healthy lifestyle. Other people will follow a diet that is based on cultural or religious commitment.

Vegetarian. People may choose to follow a vegetarian diet for health, ecological, or religious reasons. Vegetarian diets exclude all flesh foods such as meat, fish and poultry, and are high in plant foods. The lacto-ovo vegetarian diet includes milk, dairy products and eggs, while a lacto vegetarian diet excludes eggs. The vegan diet excludes all animal products and consists of plant foods only.

Religious/cultural. Certain religious or cultural groups have particular rules concerning the choice and preparation of specific items in the diet, for example:

- Adventist (7th day). A vegetarian diet is commonly followed and stimulants such as coffee, tea, and alcohol, are not permitted.
- Roman Catholic. Ash Wednesday and Good Friday are the specified days on which abstinence from meat is obligatory. In addition, Roman Catholics are required to fast for one hour prior to taking Holy Communion.
- Mormon. (Church of Jesus Christ of Latter Day Saints). Meat, although not forbidden, is eaten infrequently. Drinks containing caffeine, e.g. tea, coffee, cola, are not permitted, (Tobacco is also forbidden).
- Judaism (Jewish faith). Foods must be prepared according to Jewish law (Kosher), and only certain parts of an animal may be eaten. All pork and shellfish is prohibited; meat and dairy products are never eaten at the same time and are prepared with separate utensils. Certain periods of fasting are observed.
- Islam (Moslem, Muslim). All pork and pork products, plus alcohol, are forbidden. Any meat consumed must

Table 29.3   Vitamins and health

Vitamin	Functions	Sources	Effects of deficiency
Vitamins A (Retinol or Carotenes)	Sustains normal vision in a dim light Promotes healthy epithelial tissue—therefore raises resistance to infection Promotes growth	Cod liver oil Liver, kidney Milk Cheese Butter Cream Egg yolk Yellow fruits and vegetables	Night blindness Deterioration of epithelial tissue—therefore less resistance to infection Stunted growth
Vitamin B group Thiamine (B_1)	Nerve function Energy and carbohydrate metabolism	Wholegrain cereals Yeast extract Meats Leafy green vegetables	Polyneuritis Beriberi Wernicke-Korsakoff syndrome
Riboflavin (B_2)	Energy and protein metabolism Cellular respiration Healthy skin and mucous membrane	Liver Yeast extract Milk products Eggs Leafy green vegetables	Fissures at the corner of mouth (cheilosis) Stomatitis Glossitis Poor condition of the skin
Niacin (B_3)	Energy utilization Metabolism of fat, carbohydrate, protein Nervous system function	Liver Meat Fish Yeast extract Legumes	Pellagra
Pyridoxine (B_6)	Protein metabolism Nervous system function Formation of red blood cells	Meat Fish Offal Wholegrain cereals Bananas Avocado Peanuts	Neuritis Depression Anaemia
Pantothenic acid	Metabolism	Offal Yeast Fish Meat Egg yolk Broad beans	Fatigue Sleep disturbances Headaches
Biotin	Synthesis of fatty acids	Egg yolk Fish Offal Soya beans	Lethargy Dermatitis
Folacin	Metabolism DNA and RNA synthesis Formation of red blood cells	Citrus fruit Offal Nuts Leafy green vegetables	Macrocytic anaemia
Cyanocobalamin (B_{12})	Formation of red cells	All foods of animal origin	Pernicious anaemia
Vitamin C (Ascorbic acid)	Formation of collagen, therefore assists in wound healing and in the maintenance of healthy capillary walls Aids absorption of iron	Citrus fruits Tropical fruits Berry fruits Tomatoes Potatoes Green vegetables	Delayed healing Increased tendency to bleed. Scurvy
Vitamin D (Calciferol)	Calcium and phosphorous metabolism	Butter, margarine Egg yolk Fish oils * Sunlight on the skin	Rickets Osteomalacia

Table 29.3 (cont'd) Vitamins and health

Vitamin	Functions	Sources	Effects of deficiency
Vitamin E (Alpha-tocopherol)	Anti-oxidant Some belief (which has not been confirmed) that it is beneficial for preventing heart disease and delaying the ageing process	Wholegrain cereals. Wheat germ Nuts Legumes Vegetable oils	Not known—but thought to cause muscle degeneration, anaemias, infertility
Vitamin K (Menadone)	Formation of clotting factors	Liver Leafy green vegetables Egg yolk * Synthesized by bacterial flora in the gastro-intestinal tract	Poor coagulation of the blood and haemorrhage

* Sources other than food

Table 29.4 Mineral salts and health

Mineral	Functions	Sources	Effects of deficiency
1. Major elements			
Calcium (Ca)	Formation of bones and teeth Muscle contraction Normal blood clotting Activator for enzymes	Milk Yoghurt Cheese Sardines Salmon Sesame seed paste	Osteoporosis Severe muscle spasms
Phosphorous (P)	Formation of bones and teeth Nerve and muscle function	Milk Cheese Meat Fish Eggs	Anaemia Weight loss Abnormal growth
Sodium (Na) Potassium (K) Chloride (Cl)	Act closely together in the maintenance of osmotic pressure balance between intra- and extracellular fluid Nerve and muscle function Maintenance of acid-base balance	Salt Fruits Vegetables Monosodium glutamate	Cell and tissue fluid abnormality. Abnormal heart rhythms. Muscular weakness.
Magnesium (Mg)	Activator of enzymes Nerve and muscle function	Nuts Leafy green vegetables Dried beans	Anorexia Nausea
Iodine (I)	Formation of thyroxine	Seafoods Vegetables Iodized salt	Goitre Myxoedema
Iron (Fe)	Formation of haemoglobin which is necessary for the transport of oxygen	Liver Red meats Eggs Leafy green vegetables	Anaemia
2. Minor (trace) elements			
Zinc (Zn)	Metabolism Collagen formation Component of certain enzymes Healthy skin and hair	Wheatgerm Oysters Meat Cheese Wholegrain cereals	Impaired healing Poor condition of the skin Fatigue
Copper (Cu)	Aids iron absorption Nerve function	Offal Nuts Wholegrain cereals	Deficiency is rare — as only 2–5 mg daily is sufficient
Cobalt (Co)	Synthesis of Vitamin B_{12}	Leafy green vegetables	Pernicious anaemia
Sulphur (S)	Constituent of amino acids	Protein foods	Deficiency is rare

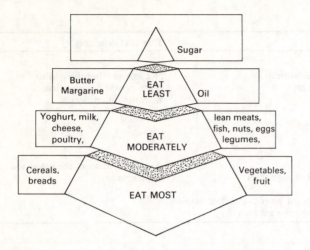

Fig. 29.1 Diet pyramid (Australian Nutrition Foundation).

be slaughtered according to strict rules (Halal). Certain periods of fasting are observed.
• Hinduism (Hindu). A vegetarian diet is commonly followed, and stimulants are forbidden.

Therapeutic diets

A specific diet may be prescribed to rectify a nutritional deficiency, to decrease specific nutrients, or to provide modifications in the texture or consistency of food. If a therapeutic diet is prescribed, it is important that the individual understands the reasons for any restrictions or modifications. Information about various therapeutic diets is provided in Table 29.5.

NURSING PRACTICE AND NUTRITIONAL NEEDS

Each institution has its own system for delivering meals and the nurse should ensure that both the individual and his immediate environment are prepared in readiness for meal times. Key aspects related to providing individuals with meals:

• Nursing care should be planned to ensure that there are no unpleasant sights, sounds, smells or treatments being performed during meal times, as these could interfere with appetite.
• Individuals should be offered the use of toilet facilities, and their hygiene needs should be attended to before meals arrive in the ward.
• Ambulant individuals may be assisted to a table, and non-ambulant persons should be assisted into a comfortable position. Tables should be cleared of unnecessary items to provide space for the meal tray.
• When the meals arrive the nurse should ensure that each individual receives the correct meal, and that all the necessary items, e.g. correct eating utensils, are provided.

• During meal times the nurse should assist as necessary, e.g. cut food, open packets, or pour fluids.
• If an individual is not able to eat what has been provided, measures should be taken to obtain some alternative nourishment for him.
• The nurse should observe the individual's intake of food, and inform the nurse in charge if his intake is poor.
• Following the meal, the nurse should ensure that the individual has an opportunity to clean his teeth.

Feeding an individual

Certain people may be unable to feed themselves for a variety of reasons which include, general weakness, paralysis, or limitations of movements, e.g. due to the presence of arm splints or casts. An individual who is dependent may experience embarrassment if he needs assistance at meal times, therefore the nurse should endeavour to make meal times as enjoyable as possible for any person who needs to be fed.

Key aspects related to feeding an individual:

• Ensure that the person is comfortable before commencing the meal. His elimination and hygiene needs should be met, he should be assisted into a comfortable position, and the table adjusted to an appropriate height.
• The individual should be provided with a serviette.
• The meal should be placed where he can see and smell it, in order to stimulate his appetite.
• The person should be asked whether he wishes to have condiments, e.g. salt and pepper, added to the food. The nurse should ascertain whether he prefers one food at a time or a combination, e.g. meat alone, or combined with the vegetables. It is also important to ensure that food or fluids are not too hot for him.
• A suitable utensil should be selected, e.g. a person may prefer to eat from a small spoon rather than a fork. The amount of food placed on the utensil should be easily managed by the individual. The utensil should be placed gently into his mouth, to avoid injury, or stimulation of the gag reflex.
• The food should be presented at a rate that meets the persons needs, giving him sufficient time to chew and swallow each mouthful.
• Sips of fluid should be offered during the meal. A flexible straw, rather than a cup or glass, may be easier for the individual to manage.
• To maintain dignity, and to promote independence, the person should be encouraged to do as much for himself as possible. He should be encouraged, but never forced, to eat his meal.
• Allow the individual to wipe his mouth with the serviette during the meal, and assist him to do so if necessary.
• On completion of the meal, the individual's hygiene and

Table 29.5 Therapeutic diets

Diet	Description	Indications
Clear liquid	No solids permitted, and only fluids that leave no residue, are non-irritating and non-gas forming are allowed, e.g. water, black tea or coffee, clear fruit drinks	Irritation of the gastro-intestinal tract. Post operatively prior to commencing on solids
Full liquid	All fluids, plus foods that become liquid at room temperature, e.g. jelly, and icecream, are permitted	Progression from clear liquids, prior to commencing on solids. Inability to chew or swallow solids
Soft	Semi-solid easily digested foods are permitted, e.g., soup, cooked cereal, milk pudding, mashed or pureed vegetables and fruit, eggs, soft meats and fish	Advance from a liquid diet. Chewing or swallowing difficulties. Certain gastro-intestinal disorders
Low fibre	Foods that can be absorbed easily and leave no residue are permitted, e.g. clear soup, tender meat, fish or chicken, eggs, refined cereal products, jelly, icecream	As part of preparation for colonoscopy. Colitis. Before and following surgery on the lower colon
High fibre	Foods that contain residue which adds bulk to the faeces, and stimulates peristalsis, e.g. fruit, vegetables, nuts, wholegrain products	Prevention and treatment of constipation. Certain disorders of the colon
Low kilojoule	The number of kilojoules is reduced below the usual daily requirement. Foods that are low in fat or refined carbohydrate are permitted	Weight reduction
High kilojoule	The number of kilojoules is increased above the usual daily requirements. Foods that are high in carbohydrate, protein and fat are included	Weight gain. To replace and repair damaged tissue, e.g. following severe burns
Low cholesterol	Foods that are high in fat and cholesterol are restricted e.g. butter, cream, whole milk, cheese, egg yolk, meat	Prevention or treatment of heart disease, atherosclerosis, high serum cholesterol levels
Low fat	Foods that are high in fat are restricted, e.g. butter, cream, whole milk, cheese, fatty meat	Liver or gallbladder disorders
Low protein	The amount of protein is restricted, and fat and carbohydrate is increased	Kidney or liver failure
High protein	The amount of protein is increased and foods high in complete protein are included, e.g. meat, fish, eggs, cheese, milk	To replace and repair damaged tissue
High iron	Foods that are rich in iron are included, e.g. liver, red meat, green leafy vegetables	Prevention and treatment of iron deficiency anaemia
Controlled carbohydrate (diabetic)	The amounts of carbohydrate, kilojoules and protein are controlled in order to meet nutritional needs, to control blood sugar levels, and to maintain an appropriate body weight	Diabetes mellitus
Controlled sodium	Foods that are high in sodium are omitted, and no salt is added to food	Cardiovascular disease. Certain kidney diseases. Fluid retention (oedema)
Gluten restricted	Foods that contain gluten are eliminated, e.g. wheat, rye, oats, malt, barley. Rice and corn are permitted	Coeliac disease
High vitamin	A well balanced diet that includes foods which are high in one or more deficient vitamin	Vitamin deficiency diseases, e.g. Night blindness Beriberi Scurvy Rickets

comfort needs should be met. The nurse should report and document the intake of food and fluid.

People who have specific needs may require further assistance.

A person who experiences difficulty with chewing or swallowing

- Modifications to the consistency of food may be necessary. Depending on the cause and degree of difficulty, the individual's needs may be met by providing meals comprised of soft foods or thick fluids.
- It may be necessary to initiate the swallowing reflex by gentle pressure on the tongue with the feeding utensil.
- All food and fluid should be offered carefully to avoid aspiration.
- If an individual has facial paralysis, the food should be placed into the unaffected side of the mouth. The nurse should ensure that food does not accumulate in the cheek of the affected side

A person who has visual impairment

- It is important to encourage independence, therefore the nurse should consult the individual about the type of assistance that would be most beneficial. For example, he may find it helpful if the nurse describes the meal by referring to the plate as a clock-face. The nurse should state where each food on the plate may be located, e.g. the meat at 2 o'clock, the potatoes at 4 o'clock, and the beans at 6 o'clock.
- To avoid injury, the individual should be made aware of the location of hot articles, e.g. pots of tea or coffee. He should be asked if he requires assistance to pour the fluids.
- If the individual is unable to feed himself, he should be made aware each time food is about to be placed in his mouth.

Further information about assisting a person with a visual impairment is provided in Chapter 50.

When a person is being fed the nurse should perform the procedure in a relaxed manner, and self feeding should be encouraged to promote independence and dignity. There are a variety of self help devices available that assist a person to feed himself. Such devices (Fig. 29.2) may be helpful for an individual who has limited arm mobility, limited grasp, or reduced co-ordination, and include:

Plate guards. A plate guard is attached to one side of the plate, and is used to assist the person to place food on the eating utensils.

Angled or swivel utensils. Utensils, e.g. forks and spoons, are designed to assist an individual who has a limited range of arm or hand movement.

Utensils with built up handles. The thicker handles are beneficial for a person who has diminished grasp.

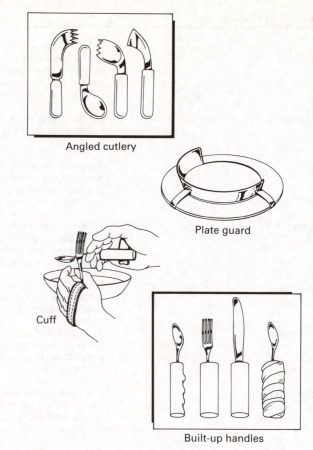

Angled cutlery

Plate guard

Cuff

Built-up handles

Fig. 29.2 Devices to assist self-feeding.

Cuffs. The cuff is placed over a patient's hand, and a spoon or fork is inserted into the slot in the cuff. A cuff may be beneficial for a who has diminished grasp.

Artificial feeding

An alternative method of meeting nutritional needs may be indicated when an individual is unable to consume food or fluid orally. Alternative methods include:

- total parenteral nutrition
- intravenous therapy
- tube feeding via a nasogastric or gastrostomy tube.

Total parenteral nutrition

Sometimes referred to as hyperalimentation, total parenteral nutrition involves the administration of solutions that contain high concentrations of essential nutrients. This method of feeding may be indicated when it is not possible for the individual's nutritional needs to be met via the digestive tract.

Hypertonic solutions are administered through a catheter that has been inserted into a large vein, e.g. the subclavian vein. The solution containing nutrients enters directly into the bloodstream. As the types of solution administered by this route provide an ideal medium for bacterial growth, and because the tubing provides access for the entry of micro-organisms, contamination and sepsis must be prevented. The catheter is inserted by a medical officer using sterile equipment and technique. Care of the equipment throughout the course of treatment requires strict asepsis.

Management of an individual who is receiving total parenteral nutrition is the responsibility of the registered nurse, and the individual must be monitored continually to prevent or detect possible complications. Complications that may result from total parenteral nutrition include:

- diarrhoea or constipation
- hyperglycaemia or hypoglycaemia
- fluid imbalance
- catheter related sepsis, e.g. swelling and inflammation at the insertion site
- air embolism.

The nurse may be required to assist with the care of a person who is receiving total parenteral nutrition, and she must be aware of the scope of her role in promoting safety and comfort.

Intravenous therapy

Intravenous therapy involves the introduction of solutions, other than those administered during total parenteral nutrition, into a vein. Information about intravenous therapy is provided in Chapter 31.

Nasogastric tube feeding

Information about tube insertion, and care of an individual with a naso-gastric tube is provided in Chapter 46, while this chapter addresses the procedure of introducing feedings via the tube.

Nasogastric tube feeding may be indicated for an individual who is unable to swallow, e.g. for a person who:

- is unconscious
- has had oral or throat surgery
- has palate or pharyngeal paralysis
- is too ill or weak to eat normally.

Prepared solutions are administered either:

- By continuous drip where the solution is delivered to the individual at a regulated rate, and allowed to flow by gravity or is administered via a controlled pump mechanism, or
- By intermittent feedings where the solution is administered at regular intervals, e.g. every four hours. A syringe is attached to the end of the nasogastric tube, solution is poured into the barrel of the syringe and allowed to flow in slowly by gravity.

The height at which the syringe is held will determine the rate of flow.

The formula is refrigerated between feedings. As the administration of cold fluids may cause abdominal discomfort, the container of solution is warmed to room temperature, and should be shaken gently to eliminate any separation of the constituents before administration.

Before any solution is introduced, the registered nurse should check that the tube is in the correct position.

A suggested procedure for intermittent nasogastric tube feeding is outlined in the guidelines.

Gastrostomy feeding

Feeding via gastrostomy may be indicated if there is an obstruction in the upper part of the digestive tract. A gastrostomy tube (Fig. 29.3) is inserted into the stomach by a surgeon, through an incision in the abdominal wall. The opening around the tube is sutured firmly to prevent leakage, and thereafter fluid feedings are introduced through the tube into the stomach. After several weeks the tube may be removed and re-inserted prior to each feeding. A prosthesis with a screw cap may be used to close the opening (stoma) between feedings.

The principles related to the introduction of formula via a gastrostomy tube are similar to those related to nasogastric tube feeding. To encourage independence, the individual may be instructed in the technique so that he is able to introduce the feedings independently.

Common disorders associated with nutrition

Although many disorders are related to a specific nutrient deficiency, the common disorders of nutrition may be classified as malnutrition, obesity, eating disorders, and nutrient loss as a result of vomiting.

Malnutrition

Malnutrition occurs as a consequence of continued poor nutrition, and may be described as the condition in which the intake and utilization of nutrients is decreased in relation to body requirements. Prevention of malnutrition, and early identification of people at risk, is an important factor in ensuring that an individual's nutritional needs are met. People who are at risk of malnutrition include those who:

- are experiencing increased metabolic demands or protracted loss of nutrients, e.g. due to burns, infection, vomiting, physical trauma and major wounds, or prolonged pyrexia.
- are not consuming oral food or fluid for more than a few days.
- have a BMI value of below 20, or who have recently

Guidelines for intermittent nasogastric tube feeding

Nursing action	Rationale
1. Ascertain the amount of formula to be administered	Correct quantities must be given to meet the individual's nutritional needs
2. Explain the procedure	Reduces anxiety
3. Assist the individual into a sitting position, unless this is contraindicated	Facilitates digestion, and reduces the risk of gastro-oesophageal reflux and aspiration
4. Wash and dry hands	Prevents cross infection
5. Assemble the equipment and place it in a convenient location	Facilitates access during the procedure
6. Remove the clamp from the nasogastric tube, attach the syringe and aspirate gently. Measure and test aspirate with litmus paper (for acid reaction)	Helps to assess tube placement. Gastric contents are aspirated and measured to establish whether the previous feed has been absorbed
If the aspirate is less than 90 ml, it should be returned through the tube to the stomach. Report to the nurse in charge if the aspirate is more than 90 ml	Aspirate is usually replaced in the stomach as it contains important digestive substances; greater than 90 ml suggests malabsorption
7. Do not introduce any formula until the position of the tube has been verified by a registered nurse	Administration of the solution through a mal-positioned tube can cause it to enter the lungs
8. Pour some of the formula into the barrel of the syringe and allow it to flow slowly, by gravity, into the tube	Rapid administration can cause distension of the stomach, nausea, vomiting, or abdominal cramps
Do not allow the syringe to empty	Prevents air from entering the tube
9. Continue to pour formula into the syringe until the correct amount has been administered	Prescribed amount must be given
10. Introduce a small amount of water, e.g. 50 ml, following administration of the formula	Maintains patency and cleanlines of the tube
11. Disconnect the barrel of the syringe and clamp the end of the tube	Prevents leakage
12. Encourage the individual to remain sitting up for approximately 30 minutes	Aids digestion, and reduces the risk of regurgitation
13. Attend to the individual's hygiene needs and position. Remove and attend to the equipment Wash and dry hands	Promotes comfort. Prevents cross infection
14. Report and document the procedure	Appropriate care may be planned and implemented

experienced a loss of more than 10% of their usual body weight.

• are alcohol or drug dependent
• are receiving medications that have antinutrient or catabolic properties, e.g. steroids, immunosuppressants, or antitumour agents.
• have a disorder that results in defective utilization of nutrients, e.g. Crohn's disease.

Malnutrition results in impaired growth and development, lowered resistance to infection, delayed healing, and anaemia. Treatment includes identification of the cause, and the provision of adequate nutrients.

Obesity

Obesity is the condition in which there is an excess of body fat, and both obesity and morbid obesity are determined by calculating the individual's body mass index using the formula shown on page 241.

Obesity results from excessive kilojoule intake, an inadequate expenditure of energy—or from a combination of both factors. Obesity may have serious consequences, e.g. cardiovascular disease, breathing difficulties, hypertension, diabetes mellitus, gallbladder disease, or psychosocial problems.

The principles of treatment include regulation of food

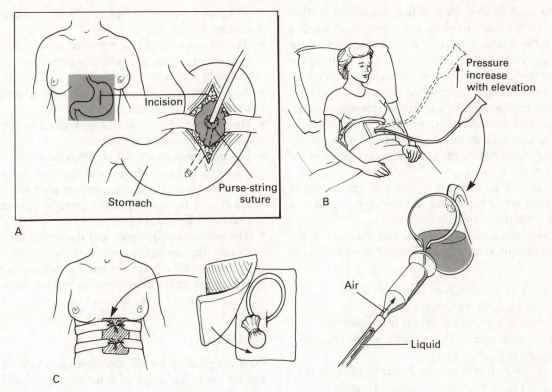

Fig. 29.3 Gastrostomy feeding. (A) Gastrostomy incision and procedure. (B) Receptacle tilted to allow escape of air. (C) When not in use the end of the tube is covered by sterile gauze, and then covered by a pad held in place with straps.

intake, exercise, behaviour modification, and medications such as appetite suppressors or oral substances containing cellulose. Surgical intervention is sometimes indicated in instances of morbid obesity. A variety of surgical procedures are available, and most are aimed at reducing the capacity of the stomach.

Eating disorders

The two most recognized disorders of eating are anorexia nervosa and bulimia.

Anorexia nervosa is characterized by self imposed starvation and consequent emaciation. Loss of weight becomes the individual's prime focus, and is the result of a belief that the body is too fat—even when extreme emaciation is evident.

Bulimia is characterized by episodes of 'binging' on large quantities of food, followed by purging with laxatives or self-induced vomiting.

The causes of both disorders are difficult to determine, but most experts agree that they result from an interaction of biological, psychological, and sociocultural factors. Treatment, which is difficult and varied, includes behaviour modification and psychotherapy.

Nutrient loss as a result of vomiting

Vomiting, if prolonged, may result in significant nutrient deficiency and dehydration. Persistent vomiting deprives the body of essential nutrients and fluids and results in electrolyte imbalance. In order to correct the imbalance, intravenous therapy or total parenteral nutrition may be indicated.

Vomiting is not a disease itself but is a symptom of disease, and may occur as a result of:

- diseases of the stomach, intestines, liver, biliary system, pancreas, or peritoneum
- hypersensitivity to certain foods
- the ingestion of irritant substances
- severe pain
- adverse reaction to, or a side effect of, certain medications
- hormonal changes during early pregnancy
- disturbances of equilibrium, e.g. travel sickness
- disorders of the nervous system, e.g. concussion
- psychological factors, e.g. fear, unpleasant sights or smells.

Vomiting (emesis) is the expulsion of the stomach contents, and is a reflex action caused by stimulation of a centre in the medulla oblongata. When this centre is stimulated the glottis and nasopharynx close, the cardiac sphincter of the stomach relaxes, and contractions of the diaphragm and abdominal muscles occur. As a result of the increased intra-abdominal pressure, the stomach contents are forced upwards and are expelled through the mouth. Vomiting may be preceded by a feeling of sickness (nausea) and accompanied by salivation, sweating and pallor. In specific conditions such as intestinal obstruction 'projectile' vomiting may occur where the vomited material is ejected with great force.

Vomiting should be assessed in terms of the nature of vomiting (effortless or projectile) and the characteristics of the material vomited (*vomitus*).

Observations made of the vomitus may assist in determining the cause of vomiting and include observations of the:

- *Consistency*. The vomitus may consist of fluid, semidigested food, or undigested food.
- *Colour*. Vomitus may vary in colour from clear to yellow, brown, or green. The presence of bile tends to colour vomitus yellow or green.
- *Presence of blood*. Blood may be present as bright red streaks or clots, or may have a 'coffee grounds' appearance. The latter occurs when blood has been partially digested by the acid gastric secretions. Vomiting of blood is called *haematemesis*.
- *Odour*. Vomitus is usually sour smelling, but a 'faecal' odour indicates reflux of bowel contents due to an intestinal obstruction.
- *Quantity*. If possible, vomitus should be measured to assess the amount of fluid being lost.

Key aspects related to care of an individual who is vomiting include:

- If he is sitting, place an emesis bowl under his chin and position a towel to protect his clothes and bedding.
- If he is lying down, lift and turn his head to one side to reduce the risk of aspiration.
- Ensure privacy, as he will feel distressed and embarrassed by the incident.
- Any dentures should be removed to prevent them becoming dislodged.
- The nurse may place her hand on the individual's forehead to provide comfort and support, or over an

abdominal wound to 'splint' it and reduce pain during vomiting.
- The vomitus should be removed as soon the episode is over, to reduce the risk of a recurrence caused by the sight or smell of vomitus.
- Any soiled linen should be changed and removed immediately from the room.
- His hands and face should be washed to refresh him and to remove any vomitus.
- His oral hygiene should be attended to by cleaning his teeth and providing a suitable mouth rinse, in order to eliminate any unpleasant after taste.
- He should be assisted into a position of comfort and permitted to rest quietly.
- The nurse should report and document the incident so that appropriate nursing actions may be implemented. An anti-emetic medication may be prescribed and administered to reduce nausea and to prevent further vomiting.

SUMMARY

Food is necessary for the development and growth of cells, and for the replacement of substances required by the cells to maintain efficient body function.

A diet that contains the essential nutrients is important throughout each stage of the life span, and people should be encouraged to follow the principles of good nutrition and to eat well balanced meals.

Food provides energy which is necessary for all the chemical and physical activities of the body, and energy requirements vary according to various factors, e.g. age, sex, and body build.

Each nutrient performs a specific function, and a nutrient deficiency may result in body dysfunction.

Many factors influence an individual's eating pattern and choice of foods, and illness may necessitate certain changes in dietary practice. Modification to the consistency of food may be indicated, or a specific diet may be prescribed for therapeutic purposes.

The nurse should assist individuals to meet their nutritional needs, and she may need to feed a person who is unable to feed himself. If an individual is unable to consume food or fluid orally, an alternative method of meeting his nutritional needs may be necessary.

Problems associated with nutrition should be identified so that appropriate care can be planned and implemented to meet the individual's nutritional needs.

30. Meeting elimination needs

INTRODUCTION

Metabolism produces wastes which must be eliminated regularly in order to maintain effective body function. This chapter addresses the elimination of urine and faeces. Observation of the individual's ability to eliminate urine and faeces, together with observation of those wastes, provides the nurse with an objective assessment of the patient's elimination status. As a result, appropriate nursing actions may be planned and implemented to assist the individual to meet his elimination needs.

Information on the structure and functions of the urinary and digestive systems is provided in Chapters 23 and 24.

Urine is produced by the kidneys as they continually filter the blood to remove metabolic waste, and conserve or release fluid and electrolytes to help maintain homeostasis. From the kidneys urine is transported by peristaltic action down the ureters into the bladder, and is then excreted through the urethra. The act of passing urine is referred to as voiding, urination, or micturition, and is normally under voluntary control by approximately two to three years of age. While the normal capacity of the adult urinary bladder is approximately 450 ml, the bladder is capable of expanding to hold larger amounts. When around 150 ml of urine has accumulated in the bladder, sensory impulses from the bladder wall travel to the brain and are interpreted as the need to void. When an individual is ready to pass urine, the urethral sphincters relax, the bladder muscles contract, and urine is expelled.

Faeces are produced in the intestines as an end result of the ingestion, digestion, and absorption of food and fluid. Following the absorption of digested nutrients and fluid, any indigestible substances are transported by peristaltic action to the rectum, and then excreted through the anus. The act of passing faeces is called defaecation or bowel action, and is normally under full voluntary control by approximately three to four years of age. When wastes reach and distend the rectum, sensory impulses from the rectal walls are transmitted to the brain and interpreted as a need to empty the bowel. When an individual is ready to pass faeces, the muscles of the abdominal wall, diaphragm, and pelvic floor are contracted. The resultant increase in intra-abdominal pressure helps to force the rectal contents down, the anal sphincters relax, and faeces are expelled.

NURSING PRACTICE AND ELIMINATION NEEDS

Assessment of the individual's elimination status is made by obtaining information about his elimination practices, and by observation of him and his excreta. The nurse should enquire about his usual pattern of voiding and defaecation, and whether he has experienced any recent alterations to this pattern. Information should also be obtained about his usual fluid and dietary intake so that whenever possible it can be maintained or improved in order to facilitate normal elimination. The nurse should observe the individual and his excreta for early signs of any problems associated with elimination, so that appropriate care can be implemented to assist him meet his elimination needs.

Providing toilet utensils

Many people will be able to walk to the toilet independently while others may require some assistance. If a person requires assistance he should be helped out of bed, and assisted into his dressing gown and slippers. Some individuals may require the nurse's support while they walk to the toilet, while others may need to be transported In a wheelchair. The nurse should remain with person who is weak, unsteady, or confused, and assist him as required. If the nurse does not need to remain with the person, she should ensure that the toilet paper is within easy reach. The individual should be shown how to use the signal device, and advised to use it if he requires the nurse's assistance. He should be provided with the opportunity to wash his hands after using the toilet, and assisted back to his room.

More dependent individuals will need to be provided with toilet utensils which include bedpans, urinals, toilet chairs and commodes.

The bedpan. A bedpan may be used by a person who is unable to get out of bed. Bedpans are made from steel or plastic and are used by females for the elimination of urine and faeces, or by males for the elimination of faeces. Bedpans are also used by ambulant females whose urine is to be measured.

The urinal. A urinal may be used by male who is unable to get out of bed, or if urine from an ambulatory male is to be measured. Urinals are made from steel or plastic, and while there are some styles available for use by females, they are more commonly used for the elimination of urine by males.

The toilet chair. A toilet chair, which is portable, has a large opening in the seat. The individual is positioned on the seat, and the chair is wheeled to and placed over the toilet.

The commode. A commode, which is portable, has a large opening in the seat under which a bed pan is placed.

In order to reduce any embarrassment associated with the use of toilet utensils, and to ensure that toilet utensils are used correctly, certain key aspects related to their provision are:

• Toilet utensils should be offered at regular intervals, and provided as soon as the individual requests them.
• Unless contra-indicated, the person should be assisted into a natural position for elimination. The elimination of urine and faeces is facilitated when an individual assumes an upright position, but this may not always be possible, e.g. if there is a spinal injury.
• Before the toilet utensil is taken to the individual, the nurse should ensure that it is clean, dry, and covered. Bed-

pans and urinals are more comfortable if they have been warmed before use.
• The nurse should assess whether the person is able to position the utensil independently or requires some assistance.
• The nurse should ensure that the individual is adequately covered and has privacy while using the toilet utensil.
• The nurse should remain with any person who is weak, unsteady, or confused, in order to promote his safety.
• If it is not necessary to remain with the individual, the nurse should ensure that the toilet paper and signal device are placed within his easy reach.
• After the toilet utensil has been used, the room should be ventilated, and the toilet utensil should be removed and covered immediately. The contents are observed, and measured or tested if necessary. The utensil is emptied, cleaned, and prepared for further use.

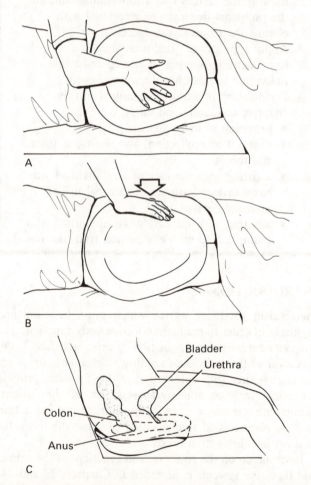

Fig. 30.1 Placing a bedpan (A) Another method of placing a bedpan is used when the individual is unable to help. The individual lies on one side, and the bedpan is placed firmly against the buttocks.
(B) The nurse pushes down on the bedpan and toward the individual.
(C) The individual is positioned on the bedpan so that the urethra and anus are directly over the opening.

• The individual's hygiene needs must be met by assisting him with the toilet paper if necessary, and by providing him with hand washing facilities.

• In order to prevent cross infection, the nurse's hands must be thoroughly washed and dried whenever toilet utensils have been handled.

Key aspects related to specific toilet utensils are:

• When a bed pan is provided, the person's night clothes and the bedding are adjusted to avoid accidental wetting or soiling. The bed pan is positioned by requesting the individual to flex his knees, press into the mattress with his feet, and raise his buttocks. Some people may require the nurse's assistance to raise the buttocks, while others may need to be turned onto one side (Fig. 30.1) to facilitate placement of the bedpan.

• In order to promote comfort and to reduce the risk of spillage, the bedpan must be positioned under the individual correctly and removed carefully.

• When a urinal is provided, the nurse hands it to the individual or places it in position. To reduce the risk of spillage the nurse holds the urinal in position if necessary, and removes it carefully.

• When a toilet chair is provided, the nurse assists the person onto the seat and wheels him to the toilet. It is important to ensure that the opening in the seat is correctly positioned over the toilet.

• When a commode is provided, a clean bed pan is placed under the seat. To promote comfort and safety, the nurse should assist the individual onto the seat, ensure his warmth, and use the safety devices, e.g. wheel brakes and lap belt. After use, the commode is wheeled from the room and the bed pan emptied, cleaned, and prepared for further use.

Elimination of urine

Normal voiding is voluntary and painless, and the frequency with which urine is passed varies with the individual. Factors that affect the frequency of voiding and the amounts of urine voided include, fluid input, the capacity of the bladder, response to the need to void, and the availability of toilet facilities. The frequency of voiding and often the amount of urine voided can be increased by, a large fluid input, fear or anxiety, exposure to a cold environment, and some disease states. The frequency of voiding and often the amount of urine voided can be decreased by a low fluid input, exposure to a hot environment, and some disease states.

Urine is composed of 96% water, 2% urea, and 2% mineral salts, and normal urine has the following characteristics:

• It is voided without pain or discomfort.

• It is clear and light amber in colour.

• It has a slight aromatic odour that increases when left to stand.

• It has a pH of between 5 and 6 slightly acidic, pH is a scale representing the relative acidity or alkalinity of a solution, with the numerical value indicating the concentration of hydrogen ions. A value of 7 is neutral, below 7 is acid, and above 7 is alkaline.

• It has a specific gravity of between 1010 and 1030. Specific gravity is a measure of the concentration of particles in the urine, and reflects the ability of the kidneys to concentrate or dilute urine.

• It is excreted in amounts of between 1000 ml and 2000 ml in 24 hours.

Collection of urine

The nurse may be required to collect urine for observation or testing in the ward, or so that a specimen can be sent to the laboratory for analysis. Key aspects related to the collection of urine include:

• Thorough washing and drying of the hands before and after collection to prevent cross infection.

• The container in which the urine is collected must be clean, and in some instances sterile, to ensure collection of a specimen free from external contamination.

• If testing or laboratory analysis is required, contamination of the container and urine must be prevented throughout the procedure.

• Adequate information about the individual and the specimen must be provided. The label on the specimen container must contain the person's name, registration number, the date and time of collection, and the method used to collect the specimen, e.g. catheter specimen of urine. When a specimen is dispatched for laboratory analysis, it must be accompanied by the medical officer's request form. The medical officer requests the collection of a specimen and indicates on the form, the specific laboratory tests to be performed.

• Specimens must be sent to the laboratory as soon as possible after collection and if there is a delay in dispatch, the specimen may require refrigeration.

• An individiual may be responsible for the collection of his urine specimen, therefore the nurse should provide him with the information necessary to ensure that the collection is performed correctly.

1. Observation or urinalysis. If urine is to be collected for observation or testing in the ward, the individual is requested to void into a clean bedpan or urinal. The urine should not be contaminated, e.g. by faeces or menstrual blood, as a false assessment may result. The urine is transferred from the toilet utensil into a clean container in preparation for observation or testing.

2. 24-hour collection. All urine excreted during a 24-

Guidelines for 24 hour collection of urine

Action	Rationale
1. Hands washed and dried before and after collecting each specimen	Prevents cross infection
2. The bladder is emptied completely and the urine discarded. Note the time	Collection begins with the bladder empty. Only the urine which is secreted during the next 24 hours is collected
3. From that time on each specimen of urine voided in the 24 hours is added to the container	All urine voided in that period is collected to ensure an accurate test result
4. The container of urine is refrigerated until the collection is complete	Keeping the urine cold will help to prevent decomposition
5. At the end of 24 hours the bladder is emptied and the urine added to the container	The last voiding empties the bladder and completes the 24 hour collection
6. Ensure that the label on the container has all the relevant information. The container and the request form are dispatched to the laboratory	Accurate documentation is necessary to avoid errors
7. If any of the urine is inadvertently discarded, the collection is abandoned and the procedure recommenced	Inaccurate results will be obtained if all urine excreted over the 24 hour period is not acquired

hour period is collected and sent for laboratory analysis in order to measure the quantity of various substances present, e.g. specific hormones. A suggested method of collecting a 24-hour specimen is outlined in the guidelines. The equipment necessary consists of a large volume screw topped labelled container and a jug to transfer urine into the container.

3. Mid stream specimen. This method of collection is used to obtain a sample of urine that is not contaminated by microorganisms from outside the urinary tract. The urine is sent to the laboratory to be tested the presence of microorganisms and their sensitivity to antimicrobial drugs. The aim is to collect the middle portion of the stream of urine, and a suggested method of collection is outlined in the guidelines.

The equipment necessary consists of a sterile container for the urine, and items to clean the urethral meatus, e.g. sterile swabs and water.

As most people will be capable of performing this procedure independently, it is important that they are provided with adequate information about the technique. The nurse performs the procedure if the person is dependent.

Guidelines for mid stream urine collection

Action	Rationale
1. Hands washed and dried thoroughly	Prevents cross infection
2. Ensure adequate privacy	Reduces embarrassment
3. Explain the procedure	The individual must be aware of the need for a specimen free from external contamination
4. The individual's genital area and urethral meatus are cleaned and dried	Prevents external microorganisms from contaminating the specimen
5. The person voids approximately 30 to 60 ml of urine into the toilet or toilet utensil	Flushes any residual microorganisms out of the urethra
6. The next 20 to 30 ml of urine is collected in the sterile container	This is the middle stream of urine and is the portion sent for analysis
7. The person completes voiding into the toilet or toilet utensil	The remainder of the urine is not required for collection
8. Hands are washed and dried	Prevents cross infection
9. The container is labelled with the required information and dispatched to the laboratory, together with the request form, as soon as possible	Decomposition and cell growth occur if urine is left standing, and may provide a false result
10. The procedure should be documented	Appropriate care can be planned and implemented

4. Using a collection bag. A urine collection bag may be used to obtain a specimen from an individual who is unable to control the flow of urine, e.g. an infant or a person who is incontinent, unconscious, or confused. A suggested method of collecting a sample of urine using a collection bag is outlined in the guidelines.

The equipment necessary consists of:

— collection bag of suitable size, i.e. paediatric or adult
— sterile labelled specimen container
— items for cleansing the genital area, e.g. soap, water, washer, towel.

5. Culture medium. A culture medium is sometimes used when the urine is to be tested for bacteria. Urine is first collected in a sterile container, and a slide containing culture medium is dipped into the urine. The culture slide is returned to its original container, and dispatched to the laboratory together with the urine in its separate sterile container. This method of collection may be necessary if there is a delay in dispatch of the specimen, and if refrigeration is not practicable.

6. Catheter specimen. A catheter specimen of urine is obtained from a person who has an indwelling catheter. The insertion of a catheter for the sole purpose of obtaining a urine specimen is generally avoided, due to the risk of introducing micro-organisms into the urinary tract. In order to reduce the risk of introducing micro-organisms

when obtaining a specimen of urine from an indwelling catheter, it is important to maintain a closed urinary drainage system. For this reason collection of a specimen from the end of the catheter which is connected to the drainage tubing should be avoided. Instead, the urine should be aspirated using a sterile syringe and needle through the

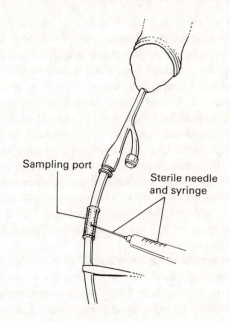

Sampling port

Sterile needle and syringe

Fig. 30.2 Obtaining a sample of urine from a catheter.

Guidelines for bag collection of urine

Nursing action	Rationale
1. Wash and dry hands thoroughly	Prevents cross infection
2. Explain the procedure	Reduces anxiety
3. Ensure privacy	Reduces embarrassment
4. Place the person in a supine position if possible	Facilitates application of the bag
5. Cleanse the perineal area, swabbing towards the anus. Ensure that the urethral meatus is clean and dry	Prevents contamination of the urine by microorganisms from the surrounding skin
6. Remove the covering from the bag's adhesive surfaces, and apply the bag. The bag should enclose the urethral meatus, but not the anus Press the adhesive surfaces onto the skin. (If necessary, the surrounding skin is shaved prior to application of the bag.)	The bag must be correctly positioned and firmly secured to avoid leakage Promotes adherence of the bag to the skin
7. Check frequently, and gently remove bag when sufficient urine is collected	Avoids damage to the skin
8. Transfer the urine into the specimen container	Prepares specimen for testing or dispatch to the laboratory
9. Reposition the individual and adjust the bed clothes to meet his needs	Promotes comfort
10. Urine for laboratory analysis should be dispatched immediately, together with the request form	Decomposition and cell growth occur if urine is left standing
11. Wash and dry hands	Prevents cross infection

sampling port (Fig. 30.2). A suggested method for obtaining a catheter specimen is outlined in the guidelines.

The equipment necessary consists of:

— sterile syringe and needle
— alcohol swabs
— sterile labelled specimen container.

If it is not possible to aspirate the urine with a syringe and needle, the catheter may be clamped to allow urine to accumulate in the bladder. The clamp is then released, and the catheter is disconnected from the drainage tubing. This must be done using aseptic technique to avoid introducing microorganisms. The area where the catheter joins the drainage tube should be wiped with an alcohol swab. The catheter is disconnected and the urine allowed to drain from it into the sterile specimen container. Avoid touching the inside of the sterile container with the catheter, and do not allow the open ends of the drainage tube or catheter to become contaminated. Both connection sites should be wiped with an alcohol swab prior to being rejoined. The nurse's hands must be thoroughly washed and dried before and after the procedure.

7. Suprapubic bladder aspiration. This procedure is not commonly performed but, when necessary, it is performed by a medical officer using sterile equipment and aseptic technique. It involves the insertion of a needle through the skin over the supra pubic area into the bladder. A quantity of urine is aspirated, placed in a sterile container, and dispatched to the laboratory. Following this procedure the nurse should observe the puncture site for bleeding, and the urine for the presence of blood.

Examination of urine

In order to detect and identify abnormalities, urine is examined by observation, by chemical testing in the ward, or by analysis in the laboratory. Abnormalities which can be detected by observation are listed in Table 30.1.

Urinalysis. Testing the urine for abnormalities is referred to as urinalysis, and is commonly performed when an individual is admitted to hospital. The frequency with which it is subsequently performed depends on the person's condition, and prescribed management. Urine may be tested for several substances at the one time, or for one specific substance. Chemical reagent tablets or strips are used to test urine, and urinalysis provides information about:

• the condition and function of the urinary system
• the presence of pathogenic microorganisms in the urinary tract or urine
• the presence of nutrient materials that are normally transported to the body cells, but which may have been excreted in the urine, e.g. glucose
• the presence of a systemic disease which is unrelated to disorders of the urinary system
• the acid-base balance of the body.

As urinalysis is an important diagnostic aid and a measure of the effectiveness of certain treatments, accuracy of performance is essential. Key aspects of performing urinalysis are outlined in the guidelines. The equipment necessary consists of:

— clean container of urine

Guidelines for catheter specimen of urine

Nursing action	Rationale
1. Explain the procedure to the patient	Reduces anxiety
2. Ensure the patient's privacy	Reduces embarrassment
3. Clamp the catheter approximately 30 minutes before the specimen is to be collected	Allows urine to accumulate in the bladder so that a specimen can be obtained
4. Wash and dry hands	Prevents cross infection
5. Wipe the sampling port with an alcohol swab	Prevents cross infection
6. Attach the needle to the syringe and insert the needle into the port. Aspirate the specimen of urine into the syringe and transfer it into the specimen container	The needle should not be inserted into the shaft of the catheter as this may result in subsequent leakage of urine
7. Wipe the puncture area on the catheter with an alcohol swab	Prevents cross infection
8. Unclamp the catheter	Allows urine to flow again
9. Dispose of the used swabs, syringe and needle safely	Prevents cross infection and injury
10. Wash and dry hands	Prevents cross infection
11. Dispatch the labelled container and request form to the laboratory as soon as possible	Prevents decomposition of urine or cell growth

Table 30.1 Abnormalities of urine detected by observation

Observation	Deviation from normal	Possible cause
Colour	Pale	High fluid intake. Other factors that dilute the urine such as diuretic medication, or disease, e.g. diabetes mellitus
	Dark or brown	Concentrated (urine) due to dehydration. Presence of bile pigment, e.g. in liver or gallbladder disease
	Smokey	Presence of occult blood
	Red	Presence of frank blood
	Bright yellow, blue, green	Specific medications
Odour	Ammonia	Decomposing urine
	Foul smelling, 'fishy' odour	Infected urine
	Sweet smelling	Presence of glucose, e.g. in diabetes mellitus
Foreign substances	Pus	Urinary tract infection
	Stones, gravel	Calculi in urinary tract
Amount	Higher than normal in 24 hours	High fluid intake
		Diuretic medications
		Diseases, e.g. diabetes mellitus
	Lower than normal in 24 hours	Obstruction to the flow of urine.
		Diseases that reduce the normal production of urine, e.g. renal failure

— paper and pen
— watch with a second hand
— test tubes and droppers (used for specific tests)
— biochemical testing agents and the manufacturer's colour comparison charts
— urinometer (one method of assessing specific gravity).

There are a variety of different chemical tablets or strips used to test urine for abnormalities, and the nurse should become familiar with their use. The abnormalities which can be detected by various tests and the possible causes of those abnormalities, are listed in Table 30.2.

Straining urine. Stones, or calculi, are insoluble sub-

Guidelines for urinalysis
Nursing action

1. Obtain urine which is free from contamination by faeces, menstrual blood or body secretions, and test within 30 minutes
2. A clean and dry container should be used to hold the urine
3. Assemble all the required equipment before commencing the test
4. Follow the manufacturer's instructions regarding the use of biochemical agents:
   - check expiry date
   - avoid unnecessary exposure to air, light or moisture
   - avoid contact with the chemical agents by the fingers
   - do not transfer agents from their original bottles into others
   - time the tests accurately

5. If abnormalities are detected do not discard the urine until the results have been reported
6. Report and document the test results immediately
7. Dispose of used chemical tablets or strips. Rinse and clean any containers. Wash and dry hands

Rationale

Test results can be affected by the presence of contaminants, or changes that occur when urine is left standing
Contaminants, e.g. disinfectant, can affect test results

The procedure should not be interrupted once the testing has commenced

out of date chemicals lose their efficiency
prevents loss of reactivity

prevents contamination

prevents deterioration and loss of reactivity

accurate timing is essential to provide quantitative results
Further testing may be indicated

Avoids errors or omissions
Prevents cross infection

Table 30.2   Urinalysis results

Test	Normal values	Deviations	Possible causes
pH	5 to 6	Elevated (alkaline)	Urinary tract infection Metabolic or respiratory alkalosis Low protein diet
		Lowered (acidic)	Metabolic or respiratory acidosis High protein diet
Specific gravity	1010 to 1030	Elevated	Low fluid input Presence of abnormal substances in the urine, e.g. protein
		Lowered	High fluid input Certain kidney diseases
Protein	Nil	Present	Kidney infections Acute febrile states Hypertension Congestive cardiac failure
Glucose	Nil	Present	Diabetes mellitus Pancreatitis Stress
Ketones	Nil	Present	Diabetes mellitus Starvation Vomiting
Bilirubin	Nil	Present	Liver disorders
Blood	Nil	Present	Urinary tract disease or trauma
Nitrite	Nil	Present	Urinary tract infections
Urobilinogen	0.1 to 1.0	Elevated	Liver disorders Congestive cardiac failure Blood disorders, e.g. anaemia
		Lowered	Obstruction of the bile duct Antibiotic therapy Cancer of head of the pancreas
Leukocytes	Very few	Increased	Urinary tract infection

stances formed of mineral salts which may develop in the kidneys. They can range in size from microscopic, through resembling sand or gravel, to several centimetres. If it is known or suspected that an individual has developed renal calculi, careful observation of the urine is achieved by straining it to detect the passage of stones. Any stones collected are sent for laboratory examination which reveals their exact composition, and helps to identify their cause. The urine is strained by pouring it through a fine substance such as gauze or filter paper.

Problems associated with elimination of urine

Problems associated with micturition may occur as a result of several factors including a change from normal routine or environment, or as a consequence of certain disease states. Any alteration in an individual's normal pattern of voiding must be recognized and reported immediately, so that appropriate actions can be planned and implemented. Problems associated with the elimination of urine include:

1. Altered amounts. The term *oliguria* used to describe a decrease in the amount of urine excreted to below 500 ml per day. This condition is caused by fluid and electrolyte imbalances, kidney dysfunction, or urinary tract obstruction.

Polyuria is the term used to describe the excretion of greatly increased amounts of urine, e.g. over 2500 ml of urine per day. It may occur as a result of a large fluid input, diuretic medications, or certain disease states such as diabetes insipidus.

2. Suppression of urine. The term *anuria* refers to the cessation of secretion of urine by the kidneys, or the production of less than 100 ml per day, and may result from kidney dysfunction or failure.

3. Retention of urine. When there is an accumulation of urine in the bladder and the person is unable to void, the condition is referred to as retention of urine. Retention of urine is commonly due to an obstruction of the bladder outlet or urethra, and it may also occur as a result of tension in the urethral sphincter caused by anxiety or pain. Retention of urine with overflow occurs when the accumulation of urine in the bladder leads to stretching of the urethral orifice and, although small amounts of urine dribble away, the bladder remains full and distended.

4. Incontinence of urine. Incontinence is the inability to control the excretion of urine, and may occur as a result of lesions in the brain or spinal cord, damage to the nerves of the bladder, injury to the urinary sphincters, and various other causes. Stress incontinence occurs when increased intra-abdominal pressure, e.g. from coughing or sneezing, is associated with a full bladder. The pressure squeezes the bladder and stretches the sphincters so that urine is expelled involuntarily.

5. Dysuria. Dysuria is the term used to describe painful micturition and is commonly due to a urinary tract infection or obstruction.

6. Frequency of micturition. When a person experiences the need to void more often than normal, and commonly voids small amounts of urine each time, he is said to have frequency of micturition. This condition is commonly associated with a urinary tract infection, or may occur as a result of anxiety or stress.

Measures to induce micturition

When a person is experiencing difficulty in passing urine, the cause must be identified and treated. Difficulty in passing urine may be as a result of an obstruction to the outflow of urine, but may also be caused by other factors such as:

- anxiety, stress, nervousness, or embarrassment associated with the need to use toilet utensils
- the need to remain in a supine position when using toilet utensils
- the effects of medications, anaesthesia, or the acute stress of surgery
- pain, which can lead to tension in the muscles controlling the urethral opening.

The nursing actions which may be implemented to induce micturition, include pain relief, privacy, a natural position, relaxation, and stimulation.

1. Relief of pain. If a person is experiencing pain, the cause should be identified and treated. The nurse should report pain immediately to the nurse in charge. Nursing actions to relieve pain include ensuring that the individual is positioned comfortably, checking any splints or dressings to detect whether they are causing the pain, and the administration of any prescribed analgesia.

2. Ensuring adequate privacy, and sufficient time for the person to void. If possible, he should be left alone to use the toilet utensils, as people are generally self conscious about the need to eliminate in the presence of others.

3. Assisting the individual to assume a natural voiding position. Whenever possible the person should be permitted to use the toilet, but if this is contraindicated an upright position may assist. Males may find it easier to pass urine if allowed to stand.

4. Helping the individual to relax by ensuring that both he and the toilet utensil are warm. Unless contraindicated, a warm shower or bath may be beneficial. The nurse in charge should be consulted as to the advisability of pouring warm water over the genitalia of a female as this action sometimes helps to stimulate micturition.

5. Stimulating the micturition response which can often be achieved by providing the sound of running water, e.g. turning on a nearby tap.

6. Unless contraindicated the individual should be encouraged to drink adequate amounts of fluids.

If these actions fail to induce micturition and the individual is uncomfortable because of a distended bladder, it may become necessary to implement further actions, e.g. the insertion of a urinary catheter.

Catheters

A catheter is a tube which is inserted into the bladder to drain urine. It is inserted through the urethra or, less commonly, through a small incision in the suprapubic area. A catheter may be inserted to empty the bladder then removed immediately, or it may be left in the bladder. A catheter that remains in the bladder may either be clamped and released at specified intervals, or connected to tubing and a bag to enable continuous drainage. A catheter which remains in the bladder is referred to as indwelling. Reasons for inserting a urinary catheter include to:

- relieve retention of urine
- closely monitor the urinary output
- obtain a sterile specimen of urine
- prevent skin maceration when a patient is incontinent
- remove residual urine when voiding does not completely empty the bladder
- allow the drainage of urine and to keep the bladder empty during or after surgery on the abdominal, pelvic, or perineal areas.
- facilitate bladder irrigation procedures.

Catheters are made from materials that cause little reaction when in contact with body tissues, and are available in a variety of styles and sizes. Some of the materials from which catheters are made include:

- polyvinylchloride (PVC), which softens at body temperature and is commonly used for short term purposes.
- silicone elastomer, which is a physiologically inert material causing few local reactions when in contact with body tissue and therefore can remain in the bladder for long periods.
- latex coated with silicone which is not as inert as silicone, but may remain in the bladder for up to 10 days.

Catheters are graded according to the French scale and the larger the number, the larger is the lumen of the catheter. Sizes range from 1 to 30 French Gauge (Fg), and the size is selected to suit the individual's needs. It is important that a suitable size is selected to avoid leakage of urine around the catheter, or trauma to the urethra or bladder.

There are a variety of styles available, which are either non self retaining or self retaining. A self retaining catheter is fitted with a device, usually a balloon, which maintains its position in the bladder. Once inserted the balloon is inflated by the introduction of sterile water, with the amount to be introduced indicated on the catheter. The two most common balloon capacities are 5 ml and 30 ml.

Insertion of a catheter. The procedure of catheter insertion is called catheterization, and is performed using sterile equipment and aseptic technique. As a catheter can cause trauma to the urethral or bladder mucosa, and is a potential source of urinary tract infection, it is inserted only when absolutely necessary. Because the male urethra is longer and more curved than the female urethra and catheterization is more difficult, male patients are usually catheterized by a person skilled in this procedure. A suggested procedure for female catheterization is outlined in the guidelines, and the nurse should refer to the institution's policy manual for information about the equipment and the protocol regarding catheter insertion. The basic requirements are:

— sterile catheters
— sterile receiver for urine
— sterile materials for cleansing the genital area
— water soluble lubricant
— sterile gloves
— sterile forceps
— sterile drapes.

In addition, if the catheter is to be indwelling:

— sterile water
— sterile 5 to 10 ml syringe
— drainage tubing and bag
— holder for drainage bag
— clamp
— hypoallergenic tape.

Male catheterization. The nurse may be required to assist with male catheterization, and the assistance includes:

- preparing the equipment
- ensuring adequate lighting and privacy
- placing the individual in a supine position with his legs extended
- promoting comfort during the procedure.

Care following the insertion of a catheter is similar for both males and females. When a person has an indwelling catheter, nursing care is planned and implemented to promote comfort, to maintain the flow of urine, and to minimize the possibility of a urinary tract infection. Key aspects related to the care include are discussed below.

- Ascertain whether the catheter is to be clamped and released at specified intervals to provide intermittent drainage, or if it is to be connected to a drainage bag for the continuous drainage of urine.
- If intermittent drainage has been prescribed the end of the catheter is clamped. At specified intervals, e.g. every 4 hours, the clamp is released to enable the urine that has accumulated in the bladder to drain. Aseptic technique should be used during this procedure, to prevent the entry of microorganisms into the open catheter. An intermittent drainage regimen is commonly implemented prior to the removal of an indwelling catheter, in order to restore any lost bladder tone.
- If continuous drainage has been prescribed, actions to promote a free flow of urine and prevention of stasis of urine include:

1. The tubing should be positioned so that it is not obstructed in any manner.
2. The tubing and drainage bag should remain below the level of the patient's bladder.
3. The individual should have a fluid input of at least 2000 ml daily, unless this is contraindicated.

- In order to prevent ascending infection, the catheter should be taped to the inner thigh to reduce any in-out

movement. If a continuous drainage system is being used the sterile closed system, comprised of the catheter, tubing, and bag, should not be disrupted unless necessary. If it is necessary to disconnect any part of the system, a septic technique must be used.

- To promote comfort, and to reduce the risk of ascending infection, the urethral meatus and catheter near the point of entry should be cleansed. At least twice daily and whenever necessary, e.g. following a bowel action, those areas should be cleansed with a non-irritating substance and sterile swabs. Cleansing should be performed by wiping in the direction away from the urethral meatus to avoid contamination of the urinary tract. An uncircumcised male's foreskin should be retracted prior to cleansing, and replaced after cleansing.
- The urine should be observed and the observations documented, for volume, colour and clarity, odour, and the presence of abnormalities such as blood, pus, or sediment. Any deviations from normal must be reported immediately.
- Any inflammation of the urethral meatus, or pain or distension over the bladder area, should be recognized and reported immediately.
- The nurse should observe for signs that urine is bypassing or leaking around the catheter. This may be caused by bladder spasm, blockage of the catheter or tubing, or insertion of a catheter of incorrect size. If leakage occurs, the cause is investigated so that the problem can be remedied.
- In order to test the patency of a catheter, or to remove clots or sediment, irrigation of the catheter or a bladder irrigation or washout may be performed. Information on this procedure is provided later in the chapter.
- When an individual has an indwelling catheter, it may be necessary to obtain a specimen of urine for laboratory analysis. A suggested technique for this procedure is described earlier in the chapter.
- Indwelling catheters are changed if contamination occurs, or if any malfunction or obstruction can not be corrected. If no complication occurs the frequency with which a catheter is changed depends on the type being used, and ranges from approximately 10 days to 6 months.
- When a catheter is being used to drain urine from an overdistended bladder, e.g. during acute retention of urine, care is taken not to allow the urine to be drained too rapidly. Decompressing the bladder too quickly may result in bladder trauma or physiological shock, therefore no more than 1000 ml should be released at any one time.
- Urine meters may be used in conjunction with drainage systems when precise measurements of urine output, e.g. 1 hourly measurements are required. The meters commonly consist of a rigid plastic container that is calibrated to measure small volumes, and are attached to the drainage system.

Collection bags. Disposable closed drainage sets consisting of tubing and bag are commonly used. The collec-

Guidelines for female catheterization

Nursing action	Rationale
1. Wash and dry hands	Prevents cross infection
2. Prepare the equipment using aseptic technique	Prevents cross infection
3. Explain the procedure	Reduces anxiety
4. Ensure adequate privacy	Reduces embarrassment
5. Ensure adequate lighting	Visualization of the urethral meatus is essential
6. Place the individual in the dorsal position, with her knees flexed and separated, and feet slightly apart on the bed. Ensure that the patient is adequately draped	Provides a clear view of the urethral meatus Reduces embarrassment
7. Place all the equipment in a convenient location	Facilitates easy access to it throughout the procedure
8. Wash and dry hands	Prevents cross infection
9. Use sterile towels to create a sterile field around the genital area	Reduces risk of equipment becoming contaminated during the procedure
10. Cleanse genital area and urethral meatus, wiping from front to back	Reduces risk of introducing microorganisms from genital/anal area into the urinary tract
11. Before inserting a self retaining catheter, inflate and deflate the balloon	Necessary to check balloon for leakage prior to insertion
12. With forceps, hold the catheter approximately 7 cm from its tip	Assists in controlling the direction of the catheter
13. Dip tip of catheter into the lubricant	Facilitates easier and more comfortable insertion
14. Place distal end of catheter into a sterile receptacle which is positioned between the individual's legs	Urine will flow into the receptacle, not onto the bed
15. Keeping the person's labia separated, insert the catheter tip into the urethral orifice. Advance the the catheter until 4–7 cm have been inserted.	Length of catheter inserted must be in relation to the anatomical structure of the urethra. The female urethra is approximately 3.8 cm long
16. If catheter is not to be left in, remove it gently when urine ceases to flow, or the required amount of urine has drained	Catheters are not left in any longer than necessary, and are removed gently to avoid discomfort
17. If a self retaining catheter is being used, inflate the balloon having first ensured that the catheter is draining adequately	Inflated balloon keeps catheter in bladder Inadvertent inflation with the balloon in the urethra causes trauma and pain
18. Connect the indwelling catheter to drainage bag and support the bag in a holder at the side of the bed. Alternatively, a clamp is placed on the end of the catheter	Urine flows from catheter, along the tubing and into the bag Intermittent drainage may be prescribed
19. Attach catheter to individual's inner thigh with hypoallergenic tape, and pass catheter over the thigh	Prevents in-out movement of the catheter Prevents tension on the urethra
20. Position tubing so that it is not obstructed by the person's weight or by tight bedclothes	Avoids blocking the flow of urine through the tubing
21. Remove excess lubricant from the individual's genital area. Replace bedding and assist her into position	Helps to promote comfort
22. Remove and attend to the equipment in the appropriate manner. Wash and dry hands	Prevents cross infection
23. Report on, and document the procedure. Document the amount of water instilled into any balloon	Appropriate care can be planned and implemented When the catheter is to be removed, it is important that the water is first withdrawn and the balloon deflated, to prevent trauma to the urethra

tion bag is emptied at specified intervals or when it is almost full, and the tubing left in position until the entire set is changed or removed. Collection bags are emptied by releasing the valve at the bottom of the bag, using aseptic technique in order to avoid introducing infection. Whenever the tubing or bag is changed, or the catheter disconnected from the tubing, the sterility of the system must be maintained. Key aspects related to emptying and changing collection bags are outlined in the guidelines. The equipment necessary consists of:

A. To empty a bag—sterile jug and cover
              —alcohol swabs

B. To change a bag—collection bag and/or tubing
              —alcohol swabs
              —sterile jug and cover
              —receiver for used items
              —clamp.

Bladder irrigation. Bladder irrigation or washout may be performed to ensure patency of the catheter, to remove sediment or blood clots, or to introduce an antibiotic or bacteriostatic agent. Bladder irrigation may be continuous or intermittent. Continuous irrigation may be prescribed if frequent irrigations become necessary, or to prevent urinary tract obstruction by flushing out small blood clots that may form after prostate or bladder surgery. Intermittent irrigation may be prescribed to remove substances blocking the catheter, or to introduce antibiotic or bacteriostatic agents.

During bladder irrigation, sterile equipment and aseptic technique are used to avoid introducing microorganisms. The procedure should be performed by a person skilled in this technique. A triple lumen catheter is needed to perform bladder irrigation. One lumen is used to introduce the irrigating solution into the bladder, a second lumen

---

Guidelines for emptying or changing collection bags

Nursing action	Rationale
To empty a bag—	
1. Wash and dry hands	Prevents cross infection
2. Explain the procedure	Reduces anxiety
3. Ensure privacy	Reduces embarrassment
4. Swab the outlet valve on the collection bag with an alcohol swab	Reduces risk of introducing microorganisms
5. Place the jug below the valve and release valve	Allows urine to drain from the bag into the jug
6. When the bag is empty, tighten the valve	Prevents subsequent drainage of urine out of the bag
7. Swab the valve with an alcohol swab	Removes any traces of urine, and prevents cross infection
8. Remove the jug, observe the urine, and measure or test it if necessary	Assists in evaluating the patient's urinary status
9. Empty and clean the jug, wash and dry hands	Prevents cross infection
10. Report any deviations from normal, and document accordingly	Appropriate care can be planned and implemented
To change a bag—	
(steps 1–6 are as previously stated)	
7. Swab the connection site where the system is to be disrupted	Reduces risk of introducing microorganisms
8. Clamp the catheter and remove the bag, and/or bag and tubing. Connect the catheter or tubing to the new bag	Prevents leakage of urine during the change
9. Swab the connection site with alcohol swab	Removes traces of urine, and prevents cross infection
10. Release the clamp, and ensure that the tubing and bag are positioned correctly	Allows urine to flow
11. Remove the soiled articles, attend to them in the appropriate manner, wash and dry hands	Prevents cross infection
12. Observe the urine, and measure or test it if necessary	Assists in evaluating the patient's urinary status
13. Report any deviations from normal, and document accordingly	Appropriate care can be planned and implemented

allows the fluid to drain out, and the third lumen allows the instillation of fluid into the balloon that holds the catheter in the bladder.

1. For continuous irrigation, a container of irrigating solution is suspended on a stand, and the tubing from the container is attached to the catheter. Drainage tubing from the catheter is attached to a urine collection bag, and the bag positioned below the level of the individual's bladder. A clamp is used to regulate the rate at which the solution flows into the bladder. During the irrigation, the inflow and outflow tubing is checked to ensure the free flow of fluid. The outflowing fluid is checked for changes in appearance and presence of blood clots. Both the inflowing and outflowing fluid must be measured and documented, and the collection bag emptied as necessary. The outflow volume, allowing for urine production, should be greater than the inflow volume.

2. Intermittent irrigation involves the gentle introduction of small amounts of prescribed solution. The solution is introduced, using a syringe, into the distal end of the catheter. A small amount, e.g. 30 to 50 ml, is introduced at a time and usually allowed to drain out by gravity. The technique is repeated until the prescribed amount of solution has been used, or until the return fluid is clear. The solution being introduced and returned is measured and documented, and the return fluid observed for changes in appearance or presence of blood clots.

Removal of a catheter. Depending on how long a catheter has been in position, the medical officer may prescribe bladder training prior to its removal. Bladder retraining involves clamping the catheter for specified periods, e.g. 2–4 hours, then releasing it to empty the bladder. This technique is repeated for several hours in order to help restore the bladder's muscle tone. Removal of a catheter requires aseptic technique and key aspects related to the procedure and after care include:-

● Ensuring that all water from the balloon is withdrawn prior to removing the catheter.
● Obtaining a specimen of urine for laboratory analysis if necessary, before the catheter is removed.
● Gently withdrawing the catheter from the urethra, using aseptic technique.
● Offering a bedpan or urinal immediately after the catheter is removed, as catheter removal often creates a desire to void.
● Encouraging the intake of fluids to stimulate urine production, to dilute the urine, and to help decrease any discomfort the individual may experience when he recommences voiding.
● Observing and documenting urine output after the catheter is removed. If the individual is voiding only small amounts his bladder may not be emptying completely, and the medical officer should be informed.

● Observing for any difficulty with voiding, incontinence or dribbling, or a distended bladder. Any problems must be reported immediately.
● Documenting the date and time the catheter was removed and the individual's response to the procedure.

Care of an individual with incontinence of urine

Incontinence is the inability to control the excretion of urine, and may result from a variety of local or generalized conditions which include:

● sphincter incompetence, e.g. as a result of urethral trauma, surgery to the bladder, or following childbirth
● urinary tract infections
● neurological lesions
● bladder tumours or stones
● impaired consciousness or awareness
● medications that increase urinary output or affect awareness
● Environmental causes such as difficult access to toilet facilities.

Incontinence of urine may be classified into four types:

1. Total incontinence, when the person experiences a constant involuntary loss of urine.
2. Stress incontinence, when the person loses urine while sneezing, coughing, laughing, or during other activities that result in increased intra-abdominal pressure.
3. Urgency incontinence, when the person experiences a strong urge to void followed immediately by loss of urine.
4. Over-flow incontinence, which is characterized by constant dribbling while the bladder remains full.

The management of incontinence depends on identifying the cause and treating any underlying conditions. Nursing care of a person with incontinence requires understanding, patience, and awareness of the need to preserve his dignity and self esteem.

There are a variety of products available which have been designed to keep the incontinent individual's skin and clothing dry. These include especially designed pants into which an absorbent pad is inserted, and absorbent sheets which may be used in place of conventional sheets.

There are also several styles of sheath or condom appliances that are fitted over the penis and attached to a collection bag. Leg bags (Fig. 30.3) are available which can be worn under normal clothing, and provide the male incontinent person with greater freedom of mobility. As there are several styles of condom fittings available, and various methods of attaching them to the penis, the nurse should follow the manufacturer's directions regarding their use.

Before any appliance is fitted, the penis must be cleaned and dried and observation made to ensure that the foreskin

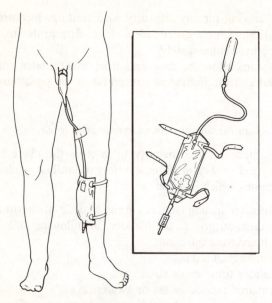

Fig. 30.3 External urinary drainage device. The urine is collected in a bag that can be attached to the calf or thigh.

is not retracted. The appliance is placed over the penis and secured in position. A special adhesive tape is commonly used, and care must be taken to ensure that it is not applied too tightly. The tubing from the appliance is connected to either a bedside collection bag, or a leg bag. The penis should be observed for oedema and discolouration; if this is detected, the appliance is removed immediately and reapplied more loosely. At least every 24 hours the appliance is removed, and the penis cleaned and dried before re application. Use of such appliances may be discontinued if there are signs of skin excoriation, persistent oedema of the penis, or urinary tract infection.

Personal clothing can be adapted if necessary to suit the individual's needs, and to facilitate easy access to any incontinence aids being used.

Incontinence of urine is a relatively common problem that affects many people of all ages and both sexes, and as a result, there are now personnel who specialize in the management of incontinence. Continence advisors are available to assess the individual and plan appropriate management. Their main aim is to promote continence, and a variety of methods may be used. Further information on bladder retraining techniques is described later in this chapter. Key aspects related to the nursing care of a patient with incontinence are described below.

1. Hygiene. As constant moisture on the skin may lead to maceration or the development of decubitus ulcers, it is essential that the skin is kept clean and dry. When the person is incontinent his skin should be washed with mild soap and water and gently dried. Particular attention is paid to the genital area, the groin, and the crease between the buttocks. A protective cream may be applied to repel moisture and prevent excoriation.

2. Clothing. Any wet personal or bed clothes should be removed immediately, and taken from the room to prevent offensive odours. The individual should be provided with clean, dry clothing.

3. Toilet facilities. The person should be encouraged to void at regular intervals, e.g. every 2 hours. Ambulant people should have easy access to the toilet, and non-ambulant people should be provided with toilet utensils. Any request for the use of toilet facilities should be responded to promptly.

4. Fluids. Unless contra-indicated, the individual should be encouraged to drink at least 1500 ml daily, as an inadequate fluid input may further decrease the functional capacity of the bladder.

5. Attitude. As a person is generally distressed and embarrassed by incontinence, the nurse should adopt a positive approach to continence management. She should demonstrate discretion, tact, and understanding in order to promote the individual's dignity and self esteem.

6. Devices/appliances. As previously mentioned there are a variety of devices available to assist in the management of incontinence, and these are used according to the person's needs.

7. Perineal exercises. The individual may be required to perform a regimen of isometric exercises designed to improve the retention of urine. These are called Kegel exercises and consist of a series of voluntary contractions of the muscles of the pelvic floor and perineum. The nurse may be required to instruct and supervise the individual in the performance of these exercises.

8. Medication. The nurse may be required to administer medications which have been prescribed, e.g. antibiotics to treat a urinary tract infection. Various other medications may also be prescribed as part of the overall management of incontinence.

Surgical intervention is sometimes indicated in the treatment of incontinence, e.g. an operation may be performed whereby the bladder is elevated into an improved anatomical position.

Planned bladder retraining regimens are commonly implemented in order to promote continence or to modify incontinence. Before a regimen is commenced, complete assessment of the person is necessary to provide accurate information about the incontinent episodes. The recording of every episode of incontinence and the time of occurrence is made for 24–48 hours. A regimen is then commenced whereby the individual is encouraged to void at specified intervals, e.g. 2 hourly, day and night. Documentation is continued and the schedule is adjusted as necessary. If the person remains continent in between the 2 hourly use of toilet facilities, the intervals may be increased to 3 and then 4 hourly. Consistency and an individualized approach are essential if success is to be achieved.

Some individuals, e.g. those who have a neurogenic bladder as a result of a neurological dysfunction, may be educated to perform intermittent self catheterization, or Crede's manoeuvre. Crede's manoeuvre involves the application of manual pressure over the lower abdomen to promote complete emptying of the bladder.

Urinary incontinence is a major but largely hidden problem in Australian society. Fortunately, recognition of the needs and problems of individuals who experience some form of incontinence is increasing.

Elimination of faeces

Normal defaecation is voluntary and painless, and the frequency with which faeces are passed varies with each individual. Factors that affect the frequency of defaecation and the quantity of faeces include, type and quantity of food consumed, level of physical activity, response to the need to defaecate, and the availability of toilet utensils. The frequency and often the amount of faeces eliminated can be increased by sufficient fibre in the diet, an adequate fluid input, anxiety or stress, medications that irritate the gastro-intestinal tract, and some disease states. The frequency and often the amount of faeces eliminated can be decreased by insufficient dietary fibre, insufficient fluid input, prolonged inactivity, medications that reduce the motility of the intestines, and some disease states.

Faeces are composed of food residue, water, bacteria and secretions from the digestive tract and liver. Normal faeces have the following characteristics:

- passed without pain or discomfort
- brown in colour
- characteristic odour
- semi solid and formed
- excreted in amounts that vary with each individual.

Collection of faeces

The nurse may be required to collect faeces for observation or testing in the ward, or so that a specimen can be sent to the laboratory for analysis. Key aspects related to the collection of faeces include:

- Thorough washing and drying of the hands before and after collection to prevent cross infection.
- The container in which the faeces are collected must be clean, and in some instances sterile, to ensure a specimen free from external contamination.
- Contamination of the container and faeces must be prevented throughout the procedure.
- Adequate information about the person and the specimen must be provided. Specimen containers are labelled with the individual's name and registration number, time and date of collection, and type of specimen. If the specimen is to be sent to the laboratory for analysis, it must be accompanied by relevant documentation, e.g. the medical officer's request form.

- Specimens must be sent to the laboratory as soon as possible after collection. Most tests require the provision of a fresh specimen, and this is of particular importance when the faeces are to be tested for the presence of parasites, e.g. amoeba. A warm specimen facilitates the isolation of such organisms.
- A person may be responsible for the collection of his own faecal specimen, therefore the nurse should provide him with the information necessary to ensure that the collection is performed correctly.

Observation or testing in the ward. The individual is requested to use a bedpan, and to avoid contaminating the faeces with urine or menstrual blood. With the aid of a disposable spatula, the faeces are transferred into an appropriate container and covered.

Laboratory analysis. The same procedure as above is followed, and approximately 20–30 ml of faeces are transferred to a labelled sterile specimen container. The specimen is dispatched to the laboratory immediately, together with the medical officer's request form.

For specific tests, e.g. to test for faecal fat, it may be necessary to collect all the faeces excreted over a specified period, e.g. 3–5 days. This test may be indicated to assist in the diagnosis of diseases such as Coeliac disease or Tropical Sprue.

Examination of faeces. In order to detect and identify abnormalities, faeces are examined by observation, by chemical testing in the ward, or by analysis in the laboratory. Abnormalities which can be detected by observation are listed in Table 30.3.

Table 9.4 lists the various types of worms that may affect humans and be present in the faeces. Most types of worms are visible to the naked eye, but confirmation of infestation requires microscopic examination of ova as the worms themselves may not be excreted.

Testing the faeces for abnormalities is generally performed in the laboratory, where the specimen is analyzed for the presence of blood, parasites and ova, bile, fat, pathogenic microorganisms, or pancreatic enzymes. Laboratory analysis of faeces provides information about:

- the condition and function of the digestive system
- the presence of pathogenic microorganisms or helminths
- the presence of blood.

One test on faeces that is commonly performed in the ward is the faecal occult blood test. This test is valuable for determining the presence of occult blood to detect any hidden gastro-intestinal bleeding, and for distinguishing between true melaena and melaena-like stools. One method of testing for occult blood involves the use of a chemical reagent tablet but as there are various methods used, the nurse should obtain information from the manufacturer's directions or the institution's policy manual about the specific testing procedure.

Table 30.3 Abnormalities of faeces detected by observation

Observation	Deviation from normal	Possible cause
Colour	Grey, pale, or clay coloured	Absence of bile due to disorders of the liver or gallbladder, or obstruction of the common bile duct
	Dark and tar-like (melaena)	Presence of digested blood due to bleeding in the upper alimentary tract
	Containing blood or streaked with bright red blood	Bleeding from the lower colon, rectum, or anus
	Black	Medications containing iron
	Green	Gastrointestinal infections
Consistency	Hard and dry	Insufficient fluid or fibre
		Medications that reduce the motility of the intestines
		Prolonged inactivity
	Loose and watery	Reaction to certain foods or fluids
		Medications that increase the motility of the intestines
		Gastrointestinal infections
Foreign substances	Pus or mucus	Infection or irritation of the intestines
	Undigested food substances	Malabsorption states
	Worms (Refer to Table 9.4)	Helminth infestation
Odour	Foul smelling	Steatorrhea
		Coeliac disease

Problems associated with elimination of faeces

Problems associated with elimination from the bowel may occur as a result of several factors including a change from normal routine or environment, or as a consequence of certain disease states. Any alteration in the individual's normal pattern of defaecation must be recognized and reported immediately, so that appropriate actions can be planned and implemented. Problems associated with elimination from the bowel include:

1. Altered frequency. Constipation is the infrequent passage of dry hard stools, and diarrhoea is the frequent passage of loose unformed stools.

2. Impaction. If the faeces remain in the rectum for a long time, a large hardened mass develops that is difficult to expel. Impacted faeces is the term used to describe this condition.

3. Flatulence. The excessive formation of gas in the stomach and intestines is called flatulence. If the gas is not expelled, the intestines become distended and the person may experience abdominal discomfort and swelling. Flatus is the term used for gas in the intestine that is expelled through the anus. Flatulence may result from swallowed air, the consumption of gas forming food or liquid, or bacterial action within the intestines.

4. Incontinence. Incontinence of faeces is the inability to control the expulsion of faeces, and may occur as a result of lesions in the brain or spinal cord, impaired consciousness or awareness, or various other factors.

5. Painful defaecation. Pain on defaecation may be due to the presence of lesions such as haemorrhoids or anal fissures. Tenesmus is the term used to describe persistent ineffectual spasms of the rectum accompanied by the desire to empty the bowel, and may be associated with disorders such as inflammatory bowel disease.

6. Artificial openings into the intestine. As a result of certain disorders such as obstruction or tumours in the bowel, the passage of faeces through the rectum and anus may not be possible. In these instances, the surgical creation of an artificial opening from the colon to the surface of the abdomen may become necessary. Care of an individual with an artificial opening (stoma) is described in Chapter 46.

Constipation

Whenever a person is experiencing problems with elimination from the bowel, the cause must be identified and treated. Two of the more common conditions which may require nursing intervention to assist the individual to meet his bowel elimination needs, are constipation and diarrhoea.

Constipation is a relatively common problem and is often the result of some deficiency in the three elements necessary for normal bowel activity: dietary fibre, adequate fluid input, and sufficient physical activity. Other causes include disregarding the urge to defaecate, chronic use of laxatives, or certain disease states. When constipation occurs, the individual often strains to produce hard dry stools, and such straining may aggravate pre-existing rectal conditions, e.g. haemorrhoids. Constipation is often accompanied by abdominal distension and discomfort, nausea, headache, and diminished appetite.

Natural measures to prevent constipation include:

- Sufficient dietary fibre. Foods such as wholegrain

cereals, fruit, and vegetables, contribute bulk and induce peristalsis.

● Adequate fluid input. At least 1500 ml daily is necessary to help keep the intestinal contents in a semi solid state for easier passage and excretion.

● Responding to the desire to empty the bowel as soon as practicable.

● Maintaining a routine where a regular time for bowel movement, e.g. after breakfast, is established.

● Incorporating sufficient exercise, e.g. walking, into the daily routine.

● Relaxing and assuming a natural position when having a bowel action. Some people find the use of a small foot-stool, to promote thigh flexion, helpful.

● Avoiding undue anxiety about bowel habits. While some individuals have a bowel action every day, it is quite normal for others to have a 2–3 day interval between bowel actions.

Other measures to assist elimination from the bowel may be necessary, and these include:

● Laxatives. Laxatives are substances taken orally, that promote evacuation of the bowel by increasing bulk, by softening the faeces, or by lubricating the walls of the colon.

● Suppositories. A suppository is a small solid mass which melts at body temperature when inserted into the rectum.

● Enemas. An enema involves the introduction of fluid through the anus into the lower colon.

Suppositories

Suppositories may be ordered and inserted into the rectum to promote the evacuation of faeces, or to administer a drug rectally. A suggested method for the administration of rectal suppositories is outlined in the guidelines. The equipment necessary consists of:

Guidelines for inserting a rectal suppository

Nursing action	Rationale
1. Explain the procedure	Reduces anxiety
2. Assemble the equipment, and follow the nursing policies related to checking medications	The correct type, size, and quantity must be administered
3. Ensure adequate privacy	Reduces embarrassment
4. Place the individual in a left lateral position	Anatomical site of the lower colon means that this position is the most effective for the introduction and retention of suppositories
5. Ensure that the person is adequately covered with only the buttocks exposed	Promotes warmth and comfort
6. Wash and dry hands, and put on the finger cot or glove	Prevents cross infection
7. Lubricate finger cot and suppository	Facilitates insertion of suppository
8. Gently insert the suppository by directing it with the finger, through the anus approximately 3.5 cm into the rectum	Suppository must pass the internal anal sphincter and come in contact with rectal mucosa
9. During insertion, encourage the individual to take deep breaths through his mouth	Helps to relax the anal sphincters
10. Encourage the individual to retain the suppository for the correct length of time. A suppository administered to cause a bowel action should be retained for at least 20 minutes	He must be aware whether the suppository is to be retained to allow any medication to be dissipated, or whether to expect a bowel action. Suppositories to promote a bowel action must be retained long enough to be effective
11. Ensure the person has easy access to toilet facilities and the signal device	Reduces anxiety related to accidental expulsion of the suppository or faeces
12. Dispose of used equipment appropriately, wash and dry hands	Prevents cross infection
13. If a bowel action results, the faeces are observed and the observations reported and documented	Helps to assess the effectiveness of the treatment, and detects any abnormalities
14. Attend to the individual's hygiene and position	Helps promote comfort
15. Report and document the procedure	Appropriate care may be planned and implemented

— Prescribed suppository/suppositories
— disposable finger cot or glove
— water soluble lubricant
— receiver for used articles
— extra equipment as listed in the institution's policy manual.

Before the suppository is administered, the nurse should ascertain whether it is being given to administer a drug and is to be retained, or whether it is being given to promote evacuation from the bowel. Types of medications that may be administered rectally by suppository include those which relieve nausea, or those which relieve bronchospasm, e.g. during an asthma attack. Suppositories prescribed to promote a bowel action are composed of various substances, e.g. glycerine. Evacuant suppositories act by softening and lubricating the faeces to facilitate easier passage and excretion, or by increasing peristalsis through the irritation of intestinal sensory nerve endings.

Enemata

An enema may be ordered and administered to promote the evacuation of faeces and flatus, or to administer a drug rectally. When a solution or medication is introduced and retained it is referred to as a retention enema. When a solution is administered to promote evacuation of the bowel, it is referred to as an evacuant enema. Prior to administration, the nurse should ascertain the type and purpose of the enema which has been prescribed.

An evacuant enema acts by distending the bowel and stimulating the nerves in the rectal wall, thus promoting peristalsis. An evacuant enema may be administered to relieve constipation, or to empty the lower colon prior to examination, radiological investigation, or surgery.

Enema solutions may be commercially prepared and packaged in disposable sets, or be prepared in the ward immediately prior to administration. Substances used include a solution of enema soap and water, emollients such as olive or mineral oil, and hypertonic solutions. The quantities administered range from 5–1200 ml, depending on the substance used and the age of the patient. A suggested method of administering an enema is outlined in the guidelines. Disposable or re-usable equipment may be used to administer the solution, with a basic set consisting of:

— container of solution
— funnel
— length of tubing with a clamp
— rectal catheter
— water soluble lubricant
— lotion thermometer
— disposable gloves
— extra equipment as listed in the institution's policy manual.

Bowel lavage

The introduction of fluid to irrigate the lower colon is sometimes performed following an evacuant enema to thoroughly cleanse the colon prior to examination, radiological investigation, or surgery of the bowel. This procedure is referred to as a bowel lavage, irrigation, or washout. It involves the introduction of fluid, e.g. water, into the rectum, then siphoning it off, and is continued until the return fluid is clear. Siphoning off the fluid is achieved by gravity, and involves lowering the tubing below the level of the patient. A suggested method of performing a bowel lavage is outlined in the guidelines. The equipment necessary consists of:

— container holding approximately 4 litres of water
— rectal tube
— clamp
— tubing and connection
— water soluble lubricant
— lotion thermometer
— funnel
— disposable gloves
— bucket
— extras as listed in the institution's policy manual.

Prior to commencing the procedure, the water is warmed to 38–40°C.

Rectal tube

Gastrointestinal hypomotility, may result in an accumulation of gas and abdominal distension. Hypomotility may result from various medical or surgical conditions or medications that decrease peristalsis. In these instances, the bowel fills with gas and distends, and it may be necessary to insert a tube through the anus into the rectum to facilitate the release of gas. A suggested method of inserting a rectal tube is outlined in the guidelines. The equipment necessary consists of:

— rectal tube
— water soluble lubricant
— receiver, e.g. a sealed plastic bag or a container of water
— hypoallergenic tape
— disposable gloves
— extra equipment as listed in the institution's policy manual.

Impacted faeces

The term faecal impaction refers to the presence of a large hard dry mass of faeces in the lower colon. When the condition occurs it is a result of prolonged constipation. If measures to promote a bowel action, e.g. a suppository or

Guidelines for administration of an enema

Nursing action	Rationale
1. Explain the procedure	Reduces anxiety
2. Assemble the equipment. Follow the nursing policies related to checking medications. If a soap and water solution is used, the ratio is 30 g of enema soap to 600 ml of water	The correct substance and amount must be administered
3. Solutions which are to be warmed are administered slightly above normal body temperature	Cold solutions may cause discomfort, and overheated solutions may damage the rectal mucosa
4. If a soap solution is used, all air bubbles must be removed before it is administered	The introduction of air causes abdominal distension and discomfort
5. Ensure privacy	Reduces embarrassment
6. Place the individual in a left lateral position	Anatomical site of the lower colon means that this position is the most effective for the introduction and retention of fluid
7. Ensure that the individual is adequately covered with only the buttocks exposed	Promotes warmth and comfort
8. Wash and dry hands, put on gloves	Prevents cross infection
9. Ensure the equipment is assembled and functional. Pour some fluid into the funnel and tubing. As soon as solution reaches the end of the catheter clamp the tubing	Eliminates any air that would cause distension and discomfort. Prevents funnel from emptying
10. Lubricate the tip of the catheter	Facilitates insertion
11. Without force, gently insert the catheter through the anus into the rectum. The catheter should be inserted 7–10 cm for an adult, and depending on age, from 2.5–7 cm for a child	Catheter must be inserted past both anal sphinchers so the tip lies in the rectum. Gentle insertion prevents damage to the mucosa
12. During insertion, encourage the individual to take deep breaths through his mouth	Helps to relax the anal sphincters and facilitates insertion
13. Unclamp the tubing and administer the solution slowly by raising the container no higher than 45 cm above the level of the patient's hip	The solution is more easily retained, and less discomfort results, if it is administered slowly
14. Encourage the individual to retain the solution for the correct length of time. If it is an evacuant enema, the solution should be retained for at least 15 minutes	He must be aware if the solution is to be retained for medicinal purposes, or whether to expect a bowel action. Solutions to promote a bowel action must be retained long enough to be effective
15. Ensure the person has easy access to toilet facilities, and the signal device	Reduces anxiety related to accidental expulsion of the fluid or faeces
16. Remove and attend to the equipment, wash and dry hands	Prevents cross infection
17. If a bowel action results, the faeces are observed, and the observations reported and documented	Helps to assess the effectiveness of the treatment, and detects any abnormalities
18. Attend to the individual's hygiene and position	Helps promote comfort
19. Report and document the procedure, and the person's response including any adverse reactions such as faintness or dizziness	Appropriate care may be planned and implemented

enema, are ineffectual, digital removal of the mass may be prescribed. As this procedure is contraindicated in many instances and because a variety of adverse reactions, such as stimulation of the vagus nerve and subsequent faintness, may result, it should be performed only by people who are skilled in this technique. The technique involves inserting a gloved finger past the anal sphincters into the rectum, and rotating the finger in order to dislodge and break the

Guidelines for administration of a bowel lavage

Nursing action	Rationale
1. Explain the procedure	Reduces anxiety
2. Prepare the equipment and place it near to the bed	Facilitates access to it during the procedure
3. Ensure privacy	Reduces embarrassment
4. Place the individual in a left lateral position	Anatomical site of the lower colon means that this position is the most effective for the introduction of fluid
5. Ensure that the individual is adequately covered with only the buttocks exposed	Promotes warmth and comfort
6. Wash and dry hands, put on gloves	Prevents cross infection
7. Assemble the equipment Pour some water into the funnel and tubing. As soon as water reaches the end of the tube, apply the clamp	Expels air from the tube Prevents funnel from emptying
8. Lubricate the tip of the rectal tube	Facilitates insertion
9. Gently insert the tip of the rectal tube through the anus into the rectum for approximately 7–10 cm	Tip of the tube must pass both anal sphincters and enter the rectum
10. Pour water into the funnel, unclamp the tubing and hold the funnel approximately 45 cm above the individual	Enables fluid to begin flowing slowly into the rectum
11. When approximately 500 ml has been administered, lower the tubing and funnel over the bucket	Allows the fluid to siphon off into the bucket
12. When fluid return ceases, keep funnel low, refill it with fresh water, raise it slowly to the correct height again	Prevents air from entering the funnel. Raising the funnel then enables the fluid to flow into the rectum again
13. Continue steps 10–12 until the return fluid is clear	All faecal material must be cleansed from the lower colon
14. If the individual becomes distressed at any stage, stop the procedure and report to the nurse in charge	The procedure may be discontinued and recommenced later, after the person's condition has been assessed
15. On completion withdraw the tube and offer the use of toilet facilities	There may be fluid remaining in the rectum for the person to expel
16. Remove and attend to the equipment in the appropriate manner, wash and dry hands	Prevents cross infection
17. Attend to the individual's hygiene and position	Promotes comfort
18. Record and document the procedure. Include the observations made of the return fluid	Evaluates the effectiveness of the procedure, and appropriate care can be planned and implemented

mass into small pieces. The finger is used to remove the pieces of stool from the rectum.

During the procedure the individual is observed for adverse reactions and the procedure is stopped if he experiences pain, nausea, rectal bleeding, faintness, pallor and sweating, or changes in the pulse rate. Following the procedure the person's hygiene needs are attended to. The procedure, the observations made of the faeces, and the individual's response, are documented.

Diarrhoea

Diarrhoea is the discharge of frequent loose unformed stools due to the rapid passage of contents through the intestines. The person with diarrhoea may be exhausted due to frequent defaecation, and the presence of accompanying abdominal distension and pain. If diarrhoea is prolonged, the absorption of nutrients and fluids is impaired and the person shows signs of fluid and electrolyte

---

Guidelines for insertion of a rectal tube

Nursing action	Rationale
1. Explain the procedure	Reduces anxiety
2. Place the equipment near the bedside	Facilitates easy access during procedure
3. Ensure adequate privacy	Reduces embarrassment
4. Place the individual in a left lateral position	Facilitates insertion of the rectal tube
5. Ensure the person is adequately covered with only the buttocks exposed	Promotes warmth and comfort
6. Wash and dry hands, and put on the gloves	Prevents cross infection
7. Lubricate the tip of the tube	Facilitates insertion
8. Gently insert the tip of the tube through the anus and advance it approximately 5–8 cm into the rectum. Tape the tube to the individual's left thigh	Gentle insertion avoids damage to the rectal mucosa, and the tip of the tube must enter the rectum
9. Attach the tube to the bag or container of water	Any escaping gas will be observed as inflation of the bag, or bubbles in the water
10. Leave the tube in position for the prescribed time, e.g. 15–20 minutes, and observe for escaping gas and a reduction in abdominal distension	Assesses the effectiveness of the procedure
11. Remove the tape and withdraw the tube, attend to equipment appropriately, remove gloves, wash and dry hands	Prevents cross infection
12. Attend to individual's hygiene and position	Promotes comfort
13. Report and document the procedure	Appropriate care may be planned and implemented

---

loss. Diarrhoea is a symptom of various conditions that include:

- irritation or inflammation of the gastrointestinal tract, e.g. due to pathogenic infection, highly spiced foods, or medications that increase intestinal motility.
- disorders of digestion or absorption
- disorders that affect secretion and utilization of bile or pancreatic juice, e.g. obstructive jaundice
- emotional states such as anxiety or stress

Diarrhoea should be assessed in terms of the frequency of defaecation, and the characteristics of the faeces. The cause of diarrhoea must be investigated and treated. Key aspects related to the care of an individual with diarrhoea include:

- Reduction of intestinal peristalsis. Dietary management involves the withholding of food until the diarrhoea diminishes, then the gradual resumption of food. Foods low in fibre may be provided initially to reduce stimulation of the intestines.
- The administration of any prescribed medications. Anti-diarrhoeal medications such as codeine phosphate may be prescribed, as may anti-spasmodic preparations to reduce abdominal cramps and pains.
- The fluid input must be maintained in order to replace lost fluids and to prevent dehydration. Oral fluids are given if tolerated, or fluids may be administered intravenously.

Input and output should be observed and documented as part of the individual's fluid balance assessment.
- The person's hygiene needs must be met. After each bowel action, the anal area and buttocks should be cleansed with a mild soap, and thoroughly dried. A protective cream may be applied to reduce discomfort, and the area should be observed for signs of excoriation.
- As the individual may be embarrassed by the odours associated with diarrhoea, measures to eliminate odours should be taken. Any soiled linen should be changed and removed from the room immediately. The room should be well ventilated, and room deodorants may be used with discretion.
- Whenever toilet facilities are being used the person should have adequate privacy, and used toilet utensils should be removed from the room immediately.
- If the diarrhoea is due to a pathogenic infection, isolation precautions must be implemented to prevent cross infection. Information on isolation protocol is provided in Chapter 61.

Faecal incontinence which is the inability to control the excretion of faeces, may sometimes occur in conjunction with urinary incontinence. Some people may be continent of urine but develop faecal incontinence due, for example, to severe and prolonged diarrhoea. The principles of management of an individual with faecal incontinence are similar to those for the management of urinary incontinence. The cause must be identified and treated, the person's hygiene needs attended to, and measures taken to maintain dignity and esteem.

SUMMARY

Urine, which is excreted from the urinary system, and faeces, which are excreted from the digestive system, are two of the wastes resulting from metabolism. Regular elimination of both waste products is necessary for the maintenance of normal body function. Elimination of urine and faeces is affected by various factors ranging from the intake of food and fluids, to the changes that occur as a result of certain disease states.

As part of the assessment of an individual's elimination status, urine and faeces are observed and, if necessary, tested in the ward or sent to the laboratory for analysis. The nurse must ensure that specimens are collected and tested correctly so that accurate results are obtained.

Problems associated with the elimination of urine or faeces may occur, and the implementation of certain nursing actions may be necessary to assist the individual to meet his elimination needs. Any procedure which is to be performed must be thoroughly understood, so that the desired effects are achieved and safety and comfort are promoted.

31. Meeting fluid and electrolyte needs

INTRODUCTION

Fluid and electrolyte balance is an essential component of the body's homeostatic processes, and must be maintained for the body to function effectively. In health the body maintains a precise fluid balance with the volume and constituents of body fluids varying only slightly in order to maintain a stable internal physical and chemical environment. When there is a disturbance in fluid and electrolyte balance, the body attempts to compensate by various adaptive mechanisms. If the imbalance is too great or prolonged, the body's adaptive mechanisms will not be able to cope and serious consequences will occur.

The physiological processes involved in the maintenance of fluid and electrolyte balance are:

- the distribution of fluid and electrolytes within the body
- the movement of fluid and electrolytes
- the balancing of fluid input and output
- the mechanisms which regulate fluid and electrolyte balance
- the maintenance of the body's acid-base balance.

Distribution of fluid and electrolytes

Body fluid is divided between two major compartments, being present either inside the cells or outside the cells. Intracellular fluid makes up approximately 50% of total body fluid, while the remainder is comprised of extracellular fluid. Extracellular fluid consists of interstitial fluid which surrounds the cells and supplies them with substances needed for cellular function, intravascular fluid which is the fluid part of blood, and transcellular fluid which is comprised of the body's secretions and excretions.

Intracellular and extracellular fluid contains both electrolyte and non-electrolyte substances. Electrolytes are substances such as salts and minerals, whose molecules dissociate in water and disintegrate into electrically charged particles (ions) which are capable of conducting a weak electrical charge. Non-electrolyte substances such as glucose and urea do not dissociate in water nor develop electrical charges. The predominant electrolytes in extracellular fluid are sodium and chloride, while the major electrolytes in intracellular fluid are potassium and phosphate.

Movement of body fluids and electrolytes

Fluid and electrolytes are constantly moving between the cells and the extracellular compartments through the processes of osmosis, active transport, and diffusion (see Figs 15.3 and 15.4). *Osmosis* is the movement of water through a semipermeable membrane (e.g. the cell wall) from a solution that has a lower solute concentration to a solution that has a higher solute concentration, the movement continuing until the concentrations of both solutions equalize. Electrolytes do not move between the cell walls and capillaries as readily as water, and so the mechanism of *active transport* occurs. A chemical substance known as

ATP (adenosine triphosphate) is released from the cell which gives the electrolytes the energy required to pass through a semipermeable membrane. *Diffusion* is the process in which ions and molecules move from an area of greater concentration to an area of lower concentration, resulting in an even distribution of the particles in the fluid.

Balancing of fluid input and output

The body maintains fluid equilibrium by equalizing its input and output. A healthy adult body requires approximately 2500 ml of water daily which is obtained:

1. By ingestion. Approximately 2200 ml is obtained from ingested liquids and from the water content of meat, fruit, and vegetables.
2. By metabolism. The oxidation of food during metabolism yields approximately 300 ml.

Fluid input is balanced by the body's water losses, the total amount being largely dependent on the amount of fluid input. Water is lost from the body, with the average loss per day being via:

- urine, approximately 1500 ml
- faeces, approximately 200 ml
- the skin (in perspiration), approximately 400 ml
- the lungs (in expired air), approximately 300 ml.

The primary regulator of fluid intake is the body's thirst mechanism. The thirst centre is located in the hypothalamus and is highly sensitive to changes in body fluid osmotic pressure. Thirst is stimulated by lower extracellular volume and by a higher plasma osmolarity. These two conditions stimulate the production of ADH (antidiurietic hormone), therefore the thirst mechanism controls fluid input at the same time that ADH controls fluid output. Thirst results from decreased fluid input, excessive fluid loss, or excessive sodium input.

The balance between fluid input and fluid output is maintained within a narrow range, unless body dysfunction causes an imbalance.

Mechanisms regulating fluid and electrolyte balance

Homeostatic regulation of the body's fluid volume, electrolyte concentration, and the electrolyte composition of body fluids is maintained by the cardiovascular system, the kidneys, the pituitary gland, the lungs, the parathyroid glands, the adrenal glands, and the hypothalamus.

- The cardiovascular system provides the kidneys with sufficient plasma to allow regulation of water and electrolyte content of body fluids. The volume of urine filtered by the kidneys is decreased as a result of decreased blood pressure caused by cardiovascular dysfunction.
- The kidneys maintain the volume and regulate the acid-base balance of extracellular fluid through selective reabsorption of water and electrolytes, and through the removal of waste.
- The pituitary gland secretes an antidiuretic hormone (ADH) which stimulates reabsorption of water in the renal tubules, and secretes a diuretic hormone which directly increases urine output.
- The lungs maintain the composition of the blood's oxygen and carbon dioxide levels, and therefore play an important role in regulating the acid-base balance in extracellular fluid. The lungs also influence the loss of fluid through ventilation.
- The parathyroid glands maintain the level of ionized calcium in the blood and regulate calcium and phosphorous metabolism.
- The adrenal glands secrete hormones, e.g. aldosterone, which promote reabsorption of sodium and water, and the excretion of potassium.
- The hypothalamus influences the production of pituitary hormones, and therefore indirectly plays an important role in body fluid balance and electrolyte content.

Maintenance of acid-base balance

Acid-base balance depend on the hydrogen ion concentration in body fluids. A balance exists when the rate at which the body produces acids or bases equals the rate at which acids or bases are excreted. The result is a stable concentration of hydrogen ions in body fluids.

Normally the body's internal fluid environment is maintained at a pH of 7.35–7.45 by the buffering capacity of the body fluids. A buffer is a chemical substance that prevents changes in pH by neutralizing added acids or bases. A simple buffer consists of a weak acid and its salt. Reaction of the buffer with hydronium ions produces more of the acidic component, while the addition of base results in formation of more of the acid salt. Basic physiologic processes produce an excess of acid, and to keep the acidity of body fluids at a constant level, acid must be eliminated and base must be conserved. For example, CO_2 is an end product of metabolism and frequently combines with water to form carbonic acid ($CO_2 + H_2O = H_2CO_3$). Excess carbonic acid is decomposed into carbon dioxide and water which are excreted, and a change in pH is prevented. Conversely, if hydronium ions are being lost from the blood, they are replaced by the ionization of carbonic acid and a rise in pH is prevented. An example of the buffering action of bicarbonate ion is its reaction with lactic acid. Lactic acid is produced from glucose during muscle contraction, and the dissociation of lactic acid tends to lower the pH. As lactic acid is stronger than carbonic acid, its conjugate base (lactic ion) is weaker. The stronger base (bicarbonate ion) combines with the hydrogen from lactic acid forming dissociated carbonic acid.

The renal, respiratory, and circulatory buffer systems act

as part of the body's response to rid itself of carbonic and other acids. An acid-base imbalance occurs where there is a deficit or excess of carbonic acid or base bicarbonate. When the body is subjected to stress, e.g. prolonged muscle contraction, the buffer system may be unable to keep the pH within the normal range. If the pH rises above 7.45 the condition is called *alkalosis*, and if the ph falls below 7.35 the condition is called *acidosis*.

Alkalosis results from accumulation of base, or loss of acid without comparable loss of base, and is characterized by a decrease in hydrogen ion concentration.

Acidosis results from accumulation of acid or depletion of alkaline reserve (bicarbonate content), and is characterized by an increase in hydrogen ion concentration.

Factors affecting fluid and electrolyte balance

There are several factors that may disturb the body's fluid and electrolyte balance resulting in overhydration or underhydration. Imbalances can be categorized into two types of conditions according to the cause, as follows:

1. a deficit or excess of essential body substances such as water, sodium, potassium, or calcium.
2. an abnormal shift of fluid from one fluid compartment to another.

Water deficit syndromes result from either water depletion or extracellular solute excess, and both cause cell shrinkage and dehydration. The causes include:

- decreased input of fluids
- increased output of fluids, e.g. due to diarrhoea, vomiting, excessive urine output, hyperventilation, excessive perspiration, prolonged fever, burns or haemorrhage.
- excess of solutes, e.g. due to uncontrolled diabetes mellitus with hyperglycaemia, or excessive intravenous administration of glucose or sodium bicarbonate.

Water excess syndromes result from either fluid overload or solute deficit, and both result in cellular oedema. The causes include:

- excessive ingestion of water in a short time
- excessive administration of intravenous fluids
- disturbance of the homeostatic mechanisms, e.g. water retention resulting from kidney failure
- insufficient sodium, e.g. due to a low salt diet or diuretic medications.

Fluid volume imbalance occur as a result of the movement of sodium and water between the plasma and the interstitial fluid, and include:

- extracellular volume depletion caused by a shift of sodium and water from the plasma to interstitial fluid. This condition can result from severe burns, fever, haemorrhage, diarrhoea, or vomiting.
- extracellular volume excess caused by a shift of sodium and water from the interstitial fluid to the plasma. This condition can result from cardiac, renal, or hepatic failure, or excessive intravenous administration of normal saline.

When fluids are lost or retained in excessive amounts there is an accompanying loss or retention of electrolytes, so that both fluid and electrolyte balances are disturbed. As a result of fluid and electrolyte imbalance:

- The cells do not receive adequate nourishment
- There is an accumulation of waste products due to inefficiency of the mechanism for their removal
- The acid-base balance is upset
- Temperature regulation is impaired
- Activities that depend on the transmission of electrical energy, e.g. muscle contraction, are impaired.

NURSING PRACTICE AND MEETING FLUID AND ELECTROLYTE NEEDS

Assessment of an individual's fluid and electrolyte status is essential so that appropriate care can be planned to prevent or correct an imbalance. Assessment is made by obtaining information from the individual about his usual pattern of fluid input and output. The nurse should ascertain the types of fluid he prefers and the amount he usually consumes. She should also note any recent alterations in his intake of fluids, or loss of fluids through, e.g. vomiting or diarrhoea. The nurse should observe for early signs of fluid retention or dehydration so that appropriate therapy can be implemented. Information on the signs and symptoms of fluid retention and dehydration is provided later in this chapter.

Key aspects related to helping an individual to meet his fluid and electrolyte needs, and therefore maintain fluid balance are:

- ensuring an adequate intake of fluid and food
- monitoring his fluid input and output
- observing for the signs and symptoms of imbalance.

Ensuring an adequate intake of fluid and food

In order to maintain normal fluid and electrolyte balance, adequate nutrition is essential. Information on helping an individual to meet his nutritional needs is provided in Chapter 29.

Sufficient fluid intake must be maintained throughout all stages of development in the life cycle. Infants and young children have a higher percentage of total body water than adults, and a higher metabolic rate, therefore they require a larger fluid intake proportional to body weight. In adolescence there is maturing of all body systems, and the homeostatic mechanisms that regulate fluid and electrolyte balance begin to function as they do in adulthood. With increasing age there is a gradual decrease in efficiency of the fluid and electrolyte regulating mechanisms. As a result, the older person recovers more slowly from an imbalance than does a younger person.

Fluid requirements increase in response to various factors including a high environmental temperature, strenuous physical activity, fever, and body dysfunction, e.g. burns or prolonged vomiting. Fluid input may need to be restricted to below the normal daily requirements as part of the management of specific renal or cardiac diseases. If fluid intake is unrestricted, the nurse should ensure that an individual is provided with adequate amounts. Some people may need encouragement to consume sufficient fluid, and assistance should be provided for a person who experiences any difficulty in pouring fluid or holding a cup or glass.

A person may be required to increase his normal daily fluid requirements, and the consumption of copious amounts of fluid may be prescribed. For example if a person's fluid output exceeds his fluid input, extra fluids may be prescribed to correct the negative fluid balance. A person may be encouraged to drink at least 3000 ml in a twenty four hour period by:

- explaining the importance of consuming increased amounts
- providing the types of fluids preferred and presenting a variety
- ensuring that all fluids are presented attractively
- advising him to drink small amounts of fluid at frequent intervals
- ensuring that approximately 75% of the total volume of fluid is taken by early evening so his sleep is undisturbed
- ensuring that toilet facilities are easily accessible.

An individual may be required to restrict his daily intake of fluids to 1500 ml or less, and it is important that the specified amount is known by him and all those involved in his care. For example, a person who is experiencing retention of fluid may have a reduced fluid intake prescribed as part of his management. He may be assisted to restrict his fluid intake by:

- explaining the importance of consuming restricted amounts
- planning to distribute the fluid evenly throughout the day, ensuring that an adequate amount is reserved for his needs during the night
- encouraging him to drink small amounts at regular intervals to avoid thirst
- providing thirst quenching fluids, e.g. fruit juice, and avoiding sweetened drinks that increase thirst

- ensuring, by regular attention to oral hygiene, that his mouth does not become dry.

If not contra-indicated, the individual may be permitted to suck acid sweets or chew gum to stimulate production of saliva and thereby keep the mouth moist.

When a person is required to drink either copious or restricted fluids, it is important to construct a plan which indicates the distribution of fluid throughout the 24 hour period. Documentation of input and output is necessary to assess his fluid balance status.

Monitoring fluid input and ouput

It may be necessary to monitor fluid input and output if an individual has an existing or potential problem related to fluid balance. Fluid status may be monitored by weighing him daily, by measuring and recording his fluid input and output, and by observing for the signs and symptoms of imbalance.

Weighing

Weighing, together with maintaining a record of fluid input and output, is a commonly used method of assessing fluid status. Weight gain results when fluid input exceeds fluid output and, conversely, weight loss occurs when fluid output exceeds fluid input. 1 ml of water weighs 1 g, therefore if a person's fluid intake exceeds his fluid output by 1000 ml in 24 hours, his body weight will increase by approximately 1000 g (1 kg).

The individual should be weighed daily at the same time, wearing the same type of clothing, and using the same set of scales. Weight can be measured with a standing, chair, or bed scale; and the measurement should be recorded on the appropriate form.

Fluid balance charts

The function of a fluid balance chart (Fig. 31.1) is to show an accurate record of all fluid input and output over a 24 hour period. Accurate recording is essential as this record may be used to assess the individual's condition and progress, and as a guide for prescribing treatment. Key aspects related to maintaining an accurate record of fluid balance are:

- Measuring all fluids in millilitres (ml).
- Measuring and recording the total amounts of all fluid input, including fluids taken orally and those administered by an alternative route, e.g. intravenously.
- Measuring and recording the total amounts of all fluid output. It is possible to measure accurately urine, vomitus, gastric aspirate, and wound drainage if the individual has a drain tube connected to a bag or bottle. Although signi-

24 HOUR FLUID BALANCE CHART

Date:				Ward:						(Identification label)				
			INPUT							OUTPUT				
Time	OR	E	IV	IV	IV			Time	U	G/A	V	W	O	
Totals								Totals						
	Total intake =					ml			Total output =				ml	

Total 24 hr 12 M.N balance = ml±

KEY: Or = Oral
        E = Enteral
        IV = Intravenous

U   = Urine
G/A = Gastric aspirate
V   = Vomitus
W   = Wound drainage
O   = Other (specify)

Fig. 31.1 Sample 24-hour fluid balance chart.

ficant amounts of fluid may be lost in faeces, perspiration, incontinent episodes, and into wound dressings, it is not possible to measure these losses accurately. Instead, an explanatory note is entered on the chart.

• Recording measurements on the chart immediately fluids have been administered or excreted, to avoid omission or errors.

• Requesting an ambulant person to use a bedpan or urinal so that his urine output can be measured. A female who also wishes to use her bowels should be provided with two bedpans, so that an accurate measurement of her urine

may be more easily obtained.

• Emptying and measuring urine from urinary drainage bags at regular intervals, e.g. every four hours.

• Recording each entry in the appropriate column on the chart.

• Determining the total input and output in a given period, by adding up the columns at the end of 24 hours.

• Indicating on the chart whether there is a negative or positive fluid balance. If the total output exceeds the input there is a negative balance, and conversely, a positive fluid balance occurs when the total input exceeds the output.

Observing for signs and symptoms of imbalance

The individual is observed for signs or symptoms that indicate a fluid and electrolyte imbalance, which can result in either overhydration or underhydration.

Overhydration is an excess of water in the body and may result from an increased fluid input or a decreased fluid output, e.g. due to a specific cardiac or renal disease. Cellular oedema occurs which results in:

- rapid weight gain
- peripheral and periorbital oedema
- bounding pulse and distended neck veins, due to an increased volume of fluid in the blood
- diluted urine that has a low specific gravity
- headaches, and sometimes personality changes, due to cerebral oedema
- shortness of breath, and sometimes pulmonary rales.

The excess fluid in the body may accumulate in the lungs (pulmonary oedema), in the peritoneal cavity (ascites), or in dependent parts of the body. Body parts where dependent oedema is likely to occur are related to the individual's position. For example, in a recumbent position fluid tends to accumulate in the sacral area which is the lowest point. If the person is sitting in a chair, the lower legs and feet will become oedematous. If oedematous tissue remains indented following digital pressure, the condition is referred to as 'pitting' oedema.

Underhydration (or dehydration) is a deficit of water in the body and may result from a decreased fluid input, an increased fluid output, or the inability of the kidneys to concentrate urine. Cellular dehydration occurs which results in:

- loss of weight
- dry skin and loss of tissue turgor
- elevated temperature and lowered blood pressure
- thirst
- sunken eyes
- sunken anterior fontanelle in a baby
- dry mouth and tongue
- oliguria, with concentrated urine which has an increased specific gravity
- irritability and confusion.

Nursing management of an individual with fluid and electrolyte imbalance

As previously described, the major manifestations of fluid and electrolyte imbalance are overhydration or underhydration. When either of these conditions occur, nursing care must be planned and implemented to help restore homeostasis and to promote comfort.

Care of an individual with fluid retention

Oedema impairs the function of cells and vital organs and increases the possibility of cell death. The accumulation of excess fluid makes oedematous tissue vulnerable to pressure and damage. Key aspects related to the care of an individual with oedema are:

- The implementation of prescribed treatment of the underlying disease process that is causing retention of fluid. Nursing actions may include administration of prescribed medications such as diuretics which promote the formation and excretion of urine.
- Restricting fluid input until homeostasis has been achieved.
- Monitoring his fluid status by measuring and recording all fluid input and output, and by weighing him daily.
- Placing him in a position of comfort and, where possible, elevating the oedematous part to facilitate fluid drainage.
- Maintaining skin integrity. As oedema can restrict blood circulation and therefore lead to the formation of decubitus ulcers, his position should be changed every two to four hours. Pressure-relieving devices, e.g. a sheepskin, may be used to reduce pressure on oedematous areas. Oedematous parts of the body should be handled and moved carefully to avoid skin damage.
- Ensuring that he receives a restricted sodium diet if prescribed. If sodium intake is reduced, the sodium and water already in the tissues tend to enter the blood to be excreted in the urine, and thus oedema is reduced.

The nurse should continue to assess the individual's fluid status in order to evaluate the effectiveness of the actions that have been implemented.

Care of an individual with fluid deficit

Excessive loss of fluid from the body causes dehydration. Dehydration, which occurs as a result of a variety of disorders, may be mild and readily corrected by oral fluid replacement; or may be severe leading to shock, acidosis, and the accumulation of waste products. Key aspects related to the care of an individual with dehydration are:

- The implementation of prescribed treatment of the underlying disease process that is causing dehydration. Nursing actions may include administration of prescribed medications, e.g. anti-emetics to prevent vomiting.
- Replacing lost fluids as prescribed. Oral fluids are administered if tolerated, but in some instances intravenous administration will be necessary. Information on intravenous therapy is provided later in this chapter.
- Monitoring his fluid status by measuring and recording all fluid input and output.

● Maintaining the integrity of skin and mucous membrane. The skin and mucous membranes become dry and are more susceptible to breakdown, therefore careful attention to his skin and oral hygiene needs is essential.

Two of the common causes of dehydration are excess loss of fluid through vomiting and diarrhoea. Information on the care of an individual who is vomiting is provided in Chapter 29, while information on care of an individual who has diarrhoea is provided in Chapter 30.

Maintenance of fluid and electrolyte balance is essential for homeostasis, and when an imbalance occurs actions must be taken to restore homeostasis. The major sources of fluid and electrolytes are the foods and fluids a person consumes, and if a mild imbalance occurs adjustments to the diet or fluid intake may be sufficient to rectify the imbalance.

If the loss of fluid and electrolytes is too great to be corrected by oral intake, or if the ingestion of substances orally is contra-indicated, administration by an alternative route is necessary. Intravenous infusion into a peripheral vein can provide the individual with the fluids and electrolytes necessary to maintain normal body function. Intravascular therapy may also be used to administer nutrients parenterally (TPN), blood or blood products, and drugs. Information on TPN is provided in Chapter 29, and information on drug administration is provided in Chapter 58. This chapter addresses the techniques involved in the intravenous administration of fluids and electrolytes.

Intravenous therapy

Management of an individual who is receiving intravenous therapy is the responsibility of the registered nurse, and part of her role is to maintain the intravenous equipment and to prevent complications occurring during the infusion.

Insertion of an intravenous infusion is performed by a medical officer, but as the nursing care of an individual with an infusion is an important function, it is the nurse's responsibility to be fully aware of the nursing regulations and policies regarding all aspects of intravenous therapy.

The medical officer inserting the intravenous infusion first assesses the individual to select the most appropriate insertion site. The choice of site is dependent on several factors, including the condition of the person's veins and consideration of his general comfort. A vein in the non-dominant arm is commonly used and the infusion is not inserted in a limb that is oedematous or otherwise impaired. If the site chosen is near a joint, extension of the limb by splinting may be necessary. A site which is commonly selected is one of the superficial veins on the back of the hand.

The medical officer determines the type and amount of fluid to be administered according to the needs of the individual. Intravenous solutions are packaged in plastic containers which collapse as they empty, or in glass bottles which require an airway to vent the bottle as the fluid runs through the tubing to the person. There are several types of fluids which can be administered intravenously, and most consist of water with added glucose and electrolytes such as sodium chloride, potassium, calcium, or sodium bicarbonate.

Types of intravenous solutions

Isotonic. These solutions do not promote osmosis, but increase the extracellular fluid volume. Two examples of isotonic solutions are 0.9% w/v sodium chloride solution, and 5% w/v glucose solution.

Hypotonic. These solutions promote osmosis of some of the water in extracellular fluid into the cells. An example of a hypotonic solution is sodium chloride solution of less than 0.9% w/v concentration.

Hypertonic. These solutions promote osmosis of water out of the cells into the extracellular fluid. An example of a hypertonic solution is sodium chloride solution of greater than 0.9% w/v concentration.

Insertion of a peripheral intravenous infusion

Equipment. As there is a variety of equipment available for the intravenous administration of fluids and electrolytes, the nurse should refer to the institution's policy manual for information about the type of equipment currently in use. The basic equipment necessary for the insertion of a peripheral intravenous infusion includes:

— flask or bottle of intravenous solution
— pole or stand to hang the flask
— intravenous administration set
— selection of intravenous needles, catheters and cannulae
— skin preparation (antiseptic and swabs)
— local anaesthetic, syringe, and needle
— gauze swabs
— hypoallergenic tape
— scissors
— arm board and bandage
— tourniquet.

Procedure. Prior to the insertion of the infusion, the nurse should ensure that the individual is positioned comfortably with the insertion site exposed. She should ensure that adequate lighting is available, and that all the equipment has been assembled in a convenient location. The nurse's hands should be thoroughly washed and dried, in preparation for assisting the medical officer with the equipment. The information on the label of the intravenous solution container must be checked carefully to confirm the correct infusion. The nurse must adhere to the nursing regulations and policies which relate to the checking of intravenous solutions. The procedure is performed using aseptic technique and sterile equipment.

The administration tubing is attached to the flask which is then hung on the pole or stand. A small quantity of fluid from the container is run through the tubing, then the tubing is clamped. The torniquet is applied approximately 10–20 cm above the intended puncture site to dilate the vein. The site is prepared by swabbing the skin with antiseptic. Sometimes the medical officer will inject local anaesthetic into the area surrounding the site prior to inserting the infusion. The intravenous needle, cannula, or catheter is inserted into the vein and once its position has been verified, the torniquet is released and the tubing connected. The clamp is released and the rate at which the solution is to flow is established. The needle and tubing are attached to the skin with hypoallergenic tape. If necessary the limb may be supported on a board which is secured in position with a bandage. A board is commonly used when the puncture site is close to a movable joint, to provide stability and reduce the risk of the needle becoming dislodged.

The flow rate may be controlled by use of the clamp, or by threading the tubing through a peristaltic pump which can be set to deliver the fluid at a predetermined rate. Once the infusion has been established the nurse should promote the individual's comfort. He should be positioned comfortably, and if necessary the limb in which the infusion is inserted should be supported on a pillow. His signal device and other items he may require should be easily accessible. Superfluous equipment is removed and attended to in the appropriate manner. The procedure is documented, recording details that include the type and flow rate of the intravenous solution.

Care of an individual with an intravenous infusion

The nurse caring for the individual has a responsibility to promote his general comfort, to ensure that the infusion is administered as prescribed, and to observe for and prevent complications. Key aspects related to the care of an individual with an intravenous infusion are described in the next paragraphs.

• Ensuring that the flow rate is set as prescribed and adjusted when necessary, to deliver the correct amount of fluid within the prescribed time. Various methods of determining the number of millilitres per minute are used, in order to distribute the total amount of solution equally over the time period prescribed for the infusion.

A calibrated burette or microdrip volume control set may be incorporated into the infusion system. Such devices enable very small or precise amounts of fluid to be administered, and may also be used when medications are to be given intravenously.

A formula is used to determine the number of drops per minute at which the solution should flow. To calculate the flow rate, the formula used is:

$$\frac{Volume\ of\ infusion\ (in\ ml)}{Time\ of\ infusion\ (in\ minutes)} \times drops\ per\ ml = drops\ per\ minute$$

When calculating the rate it is essential to know the calibration of the drip rate for each manufacturer's product, as these vary from 10 drops per ml to 60 drops per ml.

The flow rate should be checked every 15 minutes until it is stable, then every hour, or at the time intervals specified in the institution's policy on intravenous infusions.

• Checking the level of solution to determine the volume of fluid in the flask. It is important to ensure that a flask does not empty completely, as this permits air to enter the tubing which could lead to an air embolism.

An air embolism results in decreased blood pressure, rapid weak pulse, cyanosis, and loss of consciousness.

• Checking the insertion site for signs of inflammation or infiltration. Infection at the insertion site can occur and is indicated by redness, swelling and tenderness. The vein may become injured or irritated and phlebitis may occur. Signs and symptoms which indicate phlebitis are pain, swelling, and inflammation along the course of the vein. The vein feels hard and warm to touch. Infiltration occurs if the needle becomes displaced causing intravenous solution to flow into the surrounding tissues. Signs and symptoms of infiltration are cool skin in the site area, swelling and discomfort at the site, oedema of the limb, sluggish flow rate, and absence of blood in the tubing when it is lowered.
• Checking the tubing for air bubbles that can interfere with the flow rate; if large quantities of air enter the vein an air embolus may result.
• Observing the individual for signs of overhydration or circulatory overload, caused by excessive or too rapid fluid administration. Signs and symptoms of circulatory overload are elevated blood pressure, venous dilation especially of the neck veins, rapid ventilations and shortness of breath.
• Checking the information on the label of the flask when a new flask is being commenced. It is essential that the individual receives the prescribed solution, therefore the nurse should follow the nursing protocol regarding checking of intravenous solutions.

The type, volume, and expiry date of the solution is checked. Glass containers are inspected for chips and cracks and the seal over the opening is observed to ascertain if it is intact. Plastic containers should be squeezed gently to detect leaks. The solution is examined for particles, abnormal discolouration, and cloudiness. The container is not used if there are any deviations from normal.

• Documenting, throughout the course of the infusion, details of the flow rate, the type and amount of fluid being administered, and the individual's fluid output. The vital signs (temperature, pulse, ventilations, and blood pressure) are also measured regularly and documented.

Nurses must be aware of the scope of their role in relation to the management of intravenous infusions. Of prime importance is careful observation of the individual and the intravenous equipment used during the infusion, and accurate reporting of the observations to the nurse in charge.

The complications that may occur when an individual has an intravenous infusion, and which must be recognized and reported immediately, are:

• a flow rate which is too slow or too fast, or cessation of flow
• infection or infiltration at the insertion site
• phlebitis of the vein being used for the infusion
• circulatory overload
• air embolism.

Discontinuation of an intravenous infusion. An intravenous infusion is discontinued when ordered by the medical officer on completion of therapy, if infection or infiltration occurs, or if it is necessary to recommence the infusion in another site. The flow of solution is stopped and all tape removed from the individual's skin. The needle is gently and smoothly withdrawn from the vein, a swab placed over the insertion site, and digital pressure applied until the bleeding stops. The site is cleansed with antiseptic and an adhesive bandage applied. The tip of the needle, cannula, or catheter, is inspected and may be sent for culture in the laboratory if this forms part of the institution's policy. The appearance of the insertion site and the time the infusion was discontinued are documented.

SUMMARY

An essential part of the body's homeostatic processes is the maintenance of fluid and electrolyte balance. Water is distributed throughout the body as either intracellular fluid or extracellular fluid.

Body fluids and electrolytes are constantly moving between the two fluid compartments through the processes of osmosis, active transport, and diffusion.

Water and electrolytes are obtained from the ingestion of fluids and food, and water is also obtained from the oxidation of food during metabolism. Fluid is normally lost from the body in urine, faeces, perspiration, and expired air.

The body's regulating mechanisms maintain fluid balance within a normal range. Body dysfunction can cause an imbalance resulting in either overhydration or underhydration.

Assessment of fluid and electrolyte status is necessary for the planning and implementation of appropriate nursing care.

The nurse assists the individual to meet his fluid and electrolyte needs by ensuring an adequate intake of food and fluid and by monitoring his fluid input and output. The nurse should recognize the signs and symptoms of fluid and electrolyte imbalance, and understand the key aspects of caring for an individual with an imbalance.

Certain individuals may need either more of less than the normal amounts of fluid, and patients who are unable to have fluids orally may require an intravenous infusion.

The nurse caring for an individual with an infusion must be aware of the extent of her role and function, in order to promote safety and comfort during insertion and while the infusion is in progress. Continued assessment of the individual and his need for fluids and electrolytes is made, so that appropriate nursing actions may be planned, implemented and evaluated.

32. Meeting oxygen needs

OBJECTIVES

1. State the factors necessary for an adequate supply of oxygen to the cells.
2. State the factors that affect respiratory function.
3. Describe the observations to be made of the ventilations.
4. Identify the deviations from normal ventilation.
5. Demonstrate the ability to measure, report on, and document ventilations accurately.
6. Apply relevant principles in the planning and implementation of nursing actions to assist the patient receiving oxygen therapy.

INTRODUCTION

Oxygen, which is a colourless and odourless gas, makes up approximately 20% of the atmosphere, and is essential in sustaining most forms of life. Every cell in the human body requires oxygen for metabolism, and must get rid of the metabolic waste product—carbon dioxide. The intake of oxygen and the elimination of carbon dioxide is achieved through the respiratory system, and further information about the structure and function of this system is provided in Chapter 22. The respiratory system delivers oxygen from the atmosphere to the blood stream, and carbon dioxide from the blood stream to the atmosphere, through the act of breathing or ventilation.

The cardiovascular system is the means by which the gases are transported to and from the cells. From the lungs oxygen, in combination with haemoglobin, is transpsorted in the blood to the cells. Carbon dioxide from the cells is transported in the blood to the lungs for excretion.

During breathing the lungs inflate and deflate approximately 20 times every minute. Inspiration of air occurs as the diaphragm contracts and flattens, thus enlarging the thoracic cavity. At the same time the ribs are pulled up and outward by the action of the intercostal muscles. As the chest expands air enters the lungs. Exhalation occurs as the ventilatory muscles relax and the chest returns to its minimum size, thus expelling air from the lungs.

Respiration is the exchange of oxygen and carbon dioxide. External respiration is the exchange of oxygen and carbon dioxide between the external environment and the blood, by the process of diffusion in the lungs. Internal respiration is the exchange of oxygen and carbon dioxide between the blood and the body tissues, by the process of diffusion between the capillaries and the cell membrane. The mechanisms whereby oxygen and carbon dioxide are exchanged are illustrated in Figures 22.2 and 22.5.

Factors necessary for respiration

The passage of oxygen from the atmosphere to the alveoli in the lungs and the passage of carbon dioxide from the alveoli to the atmosphere, requires an unobstructed airway. In addition, the entire process of respiration requires:

- adequate oxygen in the atmosphere
- a functioning respiratory tract
- functioning thoracic muscles and nerves to control the thoracic cage
- blood to transport the gases
- capillaries in close proximity to the cells to allow the exchange of gases.

Regulation of ventilation

The automatic control of breathing stems from the respiratory centres located in the brain stem. From these sites, impulses travel along the spinal cord to the nerves that control the diaphragm and intercostal muscles. Reflex responses and chemical signals control these nerve centres and thus the rate of breathing. During actions such as speaking and swallowing, impulses from the throat are conveyed to the respiratory centre and breathing stops temporarily. The chemical control of breathing is mainly dependent on the level of carbon dioxide in the blood. The presence of excess carbon dioxide causes the ventilatory rate to increase until the excess carbon dioxide is eliminated. Conversely, a decreased carbon dioxide level slows the ventilatory rate.

Factors affecting respiratory function

Factors that affect the process of respiration include:

1. Availability of oxygen

Oxygen makes up 20% of the air and normally this is sufficient to meet the needs of the body, but a decrease in this amount of oxygen can cause problems. Two instances where the available oxygen may be deficient are:

High altitude. The total pressure of all gases in the air decreases at high altitude. As the total pressure decreases, the oxygen pressure decreases proportionately, and the individual will experience difficulty in obtaining adequate oxygen until he becomes acclimatized. As a result, the ventilatory rate is increased in an attempt to supply the body with sufficient oxygen.

The presence of noxious gases. Noxious gases in the air displace the oxygen, and reduce the amount normally available for inspiration.

2. Regulating mechanisms

Any factor that interferes with the control mechanisms for breathing may cause ventilatory difficulties. Ventilations may be depressed by factors that reduce the activity of the respiratory centre, e.g. cerebral oedema, or medications such as morphine. Ventilations will be increased when the pH of the blood is lowered, as a respiratory response to rid the body of the excess acid.

3. Passage of oxygen and carbon dioxide

The efficiency of respiration can be affected by any factor that obstructs the patency of the respiratory tract or the actions of the ventilatory muscles. For example, an accumulation of secretions resulting from a reduced cough reflex. Ventilations may be reduced by factors which affect the actions of the ventilatory muscles; for example, injury or disease which restricts the movements of the diaphragm.

4. Diffusion of oxygen and carbon dioxide

Any dysfunction of the lungs e.g. pulmonary oedema, asthma, or chronic obstructive airways disease may impede the transfer of oxygen and carbon dioxide.

Information on these, and other, respiratory disorders is provided in Chapter 45.

5. Transport of oxygen and carbon dioxide to and from the cells

Any condition affecting the efficiency of the heart, the blood vessels, or the blood, can interfere with the transportation of oxygen to the cells and carbon dioxide away from the cells. Such conditions include congestive cardiac failure, atherosclerosis, and anaemia.

Information on these, and other, cardiovascular disorders is provided in Chapter 44.

6. Influences on the rate, depth, and rhythm of breathing

A number of factors influence the characteristics of breathing, e.g. the degree of physical activity. Oxygen requirements are greatest during exertion and least during sleep. The ventilatory rate and depth vary in response to the body's demand for oxygen, e.g. during strenuous exercise the volume of air drawn into the lungs with each breath may be increased from the usual 500 ml to as much as 4000 ml. Changes in mood or emotion may also affect the rate, depth, and rhythm of ventilation. For example the ventilation rate is commonly increased during anxiety, pain, or anger. Smoking also affects breathing and often causes short term effects such as coughing and shortness of breath, or long term effects such as severe dyspnoea resulting from emphysema.

NURSING PRACTICE AND OXYGEN NEEDS

Assessment of an individual's respiratory status is made to ascertain whether he is receiving an adequate supply of oxygen to meet his body's needs. Assessment is made by observing him for signs and symptoms of an inadequate oxygen supply, identifying any deviations from normal, and by assessing his ventilations. Assessment of his respiratory status, and the identification of any actual or potential problems, is assisted by obtaining information from the individual regarding:

- allergic reactions, such as coughing, sneezing, or shortness of breath, that occur as a result of exposure to allergens such as dust, pet hairs, or pollen
- exposure to environmental air pollutants such as chemical wastes
- smoking habits
- presence of a cough and/or the production of sputum
- chest pain.

It is important to observe the skin colour for signs of *cyanosis*. Cyanosis is a bluish discolouration of the skin and mucous membranes due to inadequate oxygenation, and can be either peripheral or central. Peripheral cyanosis is caused by local vasoconstriction and is usually visible only in the nail beds and sometimes the lips. Central cyanosis is the result of prolonged hypoxia and affects all body organs. It is most visible in highly vascular areas such as the lips, nail beds, tip of the nose, the external ear, and the underside of the tongue. In people with naturally dark brown or black skin, cyanosis can be most readily detected by inspecting the mucosa inside the lips.

The individual should be observed for signs and symptoms of *hypoxia*, which is a diminished availability of oxygen to the body tissues. Hypoxia may result from disorders that limit the volume of air entering the lungs, or from obstructive lung diseases such as asthma and emphysema. The signs and symptoms of hypoxia, and respiratory distress, include:

- elevated blood pressure and pulse rate
- shortness of breath and fatigue
- cyanosis
- abnormal ventilations
- use of accessory muscles during breathing and flaring of the nares
- retraction of the sternum and intercostal muscles
- apprehension or agitation
- confusion or reduced level of consciousness
- visible perspiration.

A person who has a chronic respiratory disorder should also be observed for a barrel shaped chest, which is a thoracic deformity commonly associated with chronic obstructive airways disease. When chronic hypoxia exists the individual experiences general fatigue, intolerance to exercise, and may have clubbing of the fingers. (The mechanism whereby diminished oxygen tension in the blood causes finger clubbing is not well understood.)

Assessment of ventilations

Assessment of ventilations, provides information about the individual's respiratory status and aids in the evaluation of airway patency, the status of the ventilatory muscles, and the individual's metabolic state. Patients have their ventilations assessed, together with the other vital signs, when they are admitted to hospital. The frequency with which ventilations are subsequently assessed depends on how closely the patient's condition needs to be monitored. Residents in long term care facilities commonly have their ventilations assessed less often than acutely ill patients whose condition may need to be monitored at intervals ranging from every 30 minutes to 6 times a day.

Ventilations are assessed without the person's knowledge, by noting the rise and fall of his chest. If an individual is aware that his ventilations are being assessed, he will become conscious of them and may unintentionally change their character. The nurse may assess the ventilations by observing the person, or by placing her hand on his chest to feel the rise and fall. To avoid making the person aware that his ventilations are being assessed, the nurse may place her fingers on his radial pulse site and continue as if she were counting the pulse.

Normal ventilation

Ventilations are assessed for rate, rhythm, depth, and sound.

1. Rate. The ventilatory rate is the number of ventilations per minute. One inhalation and one exhalation equals one ventilation. The rate of ventilation varies according to age, level of activity, and emotions. The normal ventilatory rates according to age are approximately:

- 28–40 ventilations per minute for an infant
- 20–28 ventilations per minute for a child
- 16–20 ventilations per minute for an adult.

2. Rhythm. The rhythm of ventilation is the pattern or regularity of breathing. Normal ventilations are evenly spaced with little variation from one breath to another.

3. Depth. Depth of ventilations depends on the volume of air being inhaled and exhaled with each ventilation. The depth should be constant with each breath, and is assessed by observing the patient's chest movement for adequate expansion. Ventilations are described as being normal, shallow, or deep.

4. Sound. Normal ventilations are inaudible.

A suggested procedure to assess ventilations is outlined in the guidelines.

Abnormal ventilation

Many factors may cause alterations to the rate, rhythm, depth, and sound of ventilations and deviation from the normal pattern.

1. Rate. An increase in the rate above normal is called *tachypnoea* and may occur as a result of:

- physical exercise
- states such as fear, pain, anxiety, excitement, or anger,
- disease states such as fever, infection, respiratory disorder, thyrotoxicosis, congestive cardiac failure.

A decrease in the rate below normal is called *bradypnoea* and may occur as a result of:

- absolute rest or sleep
- trauma to the brain, uraemia, diabetic coma, or medications that depress the respiratory centre, e.g. morphine.

2. Rhythm. The normal regular pattern of breathing may be altered by a variety of disease states. In obstructive

Guidelines for assessing ventilations
Nursing action

1. Ensure that the individual is resting in a position of comfort

2. Using a watch with a second hand, and without the person's knowledge, count the ventilations for 1 minute
   While measuring the rate, also observe the rhythm, depth, and sound of ventilations

3. Document the time of measurement, and the rate and character of the ventilations on the appropriate chart using numbers or dots
   Report any deviations from normal

Rationale

Exercise or discomfort alters the nature of ventilations

The intervals between ventilations may be inconsistent, and counting for a full minute enables an accurate measurement of rate
A complete assessment of ventilations is necessary

A record of the ventilations provides information about the person's condition to members of the health team
Appropriate care may be planned and implemented

---

airways disease, e.g. asthma, chronic bronchitis, or emphysema, there is a prolonged expiratory phase. In heart failure or increased intracranial pressure Cheyne-Stokes breathing may occur. This is an abnormal pattern characterized by periods of apnoea. The cycle of Cheyne-Stokes breathing begins with slow shallow breaths that gradually increase in depth and rate. Breathing then gradually becomes slower and more shallow culminating in a 10–60 second period without ventilation (apnoea), before the cycle is repeated.

3. Depth. If an individual inhales and exhales only small amounts of air the ventilations are described as shallow.

Hypoventilation is the term used to describe a reduced rate and depth of ventilation, and may occur as a result of a decreased response of the respiratory centre to carbon dioxide, or in respiratory disorders such as bronchitis or atelectasis. Unresolved hypoventilation results in hypoxia and increased amounts of carbon dioxide in the blood.

When large amounts of air are inhaled and exhaled the ventilations are described as deep. Kussmaul's breathing is the term used to describe abnormally deep, very rapid, sighing ventilations. This pattern of breathing may occur as a result of disorders such as renal failure or metabolic acidosis.

Dyspnoea is the term used to describe shortness of breath or difficulty in breathing, and may occur after strenuous exercise (temporarily) or as a result of certain respiratory or cardiac disorders. Dyspnoea is commonly accompanied by hypoventilation or hyperventilation.

Hyperventilation is the term used to describe rapid deep breathing. Sustained hyperventilation, which is sometimes a consequence of extreme anxiety, causes loss of carbon dioxide and a decrease in carbonic acid—so that alkalosis occurs.

Orthopnoea is the term used to describe the condition when an individual must sit up or stand in order to breath deeply or comfortably. The condition occurs in various respiratory or cardiac disorders, e.g. emphysema, pulmonary oedema, and asthma.

Pursed lip breathing is a technique which is commonly employed by an individual with severe dyspnoea or orthopnoea, e.g. as a consequence of emphysema. This technique of breathing funnels expired air through a narrow opening, thus creating a positive back pressure on the airways to keep them open.

4. Sound. Abnormal breath sounds can occur when air passes through narrowed airways or moisture, or when there is inflammation of the lungs or pleura.

- Stertorous breathing. This is the term used to describe laboured ventilations that have a snoring sound, which commonly result from an obstructed airway.
- Wheezing. As a result of narrowed airways, e.g. in asthma, the ventilations sound high pitched and squeaking.
- Rales. When air passes through moisture, e.g. in pulmonary oedema, the ventilations sound bubbly or crackly.
- Rhonchi. As a result of fluid or secretions in the large airways, or if there is narrowing of the large airways, the respirations sound coarse and rattly.
- Stridor. As a result of an obstruction or spasm in the trachea or larynx, e.g. laryngotracheobronchitis (croup), the ventilations have a high pitched musical sound particularly on inspiration.

When the nurse is assessing an individual's breathing, any deviations from normal should be reported immediately so that appropriate actions can be planned and implemented. Ventilation rates are documented, using numbers or dots, on a chart similar to the one illustrated in Figure 33.2.

In certain circumstances an instrument called a spirometer is used to assess pulmonary function, by measuring and recording the volume of inhaled and exhaled air. Information on this technique is provided in Chapter 45.

Meeting an individual's need for oxygen

Breathing is an automatic activity, and normally an adequate supply of fresh air is all that is required to ensure that an individual's need for oxygen is met. However, admission to hospital may affect an individual's normal pattern of breathing. For example, if a person is anxious or unaccustomed to an air conditioned or centrally heated environment, he may experience temporary breathing difficulties. In these instances measures to promote the return of normal breathing include providing the patient with adequate information to allay some of the anxiety of hospitalization. The nurse should also attempt to ensure that the room is ventilated adequately and at a comfortable temperature.

People who experience breathing difficulties due to body dysfunction may require assistance to meet their oxygen needs. As well as other methods used to assist, e.g. correct positioning, individuals who suffer from an oxygen deficiency will commonly require administration of oxygen to supplement that being obtained from the atmosphere.

Administration of oxygen

Oxygen may be administered by cannula (nasal prongs), catheter, mask, or tent, in order to prevent or reverse hypoxia and to improve tissue oxygenation. It is generally agreed that oxygen should be regarded as a drug, therefore the administration of oxygen is prescribed by a medical officer who determines the concentration and the length of time oxygen is to be administered.

To promote the safety and comfort of the individual who is receiving oxygen therapy, the nurse should be aware of certain principles relevant to the administration of oxygen:

• Hypoxia can result from insufficient oxygen, flow or delivery, and the equipment must be checked at regular intervals to ensure that it is functioning properly. If signs or symptoms of hypoxia occur they must be reported immediately, as adjustment to the concentration being administered may be necessary.

• Because oxygen supports combustion, it is essential to implement safety precautions to reduce the risk of fire. Smoking is prohibited in the vicinity, and measures are taken to prevent sparks which may be given off by electrical or mechanical items. Inflammable substances such as oil or alcohol should not be used near or on the oxygen equipment.

• Because oxygen may dry and irritate the mucous membranes, it should be humidified prior to administration.

• Because oxygen cannot be seen or smelt, gauges on the equipment indicate that oxygen is being delivered.

These should be observed closely while oxygen is being administered.

• Because oxygen toxicity may occur, especially if a high concentration of oxygen is being administered, the patient's arterial blood gases are commonly measured during oxygen therapy and the concentration of oxygen adjusted as prescribed.

The nurse must know how to check that the equipment is functioning correctly, how to clean or dispose of the equipment, and how to promote the individual's comfort and safety during oxygen therapy.

Delivery of oxygen

Oxygen which is piped to a wall outlet or, less commonly, is supplied via a portable cylinder, may be delivered to the individual using one of several devices (Fig. 32.1).

1. Nasal cannula. A nasal cannula, or nasal prongs, is made from a soft plastic material and contains two short tubes that fit into the nostrils. It is secured in position by an elastic strap around the back of the head. Because it does not enclose the nose or mouth, the cannula is comfortable and convenient for the person. Before insertion, the cannula is connected to the oxygen supply and the oxygen turned on at a low flow rate. The prongs are inserted following the natural curve of the nostrils, and the elastic

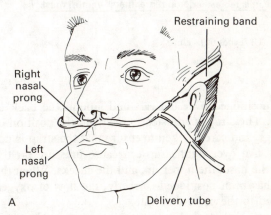

Fig. 32.1 Oxygen delivery devices. (A) Nasal cannula.

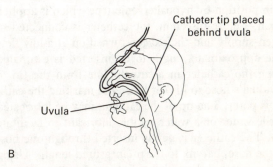

Fig. 32.1 (B) Nasal catheter.

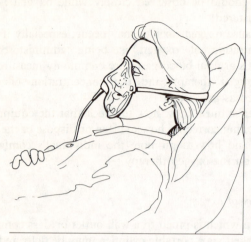

C A plastic oxygen mask

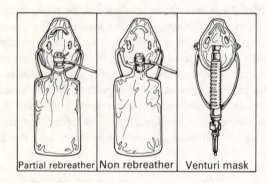

Partial rebreather Non rebreather Venturi mask

Fig. 32.1 (C) Types of face mask.

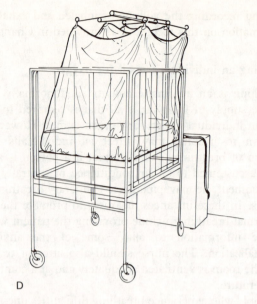

D

Fig. 32.1 (D) Oxygen tent.

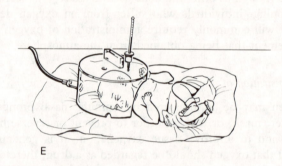

E

Fig. 32.1 (E) Head box (oxyhood).

strap is positioned over the ears and around the back of the head. The strap is adjusted to maintain the position of the prongs, and care is taken to ensure that the strap is not too tight. An over tight strap can cause pressure on the nostrils, the nose, the upper lip, and the cheeks. When the cannula has been positioned correctly, the flow of oxygen is adjusted to the prescribed rate.

2. Nasal catheter. An intranasal oxygen catheter is made from a soft plastic material and contains a series of holes along the sides. It is inserted into one nostril and secured in position by hypoallergenic tape which is applied to the skin. Before insertion, the catheter is connected to the oxygen supply and the oxygen turned on at a low flow rate. The approximate length to be inserted is estimated by holding the catheter in a straight line from the tip of the individual's nose to his ear lobe, and marking the catheter at this point. The tip of the catheter may be lubricated with sterile water or a water soluble lubricant to facilitate insertion. The catheter is gently inserted through one nostril into the nasopharynx to the premeasured length. Using hypoallergenic tape, the catheter is secured to the nose and cheek, avoiding traction on the nostril which could cause

skin breakdown. When the catheter has been positioned correctly, the flow of oxygen is adjusted to the prescribed rate.

As it is an invasive device the catheter may cause irritation of the mucosa, therefore it is usual to remove it after approximately 8 hours and to insert a clean one into the other nostril. Rotating the site reduces the risks of mucous membrane irritation and skin breakdown at the tip of the nose.

3. Face mask. Face masks are available in several styles and sizes. They are made from a lightweight plastic material, fit over the nose and mouth, and are secured in position by an elastic band around the head. As the mask covers both the nose and the mouth, it is confining and impedes activities such as eating, drinking, and speaking. Depending on the style, a mask can deliver up to 100% oxygen concentration, and is commonly used when the patient requires high humidity, precise amounts of oxygen, or is able to breathe only through the mouth. Some of the styles of mask available, as illustrated in Figure 32.1, include the simple mask, partial rebreathing mask, and the

Venturi type mask. The appropriate style and size of mask is selected, connected to the oxygen supply, and the oxygen turned on at a low flow rate. The mask is placed over the nose, mouth, and chin, and the elastic strap secured around the back of the head. The strap is adjusted to ensure that the mask is firmly positioned but not uncomfortable, and the flow of oxygen adjusted to the prescribed rate.

It is important that the mask fits closely but is not uncomfortable, and the nurse should ensure that there is no leakage of oxygen from the top of the mask. Leakage of oxygen from the top of the mask can flow across the eyes, causing dryness and irritation of the delicate tissues.

4. Tent. An oxygen or mist tent such as the 'Croupette' is sometimes used to deliver oxygen and humidity to a child. Tents can be used to deliver oxygen and humidity or humidity only, and are used in place of nasal catheters or face masks which pose difficulties for children. Tents commonly consist of a plastic canopy that fits over the bed. The oxygen supply should be connected to the tent and the flow regulated, before the tent is placed over the bed. The temperature, humidity, and oxygen content of the air inside the tent are controlled. Care should be planned so that opening the tent is reduced to a minimum, as each time the tent is opened the oxygen concentration inside is reduced.

5. Head box. A head box or oxygen hood, which may be used to deliver oxygen to an infant, consists of a transparent plastic box that fits over the head. The infant can be observed easily, and high concentrations of oxygen can be administered.

The concentration of oxygen to be delivered to the individual will be specified by the medical officer, and is dependent on the delivery device used and the rate at which the oxygen flows. Oxygen concentrations vary from approximately 20% to 100%, and the flow rates from 1 litre per minute to 10 litres per minute. The flow rate is adjusted by turning the valve on the flow meter, and observing the dial that indicates the number of litres per minute at which the oxygen is flowing.

Devices used to deliver oxygen are classed as either low flow or high flow. Low flow devices such as the nasal cannula or catheter generally do not provide an exact oxygen concentration. High flow devices such as the 'Venturi mask' can deliver oxygen in precise percentages.

Whenever oxygen is to be administered the nurse should refer to the directions that accompany the device, to ensure that the correct concentration of oxygen is delivered to the individual.

Key aspects related to oxygen therapy

Measures to promote the comfort and safety of the person who is receiving oxygen include:

● Constantly monitoring the equipment to ensure that it is functioning correctly. The nurse should check the flow rate and ensure that the prescribed concentration of oxygen is being delivered to the individual. Measures should be taken to prevent the oxygen tubing becoming twisted, kinked, or disconnected, in order to facilitate a free flow of oxygen to the patient.

● Humidification of oxygen before it is administered, to prevent drying of the mucous membranes. Oxygen is humidified by passing it through distilled water. Water in the container should be renewed at least every 24 hours to prevent bacterial growth. The humidifier should be checked regularly, and water added if necessary to prevent it from emptying. Humidifiers are not used with particular masks, e.g. the 'Venturi', as significant back pressure may activate the safety pressure valve on the humidifier and may cause it to malfunction. The large openings in this style of mask allow sufficient atmospheric air to humidify the oxygen.

● Reducing any anxiety the individual, or his significant others, experiences related to the administration of oxygen. Some people may feel that the administration of oxygen is a sign that the person's condition is deteriorating, and individuals using face masks may experience anxiety related to having both their nose and mouth covered. The nurse should explain the purpose of the oxygen and the equipment that is being used. Some people may be educated to use the equipment independently and thus feel they have some control over the situation. Frequent visits to the individual, prompt attention to his needs, and efficient handling of the equipment, will help to reduce his anxiety.

● Informing the individual of the importance of maintaining the delivery device in the correct position, as changing its position may alter the amount of oxygen being delivered.

● Assisting the person meet his hygiene needs. The skin under the tubing, elastic straps, or mask, should be kept dry to promote comfort and to reduce the risk of skin breakdown caused by humidity or perspiration. Both the person's face and face mask should be wiped dry at least every 2 hours, and the skin under the delivery device checked for signs of pressure or irritation. Oral and nasal hygiene needs should be met, and a cream may be applied to the lips or nares to prevent dryness and discomfort.

● Replacing the mask with a nasal cannula if necessary, while the individual is eating or having his oral hygiene needs met.

● Measuring the person's temperature by the axillary route rather than the oral route, as placement of the thermometer in the mouth may cause further ventilatory distress.

● Monitoring the individual's condition constantly to assess the effectiveness of the treatment. The person should be observed for signs of hypoxia or oxygen toxicity. Hypoxia may occur if the oxygen concentration is inadequate, or if the equipment is not functioning properly. Oxygen toxicity is more likely to occur if the individual is receiving high concentrations, which can be detrimental to the central nervous system. Manifestations of oxygen toxicity include nausea, muscle twitching, dizziness, restlessness and irritability, convulsive seizures, and coma. Prolonged administration of high concentrations of oxygen may also cause damage to the linings of the bronchi and alveoli, resulting in pulmonary congestion or collapse of lung tissue.

Any indications of hypoxia or toxicity must be reported immediately as the concentration of oxygen being administered may need to be adjusted. It should also be noted that people with chronic obstructive airways disease, e.g. emphysema, generally should not receive more than 2 litres of oxygen per minute. Administration of an amount greater than this may inhibit their hypoxic stimulus to breathe.

• Observing the individual closely, after oxygen therapy has been discontinued, as the therapy may need to be resumed if signs of hypoxia become evident.

• Handling the oxygen equipment. The equipment used to deliver oxygen to the person should be cared for in the manner specified in the institution's policy manual. Most of the delivery devices are disposable, and thus the risk of cross infection is reduced.

In specific situations an individual may require mechanical ventilation, and oxygen may be administered via an intermittent positive pressure device or by a mechanical ventilator.

An intermittent positive pressure device pushes atmospheric or oxygen rich air into the individual's airways to promote adequate lung expansion. Commonly, intermittent positive pressure ventilation is performed via an endotracheal tube, and it allows effective control of ventilation and oxygenation. The flow of air to the lungs is set at a predetermined pressure, and as the pressure is attained the flow is stopped, pressure is released, and the person exhales.

A mechanical ventilator is a device that forces air into the lungs when a person is unable to breathe independently. A ventilator is attached to an endotracheal or tracheostomy tube, and either delivers a constant volume of air with each breath or is regulated to push air into the lungs until a preset pressure is attained.

Individuals with certain respiratory tract disorders may require a surgical opening into the trachea to provide an artificial airway so that their need for oxygen may be met. Information on care of the person with a tracheostomy is provide in Chapter 45, together with information on other aspects of care related to a person with respiratory tract dysfunction.

SUMMARY

In order to function efficiently, every cell in the body requires the supply of oxygen and the removal of the waste product carbon dioxide. External respiration is the exchange of these gases between the body and the atmosphere. The act of breathing allows the passage of oxygen and carbon dioxide to and from the lungs, while the cardiovascular system transports these substances to and from the cells. Ventilation is controlled by centres in the brain stem while certain factors such as physical activity or emotions affect the rate, rhythm and depth of breathing.

The individual's respiratory status is assessed by observing for any signs that indicate inadequate oxygenation, and by observing his ventilations. Normal ventilations, which are inaudible and regular, vary in rate according to the individual's age. The nurse should report any deviations from normal so that appropriate care may be planned and implemented.

Some people require the administration of oxygen, which can be delivered using one of the various devices available. Whenever oxygen is being administered, the nurse must promote the individual's safety and comfort, as part of assisting him to meet his need for oxygen.

33. Meeting temperature regulation needs

OBJECTIVES

1. Explain the temperature regulating mechanisms of the body.
2. State the factors affecting body temperature.
3. Demonstrate the ability to measure, report on and record body temperature accurately, using the oral, rectal, and axillary sites.
4. Apply appropriate principles when implementing nursing actions in the care of patients with disturbances of body temperature.
5. State the various methods by which heat and cold may be applied locally, and identify the safety factors involved.

INTRODUCTION

Measurement of body temperature provides the nurse with an objective assessment of the body's ability to maintain temperature regulation, identifies deviations from normal, and monitors any changes.

The human body is warm blooded with inbuilt mechanisms which maintain a balance between heat production and heat loss. As a result the internal or core temperature is stable. During ill health the balance may be upset and considerable stress may be placed on the body's adaptive mechanisms if the temperature remains abnormal.

Mechanisms for temperature regulation

Body temperature is controlled by both voluntary actions and involuntary mechanisms. The surface temperature of the body varies with changes in the environmental temperature, and people adjust to these changes by adapting their immediate surroundings. Selection of appropriate clothing, moving away from or towards the source of heat or cold, and altering the temperature of heaters or coolers can help to provide a comfortable environmental temperature.

Core temperature is maintained by inbuilt mechanisms concerned with the production of heat and its dissipation. These regulatory mechanisms, that ensure a balance between heat production and loss is achieved, are situated in the hypothalamus where neurons respond to changes in the temperature of the blood circulating through the brain. There are also temperature receptors in the skin and some internal organs, which transmit signals to the central nervous system to help control body temperature.

Balance between heat production and heat loss

Heat is continually being produced by the process of cellular metabolism and is constantly being lost to the environment through various processes.

1. Radiation. Body heat is transferred to cooler objects in the environment. Loss of heat by radiation means loss in the form of infrared rays. If the temperature of the body is higher than the temperature of the environment, more heat is radiated from the body.

2. Conduction. Only small quantities of heat are lost from the body by direct conduction from the body's surface to other objects, e.g. a bed or a chair. Loss of heat by conduction to the air represents a large proportion of the body's heat loss, unless the temperature of the air immediately adjacent to the skin is the same as the temperature of the skin.

3. Convection. Convection means the transfer of heat through a gas, or liquid, by the circulation of heated particles. As air molecules become excited by the heat energy from the body's surface, convection currents are set up which carry the heat away.

4. Evaporation. Insensible evaporation of water directly through the skin results from continual diffusion of water molecules, regardless of body temperature. When the body becomes overheated, large quantities of sweat are secreted onto the surface of the skin to provide rapid evaporative cooling of the body.

Heat balance occurs when the rates of heat production and loss are equal.

When the body temperature rises impulses from the hypothalamus to the skin arterioles are decreased causing vasodilation, with loss of heat occuring due to radiation, conduction, convection, and evaporation of sweat.

When the body temperature falls the impulses are increased causing vasoconstriction of the skin arterioles, therefore heat loss is reduced and the flow of blood to vital internal organs is increased. Shivering is an important source of heat, which is initiated by impulses travelling to the skeletal muscles. These impulses do not cause actual muscle shaking, but do increase skeletal muscle tone. The resulting increase in muscle metabolism increases the rate of heat production.

Factors affecting body temperature

In health, a number of processes and activities affect body temperature. Factors that lower the body temperature include:

- exposure to a cold damp environment
- insufficient warm clothing
- an undersecretion of the hormone thyroxine.

Factors that raise the body temperature include:

- exposure to a hot humid environment
- strenuous muscular activity
- intake of foods high in fat or carbohydrate
- strong emotions such as anger
- an oversecretion of the hormone thyroxine
- insufficient fluid intake.

Actions to assist the physiological processes of body temperature control include:

- maintaining immediate surroundings at a comfortable temperature
- adapting clothing to suit the climate
- adjusting intake of food and fluids to suit the climate
- adjusting the level of physical exercise.

NURSING PRACTICE AND TEMPERATURE REGULATION NEEDS

Assessment of an individual's temperature is made by the nurse using observational skills and an instrument, the clinical thermometer. Through use of the senses of sight and touch, the nurse can observe the individual's skin colour and temperature. Correct use of the thermometer will provide an accurate measurement of body temperature. As a result, the nurse is able to plan and implement appropriate nursing actions to assist the individual in the maintenance of body temperature.

In health the temperature varies only slightly, being lower in the early morning and higher in the evening, but remaining within the normal range.

The frequency with which an individual's temperature is measured, depends on continued assessment of each person's needs and the nursing policies of the institution. Residents of long term care facilities generally do not have their temperature measured as often as acutely ill people who require more frequent monitoring of their condition. Measuring the individual's temperature together with assessment of the other vital signs is an important method of determining his general condition. Assessment of these vital signs enables the nurse to establish baseline measurements that can be compared with future readings, and to monitor the individual's response to treatment.

Measurement of body temperature

There are several types of clinical thermometer available to measure body temperature. The most commonly used types are:

- glass
- electronic
- chemical dot.

The glass thermometer is most often used. It has a bulb at one end filled with mercury which expands and moves along a central channel when exposed to heat. The calibration that the mercury has reached indicates the body temperature. Glass thermometers are available with a long tipped bulb which is suitable for measuring oral or axillary temperatures, or with a short rounded bulb which is more suitable for measuring rectal temperature.

The electronic thermometer which is battery operated, is equipped with separate probes which can be used to measure oral, axillary, skin, or rectal temperatures. A cover is placed over the probe prior to use and disposed of after the temperature has been measured. An electronic thermometer enables an accurate temperature reading to be obtained within a few seconds, and may also be used when it is necessary to monitor a patient's temperature continuously. A signal device indicates when the temperature has registered, and the reading is obtained from either a digital display or printout.

The chemical dot thermometer contains heat sensitive dots which change colour when exposed to heat. The last dot to change colour indicates the body temperature. This type of thermometer is disposable and discarded after a single use.

All three types of thermometer are calibrated in the Centigrade scale.

Sites

Body temperature may be measured using the oral, axillary, groin, or the rectal site. Measurement of the surface temperature can also be achieved by attaching a probe to the skin.

The oral site is the most convenient and most commonly

used. The thermometer is placed under the individual's tongue to one side of the frenulum to ensure that it is in contact with a heat pocket, and the person closes his lips (Fig. 33.1).

So that an accurate measurement can be obtained safely, the individual must be:

- able to close his lips completely and retain the thermometer in the correct position

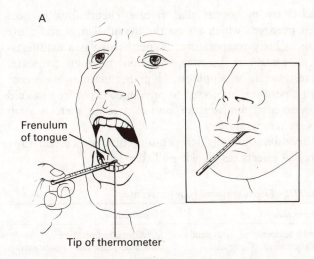

Fig. 33.1 Placement of thermometers. (A) Oral thermometer. The thermometer is placed at the base of the tongue next to the frenulum.

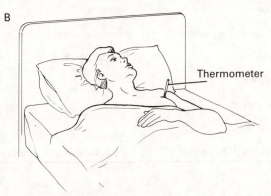

Fig. 33.1 (B) In the axilla. The thermometer is kept in place in the axilla by bringing the individual's arm over his chest.

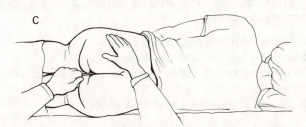

Fig. 33.1 (C) Rectal thermometer. The rectal thermometer is held in place during the measurement.

- able to breathe comfortably through his nose for the length of time the thermometer is in his mouth
- able to understand the importance of not biting the thermometer
- rested and not have consumed cold or hot fluids in the previous ten minutes.

The oral site is unsuitable for people who:

- have an oral infection or painful mouth
- have recently had oral surgery
- experience any impairment of breathing or obstruction of the nasal passages
- are confused or irrational
- are prone to seizures
- are unconscious
- are infants, or children under five years of age.

The axilla site provides a less accurate measurement of body temperature, but may be used when it is not possible to measure the temperature orally. The thermometer is placed in the axilla and in contact with two dry skin surfaces (Fig. 33.1).

The groin. Temperature may be measured by placing the thermometer in the individual's groin area, ensuring that his hip is flexed to enable contact of the thermometer with two dry skin surfaces. As an accurate measurement is difficult to obtain, this site is rarely used.

The rectal site although providing a more accurate assessment of core temperature, is embarrassing for the individual and potentially more harmful, therefore should be used with discretion (Fig. 33.1). This site is unsuitable for people who have diarrhoea, have recently had rectal or anal surgery, or who have painful anal conditions such as haemorrhoids.

To obtain an accurate measurement of body temperature and to promote the individual's comfort and safety, the nurse should:

- select the appropriate site
- check that the thermometer is undamaged, not contaminated, and is working properly
- ensure that the individual is informed of the procedure
- ensure that the individual is rested
- position the individual according to the site selected
- prevent cross infection by washing her hands, and ensuring that the thermometer has been disinfected, prior to the procedure
- ensure that the mercury level in a glass thermometer is below 35°C before it is inserted, that the thermometer is handled by the non bulb end, inserted correctly, and left in position for the recommended time
- use the correct probe for the site selected when using an electronic thermometer.

According to the site which is being used some variations

Table 33.1   Measurement of body temperature

	Oral	Axilla	Groin	Rectal
Thermometer is left in position for at least—	2 minutes	5 minutes	5 minutes	3 minutes
Normal range of temperature	36°–37.2°C	36°–37°C	36°–37°C	37°–38.1°C
Position of individual	Lying or sitting	Lying or sitting with arm across the chest	Lying with upper leg flexed and adducted	Lying in a lateral position with upper leg flexed

occur in the time the thermometer is left in position, the normal range of temperature, and the position in which the individual is placed. Details of these variations can be obtained by referring to Table 33.1.

Procedure for measuring body temperature

While the actual procedure may vary slightly in different health care settings, the general principles remain the same. The nurse should assess the needs of each individual, and refer to the institution's policy manual for information about the technique and equipment. A suggested procedure for measuring temperature using each body site is outlined in the guidelines. Temperature measurements are usually recorded on graph style charts (see Fig. 33.2 for an example). These enable the pattern of temperature variations to be observed readily.

Policies regarding the cleaning and storage of glass thermometers may vary slightly between institutions, and it is the nurse's responsibility to ascertain which protocol has been implemented.

The generally accepted measures are that:

- A separate thermometer is used for each person.
- The thermometer is stored dry in a container close to the bedside.
- The thermometer is wiped with disinfectant after each use.
- The thermometer is washed in cold water and detergent, before it is used for another person. It may also be necessary to soak the thermometer in disinfectant, e.g. if it has been used for a person with an infectious disease.

Disturbances of body temperature

Body temperature reflects body function, and a deviation from normal temperature is an indication of body dysfunction. When an imbalance occurs between the production and loss of heat, a rise or fall in normal body temperature is the result. An elevated temperature is referred to as hyperthermia, pyrexia, or fever. A temperature which is above 41°C is referred to as hyperpyrexia. A temperature which is below normal is referred to as hypothermia or subnormal. Hyperthermia occurs when cells are injured, or

invaded by pathogens that release chemical substances called pyrogens which act on the hypothalamus and cause a rise in body temperature. Hyperthermia is a manifestation of metabolic disorder, infection, neurologic disease, severe trauma, or neoplasm. Hypothermia may also occur when a person is subjected to prolonged exposure to a cold environmental temperature, and as a result there is a fall in body temperature.

Alterations in body temperature produce certain physiological effects, as shown in Table 33.2.

Table 33.2   Effects of altered body temperature

Hyperthermia	Hypothermia
Elevated temperature, pulse and ventilation rates. (Rigor may occur.)	Subnormal temperature, decreased pulse and ventilation rates.
Warm flushed skin, and sweating may be present.	Cool, pale, or mottled, dry skin
Restlessness, drowsiness or confusion.	Drowsiness Shivering
Aching muscles and joints	Muscle weakness
Headache	Mental confusion
Photophobia	
Loss of appetite	
Increased thirst	
Dehydration (if prolonged)	Unconsciousness (if prolonged)

Nursing an individual with altered body temperature

1. Hyperthermia. The aims of nursing a person with hyperthermia include:

- reducing body temperature to normal
- relieving any associated discomfort
- encouraging rest in order to decrease the production of body heat
- maintaining nutritional and fluid status.

These aims can be achieved by implementing certain nursing actions which include:

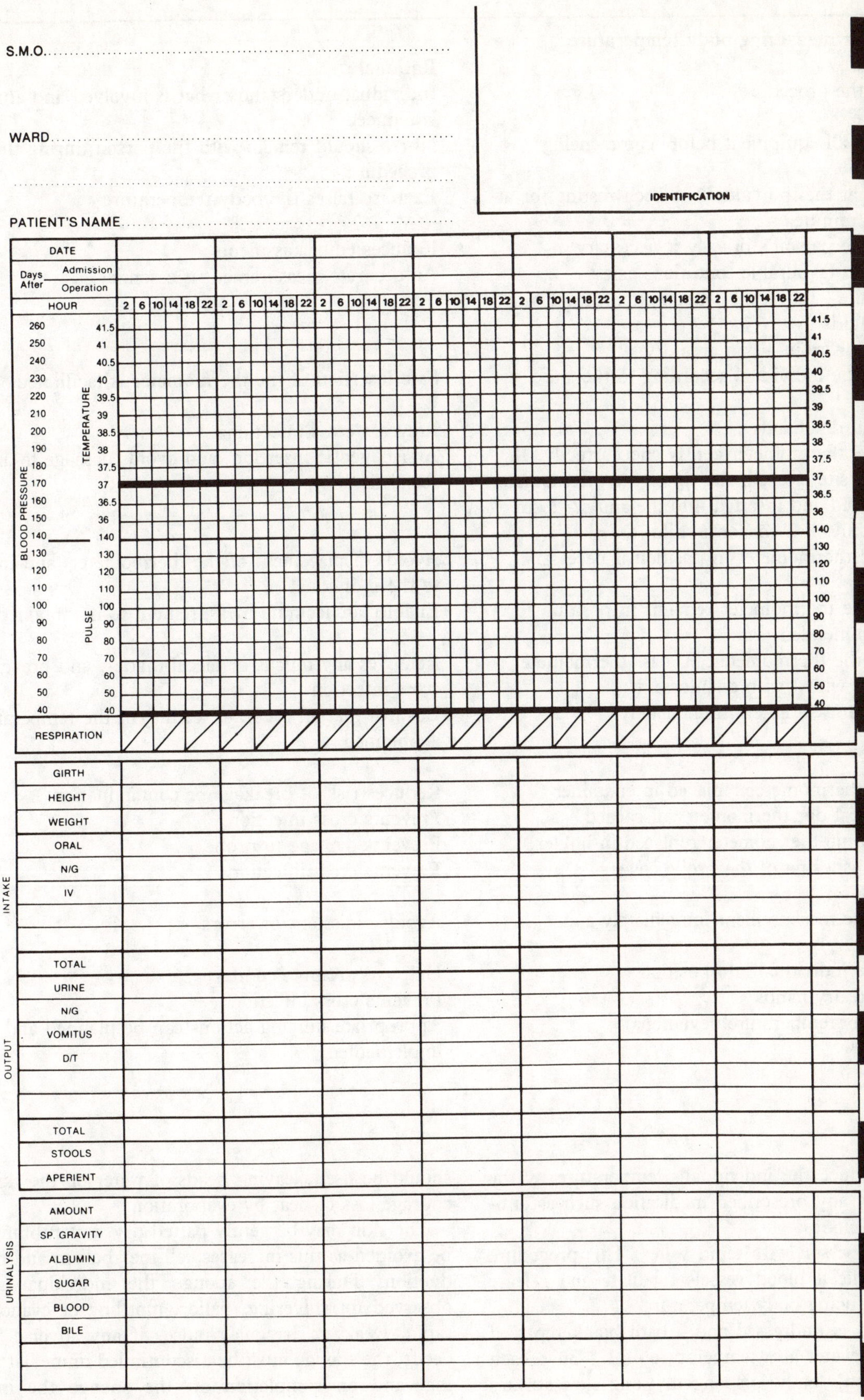

S.M.O...

WARD..

....

IDENTIFICATION

PATIENT'S NAME...

DATE									
Days After	Admission								
	Operation								

HOUR: 2 6 10 14 18 22 | 2 6 10 14 18 22 | 2 6 10 14 18 22 | 2 6 10 14 18 22 | 2 6 10 14 18 22 | 2 6 10 14 18 22 | 2 6 10 14 18 22

BLOOD PRESSURE: 260 250 240 230 220 210 200 190 180 170 160 150 140 130 120 110 100 90 80 70 60 50 40

TEMPERATURE / PULSE: 41.5 41 40.5 40 39.5 39 38.5 38 37.5 37 36.5 36 140 130 120 110 100 90 80 70 60 50 40

RESPIRATION

INTAKE
- GIRTH
- HEIGHT
- WEIGHT
- ORAL
- N/G
- IV
- TOTAL

OUTPUT
- URINE
- N/G
- VOMITUS
- D/T
- TOTAL
- STOOLS
- APERIENT

URINALYSIS
- AMOUNT
- SP. GRAVITY
- ALBUMIN
- SUGAR
- BLOOD
- BILE

Fig. 33.2 Sample vital signs graph-style chart.

Guidelines for measuring body temperature

Nursing action	Rationale
1. Explain the procedure	Individual understands what is involved and anxiety is reduced
2. Assemble all equipment before commencing	Nurse should remain with the person during the procedure
3. Check that the individual has been resting for at least ten minutes	Exercise raises the body temperature
4. Ensure the person's privacy if necessary	Reduces embarrassment
5. Check that favourable conditions exist: • Oral site—no recent consumption of hot or cold fluids • Axilla or groin—skin area dry	An accurate measurement is essential
6. Position the individual according to the site chosen	Safe insertion of the thermometer is facilitated
7. Wash and dry hands	Prevents cross infection
8. Insert the thermometer gently and correctly. If the rectal site is used, the tip of the thermometer is lubricated and inserted into the anus:2–3 cm for an adult, 1–2 cm for a child	Assists gentle insertion, and avoids damage to anal or rectal tissue
9. Hold the thermometer in position if necessary	Avoids displacement of the thermometer, and injury to the individual
10. Ensure the thermometer remains in position for the recommended time	Enables an accurate measurement to be obtained.
11. Remove the thermometer. A glass thermometer should be wiped with disinfectant	Removes any mucus or faecal matter, and prevents cross infection
12. Read the measurement immediately	Ensures that an accurate reading of the temperature is obtained
13. After use: • Glass thermometer replaced in container • Chemical dot thermometer discarded • Electronic thermometer replaced in holder, after disposing of the probe cover	Reduces risk of breakage or contamination Prevents cross infection Prevents damage to probe Prevents cross infection
14. Record the measurement immediately and accurately	Avoids omissions or errors
15. Assist the individual into position	Helps to promote comfort
16. Wash and dry hands	Prevents cross infection
17. Report any temperature deviations	Appropriate nursing actions can be planned and implemented

• Helping to reduce the individual's temperature by the administration of any prescribed medication such as antipyretics and antibiotics.

• Sponging the person with tepid water. This procedure causes the superficial blood vessels to dilate and release heat, thereby reducing body temperature.

The individual is undressed and a bath blanket placed over him. Using water at a temperature of 27°–30°C each part of the person's body is sponged. Long slow strokes should be used, leaving beads of water on the skin to encourage loss of heat by evaporation.

The skin may be gently patted dry, but rubbing should be avoided as this increases cell metabolism and heat production. During the sponge the individual must be observed for shivering, pallor, mottling or cyanosis; or a rapid, weak, or irregular pulse. If any adverse reactions occur, the sponge must be discontinued immediately. During, and on completion of, the sponge the individual should be advised to avoid unnecessary movement, as muscular activity increases heat production.

His temperature, pulse, and ventilations, should be measured 30 minutes after the sponge to assess the effectiveness of the procedure.

- Devices such as a bed cradle may be placed in the bed to elevate the upper bedclothes, and a fan may be placed in the room to provide circulation of cool air.
- Promoting the individual's general comfort by providing him with loose, light, clean and dry nightwear and bedlinen. His hygiene needs must be attended to in order to maintain a clean and dry skin. Regular mouth care including mouth rinses and the application of a lip cream, will help to reduce any oral dryness associated with hyperthermia. The room should be quiet and free from harsh light, and ventilated adequately.
- The individual should be encouraged to rest or sleep as much as possible, as a reduction in the level of physical activity will decrease the production of body heat.
- Optimal nutritional status should be maintained to cater for the increased metabolic demand associated with hyperthermia. The person should be provided with light appetizing meals which provide essential nutrients. If his appetite is poor, extra Kilojoules may be provided by adding glucose to oral fluids.

Adequate fluids are necessary to prevent dehydration, and the individual should be encouraged to drink large amounts of cool or iced fluids. If the person is unable to to tolerate fluids orally, intravenous administration of fluids may be necessary. The input and output of all fluids should be closely monitored, and the individual observed for any signs of dehydration. Information on the signs and symptoms of dehydration is provided in Chapter 31.

Continued assessment of the person's temperature and general condition should be made, to assess the effectiveness of nursing interventions.

A rigor sometimes occurs in response to the physiological processes associated with hyperthermia. The nurse should assess the individual's condition throughout the three typical stages of a rigor, and implement nursing actions necessary to promote his comfort:

1. As the body temperature begins to rise the person feels cold and may shiver violently. His comfort should be promoted by keeping him warm, but avoiding over heating. The intake of fluids should be encouraged.

2. The temperature rises to approximately 40°C and the person feels very hot and uncomfortable. Minimal clothing and bed linen should be used, and other actions to reduce the body temperature should be implemented, e.g., encouraging the individual to drink large amounts of cool fluid.

3. Profuse sweating occurs and as a result the body temperature begins to fall. Actions to reduce temperature should be ceased, and any damp clothing or bed linen should be changed to maintain a dry environment. The individual should be encouraged to rest quietly in an attempt to reduce the production of body heat.

2. Hypothermia. The aims of nursing an individual with hypothermia include:

- restoring body temperature to normal.
- relieving any discomfort associated with hypothermia.
- encouraging mobilization in order to increase the production of body heat.
- maintaining nutritional and fluid status.

These aims can be achieved by implementing certain nursing actions which include:

- Helping to increase the individual's temperature by gradually rewarming him. Rapid rewarming and the direct application of heat to the body surface should be avoided, as these actions cause peripheral vasodilation and diversion of blood away from vital internal organs. The environ- The environmental temperature should be between 26°–29°.
Lightweight warm clothing and bed linen should be provided, and a hypothermia or 'space' blanket may be used in an effort to restore normal body temperature.
- Promoting general comfort by attending to the individual's position and hygiene needs.
- Encouraging mobilization as his temperature begins to rise, in an effort to increase production of body heat.
- Encouraging the individual to consume warm food and fluids, particularly those containing carbohydrate, to assist the production of body heat.

Continued assessment of the individual's temperature and general condition should be made, to assess the effectiveness of nursing interventions.

Local applications of heat and cold

Various applications of either heat or cold may be used to promote patient comfort, or used for therapeutic purposes. Applications of heat include:

- infrared lamps
- hot compresses, packs, soaks
- poultices, counter irritants
- diathermy, ultrasound
- electric heating pads.

Applications of cold include:

- ice bags, packs
- ice compresses, soaks
- commercially prepared gel-filled packs.

Table 33.3   Effects of local applications

Heat	Cold
Increases blood circulation to the area to which it is applied, therefore: • relieves muscle spasm • relieves ischaemic pain • reduces swelling • assists healing	Slows blood circulation to, and restricts movement of body fluids in, the area to which it is applied, therefore: • reduces swelling • relieves pain caused by increased fluid in the tissues • helps to control bleeding

When heat or cold is applied to the body surface, local reactions occur. Table 33.3 lists the effects of local applications.

Applying local heat and cold

1. Before applying heat or cold the nurse should ascertain:
• the frequency and length of time it is to be applied
• whether it is to be applied directly to the skin
• whether the skin needs preparation prior to the application, e.g. a lubricating gel
• whether a cover is to be placed over the skin or appliance prior to use.
2. As complications may occur if precautions are not taken, it is necessary to observe the individual and skin area for any adverse reactions.

When heat is applied, observations should be made every five minutes for the development of:

• erythema (prolonged redness)
• blister formation
• discomfort or pain
• decreased sensation. (As the nerves in the skin are easily numbed, the individual may not feel pain if a burn is occuring.)

When cold is applied, observations of the skin should be made every five minutes for the development of:

• a pale, blue or mottled appearance
• blister formation
• decreased sensation.

3. Extra care must be taken when applying either heat or cold to people who are more susceptible to the effects, e.g.

• those with a delicate or fragile skin such as infants and young children, or the elderly.
• those with decreased sensation and awareness due to circulatory or nervous system disorders, or a decreased level of consciousness.

SUMMARY

Heat is generated in the body through cellular metabolism and lost from the body through the processes of radiation, conduction, convection, and evaporation. Both generation and loss of heat are controlled by the hypothalamus in order to maintain a balance of temperature control.

Surface temperature varies with environmental changes, while the core temperature is maintained within a narrow range.

In health, the body temperature varies slightly while remaining within the normal range; but illness may result in a temperature that is outside the normal range.

Accurate measurement of body temperature provides valuable information about an individual's condition, and any deviations from normal must be reported immediately.

Certain nursing actions may be implemented to help restore normal temperature when a person has hyperthermia or hypothermia.

Local applications of heat or cold may be used to either increase or decrease the flow of blood to a specific area of the body. Precautions must be taken to avoid adverse reactions to the application, and continued observations made to detect any complications early, to prevent permanent damage to tissue cells.

34. Meeting blood circulation needs

OBJECTIVES

1. State the factors necessary for an adequate flow of blood throughout the body.
2. State the factors involved in the maintenance of heart beat and blood pressure.
3. State the observations to be made of the pulse and blood pressure.
4. Identify the deviations from normal pulse and blood pressure.
5. Demonstrate the ability to measure, report, and document pulse and blood pressure accurately.

INTRODUCTION

Measurement of the pulse and blood pressure provides the nurse with an objective assessment of an individual's cardiovascular and fluid status. By monitoring the pulse and blood pressure, the nurse can identify deviations from normal and detect any changes.

As described in Chapter 21, the cardiovascular system transports essential substances to the tissue cells, and transports waste substances from the tissue cells to various organs for excretion. An adequate supply of blood is necessary for the cells to function effectively, and any disruption to the blood supply may have serious consequences. An adequate flow of blood throughout the body is dependent on:

- the ability of the heart to pump
- the ability of the blood vessels to transport the blood
- the quantity and quality of the blood.

The most important factor responsible for the transport of substances to the tissues is cardiac output. Cardiac output is the volume of blood pumped by each ventricle during each minute, and is dependent upon the volume of blood pumped at each beat and the number of beats during one minute. A normal heart in a healthy adult ejects approximately 5–6 litres of blood per minute. This amount can be increased by either an increase in heart rate and/or stroke volume, and can also vary according to:

- body size, as cardiac output increases in proportion to the surface area of the body
- age, as with increasing age the cardiac output decreases
- posture, as cardiac output is greater when an individual assumes a standing position
- exercise, as the greater degree of physical activity the greater the cardiac output needs to be. Strenuous physical activity can result in an increased heart rate and a cardiac output of 30 litres per minute
- a sudden increase in total blood volume, e.g. the infusion of fluid intravenously
- certain disease states. Cardiac output is increased in conditions such as pulmonary disease and anaemia, and is decreased in conditions such as shock or myocardial infarction.

The rate at which the heart beats is controlled by the nerves of the autonomic nervous system, and the Purkinje system. A key structure in the Purkinje system is the sinoatrial node which generates impulses that cause the muscle fibres of the atria to contract. Because the sinoatrial node starts each heart beat, and sets the pace for the whole heart, it is often called the 'pacemaker'.

Stimulation of the parasympathetic nerve fibres—primarily the vagus nerves—reduces the heart rate, while stimulation of the sympathetic nerve fibres increases the heart rate.

Various chemicals and ions can also affect heart activity, e.g. adrenalin inhibits the parasympathetic nerves resulting in an increased heart rate. An excess of potassium ions in the blood decreases the ability of the heart to contract.

Heart beat, and therefore the pulse rate, varies accordingly to age, sex, body build, level of physical activity, and emotions.

Blood pressure is the force exerted by the blood on the walls of the blood vessels as the heart contracts and relaxes. The pressure that the blood exerts against arterial walls during contraction of the left ventricle is called the systolic pressure. Diastolic pressure is the arterial pressure during left ventricular relaxation, and is a measurement of the minimum pressure being exerted on the arterial walls.

Blood pressure is maintained by the complex interaction of the body's homeostatic mechanisms, and is related to:

- cardiac output
- the force of ventricular contractions
- the viscosity (thickness) of the blood
- peripheral vascular resistance
- elasticity of blood vessel walls.

Blood pressure varies according to age, time of day, body posture, and emotions.

NURSING PRACTICE AND BLOOD CIRCULATION

Assessment of cardiovascular function is made by observing the general appearance of the individual and detecting the signs and symptoms of dysfunction, e.g. cyanosis, pallor, cool skin temperature, oedema, and dyspnoea.

Assessment of cardiovascular status is also achieved by monitoring the individual's pulse and blood pressure. The frequency with which the pulse and blood pressure are assessed depends on the person's condition, and how closely it needs to be monitored.

Residents in long term care facilities will commonly require pulse and blood pressure measurement infrequently, whereas people who are acutely ill may have the measurements performed at intervals ranging from every 30 minutes to six times a day.

Assessing the pulse

Assessment of the arterial pulse provides significant information about the individual's cardiac function and peripheral perfusion. As the heart beats it ejects blood from the left ventricle into the aorta. Each beat of the heart produces a wave of blood through the arteries so that there is regular recurrent expansion and contraction of the arteries. The waves of blood that cause pulsation through the arteries are palpable as a pulse.

The pulse is the wave of expansion felt when a superficial artery is compressed by the fingers, and is most easily felt over a large artery that lies close to the skin and crosses over a bone or firm tissue.

Peripheral pulse sites

The sites, illustrated in Figure 34.1, where the pulse may be palpated are:

- *Temporal*: The temporal artery is palpated immediately in front of the ear.
- *Facial*: The mandibular artery is palpated where it passes over the lower border of the mandible.
- *Carotid*: The carotid artery is palpated at the front of the neck to the side of the thyroid cartilage.

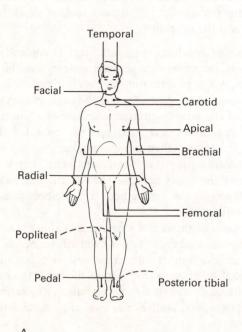

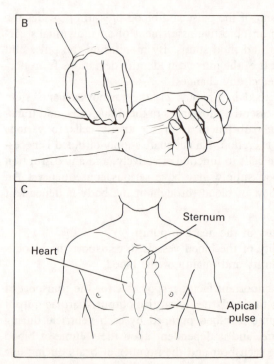

Fig. 34.1 Pulse sites. (A) Location of the pulse sites. (B) The middle three fingers are used to locate the radial pulse in the thumb side of the wrist. (C) The apical pulse is located 5 to 7.5 centimetres to the left of the sternum and below the left nipple.

- *Brachial*: The brachial artery is palpated in the antecubital fossa at the elbow joint.
- *Radial*: The radial artery is palpated in the wrist just above the thumb.
- *Femoral*: The femoral artery is palpated in the inguinal area.
- *Popliteal*: The popliteal artery is palpated at the back of the knee.
- *Posterior tibial*: The posterior tibial artery is palpated just behind the medial malleolus of the ankle.
- *Pedal*: The dorsalis pedis artery is palpated on the anterior surface of the foot.

The radial artery is the most commonly used site as it is conveniently located and readily accessible. The temporal or carotid sites maybe used if it is difficult to palpate the radial artery easily, e.g. if an individual has both arms encased in plaster.

The remaining sites are used when there are specific indications for assessing the flow of blood through a particular artery, e.g. the poplitial and pedal pulses are assessed following certain types of surgery to the leg.

The apical pulse is assessed when a more accurate estimation of heart rate or rhythm is required, or when there is any doubt about the rate or rhythm of a peripheral pulse. The apical pulse is the beat heard at the apex of the heart, and is assessed by using a stethoscope. The stethoscope is placed over the apex of the heart, in the left centre of the chest just below nipple level.

Apical-radial pulse assessment may be indicated, and is performed by two people. One person palpates and assesses the radial pulse while, at the same time, a second person assesses the apical pulses. Some heart beats which can be detected at the apex are not strong enough to be palpated at peripheral sites. Any difference between the two measurements is called the pulse deficit.

The pulse is assessed for rate, rhythm, and volume.

Rate. The pulse rate is the number of beats per minute, and the normal rate varies according to age:

- from 120–140 beats per minute for an infant
- from 90–120 beats per minute for a child
- from 60–90 beats per minute for an adult.

It should be noted that athletes and other physically fit individuals commonly have a normal pulse rate of below 60 beats per minute. A large number of elderly people also have a pulse rate that is below 60 beats per minute.

Rhythm. The rhythm of the pulse is the regularity with which the beats occur, and a normal pulse has a regular rhythm with the same intervals between each beat.

Volume. Volume refers to the strength of the beat, and a normal pulse is strong and easily palpated.

A suggested procedure for assessing the pulse is outlined in the guidelines.

Factors affecting the pulse

The pulse rate varies according to age, sex, body build, level of physical activity and emotions. The pulse may also be affected during various disease states, which result in alterations to its character.

Guidelines for assessing a pulse

Nursing action	Rationale
1. Explain the procedure to the individual	Reduces anxiety. Anxiety can cause an increased pulse rate
2. Ensure that the person is resting in a position of comfort	Activity or discomfort may increase the pulse rate
3. Wash and dry hands	Prevents cross infection
4. Select the appropriate pulse site	Site should be easily accessible, and provide an accurate assessment
5. Place the index and middle fingers over the site, and press gently until pulsation can be felt	The assessor's thumb is not used as it has a strong pulse and may be felt instead of the patient's pulse. Pressure that is too light will fail to detect the pulse, and firm pressure may obliterate the pulse
6. Using a watch with a second hand, count the pulse for one minute. While the rate is being counted, the rhythm and volume are also assessed	Allows sufficient time to detect the rate and any abnormalities
7. Document the time of assessment, the rate and characteristics of the pulse. Record the pulse measurement using numbers or dots. Any abnormalities must be reported immediately, as an apical measurement may be indicated	A record provides information about the patient's condition. An apical measurement provides a more accurate assessment of the pulse
8. Wash and dry hands	Prevents cross infection

Rate. An increase in the pulse rate above 100 beats per minute is called *tachycardia*, and may result from fear, anxiety, excitement, anger or pain. Tachycardia may also occur in conditions such as haemorrhage, shock, fever, thyrotoxicosis, or congestive cardiac failure.

A decrease in the pulse rate below 60 beats per minute is called *bradycardia*, and may occur during absolute relaxation or sleep. Bradycardia may also occur in conditions such as cerebral haemorrhage, heart block, myxoedema, or drug toxicity, e.g. digitalis.

Rhythm. An irregular rhythm, where the intervals between each beat vary, is called *arrhythmia*. Arrhythmia, or dysrhythmia, may occur in conditions such as electrolyte imbalance, or cardiac tissue damage. Patterns of irregular rhythm include:

- ectopic beats, which are premature heart beats and may be occasional or frequent
- coupled beats (or bigeminal pulse), in which two beats in close succession are followed by a pause during which no pulse is felt.
- fibrillation, in which fibrillation of a heart chamber results in inefficient random rapid contractions and, consequently, an irregular pulse.

Volume. An increased volume, when the pulse is referred to as being full and bounding, can result from strenuous physical exercise or strong emotions. An increased volume can also occur in conditions such as hypertension, thyrotoxicosis, or aortic valve incompetence.

A decreased volume, when the pulse is referred to as being weak and thready, can occur in conditions such as haemorrhage, shock, acute myocardial infarction, or cardiac failure. When the pulse is so weak that it cannot be palpated, it is referred to as being imperceptible.

When assessing the pulse, any deviations from normal should be reported immediately and documented. Pulse measurements are recorded on a chart, an example of which is illustrated in Figure 33.2. Each health care institution adopts its own printed form of graph and method for recording pulse measurements, together with the other vital signs. Commonly, the chart also provides space for recording other information, e.g. the patient's weight.

Assessing blood pressure

Measurement of blood pressure provides significant information about the individual's cardiovascular function. A series of blood pressure measurements may show the development of a trend, and is therefore more significant than a single measurement.

Blood pressure is the force exerted by the circulating blood on the walls of arteries, veins, and on the chambers of the heart. Arterial blood pressure measurement is commonly performed, and involves measuring the systolic and diastolic pressures.

Blood pressure is generally measured by a non-invasive or indirect method, using a manometer and a stethoscope. Blood pressure may also be measured directly by the insertion of a probe or catheter into a blood vessel.

Indirect blood pressure measurement is made using one of several devices (Fig. 34.2) which include:

- the sphygmomanometer, which has a calibrated column of mercury
- an aneroid manometer, which has a dial attached to the cuff
- an electronic device, where the measurement is displayed on a screen.

The sphygmomanometer is most commonly used, and consists of a cloth covered rubber bag (the cuff) from which two rubber tubes extend. One of the tubes is connected to a hand operated bulb that has a valve which can be tightened and released. The second tube is connected to the manometer which contains a calibrated column of mercury.

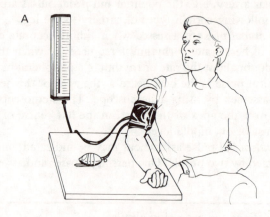

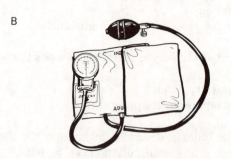

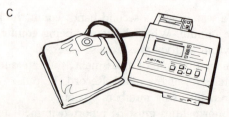

Fig. 34.2 Devices for measuring blood pressure. (A) Mercury manometer and cuff. (B) Aneroid manometer and cuff. (C) Electronic sphymomanometer.

The blood pressure is measured in millimetres of mercury (mmHg).

Blood pressure sites

The site commonly used to measure arterial blood pressure indirectly, is the brachial artery in the antecubital fossa at the elbow joint (Fig. 34.3). Less commonly, the blood pressure may be measured at the popliteal artery behind the knee.

A suggested procedure for measuring blood pressure is outlined in the guidelines.

Guidelines for measuring blood pressure Nursing action	Rationale
1. Explain the procedure to the individual	Reduces anxiety. Anxiety can increase blood pressure
2. Ensure that he is rested and in a position of comfort	Activity or discomfort may increase blood pressure
3. Wash and dry hands	Prevents cross infection
4. Remove any constricting clothing from the individual's arm. Support the arm in an extended position with the palm facing up. Position the arm so that the brachial artery is at the level of the heart	Tight clothing may reduce blood flow or create venous congestion in the arm. Correct arm placement enables an accurate blood pressure measurement
5. Select a cuff size which is appropriate	A cuff that is too small may result in a false high reading, while a cuff that is too large may result in a false low reading
6. Check for air leaks in the cuff, tubing and valves of the sphygmomanometer	Leakage of air may result in an inaccurate measurement
7. Squeeze the cuff to expel any air, then tighten the valve	Prepares the cuff for use
8. Position the cuff so that the rubber bag is centred over the brachial artery, with the lower edge of the cuff 2.5–5 cm above the antecubital fossa. Wrap the cuff smoothly and firmly around the upper arm, and secure it in position	An incorrectly placed, or loosely applied, cuff may result in an inaccurate measurement
9. Position the sphygmomanometer on a level surface	Errors in measurement can occur level surface. if the manometer is not vertical
10. Palpate the radial pulse and, with the fingers on the pulse, inflate the cuff until the palpated pulse can no longer be felt. Read the level of mercury	This measurement provides an approximation of the systolic pressure, and prevents the cuff from subsequently being over inflated
11. Deflate the cuff	Restores circulation to the arm
12. Place the disc of the stethoscope over the brachial artery in the antecubital fossa. Reinflate the cuff 10–30 mmHg above the approximate systolic pressure (point 10)	Pulse beat can be heard when the disc is placed directly over the artery Allows for precise measurement of the systolic pressure
13. Use the valve on the hand pump to release air, and slowly deflate the cuff—no faster than 5 mmHg per second	If the cuff is deflated too rapidly, there will be insufficient time to assess the pressure accurately
14. Note the level of mercury in the column as soon as the pulse beat is heard through the stethoscope	This measurement indicates the systolic pressure
15. Continue to slowly deflate the cuff. Note the level of mercury as soon as the pulse sounds muffled/or disappears	This measurement indicates the diastolic pressure
16. Deflate the cuff completely	Releases remaining air
17. Remove the cuff, and adjust the individual's clothing	Promotes comfort
18. Record the measurement immediately	Prevents errors or omissions
19. Wash and dry hands	Prevents cross infection
20. Report any deviations from normal	Appropriate care can be planned and implemented

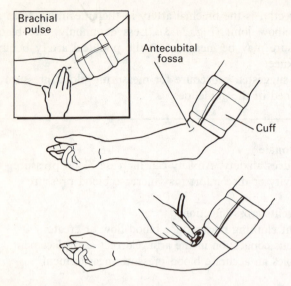

Fig. 34.3 Site for measuring blood pressure. The diaphragm of the stethoscope is placed over the brachial artery.

Blood pressure measurements may be recorded using dots on a graph similar to the one illustrated in Figure 33.2, or in longhand. If the longhand method of recording is used, the systolic pressure is recorded above the diastolic pressure, e.g. 120/70.

'Normal' blood pressure is immensely variable, therefore it is difficult to define abnormal blood pressure. It is generally considered that normal systolic blood pressure for an adult is between 100–135 mmHg, and normal diastolic pressure ranges from 60–80 mmHg. Commonly, systolic pressure is regarded as being elevated when it is higher than 150 mmHg, and diastolic pressure elevated when it is above 90 mmHg.

The significance of a blood pressure level can only be reliably assessed in the knowledge of previous levels, and in relation to the individual's current health state. For example, a person with a blood pressure of 95/60 may be perfectly healthy. Conversely, a person displaying signs of clinical shock but with a blood pressure of 135/90 may normally have a blood pressure exceeding this level.

At times it may be necessary to measure the blood pressure in both arms, or with the individual assuming first a lying then a standing position. It is important to report and document any differences observed between the two measurements.

If the blood pressure is to be measured frequently, e.g. every half hour, the cuff may be left on the individual's arm, but following each measurement the nurse must ensure that the cuff is deflated completely.

Care must be taken to avoid inflating the cuff repeatedly within a short time, as this action may result in venous congestion and cause the individual pain.

Hypertension is the term used to describe an elevated arterial blood pressure. Hypertension is a feature of many disease states, but frequently the cause of hypertension is unclear. When no cause can be detected, hypertension is described as 'essential', and the potential for onset increases with obesity, smoking, a family history of high blood pressure, or high sodium or cholesterol serum levels.

Hypertension is associated with cardiac enlargement, heart failure, coronary artery disease and cerebro vascular accidents. Sustained diastolic hypertension is associated with a high mortality rate, therefore the importance of preventing and controlling hypertension is considerable.

Hypotension is the term used to describe a low blood pressure, in relation to the individual's normal pressure. Hypotension is associated with low cardiac output states, e.g. left ventricular failure, and with hypovolaemic and cardiogenic shock. With sustained hypotension the blood pressure is not adequate for normal tissue perfusion and oxygenation, and may result in renal failure.

SUMMARY

An adequate flow of blood throughout the body is essential for normal function, and it is dependent on the ability of the heart to pump, the ability of the blood vessels to transport blood, and on the quantity and quality of blood.

Heart activity relies on the autonomic nervous system and the Purkinje system, and can be affected by various chemicals and ions.

Heart beat, and therefore the pulse rate, varies according to age, body build, the level of physical activity, and emotions. Certain disease states can cause alterations to the rate, rhythm, or volume of the pulse.

Blood pressure is related to cardiac output, the force of ventricular contractions, blood viscosity, and the condition of blood vessels. Certain disease states can result in blood pressure that is higher or lower than normal.

Measurement of the pulse and blood pressure provides the nurse with an objective assessment of the individual's cardiovascular and fluid status. Monitoring the pulse and blood pressure can detect any deviations from normal, and changes, which then enables the nurse to plan and implement appropriate actions.

Accurate measurement of the pulse and blood pressure assists in the evaluation of prescribed management, and nursing actions, which have been planned and implemented to assist the individual meet his blood circulation needs.

35. Meeting comfort, rest, and sleep needs

OBJECTIVES

1. Describe the importance of comfort, rest, and sleep to the well being of the individual.
2. State the factors that may interfere with comfort, rest, and sleep.
3. Identify the importance of a well made bed and good positioning to the promotion of comfort.
4. Apply appropriate principles to select supplementary equipment used in conjunction with bedmaking.
5. Apply appropriate principles when planning and implementing measures to promote comfort.
6. Describe the positions that individuals may be required to assume in bed, and identify the advantages and disadvantages of each position.
7. Describe the measures that may be implemented to meet the individual's needs for rest and sleep.
8. Perform the procedures described in this chapter, accurately and safely:
   - making an unoccupied bed
   - making an occupied bed
   - making an operation bed.

INTRODUCTION

Comfort may be described as ease or well being, and in order for an individual to feel comfortable his physiological and psychological needs must be met. Effective body function, which is necessary for comfort, depends on the meeting of nutritional, fluid, elimination, oxygen and temperature regulation needs. Meeting the needs of hygiene, movement and exercise, protection and safety, and freedom from pain, are also essential for promotion of comfort. In addition, comfort is promoted if the individual's need for love, self esteem, and self actualization is achieved.

Physical and emotional comfort are interdependent, and if either aspect is disrupted the other is commonly affected. For example, if an individual is experiencing some form of physical discomfort such as pain, he may develop emotional tension and become withdrawn, anxious, or depressed. Conversely, if a person is experiencing anxiety, he may develop physical symptoms such as headaches, loss of appetite, or gastro-intestinal disturbances. Therefore, for an individual to feel comfortable, he must be free from physical discomfort and emotional tension.

An important nursing responsibility is the implementation of measures that will promote the individual's physical and emotional comfort, and therefore assist him to receive sufficient rest and sleep. Discomfort can result from stimuli of physical or psychosocial origin. Where possible, the nurse should implement measures to prevent the development of situations that could be a source of discomfort. The nurse should also be aware of the appropriate actions to be taken in order to alleviate discomfort should it occur.

Some of the measures that may be implemented to promote the individual's emotional comfort are outlined in Chapters 4, 5, and 6, and are closely associated with the prevention and relief of anxiety. Freedom from anxiety is important in helping the individual to develop a sense of well being and emotional security. During the course of an illness or admission to hospital, a person commonly experiences anxiety and stress. The nurse can help to reduce a person's anxiety by providing him with adequate information about any procedures or treatments that are being performed. A trusting relationship between the nurse and the individual can help to alleviate anxiety, and the nurse's behaviour is important in developing such a relationship. Her approach and attitude towards the individual should demonstrate dependability, reliability, and respect for confidentiality. The nurse should also recognize and respect the individual's need for privacy and individualized care, both of which are essential for his emotional as well as for his physical comfort.

In order to promote the individual's physical comfort the nurse should assist him to meet all his needs, ensure that he is helped to assume a position of comfort, ensure that he is provided with comfortable clothing, and make sure that his physical environment is suitable.

A person's comfort is enhanced if he is able to wear the clothes of his choice. Many people feel uncomfortable and undignified if they are required to wear clothing provided by the health care institution, e.g. gowns or nightwear. If, however, circumstances require the person to wear hospital provided clothing, the nurse should ensure that the clothes are appropriately selected to meet the person's needs.

A suitable physical environment is one in which there is adequate lighting, fresh air, ventilation, warmth, and cleanliness it is, ideally, free from excessive noise and unpleasant sights and smells. In addition, there should be sufficient space for the individual's personal belongings, and facilities available for visitors. The physical environment can be enhanced by promotion of a psychological climate, in which the individual is encouraged to communicate any fears or anxieties. A physical environment that reduces the person's privacy and independence is unsuitable, and can be a source of discomfort to him.

This chapter addresses promotion of the individual's physical comfort through the provision of a comfortable bed, a comfortable position, and through the promotion of sufficient rest and sleep. As the need for comfort is closely associated with the need for adequate rest and sleep, the nurse should be aware of the comfort measures necessary to ensure that these needs are met. Rest and relaxation can occur only when there is freedom from physical discomfort and emotional tension, and an individual is more likely to sleep well if his normal sleeping habits are maintained.

When assessing the individual's status in relation to comfort, rest, and sleep, the nurse should obtain information regarding his usual sleeping environment. It is important to ascertain the type of bed and bedding he is accustomed to, and whether he is used to sleeping alone or in a shared bed or room. For example, if an individual is accustomed to sharing a bed, his normal sleeping pattern may be disrupted when admission to hospital necessitates a change in behaviour. Information should be obtained about his usual sleeping behaviour, such as the time he normally goes to sleep, the quality of sleep, and the time he wakes up. It is helpful to know whether he has a bed time routine, e.g. if he normally has a hot drink before bedtime, and if he requires medication to help him sleep. The nurse should also ascertain whether he is currently experiencing any discomfort that may disturb his rest and sleep, e.g. nausea or pain associated with his illness.

The information obtained, together with observation of the individual, provides the nurse with a foundation on which to plan and implement nursing actions to promote comfort, rest and sleep. When possible the person's normal bed time routine should be maintained, and his immediate environment arranged so that it is conducive to comfort, rest and sleep.

NURSING PRACTICE AND COMFORT NEEDS

To promote the individual's comfort, the nurse should ensure that he is provided with a bed that is well made and adapted to suit his needs.

Provision of a comfortable bed

The prime objective of bedmaking is the promotion of comfort, as a bed that is poorly made may disrupt rest and sleep and may be a contributing factor to the development of complications such as decubitus ulcers. Beds may be made up in a variety of ways to meet the individual's needs, and each institution commonly adopts its own method of bedmaking. Although the techniques may vary slightly, the principles of bedmaking remain the same.

Various types of bed are available, most of which can be adjusted either manually or mechanically. The majority of beds may be raised or lowered horizontally, and some can also be adjusted to alter the position of the head, foot, or centre. Some beds have a movable section which can be adjusted to form a backrest against which pillows may be placed to provide support for the patient. Beds are fitted with wheels, that enable them to be moved easily when necessary, and a brake device that prevents inadvertent movement.

Frames (Fig. 35.1) are available which may be either fitted to the bed, or used in place of the conventional bed.

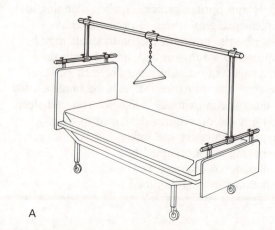

A

Fig. 35.1 Bed frames and special beds. (A) Balkan frame.

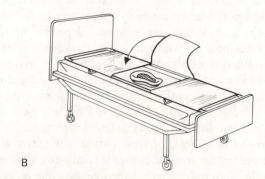

B

Fig. 35.1 (B) Bradford frame (note the removable strip in the centre to allow insertion of a bedpan).

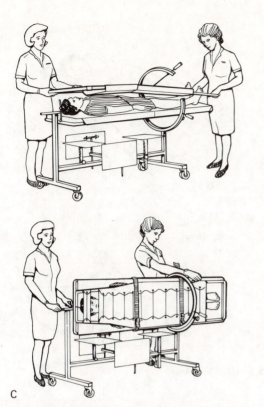

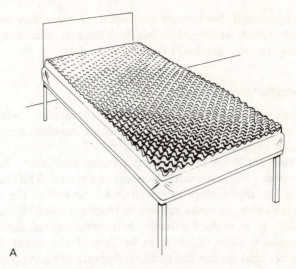

Fig. 35.2 Special mattresses. (A) The egg crate mattress.

Fig. 35.1 (C) Stryker frame. The patient is turned to the prone or supine position. Body alignment is not changed during repositioning.

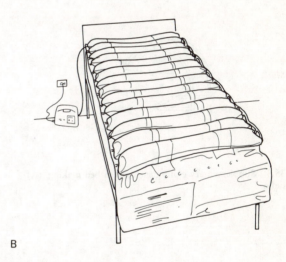

Fig. 35.2 (B) A ripple mattress.

The Balkan frame is made from wood or metal, extends lengthwise above the bed, and may be used in conjunction with traction apparatus. The Bradford frame consists of a metal frame across which canvas slings are stretched, and may be used to nurse a person who has a fracture or disease of the hip or spine. The Stryker frame consists of two canvas covered frames attached to a metal frame, and may be used to facilitate changing the position of a person who has a spinal cord injury or paralysis. The circolectric bed consists of a circular and two flat frames which are operated mechanically, and may be used to move a dependent person into various positions.

Mattresses are commonly made of rubber and covered with a waterproof material, which facilitates cleaning and therefore helps to prevent cross infection. Other styles of mattress are available, including those made from foam rubber. Individuals who have specific needs, e.g. those who are more vulnerable to the development of decubitus ulcers, may be nursed on special mattresses. These include the egg crate style (Fig. 35.2), the water mattress, the alternating pressure or ripple mattress, and a mattress that is divided horizontally into three sections. The type of mattress selected must meet the individual's needs, provide comfort and support, and should help prevent the development of complications such as decubitus ulcers.

Pillows are available in a variety of materials, most of which are enclosed in a protective waterproof covering over which a pillow slip is placed. The number of pillows used depends on the needs of the individual, and should be sufficient to provide maximum comfort and support.

Sheets are commonly available in two styles. The long sheet is similar to a conventional single bed sheet, and the draw sheet is a narrow sheet that may be placed across the bottom sheet. Because of their design, draw sheets are easy to replace under an individual without disturbing the other bed clothes. A waterproof sheet may be placed under the draw sheet to protect the bottom sheet against moisture, e.g. if a person is incontinent, or is required to use toilet utensils in bed.

Blankets are available in wool or loosely woven cotton, and should be light, warm, and able to withstand frequent laundering.

Quilts or bedspreads are commonly made from a cotton fabric that is easily laundered. Some institutions may use continental style quilts in place of blankets and a bedspread.

The frequency with which bed clothes are changed depends on the institution's policy, but they should always be replaced if they become wet, soiled, or excessively wrinkled. Clean and wrinkle free bed linen is necessary to promote the individual's comfort and safety.

Supplementary equipment

There is a variety of supplementary equipment available (Fig. 35.3) that may be used to enhance comfort, provide added support, or to promote safety.

Bed cradle. A bed cradle is a frame designed to keep the upper bed clothes off all or part of a person. The cradle may be large enough to extend from one side of the bed to the other, or small enough to place over one leg. The cradle is positioned directly above the area of the individual's body which is to be free of the upper bed clothes, and the top sheet and blankets are brought up over the cradle. A bed cradle may be used for a patient with a burn, an uncovered or painful wound, or a plaster cast.

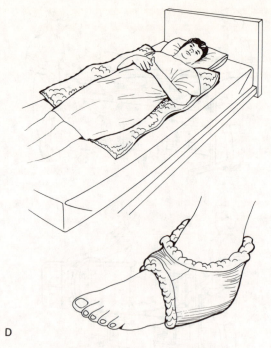

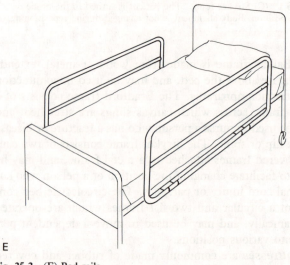

Fig. 35.3 (D) Sheepskins.

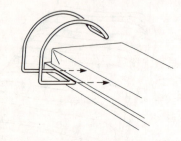

Fig. 35.3 Supplementary equipment used in bed making. (A) Bedcradle

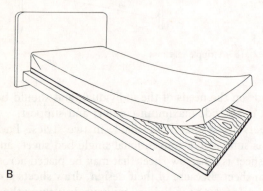

Fig. 35.3 (B) Fracture board.

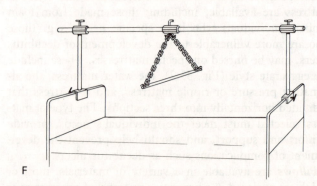

Fig. 35.3 (E) Bed rails.

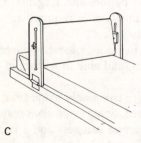

Fig. 35.3 (C) Footboard.

Fig. 35.3 (F) Overhead trapeze.

The cradle protects the area by elevating the bed clothes, and facilitates observation of the area by the nurse or medical officer.

Fracture board. A fracture or bed board is placed under the mattress to provide a firm surface and greater support for the back and legs. Fracture boards are commonly used for individuals who have an injury or disease affecting the spine or lower limbs.

Footboard. Various styles of foot board are available which are placed towards the end of the bed to support the individual's feet in a neutral position. A foot board may also be used to keep the weight of the upper bed clothes off the person's feet. For comfort, a pillow may be placed between the feet and the footboard.

Sheepskin. A sheepskin may be placed over the bottom sheet to provide a soft surface for the individual. Friction between the skin and bottom sheet is reduced, and air circulates between the wool fibres to help keep the skin dry. A sheepskin may be used to promote the individual's comfort, particularly if he has reduced mobility, and is commonly used to prevent the development of decubitus ulcers. For maximum effectiveness, the person's skin should be in direct contact with the wool surface.

Heel or elbow protectors. Made from sheepskin or foam rubber, or from inflatable plastic material, the protectors are designed to fit the shape of the heel or elbow. They are commonly used to prevent the development of decubitus ulcers on these areas as they reduce friction between the skin and the bed linen.

Bed rails. Bed or side rails may be positioned on each side of the bed to protect the individual from falls. Many beds are fitted with built in side rails which are raised when necessary. Bed rails may be used as a safety device for individuals who are irrational, confused, restless, subject to seizures, or who are experiencing altered awareness or consciousness.

Trapeze. A trapeze bar or hand grip is a swinging bar suspended from an overhead pole, and may be used by an individual to facilitate his movement in bed.

Rope. A length of rope, or similar material, may be attached to the foot of the bed, and positioned on top of the quilt. By holding on to the end of the rope, the person is able to pull himself up into a sitting position.

Bath blanket. A bath or procedure blanket is made from warm, lightweight cotton material, and is commonly used to cover the individual during a bed bath or various other procedures.

Sandbag. Sandbags commonly consist of a waterproof bag filled with sand, and are used to maintain part of the body in alignment. For example, sandbags may be used to immobilize a fractured leg prior to splinting or surgery.

Wedge shaped pillow. A wedge shaped pillow is placed between the legs to maintain abduction, e.g. following total hip replacement.

The nurse must ensure that any supplementary equip-ment is positioned and used correctly, in order to promote the individual's comfort and safety.

Making the bed

There are various styles of bed making.

Closed or open bed. When the upper bed clothes are being placed on a bed, they may be arranged in such a way as to be referred to as either a closed or an open bed. To make a closed bed, the upper bedding is tucked in at the bottom and sides. To make an open bed, the upper bedding is folded up at the bottom and sides. The advantage of the open style, is that the upper bedding can be quickly folded lengthwise or into a pack to facilitate the transfer of an individual from a trolley into the bed.

Unoccupied bed. This term is used to describe a bed that is either temporarily vacated by the individual, e.g. during his shower, or a bed that is being made up following a person's discharge from hospital.

Occupied bed. The term is used to describe a bed that is being made while it is occupied by the individual. When making an occupied bed, the nurse must be aware of any restrictions in the person's movement or position, and she should ensure that the individual's safety and comfort are maintained throughout the procedure.

Operation bed. Sometimes referred to as a surgical or post-anaesthetic bed, the operation bed is made up to receive an individual following surgery. The upper bedding is arranged into a pack (Fig. 35.4), which can be easily removed to facilitate transfer of the person from a trolley into the bed. Once the individual is in the bed, the upper bedding is unfolded and positioned over him.

Divided bed. Sometimes referred to as a split or traction bed, the divided bed involves arranging the upper bedding into 2 sections. This style of bed is commonly used for a patient who has traction equipment applied to a leg. A divided bed allows the leg in traction to be free from the weight of the upper bedding, while the rest of the individual's body is covered. A lightweight cover may be placed over the leg in traction to ensure adequate warmth.

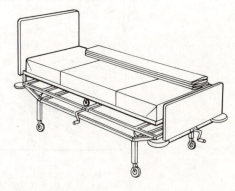

Fig. 35.4 An operation bed.

Key aspects related to bedmaking.

- All the equipment, e.g. clean linen and soiled linen container, should be collected before the procedure is commenced.
- Measures should be implemented to prevent cross infection.

The nurse's hands should be washed and dried before and after making the bed.

Any soiled bed clothes should be immediately placed into a soiled linen container.

Bed clothes should not be shaken or flicked, permitted to touch the floor, or held up against the nurse's uniform.

Beds should not be made while procedures involving the use of sterile equipment are being performed nearby.

- During bedmaking, the nurse should observe the principles of body mechanics in order to prevent strain on her back.
- When positioning the bottom sheets, the nurse should ensure that they are put on with the hem facing down. Sheets must be free from rough areas, wrinkles or creases, in order to promote comfort and to avoid damage to the individual's skin.
- To maintain bedclothes in position, the corners are mitred (Fig. 35.5). Mitred corners help to prevent the bed clothes becoming loose and uncomfortable for the person.
- To facilitate efficient bedmaking, bed clothes that are to be replaced are folded and put on a chair. Folding the bed clothes avoids excessive wrinkling, and facilitates their re-

placement. Alternately, the bed clothes may be placed over a 'bed-stripper', which is a frame attached to the foot of the bed. Bedding that is not being replaced is rolled up and placed into the soiled linen container.

- If a waterproof draw sheet is used, it must be completely covered by a cotton draw sheet to prevent its contact with the individual's skin.
- Before commencing to make an occupied bed, the nurse should assess the need for assistance. Two or more nurses may be necessary to move the individual, and to complete the procedure quickly in order to avoid the individual becoming fatigued. The person must be adequately supported, and kept warm, during the procedure.
- In some instances it may be necessary to make an occupied bed from top to bottom, rather than from side to side. It is often easier and less disruptive for an individual, e.g. one who has distressed breathing or a leg in traction, if the nurses adjust the bottom sheets in this manner.
- A vertical pleat or fold should be made in the upper bed clothes, to provide room for the person's feet. This technique prevents the bed clothes from pressing down on the feet.
- When a bed is being made up following a person's discharge from hospital, the entire bed and fittings are cleaned. The bed should be allowed to air before being made up with clean bedding.

Suggested procedures for making an unoccupied, an occupied, and an operation bed, are outlined in the guidelines.

The technique used to make an occupied bed should be

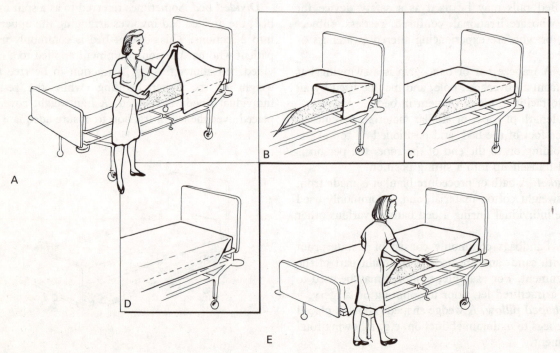

Fig. 35.5 Mitred corners.

Guidelines for making an unoccupied bed

Nursing action	Rationale
1. Wash and dry hands	Prevents cross infection
2. Place clean linen and soiled linen container near the bed	Facilitates access during the procedure
3. Ensure that there is a chair on which to place the bed clothes, or use the 'bed-stripper' attached to the foot of the bed	Bed clothes must be kept free of the floor to prevent them becoming contaminated
4. Move the bedside locker and overbed table if nesessary	Provides more space in which to work
5. Adjust the height of the bed	Appropriate height of the bed prevents strain on the nurse's back
6. Place pillows on the chair. Place any soiled pillow slips in the container	Prevents cross infection
7. Loosen the upper bed clothes	Facilitates their removal
8. Remove each item of upper bed clothes separately, fold and and place on the chair or 'bed-stripper'. Loosen the bottom bed clothes, fold and place on the chair. Any soiled items are placed in the linen container	Folding reduces wrinkling, and facilitates replacement Prevents cross infection
9. Roll, rather than fold, the waterproof sheet.	Folding may damage waterproof material
10. Turn the mattress, and pull it well up to the head of the bed	Avoids excess wear on one area Prevents gap between the head of the bed and the mattress.
11. Commencing with the bottom sheet, each item is replaced separately If a draw sheet is used, it is positioned approximately 25 cm from the head of the bed The bed clothes should be centred and, unless being made up as an open bed, tucked in around the mattress.	Bed clothes are easier to adjust, or remove, if they are replaced and tucked in separately The draw sheet needs to go under the individual's buttocks Facilitates correct placement of the bed clothes
12. Turn the top sheet back over the blankets	Protects the upper part of blankets, e.g. from spilt fluids
13. Replace the quilt, mitre the bottom corners, and allow the edges to hang freely	Provides a neat appearance
14. Replace and arrange the pillows to meet the patient's needs	Promotes comfort and support
15. If a person is to return to bed, the top corner of the upper bed clothes may be folded back Adjust the height of the bed	Facilitates easy access for the individual
16. Replace any furniture. Remove soiled linen container, wash and dry hands	Prevents cross infection

one that causes minimal disturbance to the individual. Commonly, the bed is remade following attention to the person's daily hygiene needs. It may be necessary to make an occupied bed more frequently, e.g. if the bed clothes become wet, soiled, or disarranged. When possible two nurses should work together to make the bed, for the promotion of patient comfort and safety. At times it may be necessary for more than two nurses to make an occupied bed, e.g. if the individual has an orthopedic condition requiring several people to move him.

Making an occupied bed provides the nurse with an ideal opportunity for communicating with and observing the individual. During the procedure the nurse is able to assess certain aspects of the person's condition, e.g. his ability to move, any distress associated with exertion, skin colour, the presence of pain, and his emotional state. The

Guidelines for making an occupied bed

Nursing action	Rationale
1. Wash and dry hands	Prevents cross infection
2. Explain the procedure to the individual, and ensure privacy	Reduces anxiety and embarrassment
3. Collect clean linen and soiled container before commencing to make the bed	Nurse must remain with the person during the procedure
4. Move the bedside locker and overbed table if necessary	Provides more space in which to work
5. Ensure there is a nearby chair on which to place the bed clothes, or use the 'bed-stripper'	Bed clothes should be kept free of contamination from the floor
6. Adjust the height of the bed	Appropriate height of the bed prevents strain on the nurse's back
7. Leaving sufficient pillows to support the individual, place the remainder on the chair	The individual's comfort and safety must be promoted
8. Remove each item of upper bed clothes separately. Bed clothes to be replaced are folded and put on the chair or 'bed-stripper'	Reduces wrinkling, and facilitates replacement
Cover the person with a procedure blanket before removing the top sheet	Promotes comfort
Place soiled items into the linen container	Prevents cross infection
9. Remove accessories such as a bed cradle or foot board	Facilitates bed making
10. Support the individual, and gently turn him onto one side of the bed	Provides sufficient room to adjust or change the bottom sheet/s
If only one nurse is making the bed, the side rail away from her should be elevated	Promotes safety
11. Loosen the bottom sheets on the unoccupied side, and roll each one towards the centre of the bed	Provides access to one side of the mattress.
Brush out any debris, e.g. crumbs or pieces of plaster, from the exposed mattress. Eliminate any creases from the mattress cover	Foreign objects, or creases in the cover, cause discomfort
12. Working at the unoccupied side of the bed, either: Unroll, pull the bottom sheets taut, and tuck in around the mattress OR If using a fresh sheet, place on the bed and unfold it so that the centre laundry crease lies at the centre of the mattress. Tuck in at the top, bottom, and side. Roll the excess to the centre of the bed	Provides a smooth surface under the individual
13. Carefully turn the individual to the other side of the bed, providing adequate support as he is moved	Comfort and safety must be promoted
14. From the opposite side of the bed, either: Remove any soiled sheets and place in the linen container, OR Untuck, and roll sheet/s to the centre of the bed	Prevents cross infection
15. Ensure that side of the mattress is free from debris and creases, unroll and tuck the sheet/s in around the mattress	Completes the making of the base of the bed

16. Assist the individual back into the centre of the bed, arrange the pillows to meet his needs, and assist him into position	Promotes comfort
17. Replace any accessories, put on the top sheet, and remove the procedure blanket	Promotes comfort and privacy
18. Replace the blankets and quilt, ensuring that they are positioned to cover the individual's chest and shoulders	Promotes warmth and comfort
Make foot pleats in the upper bed clothes, and avoid tucking them in too tightly	Provides room for movement
19. Place the signal device and the person's requirements within his easy reach. Adjust the height of the bed	Facilitates access
20. Replace any furniture. Remove the linen container, wash and dry hands	Prevents cross infection

observations made should be documented, and any deviations from normal should be reported immediately to the nurse in charge.

When the individual's condition permits he may be able to assist during bedmaking, by holding the over-head hand grip to facilitate his movement.

An operation bed (Fig. 35.4) is a version of an open bed, and is made up to receive an individual following surgery or anaesthesia. The nurse should refer to the institution's policy manual for information regarding the extra equipment necessary. To promote the comfort and safety of a post operative or post anaesthetic patient, it is usual for the following items to be placed at the bedside:

—oxygen and suction equipment
—emesis bowl
—sphygmomanometer and stethoscope
—thermometer and disinfectant swabs
—charts on which to record vital signs, fluid balance
—an intravenous therapy pole
—a 'nil-orally' sign.

Additional equipment may be required depending on the procedure that has been performed. To provide sufficient space for the trolley, furniture, e.g. the bedside locker, overbed table, and chair, should be moved away from the bed. Information on caring for an individual who has had surgery, is provided in Chapter 59.

A divided bed is sometimes referred to as a split or a traction bed, and may be used to nurse an individual with traction applied to a lower limb. Because the upper bedding is arranged in two sections, the person's torso and unaffected leg may be kept covered without interference to the traction apparatus. The foot of the bed is elevated to counterbalance the traction, and a fracture board is commonly placed under the mattress to provide a firm and supportive surface. A trapeze or overhead bar should be provided to facilitate the individual's movement.

When changing or straightening the bottom sheets it is sometimes easier and less disruptive for the individual intraction, to work from the top to the bottom of the bed, rather than from side to side. Information on caring for an individual who has traction applied, is provided in Chapter 42.

Certain adverse effects may be associated with prolonged bed rest and immobility, therefore it is important that the nurse implements preventive measures to reduce such effects. Information on these adverse effects, is provided in Chapter 37.

Regardless of the style of bed being made, the nurse should remember that the main aim of bedmaking is to promote the comfort and safety of the individual.

In addition to providing the person with a comfortable bed, ensuring that he assumes a comfortable position is of prime importance in meeting his comfort needs.

Provision of a comfortable position

Individuals assume, or are assisted into, the position they find the most comfortable, unless a specific posture is indicated. If an individual is able to move without assistance the nurse should ensure that his pillows are positioned for support and comfort, and that he is provided with adequate bed clothes. His signal device and personal requirement should always be within his easy reach.

A specific position may be necessary to prevent deformities, relieve pressure and strain, to assist circulation or breathing, or to enable various examinations or treatments to be performed. Some individiuals will be able to assume a position independently, while others will require the nurse's assistance. The nurse should be aware of measures to promote the individual's safety and comfort, and she should be able to assist a person into specific positions. Correct positioning can promote comfort, maintain and help restore body functioning, and help to prevent the complications associated with bed rest and immobility.

Guidelines for making an operation bed

Nursing action	Rationale
1. Wash and dry hands	Prevents cross infection
2. Collect clean bedclothes and soiled linen container	Clean bedclothes reduces the risk of post operative infection
3. Adjust height of the bed	Correct height of the bed prevents strain on the nurse's back
4. Loosen all bed clothes, remove, and place in the container	Prevents cross infection
5. Place a clean bottom, waterproof, and draw sheet on the mattress. Tuck ends and sides of the sheets under the mattress	Waterproof and draw sheet protect the bottom sheet, e.g. from wound drainage
6. Lie the top sheet and blankets on the bed, fold the top and bottom back. Fold each side to the centre, then fold in half. Fold the top and bottom to the centre, then fold in half	Creates a pack which can be be removed quickly before the patient re-enters the bed, and then unfolded over him
7. Place the pillows on a chair in the room	Pillows are placed on the bed when the individual's needs are determined
8. A heating pad may be placed in the bed under the pack	Warms the bed prior to the person's return
9. Adjust the height of the bed	Prepares the bed to receive the individual from the trolley
10. Place all the required equipment, e.g. emesis bowl, within easy reach	Prepares the room for the person's return
11. Wash and dry hands	Prevents cross infection

Key aspects related to positioning

• The nurse should observe the principles of body mechanics when helping an individual to move, in order to prevent strain on her back. Information on body mechanics is provided in Chapter 37.
• The individual should be provided with information about the importance of correct positioning, and the reasons why a specific position may be indicated. In order to provide some exercise, and to promote independence, the person should be encouraged to participate in any change of position unless active movement is contra-indicated.
• All parts of the individual's body should be maintained in proper alignment, with equal weight distribution, and the joints in a functional or neutral position. Muscle tension and strain are prevented when the joints are maintained in a slightly flexed position.
• Adequate support should be provided to maintain the natural curves of the individual's vertebral column.
• To promote safety and comfort, adequate assistance should be obtained to move a heavy or dependent person. His body should be handled gently to prevent pain or injury. Appropriate lifting devices may be used to assist an individual into position.
• Supplementary equipment, e.g. a sheepskin, may be used to enhance comfort and to relieve pressure.
• To prevent prolonged pressure on any area of the body,

the individual's position should be changed at least every four hours. Each time his position is changed, the nurse should observe the status of his skin to detect any signs of the consequences of prolonged pressure.
• The individual should be encouraged to participate in some form of exercise unless this is contra-indicated. Exercise helps to promote circulation and muscle tone and, if the person is unable to move independently, his joints should be put through the full range of motion. Information on joint movement and exercise is provided in Chapter 37.

There are various positions (Fig. 35.6) that an individual may assume, or be required to assume.

1. Supine (dorsal recumbent) position

In a supine position, the person lies flat on his back with a pillow under the head. His limbs should be positioned in normal alignment, and a footboard or firm pillow may be necessary to maintain his feet in the correct position. A supine position may be indicated:

• To facilitate relaxation of the abdominal muscles, e.g. during medical examination of the abdomen.
Following abdominal surgery, individuals may be placed in the supine position to relieve tension on the abdominal area.

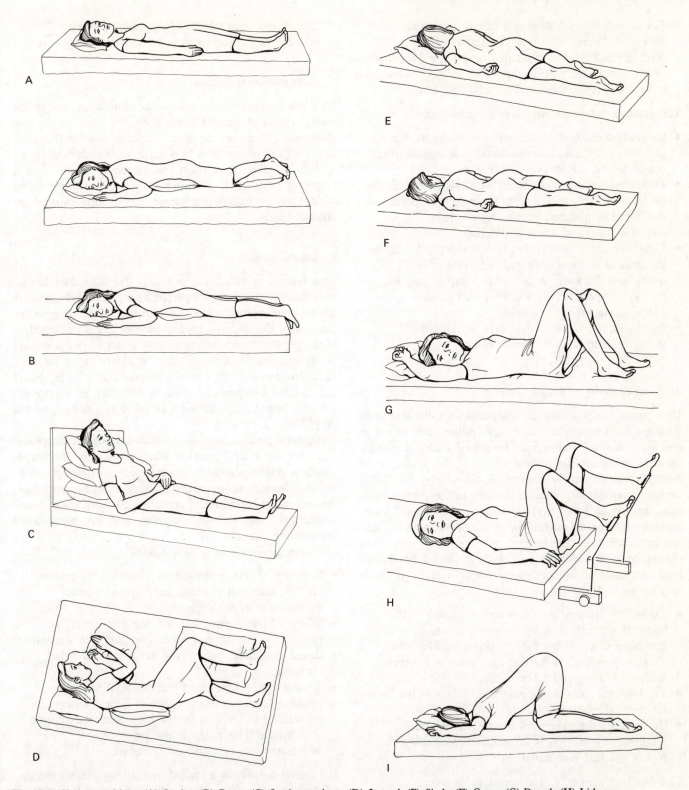

Fig. 35.6 Various positions. (A) Supine. (B) Prone. (C) Semi recumbent. (D) Lateral. (E) Sim's. (F) Coma. (G) Dorsal. (H) Lithotomy. (I) Genupectoral (knee-chest).

- For several hours following a lumbar puncture. Re-establishment of normal circulation of the cerebrospinal fluid is facilitated, and lying flat helps to prevent a severe headache which may occur from a change of pressure in cerebrospinal fluid.

The disadvantages of a supine position include:

- Restriction of chest expansion. The lungs are unable to inflate fully, and secretions accumulate, therefore congestion of the lungs may occur.
- Difficulty may be experienced when toilet utensils are being used. This may lead to incomplete emptying of the bowel or bladder, which may result in constipation or urinary tract infection.
- Depression may result from loss of independence and the difficulties associated with activities of living, e.g. eating and drinking. A person in a supine position may also experience difficulty in seeing, or participating in, ward activities.
- Increasing the work of the heart, as lying flat increases venous return (pre-load).

2. *Prone (anterior recumbent) position*

In a prone position, the individual lies on his abdomen with his head supported on a small pillow and turned to one side. A small pillow may be placed under the abdomen, to maintain the natural curve of the spine, or to relieve pressure on the breasts. A pillow may be placed under the ankles to maintain the feet in the correct position, and to facilitate slight flexion of the knees. (Alternatively, the individual may be positioned so that his toes are extended over the end of the mattress.) His arms should be positioned comfortably, e.g. flexed beside his head, or extended along side his torso. A prone position may be indicated:

- To relieve pressure on the posterior surface of the body. If a person has, for example, a burn or decubitus ulcer on his back, a prone position will alleviate pressure on the damaged area, and therefore facilitate healing and relieve pain.
- To provide access to the posterior surface of the body for medical examination.
- To promote drainage from the respiratory tract. Drainage, by gravity, is further facilitated when the foot of the bed is elevated.

The disadvantages of a prone position include:

- Restriction of chest expansion. Lung congestion is more probable, as the lungs are unable to inflate fully and secretions tend to accumulate.
- Difficulty may be experienced in performing the activities of living, e.g. eating, drinking, or using toilet utensils.

- Depression from loss of independence, and an inability to participate in ward activities, may occur.

3. *Semi recumbent position*

In a semi recumbent position, the individual lies on his back, with 3–4 pillows supporting his head, neck, and shoulders. There are no specific indications for this position, but the person may find it the most comfortable one to assume. The nurse must ensure that the individual is correctly positioned, in order to reduce shearing forces which are a predisposing factor in the formation of decubitus ulcers.

4. *Lateral position*

In a lateral, or side lying position, the individual lies on his side, with his head supported on a pillow. His arms are placed comfortably in front of him and, depending on the purpose of the position, his legs may be flexed or extended. If the person is required to assume a lateral position for a prolonged period, a pillow may be placed along his back to facilitate maintenance of the position. The limbs should not assume a dependent position and may be supported, e.g. the upper arm and leg may be flexed and supported on pillows.

A lateral position may be adapted for specific purposes, e.g. as a left lateral position where both legs are flexed, which is commonly used for examination or treatment involving the rectum or vagina. During a lumbar puncture, the individual is positioned laterally with both knees flexed and drawn towards the abdomen, and his head flexed towards the chest.

A lateral position may be indicated:

- For treatment or examination involving the rectum, e.g. the insertion of rectal suppositories, or for examination of the vagina.
- When a lumbar puncture is being performed, as placing the person in a lateral position with the spine flexed facilitates entry of the needle between the vertebrae.
- To nurse an unconscious individual. A lateral position promotes maintenance of a clear airway, by preventing the tongue from falling back and causing obstruction. This position also prevents oral secretions from entering the trachea.

If a lateral position is assumed over a long period, the disadvantages are an increased risk of postural deformities, decubitus ulcers, and various other complications associated with the prolonged use of any position.

5. *Sim's position*

In the Sim's, or semi-prone, position the individual lies on the side with the upper leg drawn up towards the chest and the buttocks towards the edge of the bed. The lower arm is placed behind the person, and the upper arm is positioned comfortably in front. The head is supported on a small pillow. The Sim's position may be indicated for:

- vaginal examination, as it facilitates the insertion of a speculum and visualization of the vagina and cervix.

This position is considered to be less embarrassing than the dorsal position, when a vaginal examination is being performed.

6. Coma position

In the coma position, the individual is placed in a position that is basically the Sim's, but without a pillow under the head. Correct positioning of the head is essential to promote a clear airway, and a pillow may impede breathing. A coma position may be indicated:

- Temporarily during unconsciousness, e.g. following an episode of fainting. A clear airway is facilitated with the head on one side, as this prevents the tongue or oral secretions from obstructing the trachea.

If used for an extended time, the disadvantages of the coma position include:

- Restriction of chest expansion. The lungs are unable to inflate fully, secretions accumulate, and the risk of lung congestion is increased.
- Postural deformities such as limb contractures are more likely to occur. In addition, prolonged pressure on the shoulder and arm that is placed behind the individual may result in damage to the brachial plexus.

7. Dorsal position

In a dorsal position, the individual lies on the back, with knees flexed and apart, and the soles of the feet flat on the bed. The head is supported on a pillow, and the arms are positioned comfortably. A dorsal position may be indicated:

- to introduce a urinary catheter into a female, as the urethral meatus is made visible and accessible.
- to perform vaginal examinations or treatments, e.g. insertion of vaginal ointment.
- to administer an enema or rectal suppositories, if the person is unable to assume a lateral position.

The disadvantage of a dorsal position is that it is embarrassing for the individual.

The dorsal position may also be adapted to form the lithotomy position, where the person's legs are elevated and supported by stirrups. A lithotomy position may be used during gynaecological surgery, or during the birth of a baby.

8. Sitting positions

There are three variations of a sitting position (Fig. 35.7).

A. The semi-upright position where the individual sits at an angle of approximately 30°, supported by pillows which are placed against the back-rest of the bed.

B. The upright position where the individual is in a full sitting position, with pillows placed to support his upper body.

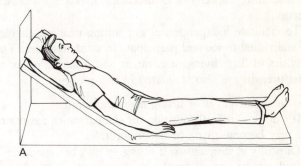

Fig. 35.7 Sitting positions. (A) Semi upright.

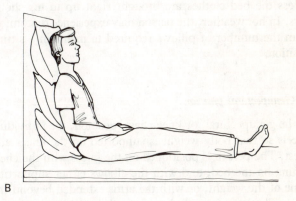

Fig. 35.7 (B) Upright.

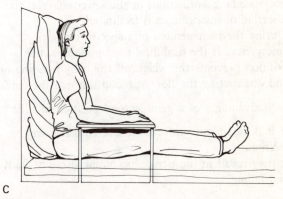

Fig. 35.7 (C) Orthopnoeic.

C. The orthopnoeic position where, from an upright position, the individual leans on to an overbed table.

A sitting position may be indicated:

• Following abdominal or thoracic surgery. Less tension is exerted on an abdominal wound, therefore comfort is promoted. Drainage by gravity from body cavities is facilitated, e.g. when there has been a drainage tube inserted following surgery.

• To facilitate breathing and reduce dyspnoea. Because the diaphragm is able to flatten, maximum chest expansion is promoted and the risk of lung congestion is decreased. Leaning forward, as in the orthopneic position, helps to increase lung capacity and therefore alleviate distressed breathing.

• To facilitate independence, as a sitting position enables the individual to see and participate in ward activities. The activities of daily living, e.g. eating and drinking or using toilet utensils are also facilitated in this position.

The disadvantages of a sitting position include:

• It can be a difficult position for the person to maintain, and may become tiring or uncomfortable.

• Difficulty in sleeping while sitting up may be experienced.

• Prolonged pressure on the buttocks and sacral area increases the risk of decubitus ulcers.

• It may be difficult to ensure the individual's warmth, unless the bed clothes are brought right up to his shoulders. In hot weather, the person may experience discomfort from the number of pillows required to maintain a sitting position.

9. Genupectoral position

In the genupectoral, or knee-chest, position, the individual kneels so that body weight is supported on the knees and chest. The person is positioned on the knees with the chest resting on the bed, and with the elbows either supporting some of the weight, or with the arms extended beyond the head. The head is turned to one side and supported on a pillow. A genupectoral position may be indicated:

• For specific examinations of the lower colon as the insertion of instruments is facilitated.

• During the management of a specific obstetric emergency. If the umbilical cord prolapses, this position prevents the weight of the baby pressing on and obstructing the flow of blood through the cord.

The disadvantages of a genupectoral position include:

• It is difficult, uncomfortable, and embarrassing to maintain.

• It may result in the person becoming dizzy or faint, and falling.

Whatever position the individual assumes, the nurse should implement measures to promote comfort and safety. Pillows should be arranged for maximum comfort and support, and placed so that the person's head, neck, shoulders and spine are supported at a comfortable angle. The pillow behind the head and neck should be placed so that the individual's head is not pushed forward. Supplementary equipment, e.g. sheepskins, should be used to enhance comfort and to relieve pressure. Upper bed clothes should be arranged for maximum covering and warmth, and tucked in loosely to allow room for movement. A footboard or firm pillow may be placed in the bed to help sustain the individual's position, and to help maintain the feet in a neutral position. To reduce development of decubitus ulcers or postural deformities, the position of the individual should be changed at least every four hours. When a person is required to assume a specific position for examination or treatment purposes, the nurse should ensure adequate draping and privacy to reduce embarrassment and promote comfort.

It is also important to ensure that the individual is correctly positioned when he is sitting in a chair. A variety of chairs is available, and a style should be chosen to meet the person's needs. A chair should be comfortable and support the individual adequately. Specially designed chairs may be indicated for some people, e.g. a chair with an elevated seat is used following hip surgery, to prevent strain on the joint.

When sitting in a chair, the individual's spine and buttocks should be well aligned to the contours of the chair. Both feet should be flat on the floor, or (at times) it may be necessary to support one or both feet on a footstool or chair. Limbs should be supported in a position of comfort, and pillows used when necessary, e.g. to support an arm when an intravenous infusion is in progress, or a plaster cast has been applied. The individual should be adequately dressed, and light coverings should be provided to promote his warmth and privacy. Some people may require a postural support device to help maintain their upper body in alignment. Postural support devices include a style of vest which is placed over the individual's clothes, and it contains straps which are attached to either side of the chair. This type of support device, and any others used, must be applied correctly to promote the person's comfort and safety. Further information on the use of support devices is provided in Chapter 38. Adequate explanation should be given to the individual, and, if necessary, to the significant others that such a device is being used to assist the individual maintain his position.

Rest and sleep

The need for comfort is closely related to the need for sufficient rest and sleep. Rest is dependent on relaxation, and in order to be relaxed, an individual must be physically comfortable and free from emotional tension. Relaxation does not necessarily mean inactivity, e.g. a person who has a sedentary occupation may find the physical activity of a brisk walk relaxing. People who are confined to bed may find it more relaxing if they are reading or watching television, rather than lying in bed with nothing to do.

An individual may find it difficult to rest in a hospital environment due to the constant activity around him, or due to the disturbing sights and smells that may be associated with illness. A person may be subjected to bright lights or disruptive noises, and his rest may be disturbed by members of the health care team constantly attending to him. Anxiety related to his illness, and its consequences, may prevent relaxation and interrupt his sleep. Being in hospital involves a number of potential stressors, therefore the nurse should implement measures to provide as stress free an environment as possible.

Nursing care should be planned so that repeated disturbance to the individual is avoided. Emotional tension may be reduced by providing the person with adequate information before any treatment or procedure is commenced. The nurse should promote a climate that is conducive to communication, by spending time with the individual and his significant others to provide opportunities for questions to be asked and answered. Unnecessary noise should be eliminated, and the reasons for unavoidable noises should be given.

Some regulation regarding visiting times may be necessary to avoid over tiring the individual. Many institutions have specified times during the day that are regarded as rest periods. Throughout these periods visitors to the ward, and activities in the ward, are kept to a minimum to provide a quiet, relaxed environment. During rest periods people should be encouraged to try to sleep, or to engage in some relaxing, non-stressful activity. To facilitate rest and relaxation the individual's physical comfort should be promoted, as it is difficult to rest in the presence of discomfort, e.g. pain, or an uncomfortable position.

The many stressors associated with illness may have a detrimental affect on a person's well being, and some individuals may find various relaxation techniques helpful. For many people, physical exercise is an effective method of relieving stress, but as this is not always practical, relaxation techniques may be used instead. There are a number of techniques available for stress reduction and the promotion of relaxation, all of which aim to help an individual to control his reaction to stress. Stress is the body's response as it attempts to adapt to changes, and the subject of stress is outlined in Chapter 6.

In order to promote relaxation so that the need for rest and sleep may be met, the teaching of a constructive method of coping with stress may be indicated. Relaxation techniques should initially be learned in a quiet restful environment and, with practice, may then be used in most situations to reduce stress. In order to practice these techniques, the individual should be lying or sitting comfortably, with the limbs relaxed, the eyes closed, and with sensory stimulation reduced to a minimum.

Relaxation techniques

Yoga and meditation. Both are forms of relaxation that are helpful to many people, and while neither is difficult, they should be taught by people who have specialized in these methods.

Relaxation breathing. This technique consists of controlled breathing, performed while the individual assumes a comfortable position. The person is encouraged to concentrate on his breathing, and may find it helpful to visualize each breath as providing his muscles with energy-giving oxygen. He is encouraged to take a deep breath, hold it briefly, then exhale slowly. Each time he exhales, he is encouraged to say 'relax' to himself and, as the technique is repeated, he should feel progressively more relaxed.

Progressive muscular relaxation. The theory behind this technique is that a relaxed body leads to a relaxed mind. The technique consists of consciously tensing and relaxing the major muscles of the body in sequence. The individual is encouraged to tense one or a group of muscles, feel the tension, then slowly ease the tension by relaxing the muscles. As the technique is repeated, he should become aware of the sensation of relaxation in the muscles.

Visual imagery. This technique involves encouraging the individual to imagine a restful scene. By imagining the scene, together with the associated sounds and smells, it is possible to become quite relaxed.

Touch/Massage. It is generally considered that the sense of touch is as important a contact with reality, as the senses of sight and sound. Massage is a method of communication without words, and a good massage can induce a feeling of physical and mental relaxation. There are many types of massage and, while most are relatively easy to learn, the basic techniques should be taught by people with experience. Muscles contract and become tense in stressful situations, and massage can be an effective method of promoting muscle relaxation. Some of the key aspects of massage are:

- Provision of a quiet, private environment, free from harsh lighting.
- Provision of warmth. The room, the person receiving the massage, and any oils being used should be comfortably warm.
- The person who is giving the massage should have short finger nails, and clean warm hands.
- Verbal communication should be limited, and the recipient encouraged to concentrate on the sensation of physical contact.
- The person giving the massage should convey, in her

touch, an impression of confidence and ability. Remembering that the recipient is a person with dignity will influence the quality of touch.

● Following the massage, the recipient should be encouraged to remain resting, quiet, and relaxed.

Although a massage can be most beneficial, some people may not feel comfortable about being massaged. In addition, the physical condition of an individual may contra-indicate the use of massage. In the right situation, however, massage—particularly of the neck and back—can be very relaxing and promote rest.

Sleep

Sleep may be defined as a period of reduced consciousness, diminished muscular activity, and depressed metabolism. Sleep provides the greatest degree of rest, with all body systems functioning at a reduced level. Although sleep is a state of reduced consciousness, certain stimuli, e.g. a sudden loud noise, will usually rouse the person.

There are individual variations in the optimum amount of sleep required, with approximately 7 hours per night being the average. The quality is equally as important as the quantity of sleep achieved. Sleep patterns change throughout the life cycle, and the quantity of sleep diminishes from approximately 20 hours per day in infancy to as little as 4 hours in old age.

There are several theories about the purpose of sleep, with the most commonly accepted concept being that sleep promotes the growth and repair of body cells. It would seem that, during sleep, there are variations in the amount of circulating hormones, e.g. the growth hormone and those secreted by the adrenal glands. The alteration in the amount of these hormones circulating during sleep is considered to facilitate cell growth and repair. It is therefore of particular importance that the person who is hospitalized has the opportunity to benefit from the restorative nature of sleep.

There are two types of sleep—non rapid eye movement sleep, and rapid eye movement sleep. Normally a period of sleep consists of approximately 4—6 cycles, each lasting around 100 minutes. It is generally recognized that each sleep cycle consists of five stages. The first four stages are described as the stages of non rapid eye movement (NREM) sleep, while the final stage is described as that of rapid eye movement (REM) sleep. The five stages of sleep are:

1. General relaxation and drowsiness. During this stage, which lasts approximately 15 minutes, the person can be awakened by any slight stimulus, e.g. the sound of a dog barking in the distance.
2. During this stage, the person can still be awakened easily but there is greater relaxation.
3. Stage 3 occurs approximately 30 minutes after the

person goes to sleep, during which he is not roused by familiar noises. There is complete relaxation where most body systems slow down, e.g. the pulse rate is reduced.
4. The individual is in a deep sleep, his body is relaxed, and he is difficult to rouse.
5. This is a period of light sleep during which dreaming occurs, and the eyes move rapidly back and forth (REM). If awakened during this stage, the individual may recall vivid dreams.

The act of dreaming, while not fully understood, is considered by some as necessary for the promotion of psychological integration. Dreams can be described as a sequence of thoughts, images, and emotions, that pass through the mind during the REM stage of sleep.

Sleeping is influenced by a variety of factors that may be described as physical, psychological, or environmental. The physical factors that influence sleep include the amount of exercise achieved during the day, and the consumption of certain types of food or fluid. Generally exercise induces sleep, while substances containing caffeine have a stimulant effect that may inhibit sleep.

During a 24-hour period there is a cycle of physiological functions that tend to be highest during the early evening, and to be lowest during the early morning. Examples of these functions are metabolic rate, heart and ventilation rates, and body temperature. A pattern based on this 24 hour cycle is referred to as a circadian rhythm, in which certain actions such as eating and sleeping are repeated regularly. It would appear that the 24 hour cycle of light and dark is the pattern to which humans synchronise their body rhythms and is an important factor in the cycle of sleeping and waking. Any disruption to an individual's circadian rhythm can cause discomfort, e.g. disturbed sleep patterns. One example of the consequences of disrupted circadian rhythm, is the state known as 'jet lag'. This condition occurs when the individual's circadian rhythm is disrupted by travel across several time zones in a relatively short time, and is characterized by fatigue, insomnia, and sluggish physical and mental function. People who are being nursed in intensive care units may experience the same phenomenon. Intensive care units are usually brightly lit during the night as well as during the day. Without a regular pattern of light and dark, together with the disturbing sights and sound, an individual in I.C.U. may experience disruption to his normal 24 hour rhythm. An individual who engages in shift work may experience symptoms similar to jet lag, as his body adapts to changes in his 24 hour biological clock. For example, working on night shift removes sleeping from the normal night time activities, and renders it out of order with his body time.

Any interruptions to sleep may cause interference with an individual's ability to carry out normal activities. A person who experiences a sleep pattern disturbance may exhibit changes in behaviour and performance. He may show signs of increased irritability, lack of energy, and fatigue. Sleep pattern disturbances include difficulty in falling asleep, periods of wakefulness during the night, wakening earlier than usual, and not feeling rested after sleep.

Some individuals experience nightmares or sleep walking. A nightmare is a dream that arouses feelings of intense fear or extreme anxiety, and usually wakens the sleeper. Sleep walking is a state that culminates in walking about, and although in full possession of his senses, the individual has no recollection of the episode.

Nursing practice to promote sleep

As a result of illness and/or hospitalization, e.g. due to physical discomfort, anxiety, or environmental disturbances such as distressing sounds, a person may experience difficulty in maintaining his normal sleep pattern. Individuals should be encouraged to maintain their normal routine which may include adopting the natural measures to promote sleep.

Natural measures that facilitate sleep

- Sleeping in a room that is quiet, at a comfortable temperature, and which has sufficient fresh air.
- Engaging in physical exercise during the day to promote rest at night.
- Spending some time relaxing and unwinding before going to bed. Sleep may also be more easily achieved, if people are able to resolve any problems before going to bed.
- Resisting stimulants such as tea, coffee or cocoa, immediately before going to bed. People may find it easier to sleep if they avoid going to bed feeling hungry or overfed.
- Adopting a pre-sleep routine, e.g. warm bath or shower, warm drink, and some peaceful music or relaxing reading.

The nurse should assist a person in preparation for sleep, by ensuring that his key physiological and psychological needs are met.

Hygiene needs. The person should be assisted to meet his hygiene needs, e.g. washing his face and hands and cleaning his teeth. An ambulant individual may like to have a warm shower or bath before settling to sleep, and pressure area care should be provided for the non-ambulant person.

Nutritional and fluid needs. A warm drink and snack should be offered to the individual, unless this is contra-indicated. A person may prefer a non stimulating milk-based drink, rather than tea or coffee which can have a stimulating effect. A person who is permitted oral fluids should also be provided with fluid which can be consumed during the night if desired.

Elimination needs. The individual should be provided with toilet facilities before settling for sleep. The nurse may need to assist an ambulant person to the toilet, or provide a non-ambulant person with the appropriate toilet utensil. Urinary drainage equipment should be checked, and the collection bag emptied if necessary.

Comfort needs. The room should be prepared by ensuring that there is adequate ventilation and warmth, and that lighting is reduced to a minimum. The individual's signal device and any other items he may require during the night, should be placed within easy reach. The nurse should ensure that he is positioned comfortably, and that the bedclothes and pillows are arranged to meet his needs. The bottom sheets should be free of wrinkles or creases, and supplementary items such as a sheepskin may be used to enhance his comfort. Any splints or dressings should be checked and, if necessary, adjusted or changed. If possible, treatments and procedures should be completed before the individual settles for sleep.

Protection and safety needs. Measures should be taken to promote the individual's safety during sleep. If a person is restless or confused, the use of bed rails may be indicated. For some individuals, it may be appropriate to adjust the height of the bed to its lowest level. (As an alternative safety measure, the person's bed may be made up on the floor for the night. This measure may be indicated for an individual who is disorientated, and inclined to get out of bed and wander.)

Adequate lighting should be provided, particularly if the person needs to get out of bed during the night. The individual should be monitored regularly throughout the night, to assess his condition, and to ensure that any equipment, e.g. intravenous infusion apparatus, is functioning properly.

Pain avoidance needs. The nurse in charge must be notified immediately if an individual is experiencing pain, or any other distressing symptoms such as a troublesome cough.

Psychological needs. The nurse should explain to the individual that there will always be some one there during the night to attend to his needs. If the person is anxious or worried, the nurse should try to ascertain the reason and notify the nurse in charge. For example, a person may be concerned about some aspect of his treatment such as forthcoming surgery, and providing him with further information may help to alleviate his anxiety.

An individual may be prescribed medication to promote sleep, e.g. a sedative. Once this has been administered, the person should be encouraged to relax and allow it to take effect. When the individual has settled for sleep, all activity, noise, and light should be reduced to a minimum.

During the night, the nurse continues to observe the individual, and to perform procedures or treatments as necessary. The person should be disturbed as little as possible, and if he wakes and experiences difficulty in re-settling, measures such as a change of position, adjustment to the bedding, or a warm drink, may help him to resume sleep. The nurse in charge must be notified if the individual does not re-settle after these measures have been implemented.

The nurse on night duty must ensure that the individual's comfort and safety are promoted. Continuity of care is essential, and as there are usually fewer staff working at night, the nurse's observational skills are vital in detecting any change in a person's condition. The nurse has a responsibility to become aware of the institution's policies with regard to her role during the night shift.

SUMMARY

Comfort is dependent upon having both the physical and psychological needs meet, and upon freedom from physical discomfort and emotional tension. Discomfort can result from either physical or emotional stimuli, and the nurse should implement measures to prevent or alleviate discomfort. Relief of anxiety, or emotional tension, can be facilitated by providing the individual with sufficient information prior to any procedures or treatment. The person's physical comfort can be promoted by ensuring that all his needs are met, and the provision of a well made bed will enhance comfort. A bed is made up to meet the individual's needs, and supplementary equipment, e.g. a sheepskin, may be used as an additional comfort measure. Other equipment used in conjunction with bed making is available to facilitate the individual's movement, to provide added support, to promote safety, or to prevent complications associated with immobility.

Individuals assume, or are assisted to assume, positions of comfort or specific positions for therapeutic purposes. Correct positioning is necessary to promote the person's safety and comfort, and poor positioning can lead to discomfort or certain complications, e.g. decubitus ulcers.

Comfort is necessary for relaxation, rest, and sleep. A person's ability to relax, and therefore to receive sufficient rest and sleep, may be disrupted during illness or hospitalization. The measures which are implemented to promote rest, may include certain techniques that facilitate relaxation. Sleep can be promoted by allowing the individual to maintain his normal pre-sleep routine, and by ensuring that the person's safety and comfort are promoted during the night, as at any other time. Assisting the individual to meet his need for comfort, rest, and sleep, is essential in the promotion of his physical and psychological well being.

36. Meeting pain avoidance needs

OBJECTIVES

1. Describe the physiological processes whereby pain sensations are received, transmitted, and interpreted.
2. State the factors influencing an individual's perception of, and reaction to, pain.
3. Describe the observations made to assess pain.
4. State the methods of pain management.
5. Apply appropriate principles in planning and implementing nursing actions to prevent and to alleviate an individual's pain.

INTRODUCTION

Pain is both an unpleasant physical sensation and an emotional experience, and each episode of pain is a unique personal event. Because no one can fully appreciate the pain of another person, pain is always a subjective experience.

Pain may be mild or severe, acute or chronic. Pain is difficult to define as it is an individual experience with varying levels of intensity, and it may be physical, psychological, or emotional in origin. Pain is often described as being a sensation of distress or suffering caused by a stimulus, but a more appropriate definition is that 'pain is what the person says it is'.

Pain is one of the most common causes of discomfort, and both Maslow and Kalish included pain avoidance as first priority physiological needs (refer to Ch. 28). Pain avoidance appears to be an instinctive reaction to harmful factors in the environment, e.g. a newborn will draw away from a painful stimulus if possible. Throughout the life cycle, individuals avoid painful stimuli or take actions to withdraw from the stimulus.

Causes of pain

Pain is often a useful protective signal, as it can be a warning of actual or impending tissue damage. The sensation of pain can also warn the individual of emotional or stress-related problems, e.g. a headache caused by tension or anxiety. Pain can result from mechanical trauma, chemical irritants, extremes of temperature, ischaemia, and psychological factors.

Mechanical trauma. Pain may result when body tissues are stretched, e.g. distension of a hollow organ such as the stomach or bladder. When tissues are contracted, e.g. in muscle spasm, pain occurs as a result of local ischaemia, stretched nerve endings, and from an accumulation of metabolic wastes. Prolonged pressure on tissues causes local ischaemia and pressure on nerve endings, and consequently pain. Physical force, e.g. a hard blow, to the tissues results in initial pressure on the nerve endings and subsequent irritation from substances released by the damaged cells.

Chemical irritation. Stimulation of sensory nerve endings by irritant chemicals from an external source, e.g. acid, or by chemical substances released by damaged cells will cause pain. Substances may leak from an organ into the peritoneal cavity and stimulate large areas of pain fibres causing severe pain, e.g. gastric juice may escape as a result of a perforated gastric ulcer.

Extremes of temperature. Extremes of heat or cold, as in a burn or frostbite, damage tissues and cause pain. In many burns, or scalds, the nerve endings are damaged, and frostbite causes local blood vessel constriction and ischaemia.

Ischaemia. Decreased blood supply, or ischaemia, causes cell damage or death with the subsequent release of irritating chemical substances that stimulate the pain nerve endings.

Psychological factors. Pain may be experienced in the absence of any physiological cause, or as a result of the physical manifestations of psychological disorders, e.g. abdominal cramp resulting from stress or anxiety.

Physiology of pain

The ability to relieve or to control pain depends on an understanding of how it occurs and how it is controlled by the brain.

Pain receptors in the skin and other tissues are free nerve endings, some of which are the peripheral terminations of small diameter C fibres, while others are the slightly larger diameter A fibres. The A fibres transmit pain impulses more rapidly than do the slow conducting C fibres. When histamine and other naturally occurring chemical substances are released, e.g. as a result of tissue damage, pain sensations travel along the nerve fibres. Pain sensations are transmitted to the dorsal root ganglia of the spinal cord (Fig. 36.1), and synapse with certain neurons in the posterior horns of the grey matter. Pain sensations are then transmitted to various areas of the brain, by synapses at the thalamus, where they are perceived and interpreted.

Pain causes both reflex motor reactions and psychic reactions. Some of the reflex actions occur directly from the spinal cord, where small neurons in the grey matter transmit an impulse straight from the skin to the muscles—without brain involvement. For example a painful stimulus to the hand, such as extreme heat, initiates reflex contraction of the flexor muscles which cause withdrawal of the arm.

Although the complex mechanisms of the physiology and psychology of pain are not understood completely, the Gate Control Theory of pain suggests that neural mechanisms in

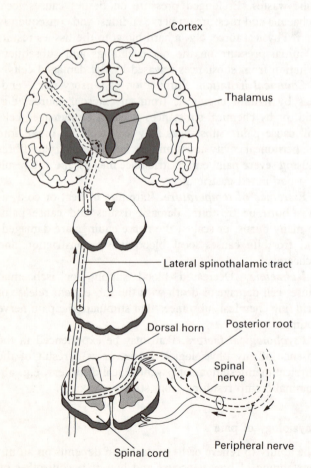

Fig. 36.1 The pathway of pain.

the dorsal horns of the spinal cord can act like a gate. This theory suggests that activity in the large diameter nerve fibres can close the gate and block pain impulses, resulting in a decrease or elimination of pain sensation. Therefore, according to the Gate Control Theory, it is possible to block pain impulses travelling to the brain by stimulating the large A nerve fibres and closing the gate. This theory may help to explain the reason why acupuncture can relieve pain; as in acupuncture, stimulation of non-painful nerve fibres can suppress pain signals. It is acknowledged that pain can be inhibited along the course of transmission, and that endorphins play a complex role in closing the gate to pain. Some of the pain-inhibiting neurons in the dorsal horn produce endorphins, which are neuro-transmitters that mediate the transmission of pain information.

Endorphins are substances with opioid qualities that combine with the same receptors as do morphine and other narcotics, producing the same effect, i.e. analgesia. As a result of pain or stress, an impulse from the brain may trigger the release of endorphins which block transmission of the pain impulse before it reaches the brain. Various studies have shown that plasma endorphin levels increase in states of stress, and also that acupuncture and transcutaneous electrical nerve stimulation (TENS) increase endorphin release. Therefore, although incompletely understood, it is known that the body has some internal mechanisms that help to control pain and its perception.

Types of pain

1. Acute pain is usually of rapid onset, varies in intensity, is self limiting, and lasts for varying lengths of time. Acute pain, if mild, may require no specific intervention, and more severe acute pain can usually be managed successfully. Acute pain may result from injury, infection, or following surgical intervention; and when tissue damage is the cause, pain declines as the tissues heal.

2. Chronic pain is considered to be pain that has lasted for at least six months, and is an on-going experience that fails to resolve naturally or does not respond well to intervention. The pain from arthritis may be regarded as chronic pain. An individual who experiences unrelieved pain for an extended period often feels trapped and helpless. His anxiety increases as he becomes preoccupied with the pain and his state of health. He may experience sleep disturbances and fatigue, and as a result, he may become increasingly irritable, aggressive or withdrawn, or he may feel depressed.

3. Superficial (cutaneous) pain originates in the skin or mucous membrane as a result of stimulation of receptors in those areas. Because there are large numbers of sensory nerve endings on the surface of the body, an individual is usually able to localize surface pain accurately.

4. Deep (visceral) pain originates in internal body structures as a result of stimulation of receptors in those areas. As there are fewer sensory nerve endings in the viscera than in the skin or mucous membrane, it is more difficult to localize visceral pain. Localized damage to the viscera rarely causes severe pain, whereas widepread damage causing diffuse stimulation of the nerve endings produces extreme pain. For example, occlusion of the blood supply to a large section of the intestine stimulates many diffuse fibres and can result in severe pain. Visceral pain may be felt at a site far removed from the affected area, through the mechanism of referred pain.

5. Referred pain is felt in a part of the body away from the pain's point of origin, e.g. pain in the left shoulder and arm associated with myocardial infarction. Sensory neurons that transmit signals from the skin enter the same area of the spinal cord as do nerve fibres from the affected internal organ. The neurons carry pain signals from both sites to the brain and, because cutaneous pain is more common than visceral pain, the brain interprets the pain as originating in the skin. Figure 36.2 illustrates the common sites of referred pain.

6. Phantom pain is a sensation of pain felt in a body part that has been removed, e.g. when the lower leg has been amputated. Although the nerves supplying the amputated part have been severed, the remaining neurons may continue to send impulses as before—and the brain still interprets the impulses as if that part was still there.

7. Intractable pain refers to pain that is severe and constant or unrelenting, and which is unrelieved by the usual measures. For example, the extreme and constant pain often associated with cancer may not be relieved by strong analgesics alone, and the individual may also require non-drug therapy such as surgery to block the nerve fibres conducting the pain impulses.

8. Total pain. The suffering experienced by an individual with cancer pain is derived from a variety of sources, and the term 'total pain' was devised to address the complexity of pain as a somatic and psychological experience. The individual's pain threshold can be lowered by psychological factors such as fear, depression, and isolation, with the result that the pain experience is increased.

Perception of pain

The perception of pain is individual and is therefore different for each person. In addition, an individual will perceive pain differently at different times. The pain threshold is the point at which a stimulus, e.g. pressure, activates pain receptors and produces a sensation of pain. In 1982 Melzack and Wall described four identifiable levels of pain threshold.

1. Sensation threshold, which is the lowest stimulus level at which sensation, e.g. tingling, is first perceived.

2. Pain perception threshold, which is the lowest stimulus level at which the individual states that the stimulation is painful.

3. Pain tolerance, which is the lowest level at which the person withdraws from or asks to have the stimulation stopped.

4. Encouraged pain tolerance, which is the same as pain tolerance but the individual is encouraged to tolerate higher levels of stimulation.

Because the perception of pain is individual, some people will experience pain much earlier than others. Studies have shown that all people have a similar sensation threshold, but that the ways in which they react to pain vary greatly.

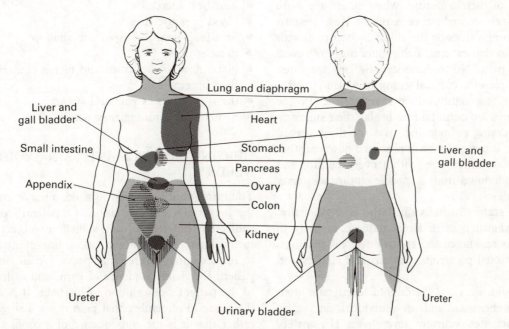

Fig. 36.2 Referred pain sites. Cutaneous areas to which pain from certain viscera is referred.

Reaction to pain

The way in which an individual reacts to pain varies tremendously, according to many factors. Behavioural manifestations of pain vary according to the individual and factors in his environment.

1. Age. As infants and young children lack the ability to express themselves verbally, their pain may not be recognized or appreciated. In addition, children are taught very early in life that they are expected to be brave, and that 'only babies cry'. As a result, a child who is experiencing pain may endeavour to hide it. Conversely, a child may invent or exaggerate pain as a method of gaining attention.

When an older child or adolescent experiences pain, he tends to think of it in terms of how it will affect his activities and the attainment of goals. Young patients sometimes harbour distressing fantasies about the significance of pain, as a result of misunderstanding about their body and illness. Consequently, both anxiety and pain are increased.

The ability to tolerate pain generally seems to increase with age, and this may be partly due to an increased ability to cope with pain and partly to expectations about what constitutes 'adult' behaviour.

2. Sex. It is a common belief that males are more able to tolerate pain than females. It is important to be aware that many males have been conditioned by society to be brave. Many people consider that any display of emotion, e.g. crying, by a male is a sign of weakness. As a result of society's expectations of acceptable behaviour, a male may suppress his expressions of pain.

3. Culture. An individual's culture, e.g. race and status, plays an important role in the way he reacts to pain. Some people have a matter of fact attitude to pain with little outward expression of their suffering, while others are more expressive and seek immediate pain relief. Most western cultures place strong values on the ability to bear pain with silent fortitude, so that external behaviours may not reveal the intensity of pain. North American Indians are often cited as an example of a cultural group in which stoic indifference to pain is a highly valued characteristic. People from Latin cultures are permitted to display their suffering openly, e.g. by crying or moaning, as a socially accepted response to pain. It must also be appreciated however, that there are enormous differences within every culture and that not every individual from a specific culture will react in the same manner.

4. Emotional state. An individual who is emotionally, or physically, exhausted often has a reduced capacity to tolerate pain. His resistance and control over his reactions is lessened. Continual pain results in anxiety; anxiety and fear aggravate pain.

5. Previous pain. Previous episodes of severe pain often cause great apprehension, and an individual can suffer greatly if he anticipates recurrent severe pain. His anxiety is increased if his previous experience of severe pain was poorly managed.

6. Self image. How an individual perceives himself can influence his reaction to pain. For example, a person who has a low self esteem may try to bear his pain stoically in order to be regarded highly by others. Conversely another person with a poor self image, and feelings of worthlessness, may tolerate pain poorly in an attempt to gain attention and recognition.

7. Time of day. Night, with accompanying darkness and reduced sensory input, often increases an individual's sensation of pain. Fear and anxiety may be increased and, as a result, so too is the sensation of pain.

8. Environment. There is a relationship between anxiety and pain, and environmental factors can either contribute to or reduce anxiety levels. The environment can act as an anxiety-provoking stressor, e.g. if it is ugly, if there is an atmosphere of tension, or if there is a lack of privacy. Privacy allows an individual uninhibited expression of pain, e.g. crying or moaning. The continued presence of other people, e.g. in a shared ward, results in a sense of loss of privacy. This may be a cause of anxiety and a contributing factor in the perception of, and reaction to, pain.

It is, therefore, important to recognize the many factors that influence pain reactions, and to appreciate that each pain experience is unique and personal. Anyone who is caring for a person experiencing pain should not judge the appropriateness of that person's reaction to pain, and must be sensitive to individual needs.

Although behavioural reactions to pain are individual, the physiological manifestations of pain can be observed in all people. When pain occurs the stress response is activated, with the result that:

- heartbeat increases
- blood pressure rises
- breathing becomes rapid and shallow
- muscles tense
- blood flow to the hands and feet is constricted, and they become cold
- the skin becomes pale and sweaty
- nausea and vomiting may occur.

NURSING PRACTICE AND PAIN AVOIDANCE NEEDS

The nurse is in a position to make a major contribution to the prevention and alleviation of a patient's pain. Pain is a subjective experience, not subject to objective measurement. Therefore the nurse has an important responsibility to implement measures that prevent pain, to observe the patient for visible evidence of pain, and to listen carefully to the patient's description of his pain. It is important for the nurse to remember that pain is not a single entity, but rather that it is the consequence of a conflict between the stimulus and the whole individual. The nurse has a responsibility to the patient, firstly not to cause or allow him to experience unnecessary pain; and secondly, if pain is experienced, to do all that is possible to relieve his pain and suffering. The nurse also has a responsibility to monitor the efficacy of any prescribed pain management.

Assessment of pain

In addition to observing the patient for the physiological and behavioural manifestations of pain, the nurse should ask questions that enable the patient to describe his pain in his own words. The nurse must never ignore a patient's statement that he has pain, and she should remember that 'pain is what the patient says it is'. A patient can usually sense that he is not believed about pain, and this increases his sense of helplessness. As a consequence, he may compensate by under-reporting pain or by anxiously over-reporting. Either reaction aggravates the circle of mistrust–anxiety–more pain. When assessing a patient's pain the nurse should make certain she obtains sufficient information by observation and questioning.

1. Location. The patient may be able to locate the area specifically, e.g. the tip of the thumb on the left hand, or he may describe the painful area more generally, e.g. all over the abdomen.

2. Time it occurs. Information should be obtained regarding the onset of pain, e.g. whether it was sudden or gradual. The patient should also be asked if the pain increases or decreases at specific times of the day or night. For example, a patient who has arthritis may experience severe joint pain on waking but the pain may become less severe throughout the day.

3. Duration. It is important to establish how long the pain lasts, e.g. whether it is continual, or seems to come and go.

4. Precipitating factors. Certain physical activities or psychological factors may precipitate pain. For example, chest pain may occur following physical exercise, or abdominal pain may occur after eating. A change of posture may aggravate or relieve pain, and factors such as anxiety or fear may also precipitate pain.

5. Impact on activities. The patient should be asked if the pain interferes with the activities of living, e.g. is it so unpleasant that he is unable to eat, move freely, or sleep?.

6. Character/type. This is the way the pain is described by the person who is experiencing it, and it is important for the nurse to report and record the patient's own words. Some of the terms used to describe pain are gripping, knife-like, burning, prickling, tingling, dull, aching, cramping, gnawing, constricting, throbbing, vise-like, crushing, stabbing, shooting.

7. Intensity. The severity of pain is not always evident from the individual's reaction, and must therefore be assessed as the patient's own perception. Several

measurement tools have been designed to assist a patient to describe the intensity of pain. Health care institutions may devise their own measurement tool, or may use a standard tool. One method of assessment is a linear scale from 1–10, on which the patient indicates the intensity of his pain (Fig. 36.3). This type of measurement device facilitates both assessment and management of pain.

8. Associated signs or symptoms. The painful area should be observed for signs of distension or oedema, discolouration e.g. bruising or inflammation, change in skin temperature, and any loss of function or mobility. The nurse should also ascertain whether there is any accom-panying nausea e.g. with abdominal pain, cyanosis e.g. with chest pain, or skin pallor and sweating.

9. Posture and facial expression. The patient's posture and facial expression may indicate that he is experiencing pain. He may assume a certain position in order to minimize the pain, e.g. a patient may lie on his side with the knees drawn up in order to relieve abdominal pain. Severe pain may cause a patient to lie rigidly, as any movement increases the pain. The patient's facial expression is not always a reliable guide to the presence or severity of pain, as facial expressions are varied and may be misleading. A patient experiencing acute pain may grimace and look anxious, whereas a patient with chronic pain may show few signs of distress and his suffering may be masked by a brave or exhausted facial expression.

10. Vital signs. The patient's temperature, pulse, ventilations, and blood pressure should be measured when pain is first experienced. The results should be documented, and repeated measurements made to detect any alterations. Any abnormal result is reported to the nurse in charge immediately.

11. Signs of emotional tension. The patient should be observed for signs of increased emotional tension, e.g. irritability, anxiety, depression, aggression, exhaustion, or sleeplessness.

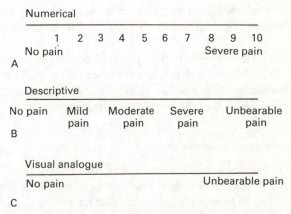

Fig. 36.3 Scales for measuring pain intensity. The individual identifies a point on the scale that corresponds to his perception of the severity of the pain.

When a patient experiences pain the nurse should make the observations as described, report them to the nurse in charge immediately, and document them.

Pain management

The management of pain includes treating the underlying disease to remove or diminish the cause; treating any other symptoms, e.g. nausea or constipation, that may increase the perception of pain; and pharmacological and non-pharmacological therapy. Specific nursing interventions, as described later in this chapter, include minimizing the stimulus that is causing the pain, alleviating pain, and assisting the patient to cope with pain.

Pharmacological therapy

Medications prescribed by the medical officer to relieve pain may be either local or systemic, analgesic or co-analgesic. Information about medications and the nurse's role in their administration is provided in Chapter 58.

Counter-irritants. Counter-irritants, e.g. mentholated ointments, applied locally to the skin produce an inflammatory response thereby relieving congestion in underlying tissues and reducing pain.

Analgesic, or pain relieving, medications may be non-narcotics such as acetylsalicylic acid (aspirin), or narcotics such as morphine. Analgesics may be administered orally, intramuscularly or intravenously, or in some instances they may be applied topically. The route, type and dosage of analgesic medications will be prescribed by the medical officer according to the patient's needs. Effective analgesia is achieved by administering sufficient amounts of the most appropriate medication at regular intervals.

Co-analgesics, while not true analgesics in the pharmacological sense, act to relieve pain alone or in combination with analgesics. Examples of co-analgesic medications are corticosteroids that decrease inflammation and oedema, and tranquilizers that reduce anxiety. Sometimes a small dose of a tranquilizer together with an analgesic, can produce greater pain relief than a higher dose of an analgesic alone.

When medications have been prescribed, it is the nurse's role to administer them if it is within her ability and legal responsibilities. It is also her responsibility to monitor the patient to assess the effectiveness of the treatment.

Non-pharmacological therapy

Pain management and control may be achieved by a variety of measures other than medication. Non-drug approaches to pain management include heat or cold, massage and psychological methods.

Application of heat or cold. Information about the local application of heat or cold is provided in Chapter 33. Heat applied to the skin causes dilatation of the local blood vessels and, as a result, swelling is reduced, healing is promoted, and pain is relieved. Cold applications may also be used to relieve pain, as cold has a numbing effect which helps to reduce pain in the part.

Massage. Information about massage is provided in Chapter 35. Massage involves the manipulation of soft tissue and can increase circulation, reduce muscle tension, relax the individual, and relieve pain.

Psychological methods. Various techniques may be used to promote general relaxation of the patient, and therefore reduce anxiety and relieve pain. Music may be used as a sensory distraction or as a soothing method of reducing stress. Other methods of distraction may be helpful to lessen the individual's awareness of painful stimuli, e.g. encouraging him to concentrate on slow rhythmic breathing exercises.

Other approaches

Several other methods of pain management may be prescribed and while it is not the role of the nurse to implement them, she may be required to be present while they are being performed.

Acupuncture. This technique involves the insertion of fine needles into the skin at selected points on the body. Acupuncture may be used to manage both acute and chronic pain, and there are several theories about how it relieves pain. Some authorities believe that acupuncture achieves analgesia by stimulating the release of endorphins, while others believe that it stimulates the large diameter nerve fibres that effectively close the gate (Gate control mechanism).

Transcutaneous electrical nerve stimulation (TENS). A specific technique of peripheral nerve stimulation, TENS involves the application of electrodes to trigger points on the skin. The electrodes are activated by a battery-powered device to produce a tingling or vibrating sensation in the painful area. The impulses block the transmission of pain impulses to the brain. TENS is well tolerated by most people, although skin irritation is sometimes experienced, but it should not be used for patients with cardiac pacemakers as it can interfere with pacemaker function.

Nerve block. Peripheral nerve transmission of pain can be interrupted temporarily by injecting a local anaesthetic, or permanently by injecting a sclerosing agent. As the latter method can result in destruction of tissue adjacent to the injected area, other pain relieving methods are usually preferred.

Hypnosis. Hypnotic analgesia may be achieved when a person enters a state of self-induced relaxation and concentration. During hypnosis, cognitive thinking is bypassed, allowing the person to become more susceptible to suggestion. The person enters a passive trance-like state which is often induced by the repetition of words and gestures while he is completely relaxed. Susceptibility to hypnosis varies from person to person.

Biofeedback. Biofeedback is a method that assists an individual to become aware of, and subsequently to control, certain autonomic physiological responses, e.g. blood pressure, muscle tension, and heart rate. Through concentration, and with the aid of instruments, the individual can learn to control these processes which are normally thought of as involuntary. The technique of biofeedback is more effective when accompanied by other relaxation techniques.

Radiotherapy and/or chemotherapy. The pain associated with malignant disease may be relieved by radiation which shrinks the tumour. Chemotherapy may often control pain if the tumour is sensitive to the medications chosen. Information on radiotherapy and chemotherapy is provided in Chapter 64.

Placebo therapy. The use of placebos poses ethical and moral problems, as it seems to involve a degree of recipient deception. Placebo therapy involves the administration of inactive substances, and seems to be effective for certain people. It is thought that placebos relieve pain or other symptoms by causing the body to release endorphins, combined with an expectation that the treatment will be effective.

Pain clinics. Individuals who experience chronic pain may be helped by attending a multidisciplinary pain clinic. Pain clinics commonly attempt to reduce pain medication, to help individuals to resume normal activities, and to help to restore a positive self image. Management includes a thorough physical and psychological examination before a programme is designed for the individual. Approaches to pain management in a pain clinic include psychological counselling acupuncture, TENS, or any of the other methods of pain relief. The individual is taught alternative ways of carrying out the activities of living, so that associated pain is minimized.

Nursing care of a patient experiencing pain

The nurse has a responsibility to try to eliminate or minimize the stimulus that is causing pain. She also observes the patient who is experiencing pain, reports and documents those observations, and implements nursing measures to alleviate pain. Continued monitoring of the patient is necessary to evaluate the effectiveness of any prescribed therapy. The nurse also plays an important role in supporting the patient's significant others, who are usually distressed by his pain experience—particularly when the pain is chronic or is a result of terminal illness.

The importance of good communication between the nurse and the patient, and his significant others, cannot be overemphasized. A positive relationship facilitates effective communication, which can affect the patient's response to pain and pain relief. The patient should be encouraged to express his feelings openly, in an atmosphere of trust. The nurse should learn to listen actively to the patient so that not only are his words heard, but any non-verbal cues are also detected. For example, a patient may state that he is not experiencing much pain—but his body language and tone of voice may indicate otherwise. To promote his peace of mind, and therefore to reduce anxiety, the patient should be provided with information about his illness and its management. He should be aware that he has a right to pain relief, and that pain-relieving measures are available. It is important to prevent or reduce the cycle of pain–stress–anxiety–pain. A variety of nursing measures minimize or alleviate pain.

Changing his position. At times pain can result from, or be increased by, an uncomfortable posture. The patient should be assisted into a more comfortable position, with pillows arranged for support. The addition of a sheepskin underneath his back and buttocks may enhance his comfort, and the bedclothes should be arranged to meet his needs. It is important to ensure that his body is in alignment, and the placement of a pillow under a painful limb may further enhance his comfort.

Meeting his needs. The nurse should ensure that all his needs are provided for, e.g. discomfort and pain can result from a distended bladder. He may feel more comfortable if his face and hands are washed, his hair brushed, and his teeth cleaned. If not contraindicated, a drink of his preferred beverage should be offered. A warm drink in the evening may help him settle to sleep.

Gentle handling. When the patient is being assisted to move, the nurse should ensure that any movements are made gently. Pain is usually increased on movement, therefore the patient should be permitted and assisted to move at his own pace. As he moves, the nurse should ensure that painful areas are supported. An incision can be supported during movement, e.g. either the patient or the nurse may place a hand over the incision to 'splint' it.

Promoting rest and sleep. Pain is very tiring, and fatigue increases reactions to pain, therefore the nurse should ensure that the patient receives adequate rest and sleep. Measures should be implemented during the day, as well as during the night, to facilitate rest, e.g. the blinds may be drawn, and all care planned so that repeated interruptions and visits to the patient are avoided. Relaxation reduces anxiety, can enhance the effect of pain relief, and facilitates sleep. The patient can be taught and encouraged to practice one of several relaxation techniques. If appropriate, massaging his neck and back may relieve tension and facilitate relaxation.

Checking dressings and splints. Any dressing, bandage, or splint should be checked, and changed or adjusted if necessary. A poorly positioned dressing can irritate a wound, a bandage may be too tight, or a splint may cause pressure and pain.

Adapting the environment. The nurse should consider the patient's immediate surroundings, and adapt them according to his needs. While some patients may prefer to rest in a darkened room, others may prefer that their room is bright and cheerful. A patient may choose to watch television or listen to music, or he may prefer to lie quietly. The presence of fresh flowers in the room may be a source of pleasure or irritation, and some patients may find it comforting if there are appropriate paintings on the wall. The nurse should ensure that there is adequate privacy and appropriate ventilation and heating, while adapting the environment to meet individual needs.

Implementing prescribed therapy. The nurse may be responsible for being with the patient during therapy, or may be involved in its implementation, e.g. administration of medications. When ever therapy is prescribed, the nurse should implement measures to promote the patient's comfort and safety. She should also monitor the patient to assess the efficacy of prescribed therapy, and report and document her observations.

SUMMARY

Pain, which is often a protective signal of actual or impending tissue damage, is both an unpleasant physical sensation and an emotional experience. Each episode of pain is unique and subjective, and it is important for the nurse to appreciate that 'pain is what the patient says it is'. Pain may be mild or severe, acute or chronic, physical or psychological.

Pain receptors transmit impulses along nerve fibres to the brain, where the impulses are perceived and interpreted. The body has some internal mechanisms that may be activated to help control pain and its perception, e.g. the Gate Control Mechanisms and the endorphin system.

The perception of pain varies with the individual, therefore some people will experience pain much sooner than others. Many factors influence an individual's reaction to pain including age, sex, culture, emotional state, history of pain, self image, the time of day, and the environment. Although each individual's behavioural reaction to pain is different, the physiological responses are the same.

The nurse has a responsibility to assess a patient's pain in terms of site, time it occurs, duration, precipitating factors, type, intensity, associated signs and symptoms, body posture, vital signs, and emotional manifestations.

The management of pain includes pharmacological and non-pharmacological therapy, and is dependent on each patient's needs. The nurse has a responsibility to eliminate or reduce painful stimuli, and to plan and implement measures to help alleviate pain or to assist the patient to cope with pain.

37. Meeting movement and exercise needs

INTRODUCTION

Exercise may be described in general terms as the performance of any physical activity that exerts the muscles in order to maintain or improve health.

Exercise may also be used for defined therapeutic purposes, e.g. to correct a musculoskeletal deformity, or to help restore body organs to a state of optimum health.

As it is the bones, muscles, and nerves that make movement possible, the systems involved in body movement are the musculoskeletal and nervous systems. The cardiovascular system is also involved as it transports the oxygen and nutrients necessary for the other body systems to function. Information on the structure and function of these systems is provided in Chapters 19, 20, and 21.

Exercise stimulates the body and the mind, and its beneficial effects include the maintenance of cardiopulmonary efficiency, muscle tone and strength, and joint mobility. Exercise can also be relaxing and therefore facilitate sleep, can combat boredom, and can be an effective means of dissipating the negative effects of stress. Strenuous or sustained exercise, such as long distance running, seems to release endorphins which are opioid-like substances in the brain, spinal cord and gastro-intestinal system. When released, endorphins combine with specific receptors to produce an analgesic effect similar to that of the drug morphine. Long distance runners or joggers commonly experience a state referred to as the 'runner's high' in which there is analgesia and a sense of euphoria.

While a certain level of exercise is necessary for efficient body function, in excess it can lead to tissue breakdown and injury. During sustained or strenuous exercise, the blood is unable to supply enough oxygen to keep pace with glycolysis (the breakdown of sugars). As a result of this anaerobic glycolysis, lactic acid accumulates in the muscle and its presence causes the pain of muscle fatigue. To reduce the risk of adverse effects strenuous exercise should be undertaken with caution. Warm up activities should precede more vigorous activity to allow the body to adjust gradually to increased demands, e.g. to allow gradual stretching of the muscles and a gradual increase in heart rate, ventilation rate, and body temperature. Following exercise, a period of gradual cooling down is recommended to allow the body to adjust to reduced physical demand. For example, after running for several minutes or longer, the individual could walk or engage in relaxation exercises for a few minutes.

Types of exercise

Exercise may be either active or passive. Active exercise involves voluntary effort by the individual to contract the muscles, whereas passive exercise involves intervention and is the movement of part of an individual's body by another person.

Active exercise

Active exercise may be isotonic or isometric.

Isotonic. In isotonic exercise the muscle fibres shorten

333

and cause movement at a joint, thus enabling a part of the body to be moved.

Isometric. In isometric exercise muscle tension is increased but the fibres do not shorten, therefore movement does not occur. For example, the quadriceps muscles can be contracted without causing movement of the leg.

Active exercise has a beneficial effect on all body systems as it:

- promotes and maintains muscle tone.
- influences the size and strength of muscles, and prevents atrophy of muscle tissue.
- stimulates circulation of the blood by the milking effect that muscular activity exerts on blood vessels.
- causes an increase in the rate and depth of breathing, which increases oxygen intake.
- aids in the prevention of constipation by maintaining muscle tone in the digestive tract.
- prevents degeneration of bone tissue which can lead to osteoporosis.
- prevents postural deformities which may occur as a result of prolonged joint immobility.
- promotes the flow of urine into and from the bladder.
- stimulates the nervous system resulting in improved co-ordination, greater awareness, and improved psychological state.

Passive exercise

Passive exercise helps to prevent contractual deformities caused by shortening of the capsule, ligaments, and muscles that control a joint. Passive exercises are performed when an individual is unable to move or exercise independently. A physiotherapist commonly designs a passive exercise programme, and participation by the nurse in implementing the programme is often required. The person who is performing the passive exercises should appreciate that:

- Only the normal range of movement in any joint is used, as an attempt to exceed the normal range may cause pain and damage to the joint.
- The part being exercised must be supported adequately without exerting pressure over the bony prominences or on soft tissues.
- Slow smooth movements are used to exercise the joint, and movement is not forced if it causes pain or meets resistance.
- As warmth facilitates muscle action, and therefore movement, the person receiving the exercises should be covered adequately throughout the procedure, and the room should be at a comfortable temperature. Certain individuals such as those affected by paralysis or cerebral palsy may benefit from having passive exercises performed on them, while they are in warm water, e.g. a heated pool.

Range of motion

Joints are capable of a wide range of movements, and range of motion (ROM) exercises involve putting the joints through those movements, which are illustrated in Figure 37.1. Terms associated with joint movement include:

- *Abduction*: movement away from the mid-line of the body
- *Adduction*: movement toward the mid-line of the body
- *Flexion*: bending
- *Extension*: straightening
- *Hyperextension*: extension beyond the normal range of motion, e.g. bending the head back toward the spine
- *Rotation*: turning around a fixed axis. Internal rotation is turning inward, and external rotation is turning outward
- *Circumduction*: circular movement
- *Pronation*: turning downward
- *Supination*: turning upward
- *Inversion*: turning a part in toward the body
- *Eversion*: turning a part out away from the body

The frequency with which ROM exercises are performed depends on the individual's condition and his prescribed management, but they are commonly performed at least twice daily. ROM exercises may be performed independently, with some assistance, or passively. When the exercises are performed it is important that the joints go through their full range of motion, but exercise should be performed for short periods only to avoid overtiring the individual. Using the appropriate movements, all the joints are exercised in a logical sequence.

In addition to physical exercise, occupational therapy is commonly used to assist an individual maintain or regain muscular strength, and to prevent loss of joint mobility. Activities are individually designed, e.g. for a person who is affected by arthritis or who is experiencing dysfunction as the consequence of a cerebrovascular accident, to encourage the use of affected muscles and ligaments.

Activities are also designed to meet the movement and exercise needs of individuals who are confined to bed and are unable to participate in normal activity. Any exercise and occupational therapy programme should be designed to meet individual physical and psychological needs.

It is important that every individual receives some form of exercise to prevent muscle atrophy. Disuse of the muscles leads rapidly to degeneration and subsequent loss of function. If muscles are immobilized, e.g. an entire limb encased in a splint, the process of degeneration begins almost immediately. As the restoration of muscle strength and tone is a slow process, preventive measures are implemented to prevent muscle degeneration and contractures —especially for any individual who is immobile. When active isotonic exercises are not possible, isometric exercises may be prescribed as part of an individual's therapy. For

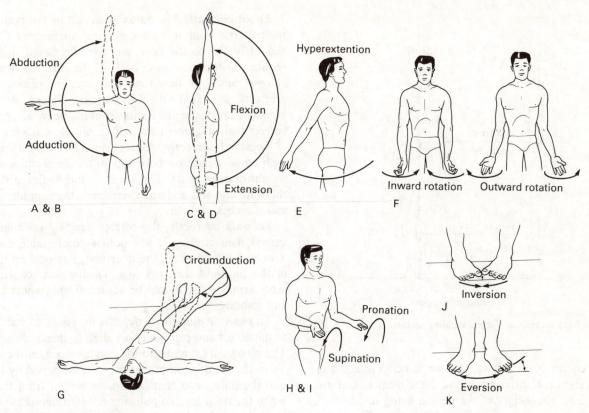

Fig. 37.1 Range of joint movements.

example, a person who has one leg in traction would be instructed however to perform isometric quadriceps exercises of the affected limb. He would be taught to contract the muscle for the count of ten, then to relax it. This exercise should be repeated approximately 10 times every 3–4 hours while he is awake.

Body posture and mechanics

Fatigue, muscle strain, and injury can result from improper use or positioning of the body during activity or rest. Good posture is achieved when all parts of the body are in correct alignment, and is important whether an individual is sitting, lying, standing, or moving. The normal spinal curves should be maintained, and the joints should be supported in their normal positions. Good posture and alignment reduces strain on all muscles and joints, and enables internal organs to function without interference, e.g. full lung expansion is facilitated.

Body mechanics is the term used to describe the physical co-ordination of all parts of the body to promote correct posture and balanced effective movement. As the nurse will be required to move and lift patients, it is important that she observes the principles of body mechanics. The practice of good body mechanics promotes economical expenditure of energy resulting in less fatigue, and reduces the risk of muscle and joint injury.

The general principles of body mechanics are based on the laws of physics applied to the human body, and include:

1. Keep the base of support wide. A wide base of support (Fig. 37.2) provides greater stability, and is achieved by placing the feet apart with the toes pointed in the direction of movement. The body weight should be distributed evenly between both feet, and the knees should be flexed slightly to provide added stability.
2. Keep the centre of gravity low. The centre of gravity (Fig. 37.2) is located in the pelvic area.
3. Keep the line of gravity vertical. The line of gravity (Fig. 37.2), or gravital plane, is an imaginary line running from the top of the head—through the centre of gravity—to the base of support. For maximum efficiency and stability, the line of gravity should remain perpendicular to the ground.
4. Large muscles do not become fatigued as quickly as small muscles, therefore when moving or lifting heavy people or objects the large and strong muscles of the body should be used. These are located in the shoulders, upper arms, hips, and thighs. To avoid using the small muscles of the back the knees should be flexed, as this action involves the use of buttock and thigh muscles.
5. Less effort is used when a heavy object is held close to the body, than when it is held with the arms extended.

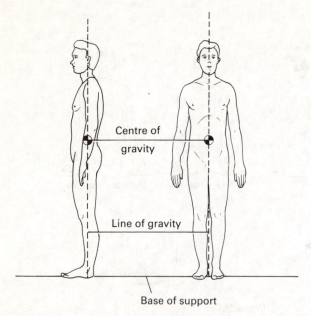

Fig. 37.2 Body mechanics. Correct standing posture.

6. Less energy is used when a person is being lifted, if the lifter's weight is transferred during the movement and used to counteract the weight of the person being lifted.

7. It is easier to push or slide an object than it is to lift it, because lifting necessitates moving against the force of gravity.

8. Friction between an object and the surface on which the object is moved, affects the amount of energy required to push or slide the object.

A knowledge of the principles of body mechanics, and skill in their application, is important so that energy is used efficiently and muscle strain is avoided. To promote safety and comfort when lifting or moving heavy people or objects it is important to apply the principles of body mechanics:

- Avoid unnecessary bending, stretching and twisting
- Face the direction in which movement is to occur
- Use both of your arms and hands
- Turn the whole body when the direction of movement is changed
- Move with smooth, even actions, and avoid sudden jerking movements
- Squat to lift heavy objects from a low level, and (keeping a straight back) push against the strong hip and thigh muscles to raise into a standing position
- Obtain adequate assistance to move a heavy person or object, either from other personnel or a lifting aid
- Stand directly in front of the person or object to be moved, with the knees flexed to minimize back flexion.

The nurse may need to assist a patient in the application of body mechanics, when sitting, standing, walking, and pushing or pulling.

To sit correctly, the buttocks should be positioned well back in the chair to promote spinal alignment. The feet should be flat on the floor, and the hips flexed slightly to reduce strain on the lower back. If the chair has arms, the elbows should be flexed and the forearms placed on the armrests to avoid shoulder strain. Several sytles of ergonomically designed chairs are available, which promote correct body alignment and reduce muscle and joint strain.

To stand correctly, the feet should be 15–20 cm apart with equal weight on both legs to minimize strain on the weight bearing joints. The knees should be flexed slightly, the buttocks and abdomen retracted, the shoulders back, and the neck straight.

To walk correctly, the correct standing position is assumed then one leg is advanced a comfortable distance. The heel should touch the floor first, followed by the ball of the foot and then the toes. During this sequence the other arm and leg should be advanced to promote balance and stability.

To push or pull correctly, it is necessary to stand close to the object and place one foot slightly ahead of the other. The elbows are flexed and the hands placed on the object. To push, smooth continuous pressure is applied by leaning into the object and transferring the weight from the back leg to the front leg. To pull, smooth continuous movement is used and the object is moved by leaning away from it. The weight is transferred from the front leg to the back leg, and once the object is moving it should be kept in motion as stopping and starting uses more energy.

When heavy people or objects are being moved or lifted, the lifter should wear suitable shoes. Shoes that have low heels, flexible non-slip soles, and closed backs promote body alignment and help to prevent accidents.

Gait

Gait is the term used to describe the manner of walking and, while varying from one person to another, there is normally a certain rhythm to an individual's walk. Gait abnormalities may occur when there is a disorder of the musculoskeletal or nervous system, e.g. unilateral hip dislocation produces a distinct 'waddle' with each step. A staggering, or ataxic, gait may be caused by a lesion in the brain or spinal cord; and a 'scissors' gait is one in which the legs cross each other in progression. An abnormal gait may also result from pain or discomfort due to a lesion on the foot, e.g. a corn, or from ill-fitting and uncomfortable footwear.

NURSING PRACTICE IN MEETING MOVEMENT AND EXERCISE NEEDS

In order to plan and implement appropriate nursing actions, the individual's ability to mobilize should be assessed. By obtaining information from him, and from the observations made of him, the nurse is able to plan and implement the measures necessary to meet his movement and exercise needs. The nurse should obtain information about his usual movement and exercise habits, and ascertain whether he requires any assistance in mobilizing. It is important to note whether the individual is experiencing any factors that limit his independence in moving, e.g. a painful hip or knee, and whether he normally requires an aid to assist him, e.g. a walking stick. The nurse should observe his body posture and gait, muscle strength and tone, and his range of movement. She should ascertain whether there are any other factors that may influence his mobility, e.g. shortness of breath on exertion. It is important to identify any potential problems that may affect his ability to move or exercise. Impaired mobility may result from a decrease in the individual's strength, presence of pain or discomfort, impaired cognition or perception, severe anxiety or depression, impaired neuromuscular or skeletal function, or as a result of imposed restrictions on movement.

A change of environment, e.g. admission to hospital, is likely to alter an individual's normal movement and exercise routine. Although there is often a degree of restriction in activities, ambulant people should be encouraged to maintain as normal a routine as possible. Non-ambulant people are deprived of independent mobility and may require assistance to move and exercise. Assistance is given to promote safety and comfort while encouraging, where possible, the return to independent function.

When planning care to meet the individual's need for movement and exercise the nurse must consider factors such as:

- maintaining and promoting normal mobility
- assisting those who have restricted mobility
- providing and assisting with use of equipment to aid mobility
- preventing and alleviating discomforts associated with reduced mobility.

Assisting individuals who have restricted mobility

While many people will be capable of independent movement, the nurse will be required to assist some individuals to move. When lifting or moving people the principles of good body mechanics must be followed, and actions implemented to promote safety and comfort. In addition to using good body posture and mechanics, key aspects related to lifting people involve preparation and teamwork.

Plan the lift. Before an individual is lifted or moved the nurse should consider his weight, the need for assistance, and the most appropriate method of lifting.

Work as a team. When more than one person is required to move an individual, it is essential that they work together. One person should control the lift and give directions. Ideally, both lifters should be of similar height.

Use a safe grip. When lifting a person, the nurse should grip with the palms and base of the fingers, keep the arms close to her body and the elbows tucked in. When two people are lifting it is sometimes necessary to join hands. A 'monkey' grip (Fig. 37.3D) is a safe and efficient method of joining hands.

Consider the individual's needs. It is important to acknowledge any specific needs of the person, e.g. any limitations or restrictions of movement, the degree to which he is able to assist, the presence of any apparatus such as an intravenous infusion, wound drainage tube, or a urinary catheter.

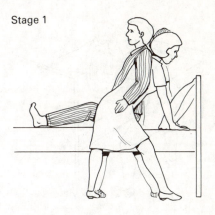

Stage 1

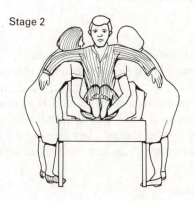

Stage 2

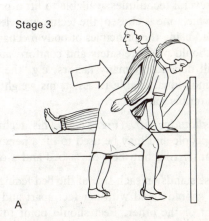

Stage 3

A

Fig. 37.3 Methods of lifting. (A) Shoulder lift (3 stages).

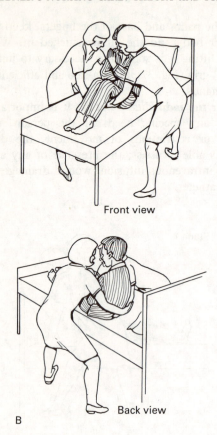

Front view

Back view

B

Fig. 37.3 (B) Orthodox (cradle) lift.

Prepare the individual and environment. The person must be informed of the procedure before it is commenced. The nurse should adjust the height of the bed, and stabilize it prior to commencing any movement. If a person is being lifted in or out of a chair that is fitted with wheels, the brakes should first be applied. Any assistive devices should be obtained as necessary, e.g. a mechanical hoist.

Lifting techniques

There are several techniques available to lift a person and, no matter which one is chosen, the technique selected must be performed using the principles of body mechanics. Each technique should promote safety and comfort, and the one selected will depend on many factors, e.g. the degree to which the individual is able to assist, his weight, and any restrictions on his movement.

1. The shoulder lift. (Fig. 37.3) This technique requires two people and may be used to lift a person in bed, or when transferring him between a bed and a chair.

• One nurse stands on each side of the bed facing its head. Each nurse should stand with her feet apart and with one foot in front of the other. Feet should point towards the head of the bed.

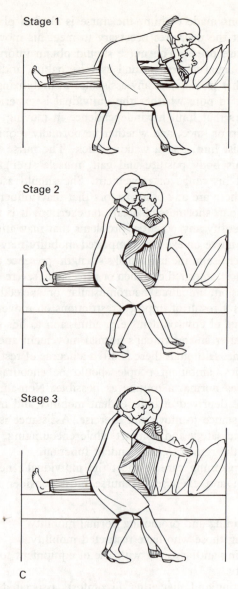

Stage 1

Stage 2

Stage 3

C

Fig. 37.3 (C) Through-arm lift (3 stages).

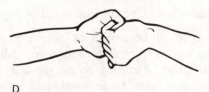

D

Fig. 37.3 (D) Monkey grip.

• The individual is assisted to lean forward and is requested to bend his knees and place his chin on his chest.
• Each nurse places her near shoulder under the person's axilla, and he is requested to rest his arms lightly on the nurses' backs.
• The nurses join hands under the individual's upper thighs, and their outer arms remain free and may be pushed into the mattress to provide extra leverage.

- At a given signal, e.g. on the count of three, the nurses lift the person by transferring their weight from back foot to front foot. The individual may be able to assist by pressing his feet against the mattress. During the move, the nurses' backs are kept straight, and the lift is made by bending at the hips and knees then straightening them.

2. The orthodox (or cradle) lift. (Fig. 37.3) This technique also requires two people, and can be adapted or modified to suit individual needs. It may be used when the person has a condition which makes a shoulder lift inappropriate, e.g. paralysis or injury to an arm.

- One nurse stands on each side of the bed facing the individual. The nurse's feet should be apart and pointed toward the head of the bed.
- The individual is assisted to lean forward and is requested to bend his knees and place his chin on his chest. He may be able to place an arm around the neck of each nurse, or fold his arms across his chest.
- Each nurse places one arm behind the person's lower back, and one arm under his upper thighs. The nurses join hands under the person's thighs, e.g. using a 'monkey' grip.
- At a given signal, each nurse lifts the individual by transferring her weight to the foot nearest the head of the bed. The person may be able to assist by pressing his feet against the mattress.

As the orthodox lift involves some actions that oppose the principles of body mechanics and safe lifting, it should only be used when an alternative method is inappropriate.

3. The through-arm lift. (Fig. 37.3) This technique may be used to assist a person who requires minimal help to move in the bed. One or two people may be required to help the individual move, and care must be taken not to pull on or injure the person's arm/s.

- A nurse stands on one side of the bed facing the head of the bed. The feet are apart, with one foot in front of the other, and both pointing toward the head of the bed.
- The individual is assisted to lean forward and is requested to bend his knees and place his chin on his chest.
- The nurse places her near arm under the individual's upper arm. The person places his arm through the nurse's and holds the back of her shoulder.
- At a given signal, the nurse assists the individual to move by transferring weight from the back foot to the front foot. At the same time, the individual assists in the move by pressing his feet into the mattress.

Moving individuals

In addition to lifting a person, one or more nurses may be required to assist him to change position. The nurse may be required to change an individual's position in bed, or to transfer him between the bed and a chair or trolley. To facilitate movement, the upper bed clothes are folded back but the nurse should ensure that the person's privacy is maintained.

There are industrial safety, health, and welfare regulations which set limitations on maximum weights which can be lifted by one person before assistance (personnel or mechanical) must be sought. It is the nurse's responsibility to ascertain current limitations regarding the maximum weights which may be lifted without assistance.

There are a variety of devices available to assist with lifting or moving individuals (Fig. 37.4), including the transfer board, the transfer belt, the Jordan frame, and mechanical hoists. Information about special beds used to facilitate movement is provided in Chapter 35.

Transfer board. A transfer board may be one piece of solid smooth material, e.g. wood or plastic, or may consist of rollers. Transfer boards facilitate safe transfer of indi-

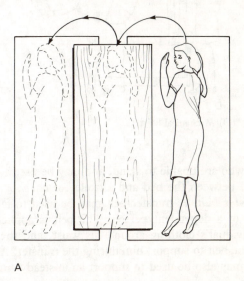

Fig. 37.4 Transfer and lifting devices. (A) Transfer board.

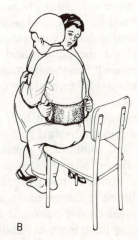

Fig. 37.4 (B) Transfer belt.

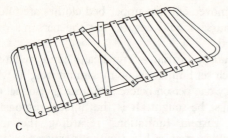

Fig. 37.4 (C) Jordan lifting frame.

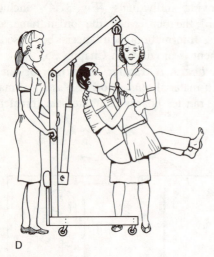

D

Fig. 37.4 (D) Mechanical hoist.

viduals who are unable to stand, and may be used to move a person between the bed and a trolley or chair.

Transfer belt. A transfer belt may be used to facilitate transfer of a dependent person. The belt is applied over the individual's clothing around his waist, and the nurse grasps the belt to support him during the transfer. A transfer belt may also be used to support an unsteady ambulant person.

Jordan frame. A Jordan frame may be used to lift a person with suspected or confirmed spinal or other major injuries, with little disturbance to the person or risk of further injury. Often used in first aid situations, the Jordan frame consists of a rigid frame with plastic gliders. The frame is placed around the person, and the individual gliders are slid underneath him then fastened to the frame. The position and tension of each glider can be adjusted under the person's body.

Mechanical hoists. A mechanical hydraulic hoist may be used to raise a supine individual to a sitting position, or to facilitate safe and comfortable transfer between the bed and a chair, bath, or toilet. Mechanical hoists are indicated for a person who is immobile, frail, or obese, and for whom manual lifting is inappropriate. Although most models can be operated by one person, it is preferable to have two people during the transfer to stabilize and support the individual. A mechanical hoist consists of an hydraulic

mechanism to raise or lower the seat, and a rigid base fitted with castors. Some models are fitted with a sling which is placed under the person, while others have a rigid seat, arms, and backrest. Because there are a variety of models, the nurse should refer to the manufacturer's instructions regarding operational, comfort, and safety aspects.

Moving a person in bed

An individual may be moved to one side of the bed during re-positioning or certain procedures. He should first be lying on his back, and is moved across to the side of the bed in three stages (Fig. 37.5):

- The nurse stands facing the person, and on the side of the bed to which he will be moved.
- The nurse places her feet apart with one foot in front of the other, and the knees flexed.
- With palm and fingers facing up, one arm is placed under the individual's neck and his far shoulder held. The nurse's other arm is placed under the person's mid-back.

A

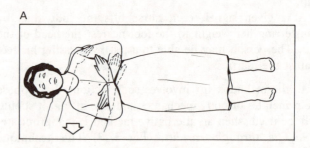

B

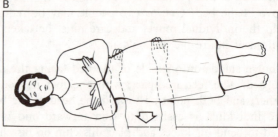

C

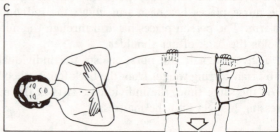

Fig. 37.5 Moving an individual across the bed. (A) The individual is moved to the side of the bed in stages. The upper part of the body is moved first, and the nurse has one arm under the individual's neck and the other under the mid-back. (B) The nurse then puts one arm under the individual's waist and the other under the thighs to move the lower body. (C) The individual's legs and feet are moved last. The nurse puts one arm under the thighs and one under the calves.

- The nurse draws the individual's upper body to the side of the bed and withdraws her arms. Then by placing one arm under his lower back and the other arm under his thighs, the nurse draws his lower body to the side of the bed. To move his legs over, the nurse places one arm under his thighs and the other arm under his lower legs.

A person may be placed on his side during repositioning or certain procedures. (Fig. 37.6).

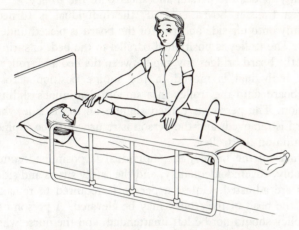

Fig. 37.6 Moving an individual onto his side. The individual is turned towards the nurse with his arms and legs crossed. The nurse has one hand on the individual's upper shoulder and upper hip.

- The nurse stands facing the individual on the side of the bed to which he is to be turned.
- The individual's far arm should be positioned across his chest, and his far leg over the other leg. His near arm should be positioned so that he does not roll on to it.
- The nurse places one hand on the individual's far shoulder, and the other hand on his far hip, and rolls the person towards her.

A person may be moved up or down in the bed using either the shoulder, orthodox, or through arm lift. If he is able to assist, he can hold the overhead hand grip and press his feet into the mattress as he is being moved.

Certain individuals may need to be turned using the 'log-roll' technique (Fig. 37.7). This technique is used to turn a person from his back to his side when it is essential to keep his spine perfectly straight, e.g. if there are spinal injuries or if the individual is recovering from spinal surgery. At least three people are required to roll the person and keep his body in alignment.

- Standing on the side of the bed to which he is to be turned, one nurse supports his head, another supports his trunk, while the third nurse supports his legs.

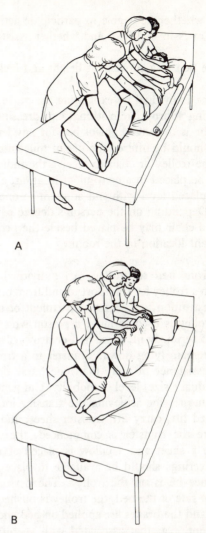

Fig. 37.7 The log-roll method of moving an individual. (A) There is a pillow between the individual's legs and his arms are crossed on his chest. The individual is on the far side of the bed. (B) A draw sheet or turning sheet may be used to log-roll an individual.

- Before commencing movement, a pillow is placed between his legs.
- At a given signal, the individual is rolled in one movement towards the nurses.

Moving a person in to or out of bed

A person may need to be transferred between the bed and a trolley or chair. Some individuals will require minimal assistance while others may require the assistance of two or more nurses. The principles of body mechanics described for lifting a person also apply when transferring him, and comfort and safety aspects must be considered. Prior to moving the individual from the bed, the nurse should:

- Determine the length of time the person is to be out of bed.

- Ascertain whether he is able to participate actively in the move or is to be lifted, and whether assistance is required.
- Adjust the bed to a convenient height and lock the wheels.
- Prepare the individual by explaining the move, and by providing appropriate clothing, e.g. dressing gown. If he is to remain out of bed for any length of time, he should be offered the use of toilet utensils.
- Prepare the trolley or chair to receive the individual. It should be placed in a convenient location, e.g. a trolley is placed level with and adjacent to one side of the bed. Depending on the person's degree of mobility, a chair may be placed beside the bed or at a convenient location in the room.

Moving from bed to trolley. An individual may be transferred to a trolley for transport to and from other areas within the institution, e.g. X-ray department or operating theatre. A trolley is used to move a person who is totally dependent, is seriously ill, is sedated or drowsy, or who is required to remain lying down. Transfer to a trolley may require the assistance of more than one nurse depending on the individual's size, level of mobility, and general condition. Techniques for achieving the transfer include the person assisted lift, carry lift, transfer sheet, and transfer board. Before the transfer is commenced, the trolley is covered with a sheet and a pillow is placed at its head. Sufficient coverings should be available to place over the individual once he is on the trolley. The person is first moved to one side of the bed, the trolley is pushed parallel to that side, and the brakes are applied on bed and trolley. Any equipment, e.g. that associated with an intravenous infusion, should be moved to the trolley before the individual is transferred. If the person is able to assist, is very light, or is a child, the nurse helps him across on to the trolley by placing her arms under his shoulders and buttocks. If he is unable to assist, he may be moved using the 3 person lift and carry technique, the transfer sheet, or transfer board.

In the 3 person lift and carry technique (Fig. 37.8) the trolley is placed at an angle of 60° to the bed, with the head of the trolley at the foot of the bed. The three team members stand on the same side of the bed as the trolley, and the person nearest the individual's head assumes the role of team leader. Standing close to the bed, one nurse places her arms under the person's upper trunk and supports his head and shoulders. The second nurse places her arms under his hips and buttocks, while the third nurse places her arms under his thighs and legs. The individual is requested to cross his arms over his chest. On the count of three, the team rolls the person towards their chests. The individual is lifted up, the team members turn and walk towards the trolley with the person on his side supported against their chests. Once at the trolley, the team

moves together to rest their elbows on it, and at the count of three lower the individual on to the trolley and slide their arms from under him.

If a transfer sheet is used it is placed under the individual, and the trolley is positioned parallel to the bed. One nurse stands at the side of the bed away from the trolley, and one or two nurses stand at the side of the trolley away from the bed. Both sides of the sheet are rolled towards the individual to promote a firm grip and stability. At a given signal the team pulls the sheet taut and, lifting slightly, slides the person and sheet onto the trolley.

If a transfer board is used, the individual is turned slightly onto his side and part of the board is placed under him. The trolley is positioned parallel to the bed, ensuring that the board bridges any gap between the bed and trolley. The individual is moved in the supine position across the board onto the trolley in a smooth continuous sliding motion. The person is turned slightly on to his side, the board is removed, and the person is returned to the supine position on the trolley.

Once on the trolley, the individual is positioned comfortably, covered adequately, and the safety straps and side rails are adjusted. Unless a person is required to remain flat, the head of the trolley may be elevated. A person on a trolley should not be left unattended, and the nurse who accompanies him to another department should remain with him until handing him into the care of another staff member.

Moving from bed to chair. An individual may be transferred to a bedside chair, wheelchair, or commode. A person may be able to stand, walk a few steps, or may need to be lifted onto the chair. If he is able to stand or walk, he should wear non-slip shoes to promote safety. A bedside chair is selected to suit his needs, and must be stable so that it does not slide as the person moves in or out. A wheelchair or commode must have the brakes applied when stationary. The number of people required to transfer the individual depends on his size, strength, and level of mobility.

To transfer an individual to a chair, the height of the bed is adjusted according to the person's needs and the chair placed in an appropriate location. Preparation of a bedside chair may include placing a sheepskin on the seat and arranging pillows to meet the individual's needs. If he is able to stand and walk, the person is first assisted into a sitting position. He is helped to swing his legs over the side of the bed. As a move from the supine to the sitting position may result in faintness, the individual should be encouraged to sit for a few moments so that his body can adjust to the change of position. While in this position he should be supported, and encouraged to breathe deeply and should move his legs to stimulate blood circulation. He should be assisted into his dressing gown and footwear. By supporting him under one or both arms, the nurse assists the individual from the bed. Once his feet are on the

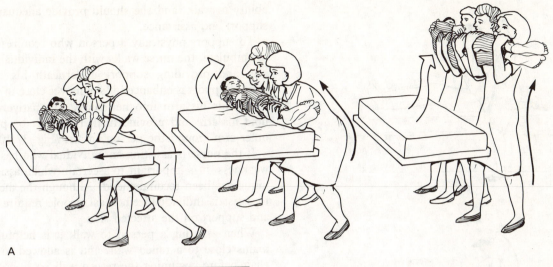

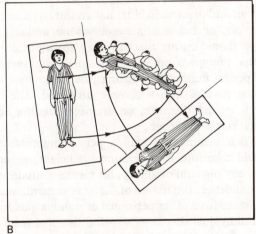

Fig. 37.8 Moving from a bed to a trolley. (A) Three person lift. (B) Three person carry.

floor, he should be encouraged to stand still for a few moments to adjust to the change of position. With adequate support, the person is assisted to move towards the chair and lower himself into it. The nurse can steady the chair by placing one foot behind a leg of the chair.

If an individual is able to stand but not walk, a pivot movement may be used to position him in the chair. The chair is placed parallel to and towards the foot of the bed, and the person is assisted from the bed into a standing position as previously described or with the aid of a transfer belt (Fig. 37.4). The nurse stands in front of the individual and requests him to place his hands on her shoulders, or around her neck. While standing in front of him, the nurse places her knees and feet so that the individual's knees and feet are blocked from bending or slipping forward. The nurse places her arms under his and around his back, or grasps the transfer belt. The person is turned (pivoted) and lowered into the chair.

If an individual is unable to stand, he is lifted into the chair (Fig. 37.9) which is positioned parallel to and towards the head of the bed. Standing behind the chair and facing the foot of the bed, one nurse places her arms around his back and under his axillae, while a second nurse, facing the head of the bed, holds his legs. At a given signal the person is lifted up and transferred into the chair.

Once the individual is seated in a chair, he should be assisted into a comfortable position which observes the principles of body mechanics and posture (p. 335). He should be covered adequately and, if he is to be out of bed for some time, any personal items he may require are placed on a table or chair beside him. It may be necessary to elevate one of his legs on a stool or another chair, e.g. if he has a plaster cast applied. An arm may need to be supported on a pillow, e.g. if an intravenous infusion is in progress, or if the arm is paralyzed.

Special safety precautions are taken when an individual is using a wheelchair or commode. Brakes are applied, and a lap belt may be necessary to stabilize the person. An individual must be warned not to stand on the foot plates of a wheelchair, as it is inclined to tip forward. When the wheelchair is in motion the brakes are released, and the person's elbows must be protected from injury, e.g. while moving through a narrow doorway.

Precautions are taken to ensure that blankets do not dangle and become entwined in the wheels.

When he is sitting out of bed, the individual's condition should be monitored. The nurse in charge must be notified immediately if he appears pale or experiences any adverse effects such as pain or discomfort, nausea, faintness, or dyspnoea.

If at any stage of the transfer out of bed the individual feels giddy, faint, or nauseated, the transfer should be halted. The person should remain on, or be returned to, the bed and the nurse in charge should be notified.

To return a person to bed, the transfer techniques are reversed.

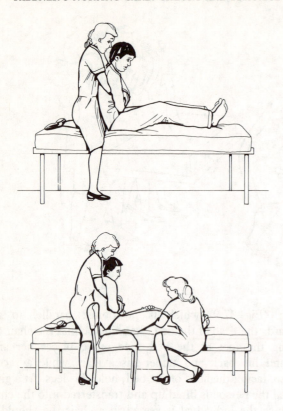

Fig. 37.9 Moving from a bed to a chair.

Ambulation

Ambulation, which is the act of walking, is encouraged and facilitated to prevent the complications associated with immobility and bed rest. In addition to preventing complications, ambulation following a period of immobility helps to restore an individual's sense of equilibrium, enhances his self confidence, and promotes independence.

Some individuals may require no assistance to ambulate while others, according to their level of independence, will require varying degrees of assistance in order to promote their safety and comfort. If a person is weak or unsteady he may be encouraged to use hand rails for added stability, or the nurse may support him using a transfer belt. Certain individuals may need to relearn how to walk, e.g. following a cerebrovascular accident or leg surgery, and may need the assistance of aids such as a walking stick, crutches, or a walking frame.

Following an extended period of immobility, the individual may need to ambulate progressively. He may move from sitting on the edge of the bed for a few minutes, through sitting in a chair, to walking a few steps, and then increasing the distance. His rate of progress will depend on his general condition and his prescribed management. Preparing a person to recommence ambulation involves both psychological and physical factors. The nurse should encourage the individual so that he gains confidence in his ability to walk, and she should provide adequate physical support and assistance.

To support physically a person who requires assistance to ambulate, the nurse walks with the individual taking his arm and providing support underneath his elbow and hand. Support is enhanced if she moves close to the person and holds his arm into her body. Alternatively, she can hold his arm and provide further support by putting her other arm around the person's waist (Fig. 37.10).

If the nurse is assisting an individual who has one-sided weakness, it is important to ascertain which assistive technique has been recommended. Although the method used to assist is individualized, most people require assistance and support on the affected side.

When assisting a person to walk it is helpful if he remains close to a railed wall, and is allowed to rest on a chair before beginning the return walk.

If an ambulant individual has an intravenous infusion in progress, or has a urinary or wound drainage bag, the nurse should ensure that any such apparatus is positioned so that therapy is not disrupted during ambulation. When the person finishes ambulating, the nurse must check any tubing in case it has become dislodged. She must also check wound dressings or drainage bags for seepage or alterations in drainage.

When planning to help a person ambulate the nurse should take into consideration his height, general condition, any physical disability, his mental attitude and degree of confidence, the nature of the environment, and whether assistance from other personnel or walking aids is required. The individual should wear well fitting foot wear with non-slip soles, and any laces should be tied securely. The individual should be allowed to proceed at his own pace. If he becomes distressed, or experiences any pain, faint-

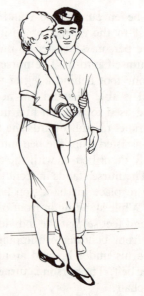

Fig. 37.10 Assisting an ambulatory individual.

ness, giddiness, or undue fatigue, he should be seated and the nurse must remain with him and notify the nurse in charge.

If a person begins to fall when walking the nurse should not try to 'catch' him, as this action could result in injuries to either person. Instead, his fall should be broken by easing him into a nearby chair or onto the floor. Care should be taken to avoid the person colliding with equipment, as he is eased down. The nurse in charge must be notified so that the individual's condition can be assessed before he is moved. Assistance should be obtained to help the person into a chair or bed, and his vital signs should be monitored. The nurse must remain with the individual, and the incident must be documented.

Walking aids

Walking aids broaden the base of support and therefore increase stability. The type of aid used depends on the individual's condition, the amount of support required, and the type of disability.

The person is commonly instructed in the use of the aid by a physiotherapist, and it is important for the nurse to know the principles involved in order to reinforce those instructions.

Walking aids that may be required on a temporary or permanent basis include crutches, walking sticks, and walking frames. Calipers or leg braces may be used to provide extra support for a weak leg, or may be used to prevent or correct deformities, or to prevent joint movement. It is important that a leg brace is applied correctly, as a poorly fitting brace is ineffective and may cause pressure and discomfort.

Crutches

Crutches enable a person to ambulate by taking the weight of his body off one or both legs. Successful use of crutches requires balance and upper body strength. Selection of crutches and walking gait depends on individual needs, and must be appropriate to be a safe and effective means of ambulation. The two types commonly used are the underarm and the forearm crutch (Fig. 37.11). Underarm crutches are often used by a person who has a sprain or leg cast, while forearm crutches are more commonly used by an individual ambulating with a swing through gait, e.g. in paraplegia.

Underarm crutches must be measured so that the person's weight is carried on his wrists and palms, and not on his axillae; the axilla bar should be 4–5 cm below the axilla and the hand bar positioned to permit 15–30° flexion of the elbows when in resting position. The height of forearm crutches must also allow 15–30° flexion of the elbows.

Before crutches are used they should be assessed for safety, by ensuring that all screws and bolts are tightened and the rubber tips are in good repair. It is important to

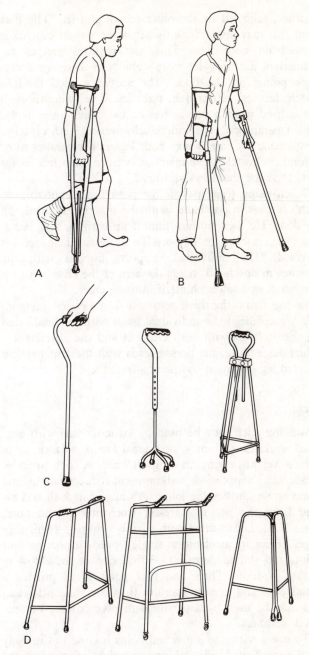

Fig. 37.11 Walking aids. (A) Underarm crutch. (B) Forearm crutch. (C) Walking sticks. (D) Walking frames.

ascertain the amount of weight-bearing allowed on the affected leg/s, i.e. partial or none.

Crutch walking gaits. The person is instructed in one of several gaits, according to his needs. The most common method is the three point gait, where the crutches are moved forward first, followed by the unaffected leg. The affected leg follows in a swinging movement because it is raised from the ground. This gait is used by individuals who cannot bear weight on the affected leg. The two point gait is used when some weight-bearing is allowed on both feet. The person advances one crutch and the opposite leg together, followed by the other crutch and leg. The four point gait may also be used when some weight-bearing is allowed on both feet. This gait requires greater co-ordination, but provides more stability as there are always three points on the floor. The sequence used is right crutch, left leg, left crutch, right leg. The swing-through gait is used when a person has no use of his lower body, e.g. in paraplegia. The individual advances both crutches simultaneously, and swings both legs either parallel to or beyond the crutches. To maintain balance the pelvis moves first, then the shoulders and head.

When rising from a chair the person is taught to hold both crutches in one hand, with the tips resting firmly on the floor. He then pushes himself up with his free hand, using the crutches for support. To sit down, the process is reversed. The individual supports himself with the crutches in one hand, holds the arm of the chair with his free hand, and lowers himself into the chair.

To use stairs, the three point gait is the easiest method. When ascending, the individual leads with his unaffected leg then follows with both crutches and the affected leg. When descending, the person leads with the crutches and affected leg, followed by the unaffected leg.

Sticks

A walking stick may be used by an individual with one-sided weakness or injury, occasional loss of balance, or to reduce weight-bearing on a hip or knee. A stick provides balance and support for walking, and reduces fatigue and strain on weight-bearing joints. A walking stick should extend from the person's greater trochanter to the floor, (Fig. 37.11) and is fitted with a rubber tip to prevent slippage. Sticks are available as single tipped, tripod, or four point, and should permit 15–30° flexion of the elbow in resting position. Three and four point sticks provide a broad base and greater stability than the standard stick, and may be used by a person with poor balance or one-sided weakness.

To use a stick the individual holds it close to the body on the unaffected side, taking the weight off the affected leg. The person is instructed to move the stick and the affected leg simultaneously, followed by the unaffected leg. Sometimes the three or four pronged stick is held on the affected side. The individual should be encouraged to keep the stride of each leg, and the timing of each step, equal. While the individual is learning to use the stick, the assistant should stand behind him to prevent falls. To ascend stairs the stick should be held in one hand and the patient encouraged to hold the stair rail, leading with the unaffected leg. To descend stairs the affected leg should lead.

Walking frames

Walkers consist of a metal frame with hand grips, four legs, and one open side (Fig. 37.11). A frame may be used by an elderly person as it provides greater support and sense of security than a stick. A frame is also useful for a person with unsteady gait, or when partial weight bearing is necessary. The height is selected to allow 15–30° flexion of the elbows when the hand grips are held. Attachments are available, e.g. baskets and trays, to meet specific needs and to promote greater independence. The individual can either pick up and advance the frame, or push it forward. Commonly, the person picks the frame up and moves it 15–20 cm in front of him. He then moves one foot, followed by the other, up to the frame. If he has one-sided weakness, the affected leg is moved first. While the individual is learning to use a frame, the assistant should stand behind him and support his hips to maintain an upright position.

To sit down, the person is instructed to stand with the back of his legs against the front of the chair, with the frame in front of him. He then grasps the arm rests of the chair and lowers himself into it. To rise from a chair, the frame is placed in front of him. He then slides forward in the chair, and pushes himself up by placing both hands on the arm rests. Once in the standing position he holds onto the frame.

When a walking aid of any type is used, the individual is assisted until he is ambulating confidently without help. He should always wear shoes with non-slip soles, and unnecessary articles or loose mats should be removed from his path.

COMPLICATIONS ASSOCIATED WITH REDUCED MOBILITY

Loss of mobility, even temporarily as a result of bed rest, affects all body systems and may have serious consequences. When an individual's condition impairs or prevents mobility, the nurse must plan and implement measures to prevent complications. Complications associated with immobility include:

- pressure on bony prominences, resulting in decubitus ulcers
- disuse of muscles and joints, resulting in contractures
- venous stasis, resulting in deep vein thrombosis
- pulmonary stasis, resulting in lung congestion
- urinary stasis, resulting in infection or calculi
- decreased intestinal peristalsis, resulting in constipation
- reduced vasomotor tone, resulting in hypotension
- decreased independence, resulting in depression, anxiety, or boredom.

Decubitus ulcers

Decubitus ulcers (also referred to as pressure sores, trophic ulcers, stasis ulcers, or ischaemic ulcers) result from ischaemic hypoxia of the tissues owing to prolonged pressure on the area. As a result of impaired blood circulation the area is deprived of essential nutrients and oxygen, and cellular death occurs. The major factors likely to interrupt local capillary blood supply are pressure and shearing forces, however these can be exacerbated by a variety of other factors. One, or a combination, of these factors increases the risk of decubitus ulcers. Predisposing factors can be classed as either intrinsic or extrinsic.

Intrinsic factors

Intrinsic factors are characteristics specific to an individual's condition.

Nutritional status. Inadequate nutrition prevents efficient cellular growth and repair, and renders the tissues more vulnerable to damage. A poorly nourished person will usually have less protection over the bony prominences and be more vulnerable to the effects of prolonged pressure.

Body type. As the sites of maximum skin compression are located over bony prominences, a thin person is more at risk. Conversely, an obese person may be at risk due to shearing forces and added pressure, caused by his body weight pressing on the skin.

Mobility. Limited mobility restricts the movements a person normally makes to redistribute pressure on weight bearing areas.

Neurological factors. Reduced sensitivity to pressure or pain may occur in certain disease states, e.g. spinal cord injury, paralysis, multiple sclerosis, or diabetes mellitus. Transmission of impulses from receptors in the skin or to the muscles may be impaired, so that the person does not receive the 'message' to move. Sometimes, although a message is transmitted, the individual is unable to move independently.

Vascular factors. Reduced local tissue perfusion may result from certain disease states, e.g. arteriosclerosis, cardiac failure, or diabetes mellitus. As reduced local tissue oxygenation and nutrition are the primary cause of decubitus ulcers, people with vascular perfusion abnormalities are at risk.

Incontinence. Incontinence of urine or faeces may result in skin excoriation or maceration. Abrasions are more likely to form due to friction between the skin and the surface under the individual, making shearing forces more severe.

Extrinsic factors

Extrinsic factors are those derived from the individual's environment.

Pressure. The greater the pressure on the skin, the more the tissues are distorted. Pressure on the skin over bony prominences can distort the blood vessels to such an extent that the blood flow is interrupted. In addition pressure can occlude lymphatic vessels, and the consequent accumulation of toxic substances can contribute to cell damage. The areas of the body where bony prominences are covered by a thin layer of tissue are those most likely to develop decubitus ulcers (Fig. 37.12(A)). However, decubitus ulcers can develop on other body areas if they are subjected to prolonged or excessive pressure.

Shearing forces and friction. When pressure is applied at an angle, the layers of the skin move over one another causing distortion of the tissue. The forces involved (shearing forces) distort and occlude the dermal capillaries resulting in tissue necrosis and the development of a decubitus ulcer. Friction between the skin and another surface, e.g. a sheet, also results in tissue distortion due to shearing forces. Friction immobilizes the epidermis while the deeper layers move, and is an important factor in a patient whose skin is friable and fragile.

Loss of skin integrity. Any skin damage increases the risk of decubitus ulcers. Actions such as excessive washing with soap, prolonged exposure to moisture, or rubbing can damage the skin's integrity.

Development of a decubitus ulcer

Development commonly passes through four stages unless measures are taken early to relieve pressure and increase local tissue perfusion. In stage one, the skin is red and does not return to normal colour with relief of pressure. The area may also be oedematous, and the person may experience tenderness or a sensation of burning. In stage two, the skin blisters, peels, or cracks. In stage three, the full thickness of skin is damaged. Subcutaneous tissue damage can also occur, and commonly a serous or bloodstained discharge is evident. A slough forms and appears as a black area, which is composed of dead tissue. Micro-organisms invade and multiply rapidly. In stage four, a deep ulcer is formed as the full thickness of skin and subcutaneous tissue is destroyed. Structures such as fascia, muscle, connective tissue, or bone underlying the ulcer are exposed and may be damaged. If any signs or symptoms of a developing decubitus ulcer are observed, the nurse in charge must be notified immediately.

Prevention of a decubitus ulcer

It is important to identify those individuals at risk of decubitus ulcers, and many assessment systems have been designed to aid identification. Health care institutions may devise their own risk assessment tool, or may use an established one, e.g. the Norton Scale (Fig. 37.12b). An assessment tool is used as a guide to facilitate the implementation of a rational preventive regimen. Thermography may also be used as a screening technique to detect incipient or actual pressure damage. Skin pressure may be

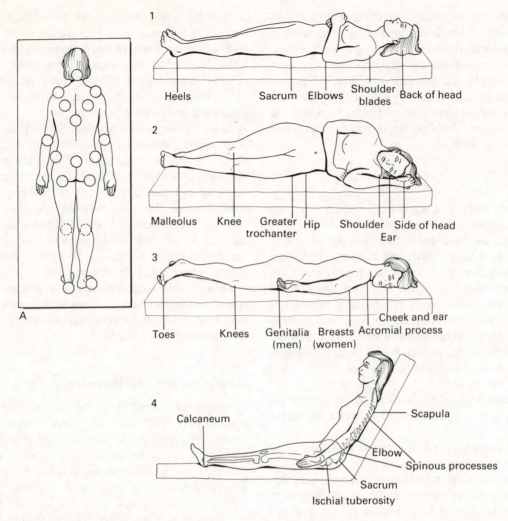

Fig. 37.12 (A) Pressure area sites (1) in the supine position, (2) in the lateral position, (3) in the prone position, and (4) in the sitting position.

measured using a specific gauge, e.g. the Denne pressure gauge, to estimate the pressure on a site.

Decubitus ulcers form in a few hours but may take many months to heal. Tissue healing is dependent on a good blood supply bringing antibodies and leucocytes to combat infection, and nutrients and oxygen for regeneration of tissues. Since a poor blood supply is both the primary cause of decubitus ulcers and of delayed healing, the prevention of decubitus ulcers is of prime importance.

Adequate nutrition. A well balanced diet is necessary to maintain the health of tissues and to prevent tissue breakdown. An adequate fluid intake is important to prevent skin dryness. If a person's appetite is poor, high protein fluids and added vitamins may be prescribed. If an individual is unable to tolerate oral food or fluids, an alternative method of meeting his nutritional needs e.g. gastric tube or intravenous feeding, may be necessary. Information on nutrition is provided in Chapter 29.

Maintenance of skin integrity. It is important to keep the skin clean and dry, supple, and intact. The skin is

washed as necessary, using a non-irritating soap sparingly to avoid causing dryness. A very dry skin may require the application of an oil or cream. Thorough drying, e.g. following a bath, is necessary to prevent skin excoriation or maceration. Particular attention should be paid to skin folds and creases, e.g. under the breasts, between the buttocks, and in the groins. Damage to the skin is prevented by careful handling, and there should be sufficient people, or a lifting device, used to move a person.

Incontinence should be prevented as far as possible, and devices used to protect the skin from constant moisture. After each incontinent episode, the skin is washed, dried carefully, and may be protected by the application of a barrier cream. Wet or soiled bed linen or clothing must be removed immediately.

The presence of any skin breaks should be reported immediately to the nurse in charge, so that early treatment can be implemented.

Prevention of pressure. Prolonged periods of pressure should be avoided, the aim being to prevent occlusion of

		Physical condition		Mental condition		Activity		Mobility		Incontinent	Total score
		Good	4	Alert	4	Ambulant	4	Full	4		
		Fair	3	Apathetic	3	Walk-help	3	Sl. limited	3		
		Poor	2	Confused	2	Chairbound	2	V. limited	2		
Name	Date	V. bad	1	Stuporous	1	Bedfast	1	Immobile	1		

B   (i)

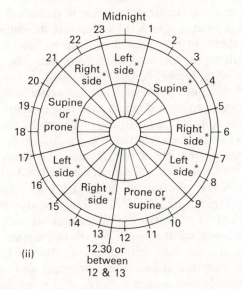

(ii)

*Normally with 2 pillows or less: if sat-up-in-bed (for meals) this should be not more than 40 minutes each meal

Fig. 37.12 (B) Prevention of decubitus ulcers. (i) Norton's scoring system. (ii) Lowthian turning clock. (Reproduced by kind permission of Peter Lowthian, Senior Nurse (Research), Royal National Orthopaedic Hospital, Stanmore.)

the blood vessels that may lead to a disruption of the blood supply. Repositioning an individual at regular intervals, e.g. every two hours, is an effective way of preventing prolonged pressure on any area. Several repositioning schedules have been designed to assist nurses in the implementation of a regular position change regimen. The Lowthian 24 hour turning clock (Fig. 37.12(B)) is one such design, and should be accompanied by documentation that records implementation of the schedule.

Special beds, e.g. a net suspension bed, may be used to relieve pressure and to facilitate position change. An overhead hand grip may be used by an individual to lift himself up and relieve pressure from the buttocks and sacral area. Pressure relieving devices such as a sheepskin may be used to reduce pressure or to distribute the person's weight evenly. For maximum effect, a sheepskin should be placed

so that it is in direct contact with the skin. Cushions or pads containing gel, foam, or water, may be placed on the seats, e.g. of a wheelchair. A person sitting in a chair is encouraged to lift himself up from the seat frequently, to relieve pressure and facilitate tissue perfusion in the buttocks and sacral area. He is assisted in this action if he is unable to lift himself independently. All splints, plasters, braces and bandages should be checked regularly and adjusted if necessary to relieve pressure.

Relief of shearing forces. Shearing may be prevented by careful positioning and lifting techniques, so that sliding in any direction is avoided. Pillows should be arranged for adequate support, and a foot board or firm pillow at his feet may assist the individual to maintain a sitting position. A person must be lifted carefully to avoid dragging his skin along any surface, and surfaces such as sheets must be kept smooth.

Topical applications may be used to reduce friction between the skin and another surface, e.g. the sheet. For instance, a transparent elastic film dressing applied over an area subjected to pressure reduces the likelihood of tissue damage from shearing forces. This type of dressing acts as a semipermeable barrier, regulating the entry and exit of substances. It permits the passage of gases, e.g. oxygen, through the film, but prevents the entry or exit of fluids. As the dressing protects the skin from contact with external moisture, e.g. urine, maceration of the skin is prevented. Because it is transparent, the dressing enables observation of the skin for signs of a developing decubitus ulcer.

Management of a decubitus ulcer

If a decubitus ulcer develops in spite of preventive measures, early detection and management increases the likelihood of successful treatment. Management aims to remove pressure from the area, treat any predisposing factors, and promote healing of the decubitus ulcer. The individual must be positioned so that the ulcerated area is free from all pressure, and management of the ulcer should follow the principles of general wound management to promote healing. Controversy exists over decubitus ulcer management, and many forms of treatment have been implemented—with varying degrees of success. Applications or techniques for which no scientifically-based explanation can be provided should be avoided. Instead nurses should refer to the results from current clinical research in order to select products or techniques that have been demonstrated as being beneficial.

Whatever treatment is prescribed, healing is promoted by relief of pressure, a diet containing adequate nutrients and fluid, removal of predisposing causes, and maintenance of a good blood supply to the area. If infection has developed, systemic antibiotic therapy may be prescribed. Information on wound healing is provided in Chapter 59.

Contractures

A contracture is an abnormal condition of a joint characterized by flexion and fixation, caused by atrophy and shortening of muscle fibres. Contractures may result from improper support or positioning of a joint, or as a result of inadequate joint movement. If a joint is allowed to remain in one position for any length of time, the muscle fibres that normally provide movement will shorten to accommodate that position. Eventually, the muscle fibres lose their ability to contract and relax.

Prevention includes encouraging the individual to be physically active and to perform active ROM exercises. A dependent person should have passive ROM exercises performed. The individual should be positioned in good body alignment so that all his joints are maintained in a functional position. Pressure relieving devices, e.g. a bedcradle, may be placed to prevent the bed clothes pressing down and forcing a joint into an abnormal position.

Foot drop

Foot drop is another term for plantar flexion, which is caused by damage to the nerve supply of the muscle responsible for dorsiflexion of the foot. If a person's feet are allowed to assume plantar flexion, they may become fixed in that position. A person with foot drop is unable to place his heels on the floor, and this severely impedes ambulation.

Prevention includes using a foot board or firm pillow in the bed to maintain the feet in dorsiflexion, i.e. the feet should be aligned as if the individual was in a standing position, at a 90° angle. Devices and techniques to keep pressure off the feet should be used, e.g. a bed cradle or foot pleat in the upper bed clothes. The person's feet should be exercised through their range of motion, either actively or passively.

If foot drop does occur, management includes the use of an orthopedic brace, intensive physiotherapy, or surgical intervention.

Venous stasis

When the flow of blood in the vessels is impeded, e.g. as a result of physical inactivity, a thrombus—or blood clot—may form. Inactivity or immobility leads to reduced muscle pump activity and a slow rate of blood flow in the legs. Slowing of the circulation allows the stream of platelets to become more peripheral, and therefore more able to become attached to the endothelial lining of a vessel. Because blood normally flows more slowly through veins than through arteries, thrombosis is more common in a vein. Venous thrombosis occurs most often in the legs or pelvis, and commonly occurs in a deep vein in the calf of the leg.

The signs and symptoms of a deep vein thrombosis may be very slight; or may present as slight pyrexia, and pain in the calf which increases on dorsiflexion. The calf becomes swollen, tender, and warm to touch.

If the thrombus detaches from the vessel wall and is transported in the blood stream, the clot is called an embolus. The embolus may eventually lodge in the pulmonary artery tree and is then referred to as a pulmonary embolus. Depending on the size of the embolus, the consequences may be very serious. Small emboli may be lysed, but massive emboli may obstruct the pulmonary vessels and cause instant or rapid death. Minor emboli may be asymptomatic or may result in retrosternal pain, haemoptysis, tachypnoea, and circulatory collapse with low blood pressure, tachycardia, and cold blue extremities. A massive embolus results in sudden collapse, severe dyspnoea and cyanosis, and commonly causes death.

Prevention of deep vein thrombosis, and consequently of pulmonary embolus, includes exercises to stimulate venous blood circulation in the legs. Active or passive two hourly exercises should be performed and consist of the individual rotating the ankles, dorsiflexion and plantar flexion of the feet, flexing and extending the knees, and raising and lowering each leg. The person should be advised not to cross his legs while lying in bed or sitting on a chair. Prolonged pressure on the backs of the legs should be avoided by careful positioning and re-positioning. The upper bed clothes should remain loose to facilitate movement of the legs.

Anti-embolic elastic stockings may be prescribed. These firm stockings expose the toes, but cover the foot and extend up the leg to the knee or groin. By supporting the blood vessels in the leg, they assist in maintaining adequate pressure on the vessels and so prevent thrombi. The individual's leg must be measured first to ensure correct fit, and the stockings are applied by rolling them slowly from the foot up the leg. Firm even pressure is essential, and the toes remain exposed so that observations can be made to check that the blood supply is not impeded. For certain individuals, e.g. those requiring surgical intervention, additional preventive measures may include antithrombotic agents pre- and post-operatively. Anticoagulants and antithrombotic medications reduce the formation of clotting factors, or reduce platelet aggregation. During surgery mechanical prophylaxis, such as intermittent electrical stimulation of the calf muscles, may be implemented if the individual is susceptible to thrombus formation.

Management of deep vein thrombosis includes supporting the limb with a one way stretch elastic bandage, elevating the foot of the bed, and thrombolytic therapy such as anticoagulant medications. Surgical intervention may be necessary to remove the thrombus.

Management of pulmonary embolus includes administration of oxygen, analgesia, and anti-coagulant therapy.

Pulmonary stasis

Lack of mobility results in decreased chest expansion, and inactivity lowers the basal metabolic rate. Carbon dioxide production is reduced and therefore respiratory stimulus is decreased. Bed rest, particularly in a horizontal position, allows pooling of secretions in the bronchial tree. The secretions may become thick and difficult to expectorate. Bronchial stasis provides a good medium for the growth of pathogenic micro-organisms, and hypostatic pneumonia may develop.

Signs and symptoms of lung congestion include a cough and production of sputum, rattling ventilations, distressed or painful breathing, and pyrexia.

Prevention of pulmonary stasis includes nursing an individual in a sitting position when possible, and the implementation of deep breathing and coughing exercises. Deep breathing exercises should be performed with the person in a sitting position, with one hand placed on the centre of his chest and the other on his abdomen just below his ribs. The individual is instructed to inhale slowly and deeply, pushing his abdomen out to promote optimal distribution of air to the alveoli. He is instructed to exhale through pursed lips, and to contract his abdomen. Exhalation through pursed lips improves oxygen diffusion, encourages a slow deep breathing pattern, and puts positive back pressure on the airways so that they stay open longer and expel greater amounts of stale air. Abdominal contraction pushes the diaphragm upward, exerts pressure on the lungs, and helps to empty them. After several breaths, the individual is encouraged to cough to expectorate any sputum.

Management of pulmonary stasis includes deep breathing and coughing exercises, and additional chest physiotherapy such as postural drainage and chest percussion and vibration. The individual's fluid intake should be increased to help liquefy mucus secretions and therefore facilitate expectoration. Oxygen therapy may be necessary, and medications such as antibiotics and analgesia may be prescribed.

Urinary stasis

Immobility can lead to retention of urine, urinary tract infection, or renal calculi. Immobility, or difficulty in using toilet utensils in bed, can result in incomplete emptying of the bladder and therefore stasis of urine. Decreased muscular activity reduces the amount of circulating lactic acid which leads to alkaline urine and precipitates calculus formation. Immobility causes loss of calcium from the skeletal system into the bloodstream, and the excess calcium which is excreted by the kidneys and may lead to the formation of calculi.

Prevention of urinary stasis includes promoting an adequate intake of fluids and ensuring that the individual understands the importance of not postponing urination and the need to empty his bladder completely.

Management of a complication resulting from urinary stasis depends on the cause, and includes increasing the person's fluid intake and treating any infection. Information on elimination of urine is provided in Chapter 30, and information on disorders affecting the urinary system is provided in Chapter 47.

Constipation

Constipation may occur as a result of decreased intestinal peristalsis due to reduced mobility, or as a result of difficulty in using toilet utensils in bed.

Prevention of constipation includes promoting the adequate intake of sufficient dietary fibre. The individual should be encouraged to maintain as normal a routine as possible to promote the elimination of faeces (refer to Chapter 30).

Management of constipation includes increasing the individual's fluid intake and dietary fibre, and the administration of any prescribed medication or procedure, e.g. rectal suppository or enema. Information on elimination from the bowel is provided in Chapter 30.

Postural hypotension

Postural, or orthostatic, hypotension is an abnormally low blood pressure occurring when an individual assumes a standing position. The condition may occur when there is some loss of vasomotor tone, e.g. as a result of prolonged bed rest or immobility. When the person assumes a standing position, the poor vasomotor tone results in widening of the peripheral arterioles, and a rapid fall in blood pressure. He experiences vertigo on assuming an upright position, and may faint.

Prevention of postural hypotension involves the gradual re-introduction of ambulation, and allowing the individual time to adjust to any change from a lying to a sitting or standing position.

Psychological effects

Psychological stress, anxiety, depression, or boredom can occur when a person's physical activity is restricted. A loss of independence occurs when he has to rely on other people or aids to be able to carry out the activities of living. Enforced inactivity, e.g. that which may be necessary during hospitalization, interferes with all aspects of normal living—including an individual's ability to engage in physical exercise or leisure activities. A person who is confined to a hospital environment, or forced to remain indoors, soon becomes tired of the monotony of his surroundings and bored by the lack of stimulation or variety. As a result of an altered daily routine, a change in level of independence, physical impairment, or isolation from family and friends, a person may feel depressed or anxious. Such states may be manifested as feelings of sadness, worthlessness, irritability, apathy, restlessness, and anxiety.

Prevention of psychological distress aims to improve the individual's self esteem. He should be encouraged to participate in any decisions regarding his care, in order to exercise some control over his life. Where possible a change of environment may be beneficial, e.g. some time spent in the day-room or outside the institution. He should be provided with newspapers, radio, television, or telephone—to maintain contact with the world outside the institution. He may be encouraged to pursue hobbies or studies, or the occupational therapy department may be able to provide alternative suitable activities. A social worker may be required to assist him with any problems about finance or his home situation. Flexible visiting hours are important,

and his family or significant others should be encouraged to maintain contact with him. The nurse can facilitate communication with the individual by showing real concern, respect, and empathy. She should actively listen to him, and provide information about his care and treatment. It is important that he be allowed to express his emotions, which may take many forms, e.g. talking or crying.

SUMMARY

Movement and exercise are necessary to maintain cardiopulmonary efficiency, muscle strength and tone, and joint mobility. Exercise also stimulates the mind and therefore enhances awareness and improves the psychological state.

Exercise may be either active or passive, and during exercise the joints should move through their full range of motion. Individuals should practice the principles of good body posture and body mechanics, in order to reduce muscle fatigue and to prevent injury. The principles of body mechanics are based on the laws of physics, and implementation of those principles facilitates economical expenditure of energy. The use of good body posture and body mechanics is important whether an individual is lying, sitting, standing or moving.

The person's ability to mobilize should be assessed in order to plan and implement the measures required to meet his need for movement and exercise. Some individuals will be able to move and ambulate independently, while others will require the assistance of personnel or aids.

Any technique or aid used to assist a person to move, should be one that promotes safety and comfort.

Immobility, e.g. as a result of enforced bed rest, can lead to complications. The nurse has a responsibility to identify those individuals who are at risk of developing complications, so that preventive measures can be implemented.

38. Meeting safety and protection needs

OBJECTIVES

1. Identify common safety hazards in the home environment and in health care facilities.
2. Identify the factors that may affect an individual's ability to protect himself against environmental hazards.
3. Apply relevant principles in planning and implementing safety precautions within a health care facility.
4. State the safety measures which should be taken to prevent mechanical accidents, fire, chemical injury, and cross infection.

INTRODUCTION

Safety is a basic need of every individual throughout each stage of the life cycle and, while Kalish regarded this need as being the third most important, Maslow classified the need for safety as second only to the physiological needs (see Fig. 28.1).

Every individual needs to maintain a safe environment in which to carry out the activities of living, and needs to protect himself from hazards. The individual's health depends on the promotion and maintenance of an environment that is as safe as possible. A safe environment is one in which an individual has a low risk of becoming ill or injured. Everyone has a responsibility to protect and improve the environment; to be informed and to inform others about the preventive measures that can be taken to avoid or reduce health hazards due to environmental factors. Every individual is being exposed constantly to a variety of environmental hazards that puts his safety at risk, and certain factors such as illness may reduce his ability to protect himself.

In a health care setting the nurse has a responsibility to protect the patient from hazards in his immediate surroundings, and therefore the patient's safety should be incorporated in all aspects of his care. While this chapter focuses on the maintenance of a safe environment in a health care setting, it is also appropriate that it briefly addresses the individual's safety outside that area.

Promoting a safe work, home and outdoor environment

An individual's safety can be jeopardized in the home, outdoors, or in the workplace. The majority of accidents are preventable and simple safety measures can help to eliminate some causes of accidental injuries.

In Australia each year, many thousands of people are either injured or killed by accidents in the home environment, on the road, or at their place of work. A large percentage of these accidents involve children, therefore those responsible for their care must be mindful of the need to promote a safe environment. While not all of the possible dangers have been included, the more common ones together with various preventive actions are outlined in this chapter.

Dangers in the home and surroundings

Glass. Injury from broken glass can be prevented, e.g. by fitting safety glass in full length doors and windows, and by ensuring that they include clear eye-level markings. Any broken glass should be cleared up immediately and disposed of safely, e.g. by wrapping it in several layers of newspaper before it is placed in a bin.

Electricity or heat. Injuries due to contact with electricity can be avoided by observing the manufacturer's instructions when electrical appliances are being used. Appliances should be turned off when not in use, and checked regularly for signs of disrepair. Electrical sockets should be fitted with safety covers when there are children in the environment.

Hot objects or articles containing hot substances should be handled carefully, and children should be prevented from coming into contact with them, e.g. saucepan handles turned in away from the edge of the stove, and cords from electrical appliances located out of their reach. Young children should not be left unattended when there is a risk of injury from heat, e.g. in the bathroom or the kitchen, and matches or lighters should not be left lying about. Open fires and radiators should be fitted with safety guards, and children should be provided with safe non-flammable clothing.

Smoking while in bed is a potentially dangerous activity and should be avoided. Occupants of the home should have a plan of action and practice what to do in the event of fire.

Chemicals. People have a responsibility to be aware of poisonous or harmful substances in and around the home, and to ensure that they are not accessible to children. For example, potentially harmful substances such as detergents, bleaches, pesticides, petrol, or kerosene should be kept in their original containers, clearly labelled, and stored in a safe place.

Medications should also be stored safely to prevent their accidental consumption by children or confused adults, and any unwanted medications should either be returned to the pharmacist or disposed of carefully, e.g. by flushing down the toilet. Care must also be taken to ensure that any medication is taken or administered correctly, e.g. the label on the container should always be checked. Many medications are packaged in safe containers, e.g. fitted with a push and turn lid or sealed in bubble packs, as an added safety precaution against accidental consumption.

Sharp objects. All sharp objects such as knives, scissors, or garden tools should be handled with care and stored safely. Children's toys should be checked for sharp edges, and the purchase of toys which can injure the user or others should be avoided.

Suffocation. Suffocation can be caused by drowning, strangulation, or choking on an object. Swimming pools should have a non-slip surface around the edge, be surrounded by a safety fence, and should be covered when not in use. Children should always be supervised when they are using the pool, and there should be a rescue device, e.g. a ring buoy, readily accessible. Occupants of the home where a swimming pool is installed have a responsibility to be able to initiate rescue and resuscitation methods. Information on resuscitation is provided in Chapter 57.

A child's cot should conform to safety standards, and have the side bars close together so that the child cannot put his head through them. Plastic bags should be stored safely, as suffocation may occur if a child places a bag over his head. Toys should be selected on the basis of safety, as a child may put small or removable parts in his mouth which may be aspirated and lodge in his trachea.

Falls. The majority of falls can be prevented by sensible thinking and preventive actions, e.g. careful use of ladders and the avoidance of highly polished slippery floors or loose floor mats. Inevitably, children will climb, therefore

adults have a responsibility to supervise them and to teach them how to climb safely.

Dangers on the road

One of the major causes of injury or death in Australia is road accidents. Preventive actions include checking vehicles for road-worthiness, responsible and safe driving, the use of seat belts, care when backing cars out of driveways, and not leaving keys in the ignition when the vehicle is unattended. Pedestrians should observe the traffic laws, and wear clothing that is easily visible. Children should be educated in road rules, and supervised until they are able to recognize dangerous situations and take safety precautions independently. Cyclists must observe the traffic laws, and should be encouraged to wear an approved safety helmet and clothing that is easily visible. The relationship between alcohol consumption and vehicle accidents has been well documented as a definite health hazard. As alcohol dulls sensory perception and slows reaction time, every individual has a responsibility to himself and to others not to drink and drive.

Dangers in the work place

Employers have an obligation to implement safety programmes to ensure that working conditions are as safe as possible. Personnel who are accountable for safety programmes have an obligation to identify existing and potential hazards, and to set safe standards. Every individual has a responsibility to observe the standards which are designed to create and maintain a safe environment, in an attempt to reduce accidents from mechanical objects, thermal hazards, and chemicals.

NURSING PRACTICE AND SAFETY NEEDS

Safety hazards exist in health care institutions just as they do in the home or the workplace, and the measures that promote safety elsewhere should also be applied in health care settings.

As part of her role the nurse has an obligation to be aware of what and where hazards exist, and she must be able to implement safe nursing practice. The nurse must also be able to recognize those circumstances that could result in an accident, i.e. she must be able to identify the potential hazards in any situation.

It is important that the nurse identifies those individuals who are most at risk from hazards and, by observing the safety regulations, implements the measures necessary to overcome or to reduce potential risks to herself or to others.

The individual should be assessed for factors that may affect his ability to protect himself. A person may be either temporarily or permanently affected by a physical, psychological, or emotional disability that impairs his ability to avoid environmental dangers.

Factors affecting self protection

The ability to avoid danger is dependent on being aware of it, and to be aware an individual must be able to perceive, interpret, and react appropriately to sensory stimuli. It is through the senses that an individual is provided with information about his surroundings, and it is the brain which interprets the impulses from the sense organs. As a result, the individual is made aware of harmful, or potentially harmful, factors in the environment. Information about the structure and function of the nervous system is provided in Chapter 20, and information about the special sense organs is provided in Chapter 27.

Any alteration to the efficiency of the senses, or to the ability to interpret impulses from the sense organs, will reduce an individual's ability to protect himself from danger.

The factors that affect an individual's independence or his ability to protect himself include age, impaired senses, mobility or awareness, psychological impairment and environmental factors.

1. Age. The level of independence changes throughout the life cycle and, although the young and the elderly are most at risk of accidents, each stage of development poses its own risks to safety.

The developing fetus depends on the mother for protection against harmful factors. Trauma to—or certain actions performed by—the mother, e.g. the consumption of alcohol, may result in damage to the fetus. The fetus is most vulnerable to the effects of teratogens (anything capable of disrupting fetal growth and producing malformation) during the first three months of development, but other hazards exist during the reminder of pregnancy which may cause abortion or premature delivery.

The infant has a limited ability to protect himself and relies on others to maintain a safe environment for him. He must be protected particularly against infection, accidents, and exposure to extremes of temperature.

The young child has not learned to distinguish between safety and danger, and is being exposed constantly to hazards as he explores and learns about the environment. The child gradually becomes independent and more aware of danger, but remains vulnerable to accidents. Many hazards are not obvious to him, and he must be protected while learning to become responsible for his own safety.

The adolescent commonly adopts an attitude of 'it can't happen to me' and engages in risk-taking behaviour. Sporting injuries are common during adolescence, although the largest percentage of injuries results from motor car and motor cycle accidents.

The adult is more likely to experience work-related injury, although the risk of being involved in a motor vehicle accident remains quite high.

The elderly person experiences changes, as a result of the ageing process, which cause diminished sensory acuity and slower perception of and reaction to hazards in the environment.

2. Impaired senses. The sensory organs and structures, as described in Chapter 27, provide the individual with information about his environment.

Thus, an impairment to any of the senses—vision, hearing, smell, touch—renders the individual more susceptible to accidents as he will be less able to identify hazards in the environment.

3. Impaired mobility. Mobility is necessary for an individual to protect himself against many environmental hazards. Impaired mobility decreases the individual's ability to maintain his safety, e.g. inability to initiate, coordinate or perform motor activities reduces his ability to physically avoid dangerous situations and injury. An individual who is unsteady on his feet, e.g. as a result of a neurological disorder, a debilitating illness, or from the effects of medication, is more vulnerable to injury as he may lose balance and fall.

4. Impaired awareness. Normal awareness and consciousness are necessary to be able to perceive, interpret and react to people, objects or places. Impaired awareness or consciousness reduce these abilities and render the individual more susceptible to injury. The risk of injury to self or to others is increased if an individual is confused, disoriented, or suffers from memory lapses. An intellectual disability may result in the individual being dependent on others for his safety.

5. Psychological impairment. Severe anxiety or stress commonly affect an individual's perception of, and his ability to react appropriately, to, harmful stimuli.

6. Environmental. Feelings of insecurity and anxiety can be experienced when an individual is in unfamiliar surroundings. Admission to a health care facility involves a significant change of environment, and the individual has to adapt to many unfamiliar elements, e.g. the height of the bed or slippery floor surfaces. Adequate orientation of a patient to his immediate surroundings is an essential safety precaution.

Many items of equipment or substances used within a health care facility are potentially harmful, therefore it is crucial that the specific safety regulations regarding their use are always implemented.

Provision of a safe environment

The goal of nursing practice, in relation to the need for safety, is to prevent injury. Commonly, health care institutions have a multi-disciplinary occupational health and safety committee, whose aim is to create and maintain a

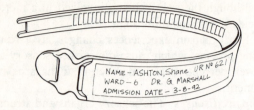

Fig. 38.1 Identification band.

safe environment. The committee identifies existing or potential hazards, and sets standards of safety for staff and patients. Safety programmes are conducted whereby staff are educated in safe practice and specific safety regulations. Health care institutions implement actions which ensure that an individual is correctly identified prior to the commencement of any treatment. The individual is provided with an wrist band (Fig. 38.1) which includes identifying information such as his full name and unit registration number. Before any treatment is commenced, the information on the wrist band is compared with other documented information, e.g. the medication order sheet. As an additional safety precaution, the individual should be addressed by name while checking his wrist band. Checking the wrist band is of particular importance if the person is unable to identify himself, e.g. if he is an infant, disoriented, or unconscious.

Provision of a safe environment includes prevention of mechanical accidents, fire, chemical injury, and cross infection.

Prevention of mechanical accidents

Mechanical accidents include falls, injury from sharp objects, and thermal injuries.

*1. **Falls**.* A person is more susceptible to falling if he is weak or unsteady, or if he is not provided with adequate assistance or supervision. Prevention of falls includes:

• Keeping floors free of slippery substances and loose mats. Any spills should be wiped up immediately, floor coverings should be kept in good repair, and mats should have a non-slip backing. Large, clearly worded warning signs should be displayed when water or polish is being applied to a floor.

• Using side rails if an individual is at risk of falling out of bed. Side rails may be necessary to promote the safety of people who are unconscious, disoriented, sedated, or restless. An adult may find the use of side rails degrading therefore, while protecting him from physical harm, the nurse should not forget his need for self esteem and dignity. It is essential to explain to the individual, and to his significant others, that the side rails are being used to promote his safety. The rails on cots should remain elevated whenever an infant or young child is left unattended.

• Installing hand rails in corridors, stairways, bathrooms, and toilets. They provide support for individuals who are weak or unsteady when walking, and also provide support when a person is sitting down or getting up, e.g. sitting on the toilet, or getting out of the bath.

• Placing a non-slip mat on the floor beside the bath or shower, and a rubber mat on the base of the bath or shower cubicle. A chair should be available in the bathroom for the individual to sit on, e.g. during a shower, or while dressing or undressing.

• Observing the principles of safe lifting when transferring a person between the bed and a chair, or into and out of a bath. Information about safe lifting and transfer techniques is provided in Chapter 37. The wheels of beds, wheelchairs, commodes, or trolleys should be locked when transferring individuals to or from them.

• Adjusting the height of the bed to meet the person's needs. It is usually safer to adjust the bed to a low position for the individual who is able to get into and out of the bed independently.

• Placing any items required by the individual, while he is in bed or sitting on a chair, within easy reach. The locker and the overbed table should be positioned near the person, to avoid a fall from the bed if he attempts to reach for something.

• Remaining with an individual if there is a risk of his falling, e.g. from a trolley, a theatre table, an examination couch, or a wheelchair. Safety straps should be used, or the side rails elevated, to prevent the person from rolling off or falling.

• Ensuring that all walking aids, e.g. crutches and frames, are fitted with non-slip tips to prevent them skidding on the floor. A person who is using a walking aid should be supported adequately and supervised until he is able to use the aid safely.

• Ensuring that adequate lighting is available in all areas, and that a night light is provided in the individual's room.

• Placing the signal device within the person's easy reach so that he can summon assistance if necessary, e.g. to get out of bed.

• Keeping all areas free of items that could cause a person to fall, e.g. electrical cords, or cleaning equipment.

• Ensuring that ambulant individuals wear shoes or slippers which are well fitting and have non-slip soles. The cord from a dressing gown should not be allowed to trail as it could cause the person to trip.

• Taking care when turning a corner or going through a door, to avoid bumping into another person. Doors should remain fully open or closed, as individuals are more likely to bump into a door that is ajar.

• Using protective safety devices, e.g. restraints, if necessary to promote the individual's safety. The use of restraints is generally prescribed by a medical officer, and restraints must be used with caution as many of them pose their own risk. A disoriented person may become entangled in a restraint or, if it has been applied incorrectly, the restraint may interfere with breathing or circulation.

Restraints are prescribed for the individual's protection, e.g. to prevent falls from the bed or a chair; or to prevent a person from harming himself, e.g. a disoriented person may attempt to pull out tubing or disconnect equipment.

Restraints (Fig. 38.2) may be applied to the chest, the waist, or to the wrists or ankles. Which ever type of restraint has been prescribed, it is important to ensure that:

— The person has adequate mobility. Excessive restriction on movement may lead to feelings of frustration and confusion, and the individual may try to get out of the restraint.
— Wrist or ankle restraints are well padded and correctly applied to avoid pressure, pain, friction, or impaired circulation. They must be applied in such a manner that, although the movement of a limb or limbs is limited, the person is able to move and change his position.
— Body restraints, e.g. jacket restraints, do not impair breathing by restricting chest expansion and they should be applied to allow the individual freedom to change his position.

A restraint is used only when it is the best safety precaution for the individual. The nurse should be familiar with the health care institution's policy regarding the use of restraints, and she should always refer to the nurse in charge before a restraint is applied or removed.

2. Sharp objects. Patients and staff are at risk of cuts, puncture wounds, or exposure to infective material from needles, blades, or broken glass. Prevention of injury from sharp objects includes:

• Handling needles only when a protective covering is in place. Prior to the administration of an injection, adequate preparation and observance of safe practice is necessary to avoid accidental injury. Needles should be disposed of in a rigid puncture proof container which is appropriately labelled with an international biohazard sign. Needle-destruction kits may be used to reduce the amount of handling of needles during disposal. If it is necessary to retrieve a needle, from e.g. a container or the bed linen, it should be picked up with forceps to avoid an accidental puncture injury. When the 'used needle' container is removed from the work area, it should be sealed before being transferred to the incinerator or disposal bin.

• Storing all blades, e.g. scalpel or razor blades, in an area designated for all sharp instruments. Blades should be handled carefully to avoid contact with the sharp edges. When a scalpel blade is being inserted into or being removed from the handle, it must be held with forceps and the blade pushed or pulled in a direction away from the body. After use, all blades should be disposed of in a puncture proof container which is appropriately labelled with an international biohazard sign.

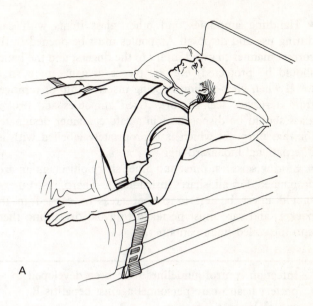

Fig. 38.2   Restraining devices. (A) Jacket restraint with the ties at the front.

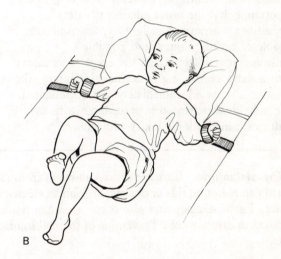

Fig. 38.2   (B) Wrist restraints are often used for individuals who are too young to understand that they should limit their movement.

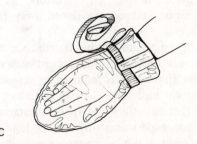

Fig. 38.2   (C) Mitten restraints can be used to keep individuals from pulling off dressings or pulling intravenous tubes out.

- Handling ampoules and other glass items with care during use and disposal. Ampoules must be opened in the correct manner to avoid injury to the fingers; and the hands should be protected, e.g. by pieces of gauze or a small towel when glass tubing is being inserted into or removed from a rubber seal or cork. Used ampoules and broken glass should be disposed of in a safe container designated for that purpose, which is appropriately labelled with an international biohazard sign.
- Storing scissors, pins, and other sharp objects in an area designated for all sharp instruments. Sharp instruments should never be left in patient areas or carried in the pocket, and care must be taken to avoid discarding them into the soiled linen container.

Infection control guidelines have been developed to protect health care personnel against hepatitis B and HIV cross infection.

As the infectious status of many patients will be unknown, health care personnel should consider all patients to be infectious unless there is a medical opinion to the contrary. Therefore it is of prime importance that the nurse adheres to safety precautions whenever handling any sharp object capable of causing injury, and possible transmission of infection. In the event of an injury from a sharp object, e.g. a needle stick injury, the incident is reported immediately and documented. The individual is treated in accordance with the health care institution's injury protocol.

---

3. Thermal injuries. Burns or scalds can result from exposure to flame, hot liquids or objects, or from an electrical appliance. Tissue damage may also occur when the tissues are exposed to extreme cold. Prevention of thermal injuries includes:

- Taking care when heat or cold is being applied to part of the patient's body for therapeutic purposes. The temperature of the application, e.g. a heat lamp or an ice-bag, must be checked before use and the individual must be monitored closely throughout the treatment.
- Ensuring that all heaters, e.g. radiators, are equipped with safety guards, and are positioned away from flammable substances.
- Checking the temperature of hot liquids, e.g. bath water and beverages, carefully before the patient comes into contact with them. Extra care is required to protect the very young and elderly individual's, as their tissues are more susceptible to thermal injury. Adequate assistance must be given if a person experiences difficulty in holding a cup, as a scald may result if hot beverages are accidently spilled. The individual must be supervised during any procedure

which involves the use of very hot liquids, e.g. a steam inhalation.
- Supervising patients to prevent their accidental contact with appliances capable of causing a thermal injury, e.g. a sterilizer or a pantry appliance.
- Ensuring that electrical appliances are checked regularly and maintained adequately, and reporting any faulty equipment or frayed cords immediately.

Prevention of fire

Fire is a constant risk in a health care institution due to the presence of many highly combustible materials. Health care institutions conduct programmes in fire prevention and the nurse has a responsibility to be aware of, and practise, fire prevention measures. She should refer to the institution's protocol regarding her responsibilities in the event of a fire.

The nurse must know the location of fire extinguishers and how to use them, the location of fire exits, the method used to sound the alarm, and how to evacuate patients from a fire area.

Fire drills are held periodically in health care institutions so that all personnel can practise the emergency procedures. Every individual should be familiar with the use of each type of fire extinguisher. Extinguishers contain water or a chemical, and act by either cooling the burning substance or by cutting off the supply of fuel or oxygen.

There are three elements necessary to start and maintain a fire: a combustible material, heat, and oxygen. A combustible material is anything that will burn, e.g. paper, textiles, flammable liquids, or furniture. Heat sufficient to ignite the combustible material may originate from a lighted match, a live cigarette, a spark, or from friction. If the other two elements are present, there is sufficient oxygen in the atmosphere to support combustion. While fire extinguishing methods are commonly aimed at the reduction of heat and the exclusion of oxygen, fire prevention is directed towards controlling combustible materials and heat. Prevention of fire includes:

- Permitting smoking only in designated areas. If a patient is permitted to smoke, he should be directed to the designated area and provided with an ash tray. If a patient is disoriented or unsteady, he must be supervised while he is smoking. Staff and visitors must be informed of the smoking regulations within the health care institution, and encouraged to practise them. Smoking is forbidden where oxygen is stored or in use, and there should be 'no smoking' signs displayed prominently.
- Keeping all areas free from accumulation of combustible materials, e.g. stacks of cardboard containers. All fire exits must be kept clear and they must be clearly labelled. Doors leading to and from emergency exits must never be locked or propped open.

• Storing all flammable liquids, e.g. anaesthetic agents, alcohol-based substances, or grease, safely in designated areas to prevent spontaneous combustion. Volatile gases and liquids must be handled, distributed, and used throughout the health care institution under strict control, and all the necessary safety precautions should be observed.

• Ensuring that electrical appliances are checked and maintained by an electrician at regular intervals. Electrical equipment must be turned off before being unplugged. To remove a plug from the outlet the plug itself should be grasped, as pulling on the cord may damage the wiring. Electrical appliances should not be operated if the cord is damaged, and the electrical outlet should never be over loaded. For safety reasons, and to avoid maintenance by unskilled persons, some electrical appliances are 'sealed' using tamper-proof means, as specified by the Standards Association of Australia. A patient may be required to have his personal electrical appliance, e.g. razor or television set, checked by the electrician before it is used in the health care institution.

Prevention of chemical injury

Accidents involving chemical substances, e.g. medications or disinfectants, usually result from incorrect use of the chemical. A substance intended for topical use may cause injury if it is ingested, and a lotion used incorrectly may result in tissue damage. Prevention of chemical injury includes:

• Strict observance of the policies and regulations regarding administration of medications. Information about the administration of medications is provided in Chapter 58.

• Storing all lotions and disinfectants separately from any substances which are intended for internal use, e.g. oral medications.

• Observing the Poisons Act. Under this act, any container which holds a poisonous substance must carry a prominent label on which a warning is clearly printed. The wording which must be used depends on the Schedule to which the substance belongs.

• Locking the cupboard in which poisonous substances are stored, to make it inaccessible to unauthorized persons.

• Recognizing that the pharmacist is responsible for the contents of most poisonous substances supplied and, as such, only he may attach or alter a label, fill a container, or transfer the contents from one container to another. If a label on a container is illegible, the container must be returned to the pharmacy department.

• Observing the safety precautions whenever a chemical substance, e.g. a lotion, is being used.

• Educating ancillary staff in the dangers of using inappropriate containers for poisonous substances, e.g. using soft drink bottles for storing cleaning fluids or disinfectants.

Prevention of cross infection

Infection is a condition which exists when pathogenic microorganisms have invaded, and multiplied in, the tissues.

Cross infection is the transmission of pathogenic microorganisms from one person to another.

Whenever there are large numbers of people congregated together the risk of cross infection is increased. In a health care institution the risk is even greater, and there is a need for constant enforcement of stringent measures to prevent cross infection. The nurse must protect herself and others by preventing the spread of microorganisms. To understand the reationale behind the measures taken to prevent the spread of infection, it is necessary to know the sources and ways by which microorganisms are spread. This information is provided in Chapter 9, which should be referred to before reading the following section.

Sources of infection include:

• secretions from the respiratory tract
• discharges from infected organs or body cavities
• excreta, e.g. faeces, vomitus, urine
• exudate from infected lesions or wounds
• blood from an individual who is infected with hepatitis B or the Human Immunodeficiency Virus (HIV).
• equipment used in the care of an infected patient.

Although patients form the largest reservoir of infection in a health care institution, microorganisms may be spread by any individual who has an infection or who is a carrier. The various modes of transmission of microorganisms are described in Chapter 9, and mentioned briefly here. Transmission may be by:

• direct contact
• fomites
• airborne droplets and dust
• contaminated food and fluids
• vectors, e.g. insects.

Prevention of cross infection includes adequate cleaning, disinfection, sterilization, aseptic practices, and isolation precautions.

Cleaning, disinfection, and sterilization

Cleaning is an important factor in preventing cross infection, but care must be taken to minimize the dispersal of dust into the atmosphere. Cleaning activities should be completed at least one hour prior to the commencement of any procedures which involve the use of sterile equipment.

Floors are generally cleaned with a vacuum cleaner which is designed to prevent dust being released into the air. All surfaces, e.g. bedside lockers and overbed tables should be cleaned daily to eliminate dust and food debris. A chemical disinfectant may be used to clean these and other items of furniture. Ward annexes and utility rooms, e.g. pantry, bathroom, toilet, pan room, should be cleaned daily. Floors and all bench surfaces are cleaned, and a non-abrasive substance is used to wipe the bath after each use. Rubbish containers should be equipped with close-fitting lids, and must be emptied frequently.

Actions should be taken to keep all areas free from flies, e.g. placing rubbish and soiled linen immediately into the appropriate containers, correct disposal of food scraps, keeping any food or fluid covered, and emptying toilet utensils immediately.

Disinfection is a process which is intended to destroy pathogenic microorganisms or to render them inert. Much of the equipment used in health care is disposable, which helps to reduce cross infection. However, non-disposable equipment must be disinfected or sterilized after each use. Disinfection is the method by which articles such as toilet utensils, wash bowls, and tooth mugs are adequately cleaned after use.

Sterilization is a process that is intended to destroy all types of microorganisms—including highly resistant bacterial spores. A sterile article is one that is free from microorganisms, and sterility is an all-or-none state—because a single living cell renders an article unsterile.

Any item which penetrates into body tissues or the blood stream, e.g. needles, invasive diagnostic instruments, fluids for parenteral administration, must be sterile. Dressing materials which come into direct contact with the body surface, e.g. gauze placed over a wound, must also be sterile.

Prior to sterilization, some articles such as surgical instruments must be cleaned thoroughly to remove all organic matter, e.g. blood, body secretions or excretions. Cleaning of such articles involves rinsing them in cold water prior to washing in warm water and detergent.

Methods of sterilization and disinfection

Agents and apparatus which are used for sterilization and disinfection are listed in Table 38.1.

Sterilization can be achieved using steam under pressure, hot air, chemical vapours, and ionizing radiation.

Disinfection can be achieved using moist heat or chemicals.

In most health care institutions there is a central sterile supply department which is responsible for cleaning, packing and sterilizing reusable equipment. If a nurse is required to operate a sterilizer she should ensure that she receives adequate information on how to use the sterilizer safely and efficiently.

Many articles are packaged prior to sterilization, which helps to ensure that sterility is maintained until they are used. Maintenance of sterility is assisted by double wrapping individual items, or by enclosing single wrapped items in a plastic bag after they have been sterilized. Industrially sterilized items should be stored in the container, e.g. carton, provided by the manufacturer. It is important to note that the porous wrappings, which are used during steam or gas sterilization, are only effective as barriers to contamination if they remain dry and intact. Before any packaged sterile item is used, the expiry date on the package must be checked.

Steam under pressure. Steam is an effective sterilizing agent because it releases a large amount of heat when it condenses on the articles being sterilized. Steam also provides moisture for destroying microorganisms—through coagulation of cellular protein. Steam under pressure is suitable for metalware, glassware, cotton fabric, specific rubber articles, nylon, polycarbonate, and polypropylene. It is unsuitable for substances that are impermeable to moisture, e.g. oils and waxes.

Materials used to wrap items for steam sterilization must be permeable to steam, and they must provide an effective barrier against external contamination. Medical grade paper, as wrapping sheets or bags, is commonly used but finely woven cloth may be required to provide mechanical strength for large or heavy items.

Hot air. Although the need to use dry heat as a method of sterilization has declined due to the availability of many commercially sterilized items, a hot air oven may still be used to sterilize non-stainless instruments, glass syringes, and various other articles. To be effective, the temperature in the hot air oven must be maintained at 160°C for a period of between 1–4 hours—depending on the type and size of the article being sterilized.

Chemical vapours. Sterilization by ethylene oxide or formaldehyde is generally restricted to articles that cannot withstand steam under pressure or dry heat, e.g. instru-

Table 38.1 Methods of sterilization and disinfection

Purpose	Agents	Apparatus
Sterilization of heat-stable equipment	Moist heat (saturated steam at 121–134°C) Dry heat (hot air at 160°C)	Pressure steam sterilizer Hot air oven
Sterilization of heat-sensitive equipment	Ethylene oxide at 45–60°C Formaldehyde at 75°C Ionizing radiation (gamma radiation or electron beam)	Specially designed sterilizer Specially designed sterilizer Industrial installations
Disinfection	Moist heat (hot water at 65–100°C) Chemical disinfectants at room temperature	Specially designed washer-pasteurizer Suitable container

ments with plastic components, electrical leads, and electronic devices.

Ionizing radiation. The industrial sterilization of pre-packaged medical devices commonly uses either gamma radiation emitted by cobalt-60 isotope, or a beam of electrons produced in a machine. As efficiency of this process depends only on *absorption* of the dose required to destroy the microbial contaminants, irradiation is extremely reliable.

Moist heat. Boiling water is not a sterilizing agent, but it is a more reliable method of disinfection than chemicals, as it destroys all types of microorganisms except bacterial spores. Specially designed washing machines are commonly used to disinfect articles such as toilet utensils, bed clothing, mops and brushes.

Chemical disinfection. As many types of microorganisms are resistant to chemicals, this method of sterilization is less reliable than moist heat. A variety of factors may reduce the effectiveness of chemicals:

- an excessive number of microorganisms
- inaccessible microorganisms, e.g. in crevices or in deposits of organic material on the article
- concentration too low or contact time too short
- inappropriate pH
- inactivation by organic matter, detergent, cotton or synthetic materials.

If an inappropriate chemical is used, or if it is used incorrectly, the article will not be disinfected. In addition, gram-negative bacteria such as *Pseudomonas* may multiply in the chemical solution. *Pseudomonas* have frequently been associated with hospital-acquired infections. Disinfectants containing phenols, quaternary ammonium compounds (QACc), or chlorhexidine have a narrow spectrum and their effectiveness is limited to non-sporing bacteria and some viruses. Chlorine and iodine compounds, gluteraldehyde and formaldehyde are broad spectrum disinfectants with activity against tubercle bacilli, hepatitis viruses and (less certain) spores.

Disinfection policy. Efficiency and economy in the use of disinfectants depend on a clearly defined and well publicized policy that covers types, brands, concentrations, and contact times for specified purposes. Health care institutions adopt their own disinfection policy based on scientific principles, and the nurse must be familiar with that policy.

In Australia, disinfectants which are labelled 'Hospital Grade' must have passed the Therapeutic Goods Act test repeatedly against four specified strains of bacteria. The final choice of a product may depend on the likelihood of inactivation during use, on the harmful effects on materials or personnel, or on cost-effectiveness.

Disinfectants should not be used if *sterilization* is required, if disinfection by moist heat is possible, or if cleaning alone is sufficient.

Disinfectants are, however, commonly used in areas where contamination with potentially infective material, e.g. blood, has occurred. Sodium hypochlorite 0.5% or 0.05% is generally effective for disinfecting environmental surfaces.

Preparations containing Chlorhexidene, povidone–iodine or hexachlarophene are commonly used to minimize the total skin flora on the hands or on the patient's skin prior to surgical intervention or other invasive procedures.

Aseptic practices

Asepsis means the absence of infection. The term covers the processes of infection control which may involve *exclusion* of microorganisms by the physical isolation of an infected individual, *removal* of microorganisms by cleansing the hands or equipment, or *destruction* of microorganisms by sterilization or disinfection.

Antisepis refers to the topical application of chemical antibacterial agents to prevent multiplication of bacterial contaminants.

Aseptic practices which are implemented in health care institutions to protect individuals against cross infection include:

- handwashing
- use of sterile equipment and aseptic techniques
- correct handling and disposal of linen
- monitoring infected personnel.

The nurse must be conscientious in the practice of asepsis, as even an isolated act of carelessness can spread microorganisms.

Handwashing. Because the hands are easily contaminated, thorough handwashing is crucial in preventing the spread of microorganisms. The hands must be washed thoroughly before and after attending to a patient, before handling food or food utensils, before handling medical equipment, and after using the toilet or handling toilet utensils. Correct handwashing technique involves:

- warm running water.
- elbow-operated taps.
- liquid soap or an antibacterial substance.
- washing the forearms as well as the hands, and paying particular attention to the skin between the fingers and the fingernails.
- washing for at least one minute using friction and rotating motions.
- thorough rinsing after washing.
- disposable towels or a hot air blower for drying.

Handwashing does not sterilize the skin, but correct handwashing reduces the number of microorganisms and inhibits their growth and reproduction.

Studies have shown that, despite good intentions, nurses frequently fail to employ an effective handwashing technique. Figure 38.3 shows areas of the hands that are most often neglected.

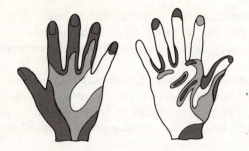

Fig. 38.3 Area most neglected when handwashing: palm (right) and back of hand (left).
Key: black = most frequently missed areas.
grey = less frequently missed areas.

In addition to washing, care of the hands involves:

- Covering any broken or infected areas of the skin with a sealed dressing.
- Keeping fingernails short and clean to prevent harbouring of microorganisms.
- Removing any rings before commencing any patient care activity. If a wedding ring is left on, care should be taken to move the ring up and down when the hands are being washed.
- Keeping the skin free from cracks. If frequent immersion in water results in skin dryness, a good quality hand cream should be used.
- Wearing gloves or using forceps when dealing with infective or potentially infective material, e.g. soiled dresssings or blood.

Use of sterile equipment and aseptic techniques. Whenever invasive procedures or dressings are being performed, aseptic techniques must be implemented to prevent cross infection.

The equipment to be used must be sterile and assembled in such a manner that it does not become contaminated. Throughout preparation of the equipment, and during the procedure, a non-touch technique is used. The sterile equipment must remain covered until it is used, and there should be no contact between sterile and unsterile items.

Any dust-raising activities in the area should not be carried out immediately prior to the performance of procedures involving the use of sterile equipment.

Prevention of cross infection during invasive techniques and wound dressings also includes thorough handwashing before and after the procedure. Further information on wound dressing technique is provided in Chapter 59.

Correct handling and disposal of linen. Linen, e.g. bedclothes, should not be flicked or shaken as these actions liberate dust and microorganisms into the air. Soiled linen should be rolled up or folded, and placed immediately into the appropriate receptacle.

Personnel should wear clean washable clothing which is changed daily. Ideally, uniforms which are worn in patient care areas should not be worn in other areas of the health care institution, e.g. the cafeteria, or outside the institution.

Monitoring infected personnel. Any member of the health care team who has an infective condition should be assessed to determine whether the infection poses a hazard to others. If precautionary measures, e.g. wearing a mask or a change of work venue are not practicable, it may be necessary for an infected individual to be given leave while his infection is treated.

In some health care institutions, routine investigations are performed, e.g. nose and throat swabbing, to ensure that team members are not harbouring pathogenic microorganisms. Such precautions are of particular importance to promote the safety of more vulnerable patients in areas such as operating rooms, burns units, or neonatal units.

Isolation precautions

To prevent cross infection, a patient with an infection or infectious disease is generally isolated from other patients. Information about source isolation and protective isolation is provided in Chapter 61.

The importance of preventing cross infection cannot be over emphasized, and to prevent cross infection in a health care institution the co-operation of all personnel is essential.

One act of carelessness can spread microorganisms and endanger safety.

A percentage of patients being treated in a health care institution develop a *nosocomial*, or hospital-acquired, infection. This means that a patient who was free of infection, contracts an infection during his period of hospitalization. As an individual is in contact with greater numbers of pathogenic microorganisms in a health care institution than he is normally, he is more likely to contract an infection. In addition, illness reduces resistance to infection, and the use of invasive devices such as a urinary catheter disturbs the normal barriers to infection. These factors increase the possibility of a hospital-acquired infection.

Elderly residents in long term care facilities are particularly vulnerable to infection. The normal process of ageing, and a decline in the efficiency of the immune response to infectious agents, contributes to their vulnerability. In a long term care facility any infection is likely to spread rapidly amongst the elderly residents—unless infection control measures are stringently implemented and enforced.

Health care institutions generally implement active infection prevention and control programmes, which aim to educate personnel in the use of techniques that prevent nosocomial infection. To promote and maintain high standards of care and safety, the nurse has a responsibility to put infection control measures into practice.

Incident reports

If an accident or incident occurs within a health care institution, the event must be reported immediately to the nurse in charge and documented. An accident or incident can be defined as any event that causes injury, or any event that has the potential to result in injury. Examples of such events are falls, medication errors, failure to carry out prescribed treatment, giving treatment to the wrong patient, loss of or damage to a patient's personal possession. The health care institution almost always requires a written report of the event. The form used is commonly referred to as an 'incident report'.

An incident report must be compiled even if there is no obvious injury, or if the incident appears to be trivial. Documentation is done as soon as possible after the event, and the incident form is used to report any event that involves a patient, staff member of visitor.

The written information must be factual, precise, and clearly written; and care is taken to avoid the use of terms that may be misinterpreted. Information provided in the report includes the name of the person/s involved, the date, the time and location of the event. The individual who is compiling the report is required to provide a written description of the event and the name of any witness. The written documentation is used to investigate the incident, and it may be used as evidence if legal action is taken.

Further information on documentation is provided in Chapter 10.

SUMMARY

Safety is a basic need of every individual throughout the life span. People are constantly being exposed to environmental hazards that endanger safety and, while many individuals are able to maintain a safe environment independently, factors such as age or illness may reduce an individual's ability to protect himself.

In a health care institution there are numerous potential hazards, and maintenance of a safe environment includes prevention of mechanical accidents, fire, chemical injury, and prevention of cross infection.

The majority of accidents are preventable, and it is important that the nurse is able to identify the potential hazards in any situation within her place of work. She must be aware of the types of patients who are more vulnerable to accidents, and she must practice the safety precautions which have been developed.

Adequate safety precautions are an integral part of all aspects of nursing care, and the nurse has a responsibility to continuously assess the patient's ability to protect himself against hazards.

39. Meeting hygiene needs

INTRODUCTION

Hygiene is the science of health and its preservation, and it can also be described as a practice such as cleanliness that is conducive to preservation of health. Personal cleanliness helps the individual to maintain a positive body image or self esteem, and helps to protect the body against disease, e.g. infection. Personal hygiene refers to the measures an individual takes to keep his skin, hair, nails, mouth, eyes, ears, and nose clean and in good condition. Detailed information about the structure and function of these areas of the body is provided in Chapters 18, 22, 23 and 27. It is important for the nurse to be aware of the function of each area and the significance of maintaining high standards of personal hygiene for efficient body function. Neglect of personal hygiene can have a detrimental effect on the physical and psychological health of an individual.

The skin is a semipermeable layer that protects underlying tissues and organs from injury or invasion by micro-organisms. It is waterproof, controls the rate at which water is lost from the body by evaporation, helps regulate body temperature, and produces keratin, melanin, sweat, and sebum. The skin also plays an important role in perception of sensation through the sensory nerve endings it contains, which are sensitive to touch, pressure, pain, and temperature.

Hair is modified epithelium and provides protection for underlying structures, e.g. the hair on the head protects the scalp and the eyelashes protect the eyes.

The nails are also derived from the epidermis, and are situated on a nail bed over the distal portion of each digit, providing protection for the underlying soft tissues.

The mouth and teeth are involved in the ingestion of food and by their role in mastication, play an important part in maintaining nutritional status. The saliva produced by the salivary glands moistens and softens food, and begins the process of chemical digestion. The tongue contains taste buds, and is also necessary for the functions of swallowing and speech.

The eyes are the organs of sight through which visual information about the environment is transmitted to the brain for interpretation.

The ears are responsible for collecting sound waves which are transmitted to the brain for interpretation, and contain receptors that react to changes in position and movement of the head.

The nose is involved in respiration, and contains receptors that detect odours.

To function efficiently these areas of the body they must be kept clean and in good condition. Neglect of personal hygiene can lead to a variety of problems or complications including:

The skin. If the skin is not washed regularly dirt, sebum, dried sweat, and dead skin cells collect, providing an ideal medium for the growth of bacteria and fungi. The bacteria decompose the dirt and dried sweat producing an unpleasant body odour. Infections such as boils are more likely if the skin is not cleansed adequately.

The hair. Hair which is not washed and brushed tends to become greasy and malodorous. The scalp can become encrusted with sebum and dried sweat which causes a feeling of discomfort. In an attempt to relieve the discomfort, the individual may scratch his scalp and cause breaks in the skin which provide a portal of entry for micro-organisms.

The nails. Nails which are not properly trimmed may become ingrown, causing infection and pain in the surrounding soft tissues. Dirty fingernails can carry microorganisms which may be transferred to food or passed to other people.

The mouth. Poor oral hygiene leads to dental decay and unhealthy mucous membranes, providing a potential source of infection as well as being a source of discomfort for the person. If food particles are not removed from the mouth and teeth, an unpleasant taste and bad breath can result.

The eyes. If the eyes are not cleansed adequately secretions may accumulate, causing discomfort and a medium for the growth of micro-organisms.

The ears. Lack of aural hygiene can lead to an accumulation of dirt and wax, which may result in discomfort and temporary hearing loss.

The nose. Secretions, from the mucous membrane that lines the nose, may accumulate causing discomfort and providing a medium for the growth of micro-organisms.

Factors affecting personal hygiene

Many factors influence people with regard to their personal hygiene practices. It is important for nurses to appreciate that emphasis on cleanliness varies according to an individual's personal preference, cultural or religious values, and lifestyle. Other factors that may affect an individual's hygiene practices include:

- stage of development
- level of independence
- physical or emotional ability or disability
- economic status
- knowlege of the significance of hygiene
- availability of facilities, e.g. water
- environment or climate.

Nurses should respect individual preferences and, whenever possible, permit a patient to follow his usual routine of personal cleansing during hospitalization or when he is receiving community nursing care.

Some patients will be unable to participate in planning their hygiene care, and in those instances it is the resonsibility of the nurse to ensure that suitable plans are devised to meet hygiene needs. Many patients will be able to attend to their own hygiene while others will require partial or total assistance from the nurse. It is important for the nurse to recognize that lack of privacy, or an in-ability to care for his hygiene needs without assistance, is usually embarrassing for the patient.

Skin changes

Skin undergoes many changes during a persons life span, and this factor is significant when meeting the hygiene needs of an individual at each stage of development.

In infancy, the skin is soft and smooth, and less resistant to injury or infection. It is very sensitive to heat or cold, therefore it is vital that the temperature of bath water is tested before bathing. Mild non irritating soaps and lotions should be used on the skin and, as the infant has no bladder or bowel control, thorough cleansing of the genital and anal areas is necessary to prevent excoriation. After washing, the infant's skin should be patted dry with a soft towel paying particular attention to skin creases and folds. Cradle cap, which may occur as a result of an accumulation of sebum, can usually be prevented by regular gentle washing and drying of the scalp and hair.

Adolescence is accompanied by many changes which are due to hormonal activity. Sweating from the axilla usually occurs at this stage and the adolescent should be encouraged to shower or bath regularly, and to use a deodorant or antiperspirant. Acne is a common problem, and skin hygiene together with a balanced diet are important ways of preventing secondary skin infection.

Middle age is often associated with further skin changes, particularly during the female climacteric. Due to a decrease in circulating ovarian hormones, the skin may become drier and the pubic and axillary hair may become sparse. Some women experience thinning and dryness of the external genitalia which may be accompanied by pruritus.

The effects of ageing on the skin are partially due to changes in the dermis, with the result that skin becomes thinner, less elastic, and dry. The decreased production of sebum and resultant dryness, means that the skin of elderly people is less able to tolerate soap. To counteract the dryness, a mild soap should be used, oil added to the bath water, or a moisturising lotion applied after a bath or shower. The nails tend to become thicker and distorted, and treatment by a podiatrist or chiropodist is often indicated.

In order to ensure that an appropriate nursing care plan is constructed, the nurse should assess the patient carefully to identify any actual or potential problems related to hygiene needs. When she is observing the patient, the nurse should remember that the characteristics of normal skin and hair vary with the individual's ethnic or racial background.

The skin

The skin should be observed for:

- Colour. Particular note should be taken of any abnormalities such as pallor, jaundice, cyanosis, and areas where pigmentation is increased or decreased.

• Hydration. Deviations from normal include excessive dryness or *oiliness*, increased sweating, and fluid retention (edema).

• Texture. The skin may be smooth and supple or contain rough scaly patches. It is also important to observe if the skin appears thin and fragile.

• Turgor. Skin turgor may be assessed by picking up a fold and releasing it. Normal skin returns rapidly to its previous state, whereas the skin of a patient who is dehydrated is slow to respond. The skin of an elderly person may also resume its shape more slowly due to poor elasticity.

• Lesions. The skin should be observed for the presence of bruises, inflammation, rashes, localized swellings such as cysts, petechiae, bites, scratch marks, or puncture marks.

The hair

The hair should be observed for thickness and texture with particular note being taken of dryness, brittleness or fragility, and patches of alopecia. Lice or nits may be present. The scalp is observed for areas of redness, heavy scaling, or flaking.

The nails

Discolouration such as pallor or cyanosis should be noted, as should the presence of inflamed areas around the nail edges. The nails should also be observed for brittleness or cracks, and any deviations from normal shape such as a spoonlike or concave appearance.

The mouth

The mouth should be inspected for obvious dental decay, pallor, inflammation, or the presence of ulcers on the mucosa. The lips should be observed for hydration, pallor or cyanosis, and the presence of cracks or vesicles. Dentures and partial plates should be noted.

The eyes

The conjuctiva should be observed for inflammation or pallor, and the sclera observed for signs of jaundice. Any discharge, discomfort or pain, and the presence of contact lenses, prostheses, or spectacles should be noted.

The ears

The ears should be assessed for any discharge, tinnitus, discomfort or pain, and the use of a hearing aid should be noted.

The nose

The nose should be assessed for the presence of any discharge other than the normal mucus secretion, for bleeding, swelling of the mucosa, or any obstruction.

In addition to these observations the nurse should assess the patient's level of mobility and independence, so that the most appropriate means of meeting his hygiene needs may be planned.

NURSING PRACTICE AND HYGIENE NEEDS

Skin care

Care of the skin includes maintenance of cleanliness and protection from injury. The skin must be protected against injury by gentle handling and the use of appropriate bed linen and equipment. Cleansing involves the use of soaps and lotions that do not cause irritation or dryness, and careful drying of the skin particularly in folds or creases. Deodorants, powders, and perfumes may be used if the patient wishes and if there is no contraindication, to enhance the feeling of freshness and to improve morale. Cleansing of the skin may be achieved by several means and is dependent on the patient's level of mobility and independence. Some patients will be able to have a bath or shower, while more dependent patients may require a bed bath. Whichever method of cleansing is used the nurse must ensure the patient's comfort and safety.

Bath or shower

A patient may have either a bath or a shower depending on his preference and general condition. Both methods of cleansing refresh the patient, stimulate circulation, and promote relaxation. They also provide an opportunity for the nurse to observe the condition of patient's body, including assessment of his mobility and strength. If the patient is able to attend to his hygiene needs independently, he may be left to bath or shower in private. It is the responsibility of the nurse to ensure that the bathroom has been prepared for use, and that the patient has all the necessary items. The nurse should ensure that the patient knows where the signal bell is and how to use it, and he should be advised not to lock the bathroom door. During the bath and shower, the nurse should check to see if he needs any assistance.

It is the nurse's responsibility to assess how much assistance a more dependent patient requires. Some patients may need help to get in or out of the bath or shower while, others will require the nurse to remain with them throughout the procedure. The nurse should remain with and provide assistance for any patient who is weak, frail, unsteady, or confused. There are several assistive devices available that facilitate bathing or showering.

Mobile hydraulic hoists. These can be wheeled to the bed, the seat lowered to bed level, and the patient transferred on to the seat. The hoist is wheeled to the bathroom and by adjusting the height of the seat, the patient can be lowered into the bath. The patient remains on the seat throughout the the procedure. This style of hoist facilitates patient transfer in and out of the bath, and eliminates strain on the nurse's back.

Fixed bath chairs. A chair equipped with a hydraulic mechanism for lowering and raising the seat, is fixed to the floor at the side of the bath. The patient sits on the seat which is swung over the edge of the bath and then lowered into the water. The patient remains on the seat while being bathed and during transfer out of the bath.

Mobile baths. Some institutions have a portable bath which can be moved to the bedside. The patient is transferred from the bed into the bath and transported to the bathroom. The bath is filled and the patient bathed in the usual manner.

Shower chairs. This type of chair is commonly made from plastic, having one or more holes in the seat which allow water to escape. The patient sits on the chair in the shower area, and the spray of water is usually directed onto him by means of a hand held nozzle. Some shower chairs have fitted wheels which enable transport of the patient to and from the shower area.

Hand rails. Rails, fixed to the wall at the side of the bath or shower, can be used by the patient to provide support.

Whenever mechanical aids are being used, the nurse must ensure that she is familiar with the operational and safety aspects of each one. Some of the types of aids available are illustrated in Figure 39.1.

Patients who are weak, frail, unsteady, or confused will require the nurse's assistance to bath and shower, and the key aspects of assisting a patient are outlined in the guidelines.

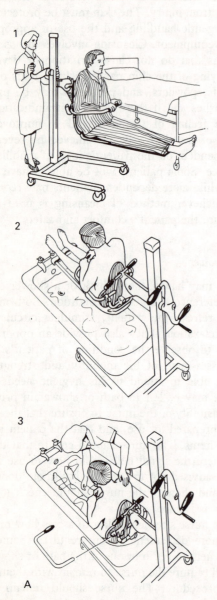

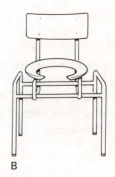

Fig. 39.1 (B) Shower chair.

Fig. 39.1 Devices to assist bathing and showering. (A) Mechanical hoist. (1) Lower individual, transport to bathroom in this position and raise clear of bath. (2) Position over bath. (3) Lower individual and perform bathing.

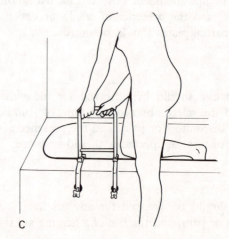

Fig. 39.1 (C) Hand rail attached to the side of the bath.

Guidelines for assisting a patient to bath or shower

Nursing action	Rationale
1. Explain the procedure to the patient	Reduces anxiety
2. Prepare the bathroom:	
• adjust temperature and exclude draughts	Avoids chilling
• ensure bath or shower is clean	Prevents cross infection
• ensure there is a non-slip mat or strips in the bottom of the bath or shower recess, and a bathmat on the floor	Provides non-slippery areas, thus preventing falls
• place a chair beside the bath or shower (unless a mechanical hoist is used)	Provides a seat for the patient while undressing and dressing
3. Ensure that all the required items are assembled in the bathroom and within easy reach	Avoids the nurse having to leave the area at any stage
4. Assess the patient's mobility and strength, and gain assistance if necessary to transport him to the bathroom	Adequate assistance is necessary to promote his safety and comfort
5. Offer the patient use of toilet facilities	Helps to promote comfort
6. Adjust the water flow and temperature before patient begins cleansing. Water temperature of between 38°C and 41°C is comfortable and safe for most patients	Prevents scalds Water which is too hot may cause peripheral vasodilation and faintness
7. Help the patient sit down and undress. Observe the condition of his skin.	Reduces the risk of falls Detects any abnormalities
8. Using mechanical devices as indicated, assist the patient into the bath or shower	Promotes his safety and prevents falls
9. Ensure that the patient is positioned away from the taps	Reduces the risk of injury
10. Encourage the patient to participate as much as he is able, ensuring that all body areas are washed and that the skin is rinsed free of all soap.	Promotes independence Promotes adequate cleansing Prevents skin dryness
11. When the patient has completed washing, drain the bath or turn off the shower	Facilitates easier and safer exit from the bath or shower
12. Assist the patient from the bath or shower, and ensure that he is dried completely While drying him, the patient should be seated	Skin must be thoroughly dried to prevent excoriation Reduces the risk of falling
13. Enquire if the patient wishes to use powder or deodorant. Avoid excessive amounts of powder	Helps to promote comfort Powder can accumulate and 'cake' on the skin
14. Ensure that the patient is dressed without delay	Prevents him becoming chilled
15. Ensure that the patient's oral hygiene and hair care needs are attended to Assist a male patient with a facial shave as required	Helps to promote comfort Promotes comfort
16. Escort the patient back to his room and allow a rest period if required	Restores energy after the exertion of the bath
17. Ensure that he is comfortably positioned, with all requirements within reach	Helps to promote comfort and safety
18. Attend to the bathroom:	
• air room if possible	Ventilates the room and removes steam
• ensure bath or shower is clean	Prepares them for further use and helps to prevent cross infection
• remove any soiled linen	
• return personal articles to the patient's unit.	
19. Report and record the procedure	The patient's condition is evaluated so that appropriate care can be planned and implemented

Some patients will require special consideration when they are bathing or showering, including:

● A patient who has a urinary catheter, wound drainage tubing, or intravenous tubing. Careful handling is necessary to avoid kinking or dislodging the tubing. Intravenous tubing and flask should be positioned above the level of the patient's heart, to maintain flow of the fluid. Precautions must be taken to prevent the intravenous insertion site becoming wet. Drainage tubing, and containers, must be positioned below the area where the tubing is inserted to promote drainage and to prevent back flow.

● A patient who has a wound dressing or bandage. The nurse should ask the nurse in charge if the dressing or bandage is to be removed prior to the bath or shower. If they are to remain in position, the dressing of bandage must be protected from moisture.

● A patient who has a plaster cast on a limb. The plaster must be protected from moisture by applying a waterproof cover over the limb.

● A patient who has a skin disorder, or who has had perineal or rectal surgery. A substance to be added to the bath water may be prescribed, e.g. salt or a pine-tar preparation. The nurse should also ascertain whether a lotion or cream has been prescribed for application following the bath.

A patient may feel faint and collapse in the bath or shower. If this occurs, the nurse should immediately drain the bath or turn off the shower. Towels should be placed over the patient, and he should be supported—keeping his head low. The nurse should summon assistance and remain with the patient.

Patients who are confined to bed or whose condition does not enable them to have a bath or shower may either be provided with equipment for washing in bed, or may be given a bed bath by the nurse. If the patient is able to wash himself, he is provided with all necessary items, the upper bedclothes removed, and a bath blanket placed over him for warmth and privacy. The nurse provides assistance by washing and drying his back, and any other parts of the body he is unable to attend to independently. When the bath is completed and the patient has attended to his hair and teeth, the nurse remakes the bed.

A complete bed bath involves washing the entire body of a patient in bed, and is performed by the nurse when a patient is unable to wash himself. Patients who may require a bed bath include those who are weak from surgery or illness, unconscious, paralyzed, or confused. Depending on the patient's level of mobility, either one or two nurses perform the procedure.

Institutions commonly adopt their own particular method for performing a bed bath, therefore one suggested method is outlined in the guidelines.

The basic equipment required for a bed bath is:

— wash bowl of hot water
— soap (on a soap dish)
— 2 bath towels
— 2 face washers
— bath blanket
— items for oral hygiene, e.g. tooth brush, tooth paste, water
— hair brush and/or comb
— powder, deodorant, body lotion (optional)
— as indicated:
  ● clean bed linen
  ● clean night clothes
  ● nail brush
  ● shaving equipment
  ● container for soiled linen.

Key aspects related to performing a bed bath

● During the bed bath, the nurse should assess the status of the patient's skin, hair, nails, and level of mobility. The bed bath also provides an opportunity for conversation with the patient and therefore helps to facilitate nurse-patient interaction.

● The patient should be encouraged to help himself as much as he is able, to promote independence.

● A patient may not have been bathed in bed before and may be embarrassed about the exposure of his body and loss of independence, therefore it is the responsibility of the nurse to ensure adequate privacy throughout the procedure.
Maintain the patient's privacy and warmth throughout the procedure by exposing only the area which is being washed, and by keeping the bath blanket over the rest of the patient.

● The nurse who is to perform the bed bath, must be aware if there are any limitations of movement or position for the patient. For example, a patient who has had a total hip replacement must not lie on the affected side, and a team of 3–4 nurses is required to move him onto his unaffected side using the 'log-roll' method. A patient who is experiencing difficulty in breathing may need to remain sitting up throughout the bed bath, to prevent further respiratory distress.

● When dressing a patient who has some impairment of an arm of leg, e.g. paralysis, the affected limb should be placed into the garment first so that maximum use may be made of the flexibility of the unaffected limb.

● If a patient is experiencing pain, e.g. following surgery, ensure that prescribed analgesia has been given before the bed bath is performed.

● Ensure that the water is warm enough, and changed throughout the procedure when it becomes cool, too soapy, or dirty.

● If the patient's range of movement permits, it may be helpful to place his hands and/or feet in the bowl of water. This is more refreshing for the patient and enables the nails

Guidelines for performing a bed bath

Nursing action	Rationale
1. Explain the procedure to the patient	Reduces anxiety
2. Offer the patient use of toilet facilities	Helps to promote comfort during the procedure
3. Clear the top of the locker or overbed table	Provides space for bath equipment
4. Shut windows and doors, and/or draw the screens around the bed Close blinds	Promote privacy and warmth
5. Adjust the bed to a suitable height	Facilitates the procedure and prevents strain on the nurse's back
6. Assemble all the items necessary at the bedside	Nurse must remain with the patient throughout the procedure
7. Ascertain whether the assistance of a second nurse, or a mechanical lifting device, is necessary	Promotes comfort and safety
8. Wash and dry hands	Prevents cross infection
9. Remove the upper bed clothes and place them on a chair Place a bath blanket over the patient	Facilitates the procedure Promotes warmth and privacy
10. Remove the patient's night clothes	Exposes the body for adequate cleansing
11. Position the patient lying back on 1–2 pillows, unless this position is contra-indicated	Relaxing position, and facilitates the procedure Position must not cause discomfort or distress
12. Begin to wash and dry the patient in the suggested order: face and neck arms and hands axillae, chest and breasts abdomen legs and feet genitals and groin back and buttocks	Logical progression which ensures that all areas of the body are washed
13. While the patient is on his side after having his back washed, remake that side of the bottom part of the bed	Avoids moving him again unecessarily
14. Turn the patient onto his other side and finish making the bottom part of the bed	To complete making the bottom part of the bed
15. Dress the patient in his night clothes	Promotes warmth and comfort
16. Replace pillows and assist the patient into position	Promotes comfort
17. Attend to the patient's hair and oral hygiene, also facial shave if necessary	All hygiene needs must be attended to
18. Replace the upper bed clothes and remove the bath blanket	Promotes comfort and warmth
19. Replace equipment, e.g. the patient's personal items in the locker, and the signal device in easy reach	Ensures his surroundings are tidy, and access to his belongings
20. Disinfect, wash bowl, tooth mug Remove soiled linen container Wash and dry hands	Prevents cross infection
21. Note the patient's response, document the procedure and report observations	Appropriate care can be planned and implemented

to be more adequately cleansed. If necessary the nails may be cleaned with an orange stick or nail brush.

• Ensure that all soap is rinsed off the skin, as residual soap may cause dryness.

• If using powder it should be applied sparingly to avoid caking and irritation.

• Special care should be taken to ensure that all skin folds and creases are washed and thoroughly dried, e.g. under breasts, in the groin area, between the buttocks, fingers and toes. If these areas are not dried properly, the skin may become excoriated and painful.

• If the patient's skin is very dry bath oil may be used instead of soap, or a moisturising lotion applied after the bed bath.

• Throughout the bed bath the patient's skin should be observed for areas of redness, breaks, bruises, and other deviations from normal. The nurse should inspect areas of the skin for signs of developing decubitus ucers. Information about decubitus ulcers is provided in Chapter 37.

• If the patient has an indwelling urinary catheter, or has had certain types of perineal or vaginal surgery, special perineal care should be provided. Information on perineal care is provided in Chapters 30 and 49.

• During the bed bath, the patient's joints should be put through their full range of motion, unless this is contraindicated. Movement improves circulation, maintains joint mobility, and preserves muscle tone.

• Maintain the patient's privacy and warmth throughout the procedure by exposing only the area which is being washed, and by keeping the bath blanket over the rest of the patient.

• Throughout the bed bath the nurse should promote the safety and comfort of the patient, while ensuring that all his hygiene needs are met.

Hair care

Care of the hair includes brushing and combing to stimulate scalp circulation, remove shed skin cells, and to distribute the natural oils which give the hair a healthy sheen. Care also includes shampooing to remove dirt and to prevent offensive odour. Hair that is well cared for improves self image and assists an individual's feeling of general comfort. The frequency of hair care depends on the length and texture of the hair, the patient's usual practice and his general condition. Hair should be brushed or combed at least twice daily and shampooed according to personal preference or as necessary.

During long periods of hospitalization, patients may desire the services of a hairdresser to cut or style their hair, but hair should not be cut or restyled unless the patient gives permission. Brushes and combs should be washed regularly and should not be shared between patients. As part of patient assessment, the nurse should observe for and report any abnormalities such as excessive dandruff,

hair fragility or loss, sores on the scalp, or infestation with lice. Some patients will be able to care for their hair independently, while others will require the nurse's assistance. Patients may have their hair shampooed during a bath or a shower, but if confined to bed the shampoo may be performed with the patient in bed or lying on a trolley. Certain devices are available to facilitate hairwashing in bed, such as a shampoo tray as illustrated in Figure 39.2(A). If these are not available, a waterproof sheet can be placed under the patient's head (Fig. 39.2(B)), and arranged so that the water can drain into a bucket at the side of the bed. Patients who can be moved from the bed onto a trolley may be wheeled to a sink, and positioned (Fig. 39.2(C)) so that the neck is supported on a pillow and the head extended over the sink.

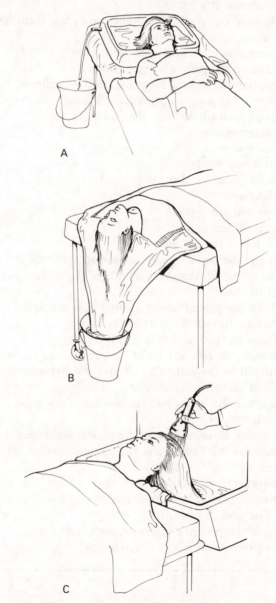

Fig. 39.2 Devices to assist hairwashing. (A) Using a shampoo tray. (B) Making a trough from a waterproof sheet. (C) Individual on a trolley with head over a sink.

The method of giving the patient a shampoo is usually determined by the facilities available and the patient's condition. A suggested procedure for shampooing the hair of a patient confined to bed is outlined in the guidelines. The basic equipment for shampooing the hair consists of:

— shampoo of the patient's choice
— conditioner if desired
— 2 bath towels
— 1 face washer
— protection for the bed, e.g. waterproof sheet
— warm water (directed with hand held nozzle or jug)
— brush and comb
— hair dryer if available
— shampoo tray or equipment for fashioning a trough
— receptacle for soiled water

If a patient is too ill or cannot tolerate a shampoo with water, a dry shampoo may be used. There are several commercially prepared substances available which are applied to the hair then brushed out.

Pediculosis is a condition in which the hair is infested with lice. Lice (or pediculi) are minute parasites that suck blood from the skin and inject a toxin which causes itching, that may result in excoriation from scratching. The lice lay eggs (or nits) which attach themselves along the shaft of the hair with a cement like substance that makes their removal difficult. Pediculosis can occur wherever there is hair, and the three varieties of lice are 'pediculi corporis' infesting body hair, 'pediculi pubis' infesting pubic hair, and 'pediculi capitus' infesting head hair. Signs and symptoms that pediculi have infested the hair include pruritis, excoriation of the skin from scratching, and visible lice or nits. Untreated pediculosis can result in secondary skin infection such as dermatitis. The lice also spread from person to person on clothing, bedding, combs and brushes. It is important to note that pediculosis is not necessarily a sign of poor personal hygiene, as the parasites survive equally well on clean hair. The nits and lice can be destroyed by the use of a prescribed lotion or shampoo, e.g. 'Quellada'. With the preparations that are available, one single application is often effective. Sometimes a second treatment is recommended approximately one week later, in case any remaining nits have hatched into lice. The bed linen, personal clothing, hair brush and comb belonging to the

Guidelines for giving a shampoo

Nursing action	Rationale
1. Explain the procedure to the patient	Reduces anxiety
2. Arrange the equipment in a convenient location	Facilitates the procedure
3. Ensure privacy for the patient	Reduces embarrassment
4. Position the patient lying flat if not contraindicated	Facilitates the procedure
5. Wash and dry hands	Prevents cross infection
6. Protect the patient and bed linen with waterproof sheet and/or towels	Prevents patient and bed from becoming wet
7. Place shampoo tray under the patient's head, or fashion a trough (as in Fig. 39.2)	Facilitates drainage of water
8. Place a facewasher across the patient's eyes	Protects eyes from water and shampoo
9. Wet the hair thoroughly, apply shampoo, and work it into a lather	The hair needs to be adequately cleansed and the scalp stimulated
10. Rinse the hair thoroughly	Shampoo must be rinsed off the hair and scalp to prevent dryness
11. Repeat the shampoo and rinsing if necessary	Hair must be adequately cleansed
12. Apply conditioner if the patient wishes, and rinse off	Conditioner helps to keep the hair soft and glossy
13. Remove the tray or trough, and wrap a towel around the patient's head. Rub the hair dry, or use a hair dryer.	It is important to dry the hair quickly to avoid chilling the patient
14. Comb or brush the hair	Removes any tangles and helps promote comfort
15. Change any wet bed linen or night clothes, and assist the patient into position	Help promote warmth and comfort
16. Disinfect used equipment, wash and dry hands	Prevents cross infection
17. Note the patient's response, document the procedure and report observations	Appropriate care may be planned and implemented

person infested with lice must also be treated to prevent re-infestation. To avoid transmitting the parasites to others, thorough handwashing after treatment is essential.

Shaving

Shaving is often part of the male's usual daily hygiene practices, and if so, should be continued as part of meeting his hygiene needs during illness. Shaving promotes patient comfort by removing whiskers that may itch and irritate the skin. A facial shave can be performed using an electric or blade razor. Because the skin can be cut or nicked with a blade razor, an electric one is usually safer to use. If a patient is unable to shave himself the nurse may be required to shave him. Electric razors should be checked for function and cleanliness prior to use, and brushed free of whiskers following use. If the razor head is adjustable, select the appropriate setting. Use the razor in a circular motion pressing it firmly against the skin, and shave each area of the patient's face until it is smooth.

If a blade razor is used the blade should be checked to see that it is clean, sharp, and rust free. Many blade razors are used only once and then disposed of. Use soap and hot water or shaving cream to lather the skin, hold the skin taut and draw the razor over it in firm strokes. Shave in the direction the hair is growing, rinsing the razor frequently to remove soap and whiskers. Use short gentle strokes around the nose and mouth to avoid irritation of those sensitive areas. If the patient wishes an after shave lotion may be applied.

Some females develop a growth of facial hair, and this is usually removed by depilatory creams, tweezers, or wax. Shaving should be avoided as it encourages the growth of hair.

Nail care

Care of the nails involves keeping them clean, shaped, and trimmed. Dirty nails can spread infection, torn cuticles provide a portal of entry for micro-organisms, and jagged nails can scratch the skin. Many patients will be able to care for their nails independently, while others will require assistance. In many institutions the care of patients' toe nails is the responsibility of a podiatrist or chiropodist who specializes in treating the feet for conditions such as corns and callouses. Patients who are particularly prone to infection, e.g. those with diabetes mellitus or circulatory problems, usually have their nails attended to by a podiatrist or chiropodist. Nails can be kept clean by removing any visible dirt with a blunt instrument such as an orange stick, then using a nail brush. After washing, the cuticles should be gently pushed back and cuticle cream applied to keep them soft. Whether finger nails are long and pointed, rounded, or cut square, is largely an individual preference or determined by the person's occupation. Toenails should

be cut straight across to avoid ingrown nails, and nails should be filed to keep them smooth and free from rough edges that can catch and tear.

Some patients have very tough nails and cutting them may be facilitated if the patient soaks his hands or feet in warm water first. Whenever nails are being trimmed, extreme care must be taken to prevent any damage to surrounding tissues. Nail clippers commonly used in preference to scissors, as a safety measure. The nurse should ascertain whether it is part of her role and function to care for the patient's nails.

Mouth care

Oral hygiene involves measures to keep the mouth and teeth clean and in good condition. Care of the mouth includes brushing the teeth, mouth rinses, and regular visits to the dentist. The measures necessary to maintain the mouth and teeth in a healthy condition include:

- An adequate fluid intake, including citrus juices when possible to stimulate the flow of saliva. Saliva helps to maintain a healthy mouth by washing away shed epithelial cells, food debris, and microorganisms. Saliva also keeps the mouth lining moist and acts as a mild antiseptic which inhibits the growth of microorganisms.
- A well balanced diet that provides the tissues with the nutrients necessary for growth and repair. Foods that require chewing stimulate blood circulation to the gums and should be included when possible.
- Brushing and flossing the teeth to remove plaque and food debris, massage the gums, prevent mouth odour, and to prevent infection.
- Rinsing the mouth to remove unpleasant tastes or odours.
- Regular visits to the dentist to allow inspection of the teeth for decay, for cleaning, and for treatment of any cavities and other abnormalities.

If oral hygiene is neglected several complications may occur including:

- dental decay and halitosis
- coated tongue and subsequent dulling of taste, which may lead to loss of appetite
- inflammation of the oral mucosa (stomatitis). Inflammation of the tongue (glossitis) and inflammation of the gums (gingivitis) are forms of stomatitis.
- an accumulation of food particles, dead epithelial cells, and micro-organisms on the teeth, tongue and lips (sordes)
- the spread of oral infections to other parts of the body such as the parotid glands, eustachian (auditory) tubes, and respiratory tract
- dryness of the mucosa resulting in cracking or ulcers.

Patients who are particularly prone to develop an unhealthy condition of the mouth, are those who have a reduced flow of saliva or those whose normal chewing or swallowing actions are impaired, for example, patients who:

- experience dyspnoea, which results in mouth breathing and consequently a dry mouth
- are febrile or dehydrated
- who are not taking food or fluids orally, or whose fluid intake is restricted
- are receiving certain medications which cause dryness of the mouth
- have impaired movement of the mouth, such as facial paralysis or surgical immobilization of the jaw.
- have a nasogastric tube or airway in position which may irritate or damage the mucosa, or lead to an accumulation of debris in the mouth
- wear partial or full dentures which allow food particles to accumulate in the mouth
- because of their physical or emotional state are unable to care for their oral hygiene adequately.

Assisting the patient with oral hygiene

Independent patients are usually able to attend to their mouth oral hygiene, but may require encouragement and some assistance. The nurse should offer patients the opportunity to brush their teeth after meals and in the evening. The nurse should ensure that each patient has a toothbrush and toothpaste, and should assist them to the bathroom if necessary. More dependent patients will require greater assistance with their oral hygiene. For patients who are confined to bed, the nurse should provide teeth cleaning equipment consisting of toothbrush, toothpaste, mug of cold water, a container for used water, and a towel. Patients who are accustomed to using dental floss as part of their normal hygiene practices should be encouraged to continue the practice.

Patients who are unable to brush their teeth will require the nurse's assistance with this procedure. Patients are taken to the bathroom or teeth cleaning equipment is brought to the bed side. The patient should be assisted into a comfortable sitting position, and his clothing protected by a towel. The nurse should apply paste to a dampened toothbrush and gently but thoroughly brush the patient's teeth using an up and down movement. Water is provided for the patient to rinse his mouth, and a container is positioned for him to receive the used rinsing water. Encourage adequate rinsing so that all traces of toothpaste are removed. His mouth should be wiped dry, the toothbrush and toothpaste replaced, and the tooth mug and container removed for cleaning.

Some patients wear partial or full dentures which, like natural teeth, require proper care to remove deposits and to prevent mouth odour. Care of dentures involves remov-ing, brushing and rinsing them after meals. If it is the patient's usual practice his dentures may be soaked in a commercial denture cleaner. Some people remove their dentures at night, and if so, the nurse should ensure that they are put in a container and placed in a safe position. Patients may not be able to care for their dentures independently, therefore it is the nurse's responsibility to attend to the dentures. To remove a partial denture equal pressure is exerted on the border of each side of the plate, and not on the clips which may easily bend or break. A full upper denture may be removed by breaking the seal of the denture from the palate. This can be achieved by taking hold of the denture at the front or side with the thumb and index finger. A lower denture is removed by holding it in the centre, and turning it slightly before lifting it out of the mouth. A gauze square may be used to provide a firmer grip on the dentures.

Dentures should be gently placed in a denture container and taken to the bathroom for cleaning and rinsing. When handling dentures care must be taken to avoid damaging them. Before they are replaced the patient should be encouraged to rinse his mouth to remove any debris. If the patient is unable to insert his dentures the nurse should do it for him. Moisten the dentures to facilitate easier insertion, and carefully position them firmly in place. Patients should be encouraged to wear their dentures to enhance appearance, facilitate eating and speaking, and to prevent changes in the gum line that may affect denture fit.

If normal oral hygiene practices are not possible, the mouth and teeth must be cleaned by other means. Special mouth care is often required if the patient:

- is unconscious
- is not taking oral food or fluids
- experiences any impairment to mouth movement, e.g. facial paralysis
- has developed sordes
- has a mouth infection
- has a very dry mouth, e.g. as a result of mouth breathing, dehydration, or the effect of certain medications

In these instances the patient's mouth is cleansed either by the use of mouth rinses or by carefully swabbing all areas. The latter procedure is often referred to as a 'mouth toilet'. A variety of substances may be used to clean and refresh the mouth including a sodium bicarbonate solution, or lemon-glycerine swabs. The nurse should refer to the institution's policy manual for information on the equipment, substances, and method. Special care by swabbing the mouth is performed according to the patient's needs, and carried out at intervals ranging from every 2 hours to 3 or 4 times a day.

A suggested procedure for performing special mouth care (swabbing) is outlined in the guidelines. The basic equipment consists of:

— cotton wool tipped applicators or commercially prepared swabs (e.g. lemon-glycerine)
— receiver for soiled items
— solution (e.g. sodium bicarbonate and water)
— tongue depressor
— container for dentures
— towel
— lip cream.

Eye care

Under normal circumstances, the eyes are kept clean by face washing and showering. If the eyes become irritated or infected, some patients may require extra care which consists of swabbing to remove secretions from the eyelids and to reduce discomfort. As eye bathing is sometimes required as part of the patient's hygiene needs, a suggested procedure is outlined in the guidelines in this chapter.

When bathing the eyes the nurse and use aseptic technique to reduce the risk of introducing microorganisms. The procedure must be carefully performed to prevent any injury to the eyes (Fig. 39.3). Patients who may require special eye care are those whose corneal reflex is impaired, e.g. due to unconsciousness or facial paralysis, and those whose eyes are irritated or infected. Patients with conjunc-

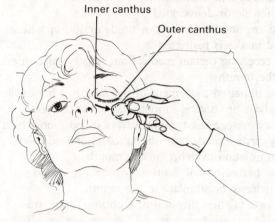

Inner canthus

Outer canthus

Fig. 39.3 Swabbing the eyes.

Guidelines for special mouth care (swabbing)

Nursing action	Rationale
1. Explain the procedure to the patient	Reduces anxiety
2. Wash and dry hands	Prevents cross infection
3. Assemble the equipment and place it in a convenient location	Nurse must remain with the patient throughout the procedure
4. Ensure adequate lighting	Visualization of the mouth is essential
5. Ensure adequate privacy	Reduces embarrassment
6. Position the patient with his head turned to one side	Reduces the risk of aspiration of fluid
If the patient is unconscious suction equipment should be available	To remove excess fluid from the mouth, and prevent aspiration
7. Place a towel under the patient's cheek	Protects patient and bedding
8. Wash and dry hands	Prevents cross infection
9. Remove any partial or total dentures	Allows access to all areas of the mouth
10. Use the tongue depressor to help keep the patient's mouth open, and inspect the mouth	The nurse must be able to see inside the mouth to detect any abnormalities
11. Gently and thoroughly swab all surfaces of the teeth, tongue and mouth.	All debris and secretions must be removed
12. Apply any prescribed substances to ulcers or infected areas	Assists healing
13. Clean any dentures before replacing them in the mouth	All aspects of oral hygiene must be attended to
14. Apply a cream to the lips	Prevents soreness and cracking
15. Wipe any excess solution from the patient's face, remove the towel and reposition him if necessary	Promotes comfort
16. Remove equipment, dispose of soiled items, wash and dry hands	Prevents cross infection
17. Report and document the procedure	Appropriate care may be planned and implemented

tivitis, which is a common condition affecting the eye caused by infection, allergies, or irritating substances such as dust or smoke may also require special eye care. Swabbing or bathing the eyes is sometimes referred to as an 'eye toilet', and the basic equipment consists of:

— sterile cotton wool swabs
— a non irritating solution, e.g. normal saline or sterile water, warmed to normal body temperature
— a receiver for soiled swabs
— a towel
— disposable gloves if there is an eye infection.

Information on the instillation of eye drops, eye ointment, and care of an artificial eye is provided in Chapter 50.

Ear care

Normally the ears are cleaned as part of normal hygiene practices, e.g. during a shower, and some people may also use small cotton wool tipped applicators to facilitate the removal of wax. Patients who are dependent on others for their hygiene needs should have their ears cleansed with the face washer during the shower or bath. If there is an accumulation of debris or wax in the orifice, this can usually be removed with cotton wool tipped applicators. Care must be taken when inserting anything into the ear to avoid sudden movements and possible injury to the ear drum. Information on the instillation of ear drops, swabbing and irrigation of the ears, and the use and care of hearing aids is provided in Chapters 50 and 58.

Nasal care

Secretions in the nostrils are usually cleared by blowing the nose. If patients are unable to perform this function, e.g. as a result of being unconscious, or due to the presence of an intranasal tube, the nurse may be required to clean the nostrils. This is commonly achieved by using small cotton wool tipped applicators moistened with a solution such as water and sodium bicarbonate. An applicator is inserted gently into the nostril, rotated and withdrawn, and the

---

Guidelines for swabbing the eyes

Nursing action	Rationale
1. Explain the procedure to the patient	Reduces anxiety
2. Wash and dry hands	Prevents cross infection
3. Assemble the equipment and place in a convenient location	Items should be readily accessible during the procedure
4. Ensure adequate lighting	Facilitates observation of the patient's eyes
5. Ensure adequate privacy	Reduces embarrassment
6. Position the patient with his head to one side	Facilitates the procedure and prevents fluid running down his face
7. Wash and dry hands	Prevents cross infection
8. Place a towel under the patient's cheek	Protects patient and bedding
9. Observe for abnormalities	Additional treatment may be indicated
10. Using moistened swabs clean the eyes, beginning with the least affected eye first	Reduces the risk of cross contamination
11. Ask the patient to close the eye, and wipe the eye lids from the inner canthus to the outer canthus	Prevents injury to the eyeball and prevents fluid and debris from entering the nasolacrimal duct
12. Use a clean swab for each wipe, and continue until the eye is clean. Repeat the procedure for the other eye	Prevents cross contamination
13. After cleansing, instill any prescribed drops or ointment. (Refer to Chapter 58 for further information)	Drops or ointment may be prescribed to treat irritation or infection
14. Wipe any moisture from the patient's face, remove the towel, and reposition the patient if necessary	Helps promote comfort
15. Remove equipment, dispose of soiled swabs, wash and dry hands	Prevents cross infection
16. Report and record the procedure	Appropriate care may be planned and implemented

technique is repeated until the nostrils are clean. Sometimes a cream is applied around the nostrils to prevent soreness.

SUMMARY

Personal hygiene needs must be met in order to keep the body clean and functioning. Continuous assessment of the patient's needs, and of the status of his skin, hair, nails, mouth, eyes, ears, and nose, is necessary so that appropriate care may be planned and implemented. Neglect of personal hygiene needs causes discomfort and may lead to infection and other serious complications. It is the nurse's responsibility to ensure that all patients have access to the facilities necessary for meeting their hygiene needs.

Dependent patients require assistance from the nurse to meet their needs, and the nurse should ensure that the patient's dignity, comfort, and safety are promoted throughout any of the procedures.

40. Meeting psychosocial needs

OBJECTIVES

1. Discuss the development of self esteem throughout the life cycle.
2. State the importance of self esteem to the individual's emotional security.
3. Discuss the three components of personal identity: self concept, body image, sexual image.
4. Discuss the development of sexuality throughout the life cycle.
5. Apply relevant principles in planning and implementing care to assist the patient meet his or her esteem, body image, sexual, and spiritual needs.

INTRODUCTION

Information on the behavioural aspects of nursing is provided in Chapters 4–7, and it should be referred to in conjunction with the contents of this chapter.

In addition to physical needs, an individual has needs that are psychological, social, and spiritual. While the basic physiological needs, e.g. the need for food, water, oxygen, are necessary for survival; the secondary needs are those which must be met to achieve or maintain a satisfactory quality of life. An outline of basic human needs is provided in Chapter 28, contrasting the physiological and secondary needs.

The needs for love and belonging, esteem and self esteem, are fundamental in the development of personal identity. Sexuality is an integral part of personality, as it involves the physical, psychological, social and spiritual aspects of the individual. Many people have some form of religious philosophy, and their spiritual beliefs, needs and practices are important in determining their behaviour and development. Fulfilment of the psychosocial and emotional needs is necessary for emotional security, and it is important for health care personnel to appreciate that the individual has needs which are complementary to the physical needs.

In the past, in some health care settings, little emphasis was placed on meeting the individual's psychosocial and emotional needs; the physical needs were viewed as having priority over the secondary needs. Changes in the concept of health care have generated an acceptance of a holistic view of the individual. Holistic care considers not only the physical needs, but the psychosocial, emotional, cultural, economic and spiritual needs of the individual.

An individual's sense of security develops in part from having the physical needs met and from being protected against environmental hazards. But, apart from physical safety, an individual also needs emotional security and a sense of belonging; and he needs to feel safe and secure in his relationships with others. In order to feel accepted as a member of society, an individual needs the love, friendship, and recognition of other people; and a sense that he is worthwhile regardless of any physical or emotional disabilities. Relationships and communication with others influence an individual's feelings of being wanted, liked, and accepted. In turn, the values an individual places on himself influence his thinking, feelings, emotions, and interactions with others.

A sense of emotional security stems from how the individual perceives himself in relation to others. Self image is the total concept that a person has of himself and of his role in society, and it depends on the components of personal identity:

- self concept
- body image
- sexual image.

Self concept

Self concept is the set of beliefs and feelings that an individual has about himself, and forms initially in childhood as he begins to interpret the reactions of other people to his behaviour. Depending on these reactions, the child begins to view himself as either a 'good' or a 'bad' person. Approval of his behaviour leads to a sense of well-being, and if the child views himself as 'good' he will generally develop self confidence and self respect. If, on the other hand, people respond to his behaviour with disapproval, the child will begin to feel anxious about himself. Constant disapproval of his actions may lead the child to view himself as 'bad', and consequently he may be unable to achieve an acceptable self concept.

Self concept, body image, and sexual image, form during childhood and continue to develop throughout the remainder of the life cycle. These three components of personal identity, which are largely gender based, consist of an 'ideal' and a 'real' self. The ideal self is the image an individual has of what or who he would like to be, while the real self is the view the individual has of what or who he really is. Relationships or experiences throughout life, e.g. illness or admission to hospital, may alter part or all of an individual's self concept, body image, or sexual image.

Self esteem

Self esteem consists of the related aspects of self confidence and self respect. Self confidence develops when an individual feels that he is competent, while self respect is a feeling that what he is doing is right and worthwhile according to his own values.

Self esteem is based on how others see the individual by parents initially and later on by other people who are significant in his life. If the individual knows that he is valued and loved, he will generally feel good about himself. If the feedback from other people communicates to him that he is not valued or respected, then the individual will often feel inadequate or worthless. As a result his self esteem will be low.

Self esteem also arises from self-referenced *internal* sources, as well as from external sources such as feedback from other people. It is generally recognized that the best regulator of self esteem is success. Thus, when an individual *feels* that he is a success, in what ever aspect of life, his self esteem is usually high.

Self esteem, which plays a significant role in the development of self concept, begins to develop during infancy in response to other people. Self esteem continues to be modified and adjusted by interactions during all stages of the life cycle. The greater the influence and significance of other people to the individual, the greater is their effect on his self esteem.

Development of self esteem. An individual's sense of emotional security, and consequently his self esteem, begins to develop from the moment of birth. Considerable emphasis is placed on the importance of *attachment* during the days immediately following birth. Attachment is the process that occurs between the infant and parents, and is significant in the formation of ties that influence his physical and emotional development. The attachment process is mutual as the infant and parents begin to interact. At-

tachment can be initiated by eye to eye contact, touching, soothing talk and other affectionate behaviour that begins to create positive emotional ties. Extensive physical contact in the newborn period satisfies the physical and emotional needs of both the infant and his parents.

Health care institutions and personnel who are involved in the birth process recognize the importance of promoting the attachment process, and are aware of the adverse effects when the process is disrupted or absent. A condition known as maternal deprivation syndrome can occur from physical or emotional deprivation, and is characterized by developmental retardation. Disruption to, or absence of, the attachment process is considered to be one of the multiple and complex causes of this syndrome.

An infant may fail to thrive as a result of either physical or emotional deprivation, and emotionally deprived children develop a very poor self esteem. These children often remain below normal in intellectual development, fail to learn acceptable social behaviour, and may be unable to form trusting and meaningful relationships later in life. To develop the trust and emotional security which are necessary for self esteem, the infant's physical and emotional needs must be met.

A young child learns to perceive himself as a reflection of how other people perceive him. Consistency in the parent's response to his behaviour, together with the freedom to develop independence, help to promote his sense of emotional security. Self esteem generally develops when the child is encouraged to learn the skills that create self confidence and self respect.

As he becomes older, the child must continue to learn to interact with a wider circle of people, e.g. at school, and encouragement and recognition of his achievements are necessary to re-inforce his self esteem. If during these interactions, the child develops a sense of insecurity he may become discouraged and withdrawn, and his self esteem may be lowered.

The adolescent's need to develop a sense of personal identity is strong, and he often identifies with a peer group that provides an identity. Adolescence is a difficult stage, during which there is a transition from childhood to adulthood; and the adolescent is commonly concerned about his appearance, personal and sexual attractiveness, and peer acceptance.

Adolescence is generally a time during which the adolescent's values are in conflict with those of adults. Positive relationships with the family, and with others, fosters self respect which is enhanced by respect for and by others. To initiate and develop satisfactory relationships, the adolescent needs a personal identity and high self esteem.

A positive self concept and sense of emotional security depends on the support the adolescent is offered, as he deals with the physical and emotional changes associated with adolescence. He needs privacy, the freedom to develop his interests, understanding, and tolerance of his frequent changes of mood and behaviour. The adolescent is acutely aware of his emerging sexuality and body image. Factors that may disrupt these aspects of his personal identity, e.g. illness and admission to hospital, commonly result in anxiety and feelings of vulnerability, and thus a reduced self esteem.

The adult is at a stage of development during which more intimate relationships with others is important. An adult who has a firm sense of personal identity, and who is comfortable in an intimate relationship, generally feels emotionally secure and has a high self esteem. Changes in, or inability to develop and sustain, an intimate relationship can greatly affect an individual's sense of security and self esteem.

During adulthood a stable individual becomes less reliant on external acclaim and reinforcement as being the main source of esteem-enhancing experiences.

Middle age is frequently accompanied by many changes, and self esteem can be affected by the physical changes associated with this stage of development. Self esteem is less likely to suffer if the individual has a positive image of his appearance, personality, relationships with other people, and the way in which he contributes to society. An individual with low self esteem is more likely to have that esteem further reduced when the physical changes of middle age occur, e.g. grey hair or wrinkles.

The elderly adult commonly experiences changes to his life that require many adjustments, e.g. retirement, loss of a partner, reduced physical abilities, or a change in living arrangements. His self esteem can be enhanced if he has good relationships with others and if he is encouraged to remain as active as possible. The elderly adult needs to feel involved, useful, and respected. Increasing dependence on others, e.g. as a result of reduced physical mobility, can produce feelings of worthlessness, dependency, and a poor self esteem.

Body image

Body image, which is a component of personal identity, is the individual's concept of the size, shape, and physical capabilities of his body. Body image begins to develop in the first few months after birth, as the infant discovers parts of his body. Development of body image continues throughout the life cycle as the individual creates a mental image of how his body appears to himself and to others.

Body image develops from self observation, and is very dependent on feedback from other people. The remarks, praise, or criticism of others becomes important in constructing a picture of how the individual views his body. Thus, body image is largely a result of socialization. An individual learns from people and from other sources, e.g. the media, whether it is acceptable to be fat or thin, tall or short, blonde or brunette. The current notion that a de-

sirable woman must have firm breasts, a small bottom, and a generally 'boyish' appearance is largely a product of commercialism derived from advertizing. Similarly, it is difficult for a male to feel satisfied with his body image unless his body conforms to the current 'ideal', i.e. tall, lean, youthful and handsome. Every individual has, however, the choice to be influenced by or to resist such idealized images. Feminism has done much to remind women that these ideals are not compulsory and can be resisted.

The first step on the way towards developing a self concept is largely concerned with building up a body image, or an integrated concept of how the parts of the body look and function. An individual tends to place considerable importance on the appraisal, approval, and acceptance of his body by others. The impact of other people's reactions to the individual's body will vary in significance depending upon how important those people are to the individual.

Consequently, an individual builds up a picture of the nature of his own body: its general attractiveness or ugliness, its impressiveness or otherwise, and its acceptability as interpreted through the feedback from other people.

There are cultural differences regarding the ideal body. While certain cultural groups regard highly a body which is plump and well rounded, other cultures place value on a body shape which is tall and lean. The perception of the characteristics that constitute an ideal and desirable body shape also changes with the times. One only has to observe the paintings by the 17th century artist Rubens, to recognize the ideal body shape of that time.

There are occasions, e.g. during the course of specific phyciatric disturbances, when the individual may experience a greatly distorted perception of his body. For instance, an individual who is suffering from anorexia nervosa commonly has a mental image of her body as being overweight—while in reality extreme emaciation may be evident. An individual who is experiencing hallucinations may see part of his body disintegrating when in fact it is not.

Adjustment to a change of body image may be easy or difficult, depending on what change has taken place. For instance, an obese individual's body image can be greatly enhanced by loss of weight, whereas adjustment to the loss of a breast or limb may be very difficult. The physical changes that accompany adolescence, e.g. pimples, menstruation, growth spurts, can make it very difficult for the adolescent to maintain feelings of wellbeing and self—assurance.

Commonly, a change in body image and self concept can result in anxiety about personal attractiveness, which can lead to low self esteem. There are many aspects which may affect physical appearance, from the loss of hair to amputation of a limb; all of which can negatively affect an individual's body image and self esteem.

An individual who has come to terms with his body, and who has a positive self-regard, may be quite able to make the necessary adjustments if some form of disablement occurs. On the other hand, it may be that just the opposite is the case. It is important to acknowledge that an individual who experiences a sense of inferiority due to an alteration in body image, needs acceptance from others. If he receives the support and understanding of other people, he can be assisted to develop and maintain a greater sense of positive self esteem.

Sexual image

Sexual image, which is another component of personal identity, is the perception of one's own sexuality. Sexual image begins to develop in the first few months after birth, as the infant begins to explore his body and observe his parent's reactions. Development of sexual image continues throughout the life cycle as the individual builds up an image of his own sexuality.

Sexuality can be described either in biological terms as the genital characteristics that distinguish male from female; or as the physical, functional, and psychological attributes that are expressed by an individual's gender identity and sexual behaviour.

Gender identity is the individual's sense of knowing to which sex one belongs. Gender role is the expression of gender identity, as it is the image that an individual presents to self and others by demonstrating maleness or femaleness.

There is a basic drive of a sexual nature in all humans, the biological purpose of which is the reproduction of the species. Human sexuality encompasses much more than the need to reproduce as it involves the whole personality, and is influenced by physical, psychological, socio-cultural, and spiritual factors. Sexuality, as part of personal identity, influences the way the individual thinks, behaves, and interacts with others. There is a direct link between sexual feelings and behaviour, body image and self esteem.

Development of sexuality. Psychosexual development is the process by which a child develops into a mature sexual being, and involves a physical as well as a psychological component. Self identity and personality, of which sexuality is a part, develop through a series of stages from infancy to adulthood.

Erik Erikson's theory of development (1963) suggests that the individual has conflicts which must be resolved at various stages in his life. Theoretically, resolution of these conflicts leads to a balanced and well adjusted person, while lack of resolution may result in personality disturbances.

According to the influential theories of Sigmund Freud (1856–1939), the formative years of childhood form the basis for later psychoneurotic disorders, primarily through the unconscious repression of instinctive drives and sexual desires.

Growth and development continues throughout life, af-
fects the total person, and passes through various stages. Each developmental stage has its own age range, characteristics, and developmental tasks. Development of sexuality is one aspect of the total development of the individual. The development of sexuality includes aspects which are physical, psychological, and social.

During infancy and childhood there is growth of the sex organs; and sex differences in body build, appearance, and rate of growth are apparent. Commonly, there are sex differences in roles and functions within the family and in community settings.

The concept of sexuality, and the values attached to it, is initially learned from the parents, as these are generally the first people the child encounters. The young child is curious and highly receptive, and large parts of sexuality learned in childhood are not erotic in nature. Children experiment with the concept of sexuality in play and through fantasy. This is natural and normal as the child begins to express an interest in his own sexuality.

The child learns from other people about attitudes towards 'sexual' behaviour, e.g. undressing in the presence of others, or handling his own genitals. Children who are reprimanded for touching their genitals or masturbating, may develop a negative attitude towards expressing sexuality. Sexual behaviour in childhood is largely self stimulatory.

The child is exposed to a sexual environment, e.g. via films, television, advertizing, books and magazines; all of which contribute to his attitude towards sexuality.

Teaching aspects of sexuality in schools remains a controversial issue, and as a result sexuality is commonly taught from a factual and biological perspective without reference to the accompanying emotional feelings.

During adolescence the development of secondary sex characteristics signal the onset of puberty and menarche, and approaching sexual maturation of the body. Females begin to menstruate and are capable of conceiving, while males experience erections and ejaculation and are capable of fertilization.

There is a great deal of experimentation in the adolescent's expression of sexuality. Sexual behaviour involves masturbation, and both heterosexual and homosexual liaisons are common. The adolescent often learns much about sexuality from the peer groups with which he relates. There can be problems associated with peer group teaching as the information imparted may be incorrect or inadequate.

During early adulthood there are continuing sex differences in body build and completion of the development of secondary sex characteristics. There is also development and modification of sexual image, and of attitudes towards sexuality, sexual relationships and behaviour. Sexual partnerships are established and/or developed, and sexual behaviour involves masturbation and sexual expression with others.

Middle age is associated with many changes and, as a result, the middle aged person may experience doubt or anxiety about his/her sexual attractiveness or adequacy. The term 'mid-life crisis' is sometimes used to describe this period which is typified by contrasts, e.g. a time of achievement and regret, of stability and change.

The major developmental change for females is the onset of menopause, which is characterized by physical and hormonal changes. The female body undergoes a number of changes in the reproductive system, perhaps the most important being that after menopause the woman is no longer able to conceive.

The term 'male menopause' is sometimes used to describe the changes occurring to a male during this stage of the life cycle. Although there is no equivalent physical basis, the term may be used to indicate the male's feelings of depression, anxiety and self-devaluation associated with middle age.

Both males and females are likely to be aware of the deterioration of their bodies. For instance, men commonly view this stage as one where their masculine virtues, strength and vigour are beginning to decline. Women commonly see their feminine characteristics of sexual attractiveness and maternal potential disappearing.

The elderly adult commonly has to adjust to the loss of a sexual partner, and may experience a temporary decline in libido and sexual behaviour. Elderly males and females may be concerned about the loss of attractiveness. The aged male remains capable of erection but may attain fewer orgasms, and the incidence of spontaneous erection declines. The aged female may experience some discomfort due to the vaginal dryness which can accompany hormonal changes. The elderly person is still a sexual being and, if intercourse is not possible or desired, sexual behaviour may involve other forms of sexual expression, e.g. touching, caressing, and embracing.

Expressions of sexuality and sexual behaviour enable the individual to declare his personality. Sexuality is expressed by personal appearance, style of dress, the use of perfume and adornments such as jewellery. Expressions of sexuality are evident in patterns of physical contact and interpersonal interactions.

Much adult sexual behaviour is dictated by what has been learned in childhood experiences and socialization. Each society adopts its own code of sexual behaviour and has laws regarding permissable sexual relationships. While there is a common prohibition against incest and rape, societies hold varying views on the acceptability of extramarital and premarital intercourse. In some societies sexual activity outside marriage is encouraged, while in others it is strongly discouraged or forbidden.

Heterosexual intercourse is the predominant sexual activity in the majority of adults in most human societies; however, homosexual behaviour of some sort is common among humans in most societies. Heterosexuality means a sexual preference or desire for a person of the opposite sex, while homosexuality means a sexual preference or desire for a person of the same sex. Some individuals are attracted to both sexes, and the term bisexuality is used to describe the pattern of sexual behaviour that alternates between heterosexual and homosexual relationships.

Transsexual is the term used to describe a person who believes that he/she is really a member of the opposite sex. Most transsexual individuals describe feelings of being 'trapped' in the wrong body, and have had those feelings since early childhood.

Transvestite is the term used to describe a person who becomes sexually excited by dressing in clothes of the opposite sex, and it is almost exclusively a male sexual activity.

Spiritual needs

Spirituality, although commonly thought of as referring solely to religion and religious beliefs, has broader implications. Spirituality may be thought of as 'being moved by some outside source'. While formalized religion is one form of spirituality, many people experience spirituality through a love of music, art, or nature.

For many people religion, through its rituals, provides an orderly progress through life into death. Religion may play an important role in an individual's life, and spiritual beliefs can help when he is facing a crisis, e.g. severe illness. Religion may provide a source of comfort and hope during illness, while spiritual beliefs and practices can influence an individual's attitudes towards health and illness. Some people may view their illness as a test of faith, and strong spiritual beliefs can help some people to prepare for death.

Religious doctrines often dictate a particular lifestyle with rules regarding various practices, e.g. diet, personal hygiene, modesty, fasting, or specific medical intervention. Such practices influence the individual's attitude towards health and health care, and may at times present an obstacle to care and recovery. For instance, the Jehovah's Witness sect refuses to allow the transfusion of blood.

It is important to appreciate also that, while many individuals may not have any religious belief, they may hold strong non-religious convictions which guide their concepts of right and wrong, and influence the way they live. However spirituality often helps a person find meaning in life, illness, suffering, pain, or death.

IMPLICATIONS FOR NURSING PRACTICE

Illness and/or admission to hospital can threaten the individual's personal identity and can result in alterations to his self esteem, body image, and sexual image. Illness can reduce independence and can result in the individual losing control over various aspects of his life. Illness and admission to hospital can disrupt interpersonal relationships as the person is separated from those he loves and from those who love him.

Real or potential threats to a person's self esteem, body image, or sexual image may result in feelings of insecurity and worthlessness. The individual may feel that others will no longer respect him, and as a result his self concept may suffer. The nurse must recognize that the individual is a total person who has a variety of needs which must be acknowledged if he is to retain his personal identity. When significant others or an individual on whom the person depends, e.g. the nurse, let him know that he is valued and respected as an individual, that person is more likely to feel good about himself.

Self esteem

Nurses will often care for a person during a critical period in his life when his vulnerability is increased, and his self esteem can be readily affected. The nurse, by her attitude and actions, can be responsible for increasing a person's self esteem—or his feelings of worthlessness.

The nurse can assist in the maintenance and promotion of the individual's self esteem by showing respect for him as a person. Unconditional positive regard for each individual is a valuable approach to all individuals, and it involves being empathic, being genuine, and being nonjudgemental. Depersonalization leads to a low self esteem, therefore the nurse should help each individual to retain the feeling that he is an important and respected person in his own right. The nurse should always address the person by the name he prefers, respect and provide privacy, regard any personal information with confidentiality, and demonstrate respect for his personal possessions. She should recognize all of his needs, and assist him to achieve them with as much independence as possible. When the nursing care plan is being developed, the nurse must consider the individual's psychosocial needs, and set goals which will either prevent, alleviate or solve any actual or potential problems.

The nurse should provide the person with sufficient information that enables him to participate in decision making. Lack of knowledge and fear of the unknown leads to feelings of insecurity and hopelessness, and a low self esteem. Giving an individual some control over his situation will generally prevent or alleviate much of the anxiety associated with illness. The nurse should help and encourage the person to make the most of his abilities and potential, and compliment his achievements.

Body image

Threats to, or alterations in, body image generally result in anxiety, and anxiety is increased when the individual does not know or understand what is happening. The nurse should be supportive to the individual who is experiencing a disturbance in body image, by permitting him to express his feelings and emotions. The person may express fear, anger, frustration and helplessness in response to body image alteration, e.g. an amputated limb, the removal of a breast, or the surgical creation of an artificial opening in his body.

The nurse should also be aware that alterations to body image may be invisible, e.g. heart attack, diabetes mellitus. Although these conditions are less obvious than the removal of a breast or limb, they do constitute a threat to normal body function. As such, they also result in an alteration to body image.

The nurse can help the individual to adjust to altered body image by assisting him to deal with the limitations or alterations caused by the change. She should help the person to recognize his own strengths and abilities, and assist him in learning to accept a disfigured body part.

Any change in body image results in a change to self concept, and the nurse can assist the individual by assuring him that he is no less a person because of the disability. The reaction of other people, e.g. of the nurse, to the manifestations of a disorder that threaten self image, will affect the person's response to his illness. Any change in self concept requires a period of adaptation, and adjustment to a change of body image is sometimes made with great difficulty.

Sexual image

The nurse should recognize that the person's opportunities for sexual expression may be restricted because of illness and/or hospitalization. The nurse should appreciate that an individual does not become asexual when he is admitted to hospital, therefore she must recognize and consider sexual needs as an integral part of total care.

While some people will be so ill that any form of sexual activity is impossible, others may desire to express their sexual needs. Admission to hospital or some other place of care does not necessarily mean that sexual needs are suppressed.

Sexuality is part of the total person and the nurse should promote, rather than discourage, expressions of sexuality. She should not be judgemental in her attitude towards the patient's sexuality and sexual behaviour, even though an individual's preferred expressions of sexuality may be in conflict with her own beliefs. The nurse should also appreciate that sexuality and sexual abilities may be affected by illness, and this aspect can be a cause of great anxiety.

The nurse can assist the expression of sexuality by encouraging the practice of normal grooming routines. This includes applying make-up and perfume, hair care and shaving. The person should be encouraged to wear clothing of his/her choice. Nightwear or gowns provided by health care institutions tend to diminish the individual's personal identity.

The nurse should ensure that privacy is provided. If a person wishes to be left in private while his/her partner is visiting, this wish should be respected whenever possible. The nurse should respect the need for privacy, and not walk into a room unannounced. Knocking before entering the room is a common courtesy.

If a couple is admitted to hospital, every effort should be made to provide them with a shared room, if this is their wish. In long term care facilities there should be no reason to separate a couple, and they should be allowed to share the same bed if their conditions permit.

The individual should be permitted to discuss any feelings about the limits imposed on sexuality or sexual expression by disability or hospitalization. If the nurse does not feel competent to discuss sexual topics, she should consult with the nurse in charge.

Sometimes, a person in her care may make a sexual overture to the nurse who may be angry or embarrassed by the situation. If the nurse is able to understand the reason for the behaviour, she is more able to deal with the situation. Looking for external and identifiable reasons is not sufficient; a basic understanding of psychology should help the nurse discern the use of unconscious coping mechanisms and other aspects of the influence of the mind on behaviour. Information on coping mechanisms is provided in Chapter 6.

For instance, sexual behaviour may be due to confusion or disorientation, so that the person confuses the nurse with his sexual partner. Or, the individual may be unable to control his behaviour because of changes in his mental function. Sexual behaviour in these situations is usually innocent.

A male may have an erection while the nurse is in his presence, which may cause embarrassment for both parties. It is important for the nurse to realize that involuntary sexual arousal is a common and natural event. For instance, adolescent males respond with an erection to a range of emotional states including fear, anxiety, anger, and pain. As the male ages he is conditioned to respond with erection only in sexual situations; although in situations of extreme fear or anxiety, an adult male may respond with an erection.

Involuntary erection may also occur when there is a neurological disorder, e.g. brain damage, or it may occur in the elderly confused person.

There are other instances where sexual behaviour towards the nurse is intentional.

The manner of dealing with any situation where a person in her care is behaving in a sexual way towards the nurse, depends on first assessing the competency of the individual. For example, it may be of little use explaining to a disoriented elderly male that his behaviour is inappropriate.

There is no ideal way for the nurse to deal with situations involving a person's sexual behaviour towards her, but she should attempt to deal with the situation in a professional manner, or seek assistance from senior nursing colleagues.

The nurse should be careful not to criticize the sexual action in a negative way, but she should address the *appropriateness* of the behaviour. If the person is able to understand, and the action was intentional she should discuss with him whether his actions are appropriate or inappropriate. The nurse could explain that this behaviour makes her uncomfortable because it is inappropriate. If the nurse does not feel able to discuss the person's behaviour with him, she should refer the situation to the nurse in charge. Personnel who are experienced in sexual counselling may be able to deal with the situation satisfactorily.

If, while attending to an individual, he becomes sexually aroused, the nurse can provide him with privacy and inform him when she will return. It is important for the nurse to remember that, in many instances, the person will be embarrassed by his sexual response to a non sexual situation.

The nurse should also be aware that she may be relating, albeit unintentionally, to a person in a sexually provocative manner, e.g. via the perfume she is wearing. A person may misinterpret her presentation and be confused about her role, e.g. 'Is she relating to me as a nurse or as a woman?'

Spiritual needs

The nurse must be careful not to assume that every person will hold traditional spiritual beliefs. Some people may find such an assumption a source of irritation. Therefore, while many may wish to have their religious needs recognized while they are in hospital, other people may react negatively to any form of spiritual counselling. Spiritual needs and beliefs are highly personal matters for many people, and the nurse must be careful not to intrude on an individual's privacy.

For a person who wishes to have his spiritual needs recognized, the nurse should provide an environment in which his religious practices can be achieved. He may request a visit from the hospital chaplain or from a member of the clergy. The nurse should inform him that a visit can be arranged if desired, and she should take the necessary steps to achieve this. If a person has spiritual needs that can be met through non-religious means, the nurse should ascertain how she may assist him to meet those needs. For instance, a person may find comfort if he is able to look outside at the trees, or he may wish to listen to the music of his choice.

It is important for the nurse to respect the right

that each individual has to his own spiritual beliefs and/or religious practices.

SUMMARY

An individual has physical needs which are necessary for survival, and secondary needs which are necessary for the achievement and maintenance of the quality of life.

Assisting the individual to meet his secondary needs, which are necessary for the promotion of emotional security, is an important aspect of total patient care.

Included in the secondary needs, are the needs for self esteem, sexual needs, and spiritual needs.

Self concept is the set of beliefs and feelings that an individual has about himself, and consists of self esteem, body image, and sexual image. Development of these components of personal identity begins in infancy, and continues throughout the life span.

Self esteem is the feelings that an individual has about himself and his place in society, and is largely dependent on the reactions of other people. Self esteem consists of self confidence and self respect.

Body image is the individual's concept of the size, shape, and physical capabilities of his body. An individual's body image develops from self observation, and from the reaction of other people to his body.

Sexual image is the perception of one's own sexuality, and is expressed by the individual's gender identity and sexual behaviour.

Spirituality can be experienced through religious beliefs or practices, or through non-religious means.

Illness and/or admission to hospital can affect an individual's self concept, self esteem, body image, or sexual image.

The nurse should consider secondary, as well as physical, needs when nursing care is being planned and implemented.

REFERENCES AND FURTHER READING

Hood G H, Dincher J R 1988 Total patient care, 7th edn. C V Mosby, St Louis
Maslow A H 1970 Motivation and personality, 2nd edn. Harper and Row, New York
Potter P A, Perry A G 1985 Fundamentals of nursing. C V Mosby, St Louis
Roper N, Logan W W, Tierney A 1990 The elements of nursing, 3rd edn. Churchill Livingstone, Edinburgh
Sorensen K C , Luckmann J 1986 Basic nursing, a psychophysiologic approach, 2nd edn. W B Saunders, Philadelphia
Suitar C J W, Crowly M F 1984 Nutrition principles and application in health promotion, 2nd edn. J B Lippincott, Philadelphia

PART 4

Care of the individual with a body system disorder

41. The individual with a skin disorder

OBJECTIVES

1. State the pathophysiological influences and effects associated with disorders of the skin.
2. Describe the major manifestations of skin disorders.
3. Briefly describe the specific skin disorders which are outlined in this chapter.
4. Describe the diagnostic tests which may be used to assess disorders of the skin.
5. Assist in planning and implementing nursing care for the individual with a skin disorder.
6. According to specified role and function, perform the nursing activities described in this chapter safely and accurately.

INTRODUCTION

Information on the normal structure and functions of the skin is provided in Chapter 18, and it should be referred to before studying the contents of this chapter.

The skin has a number of functions which are largely concerned with protection of the body, e.g. protection against infection, physical trauma, and ultraviolet radiation. Any disorder that disrupts normal skin function will affect the efficiency with which it carries out its functions, and may place the physiological integrity of the individual at risk.

The effects that disorders of the skin have on the individual range from being minor and temporary, to major and life threatening. Some serious skin disorders, e.g. burns, so affect the individual that his self concept and body image are severely impaired.

Disorders of the skin may have a single cause or may result from several interrelated factors, while for some disorders the cause is unknown.

Pathophysiological influences and effects

The major factors that affect normal structure and functions of the skin can generally be classified into six categories.

Genetic factors

Genetic factors determine skin colour and the amount and distribution of hair. Congenital skin disorders include birthmarks, hypopigmentation (albinism), and a condition called ichthyosis which involves excessive scaling or thickening of the outermost skin layer. Heredity also plays a role in predisposition to the development of acne and atopic dermatitis.

Idiopathic causes

Many skin disorders have no one known cause, e.g. vitiligo and psoriasis, while other skin disorders may be associated with emotional or physical stress and there does not seem to be any one identifiable cause.

Hypersensitivity

Some individuals have a tendency to react adversely to contact with various substances, e.g. when a substance is inhaled, ingested, or comes in contact with the skin. Some allergic reactions are manifested in alterations in the skin, e.g. reddening and itching of the skin may be side effects of certain medications.

Trauma

Damage to the skin can result from exposure to extremes of temperature, from prolonged pressure on the skin or from physical injuries resulting in lacerations, punctures, or abrasions.

Neoplasia

Any abnormal growth of new tissue, whether benign or malignant, is called a neoplasm. Calluses can develop, e.g. on the toes, from friction and chronic pressure; or keloid scarring can result after injury to the skin.

Benign or malignant neoplasms may develop from any type of cell in the skin, but the melanocytes and keratinocytes are the cells most frequently involved.

A mole (nevus), is a common type of benign skin tumour. Some benign epithelial cell lesions may develop into malignant neoplasms.

Infections and infestations

If the skin is broken, and pathogenic micro-organisms gain entry, infection may result.

Primary skin infections are commonly caused by bacteria, fungi and viruses. Secondary skin infections may occur in conditions such as stasis dermatitis, where impaired circulation damages skin cells of the lower limbs.

Systemic infections, such as measles, chickenpox, and some sexually transmitted diseases, also result in manifestations on the skin.

Skin infestations occur when parasites, such as lice or mites, invade and subsist on the skin.

Major manifestations of skin disorders

Various structural and functional changes accompany skin disorders.

Pruritus

Pruritus (itching), is one of the more common and distressing symptoms of a skin disorder. Pruritus is thought to result from a disruption in the skin nerve endings. Scratching to relieve pruritus, can result in tissue damage and infection, thereby causing further discomfort.

Lesions

Depending on the type of skin disorder, one or a variety of lesions may be present. Observation of the patient includes assessing any lesions to determine their shape, size, and distribution. Table 41.1 lists and describes the various types of skin lesions. Some types of lesions may discharge fluid, which is referred to as exudate.

Alterations in sensation

In addition to pruritus, the individual may experience other abnormal skin sensations such as numbness, tingling, burning or pain.

Table 41.1 Skin lesions

Term	Description	Examples
Bulla	Elevated, filled with clear fluid. Similar to a vesicle, but larger	Pemphigus vulgaris, drug eruptions, partial thickness burns
Comedo	A plug of secretion contained in a follicle	Acne
Crust	A superficial mass caused by dried exudate	Impetigo, eczema
Cyst	Encapsulated mass in the dermis or subcutaneous layer. May be raised or flat, and contain fluid or solid material	Sebaceous cyst
Erosion	Moist, red, depressed break in the epidermis. Follows rupture of a vesicle or bulla	Chickenpox
Excoriation	Superficial break in the skin	Scratches, abrasions
Fissure	Deep, linear, red, crack or break exposing the dermis	Tinea pedis
Macule	Small, circumscribed discolouration, e.g. red, white, tan, or brown	Freckle, rubella, scarlet fever
Nodule	Circumscribed, elevated area— usually 1–2 cm in diameter	Ganglion, acne
Papule	Circumscribed, elevated, firm, papable area	Mole, wart, pimple
Plaque	Elevated, rough, flat-topped areas	Psoriasis, seborrheic warts
Pustule	A vesicle or bulla containing pus	Acne, furuncle, folliculitis, impetigo.
Scale	Mass of exfoliated epidermis	Dandruff, psoriasis
Scar (Cicatrix)	Ranges from a thin line to thick, irregular fibrous tissue. May be white, pink, or red	Healed surgical incision or wound
Tumour	Elevated, solid formation	Lipoma, melanoma, fibroma
Ulcer	Depressed circumscribed area involving loss of the epidermis exposing the dermis, and may involve subcutaneous tissue	Decubitus ulcer, stasis ulcer
Vesicle	Circumscribed, elevated and superficial area filled with clear fluid	Blister, herpes simplex, contact dermatitis
Weal	Transitory, elevated, irregularly-shaped swelling of the epidermis	Urticaria, insect bites

Alterations in skin colour

Disorders of the skin may be accompanied by darkened areas of skin (hyperpigmentation), patches of pale skin (hypopigmentation) or inflammation. Burned skin, depending on the extent of the burn, may be reddened, blanched or charred. Cold injuries can result in red areas, e.g. as in chilblains, or in extreme pallor, e.g. as in frostbite.

Alterations in skin temperature

In certain skin disorders, e.g. bacterial infection, the skin may feel hot to touch, whereas in other conditions, e.g. frostbite, the skin is cool to touch.

Alterations in texture

Abnormalities of texture, e.g. roughness or hardness, may result from the presence of certain types of lesions such as scabs or papules. Scaling may occur, or the skin may be thick, wrinkled, or atrophied. Some skin disorders e.g. injuries from heat or cold, may result in areas of oedema.

Presence of an odour

Certain skin disorders, particularly those that are accompanied by oozing lesions, may give rise to an offensive odour.

Systemic manifestations

Certain skin disorders, e.g. acute contact dermatitis or carbuncles, may be accompanied by systemic effects such as fatigue, nausea, headaches, and an elevated body temperature.

Specific disorders of the skin

Genetic disorders

Genetic disorders are those that are present at birth, become evident soon after birth, or those that may be passed on to the next generation.

Acne vulgaris is a chronic inflammatory condition involving the sebaceous glands and the pilosebaceous follicles, particularly of the face. A blackhead forms and blocks the opening of a sebaceous gland, which becomes infected. Later, a pustule forms. This condition is most often present in adolescents and young adults. Familial tendencies are thought to contribute to the cause or exacerbation of acne. Other causative factors include endocrine imbalances, use of oral contraceptives, hormone therapy, emotional stress, and lack of personal hygiene.

Ichthyosis is any one of several inherited conditions in which the skin is dry, hyperkeratotic, and fissured—resembling fish scales. It usually appears at, or shortly after, birth. Ichthyosis vulgaris is the most common type and the least severe.

Idiopathic disorders

Idiopathic disorders are those in which no definite cause can be identified.

Psoriasis is a chronic skin disorder characterized by red patches covered by thick, dry, silvery scales. The lesions may be present on any part of the body but are more common on the extensor surfaces of the elbows and knees, and on the scalp. Psoriasis can be exacerbated by trauma, infection, stress, and the use of specific systemic medications.

Pityriasis rosea is thought to be caused by a virus, and is characterized by a scaling, pink, macular rash which spreads over the trunk and other parts of the body. The condition is self-limiting and usually disappears within 4–6 weeks.

Vitiligo is a benign disorder consisting of irregular patches of skin totally lacking in pigment.

Seborrheic dermatitis is a chronic inflammatory condition characterized by dry or moist red, scaly eruptions. Common sites are the scalp, eyelids, face, and trunk. The scales have a greasy feel and yellow crusts. Cradle cap is one form of seborrheic dermatitis.

Hypersensitivity disorders

These disorders are those which result from an immediate or delayed reaction after exposure to a certain substance.

Contact dermatitis is caused by an irritant substance which comes into direct contact with the skin, e.g. detergents, hair dye, metals, preservatives, perfumes, or specific fabrics. The resultant inflammation and skin rash may be mild or severe, depending on the individual's response. Chronic exposure to an irritant may result in the skin becoming reddened, scaly, or cracked.

Atopic dermatitis usually occurs where there is a history of asthma and/or hay-fever. The condition is characterized by pruritus, redness of the skin, papules, and thickening of the skin. Common sites are the face and neck, behind the knees and in the cubital fossae, and on the back of the hands.

Urticaria is a pruritic skin eruption characterized by transient weals with well defined red margins and pale centres. Urticaria (hives) is most frequently caused by foods, insect bites, and inhalants. Specific types of urticaria are associated with systemic diseases. Pruritus associated with urticaria is frequently intense and is commonly accompanied by stinging, numbness or prickling sensations.

Urticaria may also be a manifestation of an adverse reaction to a drug, and the skin lesions may appear almost immediately or several days after the drug has been absorbed. Drugs responsible for such adverse reaction include acetylsalicylic acid, penicillin, and codeine.

Pemphigus vulgaris is an uncommon disorder of the skin and mucous membranes, characterized by the formation of large bullae containing clear fluid. The disorder is thought to result from an autoimmune response, and may be fatal if untreated. The bullae erupt, ooze, and bleed readily, and death is often due to a secondary bacterial infection or loss of blood protein.

Trauma

A traumatic injury, which involves damage to the skin, may be due to direct force, penetration, or extremes of temperature.

Erythrocyanosis (chilblains) is redness and swelling of the skin as a result of excessive exposure to cold. Burning, itching, blistering and ulceration may occur; and the areas most commonly affected are the toes, fingers, nose and ears.

Frostbite is the traumatic effect of extreme cold on the skin and subcutaneous tissues, characterized by pallor of the exposed areas, e.g. the nose, ears, fingers and toes. Vasoconstriction and damage to blood vessels impair local circulation resulting in oedema, anoxia, and necrosis.

Immersion (trench) foot is a condition of the skin on the feet which develops from continued exposure to wetness and coldness, e.g. prolonged immersion in cold water. The feet appear pale, cold, and swollen, and the individual experiences tingling followed by loss of sensation.

Burns are injuries to the body tissues caused by heat, electricity, or chemicals. Thermal burns include injuries caused by flame, steam or hot liquids. Electrical burns result from contact with an electrical current, and chemical burns most often result from contact with caustic substances.

A burn may be minor or major, and the degree of local effects and systemic consequences depend on many factors, e.g. the severity of the burn and the age of the individual. Further information on burns, and the care of an individual with a burn, is provided later in this chapter.

Neoplasia

Neoplasms, which are abnormal growths of new tissue, may be benign or malignant.

A keloid is a benign overgrowth of fibrous tissue at the site of a wound to the skin. The new tissue is elevated, thickened and reddened, and the majority of keloids flatten and become less noticeable over a period of years. Keloids are more likely to develop if a wound has been infected, or if the edges of a wound have been poorly aligned during healing.

Sebaceous cysts are one type of epithelial cyst, and consist of a capsule containing a soft yellow-white material. These benign cysts are elevated and firm, and range in size from approximately 0.2–5.0 cm.

A lipoma is a common benign tumour composed of adipose tissue, which is generally encapsulated in the subcutaneous layer of the skin. Lipomas vary in size and most frequently occur on the neck, back, thighs or forearms.

Neurofibromatosis is a congenital condition, characterized by numerous neurofibromas of the skin and nerves, by cafe-au-lait spots on the skin, and in some cases by abnormalities of the muscles, bones, and internal organs. Many large, pedunculated soft-tissue tumours may develop.

Basal cell carcinoma is a malignant lesion, characterized by a shallow ulcer surrounded by a raised , well-defined edge. Basal cell carcinomas may also be referred to as rodent ulcers. The most common site is the face—particularly the nose, eyelids and cheeks. Basal cell carcinomas usually occur in individuals over the age of 40; and, as metastasis is rare, the prognosis is favourable.

Squamous cell carcinoma is a malignant lesion, characterized by a firm, elevated, painless nodule. The most common sites are those areas of the body most often exposed to ultraviolet rays. Squamous cell carcinoma is most frequently seen in males over the age of 55; and, as metastasis is probable, this neoplasm has a higher mortality rate than does basal cell carcinoma.

A melanoma is a malignant tumour which arises from melanocytes. The incidence of melanoma seems to be related to prolonged exposure to the sun—particularly by fair-skinned individuals. Because metastatic dissemination is relatively common, the mortality rate is high. In its premalignant stage, a melanoma appears as a flat, irregularly pigmented macule. Colour changes appear as the melanoma becomes malignant and invasive, with the colour ranging from red, brown, blue, to black. Melanoma can occur on any part of the body, but most frequently occurs in areas of the skin exposed to sunlight. There are many types of melanoma, and, because of its invasive nature, the nodular type is the most serious. Australians have the highest rate of malignant melanoma in the world, and the incidence is particularly high in Queensland and the tropics.

Infections and infestations

Because the surface of the body is constantly exposed to large numbers of pathogenic micro-organisms, the skin is a potential area for infection. In addition, dermatologic problems are often the result of infestation by parasites.

Many factors increase an individual's vulnerability to a skin infection including ill health, poor standard of hygiene, or a break in the continuity of the skin.

Bacterial skin infections include carbuncles, erisipelas, folliculitis, furuncles (boils), impetigo and paronychia.

Carbuncle. A carbuncle is a cluster of staphylococcal

abscesses or boils containing purulent matter. Eventually, pus discharges to the skin surface through numerous openings.

Erysipelas is an acute streptoccol inflammatory infection, involving subcutaneous tissue. The skin of the affected area is bright red and oedematous, with a sharply defined border. The area may develop vesicles and the individual commonly experiences pain and an elevated body temperature.

Folliculitis is a common infection of the hair follicles, caused by staphylococci. Superficial or deep pustules are evident, and the most common site is the face.

Furuncle. A furuncle (boil) is an infection caused by either staphylococci or streptococci. A furuncle starts as a painful, hard, deep follicular abscess, and the overlying skin is hot to touch. The area becomes soft and opens to discharge a core of tissue and pus.

Impetigo is an acute contagious disorder of the superficial layers of the skin, caused by either staphylococci, or streptococci. The condition begins as local erythema and progresses to pruritic vesicles which ooze, with the exudate from the lesion forming a yellow-coloured crust. Lesions usually form on the face, and spread locally.

Paronychia is a painful, inflammatory infection of the tissue around the nails.

Viral skin infections include herpees simplex, herpes zoster, and verrucae.

Herpes simplex, is an infection caused by a herpes simplex virus (HSV) which has an affinity for the skin, and usually produces small, irritating or painful fluid-filled blisters on the skin and mucous membranes. HSV-1 infections tend to occur in the facial area particularly around the mouth and nose, whereas HSV-2 infections are usually limited to the genital region. The blisters erupt and thin yellow crusts form as the lesions begin to heal.

Herpes zoster, is an acute infection caused by the varicella-zoster virus (V-ZV), and is characterized by the development of very painful vesicular skin eruptions that follow the underlying route of cranial or spinal nerves inflamed by the virus. After approximately one week the vesicles develop crusts, and the condition may last several weeks. The *pain* may last for much longer.

Verrucae. A verucca (wart) is caused by the human papilloma virus, and presents as a firm skin lesion with a rough surface. Different types of verrucae include those that commonly affect the hands, fingers or knees; and those that affect the genito-anal region.

Fungal skin infections include candidiasis and tinea.

Candidiasis, is any infection caused by a species of candida—usually candida albicans—characterized by pruritus, a white exudate, peeling, and easy bleeding. Oral or vaginal thrush are common topical manifestations of candidiasis, as are red eroded patches in the genito-anal region.

Tinea (ringworm), is a group of fungal skin diseases caused by dermatophytes of several kinds. It is characterized by itching, scaling and painful lesions. Types of tinea include tinea capitis—affecting the scalp, tinea pedis—affecting the feet, and tinea corporis affecting non hairy, smooth skin on the body.

Infestations of the skin by parasites include scabies and pediculosis.

Scabies, is a condition caused by a mite, the sarcoptes scabiei, characterized by a papular rash, intense pruritus and excoriation of the skin from scratching. The sites most commonly affected are the thin-skinned areas between the fingers, flexor surfaces of the wrists, and the inner aspect of the thigh. The mite burrows into the outer layers of the skin, where the female lays eggs. Small threadlike red streaks appear where the mite has burrowed into the skin.

Pediculosis, is infestation by blood sucking lice, which causes intense pruritus—often resulting in excoriation from scratching. Different varieties of pediculi affect the hair on the scalp, the body, or the pubic area. The lice can be seen with the naked eye, and their eggs (nits) can be seen as small pear-shaped bodies attached to the hairs.

Diagnostic tests

To diagnose specific disorders of the skin a variety of tests may be performed.

Direct examination

Examination of a lesion by the use of a magnifing lens may be performed, or a Wood's lamp may be used to determine the presence of fungal infections. Fungal infections, e.g., ringworm, show a characteristic fluorescence under black light.

Skin biopsy

The medical officer obtains a sample of skin, or part of a lesion for pathological examination. Certain lesions may be surgically excised to provide sufficient tissue for histological diagnosis.

Microscopic examination

Specimens for microscopic examination may be obtained by gently scraping the scales or crusts of lesions. Exudate from oozing lesions may also be obtained for microscopic examination.

Skin testing

Skin testing may be performed to determine which substance, or substances, causes a hypersensitive reaction. *Patch testing* provides a means for assessing contact sensitivity, where one or more suspected allergens are placed on a hairless part of the body. The test site is later examined for a visible reaction.

CARE OF THE INDIVIDUAL WITH A SKIN DISORDER

Although nursing care is planned to meet the individual's needs, according to his specific skin disorder, the nursing care of a person with any dermatosis generally involves the following aspects:

Relief of pruritus

Itching, which can be a source of considerable distress, is a feature of many skin disorders. The natural response to pruritus is to scratch, and scratching can cause further discomfort and may lead to tissue damage and infection. While medical therapy is aimed at resolving the problem responsible for the pruritus, there are certain nursing measures which can be employed to provide some relief.

- As heat tends to aggravate itching, the room should be maintained at a moderate and comfortable temperature. The bed clothes and personal clothing should be light, loose, and cool.
- Soothing, tepid baths may be helpful in alleviating the itching.
- Diversions, which are of interest to the individual, e.g. reading or watching television, may be helpful.
- The nurse should administer any prescribed medications.

Topical applications

The application of local soothing preparations, or topical medications may be prescribed. The most common mediums used to apply medications to the skin are creams, lotions, ointments and pastes, or powders. Medications that are mixed with the appropriate medium for topical application include:

- anti-inflammatory drugs such as a corticosteroid
- anti-pruritic agents such as tar or a corticosteroid
- antiseptics such as phenol
- antibiotics such as neomycin.

In addition, specific substances to be added to the bath water may be prescribed. For example, oatmeal, bath oils, or coal tar preparations may be prescribed when large areas of the body surface are affected. The nurse must ensure that the bath water is at a comfortable temperature, and she should be aware that many skin disorders result in changes in sensory perception—therefore it is essential that the water is not too hot.

Whenever topical applications have been prescribed, the nurse must observe the regulations regarding administration of medications. Each type of topical medication requires proper application, and the nurse must know the amount to use, whether gloves are required during application, and the signs of any adverse effects of the medication.

In addition to topical applications, systemic medications may be prescribed, e.g. analgesics to relieve pain, antibiotics to combat infection, or mild sedatives to promote adequate rest.

Dressings may be prescribed as part of the local treatment of skin disorders. Moist dressings may be used in the management of acute inflammatory skin disorders. Any solution that is used to soak the dressing, should be warmed to body temperature.

Occlusive dressings may be applied over a topical medication, to promote penetration of the drug into the epidermis.

Maintenance of fluid and nutritional balance

Fluid and electrolyte balance may be disrupted because of loss of fluid in exudate from the skin lesions. It is important to ensure that adequate fluid replacement is provided to compensate for any abnormal fluid loss.

A diet that is rich in protein may be prescribed to replenish losses and to promote healing. It is important to ascertain whether the individual is allergic to any specific foods, as skin disorders can be caused or aggravated by food allergies. Any known allergens must be eliminated from the diet.

Prevention of infection

Any disruption to the integrity of the skin increases the risk of infection, therefore measures should be implemented to protect the skin.

- After bathing or showering, the skin should be gently patted dry. Brisk rubbing could cause damage to the already tender skin.
- The nails should be kept short and clean to prevent damage from scratching, and the individual should be encouraged to resist scratching. It is important to explain to him that scratching increases the risk of skin trauma and infection. In some instances, e.g. with a young child or a disoriented person, mittens may be placed over the hands to reduce skin damage by scratching.
- All dressings and applications of topical substances must be performed aseptically.
- If the skin disorder is contagious, isolation precautions may be implemented to prevent the spread of infection to others.

Providing psychological support

A severe skin disorder may casue distress and embarrassment to the sufferer. He may be self conscious about his appearance, and his body image may be severely impaired. If the invididual feels that other people will avoid contact with him because of his unsightly appearance, he may experience anxiety or depression both of which may be exacerbated if his disorder is likely to result in permanent disfigurement.

To assist him, the nurse should be careful not to demonstrate any distaste or repugnance. It is important that the individual, and his significant others, are kept well informed about his disorder and its likely outcome. He should be given the opportunity to express his emotions and fears, e.g. the fear of disfigurement or alienation from his loved ones.

BURNS

Burns are one of the most serious skin injuries, as not only do they disrupt physical function—but they can result in severe emotional trauma for the injured person and his significant others.

Burns are injuries which may be caused by dry heat, moist heat, chemicals, electricity, or radiation. When a hot object comes in contact with the skin, the transfer of heat causes structural damage. Heat causes coagulation of the protein in tissue cells, and the depth of the burn is related to the amount of thermal energy dissipated in the skin.

Following a thermal injury, intravascular fluid is lost as the capillaries become more permeable. As the intravascular fluid volume decreases, the venous return and cardiac output fall. The clinical signs of 'shock' become apparent, and tissue hypoxia threatens internal organs such as the kidneys. Other changes occur in organ function, in electrolyte levels, and in metabolic function. Subsequently, complications of major burns can involve any body system because all systems are stressed during the injury and during healing.

Classification of burns

A burn is described as superficial, partial thickness, or full thickness.

Superficial burns. In superficial burns the basal layer of the epithelium remains intact; and the skin is dry, red, and oedematous. The area is painful because cutaneous nerve endings are injured. Superficial burns generally heal, often without treatment, within one week.

Partial thickness burns. In partial thickness burns there is damage to the epidermis and to the superficial dermis.

As the dermis contains blood vessels, any injured vessels exude serum—thus raising the epidermis to form blisters. The skin is painful and red and, if a blister bursts, the area beneath is pink, swollen, and wet. When the superficial dermis has been injured, the raw area is resurfaced with epithelium growing from the undamaged walls of the sweat glands and hair follicles.

Deeper partial thickness burns result in diminished sensation, as the dermal nerve endings are destroyed. Blood vessels are destroyed and, therefore, there is less leakage of serum from them.

Re-epithelization becomes slower when more skin structures, e.g. hair follicles, are destroyed. Deep partial thickness burns can heal over time, but may be skin grafted to speed recovery, reduce the risk of infection, and to minimize scarring.

Full thickness burns. In full thickness burns all layers of the skin are destroyed, and the injury may extend to underlying fat, muscle and bone. The area is painless because cutaneous nerve endings have been destroyed. The appearance of the area can vary and may be white, waxy, tan coloured, red or charred. The area is dry and feels hard.

Because all parts of the skin are destroyed, healing is only possible by epithelial proliferation from the wound edges. Skin grafting is commonly performed, unless the burn is very small.

Assessment of burn size

The severity of a burn depends more on the surface area than on the depth of tissue involved. The greater the area involved, the greater the amount of fluid lost from the body, and therefore a greater degree of shock will ensue.

To assess the size of a burn accurately, a chart is used where the size is expressed as a percentage of the total body surface. The two methods which are generally used to calculate burn size are the Lund-Browder method and the 'rule of nines' (Fig. 41.1). The Lund-Browder method is the more accurate as it allows for changes in body proportion with age. On the chart used, the numbers on each body portion indicate the percentage of body surface for that part. Both types of chart provide a rapid and accurate means of determining the extent of the burn.

Complications of burns

Following a severe burn, all body systems are involved in an attempt to maintain homeostasis. Complications are relatively common, and can involve any body system.

Shock is due to loss of fluid from circulation. The greatest loss of fluid occurs at the site of the burn, but loss also occurs throughout the body. Substances, e.g. kinins, released by the body in response to the injury increase capillary permeability, allowing serum to escape into the tissues. This loss of serum causes reduced blood volume (hypovolemia) which may lead to severe shock. As a result of hypovolemia, cardiac output decreases, blood pressure falls, and acute renal failure and death may follow.

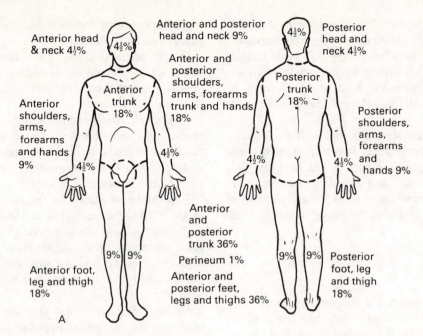

Fig. 41.1A   Assessment of burn surface area. Rule of nines (adults).

Infection may occur if microorganisms gain entry through areas where the skin has been damaged or destroyed. Although a burn wound is usually sterile initially, the area provides an ideal culture medium for a wide range of microorganisms. Necrotic tissue, oedema, and transudate all provide a nutrient medium for bacteria.

The individual's resistance to infection is reduced by factors such as shock, anaemia, and electrolyte imbalance.

Septicaemia can occur when there is bacterial invasion of the tissues and blood stream, and is a major cause of dealth in severely burned individuals.

Septic shock is a form of shock that occurs in septicaemia, when endotoxins are released from bacteria in the bloodstream. The endotoxins caused decreased vascular resistance resulting in a drastic fall in blood pressure. Pyrexia, tachycardia, rapid ventilations, confusion, and coma may also occur.

Pulmonary damage can occur from smoke, chemical inhalation or carbon monoxide intoxication. In the acute period pulmonary oedema may develop, and later pulmonary complications include pneumonia and respiratory distress syndrome.

Scarring and contractures may occur after healing has taken place. Within weeks, hypertrophic scarring results in red, itchy, raised scars which are hard to the touch. The shrinkage of these scars may cause contracture across joints, and can lead to severe disfigurement and disability unless treated. The amount of scarring depends upon the severity of the burn, the area affected, the age of the individual, and the effectiveness of treatment.

Psychological effects. An individual who has been severely burned is likely to experience depression, anxiety, and difficulty in adjusting to the consequences of his injury. In addition, his significant others are likely to experience similar emotions. If a child has been burned, his parents are also likely to experience severe guilt feelings about the incident.

Curling's ulcer is a duodenal ulcer that may develop in an individual with severe burns, and it is thought to be the result of stress.

Management of the individual with burns

The first aid management of burns is described in Chapter 57. The subsequent management of an individual with burns will depend on a number of factors, but the basic aspects of care are:

- fluid replacment
- prevention of infection
- adequate nutrition
- pain relief
- promotion of mobility
- psychological support
- promotion of healing
- preparation for discharge.

Fluid replacement

If the burned area is not too great, e.g. less than 15% in a adult, less than 10% in a child, the body generally compensates adequately for the fluid loss, and the provision of extra oral fluids only is indicated.

In more extensive or severe burns, fluid loss is a major cause of shock. Therefore, fluid replacement is of prime

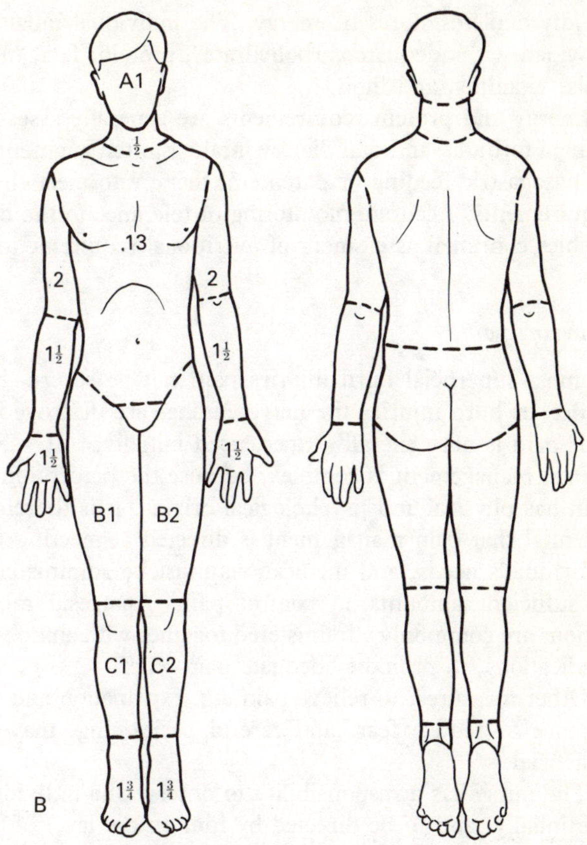

Percentage of body surface at various ages

Percent of areas affected by growth

	0	1	5	10	15	Adult age
A = ½ head	9½	8½	6½	5½	4½	3½
B = ½ one thigh	2¾	3¼	4	4¼	4½	4¾
C = ½ one leg	2½	2½	2¾	3	3¼	3½

To estimate the total of the body surface area burned, the percentages assigned to the burned sections are added. The total is then an estimate of the burn size.

Fig. 41.1B Assessment of burn surface area. Lund-Browder method.

importance. The medical officer calculates the volume of fluid replacement then prescribes the type of fluid and method of administration. Intravenous fluids are commonly prescribed and, in extensive full thickness burns, blood transfusion may be required to compensate for a reduction in erythrocytes.

Large volumes of intravenous fluids containing replacement electrolytes may be necessary, and individual fluid requirements are continually calculated and adjusted according to need. Monitoring techniques which may be performed to assess fluid requirements include:

• Insertion of a urinary catheter to enable hourly monitoring of urine output. Fluid replacement aims at maintaining a urine output of 30–50 ml/hour in an adult.
• Blood tests. Frequent, e.g. hourly, haematocrit measurements act as a guide to fluid deficit and therefore enable fluid requirements to be calculated. Measurement of electrolyte levels are also commonly performed.
• Weighing. If his condition permits, the individual may be weighed daily, as measurement of body weight provides an accurate method of assessing fluid status.

Prevention of infection

As stated previously, the burn wound provides an ideal culture medium for a range of microorganisms. Prevention of infection is directed at preventing contamination of the wound, and preventing invasion of the tissues and blood stream.

Special burns units may be available where the air is filtered, the individual is received into a bed prepared with sterile linen, and isolation techniques are used to protect him against infection. When a special unit is not available, the individual is generally nursed in a single room using protective isolation techniques. Protective isolation techniques are described in Chapter 61.

Methods of preventing infection include:

• aseptic dressing techniques
• topical antiseptic applications in dressings
• use of sterile linen on the bed
• wound excision and skin grafting
• systemic antibiotic therapy
• enhancing natural defences, e.g. by providing a high protein/kilojoule diet, and treating any anaemia.

Providing adequate nutrition

In addition to the loss of erythrocytes and protein-rich serum, the hypermetabolic response of the body to a burn rapidly depletes stores of energy. The individual must be provided with adequate carbohydrates, protein, fats, minerals, vitamins, and fluid.

Energy and protein requirements are generally assessed using a formula, and oral dietary intake is often augmented by nasogastric feeding or parenteral therapy to meet these requirements. Accurate monitoring of tolerance to the diet enables continual assessment of nutritional requirements.

Relieving pain

In most superficial burn injuries pain can be severe, but in deeper burn injuries the nerve endings are destroyed—thus pain is not generally experienced initially.

Pain management is complex, because the perception of pain has physical and psychological origins. It is therefore essential that pain management is directed at meeting the individual's needs, and medications must be administered in sufficient amounts to control pain. Analgesic medications are commonly administered together with anxiolytic medications, to promote adequate pain relief.

Other measures, to relieve pain e.g. explanation and assurance to reduce fear, and careful positioning, may be beneficial.

The nurse has a responsibility to observe the individual continually, and to be directed by him on the level of analgesia required. Further information on pain management is provided in Chapter 36.

Promoting mobility

Because of the nature of the injury, and its management, a burned person may experience prolonged periods of immobility. Thus, he is subject to the complications of immobility, e.g. venous thrombosis, pneumonia, decubitus ulcers, and contractures.

Careful positioning, and regular position changes, are essential. The person must be positioned for comfort, and also to prevent decubitus ulcers and contractures; Splints and other devices may be used to improve positioning and to prevent contractures. The patient's limbs should be correctly positioned to decrease joint flexion.

Physiotherapy is essential for an immobile person, and it involves chest physiotherapy and range of motion exercises. R.O.M. exercises may be performed actively or passively, and the degree of motion should be recorded to document progress. Ambulation is commenced as soon as possible, and the nurse may be required to assist. If skin grafting has been performed the individual will be required to increase ambulation slowly, as too rapid ambulation may destroy new grafts.

The person may be placed in a bath of warm water, e.g. prior to having dressings renewed, and the warmth and buoyancy of the water may enable him to move more freely with less pain.

Providing psychological support

As this type of injury can have devastating emotional impact on the individual and his significant others, psychological support is an extremely important aspect of the care. Following the injury, the person will experience various emotions such as the fear of death, the fear of disability, and the fear of disfigurement. Feelings of despair, anger, frustration, depression, and guilt may all be experienced at any time following the burn.

Communication between team members who are caring for the person is important to achieve adequate support for him and for his significant others.

The nurse can help to provide support by:

● Developing a trusting relationship and by being available to listen. She should encourage the individual to talk through his feelings and fears.
● Providing information about all the procedures and equipment, in a way that can be understood. Fear will be reduced if information is provided to the individual and his significant others in a way that facilitates understanding of the injury, the treatment, and the prognosis. People who are experiencing stress often have difficulty in remembering, therefore information should be repeated whenever necessary.
● Assisting the individual to adapt gradually to body changes, and by being supportive when he views his injury —particularly for the first time.
● Supporting the person's coping mechanisms for as long as necessary. The nurse should understand that any expressions of anger, aggression or intolerance, are not being directed at her. Rather, it is the individual's way of reacting to his injury and its consequences.
● Involving the person in his care as much as possible, to promote his independence and self esteem.

Promoting healing of the injury

Care of the burned area varies according to the site and severity of the injury. The aims of wound care are to prevent infection, and to promote healing with minimal scarring. Two or more methods of burn care may be used simultaneously, and methods may change during the course of healing.

The open method of treatment involves the application of antimicrobial creams without the use of dressings. The burns are left exposed to the air to allow the exuding serum to dry and form a protective crust, which prevents further fluid loss and the entry of microorganisms.

A topical antibacterial agent, e.g. silver sulphadiazine, is usually applied to the area. The cream is applied with a sterile gloved hand and, as the heat of the room and of the individual's skin melts the cream, it must be applied frequently.

The person may be nursed on a special type of bed frame which allows ventilation, and a bed cradle is used to keep the bedclothes away from the burned areas.

The open method of treatment eliminates the need for dressings, and the antibacterial agent reduces the incidence of infection. As there is rapid heat loss from the burned areas, keeping the person warm may be a problem. He is generally nursed in a room that is warm enough to maintain normal body temperature.

The closed method of treatment involves the application of a dressing which may be impregnated with petroleum jelly, paraffin or an antibacterial agent. The dressings are held in position with bandages, and may remain in place for up to 72 hours before being changed.

The outer layers of absorbent padding which cover the dressing are re-inforced if serum seeps through.

Dressing changes are performed with strict aseptic precautions. The individual is given an analgesic prior to the dressing change, or he may be given a general anaesthetic before the procedure is performed.

After the dressings have been removed, the wounds are cleansed. Warm saline baths may be used to help clean the burn, remove dead tissue, and to loosen adherent dressings.

Once the wound is free from ointment, loose *eschar* may be clipped off using sterile scissors and forceps. Following debridement, the wound is redressed rapidly to prevent hypothermia.

The frequency with which the dressings are changed depends on many factors, and may range from 3–4 times a day—to daily—to once in 2–3 days.

Surgical management of burns involves the initial cleaning and debridement before the open or closed method of treatment is used. Other surgical procedures are:

Skin grafting. Skin grafting promotes healing, prevents infection, and prevents the contraction of scars. It is performed as early as possible in the treatment of some partial thickness burns and in the treatment of all full thickness burns. *Split skin grafting* involves the removal of sheets of the epidermis and part of the dermis from a donor site, and placing them over the burned surface. In extensive burns, the sheets of skin can be 'meshed' by machine to give them a net-like appearance. By stretching the net, the skin graft can cover a greater area. *A full-thickness* graft includes the epidermis and the entire dermal layer, and is generally used when full-thickness skin loss has occurred.

Skin from a source other than the patient's own body may be used as a temporary cover for large burned areas to decrease fluid loss. A new technique has been developed whereby sections of the individual's unburned skin are grown in the laboratory, and later used to graft onto his burned areas.

In skin grafting, the *donor site* is the area from which skin is obtained for grafting onto the *recipient* area. The donor site is generally covered with a non-adherent dressing and layers of dressing material to absorb blood and serum that ooze from the wound.

To promote successful transplantation, the graft must be immobilized to prevent displacement. Immobilization is achieved by one of several methods, e.g. suturing, and the graft area is covered for protection. Successful 'take' of the graft depends on many factors, e.g. absence of infection in the area, prevention or elimination of haematomas or seromas, and adequate blood circulation.

Escharotomy. Eschar is a dry crust caused by contraction of the burned skin, and its development frequently causes increased tissue pressure which may impair circulation and lead to ischaemia. An escharotomy is a surgical procedure in which longitudinal incisions are made through the eschar to relieve pressure on the underlying tissues. As the eschar does not contain nerve endings the procedure is painless, but it does result in open wounds which provide a portal for infection.

Contractures and keloid formation following healing are always a possibility and it is important that preventive measures are implemented. Pressure placed over the healing wounds is generally successful in reducing keloid formation, and constant pressure applied during scar maturation retards the development of keloid. Tailored elastic garments (Jobst suits), which are fitted exactly over any burned body part, apply pressure to prevent and correct post-burn hypertrophic scarring and contractures. Pressure garments may be required for between six months and two years following healing.

Preparation for discharge

Before the individual is discharged from hospital, it is important that he understands that the healed burned and grafted skin is tender and will break down more easily than normal skin. He is informed that these areas are very vulnerable to extremes of temperature, irritant substances, and physical trauma. As part of his preparation for discharge the nurse should advise the individual, or the parents of the young child, to:

• Avoid sunlight on the burned areas for at least 12 months. Burned and grafted skin tans unevenly and unpredictably and burns easily. The incidence of skin cancer in burned skin is quite high.
• Use only non-irritant soaps and cosmetics on the areas.
• Exercise care if engaging in activities, e.g. sports, where there is the possibility that the burned areas may be bumped or damaged.

- Wear clothing made from soft fabrics that will not irritate the healed burned or grafted areas.
- Continue with prescribed management of the areas. Management may include the continual wearing of a tailored elastic garment, or application of a cream to the areas. The individual may also be required to follow a planned programme of exercises designed to improve mobility.
- Seek appropriate help e.g. psychological counselling, if he is experiencing difficulty in adapting to his changed physical appearance.

SUMMARY

Intact skin is a protective barrier between internal body structures and the external environment. The skin also has other important functions, e.g. regulation of body temperature, and serves as an organ of sensation and excretion.

Both the structure and functions of the skin can be disrupted by a variety of skin disorders; some of which may be minor and temporary, while other disorders may be life-threatening or chronic.

The major categories of skin disorders are genetic, idiopathic, hypersensitivity, traumatic, neoplasia, and infections and infestations.

The manifestations of skin disorders include pruritus, lesions, alterations in sensation/colour/texture/temperature, and abnormal odour.

Tests used to diagnose skin disorders include direct examination, biopsy, microscopic examination, and skin testing.

Medical management and nursing care, of an individual with a skin disorder, will vary according to the type and severity of the disorder. The care of the individual generally involves relief of pruritus, topical application of prescribed substances, maintenance of fluid and electrolyte balance, prevention of infection, and the provision of psychological support.

Burns, which are one of the most serious skin injuries, may be caused by dry heat, moist heat, chemicals, electricity, or radiation.

A burn is described as superficial, partial thickness, or full-thickness—depending on the depth of tissue involved.

The size of a burn is estimated by using either the Lund–Browder method, or the rule of nines.

Complications are common following a burn, and include shock, infection, scarring and contractures, and adverse psychological effects.

Medical management and nursing care, of an individual with burns, will vary according to the severity of the injury. The care of the individual generally involves fluid and electrolyte replacement, prevention of infection, provision of adequate nutrition, relief of pain, promoting mobility, providing psychological support, and promoting healing of the injury.

REFERENCES AND FURTHER READING

Game C, Anderson R, Kidd J (eds) 1989 Medical-surgical nursing: a core text. Churchill Livingstone, Melbourne, 754–781

42. The individual with a disorder of the musculoskeletal system

INTRODUCTION

Information on the normal structure and functions of the musculoskeletal system is provided in Chapter 19, and it should be referred to before studying the contents of this chapter. The musculoskeletal system is composed of numerous structures that function together to produce movement and support, and to provide protection for the body.

Pathophysiological influences and effects

Pathological changes in the musculoskeletal system can result from inflammation, infection, degeneration, nutritional influences, neoplasms, or trauma.

Inflammation

Inflammation of a musculoskeletal structure may result from excessive or repeated strain, or from an inflammatory disease such as rheumatoid arthritis. The inflammatory process may cause changes in the synovial membrane and destruction of articular (hyaline) cartilage resulting in pain, joint deformity, and limited joint mobility.

Infection

Bones and joints can become infected if pathogenic microorganisms enter them via the circulation or through open wounds. Proliferation of microorganisms can cause bone destruction and necrosis, resulting in pain and limited mobility.

Degeneration

Degenerative changes in musculoskeletal structures are associated with ageing, trauma, and inflammatory conditions.

The joints, and intervertebral discs, are the structures most commonly affected by degenerative conditions. The articular cartilage in joints softens and ulcerates, and the joint surfaces become rough. Intervertebral discs may become thinner and unstable, and muscle tissue may atrophy and become more fibrous.

The degenerative changes result in pain, stiffness, joint deformity, and limited movement.

Nutritional influences

Bone structure may be altered by inadequate calcium, which causes bones to become soft and deformed, and more susceptible to fracture. Joints may be damaged by deposits of urate crystals as a result of abnormal uric acid metabolism, resulting in inflammation and pain.

Neoplasms

Neoplasms, which may be benign or malignant, may develop slowly or rapidly. The effects of musculoskeletal

401

neoplasms include temporary or permanent restricted mobility, swelling, and spontaneous fractures. Other effects may occur as a result of the growth pressing on nerves, blood vessels, or organs.

Trauma

Trauma to a structure in the musculoskeletal system can cause fractures, dislocations, or muscle damage. Adjacent nerves, blood vessels, or organs may be damaged from the actual injury or as a result of the sharp edges of broken bone.

Major manifestations of musculoskeletal disorders

The major manifestations of disorders are pain, sensory changes, swelling and deformity, and impaired mobility.

Pain

Pain is a common symptom of musculoskeletal disorders as a result of trauma, inflammation, or degeneration. The individual may describe the pain as mild, aching, severe, or throbbing. The pain may be localized or generalized— depending on the specific disorder. Pain may increase with movement, be exacerbated by changes in environmental temperature, and be relieved by rest. It may be worse at certain times of the day, e.g. joint discomfort from degenerative disease is often most intense at the end of the day.

Sensory changes

A musculoskeletal disorder may be accompanied by sensory changes such as numbness, tingling, and lack of sensation. Swelling from an injury or neoplasm can cause pressure on a nerve, resulting in a loss of sensation in the area distal to the affected site.

Swelling, deformity, and impaired mobility

Swelling of an affected area may be the result of the formation of inflammatory exudate in response to injury from physical trauma, chemicals, or pathogenic microorganisms. Swelling will also occur when blood is lost from the circulation into surrounding tissues, e.g. following a fracture. A joint may become swollen if there is an increase in the amount of synovial fluid, or if blood or pus are present in the joint capsule.

Deformity may be the result of growths, fractures, dislocations, abnormal curvature of the spine, or contractures. The effects of a deformity include changes in range of joint motion, posture, and gait.

Mobility may be impaired to such an extent that the individual is unable to move without pain or be unable to carry out various activities of living, or the deformity may only cause restricted mobility at certain times, e.g. following activity or when the individual assumes a specific posture.

Specific disorders of the musculoskeletal system

Disorders may be classified as congenital, degenerative, infectious or inflammatory, immunologic, metabolic, neoplastic, traumatic, or those resulting from multiple causes.

Congenital disorders

Talipes is a congenital disorder of the lower extremities, characterized by a deformed talus and shortened archilles tendon. It may be associated with other abnormalities such as spina bifida or myelomeningocele. The disorder is associated with a combination of genetic and environmental factors which affect the developing embryo. The foot is twisted so that it points downward and turns inward. The deformity may be mild, or it may be so severe that the toes touch the inside of the ankle. The condition may be unilateral or bilateral.

Congenital hip dysplasia is an abnormality of the hip joint which may be unilateral or bilateral. The disorder occurs in varying degrees, ranging from a hip that is in normal position but which can be dislocated by manipulation, to complete dislocation in which the femoral head is totally outside the acetabulum.

Although the precise cause is unknown, the disorder is associated with placental transfer of maternal hormones which relax ligaments, and with breech delivery. Manifestations include an apparently shortened leg, and an extra skin fold on the thigh of the affected side. If the condition is undetected in infancy, the child may walk with a limp.

Osteogenesis imperfecta is a genetic disorder involving defective development of connective tissue, characterized by brittle and fragile bones that are easily fractured. The disease may be readily apparent at birth, if the infant is born with fractures or skeletal deformities reflecting healed intra-uterine fractures. Manifestations, apart from skeletal fragility, include thin skin, blue sclera, hypoplasia of the teeth, hyperextensibility of ligaments; and a tendency to bruise easily and to develop hearing loss.

Degenerative disorders

Osteoarthritis is a chronic, progressive disorder causing deterioration of the joint cartilage and the formation of new bone near the joint edges. The joint space eventually becomes narrowed, bone rests on bone, and deformity occurs. Primary osteoarthritis, a normal part of ageing, is thought to be genetically influenced. Secondary osteoarthritis occurs from joint damage caused by trauma or infection.

Osteoarthritis most commonly affects the interphalangeal joints, cervical and lumbar spine, knees, hips, and joints of the big toe. Manifestations are joint pain which is exacerbated by exercise or weight-bearing, and relieved by rest; stiffness, aching, fluid accumulation in the joint, and limited movement. Osteoarthritis of the interphalangeal joints produces bony overgrowths known as Heberden's nodes. The nodes are painless at first, but become red, swollen, and tender.

Infectious or inflammatory disorders

Tendinitis is painful inflammation of tendons and of tendon–muscle attachments to bone, which commonly affects the shoulder rotator cuff, hip, Achilles tendon, or hamstring muscle.

Bursitis is inflammation of the synovial membrane lining a bursa, and usually occurs in the subdeltoid, olecranon, trochanteric, calcaneal, or prepatellar bursae.

The cause of tendinitis and bursitis is overuse of a particular muscle group which can eventually damage a tendon or bursa. Tendinitis can also result from another musculoskeletal disorder, e.g. rheumatoid arthritis; while bursitis can also result from calcium deposits in bursae, or infection. Manifestations of both conditions are pain, swelling, and limited movement.

Occupational overuse syndrome (also known as RSI) is a collective term for a range of conditions, which are mainly work-related and characterized by discomfort, or persistent pain in muscles and tendons.

The syndrome results when activities performed on a repetitive basis cause gradual injury to specific muscles and tendons.

Osteomyelitis is pyogenic (pus-forming) infection involving bone, bone marrow, and surrounding soft tissues. The infection, which may be acute or chronic, causes bone destruction. Microorganisms which may cause osteomyelitis include staphylococcus aureus, haemolytic streptococcus, Pseudomonas aeruginosa, and Proteus vulgaris.

Acute osteomyelitis is characterized by rapid onset of severe pain in the involved bone with local heat, swelling, and inflammation. Systemic manifestations of infection include pyrexia, tachycardia, nausea, and malaise.

Chronic osteomyelitis is characterized by slight pyrexia, pain, and persistent drainage of purulent material from a sinus tract.

Infectious arthritis is inflammation of a joint resulting from microorganisms which invade the synovial membrane. Individuals most susceptible to this condition are those with existing joint destruction, diabetics, or those whose immunological status is impaired. Manifestations of infectious arthritis include severe pain, inflammation and swelling of the affected joint, accompanied by systemic manifestations of infection.

Immunologic disorders

Systemic lupus erythematosus (SLE) is a chronic inflammatory disorder of the connective tissue. The condition, which may affect one or more systems at a time, is characterized by remissions and exacerbations. While the precise cause is unknown, most theories suggest impairment of the immune system by viruses, genetic factors, hormones, or chemicals. Manifestations include arthritis and a skin rash. A rash on the cheekbone area, 'butterfly rash', is a characteristic sign of SLE. Other manifestations include pleuritic-type chest pain, signs of renal damage, signs of central nervous system involvement such as seizures and headaches, anaemia, lymphadenopathy, weight loss, and extreme fatigue.

Scleroderma is a connective tissue disorder which causes fibrous changes in various areas of the body, e.g. skin, small arteries in the digits, oesophagus, heart, lungs, and kidneys. Research suggests that immunologic mechanisms are involved in precipitating vascular changes and result in a decrease in circulation, which causes changes in connective tissue.

Manifestations include hardening of the skin, Raynaud's phenomenon, and hypomotility of the oesophagus. Other manifestations, depending on the organs affected, are dyspnoea, dysrhythmias, proteinuria, and hypothyroidism.

Rheumatoid arthritis is a systemic disease characterized by chronic inflammation of the synovial joint linings. The condition is characterized by periods of remission and exacerbation. The joints most commonly affected are those of the wrists, hands, and feet. Rheumatoid arthritis also results in muscle atrophy, osteoporosis, anaemia; and skin, pulmonary and cardiac symptoms.

The cause is unknown, but the disease involves release of antigen–antibody complexes into the joints. Research suggests that susceptibility to rheumatoid arthritis results from genetic defects that impair the autoimmune system.

Manifestations include swelling and stiffness of the joints, followed by marked deformities resulting from soft tissue weakness and joint destruction. Rheumatoid nodules may be present over the extensor surfaces of the elbows or Achilles tendons. Other manifestations include skin lesions and leg ulcers resulting from vasculitis; peripheral neuropathy, pericarditis, and pleuritis.

Juvenile rheumatoid arthritis affects children under the age of 16 and, like adult rheumatoid arthritis, the cause is unknown. In its acute febrile form, juvenile rheumatoid arthritis is characterized by pyrexia and arthralgia.

Metabolic disorders

Osteoporosis is a condition in which the rate of bone resorption exceeds the rate of bone formation—thus reducing bone mass. Bones affected by the disease lose calcium and phosphate salts, and become porous, brittle, and susceptible to fracture. The factors which contribute to excessive bone loss included diminished oestrogen levels, immobility and lack of exercise, nutritional deficiencies, and certain endocrine disorders. Manifestations include low back pain, kyphosis (rounded back), and spontaneous or pathological fractures following a minor injury.

Rickets, which is a condition caused by deficiency of Vitamin D, calcium and phosphorous, is characterized by abnormal bone formation.

Manifestations include soft, pliable bones which result in deformities such as bowlegs and knock knees, enlarged skull, spinal curvature, and chest deformities. Other manifestations include liver and spleen enlargement, profuse sweating, and generalized tenderness.

Osteomalacia is an adult form of rickets, which is characterized by a loss of calcification of the bone matrix. Manifestations include severe muscle weakness, pain, decreased height because of kyphosis, and deformities of the pelvis and femoral necks.

Paget's disease is a slowly progressive metabolic bone disease, characterized by increased resorption of bone and abnormal bone formation. The precise cause is unknown, but viral infection is suspected. There is often a family history of the disease. Manifestations vary, with some individuals experiencing no symptoms and others experiencing pain and aching. Later manifestations, which depend on the location and extent of the condition, include enlargement of the skull, hearing loss, kyphosis, changes in gait, and pathological fractures following minor trauma.

Neoplastic disorders

Tumours of the bone may be benign, primary malignant, or metastatic.

Benign bone tumours may be single or multiple, and one of several types. The most common benign form is a giant cell tumour, which is composed of multinucleate giant cells or osteoclasts. Manifestations include pain, tenderness, and localized swelling.

Osteogenic sarcoma is the most common primary malignant bone tumour. The areas most often affected are the ends of long bones, especially the distal femur or proximal tibia. The tumour may metastasize to other parts of the body, most commonly the lungs.

Manifestations include the gradual onset of pain in a limb, or the sudden onset of pain following a minor injury to the limb. A localized mass or swelling develops, and the individual may walk with a limp. Fatigue is a common symptom.

Metastatic bone tumours occur when cells of a malignant primary tumour, in another part of the body, enter the blood or lymph and are spread to the bone.

Traumatic disorders

A sprain is an injury to a ligament, caused when a joint is forced beyond its normal range of motion. The ligament may be stretched or torn. Manifestations include pain, swelling, local bleeding and bruising, and restricted movement.

A strain is an injury to a muscle and/or a tendon, resulting from excessive physical effort. Manifestations include pain, swelling, and muscle spasm.

A fracture is a break in the continuity of a bone, and is frequently accompanied by damage to nearby soft tissue structures or organs. Blood vessels near the fracture site may be torn and nerves may be damaged. A fracture is most commonly caused by injury to the bone, but stress and pathological fractures may also occur.

A *stress* fracture may occur in a bone that is subjected to repeated or prolonged stress, e.g. jogging.

A *pathological* fracture may occur in a weakened bone, e.g. as a result of osteoporosis.

Fractures are classified as open or closed, and as simple or complicated.

An *open* fracture is one which is accompanied by an open skin wound leading to the site of the fracture. The wound may be the result of an external injury to the skin, or it may be due to laceration of the skin by broken bone ends. An open fracture is also referred to as a *compound* fracture.

A *closed* fracture is one in which the skin is intact, and there is no communication between the fracture and the external environment.

A *simple* fracture is one in which the bone is the only structure involved. A *complicated* fracture is one in which other structures, e.g. blood vessels, nerves, or organs, are involved.

Table 42.1 lists the various types of fractures, according to the way in which the bone has broken.

The manifestations of a fracture vary according to its type, location, and on depending the other tissues involved. There may be pain, swelling, involuntary and painful muscle spasm, bruising, obvious deformity, abnormal mobility, and loss of function. Crepitus (grating caused by the bone fragments rubbing together) may be heard or felt. Shock may occur as a result of haemorrhage or extensive traumatic damage.

Dislocation refers to complete displacement of a joint's articulating surfaces, while *subluxation* refers to partial displacement of a joint's articulating surfaces. Both dislocation and subluxation can cause damage to surrounding soft tissue structures. Manifestations include severe pain, limited movement, and deformity of the joint.

Effusion (joint) is the accumulation of synovial fluid in

Table 42.1 Types of fractures

Type	Description
Greenstick	The fracture is incomplete and does not extend through the bone. The bone bends, and splits or cracks on one side It is common in the incompletely calcified bones of children
Transverse	The fracture line is straight across the bone
Oblique	The fracture line is at an angle across the bone
Spiral	The fracture line coils around the bone. This type of fracture generally results from twisting of the limb
Impacted	The fragments of broken bone are pushed (telescoped) into each other
Comminuted	The bone is broken into a number of fragments
Depressed	The broken edges are pushed below the level of the rest of the bone. This type of injury may occur when the skull is fractured
Avulsion	A fragment of bone, connected to a ligament, breaks off from the rest of the bone
Intracapsular	The fracture is within the joint capsule
Extracapsular	The fracture is close to a joint, but is outside the joint capsule

a joint. If blood vessels in the synovium are damaged, a haemarthrosis occurs. Joint effusions may result from severe sprains, dislocations, or fractures. Manifestations include pain and joint swelling.

Disorders of multiple cause

Ankylosing spondylitis is a chronic inflammatory disease, which primarily affects the spine and adjacent soft tissue. The cause is unknown but heredity, the immune response, and infectious agents are thought to be involved. Manifestations include gradual onset of back pain, stiffness, decreased spinal mobility, peripheral arthritis and, in advanced stages, kyphosis.

Kyphosis is an anteroposterior curvature of the spine which causes a bowing of the back, predominantly at thoracic level. Causes include growth retardation in the vertebral epiphysis during periods of rapid growth; infection, inflammation, and disc degeneration. Manifestations include mild back pain, tenderness, and stiffness. Progressive curvature may induce neurological damage, and it produces a characteristic roundback appearance. The individual is unable to straighten the spine when he assumes a recumbent position.

Scoliosis is lateral curvature of the spine, most commonly in the thoracic area. The condition may be idiopathic, but causes include poor posture, discrepancy in leg lengths, deformity of the vertebral bodies, and paraly-

sis. Manifestations, which generally appear only when the curvature is well established, include backache, fatigue, and symptoms of pulmonary insufficiency resulting from decreased lung capacity.

Lordosis is an abnormal exaggeration of the normal lumbar curve. The condition is sometimes referred to as 'sway-back'. It is usually compensatory to some other established deformity, e.g. kyphosis. Initially it causes no symptoms, but pain due to muscle fatigue may develop later.

Torticollis is a condition in which the head is inclined to one side as a result of muscle contraction on that side of the neck. The cause may be congenital, traumatic, or degenerative. Manifestations include pain, limited movement, and obvious deformity.

Gout is a condition characterized by joint inflammation due to deposits of uric acid crystals in the articular tissue. Causes include a metabolic defect responsible for increased serum uric acid production, and impaired excretion of uric acid by the kidneys. Attacks of gout may be precipitated by various factors including alcohol and diuretic medications.

Manifestations include tender, inflamed, very painful joints; and the development of tophi. Tophi are urate deposits which may be present in cartilage, synovial membrane, and soft tissue. The skin over the tophus may ulcerate and release a chalky white exudate.

Hallux valgus is a lateral deviation of the big toe at the metatarsophalangeal joint. The condition may be congenital, or develop as a result of degenerative arthritis or prolonged pressure on the foot. Manifestations include pain and the appearance of a bunion. A bunion is a red, tender swelling over the joint, caused by inflammation of the bursa.

Charcot's joints develop in the presence of a variety of neurological problems e.g. diabetic neuropathy and tabes dorsalis (a late manifestation of syphilis) that affect deep pain sensation or proprioception. Manifestations include swelling and instability of a joint or joints, atrophic and hypertrophic changes in the bone. Callus formation is common and callus breakdown can result in large ulcers.

Carpal tunnel syndrome results from compression of the median nerve at the wrist, within the carpal tunnel. Causes include trauma, arthritis, tenosynovitis, and pre-menstrual oedema. Manifestations include paresthesia in the areas supplied by the median nerve, and pain which radiates up the arm and becomes more severe at night. The pain is sometimes relieved when the individual dangles or shakes the affected hand.

Low back pain is a common symptom which has a variety of causes including poor posture, injury, inflammatory conditions, obesity, metabolic bone disorders, degenerative processes, and intervertebral disc disease. The discomfort or pain may be mild, severe, continuous, or intermittent. Pain is usually aggravated by certain movements or posture, and it may radiate into the buttocks or down the back of the legs.

Diagnostic tests

Certain tests may be performed to assist, or confirm, the diagnosis of musculoskeletal disorders.

Radiological investigation

Plain X-ray films may be taken to detect bone or joint abnormalities.

An arthrogram is an X-ray of a joint following injection of radiopaque dye into the joint space. Arthrography outlines soft tissue, e.g. the meniscus, which is not usually visualized by plain X-ray.

Bone scan

A bone scan provides imaging of the skeleton following an intravenous injection of a radioactive isotope. The radioactive substance collects in bone tissue where there is increased activity, e.g. at the site of a tumour, and scanning detects these sites. A bone scan can detect lesions at an earlier stage of disease than can a plain X-ray.

Arthroscopy

Arthroscopy is the visual examination of the interior of a joint, with a fibre optic endoscope. The knee joint is most commonly examined by this method.

The individual is given either a local or general anaesthetic prior to the procedure. A cannula is inserted into the joint, and the arthroscope is then introduced. To provide a viewing medium, normal saline is introduced through the arthroscope into the joint.

Arthroscopy can also be performed to obtain a biopsy of synovial membrane or cartilage, or to remove loose fragments from the joint.

Biopsy

Biopsies may be performed on bone, muscle, or synovial membrane. Specimens of tissue may be obtained by needle, punch, or excision.

Synovial fluid may be aspirated (arthrocentesis) and analyzed to detect infection or inflammatory joint conditions.

Serum tests

Blood may be obtained and tested for serum enzymes, antibodies and antigens, calcium and phosphorous levels, uric acid levels, and erythrocyte sedimentation rate.

CARE OF THE INDIVIDUAL WITH A MUSCULOSKELETAL DISORDER

While medical management and nursing care will depend on the specific disorder, the main aims of care are to:

- promote rest
- prevent the complications of inactivity
- maintain skin integrity
- maintain, or improve, nutritional status
- relieve pain
- prevent psychosocial problems
- promote remobilization and rehabilitation.

Promoting rest

During the acute phase of the musculoskeletal disorder rest helps to minimize pain and swelling, promotes healing of injured tissues, relieves muscle spasms, and prevents further destruction of tissues in inflammatory conditions.

Rest may be classified as general, where the individual is confined to bed, e.g. if several joints are inflamed, or if the individual is immobilized in a full body cast. Rest may also be classified as local, where a specific body part is immobilized, e.g. a limb in a splint or cast.

General care of the individual during the phase when rest is essential, involves:

1. Providing a suitable bed. The bed should have a firm mattress, and a fracture board may be necessary to ensure this. Adequate bed clothes and pillows are arranged to provide comfort, and the provision of aids such as sheepskins may further enhance the individual's comfort.

2. Assisting him to meet his basic needs. The individual who is immobilized will require assistance with most of the activities of living.

3. Preventing the complications associated with immobility. The problems associated with inactivity and bed rest, which are described in Chapter 37, include muscle atrophy, joint contractures, hypostatic pneumonia, venous stasis, pressure necrosis, urinary stasis, postural hypotension, and constipation. The nursing measures which are implemented to prevent these complications, are described in Chapter 37.

4. Assisting the individual to maintain correct posture. His trunk and limbs must be positioned in accordance with the principles of body alignment. In general, his joints should be positioned in a neutral, functional position as far as possible, preventing prolonged hyperextension or flexion of opposing muscle groups. Changes in position are important to prevent prolonged pressure on vulnerable tissues, to stimulate circulation, to facilitate lung expansion, and to permit joint movement. Supportive equipment, e.g. pillows, sand bags, or foam wedges, may be used to support functional positions. An overhead hand-grip is useful to allow the individual to shift his body weight periodically.

Maintaining skin integrity

When an individual is required to remain in bed for a prolonged period, or when appliances to ensure immobility are in place, the skin is more vulnerable to damage.

The skin must be maintained in good condition and protected from irritation, friction, and prolonged pressure. Information on general care of the skin is provided in Chapter 39, and the prevention of decubitus ulcers is described in Chapter 37.

Maintaining or improving nutritional status

Nutrition for an individual with a musculoskeletal disorder includes provision of a well balanced diet, and maintenance of recommended body weight. The diet should contain adequate amounts of protein, calcium, and Vitamin D to promote healing and maintenance of the musculoskeletal system. It should also contain adequate fibre and fluids to aid in elimination.

If the individual is overweight, a weight reduction diet may be prescribed. Loss of excess body weight helps to remove stress from inflamed or diseased joints.

Relieving pain

While the general approaches to pain management, as described in Chapter 36 are relevant to the individual with a musculoskeletal disorder, specific measures may also be indicated.

The individual may experience acute or chronic pain, depending on the specific disorder. General measures to promote comfort and minimize pain should be implemented, e.g. changing his position, performing a back massage, handling a painful limb gently, and encouraging him to rest a painful limb. If not contraindicated, elevation of the limb may relieve discomfort and pain.

Specific measures include checking to ensure that splints, casts, or dressings are not too tight or rubbing against the skin. The use of either hot or cold applications may be prescribed to provide pain relief and increased range of motion. Heat is sometimes used in chronic joint disorders, as it relaxes muscles, relieves stiffness, and provides analgesia. Heat is often applied before exercise and massage. Cold is more useful for an individual who is experiencing acute pain or acutely inflamed joints. Whenever the application of either heat or cold is prescribed, extreme caution is necessary to prevent tissue damage. Information on heat and cold applications is provided in Chapter 33.

Analgesic medications may be prescribed, and these are administered in accordance with nursing regulations and the institution's policy.

Preventing psychosocial problems

The management of a musculoskeletal disorder may require that an individual be confined to bed, or to hospital, for an extended time. Enforced inactivity may lead to boredom, frustration or depression. To prevent such problems, the individual should be encouraged to express his feelings, and he should be allowed to participate in making decisions about his care. The nurse should encourage him to become actively involved in all aspects of his care. Instructing the individual in self care techniques, and allowing him to take responsibility for some of his own care, can help to reduce some of the problems associated with dependence and immobilization.

When possible, his bed should be positioned so that he has an outside view. He can also be wheeled, in the bed, to other areas of the institution e.g. the day room or the garden. Visitors and phone calls should be encouraged, and he should be provided with facilities that enable his participation in activities that interest him. A regular programme of activity, developed with the individual and the occupational therapist, should be incorporated into the nursing care plan.

Promoting remobilization and rehabilitation

As the musculoskeletal system is crucial to functional activity, a programme of exercise and rehabilitation is developed and implemented. A planned exercise programme is generally developed by the physiotherapist, but the nurse is required to encourage and supervise regular repetition of the exercises.

During the phase of immobilization, the programme contains exercises designed to prevent muscle atrophy or joint contracture, and to prepare the individual for ambulation. Information on range of motion on (ROM) and isometric exercises is provided in Chapter 37.

After the period of immobilization a programme of graduated, non weight-bearing exercises is generally commenced. The exercises are designed to regain or increase muscle tone, to build muscle strength, and to promote joint mobility.

When the individual is able to bear weight on the affected limb, the exercise programme is directed at restoring as much mobility as possible. The individual may require instructions and supervision in the use of aids, e.g. crutches or a walking frame. Information on aids to ambulation is provided in Chapter 37.

The overall aim of rehabilitation is independence in the activities of living. Rehabilitation requires a multidisciplinary team approach. The team generally consists of nurses, medical officers, physiotherapists, and occupational therapists. Depending on the individual's specific needs, a social worker and a splint maker may be involved. Information on rehabilitation is provided in Chapter 60.

Preparation for discharge includes informing the individual of the need to continue any exercise programme, the use of splints or braces, the limits of physical activity, and the importance of attending any future appointments or on-going rehabilitation programmes.

FRACTURES

While specific medical management depends on the site and severity of a fracture, the general objectives of fracture management apply:

- Reduction, a process whereby the bone fragments are realigned.
- Immobilization, whereby the alignment is maintained.
- Restoration of function, whereby complications are prevented and the individual is prepared for mobility.

To understand the rationale behind fracture management, it is necessary to understand the stages involved in the healing of bone.

Healing of fractures

1. When a bone is broken, bleeding occurs from damaged local blood vessels and a haematoma forms.
2. Within 24 hours a blood clot develops at the fracture site, and the healing process centres on this clot.
3. Granulation tissue grows in the area, and fibroblasts produce collagen which binds the broken bone ends together.
4. Osteoblasts proliferate and osteoid tissue is laid down, forming a *callus*. The callus is a structure composed of fibrous connective tissue and cartilage, which unites the broken bone but lacks the strength of true bone.
5. Ossification of the callus occurs as calcium and phosphate salts are deposited. As ossification proceeds, the trabecular pattern is established.
6. The union strengthens, and the swelling around the fracture site created by the callus is levelled out in a process of remodelling. Remodelling involves removal of unnecessary bony tissue by the osteoclasts. *Osteoclasts* are a type of bone cell that function in periods of growth or repair, to break down bone matrix. Osteoclasts also recanalize the medullary canal thus—completing the process of reconstruction.

Efficient healing of bone depends on an adequate blood supply to the area and, in part, on several vitamins. Vitamin A is required for rebuilding activity, Vitamin D for deposition of calcium and phosphate salts, and Vitamin C is required for collagen production.

Delayed union of bone may be due to an inadequate blood supply to the area, interference with the formation of the callus, infection, the presence of foreign material or soft tissue between broken bone ends, or nutritional deficiencies.

Objectives of fracture management

1. Reduction or realignment of the broken bone, may be accomplished in three ways. *Closed* reduction is the manipulation of the bone fragments until the bone is realigned. *Open* reduction is a surgical procedure in which the fracture fragments can be directly visualized. The bone fragments are held together by the use of nails, rods, plates, screws, or pins. *Traction* involves application of a force to the limb to overcome muscle spasm and realign the fractured bone.
2. Immobilization, following realignment of the fractured bone, is essential so that healing can occur. Immobilization can be accomplished by internal fixation or by external splinting.
3. Restoration of function involves the implementation of a planned programme of exercise and ambulation which prepares the individual for mobility, and retains muscle strength and range of joint motion.

Methods of immobilization

1. Immobilization of a fracture can be achieved by strapping, e.g. for fractures of the toes or fingers; by bandaging, e.g. a figure of 8 bandage to treat a fractured clavicle; or by using a sling to immobilize fractures in the shoulder area.
2. Internal fixation immobilizes reduced fractures by means of nails, rods, plates, pins, or screws. Internal fixation is used to maintain reduction when closed treatment is inappropriate or unsuccessful.
3. External fixation holds fracture fragments in alignment, and is achieved by inserting pins into the bone above and below the fracture. The pins are attached to an external metal framework which exerts pressure on the pins to maintain the bone fragments in alignment.
4. Casts are one of the most common methods of achieving immobilization. A cast may be applied to part or all of a limb, or to the torso. A variety of cast materials are available including plaster of paris, fibreglass, and plastic.

Plaster of paris remains one of the most commonly used materials because of its low cost. Alternative materials have, however, other advantages such as quick drying, resistance to water and lightness of weight. The medical officer selects the most appropriate type of cast depending on various factors, e.g. how frequently the cast will need to be changed, if bleeding from the injury is likely to occur, and the individual's level of independence. Information on care of the individual with a cast is provided later in this chapter.

5. A variety of external splints and appliances are available to achieve immobilization, e.g. a Thomas's splint to treat a fracture of the femur. A splint may be used alone or in conjunction with traction.
6. Traction may be used to maintain alignment of bone

following fracture, to maintain joints in a functional position, to correct deformities due to contracted soft tissues, or to relieve pain caused by muscle spasm. Information on traction is provided later in this chapter.

Care of the individual with a cast

The nurse may be required to prepare the equipment for application of a cast, to assist in the individual's care following application of a cast, and to provide him with information about cast care.

Preparation for cast application

The medical officer may apply a cast in his consulting room, in the emergency department, in the operating room, in the outpatients department, or in the ward.

The basic equipment required for plaster of Paris cast application includes:

— a large waterproof sheet to protect the bed, couch, or individual
— pillows with waterproof covering
— a waterproof apron, protective boots, and gloves for the medical officer
— protection for the floor, e.g. newspapers
— a selection of plaster bandages
— cottonwool and/or orthopedic felt for padding
— tubular stockinette, to place over the affected area (The stockinette must be long enough to extend beyond both ends of the cast.)
— large bowl/s of tepid water
— scissors

Additional items which may be required include:
— shaving equipment
— plaster cutters (if an old cast is to be removed)
— walking heel (if a leg cast is being applied).

Application of the cast by the medical officer involves covering the limb with stockinette, wrapping padding around the limb, immersing the plaster bandages in water, then applying and moulding the bandages to form a cast. The ends of the stockinette are folded over the edges of the cast to create smooth edges.

The *nurse* may be required to assist during application, by helping the individual to assume a comfortable position, and by supporting the limb as the cast is being applied. The person who is supporting the limb must use the flat palms of the hands rather than fingertips, which can cause indentations in the cast—and thus pressure on the underlying tissues.

A plaster cast becomes firm to touch within approximately 10 minutes, but may take up to 48 hours to dry completely.

Care after cast application

Immediately after application, the skin above and below the cast is cleaned to remove any plaster splashes. If these are not removed, they will dry and may fall down between the cast and the skin—causing friction and discomfort.

To ensure that the cast dries evenly, without cracking or weakening, it should be exposed to the air and well supported. *Artificial* means of drying the cast are not used as they may cause cracking of the cast.

A cast on the upper limb should be supported on pillows when the individual is sitting or lying, and in a sling when he is upright. A cast on the lower limb should be supported in an elevated position on pillows; and the ambulant individual must use crutches to avoid weight bearing until the cast is completely dry. If a body cast or hip spica has been applied, the individual is nursed on a firm mattress and the curves of the cast are supported with pillows.

Even drying necessitates 2 hourly repositioning to expose the total surface of the cast to the air. The cast must be handled with the flat palms of the hands until it is completely dry.

The individual should be kept warm and adequately covered, especially if a bed cradle is in position.

To prevent stiffness and muscle atrophy, and to stimulate circulation, the individual performs a programme of planned exercises.

The two major complications which may occur, after application of a cast, are the development of pressure sores under the cast, and circulatory or nerve impairment due to constriction by the cast.

1. If the individual experiences discomfort or pain under the cast, this should be reported immediately to the nurse in charge so that appropriate action can be taken. The medical officer may make a 'window' in the cast to expose an area of underlying skin for observation or treatment. Alternatively, the cast may be 'bivalved', which involves spitting the cast along both the entire lateral surfaces. Using a cast cutter, the plaster is split throughout its length and thickness. The upper half of the cast is removed to allow assessment of the individual's skin. A bandage, or strapping, is used to fasten the two pieces of cast together again.

2. Swelling of the area encased in plaster is most likely to occur within the first 48 hours after injury. Swelling may lead to impairment of circulation or pressure on a nerve. If the early manifestations of constriction are not detected, and action taken, irreversible tissue damage may occur.

Toes or fingers of an extremity encased in plaster are assessed at regular intervals. Initially, assessment is made every 30 minutes, then at intervals, e.g. four hourly, depending on the individual's condition. Assessment is made of:

● Colour: Cyanosis or extreme pallor indicates that there

is pressure on blood vessels, resulting in circulatory impairment.
- Temperature: An abnormally cold skin suggests arterial obstruction, and abnormally hot skin suggests venous congestion.
- Mobility: Loss of movement, or excessive pain on movement, of the toes or fingers suggests that there is pressure on a nerve.
- Sensation: Loss of sensation, numbness or tingling, suggests that there is pressure on a nerve.
- Swelling: Swelling of the toes or fingers may be due to the trauma, or it may be caused by the plaster being too tight resulting in impaired circulation.
- Pain or burning sensation: Either may be due to pressure from a tight or indented plaster, or it may be a symptom of infection.
- Odour: An offensive odour may be due to a plaster sore or wound infection. It may also be caused by soiling of the plaster by urine or faeces.
- Staining of the plaster: The plaster may become stained by blood or exudate from an underlying wound. A mark should be made around the stain so that any extension may be observed.
- Condition of the plaster: The plaster may become cracked, softened, or broken at the edges.

If any deviations from normal are observed they must be reported immediately to the nurse in charge, so that appropriate actions may be taken. Elevation of the limb may restore normal skin colour and sensation. If there is no immediate improvement further action by the medical officer is necessary, e.g. cutting a window in, or bivalving the plaster.

Discharge preparation

If the individual is to return home, with a plaster cast in position, he is provided with information about cast care. Health care institutions generally develop a set of written instructions which are given to the individual, and the nurse must ensure that he fully understands them. A sample set of instructions is provided in Table 42.2.

Removal of a cast

A plaster cast may be removed with plaster shears or an electric plaster saw. If a saw is used, it is important to explain to the individual that it is a vibrating and not a cutting instrument therefore it will not cause injury.

When the cast is removed the limb may appear thin and lacking in muscle tone, the skin will be scaly and may have an offensive odour. The skin requires gentle cleansing, followed by the application of lanolin or oil.

The limb should be supported when moved, as sudden or excessive movement is painful. To control subsequent

Table 42.2 Instructions for cast care

Check the colour, temperature, movement, and sensation of all toes/fingers of the affected limb, at least twice a day.

Elevate the limb whenever possible.

Do not interfere with the cast. Do not push any objects under the cast. Do not apply powder, lotion, or any other substance to the cast.

Keep the cast clean and dry.

Inspect the skin, near the edges of the cast, every day. Assess for signs of pressure or irritation from the cast.

Inspect the cast daily for drainage, odour, cracked or softened areas.

Consult a medical officer immediately if:
- The cast becomes loose, cracked, or softened.
- There is drainage coming through the cast, or an offensive odour from the cast.
- Swelling of the toes/fingers does not resolve when the limb is elevated.
- Pain or a burning sensation under the cast is experienced.
- The skin near the edges of the cast becomes sore or broken.
- The toes/fingers become pale, blue, cold, numb; or a tingling sensation is experienced.
- There is difficulty in moving the toes/fingers.
- There is undue heat in one specific area of the cast.
- There is a rise in body temperature for no apparent reason.

Do not bear weight on the cast, unless this has been approved by the medical officer.

Continue to perform the prescribed exercises which have been designed to maintain muscle strength and tone.

Attend any scheduled appointments.

---

oedema, a supporting bandage may be applied for a short time, but joint mobility must not be restricted. If the limb swells when it is in a dependent position, the individual should continue to elevate it and continue to perform the prescribed exercises. The swelling generally subsides with continued activity and exercise.

It is important that the individual understands the amount of activity or weight bearing that is permitted. Physiotherapy may be prescribed to assist in restoring function and mobility.

TRACTION

Traction is used in orthopaedic practice to exert a force, either a direct or an indirect pull, to a particular part of the skeleton. This pulling force overcomes muscle spasm, and maintains a fractured bone in alignment. Traction can act on the limbs, or it can be applied to the pelvis or spine.

Traction apparatus

A traction set-up generally consists of a bed with a firm base or fracture board, a traction frame, pulleys, traction cord, and weights.

There are a variety of *traction frames* available, and any

frame used must be stable, secure, and equipped with overhead and cross bars and pulley attachments. The pulley attachments must allow for the cord to run smoothly and the weights to hang freely at the end of the bed.

A *pulley* is a grooved wheel on an axle over which the traction rope is passed. Pulleys are the means by which traction forces are directed. The wheel of each pulley must run freely.

Traction cord must fit exactly in the groove of the pulleys, therefore cord of approximately 3–4 mm thickness is generally suitable. As traction cord stretches and weakens with use, it should not be reused.

Weights are tied securely to the traction cord so that they hang free of the bed. A variety of forms can be used, e.g. round metal weights, sand-filled or water-filled bags. The amount of weight to be applied is prescribed by the medical officer, according to the type of fracture, and the body weight of the individual.

Types of traction

Traction may be classified as *manual, skin,* or *skeletal.*

Both skin and skeletal traction can be applied as balanced or fixed traction. Either method achieves a pull in the opposite direction to that of the traction force. This opposing pull, *countertraction,* is necessary to overcome muscle spasm, and to prevent the individual from being dragged towards the traction pull.

Manual traction is used during reduction of a fracture, as the medical officer manipulates and pulls the part to achieve realignment of the bone.

Skin traction

Skin traction (Fig. 42.1) may be exerted using halters, belts or slings for the pelvis or spine; or by applying extensions, slings, or splints to the limbs.

Traction is applied to the skin and thus *indirectly* to bone.

A halter may be positioned, so that it encircles the head, to provide a traction pull on the cervical spine. It may be used on an intermittent basis in the management of neck pain due to degenerative changes in the cervical spine.

A belt (harness) may be placed around the hips, to provide a traction pull on the pelvis. It may be used in the management of low back pain due to a prolapsed intervertebral disc, or due to degenerative changes in the lumbar spine.

A sling may be positioned under the pelvis and buttocks to suspend the individual's pelvis just clear of the mattress. It may be used in the management of some fractures of the pelvic rim.

Skin extensions to limbs are applied on both sides of the limb, and encompass a spreader to which traction cord is attached. There are a variety of commercial extension kits available, which contain of either adhesive or non-adhesive extension material—together with padding, spreader, traction cord, and retaining bandage.

Skin traction to the lower limb, which may be applied to exert either a horizontal or vertical pull, is generally used in the management of conditions affecting the hip, femur, knee, or lumbar spine. Skin traction is commonly used when partial immobilization and light traction forces are required.

A sling may be placed under the knee to cradle it and to provide a vertical pull, when two-directional lower limb traction is used. In addition to the vertical pull, a horizontal pull is exerted on the leg by means of skin extensions. This type of traction set up, (Hamilton Russell traction) may be used in the management of fractures of the femoral neck or shaft and dislocation of the hip.

A Thomas's splint may be applied to the leg or the arm. A Thomas's splint may be used to provide straight leg fixed traction, straight leg balanced traction, extended

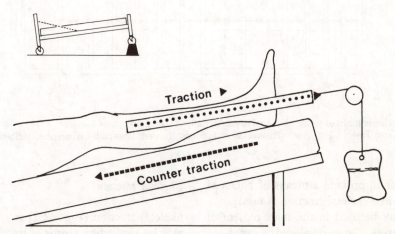

Fig. 42.1 Skin traction. (A) Balanced skin traction. (Reproduced with permission from Taylor I 1987 A ward manual of orthopaedic traction. Churchill Livingstone, Melbourne.)

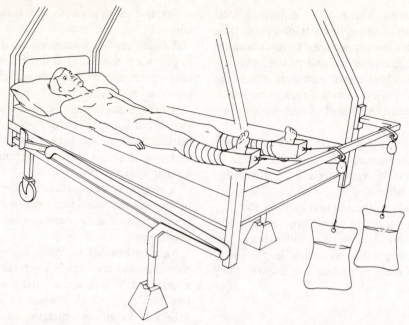

Fig. 42.1 (B) Skin traction to lower limbs (Buck's traction). (Reproduced with permission from Taylor I 1987 A ward manual of orthopaedic traction. Churchill Livingstone, Melbourne.)

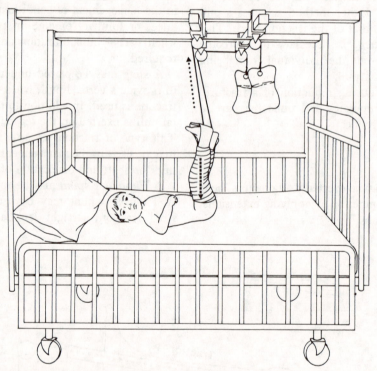

Fig. 42.1 (C) Skin traction to lower limbs of young children (Bryant's (Gallows) traction).
(Reproduced with permission from Taylor I 1987 A ward manual of orthopaedic traction. Churchill Livingstone, Melbourne.)

sidearm fixed traction, or to provide a means of balanced suspension for the leg when skeletal traction is used.

A Thomas's splint may be used in the management of femoral shaft fractures, or displaced supra-condylar fractures.

Skeletal traction

Skeletal traction (Fig. 42.2) is applied directly to bone. It may be applied by means of traction screws, wires, or pins.

As sufficient force can be transmitted directly to bone to

obtain reduction of the fracture and overcome muscle spasm, skeletal traction is effective in maintaining the position and stability of the fracture in good alignment.

Skeletal traction is established using aseptic surgical techniques, and either local or general anaesthesia. A small incision is made in the skin, and the pin or wire is inserted through the bone. Types of devices for inserting in the bone include Kirschner wires, Steinmann pins, Denham pins, and Zimmer screws. The pin or wire is connected to a device which directs the traction cord to a weight. The amount of weight used varies depending on the fracture, and on the thickness of bone at the insertion site. Weights of up to 18 kg can be used.

Skeletal traction may be used in the management of cervical spine injuries, and fractures of the pelvis, femur, tibia, humerus, radius and ulna.

Balanced traction

Balanced traction maintains traction through the use of weights and pulleys, and countertraction through the body weight and gravity. Gravity pull is exerted by elevating the foot of the bed.

Fixed traction

Fixed traction maintains traction and countertraction between two fixed points, and does not depend on gravity. For example, the *Thomas's splint* forms a complete traction unit. Traction is exerted on the leg by the pull of the extensions fixed to the end of the splint. Countertraction is exerted by the splint ring in the groin.

Balanced suspension

Balanced suspension may be added to a fixed traction system to elevate the limb, and to allow greater mobility of the individual. As such, suspension promotes comfort but does not exert any influence on the fixed traction.

Care of the individual

The overall management is directed towards maintaining the traction, supporting and promoting independence in the activities of living, preventing any complications, and promoting rehabilitation.

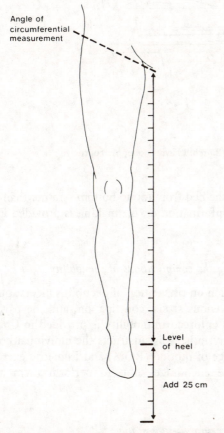

Fig. 42.1 (D) Measuring for a Thomas's splint. (Reproduced with permission from Taylor I 1987 A ward manual of orthopaedic traction. Churchill Livingstone, Melbourne.)

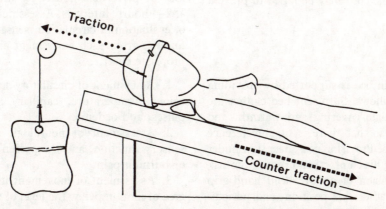

Fig. 42.2 Skeletal traction. (A) Balanced skeletal traction. (Reproduced with permission from Taylor I 1987 A ward manual of orthopaedic traction. Churchill Livingstone, Melbourne.)

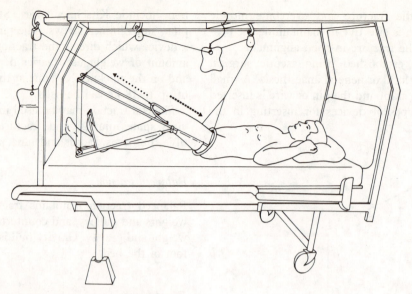

Fig. 42.2 (B) Skeletal traction in balanced suspension in Thomas's splint.
(Reproduced with permission from Taylor I 1987 A ward manual of orthopaedic traction. Churchill Livingstone, Melbourne.)

Maintaining the traction

Once the traction is established, the line and magnitude of the pull must be maintained. The nurse must check the apparatus at frequent intervals, to ensure that the traction set-up is functioning correctly. The individual must be assessed at the same time, to ensure that no damage is being caused by the traction.

The traction apparatus must not be altered without the medical officer's instructions. The weights must always hang freely and should not be lifted, as this releases the traction. If the nurse considers that lifting the weights may be necessary, she must first consult the nurse in charge.

The weights should be fastened securely, and suspended so they are not bumped by people passing by.

The spreader, or foot plate, should not touch the foot of the bed or frame. The cord is examined to see that it is not frayed, that knots are secure, that it is not rubbing against the frame, and that it is resting in the groove of the pulleys. The ends of the cord may be taped to prevent knots from slipping.

Providing a suitable bed

The individual's position in bed is supported by providing the required number of pillows. Sufficient bed clothes are provided to ensure adequate covering and warmth, and they should be arranged so that there is no interference with the traction apparatus. Provision of a sheepskin under the individual can enhance his comfort, and reduce the risk of decubitus ulcers. Provision of an overhead hand-grip enables the individual to adjust his position, and periodically relieve pressure from his buttocks and sacral area.

It is usually easier, and less disruptive for the individual,

to make the bed from top to bottom—rather than from side to side. Information on bedmaking is provided in Chapter 35.

Preventing the complications of immobility

Information on prevention of decubitus ulcers, pulmonary-/urinary/venous stasis, constipation, and the psychological effects of enforced immobility is provided in Chapter 37.

The physiotherapist instructs the individual how to perform range of motion (ROM) and isometric exercises, and the nurse encourages him to perform them at regular intervals.

Assessing neurovascular status

Regular assessment is essential to detect any impairment to nerves or blood vessels in the affected limb. Assessment may be performed hourly for the first 24 hours, and then at 2–4 hourly intervals. Assessment of an extremity consists of evaluation of circulation, sensation, and movement. The findings from each assessment are documented on an appropriate chart.

1. Assessment of circulatory status involves checking for colour, temperature, capillary refill (in the nail beds), pulses, and oedema.
2. Assessment of neurologic status involves checking sensory function; and the presence of numbness, tingling, or burning pain.
3. Assessment of movement involves evaluating the degree of motion below the level of the injury. The individual is requested to pull the toes up, and push the foot down against the assessor's hand. If the upper extremity is the

limb in traction, motion is assessed by requesting the individual to spread the fingers, move the wrist, and to bring the thumb and little finger together (opposition).

Any deviations from normal, e.g. cyanosis, pallor, reduced or absent pulses, oedema, lack of or abnormal sensation, lack of movement; must be reported immediately to the nurse in charge and documented.

Assessing skin status

If the individual has skin traction applied, 2–4 hourly assessment is necessary to detect any complications.

The limb is inspected for allergic reaction to adhesive extension material. Allergic reaction is manifested by blistering of the skin, and the individual may experience irritation or a burning sensation under the material.

The skin is also inspected for excoriation resulting from slipping extensions, and for decubitus ulcers over bony prominences. Decubitus ulcers may result from inadequate padding or from a tight encircling bandage.

If a Thomas's splint is being used, the skin under the ring must be kept clean and dry. The skin is inspected at 2–4 hourly intervals for signs of irritation or pressure from the ring.

Caring for pin sites

If skeletal traction is being used, the protruding pin or wire ends should be capped with corks. This technique prevents injury to the individual or others.

At regular intervals, e.g. 4 hourly, the pin sites and surrounding skin are checked for signs of infection. Indications of infection include inflammation, tenderness, and purulent drainage. Assessment also involves checking that the pin is not loose or slipping to one side. Care of the pin sites varies according to the medical officers instructions. The sites may be covered by an occlusive dressing, they may be left uncovered, or a gauze pad may be placed around the pin. Prior to placing a dressing or gauze pad, antibiotic or iodine preparation may be applied to the pin sites. If non-occlusive dressings are used, they are generally removed twice a day and the sites cleansed, e.g. using sterile cotton wool-tipped applicators and hydrogen peroxide. After cleansing a new sterile dressing is applied.

Assisting with remobilization

When traction apparatus and splints are removed, the individual commences a planned programme of mobilization. To avoid orthostatic hypotension, the individual must progress to an upright position gradually. The nurse should observe him for pallor, faintness, or dizzyness that may result with position change.

The affected limb will be weak and unsteady at first, therefore the nurse must ensure that the individual follows the instructions concerning the amount of weight bearing and activities permitted.

Rehabilitation, following the removal of traction or splints, involves restoration of function and promotion of independence in the activities of living. The individual may require the use of aids, e.g. to assist ambulation, and assistance such as home help services may be considered necessary.

Joint prostheses

A prosthesis is an artificial replacement for a body part. Management of a degenerative joint disease may involve the replacement of a damaged joint with a prosthesis. Joint replacement prostheses are made of inert materials, and generally consist of a ball and socket joint for the hip or a hinge-type joint for the knee. As hip replacement is a commonly performed procedure this chapter addresses the care of an individual with a hip prosthesis.

There are a variety of hip prostheses available, including the Charnley, McKee-Farrer, Ring, and Austin Moore prosthesis. Most consist of a femoral component, comprising stem and a spherical femoral head; and an acetabular lining to receive the femoral head.

Pre-operative care of the individual involves physical and psychological preparation, as outlined in Chapter 59. General post operative care is outlined in the same chapter.

Special nursing care of the individual following hip replacement involves correct positioning, gradual ambulation, assessment, and preparation for discharge.

Correct positioning to prevent hip dislocation and strain on the incisional area. The affected leg should be maintained in an abducted position for a period ranging from 48 hours to several days post operatively. To maintain an abducted position, a wedge-shaped pillow, e.g. Charnley pillow, is generally placed between the legs. The pillow is fastened with Velcro straps, which should not be placed over the upper fibula where the peroneal nerve lies. The appliance is removed to provide skin care, but the individual's leg must be maintained in an abducted position.

If the individual is permitted to lie on his side, the pillow must remain in position and he must be assisted onto his side using a 'log-roll' technique.

After 1–3 days, the individual is generally permitted to sit out of bed on a chair. An elevated chair is used to maintain alignment of the leg, and to prevent acute flexion and adduction of the hip. Similarly, an elevated toilet seat helps to prevent strain on the hip. The individual should be strongly recommended not to cross the legs, as this causes adduction and could result in dislocation of the prosthesis.

Gradual ambulation and weight bearing generally commences about 3 days postoperatively. A walking frame is used, and is later replaced by a walking stick. Information on aids to ambulation is provided in Chapter 37.

Assessing the individual for the manifestations of hip dislocation: sharp pain, and abnormal limb position such as shortening and external rotation.

Preparing for discharge includes informing the individual about restricted activities, e.g. bending the hip only to a 90° angle, keeping the knees approximately 30–45 cm apart when sitting, using a firm chair with a high seat, not bending too far or squatting. He is also advised to continue with any prescribed exercise programme, and to continue to wear elastic stockings for up to six weeks—if these have been prescribed.

Amputation

Amputation is the removal of all or part of a limb. The majority of lower limb amputations are necessary due to peripheral vascular diseases. Other indications for amputation include malignant bone tumours and persistent bone infection, e.g. osteomyelitis.

The two most common amputation sites are above the knee or below the knee.

Care of the individual immediately following amputation includes monitoring drainage from the stump, positioning the affected extremity, assisting with prescribed exercises; and bandaging and conditioning the stump.

Care of the stump will vary, depending on the amputation site, but the care generally involves cleansing and redressing the incision, and applying a bandage to prevent oedema and to shape the stump in preparation for the prosthesis. The bandage (Fig. 42.3) is applied so the greatest compression is at the distal end of the stump, with decreasing compression as the bandage is applied up the limb. The limb should be correctly positioned to prevent contractures and external rotation. When healing begins, the individual is encouraged to push the stump against a pillow and, later, against harder surfaces. These conditioning exercises help the individual to adjust to experiencing pressure and sensation in the stump.

A programme of exercises is prescribed to prevent contractures and to increase muscle strength and tone.

The stump, once healed, may be massaged with alcohol to toughen the skin.

A temporary prosthesis may be fitted and applied 2–3 weeks postoperatively. The stump shrinks as healing occurs, and the permanent prosthesis fitting is performed when shrinkage and shaping is optimal.

Ambulation may be commenced without a prosthesis or with the individual using a temporary prosthesis. An extensive programme of physiotherapy is necessary to strengthen the muscles used for ambulation, and to assist the individual to learn to use the prosthesis.

The prosthetist teaches the individual how to use and care for his prosthesis.

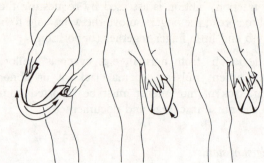

Using two 7.5 cm (3 inch) bandages, make three turns back and forth as shown; hold ends.

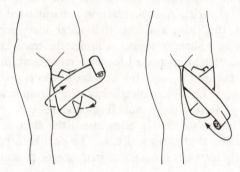

Make figure-eight turns, being sure to include the roll of flesh in the groin area.

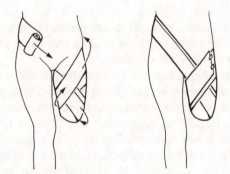

Use the 10 cm (4 inch) bandage to anchor the stump bandage about the waist as shown.
If properly applied, this bandage will not slip off stump.

Fig. 42.3 Stump bandaging (A) Bandaging an above-knee stump. One 10 cm (4 inch) and two 7.5 cm (3 inch) bandages are preferable. Always roll bandages away from you for better control.

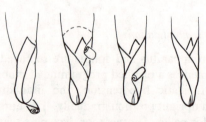

Fig. 42.3 (B) Bandaging a below-knee stump. Four inch (10 cm) elastic bandage and figure-eight turns about the knee are used.

Preparation for discharge involves ensuring that the individual is able to care for his stump, and perform the prescribed exercises. Prior to his discharge, the individual may be helped to adjust to his altered body image by a visit from an amputee who has adjusted well to a similar amputation. Referral to a community health nurse may be helpful so that she may reinforce teaching and assess the individual's progress. Community groups which consist of amputees may be able to provide the individual with information, advice, and support.

SUMMARY

The musculoskeletal system is comprised of numerous structures that function together to produce movement and support, and to provide protection for the body.

Pathological changes in the musculoskeletal system can result from inflammation, infection, degeneration, nutritional influences, neoplasms, or trauma.

Major manifestations of musculoskeletal disorders include pain, sensory changes, swelling, deformity, and impaired mobility.

Disorders of the system may be classified as congenital, degenerative, infectious or inflammatory, immunologic, metabolic, neoplastic, traumatic, or those resulting from multiple causes.

Diagnostic tests performed to assess musculoskeletal function include radiological examination, bone scan, arthroscopy, biopsy, and various serum tests.

Care of the individual with a musculoskeletal disorder includes promoting rest, preventing the complications of immobility, maintaining skin integrity, maintaining nutritional status, relieving pain, preventing psychosocial problems, promoting remobilization and rehabilitation.

The general objectives of fracture management are reduction, immobilization, and restoration of function.

Reduction, realignment of the broken bone, may be accomplished by either the closed or open method.

Immobilization may be achieved by strapping or bandaging, internal fixation, casts, splints, or traction.

Care of the individual who has a plaster cast applied includes supporting the limb, even drying of the cast, and assessment of the toes or fingers for manifestations of circulatory or nerve impairment.

Traction, which may be used in the management of musculoskeletal disorders, may be classified as manual, skin, or skeletal.

Care of the individual who has traction applied includes maintaining the traction, providing a suitable bed, preventing the complications of immobility, assessing neurovascular and skin status, caring for pin sites, and assisting with the process of remobilization.

A prosthesis may be used to replace a damaged joint, most commonly the hip or knee joint. Care of the individual following joint replacement includes correct positioning, gradual ambulation, and assessing for the manifestations of dislocation.

Care of the individual following amputation of all or part of a limb, includes care of the stump, and assisting with ambulation.

REFERENCES AND FURTHER READING

Game C, Anderson R, Kidd J (eds) 1989 Medical-surgical nursing: a core text. Churchill Livingstone, Edinburgh, 693–750

Powell M (ed) 1986 Orthopaedic nursing and rehabilitation, 9th edn. Churchill Livingstone, Edinburgh

Taylor I 1987 Ward manual of orthopaedic traction. Churchill Livingstone, Melbourne

43. The individual with a nervous system disorder

INTRODUCTION

Information on the normal structure and functions of the nervous system is provided in Chapter 20, and it should be referred to before studying the contents of this chapter.

The nervous system is comprised of three divisions: the central nervous system, made up of the brain and spinal cord; the peripheral nervous system, which is made up of nerves that connect the central nervous system to the rest of the body; and the autonomic nervous system, which regulates involuntary functioning of internal structures.

The nervous system is a communication network which initiates, co-ordinates, and regulates body responses to changes in the internal and external environments.

Pathophysiological influences and effects

The pathophysiological changes that can disrupt normal function of part or all of the nervous system can be due to congenital or developmental disorders, infectious or inflammatory conditions, trauma, neoplasia, degenerative conditions, and metabolic or endocrine disorders. Any pathophysiological change is capable of causing various types and degrees of dysfunction.

Congenital disorders

The central nervous system of the developing fetus is very vulnerable to damage. Factors which may cause nervous system damage include the passage of microorganisms and drugs across the placental barrier into the fetal circulation.

Other factors which may cause nervous system defects, and resulting physical and intellectual deterioration, include chromosomal abnormalities, metabolic disorders, cranial malformations, and structural abnormalities. The central nervous system may also be damaged during the birth process, e.g. by cerebral anoxia or cerebral haemorrhage.

Inflammatory and infectious conditions

Bacterial or viral infective processes affecting the central nervous system may result in the destruction of nervous tissue, through the action of toxins released by the living microorganisms and from the material released from dead microorganisms—which stimulates the inflammatory process. Infection and inflammation of nervous tissue may result in altered behaviour, altered consciousness, and sensory or motor deficits.

Trauma

Trauma to the nervous system may result from elements within the system, or from external forces. Trauma occurring from elements within the nervous system includes bleeding from an aneurysm or ruptured intracranial vessel, transient interruption of the cerebral blood flow causing ischaemia, and occlusion of a cerebral blood vessel by a thrombus or embolus. The most common causative factors in these conditions are hypertension, and atherosclerosis. Trauma from external forces may be caused by a direct or an indirect injury.

A *direct acceleration brain injury* occurs when the head is struck by a moving object, and a direct deceleration injury occurs when the head in motion strikes a stationary object. In an *indirect brain injury*, the traumatic force is transmitted to the head through an impact to another part of the body, e.g. the neck or buttocks.

In open head trauma, a penetrating injury damages the integrity of the skull and/or meninges and brain. Infection may occur, as the injury allows the entry of microorganisms.

A closed head injury is non-penetrating with no disruption to the integrity of the cerebral meninges. Closed head injuries can result in jarring, bruising, or tearing of brain tissue; which can cause haemorrhage, cranial nerve damage, and cerebral oedema. An important event in closed head injury is known as *coup-contrecoup*. The coup injury is cerebral bruising resulting from impact to the skull, and contrecoup refers to the rebound effect of the injury—the movement of the brain opposite to the site of impact.

The nervous system response to trauma, which may cause more damage than the actual injury, results in oedema, bleeding, and increased intracranial pressure. These factors destroy nervous tissue by compression or restriction of the circulation.

The *spinal cord* may be damaged as a result of a crushing or penetrating injury, dislocation of the spinal column, prolapsed intravertebral discs, or neoplasia. In addition to tearing of, and pressure on, the spinal cord tissues damage may be caused by haemorrhage, oedema, and disruption of the blood supply to the spinal cord.

Damage to the *peripheral nerves* may result in loss of sensory and/or motor function.

Neoplasia

Tumours of the nervous system, which may be either benign or malignant, cause symptoms related to pressure, destruction of nervous tissue, oedema, and disruption of the blood supply. The neurological manifestations of a tumour affecting the nervous system, depend on the location of the tumour and on its rate of growth.

Degenerative conditions

The causes of degenerative disorders of the nervous system are varied, and involve atrophy of neurones and nerve fibers. The course of a degenerative disorder is generally gradual and progressive over many years. The effects of degenerative disorders include progressive muscular atrophy; impaired speech, chewing, swallowing and breathing; deterioration of intellectual capacity, impaired motor function, and dementia.

Metabolic and endocrine disorders

Nervous system dysfunction may result from the effects of certain metabolic and endocrine disorders.

Some nutritional deficiencies may affect nerve cells, resulting in their damage or death. For example, degeneration of the posterior and lateral columns of the spinal cord may occur in pernicious anaemia due to a Vitamin B deficiency. Disorders of cortical function leading to confusion or coma may result from a deficiency of Thiamin.

Specific endocrine disorders such as hypothyroidism result in a decreased metabolic rate and hypothermia can develop. If the body temperature falls below 30°C, unconsciousness will result. *Myxoedema coma* is characterized by exaggeration of the signs and symptoms of hypothyroidism, with neurological impairment leading to loss of consciousness.

Major manifestations of nervous system disorders

The manifestations of a nervous system disorder will vary depending on the type and severity of the disorder.

Headaches

Headaches are common in a variety of disorders and situations, which range from functional disturbances of blood vessels to tension and stress. In neurological disorders, headaches are one of the most common symptoms. Headaches can result from compression, traction, displacement, or inflammation of the cranial periosteum, the dura mater, cerebral arteries, or branches of the cranial nerves. Headaches may also occur as a result of tension within extracranial structures such as muscles, air sinuses, and blood vessels. Headaches are commonly classified as vascular, tension, and traction-inflammatory.

Vascular headaches include migraine, cluster headaches, hypertension headaches, and headaches resulting from temporal arteritis. Although the mechanisms of *migraine* are not completely understood, migraine appears to result from an inherited predisposition and seems to be precipitated by trigger factors such as stress, abrupt falls in oestrogen levels, low blood glucose levels, and dietary intake.

One theory is that migraine results from spasm of intracranial blood vessels and dilation of extracranial blood vessels. The classic characteristics of migraine headache include throbbing, and a tendency for the attacks to be unilateral. Some attacks are preceded by a variety of visual disturbances, e.g. loss of half of the visual field, or flashing lights across the visual fields. Some individuals experience vertigo, nausea and vomiting.

Cluster headaches are a rapid succession of attacks over several days, followed by remission. Previously thought to be caused by histamine sensitization, cluster headaches are now considered to have a vascular cause. Headaches associated with severe *hypertension* may be intense, and similar to those caused by intracranial lesions. *Temporal arteritis* causes severe, throbbing headaches in the region of the temporal artery, and are sometimes accompanied by visual loss.

Tension headaches are caused by prolonged contraction (tension) of the neck, head, or facial muscles. Tension headaches are frequently associated with psychological factors such as anxiety or depression. The pain tends to be bilateral and, unlike vascular headaches, is not throbbing in character.

Traction–inflammatory headaches are related to increased intracranial pressure, which causes irritation of and traction on blood vessels and the dura mater within the skull. Inflammation of the meninges (meningitis) can also result in severe headache. Headaches of intracranial origin, related to increased intracranial pressure, vary from mild to excruciating depending on the location and cause, e.g. tumour, lesion, or cerebral oedema.

Sensory changes

Sensory changes, which can result from disorders of the brain, spinal cord, or peripheral nerves, include alterations in the sense of touch, pain, temperature sensitivity, and the loss of a sense of position. The loss of these sensations may be partial or complete.

Common sensory disturbances include neuritis, and neuralgia. *Neuritis*, characterized by pain and tenderness along the path of a nerve, can progress to complete loss of sensory and motor function. *Neuralgia* is characterized by severe stabbing pain, caused by a variety of disorders affecting the nervous system.

Other sensory changes that may accompany nervous system disorders include a loss of taste or smell, visual changes, and hearing loss.

Motor changes

Alterations in motor function include localized or generalized weakness, with difficulty in moving normally. Muscle tone may be abnormally increased or decreased. A pronounced increase in tone is referred to as rigidity. Spasticity of muscles is an increased resistance to passive stretch with rapid flexion of a joint.

Abnormal movements include:

1. Twitching: localized spasmodic contraction of a single muscle group.
2. Tremor: rhythmic, quivering movements resulting from involuntary alternating contraction and relaxation of opposing groups of muscles.
3. Myoclonus: spasm of a muscle or a group of muscles.
4. Dystonia: intense, irregular muscle spasms.
5. Athetosis: slow, writhing, involuntary movements of the extremities.
6. Chorea: involuntary, purposeless, rapid jerky movements.
7. Dyskinesia: involuntary twitching of the limbs or facial muscles.

Symptoms of *ataxia*, which is a condition characterized by impaired ability to co-ordinate movement, may be caused by a lesion in the spinal cord or cerebellum.

Dizziness or vertigo, where the individual is unable to maintain normal balance in a standing or seated position, may also be related to a disorder of the nervous system.

Unusual gait, or stance, may also result from motor or sensory deficits caused by a disorder of the nervous system, e.g. Parkinson's disease.

Paralysis, a symptom of motor disturbances, can occur in varying degrees with many nervous system disorders. Upper motor neurone lesions, in which the reflex area remains intact, generally cause spastic paralysis. Flaccid paralysis generally occurs in lower motor neurone lesions, which disrupt the reflex area.

Reflex changes

Reflex changes can provide evidence of damage to the nervous system. The absence of normal reflexes, or the presence of abnormal reflexes, generally indicate nervous system dysfunction.

Reflexes are classed as either superficial (cutaneous) or deep tendon (muscle stretch). Superficial reflexes are elicited when a stimulus is applied to the skin surface or to mucous membrane. Deep tendon reflexes are elicited when a stimulus is applied to a tendon, bone, or joint.

Altered awareness, personality, or level of consciousness

A neurological disorder, that results in altered brain structure, may cause impairment of the individual's cognitive functions. He may experience difficulty in being able to think, remember, reason, or understand.

The individual may also be confused in that his orientation to time, place, and person is impaired. He may also show signs of reduced alertness or responsiveness. Brain damage, e.g. as a result of a head injury, can cause a confusional state that is characterized by fluctuating disorientation and incoherence.

Cerebral impairment may also cause mood changes and/or inappropriate emotional responses. Diffuse brain damage, e.g. caused by a large cerebral infarction, may result in emotional instability or lability—a tendency to show alternating states of happiness and sadness, which seem to be inappropriate. The individual may also show signs of emotional flatness, or apathy, demonstrated by a reactive absence of emotions. Alternatively, the individual may become euphoric. Euphoria is a feeling of happiness and well-being.

Damage to the brain can also result in altered states of consciousness. ranging from drowsiness and difficulty in being aroused by normal stimuli, to coma. Further information on assessment of conscious level is provided later in this chapter.

Seizures

Seizures, which are paroxysmal events associated with sudden abnormal discharges of electrical energy in the neurones of the brain, may be secondary to central nervous system disease. Seizures may be focal or partial, generalized, or absence seizures. The most common type of seizure disorder is epilepsy.

Focal or partial seizures generally affect a specific body part, and the symptoms of an attack depend on the location of the cerebral focus. For example, the focal motor or Jacksonian seizure occurs from a lesion in the motor cortex or strip. Typically, it causes a stiffening or jerking in one extremity which is accompanied by numbness or tingling.

Generalized seizures are commonly described as grand mal seizures, or convulsions. This type of seizure generally consists of three phases which include generalized tonic and clonic movements.

Absence, or petit mal, seizures last only a few seconds but may progress to generalized tonic-clonic seizures. They generally begin with a brief change in the level of consciousness, which is indicated by a blank stare, eyelid fluttering or head nodding, or a pause in conversation. The individual generally retains his posture, and returns to pre-seizure activity without difficulty. This type of epilepsy usually occurs in childhood and may continue into early adolescence.

Although seizures may result from a nervous system disorder, they may be caused by many other factors, and are often idiopathic. Further information on seizure disorders is provided later in this chapter.

Specific disorders of the nervous system

Disorders of the nervous system may be congenital or genetic, due to multiple causes, degenerative, infectious or inflammatory, immunologic, neoplastic or obstructive, or traumatic.

Congenital or genetic disorders

Structural congenital abnormalities include anencephaly, spinal cord defects and hydrocephalus.

Anencephaly is the failure of normal development of the cranium and scalp. The precise cause is unknown, and babies with the disorder do not live.

Spinal cord defects include spina bifida, meningocele, and myelomeningocele. These conditions are the result of incomplete closure of the neural tube during the first three months of embryonic development. Causes are thought to include maternal exposure to viruses, radiation, and other environmental factors.

Spina bifida, in severe forms, involves incomplete closure of one or more of the vertebrae, causing protrusion of the spinal contents in an external sac. In spina bifida with meningocele, the sac contains meninges and cerebrospinal fluid. In spina bifida with myelomeningocele the sac contains meninges, cerebrospinal fluid, and a portion of the spinal cord or nerve roots.

Manifestations of congenital spinal cord defects vary and include a depression, dimple, or tuft of hair on the skin over the spinal defect. The more severe defects cause neurologic dysfunction such as paralysis of the legs, bowel and bladder incontinence, and hydrocephalus.

Hydrocephalus is an excessive accumulation of cerebrospinal fluid within the ventricles of the brain. It may result from an obstruction in cerebrospinal fluid flow, or from faulty absorption of cerebrospinal fluid. The condition can also occur after birth as a result of cerebral injury or disease.

In infants, the obvious manifestation of hydrocephalus is abnormal enlargement of the head. Other characteristics include distended scalp veins, thin and fragile scalp skin, downward displacement of the eyes, a shrill-high pitched cry, irritability, and abnormal muscle tone of the legs.

Hereditary genetic defects include muscular dystrophy, Huntington's Chorea and neurofibromatosis.

Muscular dystrophy, which is a group of congenital disorders characterized by progressive wasting and weakness of muscles.

Duchenne muscular dystrophy is the most common and severe form, which begins to manifest between the ages of 3 to 5 years. Initially, it affects the leg and pelvic muscles but there is progressive involvement of all voluntary muscles. Later in the disease, progressive weakening of cardiac and respiratory muscles results in heart or respiratory failure.

Early manifestations of Duchenne's muscular dystrophy include a waddling gait, lordosis (increased curvature of the lumbar spine) and marked difficulty rising from a supine to a standing position. As the disease progresses, facial, oropharyngeal, and respiratory muscles become involved. The incidence of mental retardation is high.

Huntington's Chorea is a disorder whereby degeneration of the cerebral cortex and basal ganglia causes chronic progressive choreiform movements and mental deterioration. Onset is generally in early middle age, and the individual gradually develops progressively severe choreiform movements and dementia. The movements usually begin slowly, with facial grimacing and jerking arm actions. Over time, the movements become frequent, erratic, and violent affecting the trunk and lower limbs. Dementia may be mild at first, but eventually severely disrupts the personality.

Neurofibromatosis is characterized by a variety of congenital abnormalities, and the condition is usually classified according to which parts of the nervous system are affected.

In the peripheral form, multiple cutaneous and subcutaneous nodules of varying size occur. Subcutaneous nodules may attach to the peripheral portion of the nerve, causing pain or pressure and, rarely, sensory loss in the distribution of the affected nerve. Neuromas, which are an overgrowth of subcutaneous tissue, may reach enormous sizes, and commonly affect the face, scalp, neck and chest.

Neurological symptoms may appear if the tumours cause pressure on the brain or spinal cord.

Disorders of multiple cause

Cerebral palsy comprises a group of neuromotor disorders resulting from prenatal, perinatal, or postnatal cerebral hypoxia or damage. The incidence of cerebral palsy is highest in premature infants, or in infants who have experienced a difficult birth resulting in cerebral damage.

Causative factors include chromosomal abnormalities; prenatal factors such as maternal infections, exposure to harmful chemicals, malnutrition; perinatal factors such as premature birth or instrumental delivery causing cerebral anoxia, and postnatal factors such as trauma, infection, and malnutrition causing cerebral damage.

The manifestations of cerebral palsy range from mild muscle inco-ordination to severe spasticity. The spastic form of the disorder is characterized by rapid alternating muscle contraction and relaxation, muscle weakness and underdevelopment, and muscle contraction in response to manipulation. The athetoid form of cerebral palsy is characterized by grimacing, writhing, and jerking involuntary movements—which become more severe during stress. Ataxic cerebral palsy is characterized by disturbed balance, inco-ordination, muscle weakness and tremor.

In addition to the range of motor deficits, the individual may experience sensory deficits, e.g. speech, visual or hearing impairment. Mental retardation accompanies cerebral palsy in approximately 40% of individuals.

A cerebral aneurysm is an abnormality of the wall of a cerebral artery, that results in a localized dilation. If the aneurysm ruptures, blood enters the subarachnoid space or cerebral tissue. Causative factors include congenital defects in the arterial walls, sclerotic changes in blood vessels, hypertension, and cerebral trauma.

Manifestations of a cerebral aneurysm do not generally appear until the aneurysm ruptures. The most common symptom of rupture is the sudden onset of a severe headache, which may be accompanied by nausea and vomiting, motor deficits, visual disturbances, and loss of consciousness.

A cerebral aneurysm may be detected before it ruptures, if the individual shows signs of occulmotor nerve compression—eyelid ptosis, and a pupil that is sluggish or non-reactive.

Transient ischaemic attacks (TIA) are recurrent episodes of neurologic deficit. The attacks, which may last from seconds to hours, are generally considered to be warning signs of an impending thrombotic cerebrovascular accident (CVA). The characteristics of a TIA, which may be caused by micro emboli or arteriole spasm, are various symptoms of neurologic dysfunction followed by a return of normal function. Symptoms include double vision, slurred or thick speech, unilateral loss of vision, staggering or unco-ordinated gait, unilateral weakness or numbness, dizziness, and falling because of leg weakness.

A cerebrovascular accident (CVA) is a sudden impairment of cerebral circulation, which causes cerebral ischaemia and infarction. The two types of CVA are ischaemic and haemorrhagic. In an ischaemic CVA, cerebral blood flow is suddenly impaired by a thrombus or embolus. In a haemorrhagic CVA, the rupture of a cerebral blood vessel causes bleeding into the subarachnoid space or brain tissue.

Factors that increase the risk of a CVA include a history of TIA, atherosclerosis, hypertension, obesity, diabetes mellitus, cigarette smoking, elevated serum cholesterol and triglyceride levels, lack of exercise, use of oral contraceptives, coagulation disorders, dehydration, rheumatic heart disease, and dysrhythmias.

Manifestations of a CVA vary depending on the artery involved and consequently the area of brain it supplies, and the severity of damage to cerebral tissue. Table 43.1 lists the clinical features resulting from specific cerebral artery occlusion or rupture. If the CVA occurs in the left hemisphere, it produces symptoms on the right side of the body. If it occurs in the right hemisphere, the left side of the body is affected.

Trigeminal neuralgia is a painful disorder, of one or more branches of the trigeminal nerve, that produces paroxysmal attacks of excruciating facial pain. While the cause is often unknown, the disorder may be associated with other neurologic conditions such as aneurysms, cerebral tumours, or multiple sclerosis.

The individual experiences excruciating, burning pain, which generally occurs suddenly in response to a stimulus, e.g. a draft of cold air, drinking hot or cold fluids, brushing the teeth, or speaking or laughing. The frequency of attacks varies from many times a day to several times a month or year.

Intellectual disability (mental retardation) is a syndrome of subnormal intellectual development, associated with impaired learning and social adjustment. The causes include:

1. Prenatal factors such as metabolic disorders, chromosomal abnormalities, cranial malformation, maternal infections, malnutrition, and anoxia.

2. Perinatal factors such as prematurity, anoxia, and intracranial haemorrhage.

3. Postnatal factors such as cerebral injury, central nervous system infections, anoxia, neoplasms, degenerative diseases, cerebral haemorrhage, nutritional deficiencies, and emotional deprivation.

Table 43.1 C.V.A. Manifestations according to involved vessel

Area	Manifestations
Middle Cerebral Artery	Hemiparesis or hemiplegia Aphasia Sensory impairment (same side as hemiplegia) Homonyous hemianopia Deterioration in conscious level from confusion to coma Headaches Inability to turn eyes toward the affected side Denial or lack of recognition of a paralysed extremity Possible Cheyne-Stokes breathing
Anterior Cerebral Artery	Hemiparesis or hemiplegia of leg and foot Paresis of the arm on the side of hemiplegia Footdrop Gait dysfunction Expressive aphasia Mental status impairments: • confusion • amnesia • perseveration • short attention span • apathy • slowness Deviation of eyes and head toward the affected side Urinary incontinence
Posterior Cerebral Artery	Peripheral signs: • homonyous hemianopia • several visual defects • memory deficits • perseveration • dyslexia Central signs: • hemiplegia or hemiparesis • diffuse sensory loss • pupillary dysfunction • nystagmus • intention tremor
Internal Carotid Artery	Hemiparesis with facial asymmetry Parasthesia on same side as hemiparesis Hemianopia Repeated attacks of visual blurring or blindness in the ipsilateral eye Dysphasia (intermittent)
Posterior Inferior Cerebellar Artery	Dysphagia Dysarthria Loss of sensation on ipsilateral side of the face Loss of sensation on contralateral side of the body Horizontal nystagmus Ataxia Vertigo Ipsilateral Horner's syndrome (miotic pupils, ptosis, and facial anhidrosis-inadequate perspiration) Paralysis of larynx and soft palate

Table 43.1 (cont'd) C.V.A. Manifestations according to involved vessel

Area	Manifestations
Anterior Inferior Cerebellar Artery	Horizontal nystagmus Sensory impairment Deafness and tinnitus Facial paralysis Horner's syndrome Ataxia
Vertebral-Basilar System	Dysarthria Dysphagia Vertigo Nausea Syncope Memory loss, disorientation Ataxic gait Double vision Tinnitus Nystagmus Facial paresis Drop attacks

Manifestations include poor motor development, impaired concepts of space and time, learning difficulties, inappropriate behaviour, and difficulty with social interactions.

Seizure disorders, as defined earlier in the chapter, may be primary and idiopathic, or secondary and symptomatic of central nervous system disorder. The international classification of seizures is illustrated in Table 43.2.

Table 43.2 International classification of seizures

I. Focal or partial seizures

   Simple (general without an impairment of level of consciousness):
   • Motor, e.g. Jacksonian seizures
   • Sensory or somatosensory
   • Autonomic
   Complex (the spread of simple or partial to a generalized convulsive form such as temporal lobe or psychomotor)

II. Generalized seizures (without a local onset, bilaterally, symmetric)

   Absences (petit mal)
   Tonic-clonic (grand mal)
   Infantile spasms (convulsions)
   Bilateral massive myoclonus
   Clonic seizures
   Tonic seizures
   Atonic seizures
   Akinetic seizures

III. Unilateral seizures

IV. Unclassified seizures (when complete data is not available)

V. Classification of paroxysmal forms
   • Benign febrile seizures
   • Convulsive equivalent syndrome
   • Breath-holding spells

A generalized seizure is commonly referred to as a tonic-clonic or a grand mal seizure. This type of seizure usually consists of three phases:

1. An aura

2. Tonic-clonic (convulsive) phase
3. Post convulsive phase.

The aura (which is not always experienced) is a warning of an impending seizure. An aura is a sensation, e.g. a specific taste or smell, experienced by the individual immediately prior to a seizure. The seizure commonly commences with a loud cry, which is precipitated by air being forced out through the vocal cords which are in spasm.

The individual then loses consciousness, and may fall. The muscles become rigid, then alternate between episodes of muscle spasm and relaxation (tonic-clonic phase), resulting in jerky spasmodic body movements. Tongue biting, incontinence of urine, laboured breathing, apnoea, and cyanosis may occur.

The seizure generally stops within 2–5 minutes, when abnormal electrical conduction in the brain ceases. The individual regains consciousness, but he may be dazed and confused or fall asleep.

Rarely, automatism may follow and violence may be exhibited. Automatism is a state whereby the individual exhibits mechanical, repetitive, and undirected behaviour that is not consciously controlled.

Status epilepticus is a condition in which the individual experiences continuous seizures without regaining consciousness in between, and it is generally accompanied by respiratory distress.

Information on the emergency management of a generalized seizure is provided in Chapter 57.

Peripheral neuritis (polyneuritis) is the degeneration of peripheral nerves, resulting in muscle weakness and atrophy, sensory loss, and decreased or absent tendon reflexes. Causes include chronic intoxication (alcohol, arsenic, lead), metabolic and inflammatory disorders (diabetes me-llitus, rheumatoid arthritis), nutrient deficiencies (thiamine), and infectious diseases (meningitis, Guillaine-Barre syndrome).

Manifestations usually develop slowly, beginning with leg pains and numbness or tingling in the feet and hands. As the disease progresses, the individual experiences flaccid paralysis, muscle wasting, pain of varying intensity, and loss of reflexes in the legs and arms. Footdrop, ataxic gait, and inability to walk will eventually occur.

Guillaine-Barre syndrome is characterized by an acute onset of ascending motor and sensory deficits, which are rapidly progressive. Although the precise cause is unclear, there is suggestion that the disorder may be viral or immunologic in origin. Approximately 50% of individuals with Guillaine-Barre syndrome have experienced a mild respiratory tract or gastrointestinal infection 1–3 weeks preceding the onset of polyneuritis.

Manifestations include paraesthesia and weakness of the leg muscles, which extends to the upper body within 24–72 hours. Respiratory distress can result from diaphragm and intercostal muscle weakness, and the cranial nerves may become involved.

Bell's palsy is a disorder of the seventh cranial nerve that produces unilateral facial weakness or paralysis. An inflammatory reaction occurs in or around cranial nerve VII, resulting in nerve compression and the onset of flaccid facial paralysis. Factors responsible for the inflammatory reaction include infection, prolonged exposure to cold temperature, and local trauma. The seventh cranial nerve can also be affected by other conditions such as a cerebral tumour, meningitis, or a middle ear infection.

Manifestations are unilateral facial weakness, which is sometimes associated with pain around the angle of the jaw or behind the ear. On the affected side the mouth droops; and the individual is unable to wrinkle the forehead, close the eyelid, or smile. There may be excessive watering from the affected eye, and drooling of saliva from the affected side of the mouth.

Degenerative disorders

Parkinson's disease is a degenerative process of nerve cells in the basal ganglia and the substantia nigra. The substantia nigra is an area in the basal ganglia considered necessary for motor control.

Although the precise cause of the disorder is unknown, research has demonstrated that a dopamine deficiency prevents affected brain cells from functioning normally. Dopamine is a neurotransmitter that plays a role in the transmission of nerve impulses between synapses. Factors which have been implicated in the development of Parkinson's disease include cerebral atherosclerosis, and long-term therapy with drugs such as haloperidol and phenothiazide.

Manifestations of Parkinson's disease are related to disturbances of movement: tremor, muscle rigidity, and dyskinesia. The most common initial symptom is tremor, e.g. 'pill-rolling' movements of the fingers, and to and fro head tremors. Tremors are aggravated by fatigue and stress, and decrease when the individual performs a purposeful activity or is asleep. The individual experiences difficulty in initiating voluntary movement and loss of posture control—so that he walks with the body bent forward. The gait consists of short shuffling steps that are slowly initiated. Facial expression becomes mask-like, and the voice is commonly high-pitched and monotone. The individual's intelligence is not affected.

Amyotrophic lateral sclerosis, which is the most common form of motor neurone disease, is a progressive degenerative condition which is generally fatal within 3–10 years after onset. The disease affects the upper and lower motor neurones of the central nervous system, resulting in progressive muscular atrophy, progressive bulbar palsy, and upper motor neurone deficits. While the cause is unknown, the disease is thought to result from viral, metabolic, toxic, infectious, and immunologic factors.

Manifestations include skeletal muscle weakness and atrophy; and impaired speech, chewing, swallowing and breathing. The cause of death is commonly respiratory muscle weakness and bulbar palsy causing respiratory failure.

Alzheimer's disease is a progressive, degenerative disorder which causes cerebral atrophy and dementia. Although the precise cause is unknown, several theories propose that the disorder may result either from a genetic factor, immunologic dysfunction, a toxin, or a virus. Recent research has focused on the role of neurotransmitters, and on the effect of a deficiency of acetylcholine in the brain—as a cause of the condition.

Manifestations of the disease generally occur in three stages:

1. Memory loss, decline in judgement and logic, disorientation, global aphasia, irritability, mood swings, and agitation.
2. Neglect of hygiene, inability to carry out deliberate voluntary movements (apraxia), inability to recognize the nature or use of objects (agnosia), repetition of a motor or verbal action (perseveration), and seizures.
3. Marked dementia, unresponsiveness, aphasia, and apraxia.

Information on the care of a confused individual is provided in Chapter 55.

Immunologic disorders

Multiple sclerosis is a disorder characterized by progressive demyelination of nerve fibres in the spinal cord and brain. Patches of demyelination throughout the central nervous system result in varied neurologic dysfunction. The cause is unknown, but the disease is thought to result from viral or immunologic factors. Manifestations vary depending on the areas of the central nervous system which are affected. Some individuals experience mild exacerbations with long remission periods, while others have frequent relapses with increasing residual deficits. The most common initial symptoms are fatigue, motor weakness, and visual disturbances. Other characteristic changes include numbness and tingling sensations, intention tremor, gait ataxia, paralysis, urinary disturbances, and emotional lability.

Myasthenia gravis is a chronic neuromuscular disorder that affects voluntary muscles, and is characterized by fluctuating muscle weakness which is exacerbated by exercise. The disease is considered to be autoimmune in origin, resulting in an acetylcholine receptor deficiency. The thymus gland is also thought to be involved in the disease as, in individuals with myasthenia gravis, the gland is abnormal and remains active after puberty.

Manifestations include progressive weakness of certain voluntary muscles, with some improvement in muscle func-

tion following rest. The eye muscles are most commonly affected, with drooping of the eyelids (ptosis) and double vision (diplopia). Other affected muscles include those involved with facial expression, speech, chewing, and swallowing. The individual may experience problems with saliva, nasal regurgitation, and choking. The shoulder and neck muscles may be affected, so that the head tends to fall forward. Weakened respiratory muscles make breathing difficult, and predispose to respiratory tract infections.

Infectious and inflammatory conditions

Meningitis is inflammation of the meninges, and it can be caused by viruses, bacteria, or fungi. The inflammation may involve one, or all three layers of the meninges. Meningitis often begins when the causative organism enters the subarachnoid space, then the infection spreads because of the open communication over the brain's convexity. The accumulation of exudate, from the inflammatory process, over the convexities or in the ventricles can obstruct the flow of cerebrospinal fluid.

Aseptic meningitis is thought to occur from meningeal irritation resulting from encephalitis, leukaemia, lymphoma, or the presence of blood in the subarachnoid space.

The major manifestations of meningitis are severe headaches, pyrexia, irritability, neck rigidity, photophobia, and pain in the back and limbs. Other manifestations are alterations in mental status, altered levels of consciousness, and restlessness. Vomiting may occur, and cranial nerve involvement causes visual disturbances, pupil abnormalities, strabismus and vertigo. There may be generalized seizures due to cerebral oedema.

Encephalitis is inflammation of the brain tissue caused by viruses, bacteria, fungi, or parasites.

Endemic encephalitis begins in a non-human host or reservoir from where the virus is transmitted to humans, e.g. through mosquito bites. Once the pathogen gains access to the central nervous system, via the bloodstream or along nerves, the white matter and meninges develop non-suppurative inflammation, and diffuse cerebral oedema results. Initial manifestations are headaches, pyrexia, vomiting, malaise, and muscular aches and pains. These are often followed by alterations in the level of consciousness, confusion, motor and sensory deficits, hyperirritability, and meningeal signs.

A brain abscess is a collection of pus, usually occurring in the temporal lobes, or the cerebellum. A brain abscess is accompanied by cerebral oedema and congestion. The majority of brain abscesses develop secondary to a primary source of infection, e.g. from mastoiditis, otitis media; or they develop from a septic focus in the respiratory tract or, less often, from a pelvic or cardiac source. A small percentage result from a penetrating head wound, e.g. a gunshot injury.

Manifestations include headache, pyrexia, vomiting, alterations in the level of consciousness, and partial or generalized seizures. Other features differ according to the site of the absess, and include motor, sensory, and speech disturbances.

Myelitis is the term which applies to a group of infective and noninfective processes which affect the spinal cord. Myelitis can be due to viruses, occur secondary to meningeal inflammation, or be of unknown etiology. The most common viral diseases causing myelitis are poliomyelitis and herpes zoster. Manifestations include a sudden onset of motor paresis, accompanied by other neurologic deficits such as loss of sensory and sphincter functions.

Herpes Zoster is a viral disorder that causes inflammation of the posterior root ganglia. Herpes zoster develops from reactivation of the varicella virus—the virus responsible for chickenpox. There is also evidence of a relationship between herpes zoster and certain systemic infections, neoplasms, and immunosuppressive therapy.

Manifestations include mild to severe neuralgic pain in the affected nerve root distribution. The pain, which may be burning, tingling, dull or sharp, may occur with or be followed by skin reddening and eruption of vesicles. The vesicles become pustules and develop a crust within 1–2 weeks. If infection or ulceration accompanies the vesicles, permanent scarring may result.

Occasionally, herpes zoster involves the cranial nerves—especially the trigeminal or oculomotor nerve. Trigeminal involvement causes eye pain and, possibly, corneal damage and impaired vision. Oculomotor involvement may result in conjunctivitis or ptosis. Rarely, herpes zoster leads to generalized central nervous system infection.

Post-herpetic neuralgia can persist for months or years, and the skin may remain hypersensitive to touch.

Poliomyelitis is an acute infectious disease caused by one of the three poliomyelitis viruses, which generally enter the body through the mouth or nose, multiply in the bloodstream, and travel to the central nervous system. The viruses are then spread along neural pathways, and destroy cells in the anterior horns of the spinal cord. The brain stem may also be damaged. The incidence of acute anterior poliomyelitis has decreased dramatically, in the Western world, since the introduction of vaccine in 1955.

The virus may cause only a minor illness, or there may be signs and symptoms of viral meningitis and paralysis. The extent of paralysis depends upon the location of the affected neurones.

The initial manifestations of paralytic poliomyelitis include pyrexia, headaches, vomiting, irritability; and pains in the neck, back, arms and legs. Approximately 5–7 days after onset, the individual experiences weakness of various muscles, paraesthesia, hypersensitivity to touch, and resistance to neck flexion. If the disease affects the brain stem, the muscles involved in swallowing, chewing, and ventilation are affected.

Neoplastic and obstructive disorders

Tumours of the nervous system may be benign or malignant, and they may be primary or metastatic. Tumours may arise in the brain tissue, the meninges, the skull, in the peripheral and cranial nerves, or in the spinal cord.

Brain tissue (cerebral) tumours include astrocytomas and, glioblastomas.

Meningiomas usually arise from the arachnoid layer of the meninges and do not invade the brain.

Skull tumours, which are rare, may be either osteomas (benign) or sarcomas (malignant).

Peripheral and cranial nerve tumours include acoustic neuromas, schwannomas, and neuroblastomas.

Spinal cord tumours may be either extradural or intradural.

Manifestations of nervous system tumours are related to invasion or compression of surrounding neural structures. Brain tumours may produce symptoms as a consequence of increased intracranial pressure, e.g. from cerebral oedema.

The neurologic manifestations of a brain tumour depend on the location of the tumour, and on its rate of growth. The clinical features associated with a brain tumour include headaches, vomiting, papilloedema (swelling of the optic disc and distension of the retinal vessels), personality or behavioral changes, seizures, visual or hearing defects, dizziness, ataxia, and hemiparesis.

Manifestations of spinal cord tumours are related to spinal cord compression and include pain, paraplegia or quadriplegia—which may be slowly progressive or acute.

Traumatic disorders

Despite being well protected by bone, meninges and cerebrospinal fluid, the brain and spinal cord are frequently injured. Serious cerebral or spinal cord damage can result from a variety of factors such as motor vehicle accidents, sports accidents, and penetrating injuries, e.g. a gunshot wound. Cerebral injury may be classified as concussion, contusion, laceration, haematomas, and tentorial herniation.

Concussion results from a blow to the head, and is characterized by a loss of consciousness for less than five minutes and memory loss of events preceding and following the injury. Other features include headaches, confusion, dizziness, visual disturbances, vomiting, and irritability.

Contusion is bruising of the brain that disrupts normal nerve function in the bruised area; and which may cause haemorrhage or oedema. Manifestations include drowsiness, confusion, behavioral changes, loss of consciousness, hemiparesis, unequal pupil response; and decorticate or decerebrate posturing.

With *decorticate posturing* (Fig. 43.1), the individual demonstrates hyperflexion of the upper extremities, and hyperextension of the lower extremities. With *decerebrate*

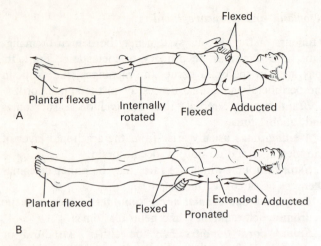

Fig. 43.1 Decorticate and decerebrate posturing. (A) Decorticate rigidity. (B) Decerebrate rigidity.

posturing (Fig. 43.1), both the upper and lower extremities are hyperextended.

Laceration is tearing of the brain tissue followed by intracerebral bleeding. Manifestations include prolonged unconsciousness, immediate neurologic deficits, and deterioration of the individual's condition.

Haematomas are collections of coagulated blood, may be epidural, subdural, or intracerebral. An epidural haematoma results from haemorrhage in the epidural space, between the skull and the dura mater. A subdural haematoma results from an accumulation of blood in the subdural space, between the arachnoid and dura mater. An intracerebral haematoma is a collection of blood within the brain tissue.

Manifestations of cerebral haematomas vary according to the location and whether the haematoma develops rapidly or slowly. Typically, an epidural haematoma causes immediate loss of consciousness, followed by a lucid interval—which eventually gives way to a rapidly progressive decrease in the level of consciousness. Accompanying features include hemiparesis, severe headaches, unilateral pupil dilation, and signs of increased intracranial pressure (decreasing pulse and ventilation rate, increasing systolic blood pressure).

Manifestations of a subdural haematoma may not occur until days after the injury. Common features include headaches, drowsiness, confusion, slow responses, and seizures. Pupillary changes and motor deficits commonly occur.

Manifestations of intracerebral haematoma include neck rigidity, photophobia, nausea and vomiting, dizziness, decreased ventilation rate, and seizures.

Tentorial herniation occurs when damaged brain tissue swells and herniates into the foramen magnum. This event constricts the brain stem, impairs vital centres and cranial nerves, and reduces the brain's blood supply.

Manifestations include drowsiness, confusion, pupil dilation, neck rigidity, hyperventilation, bradycardia, and decorticate or decerebrate posturing. Irreversible brain damage or death can occur rapidly.

Spinal cord damage may occur from traumatic injuries as a result of motor vehicle or sports accidents, gunshot or stab wounds, or falls from high places. Fracture—dislocations can occur anywhere along the spinal column and, if the spinal cord is injured, may result in temporary or permanent damage.

Apart from direct tearing of the spinal cord, the main damage is caused by haemorrhage, oedema, and disruption of the blood supply to the cord. Additional compression can result if bony fragments or disc material press on the spinal cord.

Manifestations of spinal cord damage depend on the degree and site of the injury. Complete spinal cord transection causes a total loss of motor and sensory function below the level of injury.

With cervical cord transection, there is paralysis of all four extremities (quadriplegia/tetraplegia). There are varying degrees of arm and ventilatory paralysis—depending on the injury level.

With thoracic cord transection, down to the level of the second lumbar vertebra, there is paralysis of the lower extremities (paraplegia). There is often some loss of intercostal muscle function, and loss of bladder and bowel function.

With spinal cord transection in the region of lumbar vertebrae, there is a combination of loss of sensory, motor, bowel and bladder function.

Complete cord transection results in immediate flaccid paralysis, loss of sensation, and loss of reflexes below the level of injury. As paralysis subsides reflexes usually return, and flaccidity changes to involuntary spastic movements. Recovery of any motor or sensory function is rare when there has been complete paralysis of these functions for several days.

With *incomplete* spinal-cord injuries, degrees of motor and sensory deficit below the level of damage vary. The individual may experience temporary paralysis, with function returning when any oedema subsides.

Peripheral nerve damage can result from pressure, compression, constriction, or traction on a nerve—or as a consequence of skeletal fractures, lacerations, or penetrating wounds. Nerve damage can also result from an injection of a toxic or metabolic substance into the nerve. The peripheral nerves most commonly injured are the peroneal, radial, axillary, ulnar, and the brachial plexus.

Manifestations include loss of motor function, loss of sensation, and muscle atrophy. Depending on which nerve is damaged there may be foot drop, wrist drop, limited range of motion or paralysis.

Diagnostic tests

Specific tests may be performed for diagnostic purposes, or to aid in evaluation of the individual's condition.

The neurological examination

The purpose of the neurological examination is to determine the presence or absence of disease in the nervous system; by assessing cerebral, cranial nerve, motor, sensory, and reflex function.

Evaluation of cerebral function is performed by assessing the individual's general behaviour and cognitive functions, e.g. orientation to time and place, concentration, memory, vocabulary, and abstract reasoning.

Evaluation of the cranial nerves involves assessment of:

• The olfactory nerve. The sense of smell is tested by obstructing one nostril while testing the other. A variety of substances are placed near the unobstructed nostril, and the individual is asked to identify the odour of each.
• The optic nerve. Each eye is tested to assess visual acuity and visual fields. The fundus of each eye is assessed by ophthalmoscopic examination.
• The oculomotor, trochlear and abducens nerves. These three nerves are generally tested together as they supply the various muscles that rotate the eyeball. The ophthalmoscope is used during the assessment; the pupils are observed for size, shape, and equality; and movement of the eyes is evaluated by requesting the individual to follow a finger through the six cardinal areas of vision.
• The trigeminal nerve. The sensory component of this nerve is tested with the individual's eyes closed. Test tubes of warm and cold water are brought into contact with the skin of the face to check temperature perception. Touching the face with a wisp of cotton checks perception of light touch. Pain perception is evaluated by either applying pressure or by touching areas of the face with the point of a pin.

The motor component of the trigeminal nerve is evaluated by asking the individual to clench and unclench his teeth, and by observing his ability to open the mouth against resistance.

The corneal reflex is assessed by lightly stroking the cornea with a wisp of cotton. If the corneal reflex is intact, the individual will automatically blink.
• The facial nerve. The sensory component of this nerve is assessed by placing sweet, salty, sour, and bitter substances on various areas of the tongue, and asking the individual to identify each taste.

The motor component of the facial nerve is assessed by requesting the individual to perform specific facial movements such as smiling, closing the eyes, pursing the lips, and wrinkling the forehead.
• The acoustic nerve. Generally, unless the individual has a history of vertigo, only the hearing branch of this nerve is assessed. A series of hearing tests is performed, and hearing in both ears is compared. For a more precise assessment of hearing acuity, a tuning fork is used.
• The glossopharyngeal and vagus nerves. These nerves are usually tested together, as they are closely related both anatomically and functionally. A series of tests is performed to assess the gag and swallowing reflexes.
• The spinal accessory nerve. This nerve is tested by evaluating the strength of the trapezius and sternocleidomastoid muscles, e.g. by requesting the individual to shrug his shoulders against resistance, and by asking him to turn his head to one side and push his chin against the assessor's hand.
• The hypoglossal nerve. The strength and movement of the tongue muscles are evaluated by testing the individual's ability to protrude his tongue, and also by requesting him to push his tongue against a tongue depressor.

Evaluation of motor function involves assessment of the individual's gait, posture, muscle strength and tone, balance and co-ordination. The assessor observes for abnormalities, and compares the findings on both sides of the body for asymmetry.

Evaluation of sensory function involves assessing the individual's ability to perceive various sensations, with his eyes closed. Assessment includes testing of sensitivity to touch, pain, temperature, testing of joint motion and position, and assessment of discriminative function and vibratory sensation.

Evaluation of reflexes involves testing the two types of reflex to assess the integrity of the motor and sensory systems.

1. The superficial reflexes which are evaluated include the upper abdominal, lower abdominal, gluteal, and plantar reflexes. The abdominal and gluteal reflexes are evaluated by applying a stimulus to the skin surface, e.g. stroking with a finger or pointed object, and observing for muscle contraction. The plantar reflex is evaluated by stroking the sole of the foot, with one continuous movement from the heel to the toes. Normally, the big toe curls downward in response to this stimulus. An abnormal response, *Babinski's sign*, where there is dorsiflexion of the big toe and fanning of the other toes, indicates upper motor neurone disease.

2. The deep tendon reflexes which are evaluated include the biceps, triceps, quadriceps, and Achilles. Deep tendon reflexes are elicited by using a percussion hammer, and observing the response:

• The biceps reflex is tested with the arm partially flexed at the elbow and the palm down. When the hammer is applied to the biceps tendon, the elbow should flex.
• The triceps reflex is tested with the arm partially flexed at the elbow and the palm directed towards the body. When the hammer is applied to the triceps tendon, the elbow should extend.
• The quadriceps reflex is tested with the knee flexed. When the patellar tendon is struck with the hammer, the knee should extend.
• The Achilles reflex is tested with the knee flexed. When

the Archilles tendon is struck with the hammer, the foot should plantar flex.

Radiographic examination

Plain X-ray films of the skull may be performed to detect fractures, to aid in the diagnosis of pituitary tumours, or to detect congenital abnormalities. X-ray films of the spine may be performed to detect trauma to the vertebral column, or to aid in the diagnosis of conditions that cause motor or sensory impairment.

Computerized tomography (CT) is commonly used to diagnose intracranial and spinal cord lesions. It is usually non-invasive but a contrast dye is sometimes administered to visualize blood vessels or to define lesions.

The individual lies on an X-ray table, with the head immobilized and his face uncovered. His head is moved into the scanner, and a moveable frame revolves around it while X-ray films are taken. If a contrast agent is used the individual may feel warm, and experience a transient headache, a salty taste, and nausea.

A myelogram involves fluoroscopy and radiography to evaluate the spinal cord and vertebral column, following injection of a contrast medium into the subarachnoid space.

A needle is inserted, most often in the lumbar area, into the subarachnoid space and approximately 10 ml of cerebrospinal fluid is removed. Contrast medium is then injected through the needle, and the individual is positioned to allow the medium to flow through the subarachnoid space. A series of X-ray films are taken, after which the contrast medium may be either withdrawn or allowed to remain in the cerebrospinal fluid. Water soluble agents are allowed to remain as they will eventually be excreted by the kidneys.

Cerebral angiography involves injecting a radiopaque contrast medium into an artery for radiological visualization of the intracranial and extracranial blood vessels. Common injection sites are the carotid or femoral arteries, and X-ray films are taken at various intervals after injection of the medium. Cerebral angiography may be performed using either local or general anaesthetic.

Digital subtraction angiography is a computer assisted radiographic procedure, for visualization of extracranial and intracranial vessels.

The procedure is considered to be safer than cerebral angiography and involves injection of a contrast medium through a catheter into the superior vena cava. Cerebral vessels are visualized on a screen, and pictures are taken.

Pneumoencephalography is performed infrequently since the advent of the CT scan. Pneumoencephalography allows radiographic examination of the cerebral ventricles, following injection of air or oxygen into the subarachnoid space.

Magnetic resonance imaging

Magnetic resonance imaging is a non-invasive procedure, during which the individual is placed in a strong magnetic field and is subjected to precise, computer-programmed bursts of radio pulse waves. The sharpness and detail of the images produced assist diagnosis by providing identification of abnormalities—even before structural changes have occurred.

Positron emission transaxial tomography

A non-invasive nuclear imaging technique, positron emission tomography is used to detect biochemical and physiological abnormalities. The individual is injected with a nuclide which reacts with electrons and produces gamma ray photons. A scanner detects the gamma rays and codes this data into a computer. The computer then reconstructs cross sectional images of the tissues being examined.

Radionuclide scan

This test uses a camera or scanner to provide images of the brain, following administration of a radioisotope. The rays emitted by the radioisotope are converted into images which are displayed on a screen.

Electroencephalography

An electroencephalogram (EEG) is a recording of the electrical activity of the brain (brain waves). Surface electrodes are attached to the scalp with a paste, and transmit the brain's electrical impulses to a machine which records them as brain waves on strips of paper. Brain waves are recorded while the individual is at rest, after hyperventilation, with photic stimulation, after a sensory stimulus, and during sleep.

Echoencephalography

An echoencephologram (ECHO) is a test that uses pulsating ultrasonic waves to indicate deviation of the cerebral midline structures. Since the advent of computerized tomography, echoecephalography is used infrequently.

Cerebrospinal fluid analysis

A sample of cerebrospinal fluid (CSF) is generally obtained by lumbar puncture or, less commonly, by cisternal puncture.

A lumbar puncture (Fig. 43.2) may be performed for either diagnostic or therapeutic purposes. The diagnostic indications include:

- measurement of CSF pressure

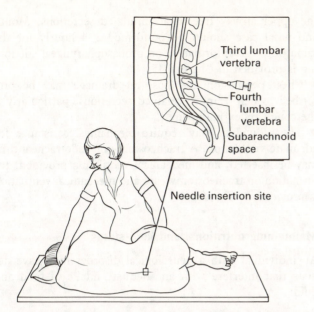

Third lumbar vertebra

Fourth lumbar vertebra

Subarachnoid space

Needle insertion site

Fig. 43.2 Lumbar puncture showing the position of the individual and the insertion site.

- examination of CSF for the presence of blood or micro-organisms
- injection of air, oxygen, or radiopaque material to visualize parts of the central nervous system radiologically
- evaluation for signs of blockage of CSF flow.

The therapeutic indications include:

- introduction of spinal anaesthesia for surgery
- intrathecal injection of medications.

For the procedure, the individual assumes a lateral position with his back arched and his knees flexed. His head should be bent forward so that his chin touches his chest.

Following preparation of the site, the medical officer inserts a spinal needle with stylus between the third and fourth lumbar vertebrae into the subarachnoid space. When the stylus is removed, CSF should drip from the needle.

If the lumbar puncture is being performed for diagnostic purposes, a manometer is attached to the needle to measure CSF pressure. Samples of CSF are then collected for visual and laboratory examination.

When the procedure is completed, the needle is withdrawn, and an adhesive dressing is applied over the puncture site.

Queckenstedt's test is sometimes performed as part of the lumbar puncture, if an obstruction of the spinal subarachnoid space is suspected. While the lumbar puncture needle is in place, an assistant manually compresses both jugular veins for 10 seconds. The CSF pressure is read and recorded at 5 second intervals, and again following release of jugular pressure.

The test is *contraindicated* if the individual has increased intracranial pressure or cerebral bleeding, because brain stem herniation or further bleeding can occur.

A cisternal puncture may be performed to obtain a sample of CSF when a lumbar puncture is contraindicated. A needle, with stylus, is inserted into the cisterna magnum, and a sample of CSF is withdrawn. Cisternal puncture is a potentially dangerous procedure, because the needle is positioned close to the brain stem.

Electromyography

This procedure involves recording the electrical activity of a muscle and peripheral nerve, and it may be performed to aid in diagnosis of neuromuscular disorders. Needle electrodes are inserted into the muscle to be examined, and recordings are made of the electrical activity of the muscle at rest and during contraction.

Nerve conduction studies

These studies involve application of an electrical stimulus to peripheral nerves, and measurement of their response by means of an oscilloscope.

Caloric testing for vestibular function

Caloric testing is a diagnostic procedure designed to evaluate the vestibular portion of the eighth cranial (acoustic) nerve. The underlying principle of the procedure is that thermal stimulation of the vestibular end organs with warm and cold water will elicit the oculovestibular reflex. This reflex, if intact, results in induced nystagmus and eye movement in response to cold or warm water irrigation of the external auditory canal.

Each external meatus is irrigated for up to 3 minutes with both cold and warm water, with a pause of at least 5 minutes between irrigations. Irrigation with cold water should result in slow nystagmic eye movements on the same side, followed by rapid nystagmus to the opposite side. Irrigation with warm water should produce rapid nystagmus on the same side.

CARE OF THE INDIVIDUAL WITH A NERVOUS SYSTEM DISORDER

Although specific nursing actions and medical management vary depending on the disorder, the main aims of care are to:

- promote a clear airway
- maintain fluid and nutritional status
- prevent and manage alterations in elimination
- promote effective communication

- promote safety
- promote mobility
- prevent complications of immobility
- provide psychological support
- assess neurological status
- provide a suitable environment
- provide pre and post diagnostic test care
- promote rehabilitation and independence.

Each individual presents specific nursing problems for which an individualized nursing care plan must be developed, implemented, and evaluated.

Promoting a clear airway

Disorders of the nervous system may affect the individual's ability to breathe normally, to cough effectively, or to prevent the tongue from obstructing the airway. Altered levels of consciousness, decreased motor function, or disrupted cranial nerve function may impair the individual's ability to maintain a clear airway. To ensure a patent airway, the individual's nose, mouth, and respiratory tract must be clear—allowing adequate oxygen and carbon dioxide exchange.

The conscious individual

- The individual should be assisted into a position which will promote effective breathing. A sitting or upright position provides better lung expansion, which improves breathing and lessens the risk of respiratory tract infection.
- The individual is instructed to take deep breaths hourly, and to cough and expectorate mucus frequently. Chest physiotherapy, e.g. percussion, may be necessary to help mobilize secretions.
- If the individual's ability to chew and swallow is impaired, care must be taken when food, fluids, or oral medications are being consumed.
- Suction equipment should be readily available if the individual is at risk of choking, or if he is unable to expectorate secretions effectively.
- Active or passive range of motion (ROM) exercises and 2–4 hourly position changes help to mobilize respiratory tract secretions.
- An adequate fluid input is provided to keep respiratory tract secretions moist.

The unconscious individual

- The unconscious individual should be nursed in a lateral recumbent position, to promote drainage of secretions and to prevent the tongue from obstructing the airway. He should be positioned on alternate sides 2 hourly, to prevent pooling of secretions in the lungs.
- Oronasopharyngeal suction should be performed to keep the upper airway free of accumulated secretions. Mouth and nasal care should be performed 2–4 hourly for the same purpose. Information on oronasopharyngeal suctioning is provided in Chapter 45.
- Chest percussion and postural drainage may be prescribed to help remove retained secretions, particularly if the cough reflex is impaired.
- The individual may require mechanical assistance for adequate ventilation. A tracheostomy or endotracheal tube may be inserted, and mechanical ventilation provided. Information on tracheostomy care and mechanical ventilation is provided in Chapter 45.

Maintaining nutritional and fluid status

An individual with a neurological disorder may have deficits that interfere with an adequate intake of food and fluid:

- altered level of consciousness
- altered mental status
- diminished or absent swallowing or gag reflex
- inability to feed self, e.g. paralysis of arm/s
- fear of choking
- paralysis of the muscles of mastication and/or the tongue
- loss of appetite due to altered sensory function, e.g. sight, smell, taste.

Information on assisting the individual to meet his nutritional and fluid needs is provided in Chapters 29 and 31. Specific nursing activities to assist the individual with a nervous system disorder include:

- Providing appropriate devices to facilitate the cutting and eating of food (refer to Fig. 29.2).
- Ensuring that suction equipment is readily available should it be needed, e.g. if the individual's swallowing or gag reflexes are impaired.
- Assisting the individual who is unable to feed himself.
- Placing the food into the unaffected side of the mouth if the individual has any facial weakness. If he is able to feed himself, the individual should be informed to feed in this manner.
- Preparing food for the individual who has motor deficits, e.g. cutting meat, spreading butter, pouring fluids.
- Redirecting the individual's attention to eating if he becomes distracted or is unable to concentrate at mealtimes.
- Assisting with the care of the individual who is being provided with nutrition and fluids by alternative methods, e.g. tube feeding or total parenteral nutrition.
- Keeping a record of fluid input and output if the individual has difficulty in feeding himself or swallowing, or if he is receiving dehydrating medications or intravenous solutions to reduce or prevent increased intracranial pressure.

Preventing and managing alterations in elimination

Many disorders affecting the nervous system can result in constipation, retention of urine, or incontinence. Factors which contribute to altered patterns of elimination include:

- loss of sphincter control
- diminished awareness of the need to empty the bladder or bowel
- altered levels of consciousness
- impaired mental status with resulting incontinence.

Information on the prevention and management of constipation, retention of urine, and incontinence is provided in Chapter 30.

Promoting effective communication

Disorders of the nervous system may affect the individual's ability to express himself verbally or non verbally, and his ability to understand the spoken or written word. The ability to communicate may be impaired by factors which include:

- damage to the speech centres in the brain
- damage to the temporal lobes, which hinders the perception and interpretation of stimuli
- damage to the cranial nerves responsible for movement of the lips, tongue, pharynx, and larynx
- limited motor function which hinders non verbal communication actions, e.g. facial expressions and gestures
- visual or hearing deficits
- altered levels of consciousness or mental status.

The two major terms used to describe communication deficits are *dysphasia* (difficulty in communicating), and *aphasia* (loss of the ability to communicate).

Aphasia

Aphasia is subdivided into three major classifications.

1. Expressive aphasia (Broca's aphasia) is inability to express oneself verbally or in writing. The degree of difficulty can range from mild hesitancy in flow of speech to limitation of expression to 'yes' and 'no'. The ability to *understand* the spoken and written word remains intact.

2. Receptive aphasia (Wernicke's aphasia) is inability to understand the spoken word. Although the individual hears the sounds of speech, comprehension of speech is impaired. The individual can speak, but he makes many errors when using words—and is often unaware of his imperfect messages. His ability to express his words in writing is also impaired.

3. Global aphasia is a combination of both expressive and receptive aphasia. The individual neither understands what he hears or reads, nor can he convey his thoughts in speech or writing.

The loss of impairment of the ability to communicate is devastating and frustrating to the individual, and to his significant others, often resulting in fear and depression.

Although the speech therapist will be the key person in the treatment of an individual with a communication problem, the nurse must be aware of prescribed therapy so that it can be continued when the speech therapist is not with the individual.

The nurse should assume a calm, reassuring, and supportive manner which conveys a sense of acceptance of the individual's behaviour. Table 43.3 illustrates guidelines which can be used when working with an aphasic individual.

Communication with the unconscious individual is very important for, although he appears to be completely unaware of his environment, it is impossible to determine his awareness of any stimulus. Many individuals have recovered from unconsciousness and given accurate details of events or conversations which took place in their presence while they were unconscious. Therefore, the nurse should assume that some stimuli will penetrate the complexities of unconsciousness. Stimuli can be provided by talking to the individual, by touch, and by playing a radio or tapes. The nurse should tell the individual what she will be doing; orient him to time, place, and person; and describe his surroundings.

Table 43.3 Assisting the aphasic individual

Expressive aphasia	Receptive aphasia
Stimulate conversation and ask open-ended questions	Speak slowly and distinctly, using a common vocabulary and simple sentences
Allow the individual time to find the words to express himself	Stand within the individual's line of vision, so that he can observe lip movements
Be supportive and accepting as the individual deals with the frustration of finding the right words	Use simple gestures as an added cue
Accept self-expression, e.g. pointing or gestures	Repeat or rephrase any instructions if they are not understood
Provide charts or books with pictures of common objects, so that the individual can point when he can't say the word	Speak in a normal voice
Reassure the individual that speech skills can be relearned, given time	Divide any tasks into small units, working with the individual to accomplish the task
Give praise for achievements and progress	Use pointing and touch to express ideas
	Eliminate background distractions
	Give praise for achievements and progress

Coma arousal is a technique whereby the unconscious individual is continuously exposed to variety of stimuli, e.g. sounds, touch, and smells in an attempt to increase his level of consciousness.

Promoting safety

The individual with a nervous system disorder is often susceptible to injury because of factors such as impaired consciousness or awareness, reduced mobility, impaired motor and sensory functions and reflexes. The individual is most at risk of skin breakdown, physical injuries, or infection.

General information on meeting the individual's need for safety is provided in Chapter 38. This chapter addresses specific nursing activities which are implemented to promote the safety of an individual with a nervous system disorder.

Maintenance of skin integrity

The nurse should assess the individual for potential skin problems and implement nursing measures to prevent skin breakdown from pressure, extremes of temperature, and physical trauma, as follows:

- The skin is kept clean and dried to prevent irritation and possible breakdown. Very dry skin should be lubricated with a suitable oil or cream to prevent cracking and breakdown.
- A protective cream or lotion may be applied to the genital area and buttocks if the individual is incontinent. Wet or soiled linen must be replaced immediately.
- The individual's position is changed every 2–4 hours to protect the skin from irritation and prolonged pressure. Pressure-relieving aids such as sheepskins may be used.
- The skin is assessed every 2 hours for colour, temperature, dryness, and the signs of impaired circulation. Any signs of skin breakdown are reported immediately, so that appropriate actions can be implemented to prevent further deterioration.
- Precautions must be taken to avoid injury to the skin by hot, cold, sharp, or rough objects. The individual is always moved correctly and gently to avoid damage to his skin.

Prevention of physical injuries

An individual who has impaired motor, sensory, or intellectual function must be protected from accidents and injuries. Protective measures include:

- maintaining the bed in a low position when not providing direct care at the bedside
- using side rails on the bed

- applying restraints, if they have been prescribed, to protect a restless or confused individual
- accompanying the individual when he ambulates, if he is unsteady or disoriented
- providing walking aids and handrails as a means of support and to promote greater safety
- providing an uncluttered environment and adequate lighting
- placing the individual's requirements, including the signal device, within his reach
- supervising individuals, who are at risk of falling, while they are performing the activities of living.

Prevention of infection

An individual with a nervous system disorder which impairs mobility, motor function, or level of consciousness is prone to infection. When an individual is ill, the body's natural defence mechanisms are stressed and, therefore, less able than usual to resist the invasion of pathogenic microorganisms. The two most common types of infection which may occur are:

1. Urinary tract infection, because of urinary stasis or catheterization.
2. Respiratory tract infection, because of inadequate lung expansion, pooling of secretions in the lungs, the presence of an artificial airway, or mechanical ventilation.

Measures to prevent a urinary tract infection include ensuring that:

- The individual receives an adequate fluid input
- Whenever possible, an external urinary drainage device or intermittent catheterization is used rather than an indwelling catheter.
- If an indwelling catheter is unavoidable, measures to prevent cross infection are implemented. These measures include maintaining a sterile closed drainage system, performing meatal and perineal care, maintaining dependent drainage, maintaining strict aseptic care, preventing cross contamination with correct hand washing technique. Further information is provided in Chapter 30.

Measures to prevent a respiratory tract infection include ensuring that:
- When possible, the individual is nursed in a sitting or upright position, to promote maximum lung expansion
- The individual performs 4 hourly deep breathing and coughing exercises
- If necessary, suction is used to remove oronasopharyngeal secretions
- Aseptic techniques are implemented when caring for an artificial airway.

The nurse must acknowledge that *correct hand washing technique* is the most effective way of preventing cross infection.

Promoting mobility and preventing the complications of immobility

Many nervous system disorders impair physical mobility through motor deficits, cerebellar dysfunction, alterations in sensory perception, and changes in conscious or mental status. Prolonged lack of physical exercise and movement can lead to many complications; including pulmonary stasis, urinary stasis, venous stasis, decubitus ulcers, constipation, and contractures. Impaired mobility varies from reductions in range of motion or unsteady gait, to total immobility. Maintaining muscle tone and preventing orthopedic disabilities are of prime importance when caring for an individual with impaired mobility. To prevent functional loss:

● Active or passive range of motion (ROM) exercises should be performed every 4 hours.
● The individual should be repositioned every 2 hours to maintain correct body alignment. Weak or paralyzed body parts must be carefully positioned to prevent deformity.
● Specific exercises, such as lifting hand weights, may be prescribed to strengthen a weakened limb.
● As soon as the individual's condition permits, balancing and sitting exercises are implemented. If the individual has been immobile for a prolonged period, it is necessary to progress slowly—to prevent orthostatic hypotension.
● Once the individual is able to balance and sit, transfer activities are commenced, e.g. from bed to chair.
● When the individual is able to stand and balance in an upright position, ambulation is commenced.
● For the individual who is unable to ambulate, wheelchair mobility may be achieved.

The individual's age, severity of illness, other neurological deficits, chronic conditions, or complications contribute to his progress. His attitude and motivation are also important factors in regaining mobility. Frequent assessment provides evaluation of the individual's needs so that rehabilitation can progress towards the greatest level of independence.

Further information on preventing the complications of immobility is provided in Chapter 37.

Providing psychological support

Many individuals who have a nervous system disorder will suffer neurological deficits resulting in loss of independence, mobility, sensory function, or speech. As a result the individual's body image and self concept may be greatly altered, and he may experience emotional lability, depression, anxiety, frustration, or hostility. The individual may undergo personality changes, which may be functional or organic in origin.

The individual may require a lengthy period to regain what were once automatically performed skills involved in the activities of daily living, or he may have to come to terms with the realization that some skills may never be regained. The emotional shock to an individual who experiences paralysis can be devastating.

The nurse has an important role in providing emotional and psychological support for the individual, and for his significant others. Some of the key aspects related to supporting the individual are:

● During his period of dependence, it is important that his dignity is preserved. Sensitivity is needed when dealing with any problems associated with loss of control, e.g. incontinence, or loss of social restraint.
● Positive feedback should be provided for his accomplishments—no matter how minor they may appear.
● He should be provided with adequate information about the disease process and its management, and he should be encouraged to participate in decision making regarding his care.
● His needs should be anticipated to decrease his frustration. He should be allowed as much self care is practicable, as a return to independence is the ultimate goal of care. The individual's significant others should be allowed to become involved in his care—if they so wish.
● The individual, and his significant others, should be encouraged to express their feelings and anxieties. If the individual is experiencing a communication problem, appropriate methods of communicating should be developed. Time, patience, and understanding are necessary to allow him to come to terms with the effects and implications of his disease.
● He should be encouraged to participate in activities of interest which will help to promote a feeling of self worth. The occupational therapist and physiotherapist generally assist the individual to find activities that interest him, and which will also provide exercise for weak or paralysed muscles.

Assessing neurological status

Assessment is of prime importance in the care of an individual with a neurological disorder. The nurse must recognize those changes which indicate a change in his condition, as changes can occur rapidly and dramatically or develop over a period of days or weeks.

Intracranial pressure

Intracranial pressure is the pressure exerted by the cerebrospinal fluid within the ventricles of the brain. However, it is more accurate to think in terms of intracranial 'pressures' rather than a single pressure as the rigid skull is filled with brain tissue, intravascular blood, and cerebrospinal fluid. If any one of these three components increases in volume, without a reciprocal change in volume of the other two, intracranial pressure will rise.

Increased intracranial pressure affects the cerebral perfusion pressure, causing hypoxia, ischaemia, irreversible neurological damage, and even death. Unless increased intracranial pressure is treated, the outcome will be herniation of a portion of the cerebrum through the tentorium—with pressure being exerted on the brain stem. The brain stem will then herniate through the foramen magnum—the only opening in the closed cranial vault.

Common causes of increased intracranial pressure include space-occupying masses such as tumours, haematomas, abscesses, or cerebral oedema; conditions that increase cerebral blood volume, and conditions that increase cerebrospinal fluid.

It is very important to identify early signs of increased intracranial pressure, so that actions can be implemented to prevent or minimize irreversible brain damage. The manifestations of increased intracranial pressure include:

1. Early signs and symptoms: deterioration in the level of consciousness (confusion, restlessness, lethargy), pupillary dysfunction, motor weakness such as hemiparesis, and possible headaches.

2. Later signs and symptoms: continued deterioration in the level of consciousness (coma), possible vomiting, hemiplegia, decortication, decerebration, increasing systolic blood pressure, bradycardia, and decreasing or irregular ventilations.

Neurological assessment

Neurological assessment includes checking the level of consciousness, the pupils, motor function, sensory function, and the vital signs. The frequency with which assessment is performed and documented will depend on the individual's condition, and on the institution's policy.

The level of consciousness is a most important factor in neurological assessment, providing valid information about changes in neurological status. Change can occur slowly over the course of many days, or it can occur rapidly in a few minutes or hours. The rapidity of change is an indicator of the severity of the neurological problem.

The individual's level of consciousness is evaluated by providing stimuli and observing his response. Sound and pain are the major stimuli used. Speaking to the individual is the most common method of applying an *auditory* stimulus, and *painful* stimuli are reserved for the individual with obviously decreased levels of consciousness.

A fully conscious individual, when spoken to, should reply with an appropriate verbal response. A person with a decreased level of consciousness may respond in a puzzled way, or he may not respond at all—showing no response even when someone speaks directly into his ear.

Painful tactile stimuli may be necessary to arouse the semi-comatose individual. Painful stimuli can be provided by exerting firm digital pressure on the nail beds, the Achilles tendon, or the gastrocnemius muscle. Pressing a hard object, e.g. a key, on the skin or running it over the skin is another technique. Response to painful stimuli can be classified into:

- Purposeful: when the individual winces, pushes the assessor away, or withdraws the affected body part.
- Non-purposeful: when the individual may move the stimulated body part only slightly, or when the application of painful stimuli causes an extensor response (a contraction of muscles) only.
- Unresponsive: when the individual shows no sign of reacting to painful stimuli.

Teasdale and Jennett's Glasgow Coma Scale (Fig. 43.3) was originally designed to assess the level of consciousness in individuals with head injuries, but it is now used in a variety of settings. It has gained increasing acceptance as an accurate and effective means of evaluating levels of consciousness.

Using the Glasgow Coma Scale, a score of 15 reflects a fully alert, well-oriented person; while a score of 7 or less is considered to indicate coma. The lowest possible score of 3 is indicative of deep coma.

Evaluation of the pupils provides vital information about central nervous system function or dysfunction. The findings in one pupil are compared with the findings in the other, and the differences between the two pupils is documented. The pupils are assessed for size, shape, and reaction to light.

Normally, the pupils are equal in size (average diameter of 3.5 mm), round, and they constrict briskly when light is shone into the eye. A pupil gauge (Fig. 43.3) may be used to estimate the size of each pupil. Abnormal responses of a pupil to light may be described as sluggish, nonreactive or fixed. Generally, any change in a pupil's size, shape or reaction is indicative of an intracranial change.

Assessment of motor function usually focuses on the arms and legs, and the identification of significant changes is important for denoting improvement, stabilization, or deterioration in the individual's condition.

The techniques used to evaluate motor function depend on the individual's level of consciousness. In the conscious individual, the assessment can be made by observing his motor responses to directions, e.g. by asking him to squeeze the assessor's hands.

If the individual is unconscious, or is unable to provide accurate responses, the assessor must rely on observational skills to evaluate motor function.

Assessment of sensory function is described on page 429 under the heading of 'The neurological examination'.

Assessment of the vital signs provides data concerning vital functions of the body. The individual's temperature, pulse, ventilations, and blood pressure are monitored and documented at a frequency which depends on his condition.

Data from neurological assessments are documented ac-

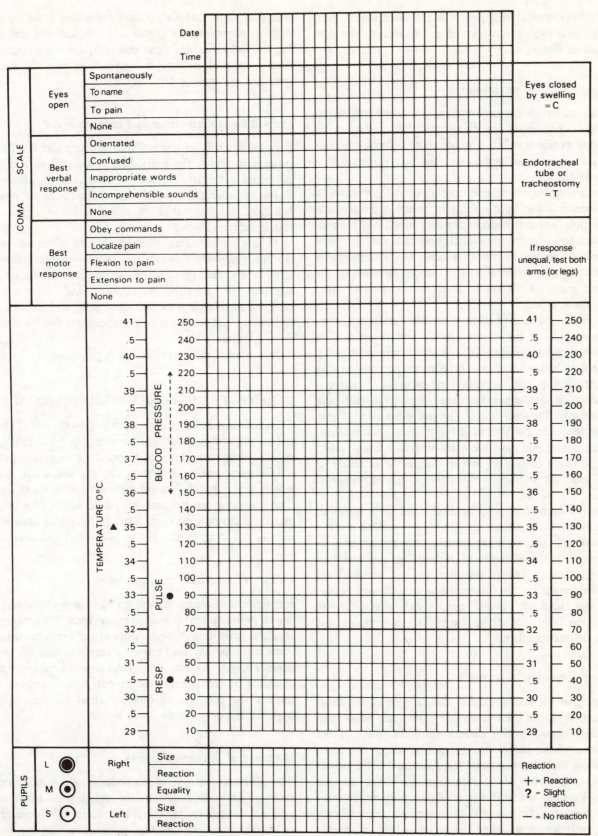

Fig. 43.3 The Glasgow Coma Scale and pupil gauge. (Reproduced with permission from Game C, Anderson R E, Kidd R J (eds) 1989 Medical-surgical nursing: a core text. Churchill Livingstone, Melbourne.)

cording to the institution's policy. Many institutions use a special neurological assessment chart, similar to the one illustrated in Figure 43.3.

Providing a suitable environment

The immediate physical environment should be adapted to meet the individual's specific needs. Items should be arranged to promote safety, e.g. adequate lighting, the signal device within easy reach, and the bed adjusted to a suitable height.

If the individual is experiencing sensory deprivation (a lack of sensory input from the environment), the nurse can provide multi-sensory stimuli. Sensory input can be provided by talking to the individual, playing a radio or tape recordings of family member's voices, touch, and *reality orientation*. Reality orientation is a process of making the individual aware of his environment, e.g. the date, time, people, place, objects.

Conversely, the individual may experience sensory overload particularly if he is critically ill and his condition requires the use of equipment such as a mechanical ventilation or cardiac monitor; or if he is receiving the constant stimuli of nursing care. Sensory overload occurs when sustained multi-sensory experiences are perceived as confusing or irritating by the individual. The manifestations of sensory overload are confusion, disorientation, restlessness, agitation, panic, and possible hallucinations. Every effort should be made to control and moderate the intensity of stimuli, e.g. the reduction of tactile and environmental stimuli.

When the individual is to be discharged from hospital, his physical home environment should be evaluated and the delivery of any necessary equipment arranged so that he can accomplish the activities of daily living and maintain his independence. The physiotherapist and occupational therapist arrange for the home use of ambulatory equipment, and identify special needs and alterations in environment that could be beneficial to support the individual's independence.

Providing diagnostic test care

Preparation of the individual for, and care following, diagnostic tests is part of the nurse's role. The nurse must refer to the institution's policy manual for information about preparation of the individual for specific diagnostic tests. Preparation includes a general explanation of the procedure, to reinforce the information provided to the individual by the medical officer. Other preparation may include dietary or fluid restrictions, administration of prescribed medications, assisting the individual into a specific position, skin preparation, and measurement of baseline vital and neurological signs.

Postprocedural care may include assessing vital and neu-rological signs, measuring and recording fluid input and output, administering prescribed medications; and assessing the individual for signs and symptoms, e.g. headaches, back pain, neck rigidity, nausea or vomiting, elevated temperature, or voiding difficulty.

Promoting rehabilitation and independence

Rehabilitation is an integral part of care, and is a dynamic process in which the individual is assisted to achieve his optimum potential. All care, throughout the individual's illness, is directed toward the maintenance of optimum function and prevention of complication—to promote as much independence as possible.

Rehabilitation of an individual with a nervous system disorder includes helping him to relearn the activities of daily living, management of neuromuscular deficits, management of impaired perception and communication deficits, bladder and bowel retraining, and educating the individual and his family in preparation for his discharge from hospital.

Information on rehabilitation is provided in Chapter 60.

CARE OF THE UNCONSCIOUS INDIVIDUAL

Consciousness is defined as a state of awareness of self and the surroundings. Consciousness implies an ability to perceive sensory stimuli and to respond appropriately to them.

Unconsciousness is defined as an abnormal state in which the individual is unresponsive to sensory stimuli. There are degrees of unconsciousness which vary in length and severity, ranging from a brief episode of unconsciousness in the form of fainting to prolonged and deep coma.

Causes of impaired consciousness

Impairment of consciousness arises from wide-spread damage to both cerebral hemispheres or from disruption of the reticular activating system in the upper brainstem. Loss of consciousness may result from a cerebral tumour, abscess, haemorrhage, haematoma, laceration, bruising, or ischaemia; or from metabolic processes that depress or interrupt the function of both cerebral hemispheres, e.g. hypoxia, hypoglycaemia, toxic agents.

Outcome of unconsciousness

The ultimate outcome of unconsciousness varies from full recovery of brain function, through a wide range of disabilities, to irreversible coma and death. The development of sophisticated monitoring techniques and life support systems has increased the survival rate for comatose individuals with severe brain damage. A small percentage of individuals emerge from deep coma to a state of wakefulness without awareness—never regaining any recognizable mental function.

Vegetative state is a term used to describe a chronic condition occurring after severe cerebral damage, which is characterized by intact autonomic functions, generally intact reflexes, presence of a sleep–wakefulness cycle, spontaneous eye opening to verbal stimuli, no localizing motor responses to verbal stimuli, and no intact cognitive functions or awareness of self or of the environment.

Brain death is a state of irreversible brain damage that is characterized by absence of cognitive functions and awareness of self and the environment, inability to maintain vital functions, and the absence of (isoelectric) activity on EEG. Brain death is a controversial, legal, ethical, and medical dilemma. Although there are no uniformly accepted criteria, the basic criteria for diagnosing brain death usually include:

- apnoea
- irreversible coma
- absence of brainstem reflexes
- isoelectric electroencephalogram
- no spontaneous breathing or movements
- evidence that brain dysfunction is the result of structural or metabolic disease—rather than the result of depressant drugs, alcohol, poisoning, or hypothermia.

Management of an unconscious individual

When an individual is unconscious a high standard of care must be provided, with the objectives of maintaining and restoring body function and preventing complications. Medical management involves establishment of a patent airway and provision of adequate ventilation, controlling intracranial pressure, and establishing the cause of unconsciousness and, if possible, reversing it. Nursing care of the individual involves:

- maintaining a patent airway
- monitoring neurological function
- positioning
- meeting hygiene needs
- meeting nutritional and fluid needs
- meeting elimination needs
- promoting safety
- preventing complications
- providing sensory stimulation.

Maintaining a patent airway

With the absence of cough and swallowing reflexes, secretions accumulate in the posterior pharynx and upper trachea. An oral artificial airway may be sufficient to maintain patency, or tracheostomy or endotracheal intubation and mechanical ventilation may be necessary. To prevent airway obstruction:

- The individual is positioned on alternate sides every 2–4 hours to prevent secretions accumulating in the airways on one side. The neck should be maintained in a neutral position.
- Dentures and partial plates are removed.
- Nasal and oral care is provided to keep the upper airway free of accumulated secretions and debris.
- Oronasopharyngeal suction may be necessary to aspirate secretions.
- Chest percussion and postural drainage may be prescribed to assist in the removal of tenacious secretions.

Monitoring neurological function

The individual's neurological signs are monitored at intervals which are determined by his condition. The results are documented and compared with previous assessments. Information on assessment of neurological function is provided on page 436.

Positioning

The individual is generally nursed in a lateral position (Fig. 35.6), with a small pillow placed under the head and neck to maintain the head in a neutral position. The upper arm is positioned on a pillow to maintain the shoulder in alignment, and the upper leg is supported on a pillow to maintain alignment of the hip. The individual's position is changed so that he lies on alternate sides every 2–4 hours.

If hemiplegia is present, the individual may be positioned on the affected side for brief periods, but care must be taken to prevent injury to soft tissue and nerves, oedema, or disruption of the blood supply. Because vasomotor tone is decreased in the affected areas, such adverse effects can develop rapidly from improper positioning.

If the correct position is maintained, secretions are able to drain from the individual's mouth, the tongue is less likely to obstruct the airway, and postural deformities are prevented.

Meeting hygiene needs

Care of the skin involves keeping it clean and dried, and protected from damage. Areas of the skin, particularly over the bony prominences, should be assessed regularly for the signs of impaired blood circulation and irritation which contribute to the formation of decubitus ulcers.

Dry skin may be lubricated with a suitable cream or lotion to prevent cracking and breakdown, and a water-repellant substance may be used to protect the skin against excreta or perspiration. The male should receive a facial shave as part of his daily hygiene care, the individual's nails are kept short and clean, and the hair is brushed, combed and washed as necessary.

Care of the mouth involves cleansing all areas at 2–4

hourly intervals to prevent a build-up of plaque, development of caries, and development of a focus of infection. Care must be taken to prevent aspiration of fluid while oral hygiene is being performed, therefore the individual's head is turned to one side and suction equipment made available throughout the procedure. The lips are lubricated with a suitable substance, e.g. petroleum jelly.

Care of the nose involves cleansing the nostrils to keep them free of dried mucus. Cotton wool tipped applicators and saline solution may be used to remove mucus and dried crusts, and a thin coating of cream may be applied to the rim of the nostrils.

Care of the eyes involves swabbing them with moistened cotton wool to remove secretions, the installation of artificial tears (or antibiotic eye drops if prescribed), and protecting the eyes from corneal abrasions. If the eyelids do not close fully, the use of eye shields or pads may be necessary to protect the corners.

Meeting nutritional and fluid needs

The nutritional and fluid needs of the individual must be regularly assessed and met to maintain body function, support tissue repair, and combat infection. The dietitian prescribes a nutritional programme based on consideration of the individual's energy needs, requirements for tissue repair, loss of fluid, and basic life functions. Methods of administering nutritional and fluid support to the unconscious individual include total parenteral nutrition, and enteral feedings administered via a nasogastric or gastrostomy tube.

Fluid input may be restricted to a specific amount of fluid in a 24 hour period. The purpose of fluid restriction is to control increased intracranial pressure, by keeping the individual slightly underhydrated. As his fluid input is correlated with his output, an accurate input and output record must be maintained.

Meeting elimination needs

An unconscious individual is incontinent, therefore an external urinary drainage appliance or an indwelling catheter may be used to manage urinary drainage. Both methods are used to keep the skin dry, since urinary incontinence can quickly lead to skin breakdown. Urinary drainage devices also enable an accurate calculation of urinary output. Information on care of the individual with a urinary drainage device is provided in Chapter 30.

Constipation and faecal impaction are common complications in an unconscious individual, because immobility and lack of a normal diet inhibit peristalsis. A programme is established whereby aperients and rectal suppositories are administered to promote regular bowel evacuation. The frequency of bowel actions, the amount and nature of faeces is documented.

Promoting safety

The provision and maintenance of a safe environment is of prime importance, because an unconscious individual is unable to perceive or react to safety hazards. Information on promoting safety is provided in Chapter 38.

Preventing complications

Because the unconscious individual is not mobile, he is at risk of developing any of the complications associated with immobility:

- muscle contractures
- decubitus ulcers
- venous stasis
- pulmonary stasis
- urinary stasis.

Information on prevention of these complications is provided in Chapter 37.

Providing sensory stimulation

The extent to which an unconscious individual may be aware of what is happening to and around him cannot usually be determined, therefore the nurse should *assume* that his brain is receiving some sensory input. When the duration of coma extends into weeks or months, it may seem meaningless to keep explaining each activity to an individual who gives no sign of comprehension. However some individuals, upon regaining consciousness, have been able to describe accurately events which happened to and around them while they were unconscious. Although they were unable to communicate their feelings, they were able to discriminate between the gentle caring manner of some people, and the inattentive ways of others. Some individuals have reported that they longed for some one to talk *to* them, rather than *about* them.

The nurse should, therefore, act as though the individual is conscious and demonstrate respect for him as a person. All activities should be explained to him, his privacy during procedures should be ensured, and he should be treated with dignity. Family members and friends should be encouraged to talk to, and touch, the unconscious individual. They should be encouraged to perform certain activities for the individual, e.g. comb his hair or apply skin lotion. Other sensory stimuli can be provided by playing a radio or tapes, or by placing perfumed flowers in the room.

Recovery from unconsciousness is a gradual process that tends to vary with each individual. Rehabilitation following a prolonged period of unconsciousness includes protecting the individual from orthostatic hypotension. Once he is able to tolerate a vertical position, an ambulation programme is developed—unless he has neurological deficits that makes it unfeasible. Information on rehabilitation nursing is provided in Chapter 60.

MANAGEMENT OF AN INDIVIDUAL WITH IMPAIRED MOTOR FUNCTION

Disturbance of motor function is common amongst individuals who experience disorders of the brain, spinal cord, or peripheral nerves, e.g. cerebral haemorrhage, spinal cord injury, or peripheral neuritis. While this chapter addresses the care of an individual who has experienced a cerebrovascular accident or a spinal cord injury, the principles of care can be applied to individuals who experience impaired motor function from other causes.

Terms related to impaired motor function

1. *Paresis*, is incomplete paralysis or muscle weakness.
2. *Paralysis*, is loss or impairment of the ability to move part/s of the body. Paralysis may be complete or incomplete, spastic or flaccid, symmetric or asymmetric, temporary or permanent.
3. *Hemiplegia*, is unilateral paralysis, or paralysis of one side of the body. Because nerves cross in the pyramidal tract before descending to the spinal cord, damage to one side of the brain causes hemiplegia on the opposite side of the body.
4. *Paraplegia*, is paralysis of the lower limbs and, sometimes, paralysis of the lower trunk and sphincters. Paralysis may be complete or incomplete, spastic or flaccid, temporary or permanent.
5. *Quadriplegia* (tetraplegia) is paralysis of the arms and legs, and of the body below the level of injury to the spinal cord.

Cerebrovascular accident

A cerebrovascular accident (CVA) is one of the leading causes of death in the Western world, and each year many thousands of individuals survive a CVA but are left with permanent disabilities. A cerebrovascular accident is classified as either thrombotic, embolic, or haemorrhagic.

A thrombotic CVA, the most common type, is associated with atherosclerosis—which causes narrowing of the lumen of arteries. A thrombus forms in one of the cerebral arteries, occluding the vessel, and resulting in cerebral ischaemia.

An embolic CVA occurs when an embolus-which may be part of a thrombus, fat, or other substance, is carried to the brain and occludes a cerebral blood vessel.

A haemorrhagic CVA, which is often associated with hypertension, occurs when a cerebral blood vessel ruptures—spilling blood into the brain tissue. Rupture of an artery may result from a degenerative change in the arterial wall, or from an anatomical defect, e.g. an aneurysm.

Risk factors

Educational programmes have been developed to inform the general public about CVA and prevention. Many factors have been identified as predisposing an individual to a cerebrovascular accident and, by increasing public awareness, high-risk individuals can seek medical advice to have any pre-existing conditions managed—thus reducing the risk of CVA. Risk factors include:

- a history of transient ischaemic attacks (TIA)
- atherosclerosis
- hypertension
- family history of CVA
- heart disease
- diabetes mellitus
- cigarette smoking
- use of oral contraceptives
- sedentary work with little other exercise
- obesity
- elevated cholesterol and triglyceride levels

Manifestations of a CVA

In all cases of cerebrovascular accident, areas of the brain are deprived of an adequate oxygen supply. If the blood supply is impaired for an extended period, the involved cerebral tissue may become necrotic—resulting in permanent neurological deficits. In instances of ischaemia, *temporary* neurological impairment may result.

The particular type and degree of neurological deficits depend on the area of the brain involved. Table 43.1 lists the clinical features resulting from specific artery occlusion or rupture. Table 43.4 lists a comparison of manifestations associated with right and left-sided hemiplegia.

Table 43.4 Manifestations of hemiplegia

Right-sided hemiplegia	Left-sided hemiplegia
Aphasia—expressive, receptive or global.	Spatial–perceptual deficits
Intellectual impairment	Tends to be distractible Impulsive behaviour
Slow behaviour	Appears to be unaware of deficits Poor judgement
Defects in right visual fields	Defects in left visual fields

Care of the individual

Medical management involves control of cerebral oedema and subsequent increased intracranial pressure, surgical intervention if indicated, and drug therapy. Nursing care of the individual involves:

- management during the acute phase
- meeting basic needs

- prevention of complications
- providing psychological support
- promoting rehabilitation.

Care during the acute phase

The acute phase begins when the individual is admitted, and continues until his condition is stable. Nursing care is directed toward maintaining a patent airway, and monitoring his vital and neurological signs.

Maintenance of a patient airway involves positioning the individual on his side, administering oxygen as prescribed, and suctioning secretions from his airway.

Care must be taken when performing oronasopharyngeal suction, as suction applied for longer than 15 seconds at a time may increase intracranial pressure.

A record of fluid input and output is kept to monitor kidney function, and to evaluate fluid and electrolyte balance.

Assessment of vital and neurological signs is performed frequently, e.g. every 15–30 minutes, to detect changes in the individuals condition. Information on neurological assessment is provided on page 436.

If the individual is *unconscious*, the principles of care described on pages 439–441 should be incorporated.

Care following the acute phase

Detailed information about the nursing measures necessary to meet the individuals basic needs for hygiene, safety, elimination, nutrition and fluid, psychological support, mobility and rehabilitation, are provided elsewhere in this text. The nurse should refer to the index.

The main aims of care for an individual who has experienced a cerebrovascular accident are to:

- assist him to meet his hygiene needs
- monitor vital and neurological signs
- maintain muscle tone and prevent contractures
- prevent skin breakdown
- prevent venous stasis (thrombus and embolus formation)
- prevent and manage alterations in elimination, e.g. incontinence, retention of urine, constipation
- maintain nutritional and fluid status
- establish an adequate means of communication
- promote reorientation, of a confused individual
- enhance self concept and body image
- institute a rehabilitation programme aimed at achieving an optimal level of independence.

Rehabilitation

Rehabilitation of the individual begins when he is admitted to hospital, and continues for as long as necessary-including after his discharge home. In some health care in-stitutions, the individual may be transferred to a rehabilitation unit following the acute phase of his illness. The focus of rehabilitation is directed at helping the individual to relearn lost skills so that he can be as independent as possible.

The individual, and his significant others, are made aware of the plan and goals of the rehabilitative phase, and their active participation is encouraged. Recovery from a CVA is a slow process, therefore the nurse must provide support and positive feedback so the individual does not become discouraged. Rehabilitation of the individual includes:

- encouraging him to participate in his own care as much as possible.
- teaching him to perform the activities of living with regard to ways of compensating for any disabilities.
- teaching, and assisting, him to perform transfer activities, e.g. bed to chair.
- assisting him to regain any lost communication skills.
- encouraging him to express his feelings, in order to decrease anxiety and to allow for correction of any misunderstood information.
- developing a bladder and bowel retraining programme (if necessary).

Further information on rehabilitation nursing is provided in Chapter 60.

Planning for discharge

Discharge planning is directed at facilitating the transition from the health care institution to the home environment. Discharge planning involves assessment of the individual and his family, identification of specific needs, planning to implement ways of meeting those needs, and evaluation of the discharge process and the results. Once the individual is discharged home, he and the family must have contact with support services, e.g. the district nurse, with whom they can rely on for continued help and support.

Spinal cord injury

Injuries involving the spinal cord result most often from motor vehicle accidents, falls, sporting and industrial accidents, and firearm or stab wounds. Injuries to the vertebral column and spinal cord result from forces applied directly or indirectly to the head, neck, or trunk. Damage to the spinal cord and nerve roots results from:

- compression by displaced bone or, ligaments, extruded disc, or haematoma formation.
- excessive stretching, crushing, shearing, or severance of neural tissue.
- swelling in response to bruising or compression.
- impaired capillary circulation and venous return.

There are four possible vectors (forces) that can be applied to the spinal column to cause injury.

1. Flexion. Excessive flexion (hyperflexion) tends to produce compression of the vertebral bodies, with disruption of the posterior ligaments and the intervertebral discs. *Hyperflexion* injuries are caused by hyperflexion of the head and neck -as in sudden deceleration.

2. Extension. Excessive extension (hyperextension) usually causes fractures of the posterior elements of the vertebral column and disruption of the anterior ligaments. *Hyperextension* injuries are caused by hyperextension of the head and neck as may occur in a rear-end vehicular accident.

3. Rotation (lateral flexion). Excessive rotation is most likely to produce rupture of the ligaments, fracture, and fracture dislocation of the vertebral facets. *Rotational* injuries are caused by extreme lateral flexion, or rotation, of the head and neck.

4. Compression. Compression can result in fractures of the vertebral body and arch, and rupture of the supporting ligaments. *Compression* injuries are caused by vertical pressure as when a person falls from a height and lands on his feet or buttocks.

Classification of spinal cord injuries

Spinal cord injuries can be classified by the type of injury and by syndromes.

Concussion. Severe shaking of the spinal cord which causes temporary loss of function, lasting approximately 24–48 hours.

Contusion. Contusion refers to bruising of the spinal cord, which includes bleeding into the cord.

Laceration. A laceration is an actual tear in the spinal cord.

Transection. A transection is severing of the cord, and it may be complete or incomplete.

Haemorrhage. Bleeding into, or around the cord. Escaped blood is an irritant to the delicate tissue.

Anterior cord syndrome. This is due to injury of the anterior part of the spinal cord, and is associated with flexion injuries and fracture—dislocations of the vertebrae.

Manifestations include loss of pain and temperature sensation, as well as motor function, below the level of the injury. The sensations of light touch, position, and vibration remain intact.

Posterior cord syndrome. This is a rare syndrome in which the senses of position and vibration are involved.

Central cord syndrome. This is due to injury and/or oedema to the central cord in the cervical region, e.g. as a result of hyperextension injuries.

Manifestations include a greater loss of motor function in the upper limbs (rather than the lower), bladder dysfunction, and varying degrees of sensory impairement.

Brown-Sequard syndrome. This results from open penetrating wounds that produce transverse hemisection of the cord.

Manifestations include loss of pain and temperature sensation on the side opposite the injury; and loss of motor function, light touch, position, and vibratory sensation on the side of the injury.

Manifestations of spinal cord injury

Generally, the degree of damage to the spinal cord at any level is described as incomplete or complete transection.

Incomplete transection of the cord produces loss or impairment of sensation and motor function that reflects the specific nerve tracts which have been damaged.

Complete transection of the cord results in permanent loss of voluntary movement, sensation, reflex and autonomic function below the level of injury.

Spinal shock

Spinal shock is an immediate response to an acute spinal cord injury, and is the temporary suppression of reflexes controlled by the segments below the level of injury.

After a period that may vary from hours to months, the spinal neurones gradually regain their excitability. Subsequent return of some function results from decompression of the cord as oedema resolves.

Functional loss from spinal cord injury

The different functions and dysfunctions associated with spinal cord injuries at specific levels, are listed in Table 43.5.

The effects of spinal cord injury on sexual response vary depending on the level and degree of injury. Sexual function is controlled by spinal levels S2, S3, and S4.

Knowledge of the physiology of alterations in sexual response following spinal cord injury is incomplete, and significant individual differences exist. Individuals with complete loss of sensation in the genitalia may still experience orgasm in response to sensations produced by stimulation of other areas of the body in which sensation is intact. Sexual pleasure can also be increased by psychological stimuli, e.g. memory, sight, sound, and odour.

Physical stimulation of the genitalia may produce reflex erection of the penis and vaginal lubrication—even though there is no sensory awareness of stimulation.

Care of the individual with spinal cord injury

The management of the individual at the scene of the accident is critical to his ultimate neurological outcome. The basic objectives of first aid management at the scene are to:

Table 43.5 Spinal cord injury—functional loss

Level of injury	Motor function	Sensory function	Bladder/bowel function	Ventilatory function
C1–C4	Loss of all function from the neck down	Loss of sensation from the neck down	No bladder or bowel control	Loss of independent ventilatory function
C5	Loss of all function below the upper shoulders	Loss of sensation below the clavicles	No bladder or bowel control	Phrenic nerve is intact, but the intercostal muscles are non-functional
C6	Loss of all function below the upper arms	Loss of sensation below the clavicles, but has some arm and thumb sensation	No bladder or bowel control	Phrenic nerve is intact, but the intercostal muscles are non-functional
C7	Incomplete quadriplegia. Loss of motor control to parts of the arms and hands	Loss of sensation below the clavicles, but has some arm and hand sensation	No bladder or bowel control	Phrenic nerve is intact, but the intercostal muscles are non-functional
C8	Incomplete quadriplegia Loss of motor control to parts of the arms and hands	Loss of sensation below the chest, and part of the hands	No bladder or bowel control	Phrenic nerve is intact, but the intercostal muscles are non-functional
T1–T6	Loss of function below the mid-chest	Loss of sensation from the mid-chest down	No bladder or bowel control	Independent phrenic nerve function, some intercostal muscle impairment
T6–T12	Loss of function below the waist	Loss of sensation below the waist	No bladder or bowel control	No interference to ventilatory function
L1–L2	Loss of most of the control of pelvis and legs	Loss of sensation to lower abdomen and legs	No bladder or bowel control	No interference to ventilatory function
L3–L4	Loss of control of part of the lower legs, and feet	Loss of sensation to part of the lower legs, and feet	No bladder or bowel control	No interference to ventilatory function
L5–S5	Loss of control of parts of the hips, knees, ankles, feet	Loss of sensation to parts of the lower limbs, and perineum	May or may not be loss of bladder and/or bowel control	No interference to ventilatory function

- prevent death from asphyxia
- prevent further spinal cord damage from torsion, flexion, or extension of the unstable spine
- transport the individual rapidly and safely to an appropriate facility.

Further information on the first aid management of spinal injuries is provided in Chapter 57.

Subsequent management of the individual involves emergency department care, early management, post acute and long term management.

Initial management

On arrival in the accident and emergency department the medical officer assesses the individual, and X-rays are taken to determine the extent of the injuries. The medical officer develops a plan of care which may include immediate surgery, a non-surgical approach with traction and immobilization; and the insertion of a nasogastric tube, indwelling urinary catheter, and intravenous infusion. Generally, glucocorticoid steroids are prescribed to reduce cord swelling.

Early management

After initial assessment and stabilization of the individual he is admitted to the intensive care or spinal unit. An individual with less severe injuries may be admitted to a general ward.

The medical management will depend on the type of spinal cord injury, and any associated injuries. Treatment may be surgical, non-surgical, or a combination of both approaches.

Surgical management may take the form of decompression laminectomy, fusion, open or closed reduction of fractures or dislocations, or the insertion of rods.

Non-surgical management involves immobilization of the spine (Fig. 43.4) using skeletal tongs with traction, halo traction, a cervical collar, or a device designed to maintain thoracic or lumbar alignment, e.g. a fiberglass body jacket.

Nursing care of the individual

Nursing management will vary according to the individual's injury and the a surgical or non-surgical approach selected. However, the major aspects of care are

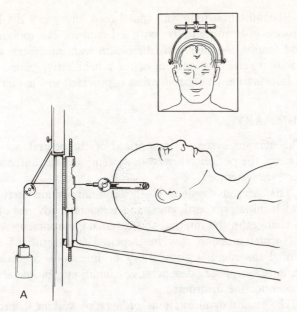

Fig. 43.4 Immobilization of the spine. (A) Cervical traction with tongs. The inset shows the position of the tongs on the bone structure of the skull.

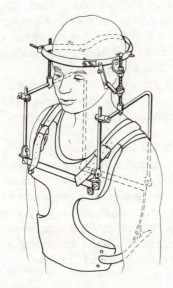

Fig. 43.4 (B) Halo traction and vest.

directed toward maintaining respiratory function, immobilization and alignment of the spine, preventing complications, meeting basic needs, providing psychological support, and rehabilitation.

Respiratory care

An individual with a spinal cord injury can develop varying degrees of respiratory difficulty, depending on the level of spinal injury. The individual will require a plan of care directed at preventing pulmonary complications. Intuba-

tion and mechanical ventilation will be required if there is impairment of respiratory muscle function. The programme of care includes:

- regular assessment for indications of inadequate ventilation
- chest physiotherapy at least every 4 hours
- maintenance of a patent airway
- use of an incentive spirometer to promote lung expansion.

Immobilization and alignment of the spine

Once alignment of the spine is achieved, immobilization serves to maintain that alignment and promotes healing at the site of injury.

For most thoracic, lumbar, or sacral injuries, the individual remains confined to bed with his back positioned and supported to achieve hyperextension of the spine at the site of injury. A bed with a firm mattress and fracture board, and correctly positioned pillows are necessary to maintain the prescribed posture.

When the injury involves dislocation or fracture-dislocation of the cervical or high thoracic spine, skeletal traction is commonly used to accomplish alignment and immobilization.

Skeletal traction may be achieved by means of cervical tongs, e.g. Crutchfield tongs, or by the halo device. The halo device may also be incorporated with the use of a body vest or jacket to stabilize the spine—thereby allowing the individual to be ambulatory. When skeletal traction is used, the individual may be nursed on a firm mattress and fracture board, or on a special bed, e.g. a Stryker frame.

Once skeletal traction is established, pain is decreased, and the individual's comfort is enhanced. He can be safely turned, using a special technique (as described in Chapter 37) to allow for skin care and a change of position. Management of the individual in cervical skeletal traction includes:

- Checking the traction equipment every 2–4 hours to ensure safety and integrity of the treatment.
- Inspecting, cleansing, and dressing the tong sites according to the institution's policy, e.g. every 4–8 hours.
- Changing the individual's position every 2 hours, to prevent the complications of immobility. The 'log-rolling' technique, or the stryker frame, is used to turn the individual, in order to maintain the vertebral column in neutral position. Information on the 'log-rolling' technique is provided in Chapter 37.
- Using various devices, e.g. pillows, a footboard, a cervical roll, to maintain good body alignment. When the individual lies supine, the arms and legs are positioned in extension with support to maintain the feet in dorsiflexion. The hands are placed in a functional position, and a cer-

vical roll is used to maintain hyperextension of the neck. When the individual is in a lateral position, the arms and legs are positioned in extension, and pillows are placed to support this position.

Preventing complications

Because prolonged immobility can lead to various complications, specific preventive measures must be implemented. Information on prevention of the complications associated with immobility is provided in Chapter 37.

Meeting basic needs

The individual with impaired motor and sensory function will require assistance to meet his needs for hygiene, safety, elimination, nutrition and fluids, temperature regulation, and pain relief. Information on assisting the individual to meet his basic needs is provided in Chapters 28–40.

Providing psychological support

A severe spinal cord injury has a devastating effect on the individual, and his significant others, and they will experience a range of emotional responses—from the time of injury through the rehabilitation process. The individual will have to adapt to the loss of motor function, and sensory deprivation—both of which severely threaten his self concept and body image.

It is important that the nurse is aware of the impact that the injury has on the individual's emotional and psychological equilibrium. She must be sensitive to the emotional and psychological response of the individual to his injury, and support him as he deals with the impact of his injury. The nurse can help to support the individual by:

- establishing a climate of trust
- accepting his behaviour, without being judgmental
- encouraging him to express feelings
- listening empathetically and attentively
- allowing him to make decisions and maintain control
- providing information as necessary
- supporting a positive self concept and self esteem
- letting him know that it will take time to adjust to the disability.

Promoting rehabilitation

In most instances of spinal cord injury, the individual will require long-term rehabilitation.

Rehabilitation following spinal cord injury is a life-long process of learning to live with a disability. The individual and family, together with the health team members, contribute to the development of the rehabilitative plans.

Information on rehabilitation is provided in Chapter 60.

SUMMARY

The nervous system is comprised of the central nervous system, the peripheral nervous system, and the autonomic nervous system.

The nervous system is the communication network which initiates, coordinates, and regulates body responses to changes in the internal and external environments.

Normal function may be impaired as a result of congenital disorders, inflammatory or infectious conditions, trauma, neoplasia, degenerative conditions, or metabolic and endocrine disorders.

The major manifestations of nervous system disorders are headaches, sensory changes, motor changes, reflex changes, altered states of awareness or consciousness, and seizures.

Disorders of the nervous system can be classified as those occurring from congenital or hereditary defects, from multiple causes, degenerative disorders, immunologic disorders, infectious or inflammatory conditions, neoplastic or obstructive disorders, and trauma.

Diagnostic tests used to assess nervous system function include the neurological examination, radiographic examination, magnetic resonance imaging, electroencephalography.

Care of the individual with a nervous system disorder includes promoting a clear airway, maintaining fluid and nutritional status, preventing and managing alterations in elimination, promoting effective communication, promoting safety, promoting mobility, preventing the complications, of immobility, providing psychological support, assessing neurological status, providing a suitable environment, and promoting rehabilitation.

REFERENCES AND FURTHER READING

Game C, Anderson R, Kidd J (eds) 1989 Medical-surgical nursing: a core text. Churchill Livingstone, Melbourne, 146–226
Brunner L S, Suddarth D S 1988 Textbook of medical-surgical nursing, 6th edn. J B Lippincott, Philadelphia
Boore J, Champion R, Ferguson M (eds) 1987 Care of the physically ill adult. Churchill Livingstone, Edinburgh

44. The individual with a circulatory system disorder

INTRODUCTION

Information on the normal structure and function of the circulatory system (cardiovascular and lymphatic systems) is provided in Chapter 21, and it should be referred to before studying the contents of this chapter.

The heart pumps the blood which is transported throughout the body in arteries, veins, and capillaries. The lymphatic system, through its action of filtering wastes and foreign substances from the lymph, plays a major role in the body's defence against infection.

Cells which are temporarily deprived of blood will not function normally, and continued disruption of blood supply causes irreversible damage or cell death. As an adequate supply of blood is necessary for the normal function of every cell, any factor that disrupts the flow of blood to or from the tissues can result in serious consequences for all body systems.

Prevention of cardiovascular disease

The nurse has a responsibility to be aware of the factors which contribute to the development of coronary heart disease and peripheral vascular disease, so that she can advise and educate people on preventive measures. Primary prevention of cardiovascular disease involves public awareness of major risk factors. Education aims to encourage people to:

- avoid cigarette smoking
- control body weight within the recommendations for height and build
- exercise regularly
- obtain adequate rest and relaxation
- follow a diet which is low in saturated fats, but which contains polyunsaturated fats; is low in salt, and high in fibre
- restrict alcohol consumption
- avoid prolonged or intense stress or use measures to help alleviate stress.

Pathophysiological influences and effects

The pathophysiological changes that disrupt the normal function of the circulatory system include those that affect the heart's ability to pump blood, those which impede the flow of blood through the blood vessels, those that impair blood formation or function and those which disrupt the return of filtered lymph to the circulation.

Changes in cardiac function

Cardiac failure occurs when the heart is unable to maintain an output of blood sufficient to meet the body's requirements and, as a result, the body tissues become ischaemic.

Cardiac failure may result from mechanical failure due to valvular disease, obstruction to the blood flow, congenital heart disease, atherosclerosis, or hypertension. Cardiac failure can also occur as a consequence of a disease process, e.g. cardiomyopathy or myocardial infarction, or as the result of normal ageing.

Consequently the heart's ability to pump blood is diminished.

When the heart fails to meet the requirements of the body, compensatory mechanisms occur in an attempt to improve cardiac output and to maintain the blood pressure. These compensatory responses are the sympathetic response, the renal response, and myocardial hypertrophy.

The sympathetic response is stimulated by reduced cardiac output, and results in increased heart rate, dilation of the coronary and cerebral arterioles, and constriction of the renal and skin arterioles. As a result, essential life functions are maintained.

The renal response results in the secretion of substances which stimulate the production of aldosterone, causing vasoconstriction and retention of sodium and water. Consequently, the increased peripheral resistance and blood volume increases the work load of the heart.

Myocardial hypertrophy results from prolonged increase in myocardial wall tension and, while this initially maintains cardiac output, eventually cardiac output and tissue perfusion are decreased.

Changes in the blood vessels

Disturbances in the ability of the arteries to stretch and recoil as blood is pumped from the heart, or changes in the ability of the veins to return the blood to the heart, result in ischaemia of the tissues.

The ability of *arteries* to stretch and recoil may be affected by conditions such as atherosclerosis, obstruction from inflammation or arterial spasms, or from excessive external pressure on an artery. When an artery is narrowed or constricted it is unable to transport sufficient blood to the area it supplies, resulting in ischaemia and possible tissue death.

The ability of *veins* to return blood to the heart may be affected by conditions such as impaired valves, lack of use of the muscles that assist venous flow, or from excessive external pressure on a vein. When blood flow through a vein is impeded, pooling of blood in the vein occurs. The pressure inside the vein increases and causes oedema in the surrounding tissues. Chronic venous insufficiency can result in thrombophlebitis, stasis cellulitis, and stasis ulcers.

The formation of an *embolus* can cause obstruction of an artery or a vein. The most common embolus is a blood clot (thrombus), although an embolus can also consist of air or fat. When the thrombus, or part of it, becomes dislodged from the vessel wall it travels in the bloodstream until it reaches a blood vessel which is too narrow for its passage. As a result blood flow beyond that area is obstructed, and the ultimate consequence may be death of the tissues which are deprived of adequate blood.

Changes in the blood

Haemoglobin in the erythrocytes is responsible for transporting oxygen in the bloodstream. Any condition that affects the normal production or function of erythrocytes may decrease the supply of oxygen to the tissues. Conditions which may impede erythrocyte formation or function include bone marrow aplasia, metabolic abnormalities, nutritional deficiencies, chronic or acute blood loss, drugs, toxins, ionizing radiation, and genetic abnormalities. Tissue hypoxia results in a compensatory high output of erythrocytes (polycythemia), which causes the blood to become viscous and less able to flow easily.

Leucocytes protect the body from infection through phagocytosis and the production of antibodies. Any disorder that decreases the production or maturation of leucocytes renders the individual susceptible to overwhelming infection. Conditions which may impede leucocyte production or function include inadequate blood cell production, proliferation of immature leucocytes, drug reactions, ionizing radiation, nutritional deficiencies, and bone marrow hypoplasia.

Thrombocytes are necessary for the clotting of blood. Any disorder that impairs thrombocyte production or function renders the individual susceptible to bleeding. A decrease, or increase, in the formation of thrombocytes generally occurs in association with other disorders.

Thrombocytopenia (decrease in thrombocytes) may be idiopathic or may result from bone marrow disease. It may also result from a condition which causes thrombocyte destruction, e.g. cirrhosis of the liver, or drug toxicity. Thrombocythaemia (increase in thrombocytes) is frequently idiopathic, but it may also accompany some disorders such as polycythaemia or chronic myeloid leukaemia.

Changes in the lymphatic system

The lymphatic system removes fluid and particles from the interstitial spaces, filters the lymph, and returns it to the circulation. Impaired lymphatic function may result from obstruction or inflammation of the lymphatic vessels or nodes, or from neoplastic disease. When lymphatic function is impaired fluid accumulates in the interstitial spaces, and oedema results.

As the function of lymphocytes is the key factor in immune responses, diseases of the lymphatic system, e.g. Hodgkin's disease, may seriously impair the immune processes. The individual with immunodeficiency is vulnerable to infection and other pathological processes that would normally be inhibited by a healthy immune system.

Major manifestations of circulatory system disorders

The manifestations of disorders of the circulatory system

vary depending on whether the disorder is one which affects the heart, the blood vessels, or the blood or blood forming organs.

Manifestations of cardiac disorders

Dyspnoea, which is difficult or laboured breathing, is the most common (and often the earliest) symptom of cardiac disease. Typically the dyspnoea occurs with exertion although, as cardiac disease progresses, the individual may experience dyspnoea at rest.

Paroxysmal nocturnal dyspnoea, which is associated with congestive cardiac failure, occurs during sleep, and the individual awakens suddenly with difficulty in breathing and a sensation of suffocation.

Chest pain may result from myocardial ischaemia or from pericarditis. Chest pain can also be caused by conditions not associated with cardiac disease, e.g. pleurisy, musculoskeletal disorders, or stress and anxiety.

Ischaemic pain is the result of a deficiency of blood to the myocardium, caused by a blocked or constricted blood vessel. *Angina* (pectoris) is pain which results from a diminished supply of oxygen to the heart, and is basically a reversible ischaemic process. *Acute myocardial infarction* represents the point where ischaemia becomes irreversible, blood flow to part of the heart is completely interrupted, and cardiac muscle necrosis results.

Table 44.1 Patterns of cardiac pain

Angina	Myocardial infarction
Gradual or sudden onset	Sudden onset
Episodic and temporary, usually lasting from 3–15 minutes	Lasts longer than 15 minutes
Substernal or anterior, not sharply localized. Radiates to back, neck, arms, jaw	Substernal, midline or anterior. Radiates to jaw, neck, back, shoulders, or one or both arms
Sensation of mild to moderate pressure. Described as tightness, squeezing or crushing	Persistant sensation of severe pressure. Described as crushing, heavy, vice-like, squeezing
Precipitated by exertion, stress, ingestion of food, exposure to cold	Not necessarily related to exertion or emotion, and may occur at rest
Accompanied by dyspnoea, diaphoresis, nausea, apprehension	Accompanied by nausea, vomiting, dyspnoea, apprehension, diaphoresis, a sensation of 'impending doom', pallor, cold clammy skin
Individual keeps still to relieve the pain	Individual moves about in search of a comfortable position
Relieved by rest and/or nitroglycerine	Not relieved by rest or nitroglycerine

Table 44.1 illustrates the characteristics of angina and myocardial infarction pain.

Palpitation is a sensation of fluttering in the chest which produces an awareness of the heart's action. The individual may describe his heart's action as racing, pounding, stopping, or skipping beats. Palpitations may be due to rhythm disturbances such as premature contractions; but they can also result from anxiety, stress, caffeine or nicotine, and fatigue.

Cough may be associated with certain cardiovascular diseases, which cause an accumulation of fluid in the lungs (pulmonary oedema).

Fatigue frequently accompanies cardiac dysfunction, and is thought to be related to inadequate cardiac output resulting in insufficient blood flow to the tissues.

Cyanosis, which is a blue discolouration of the skin or mucous membranes, appears when haemoglobin oxygen saturation is greatly reduced. Central cyanosis is evident in all areas of the body particularly in the lips, mucous membranes, and nail beds; whereas peripheral cyanosis is evident mainly in the extremities.

Syncope, which is transient loss of consciousness, may result when cardiac dysfunction causes an inadequate flow of blood to the brain. A sudden loss of consciousness due to heart block is known as a Stokes-Adams attack.

Oedema, which is a local or generalized accumulation of excess fluid in the tissues, may result from certain cardiac diseases. Oedema generally develops first in the lowest, or dependent, parts of the body, e.g. the legs and the sacral area. As venous stasis increases, oedema increases. In some forms of cardiac failure fluid accumulates in the lungs (pulmonary oedema), and in advanced cardiac failure total body oedema may develop. The severity of the oedema will depend on the degree to which venous return and/or cardiac output are reduced.

Pulse rate, volume or rhythm may be abnormal in the presence of cardiac dysfunction. Tachycardia may accompany cardiac failure, while 'heart block' commonly results in bradycardia. A low cardiac output, and therefore a reduced pulse volume, is associated with cardiac failure and acute myocardial infarction. Certain cardiac disorders cause dysrhythmias which are accompanied by an irregular pulse.

Manifestations of peripheral blood vessel disorders

Intermittent claudication is cramping pain in a muscle of the leg, and it is brought on by exercise but relieved by rest. Commonly, the pain is experienced in the calf muscle during walking, and it is thought to be due to the accumulation of lactic acid in the tissues—rather than to ischaemia of the contracting muscle.

Generally, intermittent claudication results from a blockage of the superficial femoral artery, e.g. due to atherosclerosis.

Leg pain during rest occurs when chronic arterial oc-clusive disease is advanced, or when a vessel is blocked by a thrombus or embolus. As a result the blood supply to the surrounding tissues is diminished, causing ischaemic pain.

Pale, cold extremities indicate an impaired blood flow to the limb. If an artery is suddenly occluded by a throm-bus or embolus, there will be numbness and absence of distal pulses as well as coldness and pallor.

Leg ulcers or cellulitis may be present. Chronic occlu-sion of arterioles and small arteries results in ischaemia, skin breakdown and ulceration. Pooling of venous blood in the tissues of the extremities, e.g. as a result of varicose veins, may lead to venous stasis ulcers.

Aching or a feeling of fullness or heaviness in the legs may be experienced, and is associated with venous insufficiency.

Gangrene, which is death of tissue, may occur as a result of chronic arterial insufficiency and is the consequence of severe and prolonged ischaemia. Gangrene first develops in the most distal parts of the lower limbs.

Altered peripheral pulses may be present when arterial blood flow is impeded. Diminished or absent pulses sug-gest partial or total occlusion of an artery, e.g. if the popliteal pulse is absent, the superficial femoral artery may be occluded.

Homan's sign may be positive in the presence of throm-bophlebitis. A positive Homan's sign is present when dorsiflexion of the foot (with the knee bent) produces pain in the calf.

Tenderness, firmness and swelling in the calf are also suggestive of deep-vein thrombophlebitis.

Manifestations of blood and blood-forming organ disorders

Bruising and bleeding may occur when there is abnor-mal thrombocyte production or function, or when there is absence of clotting factors in the plasma. The appearance of any bruising or haemorrhagic spots in the absence of injury is suggestive of a blood disorder. Types of bruising and bleeding include:

- *Purpura*, which are haemorrhagic areas under the skin and in the mucous membranes. If the haemorrhages are small they are termed petechiae, and larger purpuric areas are called bruises or ecchymoses.
- *Petechiae*, which are red-brown pinpoint haemorrhages in the skin. Petechiae can occur over any part of the skin, but are most common where pressure has been applied to a body part.
- *Ecchymoses*, which are haemorrhagic spots larger than petechiae. They may be precipitated by an injury or may occur spontaneously.
- *Gastrointestinal bleeding*, which appears as haematemesis and melaena. It may occur in certain

disorders of the blood, e.g. thrombocytopenia.

- *Menorrhagia or haematuria*, which may also occur in haemorrhagic disorders.
- *Neurological changes*, e.g. headaches, blurred vision, disorientation, or altered consciousness, which may occur if there is bleeding within the central nervous system.

Changes in the skin may accompany disorders of the blood or blood-forming organs. Changes which may occur include pallor, jaundice, and pruritus.

Fatigue or weakness are common manifestations of many haematologic disorders, e.g. anaemia and leukaemia. An individual with anaemia may also experience shortness of breath, particularly on exertion.

Enlarged lymph nodes may be present in disorders such as Hodgkin's disease or leukaemia.

Pain may be experienced in many haematologic dis-orders, e.g. bleeding into a joint may result in joint pain, and bone pain can occur in leukaemia or lymphoma.

Specific disorders of the circulatory system

Disorders of the circulatory system may be congenital, due to multiple causes, infectious, neoplastic or obstructive, de-generative, or may be the result of trauma.

Congenital disorders

Ventricular septal defect is an opening in the septum between the ventricles, allowing blood to shunt between the left and right ventricles. During fetal development the ventricular septum fails to close completely and, although the defect is not readily apparent at birth, manifestations of the disorder become evident approximately 4–8 weeks later. Manifestations vary with the size of the defect, and small defects may eventually close spontaneously without causing any symptoms.

Larger defects cause hypertrophy of the left atrium and both ventricles. Eventually, cyanosis and congestive car-diac failure will occur. The infant is slow to gain weight, experiences difficulties with feeding; and has a dusky skin colour, tachycardia, and rapid grunting respirations.

Atrial septal defect is an opening between the left and right atria, allowing blood to shunt between the two cham-bers. The blood shunts from left to right, which eventually causes enlargement of the right atrium and right ventricle. Sometimes the direction of the shunt is reversed, and this leads to the entry of deoxygenated blood into the systemic circulation. The condition may be undetected during child-hood, unless a large defect results in retarded growth. Manifestations during adulthood include extreme fatigue, dyspnoea on exertion, cyanosis, and clubbing of the fingers.

Coarctation of the aorta, which is a localized narrowing of the aorta, is generally associated with other congenital cardiac abnormalities. The aortic constriction results in increased pressure above the defect, and decreased pressure below the constriction. The resultant hypertension causes ventricular hypertrophy which, if untreated, may lead to cardiac failure.

The condition may be asymptomatic during infancy, or the signs of congestive cardiac failure may be evident: dyspnoea, tachypnoea, pallor, and failure to thrive. In adulthood, the defect produces dyspnoea, intermittent claudication, headaches, diminished femoral pulses, and hypertension.

Patent ductus arteriosus occurs when the lumen of the ductus arteriosus, which connects the pulmonary artery to the descending aorta, fails to close after birth. As a result, blood is shunted from the aorta to the pulmonary artery causing recirculation of arterial blood through the lungs. Initially the defect may produce no symptoms, but a large defect usually causes respiratory distress and signs of congestive cardiac failure.

Tetralogy of Fallot is a condition where there are four congenital cardiac defects:

- ventricular septal defect
- pulmonary stenosis
- right ventricular hypertrophy
- malposition of the aorta.

Blood shunts from right to left through the ventricular defect, allowing deoxygenated blood to mix with oxygenated blood. Manifestations of this complex disorder include cyanosis, with cyanotic episodes precipitated by exertion, crying, or infection. The child also experiences dyspnoea, bradycardia, and syncope. In the older child other signs of poor oxygenation, e.g. finger clubbing and increasing dyspnoea on exertion, develop.

Transposition of the great arteries is a disorder in which the arteries are reversed: the aorta arises from the right ventricle, and the pulmonary artery arises from the left ventricle. As a result, there are two noncommunicating circulatory systems; pulmonary and systemic. Within a few hours after birth, the infant experiences cyanosis, tachypnoea, and dyspnoea—each of which increases with crying. After a period of days or weeks the infant generally develops signs of congestive cardiac failure. Other manifestations include fatigue, low activity tolerance, and bouts of coughing.

Thalassemias are a group of disorders in which there is an inherited defect of haemoglobin synthesis—which causes haemolysis, anaemia, and ineffective erythropoiesis. The thalassemias are most common in individuals of Mediterranean origin, and the disorder may be either thalassemia major or thalassemia minor. Thalassemia major is the more serious form creating profound anaemia, whereas thalassemia minor may cause only mild anaemia.

Manifestations of thalassemia major usually appear 3–6 months after birth and include pallor, enlarged spleen and liver, bleeding tendencies, and anorexia. Older children with this disorder become susceptible to pathological fractures, cardiac arrhythmias, and heart failure.

Sickle cell anaemia is a disorder in which the erythrocytes are abnormally shaped.

Sickle cell anaemia is relatively common in individuals of negroid origin, and the disorder is inherited as an autosomal dominant trait. The haemoglobin in the sickle cells is abnormal which results in distortion and fragility of the erythrocytes, which become more susceptible to haemolysis. As a consequence there are widespread vascular problems due to thrombosis and infarction, and anaemia due to excessive destruction of erythrocytes.

Manifestation of sickle cell anaemia generally occurs as a result of sickle cell crisis, whereby the sickle cells cause occlusion of blood vessels, anoxia, and tissue death. Manifestations depend on which organ or part of the body is affected by an occlusive sickle cell crisis. Pain is a common symptom, and the main areas of the body which may be affected include the spleen, brain, eyes, liver, lungs, and bones.

Haemophilia is an hereditary bleeding disorder resulting from a deficiency of specific clotting factors. Haemophilia A results from a deficiency of Factor VIII, whereas haemophilia B (Christmas disease) results from a deficiency of Factor IX. The decrease of factors VIII or IX makes the individual susceptible to bleeding episodes, which may be mild to moderate or severe depending on the degree of the factor deficiency.

Typically, mild haemophilia causes easy bruising, haematomas, epistaxis, and prolonged bleeding after an injury. Bleeding into a joint (haemarthrosis) may also occur.

Severe haempohilia causes spontaneous bleeding or severe bleeding after minor injuries. Bleeding into muscles or joints causes swelling, pain, and possible permanent deformity. Bleeding near peripheral nerves causes neuropathies, pain, and paresthesia. Intracranial bleeding causes neurological symptoms, and may result in death.

Signs of hypovolaemic shock will be evident when large quantities of blood are lost from the circulation.

Von Willebrand's disease is an hereditary bleeding disorder characterized by prolonged bleeding time, deficiency of Factor VIII, and impaired thrombocyte function. This disorder results in easy bruising, epistaxis and bleeding from the gums. Severe forms of the disorder can result in haemorrhage after accidental injury or surgery, gastrointestinal bleeding, or menorrhagia. Typically, bleeding episodes occur sporadically, and the disorder decreases in severity as the individual ages.

Disorders of multiple cause

Hypertension, which means high arterial blood pressure, is generally classified as either primary (essential) or secondary hypertension.

Primary hypertension is the most common form and, while the cause is often unknown, many factors have been implicated as contributing to its development, e.g. high sodium intake, obesity, genetic factors, alcohol, cigarette smoking, and psychosocial factors.

Malignant hypertension is the term used to describe primary hypertension when there is a rapid rise of blood pressure to a high level, e.g. 250/150 mmHg. It is accompanied by severe headache, visual disturbances, and oliguria. If untreated, death may occur rapidly due to cardiac or renal failure, or cerebrovascular accident.

Secondary hypertension is caused by either disease or certain medications. Diseases which result in secondary hypertension include those where renal, vascular, endocrine, or neurological mechanisms are involved, e.g. renal artery disease, phaeochromocytoma, intracranial lesions. Medications which may lead to secondary hypertension include oral contraceptives, corticosteroids, and monoamine oxidase inhibitors.

Hypertension is frequently *asymptomatic* until the individual experiences a major problem such as cerebral haemorrhage, renal failure, or myocardial infarction. Symptoms which may be due to hypertension include dizziness, chest pain, palpitations, epistaxis, headaches, and brief episodes of memory loss (transient ischaemic attacks).

Coronary artery (ischaemic heart) disease is a disorder in which the arteries that supply blood to the heart muscle become diseased, and fail to supply the heart with sufficient blood. Atherosclerosis is the most common cause of coronary artery disease, causing disturbances of blood flow within the coronary arteries which gives rise to altered myocardial perfusion and disruption of the electrical cycle controlling heart rhythm.

Atherosclerosis is a narrowing of the arteries as a result of deposits of lipids in and around the smooth muscle, roughening of the endothelial lining, loss of elasticity with fibrosis and calcification. Eventually, the artery becomes occluded, inelastic and incapable of dilating. Although the precise cause of atherosclerosis and coronary artery disease is unclear, there is general agreement that many factors contribute to its development, e.g. genetic influences, sex (males are more commonly affected), hypertension, lack of exercise, cigarette smoking, stress, metabolic or endocrine disorders, obesity, and dietary factors. The dietary factors that are considered to contribute to coronary artery disease are salt, saturated fats, and lack of dietary fibre.

Coronary artery disease may be *asymptomatic* until the individual experiences a myocardial infarction, which may result in sudden death. Some individuals may experience *angina*, which is the classic symptom of ischaemic heart disease. Angina is described earlier in this chapter.

Myocardial infarction is the death of part of the myocardium as a result of severe or total deprivation of its blood supply. Blood flow to the myocardium may be obstructed by artherosclerosis or by thrombus formation within an atheromatous coronary artery. The most common site of infarction is the anterior surface of the left ventricle, resulting from occlusion of the left coronary artery. An infarction may affect some or all of the layers of the heart.

The two major complications of a myocardial infarction are left ventricular failure and arrhythmias, both of which account for a large percentage of deaths following myocardial infarction. It is generally recognized that the risk of death is greatest in the first few hours after myocardial infarction, with the risk decreasing after that time.

A myocardial infarction may be asymptomatic (a silent myocardial infarction). More commonly it may manifest with pain in the centre of the chest, arms neck, jaw or back lasting longer than five minutes, pallor, sweating, anxiety, shortness of breath, nausea or vomiting, or sudden collapse.

Dysrhythmias, or arrhythmias, are disturbances of the heart rate or rhythm. The many causes of dysrhythmias include ischaemia or injury to cardiac tissue, enlargement of the heart, electrolyte imbalance, and stimulants such as nicotine and caffeine. Some dysrhythmias occur as a normal physiological response, e.g. tachycardia associated with increased activity level.

Dysrhythmias are generally detected and identified by electrocardiograph (ECG) investigation, which records the pattern of electrical activity in the heart. Cardiac dysrhythmias are named for their site of origin, and include:

- Extra systoles, which are beats that occur before they are due and are followed by a longer than usual interval.
- Ventricular fibrillation, which is rapid, irregular and ineffective contractions of the ventricles.
- Atrial fibrillation, which is rapid, irregular and ineffective contractions of the atria.
- Sinus bradycardia, which is a rhythm originating in the SA node and is regular but slower than 60 beats per minute.
- Sinus tachycardia, which is characterized by normal rhythm but the heart beats at more than 100 times per minute.
- Atrial flutter, which results in a heart rate of up to 250–400 beats per minute.
- Paroxysmal tachycardia, which is an abrupt onset of very rapid heart beats up to 250 per minute.
- Heart block, which is a condition where some or all of the atrial impulses fail to reach the ventricles. The pulse rate is slow, and may be less than 40 beats per minute.

Valvular heart disease is a condition in which one or more of the valves malfunction. As a result, there is either a backflow of blood through the valves because of incompetent closure, or incomplete opening of the valves. Either condition can lead to heart failure. There are several forms of valve disease including:

- Mitral insufficiency, which results in blood flowing back through the incompetent mitral valve into the left atrium during systole. This causes the atrium to enlarge to accommodate the back flow.

• Mitral stenosis, which impedes blood flow from the left atrium into the left ventricle during diastole. This causes the left atrial pressure to rise and the left atrium to dilate.

• Aortic insufficiency, which results in blood flowing back into the left ventricle during diastole. This causes fluid overload in the ventricle, which dilates and eventually hypertrophies.

• Aortic stenosis, which results in an impeded blood flow from the left ventricle into the aorta during systole. This causes increased left ventricular pressure and, eventually, left ventricular failure.

• Pulmonary artery valve insufficiency, which results in blood flowing back into the right ventricle during systole. This causes ventricular hypertrophy and, eventually, right ventricular failure.

• Pulmonary stenosis, which results in an impeded flow of blood from the right ventricle into the pulmonary artery. This causes right ventricular hypertrophy and, eventually, right ventricular failure.

• Tricuspid insufficiency, which results in blood flowing back through the incompetent tricuspid valve into the right atrium during systole. This can eventually lead to right ventricular failure.

• Tricuspid stenosis, which results in an impeded flow of blood from the right atrium into the right ventricle during diastole. This causes hypertrophy of the right atrium, increased pressure in the vena cava, and leads to right ventricular failure.

Manifestations of valvular heart disease depend on which valve is diseased, and on the extent to which it is affected. The most common manifestations include dyspnoea, fatigue, peripheral oedema, syncope, palpitations, chest pain, and the signs and symptoms associated with heart failure.

Heart failure, or cardiac failure, is failure of the heart to maintain an output of blood sufficient to meet the body's requirements. Cardiac failure may be acute or chronic, and may be either right or left ventricular failure. It is important to realize, however, that failure of one side of the heart generally leads to failure of the other side.

The causes of cardiac failure include conditions that affect cardiac rhythm or conduction, those that overload the heart, and those that reduce the ability of the heart to contract. Cardiac failure generally develops gradually, but acute left ventricular failure may develop if the volume load is suddenly increased, or if the myocardium is suddenly impaired, e.g. as a consequence of myocardial infarction. Congestive cardiac failure is a condition in which circulatory congestion occurs as the result of heart failure.

The manifestations of cardiac failure which depend on which side of the heart is affected and on the severity of failure include dyspnoea, wheezing, expectoration of copious frothy sputum, cyanosis, fatigue, central and/or peripheral oedema, anorexia, abdominal distension, and neurological symptoms such as disorientation and dizziness.

Cardiogenic shock may be caused by any condition that causes heart failure, e.g. myocardial infarction, cardiomyopathy, or dysrhythmias. It is a condition whereby diminished cardiac output severely impairs tissue perfusion, and it has a high mortality rate. Manifestations of cardiogenic shock include cool and moist skin, urinary output of less than 30 ml per hour, systolic blood pressure of less than 90 mmHg, metabolic acidosis, and impaired consciousness.

Cardiac arrest is the sudden cessation of the heart's pumping action. Cardiac arrest may result from ventricular fibrillation, ventricular tachycardia, severe bradycardia or asystole. These disturbances of cardiac function can be caused by factors which include myocardial infarction, heart failure, electrical shock, electrolyte imbalance, acidosis, or severe haemorrhage.

Imminent cardiac arrest generally produces bradycardia and hypotension followed by loss of consciousness, cessation of ventilations and the absence of peripheral pulses and heart sounds. Further information on the detection, and management of cardiac arrest is provided in Chapter 57.

Raynaud's disease is a disorder characterized by vasospasm of the peripheral arteries and arterioles, particularly those of the hands. Factors which have been implicated as contributing to this disorder include intrinsic vascular wall hypersensitivity to cold, increased vasomotor tone, and an antigen–antibody immune response.

Manifestations of the disorder are skin changes in the fingers when the individual is exposed to cold. At first, the fingers blanch, then become blue, and finally they turn red. Numbness and tingling of the fingers generally occurs. If the disease is long-standing, trophic changes and skin ulceration may develop. Rarely, gangrene may occur.

Buerger's disease (thromboangiitis obliterans) is an inflammatory occlusive condition which leads to thrombus formation in the small to medium arteries and veins—usually of the lower limbs. This results in diminished blood flow to the legs and feet producing ulceration and gangrene. Smoking has been implicated as one of the most likely factors contributing to the disorder.

Manifestations include intermittent claudication; and coldness, cyanosis and numbness of the feet when they are exposed to low temperatures. In the later stages of the disorder ulceration and gangrene around the nails and toes may occur.

Anaemias are a group of disorders which are characterized by a reduction in the oxygen-carrying capacity of the blood. Causes of anaemia are numerous and are related to the production and destruction of erythrocytes, and to blood loss. Therefore, anaemias can be classified as those due to haemopoietic, haemolytic, or haemorrhagic causes.

Aplastic anaemia results from injury or destruction of the haematopoietic cells in bone marrow and, therefore, there is reduced or disordered erythrocyte production. In this disorder, the normal haematopoietic tissue is replaced by fatty bone marrow.

Aplastic anaemia may be idiopathic or it may be caused by medications, toxic agents, radiation, or immunologic factors. Manifestations of aplastic anaemia are related to pancytopenia (abnormal depression of the cellular components of blood). They include pallor, tiredness, repeated infections, and bleeding tendencies. Bleeding may present as petechiae, ecchymosis, haemorrhage from the mucous membranes, e.g. the gums, or gastrointestinal haemorrhage.

Pernicious anaemia is characterized by a metabolic defect involving the absence of intrinsic factor—secreted by the gastric mucosa—which is essential for Vitamin B absorption. Pernicious anaemia is thought to result from an autosomal dominant defect. Other causes include gastric cancer, gastrectomy, and malabsorption disorders involving the ileum.

Manifestations of pernicious anaemia include pallor, tiredness, sore tongue, and numbness and tingling in the extremities. Because of Vitamin B deficiency, demyelination of nerves and degeneration of nerve tissue occurs—producing neurological effects such as ataxia, altered vision, poor memory, depression or paralysis.

Iron deficiency anaemia is characterized by small and pale erythrocytes because of a reduction in haemoglobin concentration. The two most common causes of iron deficiency anaemia are chronic blood loss and an inadequate dietary intake of iron. Manifestations include pallor, chronic tiredness, tachycardia, and shortness of breath on exertion.

Folate deficiency anaemia results from an inadequate dietary intake of folate, or from a disorder of the small intestine where folate is absorbed. Manifestations are similar to those associated with pernicious anaemia.

Acute blood loss anaemia is a condition that results from sudden loss of erythrocytes and, consequently, depletion of haemoglobin and iron. Acute blood loss anaemia may result from severe trauma, postoperative haemorrhage, invasive neoplasm, ruptured peptic ulcer, ruptured aneurysm, or coagulation defects.

Acute blood loss itself produces features associated with hypovolaemia and hypoxia, e.g. pallor, faintness, restlessness, anxiety, hypotension, and a weak rapid pulse.

Disseminated intravascular coagulation (DIC) is a disorder that occurs as a complication of diseases which accelerate clotting. As a result there is small blood vessel occlusion, organ necrosis, and activation of the fibrinolytic system. This, in turn, can result in severe bleeding episodes.

Conditions which may precipitate DIC include sepsis, shock, malignancy, extensive burns or trauma, and obstetric complications such as amniotic fluid embolism or abruptio placentae.

Manifestations of DIC are bleeding tendencies, tissue damage from ischaemia, and the signs and symptoms of shock. Manifestations of thrombosis vary according to which part of the body is affected, e.g. altered consciousness if the cerebral blood flow is obstructed, or haematuria if the urinary system is affected.

Idiopathic thrombocytopenic purpura is a disorder characterized by a severe reduction in the number of thrombocytes. The disorder occurs as a result of an autoimmune response which may be stimulated by microorganisms, toxins, or chemicals. Manifestations are those associated with thrombocytopenia such as haemorrhagic episodes, purpura, petechiae, ecchymoses, and bleeding from the mucosa and gastrointestinal tract.

Agranulocytosis (granulocytopenia) is a disorder in which there is a decreased number of circulating granulocytes, with the most significantly affected cells being the neutrophils. The disorder may be caused by a decreased production of granulocytes, increased utilization of granulocytes, or medications such as cytotoxic agents. Manifestations include fatigue and weakness followed by the signs of overwhelming infection, e.g. pyrexia, tachycardia, headaches, and prostration.

Neoplastic and obstructive disorders

Tumours may occur in any of the chambers of the heart, and they may affect one or all of the layers of the heart. Secondary metastatic tumours that infiltrate the heart are more common than primary cardiac tumours. Manifestations which are related to which part of the heart is affected include signs of heart failure, dysrhythmias, angina, heart block, and infarction.

Arteriosclerosis obliterans, which most often presents in the elderly individual, is a chronic disorder where there is occlusive disease of the arteries in the extremities. Manifestations, which are related to the progressive obstruction of the arteries which results in ischaemia of the tissues, include leg pain, numbness and coldness of the feet, cyanosis and oedema of the legs and feet. Gangrene of the toes may develop.

Acute arterial obstruction is the sudden disruption of the blood supply to all or part of an extremity. The condition may be caused by embolism, thrombus formation, or injury to an artery. Manifestations include severe pain, loss of motor and sensory function, pallor and coldness of the limb. If the artery is partially occluded there may be numbness or weakness of the limb. Total occlusion causes a loss of pulses distal to the obstruction. If the obstruction is not removed, gangrene will develop.

Thrombophlebitis is inflammation of a vein with thrombus formation. It can occur in the deep or superficial veins, most commonly in the legs. In deep vein thrombosis

(DVT) the veins which are most commonly involved are the ileofemoral, popliteal, or small veins in the calf. Thrombophlebitis often begins with local inflammation (phlebitis), which then leads to thrombus formation.

Thrombophlebitis may be idiopathic but it usually results from damage to the endothelium, accelerated blood clotting, or reduced blood flow. Predisposing factors to DVT include conditions which result in localized venous stasis, e.g. prolonged immobility, varicose veins, prolonged pressure on the calf muscles, or pregnancy. Accelerated blood clotting, which can lead to thrombus formation, is associated with the use of oral contraceptives, presence of malignancy, and blood dyscrasias. Superficial thrombophlebitis may be caused by trauma, infection, and chemical irritation, e.g. from intravenous drug or fluid therapy.

Manifestations which vary with the site and length of the vein affected, include inflammation, swelling and increased warmth along the path of the vein. The individual may also experience pain, pyrexia, dependent cyanosis, an increase in the circumference of the extremity, and a positive Homan's sign (pain in the calf region on dorsiflexion of the foot).

Chronic venous insufficiency results from destruction of the venous valves, commonly as a consequence of one or more episodes of deep vein thrombosis. Destruction of the valves leaves the deep leg veins functionally incompetent, which results in dependent oedema of the leg and induration caused by cutaneous fibrosis. The skin around the ankle becomes discoloured from extravasation of blood into the subcutaneous tissue. These changes eventually lead to the formation of stasis ulcers.

Leukaemia is a neoplastic disorder characterized by an accumulation and proliferation of abnormal cells in the bone marrow. Cells fail to develop and are unable to function normally, and the accumulation of leukaemic cells in the bone marrow prevents normal haematopoiesis. The precise cause of leukaemia is unknown but several factors have been clearly implicated in its development; including chromosome abnormality, exposure to ionizing radiation or certain chemicals, and viral infection. Leukaemia occurs either in acute forms which involve the proliferation of immature cells, or in chronic forms which involve the proliferation of mature cells. The four most common forms of leukaemia are:

1. Acute myeloid (AML)
2. Chronic myeloid (CML)
3. Acute lymphocytic (ALL)
4. Chronic lymphocytic (CLL)

Although manifestations of leukaemia vary according to the particular form of the disorder, there is similarity in the signs and symptoms which are related to the lack of normal haematopoiesis in the bone marrow. Bone marrow dysfunction results in anaemia, thrombocytopenia, and leucopenia:

● Anaemia may present as pallor, lethargy, and shortness of breath.
● Thrombocytopenia commonly manifests as petechiae, easy bruising, bleeding gums, and haemorrhage, e.g. as occult haematuria.
● Leucopenia renders the individual susceptible to recurrent infections. There is generally splenic enlargement, lymphadenopathy, and bone pain.

Central nervous system involvement may be present in any of the leukaemias, giving rise to symptoms such as nausea and vomiting, irritability, headache, and blurred vision.

Hodgkin's disease is a malignant disorder of the lymph node macrophages, characterized by painless and progressive enlargement of the lymph nodes, spleen, and other lymphoid tissue. Untreated, Hodgkin's disease metastasizes via the lymphatics to sites outside the lymphatic system. The precise cause of the disorder is unknown, but both genetic and environmental factors seem to be implicated in its development.

Manifestations of Hodgkin's disease are painless enlargement of the lymph nodes-especially the cervical nodes, pruritus, night sweats, malaise, and weight loss. Other symptoms depend on the degree and location of systemic involvement.

Malignant lymphomas are a group of malignant diseases originating in the lymph glands and other areas of lymphoid tissue. Included in this group are non-Hodgkin's lymphoma and lymphosarcomas. The precise cause of malignant lymphomas is unknown, although there is suggestion that viruses or immunosuppression may be causative factors. Manifestations include painless lymph node enlargement and extranodal involvement of the skin, bone and bone marrow. Specific symptoms develop as the lymphoma progresses.

Burkitt's lymphoma is a malignant lymphoma that generally begins as a lesion in the jaw, or as an abdominal mass. The disorder is most prevalent in tropical areas, e.g. Papua New Guinea and Africa, and usually occurs in children under the age of 7. The cause of Burkitt's lymphoma is thought to be the Epstein-Barr virus. Initial manifestations of the disorder are followed by symptoms which are related to the site and extent of the tumour.

Multiple myeloma is a malignant disorder characterized by the proliferation of abnormal plasma cells in the bone marrow. Multiple myeloma disseminates throughout the skeleton, and ultimately involves the lymph nodes, spleen, liver, and kidneys. While the cause is unknown, the disorder is thought to result from a genetic stimulus.

Manifestations do not generally appear in the early stages of the disease, and the most common indication of multiple myeloma is severe and constant bone pain—which may be accompanied by spontaneous fractures. Impaired bone marrow function, as a result of skeletal infiltration, may present as anaemia, repeated infections, and bleeding tendencies. Renal function is frequently impaired as a result of tubular damage from large amounts of Bence Jones protein, which is a protein lost in the urine of an individual with multiple myeloma.

Degenerative disorders

Cardiomyopathy results from extensive damage to the myocardial muscle fibres, causing hypertrophy of the entire heart—especially of the septum. Although the heart is enlarged, the ventricular chambers are small and are resistant to filling during diastole. Cardiomyopathy leads to congestive cardiac failure, arrhythmias, and frequently to sudden death.

The cause of most cardiomyopathies is unknown, but it is thought to be genetically transmitted. Some forms of cardiomyopathy result from myocardial destruction by toxic, infectious, or metabolic agents. The most common manifestation of cardiomyopathy is dyspnoea as a result of congestive cardiac failure. Angina, fatigue, and syncope may occur because of inadequate cardiac output. As cardiac failure progresses peripheral cyanosis, oedema, liver enlargement, and jugular venous distension become evident.

Aortic aneurysm is a dilatation of the wall of the aorta. There are several types of aneurysm:

- saccular, an outpouching of one side of the arterial wall
- fusiform, a spindle shaped enlargement of the entire circumference of the artery
- dissecting, a haemorrhagic separation between the medial and internal layers of the artery.

The most common cause of an aneurysm is atherosclerosis, which weakens the aortic wall and gradually distends the lumen at the weakened area. Other causative factors include congenital defects, infection, hypertension, and trauma.

Manifestations of an aortic aneurysm depend on its location, and may not develop until enlargement of the aneurysm exerts pressure on nearby structures. Depending on the location, an aortic aneurysm may result in dyspnoea, chest pain, dysphagia, dilated superficial veins on the chest, neck, and arms; a prominent abdominal pulsation, and dull abdominal or low back pain. A *dissecting* aneurysm may produce a sudden 'tearing' pain; accompanied by pallor, shortness of breath, sweating, and syncope.

The main complication of an aortic aneurysm is rupture and, without immediate surgical intervention, the individual will bleed to death.

Varicose veins are dilated, tortuous branches of the saphenous veins. They result from incompetent valves, which cause a backflow of venous blood.

Varicose veins may result from congenital weakness of the valves, from injury or thrombophlebitis, or from conditions that produce venous stasis, e.g. pregnancy or occupations that necessitate standing for long periods.

Superficial varicose veins may be unsightly but produce no symptoms. Deeper varicose veins may produce mild to severe leg symptoms, e.g. a feeling of heaviness, cramps, dull aching and discomfort which increases with prolonged standing. Over time, dilation of the veins results in venous stasis with oedema and changes in skin pigmentation. Visible and palpable protrusions frequently occur along the veins, resulting in disfigurement of the leg/s.

Infectious and inflammatory disorders

Pericarditis, which is inflammation of the pericardium, may be an acute or chronic condition. Acute pericarditis may be accompanied by a purulent, serous, or haemorrhagic exudate which can produce further complications. Chronic pericarditis is characterized by fibrous pericardial thickening. As well as being caused by infection, pericarditis may result from trauma, radiation, neoplasms, or myocardial infarction.

The prime manifestation is chest pain which increases with deep inhalation, and decreases when the individual sits up and leans forward. Other manifestations include dyspnoea, and the signs of a systemic infection.

Myocarditis, which is inflammation of the myocardium, may be an acute or chronic condition. Myocarditis may result from viral or bacterial infections, radiation, chemicals, or metabolic disorders. Infective myocarditis usually causes non—specific symptoms that reflect a systemic infection. Myocarditis sometimes produces manifestations of severe congestive cardiac failure.

Endocarditis, which is inflammation of the endocardium, may result from invasion by microorganisms or from non-infective injury to the lining of the heart. Infective endocarditis involves the endocardium of the heart valves more frequently than the endocardium lining the heart chambers. The microorganisms stimulate the deposit of fibrin around them—producing vegetative growth on the endocardium.

Early manifestations are commonly non-specific, and the symptoms of acute endocarditis resemble those associated with influenza; pyrexia, sweats, anorexia, headaches, and musculoskeletal aches. If a heart murmur develops the pulse rate may be rapid, and if vegetations become dislodged there may be manifestations of embolization—producing the features of splenic, renal, cerebral, pulmonary, or peripheral vascular occlusion.

Rheumatic heart disease refers to the cardiac manifestations of rheumatic fever, and includes pericarditis, myocarditis, endocarditis, and chronic valvular disease. Rheumatic fever is associated with the Type A beta-haemolytic streptococcus, and is thought to be immunological in origin.

It may be as long as 10 years after an attack of rheumatic

fever before signs of heart valve disease become evident. The end result of the disease progression is stenosis of a heart valve, inability of the valve to close properly, or valve incompetence—which leads to regurgitation of blood through the valve during systole. Manifestations of rheumatic heart valve disease depend on the valve affected and on the degree of valve dysfunction. There may be signs of reduced cardiac output, pulmonary congestion, cardiac enlargement, heart failure, and the presence of heart murmurs.

Lymphangitis is an acute or chronic inflammation of the lymphatic vessels which generally results from a streptococcal infection of an extremity. The accompanying lymph node enlargement (lymphadenopathy) may be localized or generalized. Lymphangitis is characterized by red, warm, tender streaks spreading up a limb from a focal point of infection. The regional lymph nodes become enlarged and tender, and the individual experiences pyrexia and malaise.

Immunologic disorders

Polyarteritis (nodosa) is a relatively rare disorder that produces widespread inflammation and necrosis in the medium and small arteries and adjacent veins. Although the cause is unknown, the disorder is thought to be of immunologic origin. Initially, lesions develop in the tunica media of the artery and then progress into the other layers—producing palpable bead-like nodules along the course of the artery. Arterial wall changes precipitate fibrosis and weakening, resulting in arterial occlusion, thrombosis, infarction, or aneurysm.

Early manifestations of the disorder are non-specific, and include weakness, pyrexia, weight loss, and anorexia. As the disease progresses there is widespread organ involvement, and the symptoms depend on the organ or system involved. Lesions can develop in the kidneys, gastrointestinal tract, musculoskeletal system, cardiovascular system, or in the peripheral nervous system.

Agammaglobulinaemia is the complete lack of immunoglobulins in the blood, which renders the individual susceptible to recurrent infections. Although the precise cause is unknown, the inherited form is an x-linked disorder in which all five immunologic factors are absent. Acquired agammaglobulinaemia is though to be related to genetic factors and stress. Manifestations of the disorder include recurrent pyogenic infections, diarrhoea, steatorrhoea, and enlargement of the liver and spleen.

Acquired immune deficiency syndrome (AIDS) is a disease which is caused by the human immunodeficiency virus (HIV). HIV is a retrovirus which has the ability to change its genetic material (RNA) into human genetic material (DNA) through the use of an enzyme.

An individual who has the HIV infection has a defect in immunity against disease, and is prone to debilitating opportunistic infections. The immune response consists of a number of complex chemical reactions which are coordinated by the white blood cells called T helper cells. HIV infects and destroys these cells, which causes irreversible changes and a severe decrease in the number of T-lymphocytes.

Infection with HIV results in a spectrum of diseases which have been classified into 4 groups.

Group I—acute HIV infection. Approximately 50% of persons newly infected with HIV exhibit an acute transitory illness. The illness is characterized by a glandular fever-like syndrome of short duration. The test for antibodies to HIV is usually negative at first, and remains negative for 1–3 months. Individuals in this group recover from the illness, but later tests for antibodies are positive. An individual is then reclassified into group II or III.

Group II—Asymptomatic HIV infection. Group II includes those individuals who are infected with HIV and are HIV antibody positive, but who do not have any apparent illness.

Group III—Persistent generalized lymphadenopathy. Individuals in this group have persistent unexplained lymph gland enlargement in the neck, armpits, and groin.

Group IV—AIDS and related conditions. Individuals in group IV have serious illnesses associated with HIV infection. These include systemic symptoms such as pyrexia, night sweats, unexplained weight loss, persistant cough, diarrhoea, fatigue, and loss of appetite. An individual may also exhibit a neurological disorder such as dementia, or opportunistic infections. The most common opportunistic infection is pneumonia caused by infection with *Pneumocystis carinii*. An individual may also experience a form of cancer such as Kaposi's sarcoma or lymphoma.

The modes of transmission of HIV are very specific and, although HIV has been found in a number of body fluids, only blood, semen, and vaginal/cervical secretions have been implicated in transmission. In a few cases the virus has been transmitted from a mother to her baby just before or during birth or via breast milk.

HIV is transmitted through sexual intercourse (anal and vaginal) with an infected person, or through sharing of infected needles and syringes when injecting drugs. In the past transmission occurred via the tranfusion of blood or blood products, but stringent measures have since been introduced to ensure safety of these supplies.

All available evidence suggests that the virus is not spread by ordinary social contact. The reason for this is that the virus *dies rapidly* outside the human body. There is no evidence to suggest that HIV has been transmitted through air or water, sharing of crockery or cutlery, toilets, swimming pools, kissing, coughing, sneezing, or via mosquitoes and other biting insects.

The incubation period for HIV is not known and may be as long as 15 years, but recent evidence suggests that the average incubation period for people who develop AIDS is 2–5 years.

At the present time the people who are most at risk of contracting HIV infection are:

- sexually active homosexual and bisexual men
- intravenous drug users
- recepients of blood or blood products prior to 1985
- the sexual partners of the above 3 groups.

As with other sexually transmitted diseases, the more partners with whom unsafe sexual activity occurs the greater the risk of contracting the virus.

Preventing the spread of HIV includes:

- People assuming responsibility for protecting themselves against infection, which means avoiding intimate sexual contact with persons whose 'risk factor' is unknown.
- Practising 'safe sex' which involves preventing the exchange of body fluids, and avoiding contact of body fluids with mucous membranes. Condoms, properly used, significantly reduce the spread of HIV.
- Never using needles and syringes for intravenous and other injections more than once. Sharing of these items is common among users of intravenous drugs, and carries the risk of a variety of infectious diseases including HIV infection.
- People with HIV accepting the responsibility never to place another person at risk.
- Health care establishments implementing appropriate infection control guidelines to minimize the spread of HIV.
- Providing on-going research and educational programmes on HIV and AIDS.
- Ensuring that people who have engaged in or continue to practise high risk activities do not donate blood, semen, tissues, or organs.

As infection with HIV is one of the most significant health problems of the present time, further information on the condition is provided later in this chapter.

Diagnostic tests

Assessment of the individual with a suspected circulatory system disorder, or evaluation of the progress of a disorder, requires that certain tests be performed.

Assessment of cardiac function

Electrocardiography (ECG) provides a graphic record, or tracing, that represents the heart's electrical action.

Cellular activity of the cardiac muscle generates electrical impulses that flow through the heart, and this electrical activity can be measured by a system of electrodes placed at specific points on the body surface (Fig. 44.1).

The ECG displays the electrical activity as wave-forms (Fig. 44.1) which are named as P,Q,R,S, and T waves. The ECG recording illustrates the rate and rhythm of cardiac contractions, and electrical conduction through the

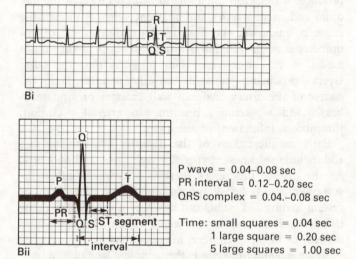

- Select flat, fleshy sites
- Avoid bony or muscular areas
- Secure electrodes to limbs and chest
  - Insert lead wires into electrodes
  - Connect LA to left arm, RA to right arm etc.
  - Select flat, fleshy sites
  - At each selected site, rub skin with electrode until skin reddens, then apply electrode pad or paste
- Relax individual
- Discuss the procedure
- Connect patient cable to cardiograph

Power cable

A

Fig. 44.1 Electrocardiogram.
(A) Placement of electrodes and leads to perform an ECG (electrocardiogram). Attaching the individual to a 12 lead ECG.

Bi

P wave = 0.04–0.08 sec
PR interval = 0.12–0.20 sec
QRS complex = 0.04.–0.08 sec

Time: small squares = 0.04 sec
1 large square = 0.20 sec
5 large squares = 1.00 sec

Bii

Fig. 44.1 (B) A normal electrocardiograph. (i) Regular sinus rhythm. (ii) Detail of ECG.

heart; and indicates enlargement of the chambers, inflammation of the pericardium, or damage to the myocardium.

Exercise electrocardiography (stress test) measures the cardiovascular effects of controlled physical stress, e.g. treadmill walking.

Ambulatory (Holter) electrocardiography records the heart's electrical activity for a specified time, e.g. 24 hours, as the individual performs his usual activities.

Echocardiography, a painless non-invasive test, directs ultra-high-frequency sound waves through the chest wall into the heart, which then reflects those waves to a transducer and a recording device. As the sound transects the various heart structures, echoes are produced and recorded. Echocardiography evaluates cardiac structure and function, and can reveal valve deformities, septal defects, cardiomyopathy, and pericardial effusion.

Nuclear cardiology involves the use of radioactive tracers to evaluate myocardial blood flow and the status of myocardial cells. An intravenous injection, e.g. of the radioisotope thallium-201, is administered and a scan performed to detect thallium uptake. Healthy myocardial tissue absorbs the radioisotope, but ischaemic or necrotic tissue does not.

Cardiac catheterization involves the insertion of a catheter into the right or left side of the heart, to obtain information on cardiac pressures, cardiac output, oxygenation, and heart valve function.

The catheter is inserted through a vein in the arm or the groin into the vena cava; the passage of the catheter is observed on a fluorescent screen and X-ray films are taken. A contrast medium may be injected through the catheter and X-ray films taken (angiography).

For *coronary angiography*, the catheter is advanced into the aortic arch and positioned into a coronary artery, then a contrast medium is injected to outline the coronary arteries as a series of X-ray films is taken.

Digital subtraction angiography is less invasive than conventional angiography, and involves injecting contrast dye into the venous system rather than directly into an artery. As the dye circulates through the heart and arterial system, a fluoroscopic image intensifier displays the vessels and focuses the image. A computer then converts the images into numbers. Several vessels can be evaluated with one injection of contrast dye.

Phonocardiography graphically records heart sounds produced as blood flows through the heart and great vessels. Microphones are placed on the chest, usually at the apex and base of the heart, and the sounds are picked up and converted into electrical impulses. The impulses are relayed to a recorder which provides a graph of the heart sounds in wave—form.

Central venous pressure (CVP) test measures the function of the right atrium. A catheter, which is threaded through the subclavian or jugular vein into or near the right atrium, is connected to a manometer. This procedure enables accurate determination of right atrial blood pressure, which reflects right ventricular pressure. CVP is also used to assess blood volume.

Intracardiac pressure monitoring involves the insertion of a balloon-tipped, flow-directed catheter, e.g. the Swan-Ganz catheter, into a large vein and then advancing it until it reaches the right atrium. Once the balloon is inflated, the flow of blood carries the catheter into the pulmonary artery. The procedure permits measurement of both pulmonary artery pressure (PAP) and pulmonary artery wedge pressure (PAWP). In addition, this procedure evaluates pulmonary vascular resistance and tissue oxygenation.

Blood tests may be performed to measure cardiac en-zymes, which helps to assess myocardial function. Cardiac enzyme measurements help detect myocardial infarction, evaluate possible causes of chest pain, and monitor the severity of myocardial ischaemia.

Assessment of peripheral blood vessels

Skin temperature studies may be performed to evaluate skin temperature of the extremities, which helps to determine adequacy of blood circulation in arterial disease.

Direct skin temperature readings may be performed and, in arterial disease, the temperature in the extremities may be lower than in other body areas.

The cold stimulation test may be used to demonstrate Raynaud's syndrome, by recording temperature changes in the individual's fingers before and after their submersion in ice water. Normally digital temperature returns to pre-test level within 15 minutes, but with Raynaud's syndrome return to pre-test level takes longer than 20 minutes.

Doppler ultrasonography involves the transmission of sound waves through the skin, which are reflected from moving blood cells in underlying blood vessels. This test evaluates blood flow in the major veins and arteries in the limbs, and helps to detect peripheral vascular aneurysms, and deep vein thrombosis.

Arteriography (angiography) is the radiographic examination of one or more arteries after injection of a contrast medium into a major artery—usually the femoral artery. Arteriography can demonstrate blood flow status, collateral circulation, vascular anomaly, tumour, and aneurysm formation.

Lower limb venography is the radiographic examination of a vein following an injection of contrast medium, and is often used to assess the condition of the deep leg veins. Venography is the definitive test for deep vein thrombosis, but it may also be used to distinguish clot formation from other forms of venous obstruction or to locate a suitable vein for arterial bypass grafting.

Impedance plethysmography is a non-invasive test for measuring venous flow in the limbs, and is helpful for detecting deep vein thrombosis. Electrodes are applied to the leg to measure changes in electrical resistance that result from blood volume variations.

Assessment of haematologic status

For information on normal blood values, the nurse should refer to Appendix 3.

Red blood cell (erythrocyte) count is the measurement of the number of erythrocytes found in a microlitre of blood. This test, together with haematocrit and haemoglobin determinations, is most often used to calculate mean corpuscular volume, mean corpuscular haemoglobin, and mean corpuscular haemoglobin concentration.

Haematocrit is a blood test used to measure the percentage of a given volume of blood occupied by erythrocytes.

Erythrocyte indices involve examination of the size, weight, and haemoglobin content of the average erythrocyte.

Total haemoglobin test measures the grams of haemoglobin (Hb) in 100 ml of whole blood.

Stained red cell examination determines abnormalities in the size, shape or structure of erythrocytes.

Reticulocyte count measures the number of reticulocytes present in a sample of blood, which is then expressed as a percentage of the total red cell count. (Reticulocytes are immature erythrocytes)

Erythrocyte sedimentation rate (ESR) measures the time required for erythrocytes, in a sample of whole blood, to settle to the bottom of a vertical tube.

Erythrocyte osmotic fragility measures red cell resistance to haemolysis when exposed to a hypotonic solution.

White blood cell (leucocyte) count is the measurement of the number of white cells found in a microlitre of whole blood.

Differential white blood cell count determines the distribution and morphology of the various white blood cells, and it provides more information about the immune system than the white blood cell count.

Coagulation function is measured by a wide variety of tests including:

1. Platelet count, which measures the number of circulating thrombocytes (platelets).
2. Bleeding time, which measures the duration of bleeding after a standardized skin incision—commonly two small punctures made on the forearm.
3. Capillary fragility test, which measures the ability of capillaries to remain intact under increased intracapillary pressure. A blood pressure cuff is placed around the upper arm and inflated to midway between the systolic and diastolic pressures. After five minutes of sustained pressure, the number of petechiae on a selected area of the forearm are counted.
4. Clot retraction test, which estimates the quantity and quality of thrombocytes and fibrinogen.
5. Prothrombin time (PT), which measures the time required for a fibrin clot to form in a citrated plasma sample.
6. Partial thromboplastin time (PTT), which evaluates the entire coagulation system—with the exception of factors VII and XIII.
7. Factor VIII activity test, which measures the amount of factor VIII in the blood and identifies a deficiency of that factor, e.g. as in haemophilia.

Immunoglobulin studies evaluate the amount and types of immunoglobin present.

Serum ferritin measurements evaluate the amount of iron stored in body tissues.

Total iron-binding capacity (TIBC) measures the amount of available transferrin (a protein that binds with iron) in the blood.

Sickle cell test detects the presence of haemoglobin S in suspected sickle cell anaemia.

Gastric fluid analysis involves measuring the acidity of secretions in the stomach, and it is used in the diagnosis of pernicious anaemia. Further information about this test is provided in Chapter 46.

Bone marrow examination provides information about the character, integrity, and production of erythrocytes, leucocytes, and thrombocytes. Bone marrow can be removed by aspiration or needle biopsy:

● Aspiration of bone marrow involves the removal of a small amount, generally less than 5 ml.
● Biopsy, performed under local anaesthesia, is done when a larger amount of bone marrow is required. A needle is inserted through the skin and tissue, e.g. over the iliac crest, until it reaches bone. The needle is then directed into the marrow cavity, and a sample of bone marrow is withdrawn.

Assessment of the lymphatic system

Lymphangiography is the radiographic examination of the lymphatic system, after the injection of a contrast medium into a lymphatic vessel in each foot. X-ray films are taken to demonstrate the filling of the lymphatic vessels and, 24 hours later, to visualize the lymph nodes.

CARE OF THE INDIVIDUAL WITH A CIRCULATORY SYSTEM DISORDER

Although specific nursing actions and medical management vary depending on the disorder, the main aims of care are to:

● promote comfort and relieve pain
● provide psychological support
● maintain skin integrity
● promote and maintain mobility
● prevent infection
● maintain fluid and nutritional status
● administer prescribed medication
● provide care before, during, and after a diagnostic test.

Promoting comfort and relieving pain

In many disorders of the circulatory system the aim is to help to individual rest comfortably, and to increase his activity progressively without pain. Comfort is promoted if the individual is provided with a bed which is made up to meet his specific needs. Ensuring that his basic needs, e.g.

hygiene and elimination, are provided for willalso help to promote the individual's comfort.

The individual may experience pain, e.g. as a result of myocardial infarction or peripheral vascular dysfunction, therefore relief of pain is an important aspect in the promotion of comfort. Pain relieving measures, e.g. the administration of adequate analgesic medication, are implemented so that the individual is able to rest comfortably, sleep without discomfort, and is able to perform the activities of daily living without experiencing pain. The individual is also advised on what precautions to take in order to avoid pain, which includes identifying any precipitating factors such as physical exertion or emotional stress. The incidence of pain can generally be reduced by careful planning of activity, modifying risk factors, and the use of prophylactic measures.

Providing psychological support

Anxiety and fear are common responses to hospitalization. An individual who is experiencing a major cardiovascular dysfunction, e.g. myocardial infarction or congestive cardiac disease, often becomes extremely anxious about pain, disability, loss of independence, and dying. An individual who has peripheral vascular disease may fear that the disorder will result in the loss of a limb, and an individual with a potentially life threatening disorder of the blood may also experience extreme anxiety.

The individual, and his significant others, may experience great concern about the alterations in lifestyle imposed by the disorder.

The nurse can provide psychological support by establishing and maintaining a trusting relationship with the individual and his significant others, and by encouraging them to express their feelings and concerns. They should be encouraged to discuss any lifestyle adjustments that may be necessary, and they should be offered guidance on how to cope with change.

Stress and anxiety can be reduced if the individual's symptoms, e.g. pain, are alleviated; and the nurse should try to provide an environment which is as stress-free as possible.

The individual should be provided with sufficient information about his illness, as knowledge helps to diminish anxiety and assists him to develop effective coping skills. The nurse should explain all the procedures, treatments, and monitoring techniques being implemented so that the individual understands his treatment.

The individual should be encouraged to participate in his care as much as possible and, when appropriate, to gradually assume responsibility for self-care to prevent loss of independence.

The individual should be informed about support groups and community resources, e.g. cardiac rehabilitation classes which may be helpful when he is discharged from hospital.

Maintaining skin integrity

An individual with a cardiac, peripheral vascular, or blood disorder is at risk of impaired skin integrity. Decreased peripheral perfusion resulting from a cardiovascular disorder, leads to hypoxia which can result in skin breakdown. With poor arterial circulation, the tissues lack adequate oxygen and nutrients and this can lead to cellulitis, ulcers, and necrosis. An individual with a blood disorder is also at risk of decubitus ulcer formation and poor wound healing.

Maintenance of skin integrity includes assessing the skin for any signs of breakdown, keeping the skin clean and dry, protecting the extremities from exposure to extremes of temperature and from trauma, position changes to avoid prolonged pressure on the skin, the use of accessories e.g. a sheepskin, to reduce pressure, and promoting mobility.

An individual with peripheral vascular disease suffers from a decreased blood supply to the legs. It is, therefore, extremely important to promote skin integrity of the legs and feet. Prevention of skin breakdown includes keeping the feet clean and dry, avoiding rough drying movements, using creams or lotions that prevent drying and cracking, avoiding scratching itchy areas on the legs or feet, nail care provided by a podiatrist or chiropodist; and protecting the feet with socks, slippers, or well fitting shoes.

Promoting and maintaining mobility

Maintenance of mobility is necessary to prevent the complications of immobility, e.g. decubitus ulcers, venous stasis, and pulmonary complications. Problems of immobility should be counteracted with position changes, range of motion (ROM) exercises, and coughing and deep breathing exercises. Ambulation of the individual as soon as possible is important to prevent the complications of immobility.

In the initial stages of illness, e.g. immediately post myocardial infarction, the individual's level of activity may be reduced to a minimum. As his cardiac tolerance increases, his level of physical activity is also gradually increased. The individual with peripheral vascular disease should understand the importance of adequate physical exercise, which provides the necessary muscle contraction for movement of arterial blood to the peripheral areas of the body.

Exercise, or activity, programmes are generally implemented gradually, and the individual is encouraged to rest after the exercise periods. As the individual's condition improves, moderate exercise is encouraged as long as pain is not induced.

Preventing infection

An individual with a blood disorder, e.g. leukaemia, is susceptible to infection. A decreased number of, or abnormal, white blood cells prevents the normal response (leucocytosis) to infection. Abnormal leucocytes do not respond to invasion by microorganisms, and are not capable of phagocytosis.

Measures to prevent infection must be implemented, e.g. good hand washing techniques, and aseptic techniques for any invasive procedure. Precautions must be taken to prevent damage to the skin or mucous membranes, as injured tissues create a portal for bacterial invasion.

If the individual's white blood cell count is low (leucopenia), it may be necessary to use protective isolation techniques to protect him against infection.

The individual whose immune system, and therefore his ability to resist infection, is impaired must be monitored closely to detect the early manifestations of infection so that appropriate treatment can be prescribed.

Maintaining fluid and nutritional status

Commonly, an individual with cardiovascular disorder will be prescribed a diet which aims to reduce serum cholesterol and triglyceride levels. The intake of sodium may also be reduced, e.g. in the control and prevention of hypertension. If the individual is obese, a weight reduction diet may be prescribed.

The diet generally should be low in total fat content—particularly saturated fats—and low in sodium. Kilojoules may be reduced to correct or prevent obesity, and alcohol should be restricted as it can raise kilojoule intake and serum lipid levels. Beverages and foods containing caffeine should be restricted, as caffeine is a cardiovascular stimulant which can cause tachycardia and dysrhythmias. If the individual is experiencing retention of fluid, e.g. as a result of congestive cardiac failure, his fluid intake may need to be restricted.

An individual with a cardiac disorder, e.g. cardiac failure, may experience fluid retention, and the nurse should assess his fluid balance by measuring his fluid input and output, and by observing for signs of oedema. Weighing the individual, e.g. each day, is another way of assessing his fluid status.

In specific blood disorders, the individual may be prescribed a diet which is high in one or more nutrients, e.g. a diet which contains foods high in iron is generally prescribed in the treatment of iron deficiency anaemia. When a specific diet is prescribed the dietitian consults with the individual to plan his diet, and to ensure that he understands any dietary modifications or restrictions.

It is important that the nurse is aware of the type of diet that has been prescribed, and she must ensure that the individual receives the correct tray at mealtimes. The nurse should encourage the individual to follow his diet and may

need to assist him at mealtimes, e.g. if he is unable to eat his meals independently. Information on assisting at mealtime is provided in Chapter 29.

Administering prescribed medications

Any medications must be administered in accordance with nursing regulations and the health care institution's policy. Information on administration of medications is provided in Chapter 58. Various medications may be prescribed in the management of disorders of the circulatory system, and include:

- analgesics
- anti-arrhythmics
- anti-angina agents
- antidiuretics
- antihypertensives
- antibiotics
- peripheral vasodilators.

Providing pre and post diagnostic test care

While some diagnostic procedures, e.g. blood tests, will require little preparation other than ensuring that the individual is informed of the procedure, other tests necessitate more extensive preparation. The nurse must understand how specific tests are performed so that she is able to reinforce the medical officer's explanation to the individual. She should refer to the institution's policy manual for information on preparation of the individual prior to each diagnostic procedure. The nurse must also know what observations, and post-test care, are required.

Preparation of the individual prior to a specific diagnostic test may include fluid or dietary modifications or restrictions, checking that written consent has been obtained, and administering any prescribed medications. Assessment of the individual following the test may include monitoring his vital signs, observing for bleeding after an invasive procedure, assessing peripheral blood circulation, and observing him for any discomfort or pain.

Planning for discharge

The individual with cardiovascular disease should be prepared carefully before discharge from hospital by:

- Explaining the importance of continuing with any prescribed medications, and ensuring that he is aware of dosages and possible side effects.
- Ensuring that he understands any dietary restrictions or modifications that must be followed.
- Advising him to seek medical attention if symptoms recur, or if he develops new symptoms.
- Advising him about the importance of not smoking, and of limiting his consumption of alcohol.

• Ansuring that he understands the level of physical activity he can engage in with safety.
• Advising him to avoid prolonged sitting or standing, and not to cross his legs if he has peripheral vascular disease.
• Ensuring that he understand how to apply anti-embolism stockings correctly if these have been prescribed. Information on the use of anti-embolism stockings is provided in Chapter 37.

TRANSFUSION OF WHOLE BLOOD OR BLOOD COMPONENTS

As part of the management of a circulatory system disorder, especially a disorder of the blood, a transfusion may be prescribed. A transfusion may consist of whole blood, or it may consist of one of the components of blood. *Whole blood* is generally transfused when decreased volumes result from haemorrhage. Blood *components* that may be transfused include:

1. Packed red cells, which are transfused when the individual's blood volume is normal but his haemoglobin and haematocrit levels are decreased.
2. Platelets, which may be transfused when the individual is bleeding and thrombocytopenic, or when his platelet count is decreased.
3. Fresh frozen plasma, which is transfused as a blood volume expander or given to an individual with a clotting deficiency. Synthetic plasma expanders are also available.
4. Plasma protein factor, which consists of selected plasma proteins in saline solution, may be transfused as a substitute if whole blood is unavailable. It may also be administered to treat hypovolaemic shock or to prevent electrolyte imbalance.
5. Albumin, which may be given to expand blood volume or, in some instances, to prevent or treat cerebral oedema.
6. Cryoprecipitate, which is obtained when fresh plasma is frozen rapidly and thawed slowly, is given to an individual with a fibrinogen deficiency, Von Willebrand's disease, or haemophilia.
7. Factor VIII concentrate, which is prepared from fresh plasma, may be given to an individual with haemophilia.

Blood donation

Blood for transfusion is generally obtained from blood donors. *Autotransfusion* is an alternative technique which involves the collection, and reinfusion of the individual's own blood at a later date.

Potential blood donors are screened to detect any factors that would disqualify them from donating blood. These precautions are necessary to protect the health and safety of both the donor and the recipient. Factors which disqualify a potential blood donor include a history of abnormal bleeding tendencies, specific pharmacological treat-

ment, recent tattoo or ear piercing; a history of viral hepatitis, syphilis or malaria; and a history of acquired immune deficiency syndrome or of being at risk of exposure to the human immuno deficiency virus (HIV).

Donated blood is obtained by inserting a needle into a peripheral vein, and allowing 500 ml of blood to flow through tubing attached to the needle into a collection bag.

All donated blood is carefully screened for the hepatitis B antigen, syphilis, and HIV. The blood is typed to determine the ABO group, and the presence or absence of Rh factors. Prior to transfusion, the blood is cross matched, which involves mixing a small amount of the recipient's blood with a small amount of the donor's blood to determine compatibility. If the wrong type of blood is transfused, the recipient could experience a severe transfusion reaction and may die.

Information on blood groups and compatibility is provided in Chapter 21.

Administration of blood or blood components

The principles of intravenous therapy, which are described in Chapter 31, also apply to the transfusion of blood and blood components. However, there are other aspects which are specific to the administration of blood or blood components.

The medical officer prescribes the type and amount of blood or blood product to be transfused, the date and rate of the infusion.

To obtain blood from the blood bank the nurse must follow the institution's policy, which specifies strict guidelines designed to prevent errors.

Prior to the transfusion, the information on each unit of blood is checked thoroughly by two nurses—one of whom must be a registered nurse. The label on the unit of blood is checked against the medical officer's order for information including the recipient's full name and registration number, the blood group and Rh factor of both recipient and donor, and the expiry date. This information is also checked against the recipient's identification wrist band.

The unit of blood, or blood component, is inspected for air bubbles and discolouration and, if these conditions are present, the product is returned to the blood bank.

The equipment required for transfusion of blood or a blood component is:

— blood administration set (tubing, filter, and drip chamber)
— container of IV normal saline solution
— blood or blood component
— IV stand
— venipuncture equipment, if necessary
— arm board and bandage
— sterile disposable gloves
— blood-warming device, if necessary.

Key aspects related to transfusions

- The recipient's vital signs are measured before the transfusion is commenced. This set of measurements is used as a baseline against which subsequent measurements are compared. An elevation of vital signs during the transfusion indicates a probable transfusion reaction.
- The nurse must remain with the recipient for at least 10 minutes after the transfusion has been commenced—to assess for signs of transfusion reaction. If such signs develop, the transfusion is ceased immediately. Information on transfusion reactions is provided later in this chapter.
- The nurse must thereafter monitor the recipient, and the transfusion, at regular intervals, e.g. every 15 minutes. Monitoring is necessary to assess for signs of transfusion reaction, and to ensure that the transfusion equipment is functioning correctly. Each time an assessment is made the results, e.g. vital signs, are documented on the appropriate chart.
- The rate of flow must be checked every 15 minutes to ensure that the solution is flowing at the prescribed rate. As blood is a thick solution, it may obstruct the tubing and alter the flow rate.
- Urine tests should be performed throughout the transfusion to detect evidence of the lysis of red blood cells—which occurs when there is incompatibility of donor and recipient blood.
- Termination of a blood transfusion is similar to termination of an intravenous infusion. Refer to Chapter 31 for further information. After completion of the transfusion, the filter and tubing are generally flushed with IV saline solution. The empty blood bag is returned to the blood bank, and the filter and tubing are discarded.

Transfusion reactions

As blood is a protein substance it has the potential for initiating an antigen–antibody reaction.

A transfusion reaction may be mild or it may be severe enough to result in anaphylaxis. In general, the greater number of transfusions the individual receives, the greater is the risk of developing antibodies against blood or blood components.

With any transfusion reaction, or suspected adverse reaction, the nurse must report the incident immediately to the nurse in charge. Steps are then taken to:

- Stop the transfusion. The container of blood is saved and sent to the blood bank for testing to assist in determining the cause of the reaction
- Start a saline infusion to maintain venous access
- Notify the medical officer
- Measure the vital signs, e.g. every 5 minutes
- Document the sequence of the reaction
- Notify the blood bank of a possible transfusion reaction

- Obtain a specimen of urine for examination. Laboratory analysis may detect the presence of haemoglobin, which would indicate a haemolytic reaction.
- Observe for oliguria or anuria, as haemoglobin deposits in the renal tubules can cause renal damage
- Make the patient as comfortable as possible, and administer oxygen or medications as prescribed.

The types of transfusion reactions are listed in Table 44.2.

THE INDIVIDUAL WITH ACQUIRED IMMUNE DEFICIENCY SYNDROME

AIDS is one of the most serious health problems of this time, and the nurse is in a key position to play a vital role in the care and support of an individual with HIV infection.

The nature of the disease is such that it places considerable stress on all those involved. Much of the stress related to caring for an individual with HIV infection can be reduced through education. Education is the most effective tool for reducing fear and anxiety about the disease, therefore it is important that the nurse keeps informed about current research, prevention, and management of acquired immune deficiency syndrome. She must also keep informed about the health care institution's policies related to infection control.

The nurse must prepare herself to accept an educational role, and to become a resource person both in the hospital and in the community.

Care of the individual with HIV infection

Many individuals will choose to remain at home, and most regions now provide home nursing care for people with AIDS. Other individuals may require admission to hospital, and the type and extent of physical care required by the individual will depend on his condition and on his specific needs.

Some of the physical aspects of care, both in the home environment and in hospital, involve the practice of infection control techniques. It is important for the nurse, and for other personnel involved in the care of the individual, to realize that the virus that causes AIDS is not *easily* transmitted. However, care must be taken to prevent coming in contact with blood and all other body fluids. Strict isolation of the individual is not generally necessary, unless it is to protect him against opportunistic infection.

The basic principles of hygiene and infection control that apply to the care of all patients are generally sufficient when caring for an individual with HIV infection. The nurse should be aware that it is not the individual she is caring for who places her at risk of contracting any infec-

Table 44.2 Transfusion reactions

Type	Cause	Manifestations
Haemolytic	Antibodies in the recipient's plasma react with antigens in the donor red blood cells	Onset is generally immediate Pyrexia of 40°C or higher Shivering Chest pain Dyspnoea Headache Low-back pain Tachycardia Hypotension Shock
Allergic	Thought to result from the reaction of allergens in donor blood with antibodies in recipient's blood	Urticaria Pruritus Wheezing Pulmonary oedema Laryngeal oedema Anaphylactic shock
Febrile	Recipient sensitivity to donor leucocytes or platelets	Onset occurs within approximately 1 hour Pyrexia Shivering Flushed skin Headache Tachycardia Malaise Nausea and vomiting
Bacterial	Bacterial contamination of donor blood	Pyrexia Shivering Dry, flushed skin Abdominal pain Extremity pain Vomiting Diarrhoea with passage of blood
Circulatory overload	Volume or rate of transfusion exceeds circulatory system capacity	Chest pain Dyspnoea Cough Pulmonary oedema Pleural rales Cyanosis Frothy sputum Tachycardia

tion, but that it is the practices that are carried out on or with the infected person which pose a risk.

As it is not always possible to know the status of an individual in regard to HIV, or hepatitis B, infection control precautions should be practised at all times with all patients. *Precautions* that should be taken include:

- Using disposable equipment for invasive procedures
- Decontaminating reusable equipment and subsequent sterilization. Cold water and detergent should be used to remove blood and other materials containing protein
- Incinerating waste

- Double bagging linen that is soiled with blood or body fluids
- Wearing gloves if contact with body fluids is anticipated
- Handling specimens with care
- Wearing a mask when there is direct contact with a patient who is coughing, or when suction is used to clear airways. Masks should also be worn during any invasive procedure, particularly where the procedure results in splashing and generation of drops of blood or other body fluids. Protective eyewear may be worn to prevent exposure of the mucous membranes of the eyes to blood or body fluids
- Disposing of needles and syringes into a rigid-wall, puncture-resistant container
- Applying sodium hypochlorite solution to areas that have become soiled with blood or body fluids. Spills may be wiped up with a pad of absorbent material soaked in sodium hypochlorite solution. The contaminated pad must be discarded into a container for subsequent incineration.

Careful and thorough washing of hands is one of the simplest and most effective infection control precautions. Hands should be washed and dried before and after contact with the individual, and after contact with body fluids. Information on handwashing technique is provided in Chapter 38.

The nurse should also practise any other infection control measures which have been implemented by the health care institution.

Psychological support for the individual with HIV infection is equally as important as meeting his physical needs. The individual may have many needs as a result of e.g. feelings of guilt about his sexual orientation or behaviour, fear of rejection by his family and friends, anxiety about the implications of the disease, and fear of dying.

The individual with HIV infection may demonstrate signs of depression, denial, anger, grief and mourning, lowered self esteem and worth.

It is important for the nurse to accept and encourage the expression of feelings that the individual may be experiencing, in order to help him to cope with the disease and its implications. The nurse can best help the individual by adopting an unconditional supportive approach. She should not be afraid to talk with the individual about his fears and uncertainties. The nurse needs to be broad minded, and to be able to accept that the individual's behaviour and lifestyle is his choice—and his responsibility. The nurse must not attempt to moralize, judge, or lecture the individual whose lifestyle is in variance with her own. A friendly approach that offers support and an opportunity for the individual to freely discuss aspects of his illness, is the most helpful.

Some nurses may not have the time or the appropriate

skills to provide adequate psychological support. Referral of the individual to AIDS programmes which provide counselling and referral services may be indicated. Such services employ people who are skilled in providing support and information for the individual with HIV infection, and for his significant others. Therefore, it is important that the nurse keeps informed of the support services that are available, and how they can be contacted.

Confidentiality is crucial and must be maintained, e.g. by being discreet regarding names and personal details, and the careful storage of documentation.

PACEMAKER IMPLANTATION

When the natural cardiac pacemakers fail to maintain a normal heart rate, and when medications prove ineffective, an artificial pacemaker may be required.

A pacemaker, which may be temporary or permanent, stimulates cardiac contraction by means of wires connected to electrodes which are inserted into the heart. The other ends of the wires are attached to a pulse generator which is implanted under the skin in the chest or abdomen (Fig. 44.2).

Permanent pacemakers may be one of several types. The fixed-rate pacemaker paces continuously, while the demand (self-adjusting) pacemaker is programmed to pace the heart when required, altering the pulse rate slowly and smoothly, as the heart normally does.

Post-operative care following the insertion of a pacemaker includes:

- Assessing the vital signs frequently, e.g. every $\frac{1}{2}$–1 hour for the first 24 hours, then at intervals determined by the individual's condition.
- Monitoring pacemaker function on the ECG (electrocardiograph).
- Checking the wound for signs of bleeding, infection, swelling or inflammation. Changing the wound dressing in accordance with the medical officer's orders or the institution's policy.
- Administering any prescribed medications, e.g. analgesics and antibiotics.
- Assessing the individual for signs of pacemaker failure: hypertension, chest pain, dizziness, light-headedness.
- Assessing the individual for signs of cardiac tamponade, which may result from a perforated ventricle: muffled heart sounds, distended neck veins, cyanosis, hypotension, restlessness, and pulsus paradoxus. *Pulsus paradoxus* is an abnormal decrease in systolic blood pressure during inhalation.

Education of the individual prior to his discharge from hospital includes teaching him how to assess his pulse; advising him on how the pacemaker works, how long any batteries should last, and the signs of pacemaker failure. The individual should also carry a card with him that contains information about his pacemaker, e.g. the model, serial number, and date of implantation. An individual with a pacemaker must also know those situations which could result in malfunction, e.g. close proximity to microwave ovens, large electrical generators, or high-voltage fields created by overhead power lines. He should always inform his dentist or medical officer that he has a pacemaker, as any procedure which involves the use of electricity, e.g. diathermy, could result in pacemaker malfunction.

The individual with a pacemaker can use a special telecommunications device to transmit his heart rate and rhythm to the hospital, where it is transformed onto ECG paper for interpretation.

HEART TRANSPLANTATION

In recent years heart transplantation has been performed to enable the individual with intractable cardiac disease, for which there is no alternative therapy, to lead a healthy and productive life.

Transplantation requires the heart of a young person in good general health, who has died in such a way that the heart is not injured, e.g. as a result of a motor vehicle accident. The donor heart is transplanted into a recipient when there is ABO compatibility and a negative lymphocyte crossmatch—to reduce the possibility of rejection.

Centres where transplants are performed set their own criteria for the selection of a suitable recipient. A lack of donor hearts remains the limiting factor in transplant programmes, and many potential recipients may die while waiting for a donor.

The surgical procedure involves attaching a heart-lung machine to the recipient and placing him on cardiopulmonary bypass. His heart is removed, leaving the posterior parts of the atria, and the openings of the aorta and pulmonary artery, intact. The donor heart is placed in the recipient's pericardial cavity, the atria are sutured into position, and the major blood vessels are anastomosed. Resumption of cardiac contraction may be spontaneous, or defibrillation may be necessary. Temporary pacing wires and drainage tubes are inserted, and the heart-lung machine is disconnected from the recipient.

The physiological implications for the recipient following transplantation include the risk of infection, and rejection of the donor heart.

Immunosuppressive therapy begins immediately after surgery and continues for the individual's lifetime. Regular biopsies and laboratory tests are performed to detect any signs of rejection. Because of immunosuppressive therapy the individual remains at high risk of infection, and must take precautions to prevent contracting an infection. The individual must visit his medical officer frequently, and he must follow a diet that is low in saturated fat and cholesterol.

Many individuals have been able to resume an active and productive life following a successful heart transplant.

BONE MARROW TRANSPLANTATION

Bone marrow transplantation is the replacement of deficient or diseased bone marrow with healthy marrow from a donor. This technique may be used in the treatment of blood disorders such as leukaemia and aplastic anaemia. A suitable donor must be located, and compatibility tests performed to determine whether the donor tissue is a suitable match. Siblings are the most common donors, and identical twins are ideal donors as they are genetically similar.

The surgical procedure to obtain the donor marrow involves the removal of up to 700 ml of bone marrow from the anterior and posterior iliac crests. The donor marrow is mixed with anticoagulant, strained, cultured, mixed with saline, and transferred to a blood bag. The recipient is prepared for the infusion of bone marrow by a course of chemotherapy and irradiation, to suppress his tissue-rejection potential. The bone marrow is infused through a vein over a period of approximately 4 hours.

The physiological implications for the recipient following bone marrow transplantation include the risk of infection, and graft-versus-host disease (GVHD). GVHD is a tissue incompatibility syndrome in which donor T-lymphocytes attack host tissue. It generally occurs within 1–2 weeks following transplantation, but it may develop as late as 12 months afterwards.

A successful transplant is often life-saving, as it restores haematologic and immune functioning.

SUMMARY

The functions of the circulatory system are to pump blood and transport it through the body in a system of arteries, veins, and capillaries. The lymphatic system filters wastes and foreign substances and plays a major role in defence against infection.

Normal function can be impaired by factors which affect cardiac pumping ability, impede the flow of blood through the blood vessels, impair blood formation or function, or disrupt the return of filtered lymph to the circulation.

The major manifestations of circulatory system disorders are dyspnoea, chest pain, palpitation, cough, fatigue, cyanosis, syncope, oedema, alterations in the pulse, pain in or impaired circulation to the lower extremities, bruising and bleeding, and enlarged lymph nodes.

Disorders of the circulatory system can be classified as congenital defects, hereditary disorders, of multiple cause, infectious or inflammatory, neoplastic or obstructive, degenerative, or those resulting from trauma.

Diagnostic tests used to assess circulatory system function include tests to assess cardiac function, peripheral blood vessels, haematologic status, and lymphangiography.

Care of the individual with a disorder includes promoting comfort and relieving pain, providing psychological support, maintaining skin integrity, promoting and maintaining mobility, preventing infection, maintaining fluid and nutritional status, and administering prescribed medications.

Nursing activities also include assisting in the care of an individual who is receiving a transfusion of blood or blood components.

Acquired immune deficiency syndrome (AIDS) is one of the most serious health problems of the time, and the nurse is in a key position to play a vital role in the care and support of an individual with HIV infection.

Specific disorders of the circulatory system may require surgical intervention which includes pacemaker implantation, heart transplantation, or bone marrow transplantation.

REFERENCES AND FURTHER READING

Brunner L S, Suddarth D S 1988 Textbook of medical-surgical nursing, 6th edn. J. B. Lippincott, Philadelphia
Boore J R P, Champion R, Ferguson M C (eds) 1987 Nursing the physically ill adult. Churchill Livingstone, Edinburgh
Ford R D (ed) 1984 Cardiovascular disorders: nurse's clinical library. Springhouse, Pennsylvania
Game C, Anderson R, Kidd J (eds) 1989 Medical-surgical nursing: a core text. Churchill Livingstone, Melbourne, 276–332
Hampton J R 1986 The ECG made easy, 3rd edn. Churchill Livingstone, Edinburgh

45. The individual with a respiratory system disorder

INTRODUCTION

Information on the normal structure and function of the respiratory system is provided in Chapter 22, and it should be referred to before studying the contents of this chapter. The function of the respiratory system is to deliver oxygen from the atmosphere to the bloodstream, and to deliver carbon dioxide from the blood stream to the atmosphere. Any disorder that disrupts respiration injures body cells, and may have permanent effects on a part or all of the body. Although disorders of the respiratory system are common in most communities , the incidence of respiratory disease is controlled to some extent by:

- immunization against infections such as pertussis and tuberculosis.

- legislation to control environmental pollution, which aims to ensure that individuals in their place of work are not exposed to high levels of respiratory tract pollutants and irritants.
- legislation to control the processing, handling, and sale of foods which may otherwise be responsible for the transmission of respiratory diseases.
- public health education about smoking and its relationship to lung cancer and chronic obstructive pulmonary disease; the means of preventing droplet-spread infection; and the effects of air pollutants on the respiratory tract.

The community health nurse, who plays a major role in illness prevention, health maintenance and health promotion, can make a significant contribution in reducing the incidence of respiratory disease—through the planning and implementation of community education programmes.

Pathophysiological influences and effects

Some diseases of respiration result from inadequate ventilation, while other diseases result from abnormalities of diffusion through the pulmonary membrane or inadequate transport of oxygen from the lungs to the tissues.

Inadequate ventilation (hypoventilation)

Hypoventilation is ventilation below the level necessary to maintain normal carbon dioxide tension (PCO_2). If hypoventilation occurs the arterial blood levels of carbon dioxide will be above normal (hypercapnia). Hypoventilation occurs when the volume of air entering the alveoli is not adequate for the metabolic needs of the body.

Hypoventilation has many causes including obstruction of the airways by oedematous mucous membrane lining, polyps or tumours, retained secretions, bronchospasm and obstructive diseases such as emphysema. Hypoventilation can also result from abnormalities of the central nervous system, as well as from neuromuscular or skeletal abnormalities.

Impaired diffusion

Diffusion is the process by which oxygen and carbon dioxide molecules are transported between the alveoli and the capillary network. Diffusion abnormalities can interfere with the passage of oxygen into the blood. Such diffusion abnormalities can result from pulmonary oedema, a reduction in the amount of functioning lung tissue, or fibrosis of the alveolar walls.

Impaired perfusion

Not only is an adequate intake of oxygen by ventilation essential, but for oxygenation of the body tissues to occur adequate perfusion of lung tissue with blood is necessary. Any condition that decreases circulation to lung tissue may lead to *hypoxia*, e.g. a decrease in total blood volume pulmonary embolism and chronic obstructive pulmonary disease.

In addition to abnormalities of the lungs or respiratory structures, dysfunction of other body systems can adversely affect respiratory function. For example, a disease process that affects the nervous system may adversely affect respiration. One instance where a disorder of the nervous system greatly impairs respiratory function, is when the spinal cord is damaged.

Cardiovascular dysfunction can affect respiratory function, e.g. right-sided heart failure may affect the volume of pulmonary blood circulation. A deformity of the skeletal system, e.g. scoliosis, may restrict movement of the thoracic cage and thus alter respiratory function. Inadequate lung expansion can also occur following abdominal surgery, as pain in the operation site may inhibit deep breathing and coughing.

Not only can abnormalities of other body systems adversely affect the respiratory system, but respiratory abnormalities generally affect all other body systems.

Major manifestations of respiratory disorders

The signs and symptoms manifested by the individual with a respiratory disorder vary with the location and severity of the disorder.

Chest pain

Disorders of the respiratory system, e.g. pleurisy, can result in chest pain. During ventilation, friction occurs between the inflamed layers of serous membrane (pleura) covering the lungs and lining the thoracic cavity. Chest pain may be localized, or may be experienced only when the individual breathes deeply, and can vary from a continuous aching pain to a stabbing knife-like pain. Pain associated with respiratory disorders may be retrosternal, lateral or posterior.

Cough

A cough is a common symptom of many respiratory disorders, and it may result from irritation or from retained secretions that obstruct some part of the airway. If sputum is expelled the cough is described as 'productive', and a 'non-productive' or dry cough is one which is not accompanied by the expectoration of sputum. Sputum is not normally produced, but sputum production can result from inflammation, infection or congestion.

Haemoptysis, which is the expectoration of blood, may occur in some lung diseases. Blood-streaked sputum frequently occurs in minor upper respiratory tract infections or in bronchitis. The expectoration of bright red frothy blood indicates a more serious disorder, e.g. bronchogenic carcinoma, lung abscess, or tuberculosis.

Voice change

Voice changes, e.g. hoarseness, may accompany upper respiratory tract infections or may be due to more serious disorders such as a laryngeal tumour. Disorders of the upper respiratory tract, e.g. laryngitis, can sometimes result in loss of voice.

Dyspnoea

Dyspnoea, which is difficult or laboured breathing, may result from disorders affecting either the upper or lower respiratory tract. Disorders of the upper respiratory tract which may cause dyspnoea include obstruction of the airway by inflammation, a tumour, or a foreign body. Disorders of the lower respiratory tract which cause dyspnoea include carcinoma of the lung and chronic obstructive pulmonary disease. A disorder affecting the thorax, e.g. trauma to the chest wall, commonly causes dyspnoea. Laboured breathing may be accompanied by nasal flaring, the use of the neck and accessory chest muscles, and an increased ventilation rate.

Changes in breathing patterns

Certain disorders of the respiratory system produce characteristic changes in breathing patterns. An acute respiratory disorder can produce rapid, shallow breathing (tachypnoea); and airway obstruction e.g. due to emphysema, can result in prolonged forceful expiration and pursed lip breathing. Certain disorders also result in abnormal breathing sounds, e.g. wheezing, or 'grunting' ventilations. Information on abnormal breathing sounds is provided in Chapter 32.

Hypoxia

Hypoxia is an oxygen deficiency in the tissues, and it may

be due to lung disorders which prevent adequate supplies of oxygen from reaching the blood. Hypoxia may also be due to hypoventilation, anaemia, and impaired tissue utilization of oxygen. The manifestations of hypoxia include tachycardia, tachypnoea, breathlessness, pallor or cyanosis. Cerebral signs such as lethargy, confusion, or agitation may result.

Thoracic abnormalities

Chronic respiratory system disorders may alter chest configuration, e.g. a 'barrel chest' is characteristic of emphysema. Asymmetrical chest expansion can result from trauma, e.g. 'flail chest' and pneumothorax.

Other manifestations

Depending on the type and severity of the disorder, other manifestations may be evident. For example, infections of the respiratory tract generally result in pyrexia, headaches, aching muscles, and lethargy. Difficulty in swallowing (dysphagia) may be present in disorders such as pharyngitis and tonsillitis.

In certain chronic disorders of the respiratory system, clubbing of the fingers may be evident. The distal portions of the fingers are abnormally enlarged, and the nails show increased curvature. The mechanism whereby diminished oxygen tension in the blood causes clubbing is not well understood.

Specific disorders of the respiratory system

Disorders of multiple cause

Certain disorders of the respiratory system have more than one cause, and may be related to structural or functional changes, to environmental conditions, or to a combination of factors.

Epistaxis is bleeding from the nostrils, and is an indication of a physiological abnormality or underlying trauma. The most common cause is trauma, but epistaxis may be related to local nasal infections, tumours of the nose, or it may be associated with certain systemic disorders, e.g. leukaemia. Bleeding from the nose may be unilateral or bilateral, and the amount of blood loss varies. Information on the first aid management of epistaxis is provided in Chapter 57.

Rhinitis is inflammation of the nasal mucous membranes, usually accompanied by mucosal swelling and nasal discharge. Acute rhinitis, also known as the common cold or coryza, is the most common cause of nasal airway obstruction. Allergic rhinitis is often referred to as hay fever, and is related to sensitivity to pollens from grasses, flowers or trees, or to atmospheric pollutants.

Laryngeal oedema may result from an infection, neoplasms involving the neck, trauma, or as an allergic response of the tissue of the larynx. Mild oedema may result in hoarseness; but in more severe cases the airway becomes obstructed, and dyspnoea, cyanosis and tachypnoea may occur.

The pneumoconioses are diseases of the lungs caused by chronic inhalation of inorganic dusts of occupational or environmental origin. Included in the pneumoconioses are asbestosis and silicosis. As a result of chronic inhalation the lungs become non-elastic, lung volume is reduced and gas exchange is impaired. The individual develops shortness of breath, cough, and production of sputum. As the condition progresses, respiratory impairment becomes severe. Mesothelioma, a cancer of the pleura is associated with asbestosis and is often the cause of death of the individual with asbestosis.

Sarcoidosis is a chronic disorder of unknown cause characterized by the formation of granulomas in many organs. The most common site is the lungs, but it also affects the liver, spleen, skin and mucous membranes. There can be spontaneous remission, or the condition can progress to wide spread granulomatous inflammation and fibrosis.

Pleurisy is inflammation of the pleura, and is a symptom of many disorders, e.g. pneumonia, tuberculosis, and bronchial carcinoma. Pleurisy is characterized by dyspnoea, coughing, and stabbing chest pain which increases during deep inhalation.

Adult respiratory distress syndrome (ARDS) is a cause of respiratory failure due to impaired gas diffusion, and may result from shock, inhalation of gastric contents, fat embolus, toxaemia, oxygen toxicity, or excessive fluid administration. Diffuse damage to either side of the alveolar–capillary membrane occurs, resulting in increased vascular permeability with oedema and haemorrhage. The main features of the condition are increasing hypoxia and pulmonary oedema. As the condition worsens severe dyspnoea, grunting ventilations, cyanosis and confusion become evident. Unless corrected, respiratory acidosis and terminal respiratory failure may occur.

Infectious disorders

Infectious disorders can be classed as upper or lower respiratory tract infections. Infections of the upper respiratory tract are caused by bacteria or viruses, while a variety of microorganisms can cause lower respiratory tract infections.

Sinusitis is inflammation of one or more of the paranasal sinuses. Although the condition may be caused by an allergy, a change in atmosphere, or a structural nasal defect, sinusitis generally refers to a suppurative infection involving bacterial invasion of the mucosa. The initial symptom is nasal congestion, followed by a sensation of pressure over the infected sinus. Later, the individual experiences localized pain and tenderness, headache, and pyrexia. Nasal discharge may be blood stained at first, becoming purulent and copious later.

Influenza is a contagious infection of the respiratory tract transmitted by airborne droplets. The onset is sudden, starting with headaches, backache, joint pain, lethargy, and pyrexia. There may be a painful unproductive cough, conjunctivitis, sore throat, and enlarged lymph glands. Influenza commonly occurs in epidemics, and is caused by one of the many influenza group viruses.

Pharyngitis is inflammation of the pharynx, and may be acute or chronic. Acute pharyngitis is usually viral in origin, but it may be due to a bacterial infection. Symptoms include sore throat, slight dysphagia, cough, and low grade pyrexia. Chronic pharyngitis is usually associated with a nasopharyngeal obstruction or inflammation, frequently resulting from constant exposure to an allergen or to factors which cause excessive dryness of the mucosa, e.g. air conditioning.

Tonsillitis is inflammation and enlargement of the tonsil tissue, and may be acute or chronic. Acute tonsillitis is frequently caused by streptococcal infection, and is characterized by a very sore throat, dysphagia, headaches, muscular discomfort and pyrexia. Enlarged lymph glands in the neck are frequently evident, and the individual may experience referred ear pain.

Chronic tonsillitis produces a recurrent sore throat and purulent drainage, and frequent attacks of acute tonsillitis may also occur. Removal of the tonsils may be the most effective treatment for proven chronic tonsillitis.

Quinsy, peritonsillar abscess, is an infection of tissue between the tonsil and pharynx, which may occur following acute follicular tonsillitis. Manifestations include dysphagia, pain radiating to the ear, pyrexia, redness and swelling of the tonsil and adjacent soft palate.

Laryngitis is inflammation of the mucous membrane lining of the larynx, commonly accompanied by oedema of the vocal cords and hoarseness. Laryngitis may be caused by an infection, or it may be related to excessive use of the voice, exposure to irritating fumes, or an allergy. In addition to hoarseness, or loss of voice, the individual may experience a tickling sensation in the throat, and the general symptoms of an upper respiratory tract infection are commonly present.

Epiglottitis, which is inflammation of the epiglottis, is considered an emergency because it can rapidly lead to total airway obstruction. Although it is more common in children, epiglottitis also affects adults. Acute epiglottitis is characterized by a sore throat, dysphasia, pyrexia, and 'drooling' of oral secretions. Respiratory obstruction, with stridor and cyanosis, becomes evident as the inflammation progresses.

Acute bronchitis is an infection of the bronchi, frequently caused by a virus. It is characterized by a productive cough and chest pain. The general symptoms of

infection, e.g. headache, muscular pains, lethargy, are common, and pyrexia may be present.

Pneumonia is inflammation of the lung tissue and may be caused by bacteria, viruses, rickettsiae or fungi. Characteristics of pneumonia are pyrexia, chills, pleural pain; and a cough that produces purulent sputum is common. Ventilations usually become more difficult, painful, shallow, and rapid.

Aspiration pneumonia is an inflammatory condition which may occur if an individual's gag or swallowing reflexes are impaired—resulting in the inhalation of vomitus containing acid gastric contents. Aspiration pneumonia most often occurs during general anaesthesia—or during recovery from anaesthesia, or when an individual has a condition characterized by a decreased level of consciousness and vomiting.

Pertussis (whooping cough) is an infectious respiratory condition caused by *Bordetella pertussis*. Pertussis occurs more commonly in children, and manifestations develop throughout a period of approximately 6 weeks. Typically, the illness can be divided into three phases: catarrhal, paroxysmal, and convalescent. The first (catarrhal) phase is characterized by an irritating nocturnal cough, sneezing, conjunctivitis, anorexia, pyrexia, and fatigue. The second (paroxysmal) phase begins approximately 7–14 days afterwards. The individual experiences a series of violent sharp coughs. Each paroxysm of coughing typically ends in a loud high-pitched inhalatory whoop, which is caused by spasmodic closure of the glottis. Choking on mucus, which causes vomiting, is common, and the individual may become cyanotic and apnoeic. During the convalescent phase, paroxysmal coughing and vomiting gradually subside. For some months afterward, even a mild upper respiratory infection may trigger paroxysmal coughing.

Croup (acute laryngotracheobronchitis), which is severe inflammation and obstruction of the upper airway, usually affects children between the ages of 3 months and 3 years. It generally results from a viral infection, with its onset following an upper respiratory tract infection. Manifestations include stridor on inhalation, respiratory distress, and a characteristic sharp 'barking' cough. As the condition progresses it causes inflammatory oedema and spasm—which can obstruct the upper airway and severely compromise breathing.

Tuberculosis is an infectious disease caused by *Myobacterium tuberculosis*, generally transmitted by inhalation or ingestion of infected droplets, and usually affecting the lungs. Tuberculosis of the lungs commonly develops as a chronic illness with symptoms appearing over weeks or months. Symptoms include weight loss, fatigue, anorexia, vague chest pain, low grade pyrexia, and night sweats. As the disease progresses, there is some dyspnoea, expectoration of sputum, and haemoptysis. Tuberculosis may spread from the lungs, via the lymphatic and blood vessels, to the liver, spleen and other organs.

Empyema is the accumulation of pus in the pleural space, or a purulent pleural effusion. It can result from a lung infection or, less commonly, from a penetrating chest wound. Common symptoms are pleuritic chest pain, dyspnoea and pyrexia. There may be a productive cough and blood stained sputum.

Obstructive disorders

Obstructive disorders are lung diseases that cause a persistent obstruction of bronchial air flow. Airway obstruction can also be due to the inhalation of a foreign body, or one or both bronchi may become obstructed by a benign or malignant tumour. Some of the more common types of airways obstruction are grouped under the heading of chronic obstructive pulmonary disease, (COPD) or chronic obstructive airways disease. Common forms of chronic obstructive airways disease include asthma, bronchiectasis, chronic bronchitis, and emphysema.

Asthma is a disease manifested by difficulty in breathing caused by generalized narrowing of the airways. Asthma is characterized by recurring episodes of paroxysmal dyspnoea, wheezing on exhalation, coughing, and tenacious mucoid bronchial secretions. The individual having an asthma attack commonly experiences anxiety, diaphoresis, tachycardia and an elevated blood pressure. The increased effort of breathing can cause marked fatigue.

Episodes of asthma may be precipitated by inhalation of allergens or pollutants, infection, vigorous exercise, cold air, or emotional stress. The severity and duration of asthma attacks vary; treatment may control the attack rapidly or the symptoms can become increasingly severe and prolonged.

A severe and prolonged asthma attack that resists treatment is referred to as *status asthmaticus*. Unless treatment reverses the condition, the individual may develop respiratory failure.

Bronchiectasis is a condition characterized by irreversible dilatation of the bronchial tree and destruction of the bronchial walls. It is most often the result of repeated bronchial infections and prolonged bronchial obstruction. The main feature of bronchiectasis is a chronic, loose cough that produces large amounts of mucopurulent sputum. Haemoptysis is a common occurrence, as are bronchopulmonary infections. The individual can experience dyspnoea, fatigue, and chronic sinusitis.

Advanced bronchiectasis can lead to pulmonary hypertension, hypoxaemia, and finger clubbing. Complications of bronchiectasis include pneumonia, lung abscess and empyema.

Chronic bronchitis is a condition characterized by an excessive secretion of mucus in the bronchi, accompanied by a chronic or recurrent productive cough. Additional symptoms include frequent respiratory tract infections, cyanosis, and hypoxia. An individual who has advanced chronic bronchitis may have central cyanosis, pulmonary hypertension, general oedema, and clubbing of the fingers.

Chronic bronchitis is associated with cigarette smoking, atmospheric pollution and occupational pollutants. Complications include bronchopneumonia, emphysema and cardiac failure.

Emphysema (pulmonary) is a chronically progressive disease characterized by overdistension and destruction of alveolar walls, resulting in a loss of lung elasticity. The predisposing causes are the same as for those chronic bronchitis, with cigarette smoking being the major factor.

Initially the peripheral bronchioles become inflamed and the subsequent narrowing of the airways traps air in the alveoli. As the disease progresses the alveolar walls become over-inflated and rupture. Because of loss of lung elasticity the terminal bronchioles tend to collapse prematurely during exhalation, making expulsion of air from the lungs more difficult.

Symptoms of chronic emphysema include shortness of breath, dyspnoea, cyanosis, and cough. Individuals will commonly exhale through pursed lips to prolong expiration and reduce the tendency of the airways to collapse. As the disease becomes more severe, the individual uses his accessory muscles to breathe.

The anterior-posterior diameter of the chest usually increases, due to expansion of the chest wall and loss of lung elasticity, giving the chest a barrel-shaped appearance. Distension of the neck veins may be present, as may clubbing of the fingers. In advanced emphysema, the individual fights for every breath of air.

Acute respiratory failure is the sudden failure of the respiratory system, and heart, to meet the demands of internal (tissue) respiration. It can result from chronic obstructive pulmonary diseases, from certain neuromuscular diseases, cerebral disorders, or an overdose of drugs that depress the respiratory centre. Any condition that alters the mechanisms of ventilation, diffusion, or circulation, impairs gas exchange and may result in respiratory failure.

The condition may occur gradually or very suddenly, and the signs and symptoms are those associated with hypoxia and/or hypercapnia. Neurological symptoms include headache, confusion, restlessness, drowsiness or coma; cardiovascular symptoms include tachycardia, hypertension, and dysrhythmias; respiratory symptoms include dyspnoea, tachypnoea and cyanosis. If the condition is not detected and treated promptly, congestive cardiac failure and respiratory acidosis may result.

Neoplastic disorders

Benign or malignant neoplasms may affect the upper or lower respiratory tract. Tumours can affect the normal functioning of the respiratory tract and, if malignant, can cause extensive tissue damage by infiltration. The signs and symptoms of neoplastic disease vary depending on the location and extent of the lesion.

Nasal polyps are masses of hypertrophied mucosa which commonly form in response to recurrent swelling of the nasal mucosa. Obstruction of the nasal passages develops gradually as the benign polyps multiply and enlarge. The individual experiences difficulty in breathing through the nose, and the voice may have a nasal quality.

Laryngeal polyps are growths that arise from the mucous membrane of the vocal cords, and the major symptom is hoarseness. Laryngeal polyps are usually benign, but they may become malignant.

Laryngeal carcinoma is a malignant neoplasm arising from or around the vocal cords. Persistent hoarseness is the major symptom, and heavy cigarette smoking is believed to be a major factor in the development of laryngeal cancer. If the lesion is large, dysphagia may be present.

Lung cancer commonly affects the bronchus. It arises from the bronchial epithelium and rapidly invades lung tissue, causing parts of the lung to collapse. It may spread through the lymphatic network and bloodstream to form metastases in other parts of the body, e.g. the liver, bones, or brain.

The incidence of lung cancer is related to several factors, the most important being the inhalation of cigarette smoke. Other factors include exposure to atmospheric pollution and occupational pollutants.

Unfortunately, the physical manifestations of lung cancer do not generally appear until lung cancer is well advanced. Symptoms include persistent cough, dyspnoea, purulent or blood streaked sputum, chest pain, and repeated attacks of bronchitis or pneumonia. Sometimes, the initial symptoms are associated with organs that are the sites of metastasis, e.g. the liver, bones, or brain. Cancer of the lung may also occur secondary to a primary malignant tumour elsewhere in the body, as a result of metastasis.

Further information on cancer is provided in Chapter 64.

Traumatic disorders

Injury to part of the respiratory tract can result from a variety of causes.

Laryngotracheal trauma can be minor and cause hoarseness and some dysphagia, or it may be as severe as a layngeal fracture. In a severe injury, oedema of the larynx may occur and be accompanied by signs of respiratory distress.

Flail chest occurs when multiple rib fractures result in 'floating' of a segment of the rib cage. As a consequence there is instability in part of the chest wall and paradoxical breathing. Paradoxical breathing is characterized by the injured chest wall collapsing in during inhalation, and moving out during exhalation. The lung underlying the injury contracts on inhalation and bulges on exhalation. If uncorrected, ventilation is impaired, which may lead to hypoxia and respiratory failure. Manifestations of a flail chest are paradoxical motion of the chest wall during breathing, severe pain, dyspnoea, tachycardia, and cyanosis.

Pneumothorax is a collection of air in the pleural space causing the lung to collapse. A pneumothorax may be open or closed. In an open pneumothorax, an injury creates an opening in the chest wall—allowing air to flow into the pleural cavity. In a closed, or spontaneous, pneumothorax, the chest wall is intact and air enters the pleural space from an opening on the surface of the lung.

A pneumothorax causes pain, dyspnoea and tachypnoea, and unilateral diminished breath sounds. There may be subcutaneous emphysema in the neck and upper chest, and a 'sucking' sound may be heard in the region of an open pneumothorax.

Tension pneumothorax is a particularly severe form that occurs when air escapes into the pleural cavity. As a result, continuously increasing air pressure in the pleural cavity causes progressive collapse of the lung tissue. Emergency aspiration of air from the pleural cavity is necessary.

Haemothorax is the accumulation of blood in the pleural space, usually as a result of trauma. Manifestations of haemothorax include dyspneoa, chest tightness, haemoptysis, and signs of hypovolemic shock. If not treated, haemothorax can lead to shock from haemorrhage, severe pain, or respiratory failure.

Diagnostic tests

Certain tests may be used to assist, or confirm, the diagnosis of respiratory disorders.

Pulmonary function tests

These tests measure the functional ability of the lungs. A spirometer is used to assess the individual's lung volume, by measuring and recording the volume of inhaled and exhaled air. The values are then compared with the normal values expected for an individual of the same sex, weight, height, and age. Table 45.1 lists types of pulmonary function tests and the normal expected values.

Chest X-ray

A chest X-ray is one of the most common procedures used to evaluate the lungs, and generally involves posterior—anterior and lateral views. Abnormal findings that may be evident on chest X-ray include areas of density, presence of a mass, and accumulation of fluid.

Lung scan

A lung scan may be performed by administering radio-

Table 45.1 Pulmonary function tests

Tests	Explanation	Normal value*
Tidal volume	Amount of air inhaled or exhaled during normal breathing	500 ml
Total lung capacity	Total volume of the lungs when maximally inflated	5800 ml
Vital capacity	Total volume of air that can be exhaled after maximum inhalation	3000–6000 ml
Functional residual capcity	Amount of air remaining in the lungs after normal exhalation	2300 ml
Inspiratory capacity	Amount of air that can be inhaled after normal exhalation	3500 ml
Expiratory reserve volume	Amount of air that can be exhaled after normal exhalation	1100 ml
Forced expiratory volume	Maximum amount of air that can be forcibly exhaled, in one second, after full inhalation	3000–5000 ml
Residual volume	Amount of air remaining in the lungs after forced exhalation	1200 ml

*Values given are the average for a young adult male.

active dye. The radioactive particles are distributed and trapped in the pulmonary capillary bed, and the lung scan produces a visual image of pulmonary blood flow. Conditions such as pulmonary oedema, lung cancer, or COPD, may cause abnormal perfusion.

Blood gas analysis

Blood gas analysis shows how well the individual's lungs are delivering oxygen to the bloodstream, and eliminating carbon dioxide. Blood is collected for analysis of pH, PCO_2, PO_2, bicarbonate and base levels.

Cultures

A specimen of secretions, is obtained e.g. via a nose or throat swab, and sent to the laboratory so that any microorganisms present can be identified. Sensitivity studies are then done to determine which drug is effective against the specific microorganism.

Sputum cytology

A specimen of sputum is obtained and sent to the laboratory, where it is examined to detect the presence of pus, pathogenic microorganisms, or malignant cells.

Skin tests

The most common skin test performed is the Mantoux test. This test is used in the detection of tuberculosis, and is performed by injecting intradermally 0.1 ml of solution containing old tuberculin. A positive reaction, which shows as an area of induration of at least 5 mm in diameter within 48–72 hours, indicates the presence of antibodies to the tubercle bacillus.

Bronchoscopy

Bronchoscopy involves the direct viewing of the trachea and bronchi by means of an instrument called a bronchoscope. Bronchoscopy is used in the diagnosis of respiratory tract disorders, and may be used to remove foreign bodies or to obtain a specimen of secretions or tissue for microscopic examination.

Thoracentesis

In this procedure, the thoracic wall is punctured with a needle to obtain a specimen of pleural fluid for analysis. The procedure may also be performed to relieve pulmonary compression caused by a pleural effusion. A local anaesthetic is injected into the skin before the thoracentesis needle is inserted.

Other diagnostic tests which may be performed include fluoroscopy, tomography, bronchography and pulmonary angiography. Blood tests may also be carried out to detect and identify the source of bacterial or viral infections.

CARE OF THE INDIVIDUAL WITH A RESPIRATORY SYSTEM DISORDER

Although specific nursing actions and medical management vary depending on the individual's respiratory disorder, the main aims of care are to:

- maintain airway patency
- facilitate normal and effective breathing
- promote efficient gas exchange.

The individual who has a respiratory system disorder will commonly experience problems such as a change in breathing habit, and discomfort associated with breathing. Nursing activities include alleviating discomforts associated with breathing, administering oxygen, and helping the individual with breathing exercises. As well as planning care to meet specific respiratory needs, the nurse must also consider the individuals other needs, e.g. nutritional, elimination, and the need for comfort.

Promoting a clear airway

One of the most important aspects of care is the maintenance or restoration of a clear airway, which includes measures directed at removing secretions. Commonly, an inflammatory respiratory tract disorder results in the production of excessive, tenacious secretions. The individual may experience some difficulty in expectorating secretions, and the measures which will assist him are as follows:

Adequate hydration

Dehydration will make any secretions more viscid and difficult to expectorate, therefore an adequate fluid input is important. Unless contraindicated, the individual should be encouraged to drink at least 2–3 litres in each 24 hours. If he is unable to tolerate sufficient oral fluids, the administration of fluids intravenously may be necessary.

Cessation of smoking

If the individual is a smoker, he should be encouraged to stop smoking. Cigarette smoke causes impaired function of the cilia, and smoking generally aggravates any existing respiratory tract disorder.

Local hydration

As well as an adequate fluid input, local hydration by means of humidifiers, inhalations, or nebulizers may be necessary. Local hydration facilitates removal of respiratory secretions, by loosening them so that expectoration is less difficult. Information on the use of humidifiers and nebulizers is provided later in the chapter.

Positioning

The individual should be assisted to assume a position that will facilitate lung expansion and effective breathing. A sitting position, as described in Chapter 35, will provide for better expansion of the lungs which improves breathing. The nurse should ensure that pillows are placed so that the individual's back, neck, and head are well supported.

Medication

Medications may be prescribed to loosen secretions, relieve bronchospasm, combat infection, control coughing, or relieve pulmonary oedema.

Medications may be given by inhalation, orally, or by injection. The types of medications prescribed may include decongestants, antihistamines, antibiotics, bronchodilators, or expectorants.

The nurse must ensure that any medication is administered in accordance with nursing regulations and the institution's policies.

Oronasopharyngeal suction

If coughing is ineffective in removing secretions, suction may be necessary. Oronasopharyngeal suction removes secretions from the pharynx by means of a suction catheter inserted through the mouth or nostril. This technique is used to maintain a patent airway, and is indicated for the individual who is unable to clear his airway effectively with coughing and expectoration. Information on this procedure is provided later in the chapter.

Chest physiotherapy

The techniques of chest physiotherapy mobilize and eliminate secretions, re-expand lung tissue, and promote the efficient use of the muscles of ventilation. Chest physiotherapy includes postural drainage, chest percussion and vibration, and coughing and deep breathing exercises.

Postural drainage encourages pulmonary secretions to empty by gravity into the bronchi or trachea, so that they may be expectorated. The individual is assisted to assume positions that promote drainage from the affected parts of the lungs. Effectiveness of the technique largely depends on positioning that allows drainage by gravity (Fig. 45.1). Postural drainage should be avoided immediately before or after meals, to prevent nausea and aspiration of food or vomitus.

Percussion and vibration are techniques employed to help loosen respiratory secretions, and are commonly used in conjunction with postural drainage. Percussion is performed by rhythmic tapping using cupped hands over the affected segments of the lungs. It is begun gently and is increased in forcefulness as the individual tolerates increased percussion. Vibration is performed by placing the hands over the affected area, and shaking—so that the chest wall is vibrated.

After postural drainage, percussion and vibration, the patient is instructed to cough to remove the loosened secretions. Oral hygiene should be attended to following the procedure, because the expectorated secretions may have an offensive taste or odour.

Promoting effective breathing and aeration

In addition to the measures employed to promote a clear airway, other measures may be necessary to maintain ad-

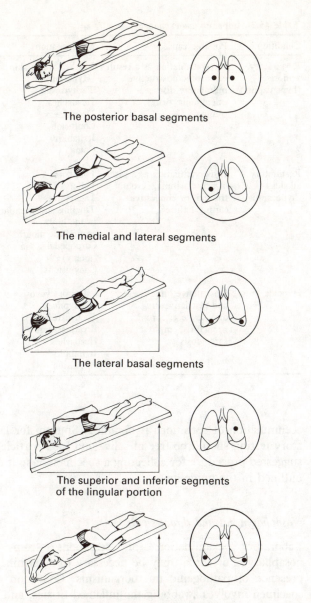

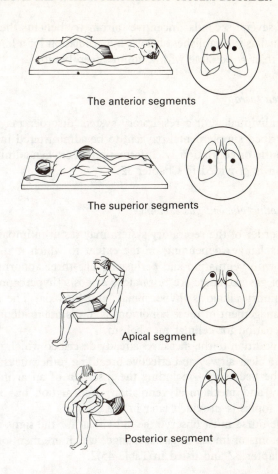

Fig. 45.1 Positions for postural drainage from various parts of the lungs.

equate ventilation. Breathing exercises may be used by the individual to promote and maintain optimal pulmonary ventilation, and oxygen may be prescribed to supplement that being obtained from the atmosphere.

Breathing exercises

When respiratory system disorders produce ineffective breathing patterns and inadequate ventilation, the individual will be instructed in breathing exercises.

Deep, or diaphragmatic, breathing uses the diaphragm and abdominal muscles to fully aerate the lungs. The in-

dividual should be assisted into a sitting position to promote optimal lung expansion. One hand is placed on the chest, and the other hand is placed on the abdomen. If the individual is breathing correctly the hand on the abdomen should rise with inhalation and fall with exhalation; the hand on the chest should remain still. The individual is instructed to inhale deeply and slowly, pushing his abdomen out—to promote optimal distribution of air to the alveoli. He is instructed to exhale through pursed lips, while contracting his abdomen. Exhalation through pursed lips improves oxygen diffusion and encourages a slow, deep breathing pattern. Abdominal contraction pushes the diaphragm upwards, exerts pressure on the lungs, and helps to empty them.

Breathing exercises are performed according to the individual's condition, e.g. short sessions may be indicated if the individual becomes fatigued easily. The duration and frequency with which deep breathing exercises are performed vary, e.g. they may be performed for one minute with gradual progression to a ten minute exercise period, four times daily.

Incentive spirometry uses a breathing device to encourage the individual to achieve maximum ventilation. The device measures respiratory flow or respiratory volume, and induces the individual to take a deep breath and hold it for several seconds. Incentive spirometry benefits the individual as it establishes alveolar hyperinflation for a longer time than is possible with a normal deep breath.

Oxygen therapy

An individual with a respiratory system disorder may be prescribed supplemental oxygen, to be administered intermittently or continuously. Information on oxygen administration is provided in Chapter 32.

Promoting efficient gas exchange

A disorder of the repiratory system may result in impaired gas exchange, depending on the extent to which it interferes with ventilation and perfusion. The three abnormalities of gas exchange are respiratory acidosis (hypercapnia), respiratory alkalosis (hypocapnia), and hypoxia. The aim of management of these conditions is to maintain adequate oxygenation for cellular metabolism.

In addition to the measures already described which promote a clear airway and effective breathing, other measures may be necessary—including the insertion of an artificial airway and mechanical ventilation. Information on both these topics is provided later in the chapter.

The nurse must observe the individual for the signs and symptoms of impaired gas exchange, which are mentioned in Chapter 32 and listed in Table 45.2.

Nursing activities

Specific nursing activities relevant to caring for an individual with a respiratory system disorder include:

- collection of a specimen of sputum
- obtaining nasal or throat swabs
- administration of oxygen
- oronasopharyngeal suction
- inhalation therapy.

Collection of sputum

Sputum is a mucus secretion produced by the mucous membranes that line the respiratory tract in response to inflammation, infection or congestion. Laboratory examination of sputum may be necessary to determine whether any microorganisms, blood, or malignant cells are present.

The nurse should observe any sputum, noting the amount, the consistency, the colour, and the presence of an odour. Sputum varies in colour from clear to white, yellow, rust-coloured, or green. It may be tinged with blood, or contain streaks of blood. The consistency varies from watery to mucoid to tenacious.

When a specimen of sputum is required it is best collected early in the morning, so that the overnight

Table 45.2 Impaired gas exchange

Condition	Possible cause	Manifestations
Respiratory acidosis (hypercapnia)	Hypoventilation as a result of chronic obstructive pulmonary disease, pneumonia, drugs, or trauma	Flushed warm skin Hypertension Tachycardia Headaches Drowsiness Confusion Irritability Coma
Respiratory alkalosis (hypocapnia)	Hyperventilation as a result of acute asthma, cerebral trauma, or congestive cardiac failure	Diaphoresis Pallor Tachypnoea Tingling and numbness in the limbs, or around the mouth Carpopedal spasm (tetany) Convulsions
Hypoxia	Obstructive lung diseases, and restrictive lung diseases, e.g. chronic bronchitis, emphysema, sarcoidosis	Pallor or cyanosis Tachypnoea Tachycardia Breathlessness Headaches Irritability Confusion

accumulation of secretions is obtained. Sputum for laboratory testing should be free of saliva and food particles. A suggested procedure for collecting a specimen of sputum is outlined in the guidelines.

Nasopharyngeal and throat swabs

Laboratory examination of secretions from the nosapharynx or throat may be necessary to determine the presence of pathogenic microorganisms. Collection of a specimen involves swabbing the inflamed tissues, and collecting exudate, with sterile cotton wool-tipped applicators. The nurse should refer to the institution's policy manual for information about the type of applicator, culture tube and transport medium to use. A suggested procedure for collecting a nasopharyngeal or throat swab is outlined in the guidelines.

Administration of oxygen

Information on oxygen administration is provided in Chapter 32.

Oronasopharyngeal suction

Oronasopharyngeal suction may be required when secretions or foreign substances are causing an obstruction to the patient's airway. Suction is indicated for the patient

---

Guidelines for collection of sputum

Nursing Action	**Rationale**
1. Explain the procedure to the individual, ensuring that he understands it is sputum and not saliva that is required	Reduces anxiety Saliva will produce inaccurate test results
2. Assist the individual to assume a sitting position.	Facilitates coughing and expectoration
3. Instruct the individual to cough, and to expectorate into a sterile container	A sterile container ensures that the specimen is not contaminated
4. Place the lid on the container, wipe the outside of the container, and wash hands	Prevents cross infection
5. Despatch the specimen, together with the request form, to the laboratory as soon as possible. Ensure that the container is clearly labelled with the relevant information	Proliferation of microorganisms occurs if the specimen is not dispatched as soon as possible after collection Avoids errors

---

Guidelines for nasopharyngeal and throat swabs

Nursing action	**Rationale**
1. Explain the procedure to the individual. Inform him that he may experience the urge to sneeze or gag during the swabbing	Reduces anxiety
2. Assist him to assume a sitting position, if possible.	Facilitates collection of the specimen
3. Wash and dry hands	Prevents cross infection
4. If a nasopharyngeal swab is to be obtained, request the individual to blow his nose	Clears the nasal passages
5. Request him to tilt his head back	Facilitates collection of the specimen
6. To obtain a swab of the nasopharynx, gently pass the swab through the nostril until it reaches the posterior pharyngeal wall. Rotate, then withdraw the swab	Gentle insertion prevents tissue damage
To obtain a swab of the throat request the individual to open his mouth, depress the tongue with a tongue depressor and use a torch to illuminate the throat	Facilitates access and visualization
Ask him to say 'ah'	Raises the uvula
Pass the swab over the tonsils, posterior pharyngeal wall and posterior edge of the soft palate	
7. Place the swab in the culture tube immediately, and close the end of the tube. Wash and dry hands	Prevents cross infection
8. Despatch the specimen, together with the request form, to the laboratory as soon as possible	Proliferation of microorganisms occurs if the specimen is not dispatched and refrigerated as soon as possible after collection
Ensure that the container is clearly labelled with the relevant information	Avoids errors

---

who is unable to clear his airway effectively with coughing and expectoration, e.g. the severely debilitated or unconscious patient.

The removal of excess secretions and mucus from the airway aids breathing, promotes pulmonary gas exchange, and prevents the accumulation of secretions which may cause pneumonia.

Suctioning is achieved by means of a catheter which is introduced into the pharynx, through the mouth or nose. A suggested procedure is outlined in the guidelines.

The basic equipment consists of:

— wall suction or portable suction apparatus
— collection bottle
— connecting tubing
— connector
— water in a small container
— sterile suction catheters
— disposable gloves
— tongue depressor.

Suction equipment is usually kept in readiness at the bedside if there is an indication that it may be needed frequently, or as an emergency measure.

The nurse should ensure that she is aware of the suction pressure to use. In general, the pressure may be set at 80–120 mmHg for an adult and considerably lower for a child.

If using the nasal route, suctioning should be alternated between the left and right nostrils to reduce trauma to one nostril. It may also be necessary to lubricate the tip of the catheter with a sterile water-soluble lubricant, before insertion into the nostril.

Inhalation therapy

There are various forms of inhalation therapy which may be prescribed for a patient who has a respiratory system disorder. These include:

• steam inhalations
• humidified air
• aerosols via a nebulizer or an intermittent positive pressure ventilator.

Guidelines for oronasopharyngeal suction

Nursing action	Rationale
1. Explain the procedure to the individual, and provide privacy	Reduces anxiety and embarrassment
2. Position him in a sitting position if possible; or with his neck extended	Promotes lung expansion and effective coughing Facilitates catheter insertion
3. Wash and dry hands. Put on gloves	Prevents cross infection
4. Attach collection bottle to the suction unit, attach connecting tubing, connector, and catheter Turn on the suction and dip the tip of the catheter into the water	Equipment must be assembled and checked for function before the procedure is commenced Lubricates the catheter to facilitate insertion
5. With the suction off, e.g. by using the Y-connector, gently introduce the catheter into the mouth or nostril If the oral route is used, the individual's tongue may be depressed with a tongue depressor	Suction during insertion may damage the mucosa Facilitates insertion of the suction catheter
6. Ensure that suction pressure is below 120 mmHg. Apply suction as the catheter is withdrawn, rotating the catheter as it is being withdrawn	Pressure above 120 mmHg may damage the mucosa Rotating motion prevents tissue trauma
7. Apply suction for only 8–10 seconds at any one time Allow the individual time to rest between suctionings	Suctioning for longer than 10 seconds can cause tissue trauma and hypoxia
8. If secretions are tenacious, dip the the tip of the catheter in water and apply suction	Clears the lumen of catheter
9. Repeat the procedure, if necessary, until all mucus has been removed	Promotes a clear airway
10. After suctioning instruct the individual (if he is able) to take several slow, deep breaths	Relieves hypoxia and promotes relaxation
11. Dip the catheter into the water and apply suction	Clears catheter and connecting tubing
12. Discard the catheter, water and gloves. Attend to the rest of the equipment. Wash hands	Prevents cross infection
13. Assist the individual into a position of comfort	Promotes rest and relaxation
14. Document and report on the procedure, including observations of the aspirate	Appropriate care can be planned and implemented

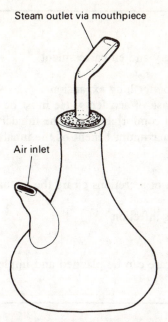

Steam outlet via mouthpiece

Air inlet

Fig. 45.2   Nelson inhaler. (Reproduced with permission from Chilman A M, Thomas M (eds) 1987 Understanding nursing care, 3rd edn. Churchill Livingstone, Edinburgh.)

Inhalation therapy may be prescribed to:

- relieve inflammation of the air passages
- loosen secretions to facilitate expectoration
- reduce drying and irritation of the mucous membranes
- deliver medications, e.g. to relieve bronchospasm.

Steam inhalations may be prescribed for a patient with an upper respiratory tract disorder, e.g. sinusitis, laryngitis or tracheitis. A steam inhalation may be administered continuously via a steam tent, or periodically by means of steam from hot water in a jug or a Nelson inhaler (Fig. 45.2).

In some instances a substance may be added to the hot water to provide medicated steam. Substances which may be used to medicate the steam include:

- menthol
- eucalyptus
- tincture of benzoine.

If these, or any other, substances are to be administered the nurse must ensure that the correct amount is added to the water. The temperature of the water for a steam inhalation should be between 71°–82°C.

If a steam inhalation is to be administered, the nurse must implement preventive measures against burning. Safety precautions include:

- Standing the container of hot water in a bowl and placing it on a firm even surface.
- Assisting the patient to assume a sitting position, and ensuring that his back is well supported.
- Warning the patient not to touch the outside of the con-

tainer of hot water, or to tilt it towards him. A towel may be wrapped around the container for added safety.
- Remaining with a patient who is debilitated, disoriented, or unsteady.
- Ensuring that, if a Nelson inhaler is used, the level of water is below the air inlet and ensuring that the air inlet is facing away from the patient. The mouthpiece of the inhaler should be covered with gauze to protect the patient's mouth from heat.

A suggested procedure for administering a steam inhalation, using a Nelson inhaler, is outlined in the guidelines. If an inhaler is unavailable, a steam inhalation can be administered using a jug of hot water. In this instance, the patient leans over the jug and inhales the steam. A towel is draped over the patient's head to reduce the amount of steam escaping into the environment. The disadvantages of using a jug include the discomfort of having the head covered, irritation of the eyes by steam, and impregnation of the patient's hair and clothing by medicated steam.

The basic equipment for a steam inhalation is:

— Nelson inhaler (or a 1 litre jug)
— bowl in which to stand the inhaler or jug
— piece of gauze (for Nelson inhaler)
— prescribed medication
— hot water
— towel to wrap around inhaler or jug
— extra towel (if jug is being used)
— paper tissues and a sputum receiver
— lotion thermometer.

Humidifiers add water vapour to inspired air to prevent drying and irritation of the respiratory mucosa, and to help loosen secretions for easier expectoration. Humidifiers provide either cold mist or steam.

Humidification must be provided when oxygen is being administered, and this is achieved by connecting a humidifier containing distilled water to the oxygen equipment. As the oxygen passes through the water it is humidified to prevent dryness and irritation of the mucous membranes.

Humidity may be provided by means of a humidity tent or croupette, or a humidifier (Fig. 45.3) may be positioned in the room so that the moist air is directed towards the individual. The moist air may be passed over a prescribed medication, which is then inhaled by the individual.

When a room humidifier is being used the windows and doors of the room should be closed to maintain a constant correct humidity level. After the humidifier has been plugged in, the nozzle should be directed toward the individual to promote effective treatment. A fine mist should be visible at the nozzle. The unit is refilled with distilled water as necessary, to provide a continuous supply of mist.

The bedding and clothing are changed as soon as they become damp, and the temperature of the room should be maintained at a comfortable level.

Guidelines for administering a steam inhalation

Nursing action	Rationale
1. Explain the procedure to the individual and provide privacy	Reduces anxiety and embarrassment
2. Assist him to assume a sitting position	Provides for better lung expansion
3. Place the inhalation equipment on a firm surface, at a suitable height, in front of the individual	Reduces the risk of accidents. He must be able to bend his head comfortably over the inhaler
4. Instruct the individual to close his lips around the mouthpiece, to inhale through the mouth and exhale through the nose	Provides for maximum benefit of the inhalation
5. Encourage him to expectorate any loosened secretions into the sputum receiver	Expectoration of secretions clears the air passages
6. After 10–15 minutes, remove and attend to the equipment, attend to individual's comfort needs, wash hands	Prevents cross infection
7. Document and report on the procedure, including the observations of any expectorated secretions	Appropriate care can be planned and implemented

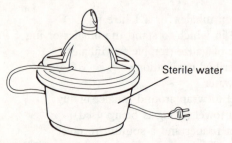
Sterile water

Fig. 45.3 Room humidifier (cool mist or steam vaporizer).

Nebulizers, or atomizers, are devices which are used to deliver moisture or medication, and dispense their contents in a fine spray. Aerosol bronchodilators are commonly prescribed in the management of asthma. Information on the use of hand held inhalers is provided in Chapter 58. Aerosols may also be used with positive pressure ventilators, e.g. Bird or Bennet ventilators, to deliver medication to a patient on a ventilator or during intermittent positive pressure breathing therapy.

Nebulizers may also be used with compressed air or oxygen to deliver aerosolized medication. The prescribed medication is inserted into the nebulizer together with the prescribed amount of sterile water or saline, and one end of the oxygen tubing is attached to the nebulizer. The other end of the tubing is attached to the pressurized gas source, which is turned on to check for proper misting. In order to produce particles of the correct size, a flow rate of 8 litres per minute is generally required. The individual is instructed to breath deeply, slowly, and evenly through the mouthpiece or mask. He is instructed to hold his breath for 2–3 seconds on full inhalation, to receive the full benefit of the medication. He should be encouraged to cough and

expectorate, and the treatment should be stopped briefly if he needs to rest.

Mechanical nebulization is generally performed when a patient has a tracheostomy or is being mechanically ventilated. A range of commercially assembled sterile closed systems are available which provide protection against cross-contamination, and precise control of oxygen delivery. Adapters are provided for connection to sterile, prefilled containers of solution, e.g. sterile water or normal saline.

Mechanical ventilation

Mechanical ventilation is sometimes indicated for a patient with a respiratory system disorder. Mechanical ventilation artificially assists or controls respiration, and it is indicated to correct or prevent gas transport abnormalities. To maintain adequate pulmonary blood gas exchange, an endotracheal or tracheostomy tube is inserted and connected to the ventilator.

There are a variety of ventilators available which may be one of two main types; pressure controlled or volume controlled. With the pressure controlled ventilator, the gas is delivered to the lungs until a predetermined pressure is reached, then inspiration is terminated. With a volume controlled ventilator, a set volume of gas is delivered with each inspiration. The ventilation rate may be pre-set, controlled by the patient, or may be a combination of both.

The care of a patient who is receiving mechanical ventilation should be provided by personnel who are qualified and experienced to provide it. A patient who requires mechanical ventilation is generally nursed in an intensive care unit, as he requires constant physical attention and emotional support.

The individual with an artificial airway

The placement of an artificial airway is indicated to relieve obstruction, to facilitate suctioning of the lower respiratory tract, to prevent aspiration, or to allow for mechanical ventilation. Artificial airways include the oropharyngeal airway, the endotracheal tube, and the tracheostomy tube.

Oropharyngeal airway

An oropharyngeal airway is a curved rubber or plastic device (Fig. 45.4) which is inserted into the mouth to the posterior pharynx, to establish or maintain a patent airway. The airway allows air to pass around and through the tube, and facilitates oropharyngeal suctioning. It is used for a short term only, e.g. in the immediate post anaesthetic period. If a patient requires respiratory assistance for a longer period an endotracheal tube is generally used.

Endotracheal tube

An endotracheal tube (Fig. 45.4) is a flexible cuffed tube which is inserted via the mouth or nostril through the larynx into the trachea. Endotracheal intubation establishes and maintains a patent airway, prevents aspiration by sealing the trachea off from the digestive tract, facilitates the removal of tracheobronchial secretions, and provides a means whereby optimum ventilation can be achieved.

Endotracheal intubation may be required in an emergency or short term situation, or long term intubation may be necessary. The tube is inserted by a medical officer, who uses a laryngoscope to visualize the trachea and facilitate the passage of the tube. The majority of endotracheal tubes have a cuff (Fig. 45.4), which is inflated with air to provide a seal which prevents the leakage of air around the tube when the patient is ventilated. To avoid inadvertent removal or displacement of the tube, tapes are applied to secure the tube in position.

Continuous expert care is required following endotracheal intubation, to ensure airway patency and to pre-

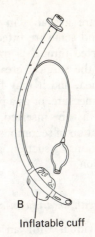

B

Inflatable cuff

Fig. 45.4 (B) Endotracheal tube.

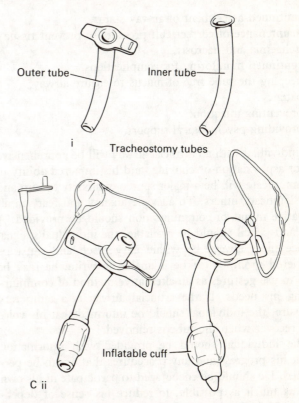

Outer tube   Inner tube

i   Tracheostomy tubes

Inflatable cuff

C ii

Fig. 45.4 (C) Tracheostomy tubes. (i) metal tube (for permanent tracheostomy). (ii) Cuffed synthetic tube.

vent complications. A patient who has been intubated is generally nursed in an intensive care unit, as he requires constant physical attention and emotional support.

Tracheostomy tube

A tracheostomy tube is a short, curved tube which is fitted with a flange that assists in stabilizing the tube (Fig. 45.4).

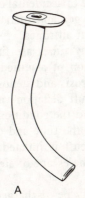

A

Fig. 45.4 Artificial airways. (A) Oropharyngeal airway.

Tracheostomy tubes are available in a range of styles, materials, and sizes; and some are fitted with an inflatable cuff. The tube is inserted through a tracheostomy.

A tracheostomy is the surgical creation of an external opening into the trachea, and it may be performed as an emergency temporary measure, or as a permanent measure. A tracheostomy, with a tube inserted, provides a patent airway, prevents aspiration of secretions, allows removal of tracheobronchial secretions by suction, and permits the use of mechanical ventilation.

Care of an individual with an artificial airway

The care of an individual with an artificial airway—whether it has been inserted for a short or long term—involves many physical actions and the provision of emotional support. The main aspects of care include:

- continued assessment of airway status.
- maintenance of correct cuff pressure to prevent tissue ischaemia and necrosis.
- continued monitoring for complications.
- keeping the tube free of mucus to ensure airway patency.
- preventing infection.
- providing psychological support.

An individual with an artificial airway will be apprehensive about asphyxiation or choking, and his impaired ability to communicate will be a major source of anxiety to him and his significant others. To alleviate anxiety and fear, an alternative means of communication should be provided. A pad and pencil should be available, the individual's signal device must always be within easy reach and must be answered promptly. If he is unable to write, he may be able to use gestures as an alternative method of communicating his needs. If the artificial airway is a temporary measure, the individual should be informed that his voice will recover when the tube is removed.

The individual should be provided with information about his progress and any procedures that are to be performed. He should be encouraged to participate in his own care as much as possible, to reduce his sense of dependency. His significant others should be involved in his care, and be encouraged to talk to him.

It is important for the nurse to remember that the individual's ability to remove secretions effectively is impaired. When he is unable to cough and expectorate secretions, suctioning must be performed. This procedure is uncomfortable and frightening, and the individual must be provided with an explanation of the suctioning technique before it is performed. Two people should be present during the procedure: one to aspirate, and the other person to assist. A suggested method of tracheostomy suctioning is outlined in the guidelines. The basic equipment for tracheostomy suctioning is:

- sterile suction catheters
- wall or portable suction apparatus
- Y-connector if the catheter has no control valve
- connecting tubing
- sterile gloves
- container of sterile water
- receiver for soiled items
- items for the administration of oxygen.

Care of the tracheostomy and tracheostomy tube is performed to minimize bacterial contamination, and to decrease the possiblility of obstruction by secretions. Tracheostomy care, which is performed using sterile equipment and asepic technique to prevent infection, involves cleansing of the inner cannula and the area around the stoma. The frequency with which the care is provided may vary depending on the amount of secretions present, and may be as frequent as every $\frac{1}{2}$–1 hour or may only be required once every eight hours.

A suggested procedure for tracheostomy care is outlined in the guidelines. The basic equipment for tracheostomy care is:

- sterile container of solution for cleansing the stoma, e.g. normal saline
- sterile container of solution for cleansing the tube, e.g. hydrogen peroxide
- sterile container of sterile water for rinsing the tube
- sterile gloves
- sterile pipe cleaners and/or tube brush
- sterile gauze squares
- sterile tracheostomy dressing
- tracheostomy tapes
- scissors
- receiver for soiled items
- spare tracheostomy tube
- sterile suction catheter and suction source
- tracheal hooks and dilators.

When caring for an individual with a tracheostomy, a spare sterile tube and tracheal dilator should be available at the bedside in case of accidental dislodgment or obstruction of the tube. Oxygen and suction equipment must also be readily available at all times.

Many tracheostomy tubes are fitted with an inflatable cuff. Regular deflation of a cuffed tube is performed to prevent tracheal necrosis and stenosis. The frequency and length of time for cuff deflation varies depending on the type of tube used and the condition of the patient.

Prior to deflation, the tube and oronasopharynx are aspirated. When the cuff is inflated, only sufficient air is inserted to occlude the escape of air from around the sides of the tube.

The individual may be discharged from hospital with a tracheostomy tube in position. As soon as possible he is instructed in self care so that he feels comfortable and con-

Guidelines for tracheostomy suctioning

Nursing action	Rationale
1. Explain the procedure and provide privacy The individual should be informed that suctioning may cause transient coughing or gagging	Reduces anxiety and embarrassment
2. Place the equipment within easy reach	Facilitates performance of the procedure in an organized manner
3. Remove any humidification (or ventilation) device	Allows access to the tracheostomy tube
4. Wash and dry hands and put on gloves	Prevents cross infection
5. Attach the catheter to the suction tubing and set suction pressure to between 80–120 mmHg	Pressure above 120 mmHg may damage the tracheal mucosa
6. Ask the individual to cough and breathe slowly and deeply	Coughing helps loosen secretions, and deep breathing helps to minimize hypoxia
7. If necessary, or prescribed, the individual's lungs are hyperoxygenated prior to aspiration	Helps to prevent hypoxia
8. Insert the catheter *without suction* into the tracheostomy tube	Prevents tracheal mucosa trauma
9. Apply suction and withdraw the catheter, rotating it gently	Rotating motion avoids tissue trauma
Suction for no longer than 10 seconds at a time	Short term suctioning limits the amount of oxygen removed
Allow the individual to take 4–5 breaths between each aspiration	Prevents hypoxia
If secretions are thick, dip the catheter into sterile saline and apply suction	Helps to clear the lumen of the catheter
10. Report immediately if there is any difficulty in inserting the catheter into the tube	The tube may be blocked with secretions
11. When suctioning is completed, the individual may need to be hyperoxygenated again	Prevents hypoxia and promotes relaxation
Replace any humidification device	Re-establishes delivery of humidity
12. Dispose of the gloves and suction catheter appropriately, wash and dry hands	Prevents cross infection
13. Document and report on the procedure	Appropriate care can be planned and implemented

fident about caring for his tracheostomy. The individual should be provided with information about relevant support groups, e.g. Tracheostomy associations, that he may wish to contact.

Prior to the permanent removal of a tracheostomy tube the individual will require sufficient information and emotional support, as he may feel that he will not be able to breathe without the tracheostomy tube. The tube may be removed when the individual is able to maintain independent respiratory function, is able to breathe through the upper respiratory tract, and has satisfactory protective reflexes, e.g. cough reflex.

To prepare the individual for permanent removal of the tracheostomy tube a fenestrated tube may be inserted. This type of tube has an opening in the outer cannula which allows the individual to breathe around as well as through the tube. Thus, he is able to adjust gradually to removal

of the tube. By covering the tube, he is able to speak, breathe normally through the upper airway, and expectorate secretions.

Before the tube is removed, suction is applied to remove tracheal and pharyngeal secretions. The cuff is deflated, and the tube is removed. Generally a dry dressing is placed over the stoma until healing occurs.

The insertion of an artificial airway can result in several complications:

• infection due to altered ciliary function or colonization of the airway with bacteria.
• tracheal necrosis and stenosis due to excessive pressure on the trachea from the cuff.
• tracheo-oesophageal fistula.
• partial or complete airway obstruction, e.g. due to an accumulation of secretions in the tube.

Guidelines for tracheostomy care

Nursing action	Rationale
1. Explain the procedure and provide privacy	Reduces anxiety and embarrassment
2. Place the equipment within easy reach	Facilitates performance of the procedure in an organized manner
3. Wash and dry hands	Prevents cross infection
4. Remove any humidification (or ventilation) device	Allows access to the tracheostomy tube
5. Suction the tracheostomy tube. (Refer to guidelines on suctioning)	Removes secretions from the airway
6. Remove and discard the tracheostomy dressing into the receiver	Correct disposal prevents cross infection
7. Place sterile drape or towel around the tracheostomy site	Provides a sterile field around the stoma
8. Put on sterile gloves	Prevents cross infection
9. Remove inner cannula of the tracheostomy tube, and place it in solution	Remove secretions from the cannula
10. Cleanse the skin around the stoma and the flanges of the tube using gauze and appropriate solution	Removes accumulated secretions and crusts
Take care not to let solution or strands of gauze enter the stoma	These may be aspirated into the lungs
11. Remove the inner cannula from the solution, clean the inside with a pipe cleaner, and rinse it thoroughly	Removes all secretions and solution from the cannula
12. Reinsert the cannula into the tracheostomy tube, and lock it into place	Ensures correct placement of the cannula
13. Inspect the surrounding area and stoma site for inflammation or skin breakdown	Signs of impaired healing or infection require immediate attention
14. Apply a sterile tracheostomy dressing	Protects the stoma site
15. Replace the tracheostomy tapes if they are soiled or loose	Tracheostomy tube must be secured in position. Soiled tapes predispose the individual to infection
Whenever possible, two people should be present to change the tapes	Prevents accidental dislodgement of the tube
16. Replace any humidification device	Re-establishes delivery of humidity
17. Remove gloves, dispose of the equipment appropriately, wash and dry hands	Prevents cross infection
18. Assist the individual into position, and place his signal device within reach	Promotes comfort and relaxation
19. Document and report on the procedure	Appropriate care can be planned and implemented

- subcutaneous emphysema.
- psychological effects, such as frustration at being unable to communicate normally.

The individual with thoracic drainage tubes

The insertion of chest drainage tubes permits the drainage of air or fluid from the pleural space which, if not removed, alters intrapleural pressure and causes lung collapse. Ventilation is adversely affected by any disruption of the intrapleural pressure which may be caused by surgery, trauma, and pulmonary disease. Insertion of chest tubes drains the excess air or fluid and enables the lungs to function normally.

Chest drainage tubes may be inserted at the time of surgery while the individual is anaesthetized, or may be inserted following a local anaesthetic. Because the procedure is painful, a conscious person is generally given analgesic medication approximately 30 minutes prior to tube insertion. The procedure is performed by a medical officer using sterile equipment and aseptic technique. The insertion site is selected according to the individual's condition, and one or more tubes may be inserted at the same time.

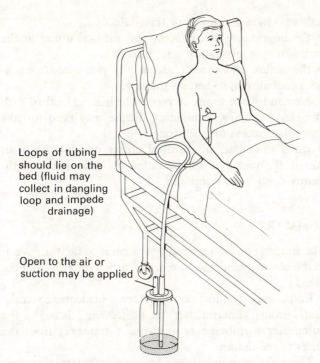

Loops of tubing should lie on the bed (fluid may collect in dangling loop and impede drainage)

Open to the air or suction may be applied

Fig. 45.5 Underwater-seal thoracic drainage.

Following insertion, the chest tube is connected to a drainage system that permits drainage out of the pleural space—and prevents backflow into that space. The tubing leads to a collection system (Fig 45.5) which is positioned well below the level of the patient's chest. This dependent position facilitates the the removal of air or fluid from the intrapleural space, and prevents the backflow of fluid into the intrapleural space. To prevent the entry of air into the intrapleural space, the distal end of the tubing is submerged under water. This provides a closed water-seal drainage system.

Some systems of underwater seal drainage, e.g. the Pleur-evac system, are available already assembled and are disposed of after use. Such systems provide a water seal and can be connected to suction. Other types of thoracic drainage systems include the one, two, or three-bottle systems. The one and two bottle systems are primarily gravity systems, while the three-bottle and commercially prepared systems also provide for mechanical suction. In most of health care institutions, the sterile supply department provides thoracic drainage systems partially assembled.

The aim of closed chest underwater seal drainage is to promote lung expansion by facilitating drainage of air and fluid. Care of the individual includes:

• Nursing him in an upright position, where possible, to facilitate optimal lung expansion and to promote drainage by gravity.
• Providing adequate explanation and emotional support to reduce anxiety. He may tend to restrict his breathing and movement for fear of dislodging the tube, therefore it

is essential to explain that the tube is secured in position with tape and/or sutures.

• Administering adequate analgesic medication to decrease discomfort. It may be necessary to administer analgesic medication 30–45 minutes before physiotherapy in order to promote pain relief and relaxation.
• Encouraging the individual to breathe deeply, and cough frequently to help drain the pleural space and expand the lungs.
• Regularly assessing his respiratory status. The individual should be observed for discomfort and any difficulty in breathing, and it is important to observe whether his chest is expanding symmetrically. His ventilations are assessed at regular intervals, e.g. every 1–4 hours, for rate, rhythm, and character.
• Maintaining the water seal and preventing air leakage is essential to prevent entry of air into the pleural space. The fluid level in the drainage bottle should be checked frequently, and sterile water added if necessary to ensure that the distal end of the water seal tube is submerged.

Precautions must be taken to prevent separation of the connections and breakage of the drainage bottle/s.

If the system is accidently disconnected, air will enter the pleural space and the lung may collapse. In the event that the system is accidently disconnected, it is general practice to place two clamps on the chest tube, and summon assistance immediately. There is some controversy surrounding this emergency measure, as some authorities believe that clamping a chest tube could result in a tension pneumothorax. It is essential that the nurse be aware of the institution's measures to be taken should accidental disconnection of the system occur.

If a chest tube is accidently dislodged, or falls out, the individual is asked to exhale forcefully and the opening in his chest must be covered until the tube can be re-inserted.

• Maintaining patency of the drainage system is essential to facilitate expansion of the lung. The system must be frequently observed for loose connections and for fluctuation in the water-seal bottle. As the patient inhales the fluid should rise in the water-seal tube, and as he exhales the level should fall back. If the system is connected to suction, the fluid line in the water-seal tube should remain constant. During exhalation, bubbling is normally present in the water-seal bottle. Gently bubbling in a suction control bottle indicates that the correct level of suction has been achieved.

The tubing must be observed for, and kept free from, kinks. Kinking of the tubing will obstruct the flow of air or fluid. To prevent kinking, or dependent loops of tubing, the tubing should be coiled flat on the bed and may be attached to the edge of the bed with tape and a safety pin. The tubing should fall in a straight line from the coil to the drainage bottle, to facilitate flow. The nurse must ensure that the individual is able to move freely without pulling or lying on the tubing.

The drainage bottles must always remain below the level of the individual's chest to prevent aspiration or backflow of fluid. Generally, a rack in which the bottle/s is placed, is attached to the side of the bed. When it is necessary to replace a drainage bottle, the chest tube is double clamped near the site of insertion. The bottle, and if necessary the connection tubing, is replaced and the clamps are removed. The tubes should not be clamped for longer than two minutes, as a tension pneumothorax may result when air or fluid is prevented from escaping. As a safety precaution, two nurses should be present whenever a drainage bottle or system is being replaced.

● Using sterile equipment and aseptic techniques to prevent infection. The insertion site is protected by a dressing, e.g. petroleum impregnated gauze covered by an occlusive dressing. The dressing is renewed in accordance with the institution's policy.

● Assessing and documenting the colour, amount, and type of drainage. Any alteration in the amount, colour, or flow of drainage must be reported immediately. Sudden cessation of flow of drainage may indicate a malfunction of the system.

Removal of a chest tube is performed by the medical officer. Generally, the tube is clamped for up to 24 hours prior to removal, and a chest X-ray is performed to determine full lung expansion. If the individual develops respiratory distress or a pneumothorax, the clamps are removed, and the tube is left in place.

Analgesic medication is usually administed 30–45 minutes prior to tube removal. Once the tube has been removed the insertion site is covered with an occlusive dressing to provide an airtight seal.

Following removal of the tube the insertion site is checked regularly for sounds of air leakage, and the individual is observed for manifestations of pneumothorax, infection, subcutaneous emphysema, and respiratory distress.

Education

Planning for an individual's discharge from hospital is of particular importance if his respiratory disorder is chronic or recurrent. The individual must be provided with sufficient information because, by understanding his condition and how to manage his symptoms, he will be better able to cope with chronic respiratory disease. He should be encouraged to pursue as normal a lifestyle as possible, and should be given information about:

● the importance of avoiding factors which may precipitate or exacerbate his condition, e.g. extremes of temperature, exposure to allergens or environmental irritants, fatigue, or emotional stress.
● the importance of avoiding close contact with individuals who have a respiratory tract infection.
● the importance of contacting his medical officer at the first sign of a respiratory tract infection.
● the nature and correct use of any prescribed medications, nebulizers, or aerosal therapy.
● how and when to use oxygen, which an individual with chronic obstructive pulmonary disease may need to have immediate access to at all times.
● when to contact his medical officer or go to hospital, e.g. if the measures implemented at home fail to sufficiently control his symptoms.

SUMMARY

The function of the respiratory system is to deliver oxygen to the bloodstream, and to remove carbon dioxide from the blood.

Respiratory dysfunction results from inadequate ventilation, from abnormalities of diffusion through the pulmonary membrane or inadequate transport from the lungs to the tissues.

The major manifestations of respiratory system disorders are chest pain, cough, voice change, dyspnoea, altered ventilations, hypoxia, and thoracic skeletal abnormalities.

Disorders of the respiratory system can be classified as those occuring from multiple causes, from infection, as a result of neoplasms or obstruction, or as a result of injury.

Diagnostic tests used to assess respiratory function include pulmonary function tests, chest X-ray, lung scan, blood gas analysis, cultures, sputum cytology, skin tests, bronchoscopy, and thoracentesis.

Care of the individual with a respiratory system disorder includes promoting a clear airway, promoting local hydration, proper positioning, administration of medications, oronasopharyngeal suction, chest physiotherapy, and the administration of oxygen. The nurse may be required to obtain a specimen of sputum for laboratory examination, to obtain a nasal or throat swab, or to administer inhalation therapy.

An individual with a specific disorder of the respiratory system may require the insertion of an artificial airway, and/or mechanical ventilation.

The insertion of chest tubes may be necessary to promote the drainage of air or fluid from the pleural space.

REFERENCES AND FURTHER READING

Boore J R P, Champion R, Ferguson M C (eds) 1987 Nursing the physically ill adult. Churchill Livingstone, Edinburgh
Brunner L S, Suddarth D S 1988 Textbook of medical-surgical nursing, 6th edn. J B Lippincott, Philadelphia
Game C, Anderson R, Kidd J (eds) 1989 Medical-surgical nursing: a core text. Churchill Livingstone, Melbourne, 336–374

46. The individual with a digestive system disorder

INTRODUCTION

Information on the normal structure and function of the digestive system is provided in Chapter 23, and it should be referred to before studying the contents of this chapter. The functions of the digestive system are to ingest and digest food so that nutrients can be absorbed into the bloodstream, and to eliminate wastes from the body. All body cells rely on a constant supply of nutrients in order to function effectively, therefore any dysfunction of the digestive system has some effects on all the other systems.

Pathophysiological influences and effects

Alterations in normal function of the digestive system can be classified as changes in swallowing, secretory function, motility, digestion, absorption, and elimination. Any of these disturbances of normal function can have significant consequences on the assimilation of nutrients or on the elimination of wastes.

Changes in swallowing

Swallowing is a complex mechanism, beginning with a voluntary action as the food is rolled to the back of the mouth, followed by a reflex action which passes the bolus of food through the pharynx into the oesophagus. Alterations in swallowing include dysphagia, which is difficulty in swallowing, and regurgitation which is the reflux of partially digested food back into the mouth. When the swallowing mechanism is impaired the individual may be unable to swallow at all, food may pass into the trachea, or food may reflux into the nose.

Difficulty in swallowing can result from physical abnormalities, obstruction or inflammation of the mouth, pharynx, or oesophagus. Emotional factors such as severe anxiety may also affect the first phase of the swallowing mechanism.

Changes in secretory function

Changes may involve an increase or decrease in the secretions produced by the alimentary tract. Alterations in normal production of mucus or digestive secretions may severely affect the digestion and absorption of nutrients. Changes in normal secretion may be related to inflammatory disorders, infection, mechanical trauma, malnutrition, neoplasms, neurohormonal disorders, or psychological states.

A decrease in mucus secretion can reduce the protective mechanisms, leading to irritation or ulceration of the alimentary tract. If the production of specific digestive enzymes is reduced or absent, certain nutrients will not be absorbed. An excess of certain digestive secretions, e.g. hydrochloric acid, may result in diarrhoea and a subsequent loss of fluid and electrolytes.

Changes in motility

Motility, or movement in the digestive tract, may be increased or decreased as a result of trauma, neurohormonal or inflammatory factors. Hypermotility, or increased motility, results in the rapid passage of contents through the digestive tract and, as a result, digestion and absorption of nutrients is impaired. Hypomotility, or decreased motility, results in the sluggish passage of contents through the digestive tract and, as a result, distension, nausea, vomiting, constipation or faecal impaction can occur.

Changes in digestion

Digestive enzymes, and mechanical actions, are necessary for food to be broken down into absorbable forms. Alterations in the normal production of digestive enzymes and other secretions result in the inadequate digestion of nutrients and, therefore, impaired absorption. Alterations in normal enzyme production and activity may result from trauma, e.g. surgery on the bowel, from inflammatory disturbances, from malnutrition, or from disturbances of secretion.

Changes in absorption

Most absorption of fluids, electrolytes, and nutrients occurs in the small intestine; while both water and electrolytes are also absorbed by the large intestine. Factors which may result in malabsorption include maldigestion, trauma, neurohormonal disorders and inflammatory disturbances. The consequences of malabsorption include fluid and electrolyte imbalance, nutrient deficiency, and steatorrhoea.

Changes in elimination

Alterations in elimination of wastes from the digestive tract include increased or decreased frequency of elimination, painful or difficult defaecation, and the presence of abnormal substances in the faeces.

Increased frequency of defaecation (diarrhoea) results in the loss of fluids and electrolytes, while decreased frequency (constipation) causes abdominal discomfort and painful defaecation. Diarrhoea may be caused by factors including hypermotility, inflammatory disturbances or disturbances of digestion or absorption.

Constipation may result from hypomotility, lack of dietary fibre or fluids, immobility, or certain medications.

Painful defaecation is commonly related to abnormalities of the rectum or anus, e.g. neoplasms or haemorrhoids. Painful defaecation often results in constipation—as the individual avoids defaecation. Blood in the faeces may be due to factors such as gastrointestinal bleeding or haemorr-

hoids; and it may be present as bright red blood, or the faeces may be dark and tar-like (melaena).

Major manifestations of digestive system disorders

The signs and symptoms manifested by the individual with a digestive system disorder vary according to the location and severity of the disorder.

Pain

The pain experienced will vary in type and intensity depending on the disorder. Pain may be associated with gaseous distension, pressure caused by neoplasms, inflammation, strong contractions of the intestine, or obstruction of part of the digestive tract.

Visceral pain from the stomach or intestines, may be localized or referred to other parts of the body. Pain receptors in the viscera are most responsive to stretch stimuli, therefore pain caused by distension is often the most severe. Pain may be spasmodic or continual, and may either increase or decrease when the individual moves. Commonly, visceral pain is intensified with movement therefore a patient with abdominal pain will often lie still, and may curl up in an attempt to minimize the pain. The individual may describe his pain as indigestion or heartburn, or he may describe the pain as being stabbing, colicky, or burning.

Flatulence

Flatulence is the accumulation of gas in the digestive tract which may cause pain and/or abdominal distension. Gases enter the gastro-intestinal tract from swallowed air or are formed as a result of bacterial action. Gas may either be eructated from the oesophagus and stomach, or expelled as flatus through the rectum. Excessive motility of the large intestine is the most usual cause for the expulsion of large amounts of gas. In some disorders of the digestive system excessive amounts of gas are produced and expelled easily, while in other disorders the gas becomes trapped causing distension and discomfort.

Borborygmi is the term used to describe the sounds produced by the movement of gas and fluids in the intestine—usually by hyperactive intestines.

Altered eating habits

In many disorders of the digestive system, the desire to eat is reduced. The individual may decline food totally or may omit certain items from the diet which appear to cause or aggravate symptoms. The individual may reduce the amount of food usually consumed, especially if the ingestion of food results in pain, distension, nausea, or vomiting. Loss of appetite (anorexia), if persistent, will result in malnutrition and weight loss. Anorexia nervosa and bulimia, two complex disorders of eating, are described in Chapter 29.

Nausea and vomiting

Nausea may accompany many disorders of the digestive system, e.g. distension or irritation of the stomach or small intestine. Nausea which commonly precedes vomiting, is frequently accompanied by sweating and pallor. Vomiting is a reflex act which is caused by a variety of stimuli, and is the means by which the upper digestive tract rids itself of its contents, e.g. when it is irritated or overdistended. Information on vomiting is provided in Chapter 29.

Altered bowel function

Changes in normal bowel function include diarrhoea, constipation, painful defaecation, faecal incontinence, rectal bleeding, increased or decreased flatulence, and abnormalities in the faeces, e.g. the presence of increased mucus, or steatorrhoea.

Dysphagia

Dysphagia related to disorders of the digestive system is most commonly due to an obstruction of the oesophagus, e.g. by a neoplasm.

Other manifestations

Although halitosis (offensive breath) has numerous causes, e.g. poor oral hygiene or insufficient oral fluids, it can be a symptom of some digestive system disorders such as appendicitis. In some disorders, e.g. hepatitis, the individual may be jaundiced, while in malignant disease the individual's skin may appear pale or grey. Loss of weight may occur if the disorder causes malnutrition or dehydration. Abdominal distension, or asymmetry, may be a feature of specific disorders.

Specific disorders of the digestive system

Disorders of multiple cause

Certain disorders have more than one cause, and many disorders may be due in part to the individual's life style, e.g. dietary habits.

A hiatus (diaphragmatic) hernia is the herniation of the stomach through the diaphragm into the thoracic cavity. The incidence of hiatus hernia increases with age and is more common in females. It may be the result of muscular weakening or diaphragmatic abnormalities, or herniation may occur when the intra-abdominal pressure is raised, e.g. by pregnancy, obesity, malignancy, trauma, persistent coughing or sneezing.

There may be no symptoms, or the individual may experience reflux, regurgitation, heartburn, eructation and flatulence. The individual may also experience a feeling of fullness after eating, and some chest discomfort. Chest discomfort, or pain, commonly occurs after meals and is frequently aggravated when the individual lies flat.

Diverticular disease. Diverticulosis is the presence of bulging pouches (diverticula) in the intestinal mucosa. Faecal matter becomes trapped in the pouches, and the resulting inflammation is called diverticulitis. It is thought to be due to high intraluminal pressure on areas of weakness in the intestinal wall, and a lack of dietary fibre is considered to be a contributing factor. Diverticulitis causes mild to severe abdominal pain, some nausea, and altered bowel habits. In severe cases, the diverticula can rupture producing abscesses or peritonitis.

A Meckel's diverticulum which is a congenital abnormality, is a blind tube which opens into the distal ileum near the ileocaecal valve.

Irritable bowel syndrome is a relatively common disorder. The condition is thought to result from food intolerance, psychological distress, or in the presence of increased gastrin levels. The individual experiences alternating bouts of diarrhoea and constipation, which may be accompanied by abdominal distension or pain. The faeces usually contain excessive amounts of mucus.

Peptic ulcer disease encompasses gastric ulcer, duodenal ulcer, and stress ulcer.

1. Peptic ulceration is related to erosion of the gastric or duodenal mucosa by acidic digestive juices and, in severe or chronic cases, erosion may penetrate the muscle tissue and serosa—allowing acidic juices to enter the abdominal cavity. Although a precise cause has not been determined, factors that have been implicated in gastric ulcer development are smoking, and certain medications which render the mucosa susceptible to damage.

2. A duodenal ulcer results from excessive gastric acid secretion—possibly due to an overactive vagus nerve. Factors that appear to be related to duodenal ulcer development are the ingestion of caffeine, alcohol, certain medications, and smoking.

3. A stress ulcer may affect either the stomach or the duodenum, and occurs in a high percentage of individuals who have experienced severe trauma, shock, burns, or infection.

The manifestations of an ulcer vary according to the site, and whether it is a chronic or acute condition. The individual with chronic ulcer disease may experience burning epigastric pain, which may be aggravated by stress or fatigue. The pain of a gastric ulcer tends to occur sooner after eating, than does the pain of a duodenal ulcer. Eating, or taking an antacid, tends to relieve the symptoms of a duodenal ulcer.

Complications of peptic ulcer disease include perforation, haemorrhage, intestinal obstruction, and peritonitis. If gastro-intestinal bleeding occurs it may be manifested by *haematemesis* and *melaena* and, if severe, by signs of hypovolaemic shock.

An intestinal hernia is the protrusion of part of the intestine through the abdominal wall. Various types of hernias are named according to their location; umbilical, inguinal, and femoral. A ventral, or incisional, hernia occurs at the site of an abdominal incision. An intestinal hernia may occur as a result of factors which increase intra-abdominal pressure or which cause weakening of the abdominal wall, e.g. obesity, constipation, or pregnancy.

The hernia appears as a lump in the affected area and tends to disappear when the individual is supine. The swelling increases in size of when a standing position is assumed, or during exertion.

The major complication of a hernia is strangulation, where the blood flow to the protruding loop of bowel may be so obstructed that necrosis occurs.

Gastro-intestinal haemorrhage may occur as a result of a variety of disorders. Common causes of bleeding from the upper digestive tract are peptic ulcer disease, oesophageal varices, malignancy, and erosive gastritis. Causes of bleeding from the lower digestive tract include haemorrhoids, fissures, inflammatory bowel disease, polyps, diverticular disease, and malignancy. Gastro-intestinal bleeding is sometimes associated with disorders of the blood, e.g. leukaemia.

Upper gastro-intestinal haemorrhage may be accompanied by haematemesis, melaena, or occult blood in the faeces. Haemorrhage from the lower intestinal tract may present as bright red blood excreted through the anus, or as occult blood present in the faeces. If blood loss is severe, the signs and symptoms of hypovolaemic shock will be evident.

Haemorrhoids which are distended veins in the anal area, may be internal or external. Internal haemorrhoids remain within the anal area, while external haemorrhoids prolapse through the anal canal. Haemorrhoids commonly result from increased pressure in the anal area related to constipation, straining to defaecate, obesity, pregnancy, and prolonged sitting or standing.

The individual commonly experiences pain in, and bleeding from, the anus particularly during defaecation. Pruritus of the anal area may occur in the presence of external haemorrhoids. Thrombosis of external haemorrhoids produces sudden anal pain, and the appearance of a palpable firm lump protruding from the anus.

An anal fissure is a crack in the lining of the anus and, like haemorrhoids, is associated with increased pressure in the anal area. Sudden occurrence is characterized by a tearing or burning pain during or immediately following defaecation, and by the appearance of a few drops of blood. An anal fissure may heal spontaneously, or it may partially heal and recur. A chronic fissure produces scar tissue which may impede normal defaecation.

A rectal prolapse is the protrusion of one or more layers of the mucous membrane of the rectum through the anus. Prolapse may be partial, or complete with displacement of the anal sphincter and rectum. Rectal prolapse is associated with increased intra-abdominal pressure from, e.g. straining to defaecate or malignancy. It may also result from weak rectal sphincters or muscles. Protrusion of tissue from the rectum is evident, and the individual may experience a sensation of rectal fullness, bleeding, and pain due to ulceration of the exposed tissues.

Cirrhosis of the liver is a chronic disease which is characterized by diffuse destruction and fibrosis of hepatic cells. The fibrosis impairs blood and lymph flow and eventually causes hepatic insufficiency, hepatic failure, and portal hypertension. Causes of cirrhosis of the liver include malnutrition resulting from chronic alcohol abuse, diseases of the bile ducts and hepatitis. Early manifestations include anorexia, nausea, altered bowel habits, and dull abdominal pain. Late symptoms develop as a result of hepatic insufficiency and portal hypertension, e.g. abdominal ascites, jaundice pruritus, emaciation, bleeding tendencies, and bleeding from oesophageal varices.

Inflammatory and infectious disorders

Inflammatory and/or infectious disorders of the digestive system may be related to internal or external irritation, or to the proliferation of pathogenic micro-organisms.

Stomatitis is a term which refers to inflammation of the mouth, and it may be a primary condition or a symptom of another disease. Inflammation may affect the lips, tongue, gums, mucous membranes, or palate. Stomatitis is characterized by pain, bleeding, swelling, ulceration, and halitosis.

Parotitis is inflammation of the parotid glands which may be related to poor oral hygiene or dryness of the mouth, or it may be caused by a micro-organism. Infectious parotitis (mumps) is an acute viral disease. Parotitis may also result from a calculus in the parotid gland. Symptoms of parotitis include tenderness and swelling of the gland, and pain associated with the ingestion of food or sour fluids.

Gastritis, which is inflammation of the gastric mucosa, may be acute or chronic.

Acute gastritis is associated with irritation of the mucosa related to the ingestion of irritating foods, alcohol, caffeine, and certain medications. Acute gastritis may also be caused by food poisoning, micro-organisms, or psychological stress.

Chronic gastritis is commonly associated with an underlying disorder, e.g. peptic ulcer, chronic alcohol abuse, or malignancy. Many individuals with chronic gastritis have no symptoms, while others experience anorexia, a feeling of fullness, eructation, and vague epigastric pain.

The same symptoms appear in acute gastritis, and the individual may also experience abdominal cramps, nausea and vomiting, and diarrhoea. Haemorrhage may occur, presenting as haematemesis, occult blood in the faeces, or melaena.

Gastroenteritis, which is inflammation of the stomach and intestines, is an acute disorder characterized by diarrhoea, nausea, vomiting, and abdominal cramps. Gastroenteritis has many causes including the ingestion of bacteria, amoebae, parasites, viruses, toxins or food allergens, and drug reactions. The symptoms vary according to the cause, the extent to which the digestive tract is involved, and the age of the individual. Infants, aged, and debilitated individuals are more vulnerable to the rapid loss of fluid and electrolytes which occurs with the condition.

Appendicitis which is inflammation of the appendix, may occur as a single attack or as repeated episodes. The condition commonly results from an obstruction of the lumen of the appendix, e.g. by a faecal mass, or as a result of inflammation and oedema due to a viral infection. The obstruction causes inflammation which can lead to infection, necrosis and perforation. If the appendix perforates, the contents spill into the abdominal cavity, causing peritonitis.

Commonly, the manifestations of appendicitis are anorexia, nausea, vomiting, and diffuse abdominal pain. The pain eventually localizes at McBurney's point in the right lower quadrant of the abdomen. Pyrexia and leukocytosis are generally present.

Peritonitis is inflammation of the peritoneum and it may be associated with many conditions. Causes of peritonitis include a perforated peptic ulcer, appendix, or diverticulum; abdominal trauma, or as a complication of abdominal surgery. The peritoneum becomes inflamed and oedematous, which generally results in decreased intestinal motility and intestinal obstruction.

The onset of peritonitis may be acute, or slow and progressive. The inflammatory process causes accumulation of fluid in the abdominal cavity leading to abdominal distension and rigidity, severe pain, nausea and vomiting. As a result of loss of fluid and electrolytes into the abdominal cavity, the individual displays signs of hypovalaemic shock. Abdominal distension results in upward displacement of the diaphragm and, typically, the individual's ventilations become shallow.

Pancreatitis, which is inflammation of the pancreas, may be acute or chronic. In both forms, inflammation may cause extensive tissue changes and damage. Pancreatitis may result from any disorder that interferes with the flow of biliary or pancreatic secretions, or which causes the secretions to become more viscous. Pancreatitis may be associated with chronic alcohol abuse, trauma, infection, metabolic disorders, malignancy, biliary tract disease, and certain medications.

The manifestations of pancreatitis include anorexia, nausea and vomiting, and severe upper abdominal pain. Pyrexia is usual and, if the common bile duct is obstructed, jaundice occurs. The individual is generally unable to tolerate fatty foods, and diarrhoea with steatorrhoea commonly occurs. If pancreatitis damages the islets of Langerhans, diabetes mellitus may develop. Extensive tissue damage may lead to necrosis and haemorrhage from the pancreas.

Inflammatory bowel disease is the term generally used to describe ulcerative colitis and Crohn's disease, both of which are chronic and recurrent disorders. Although the precise cause of inflammatory bowel disease is unknown, the factors which have been implicated include a familial tendency, infection, autoimmune reactions, and psychological stress.

1. Ulcerative colitis primarily affects the superficial mucosal layers of large areas of the colon. The inflammation associated with the disorder destroys tissue, causing ulceration and necrosis. Symptoms may be intermittent or continuous, and include abdominal pain and diarrhoea. The faeces are generally watery and may contain blood and mucus. Complications of ulcerative colitis include haemorrhage, formation of abscesses or fistulas, and bowel obstruction.

2. Crohn's disease (regional enteritis) affects all layers of the ileum and/or the colon. Sometimes the regional lymph nodes and the mesentery are also involved. Symptoms vary according to the site and extent of the lesions and, in acute episodes, the individual experiences lower right abdominal pain and cramps, flatulence, diarrhoea, nausea and vomiting, and pyrexia. The faeces may contain large quantities of blood and mucus. Complications of Crohn's disease are similar to those of ulcerative colitis.

Chronic or prolonged episodes of inflammatory bowel disease lead to nutritional imbalances and marked weight loss.

A pilonidal cyst forms in reaction to ingrown hair, and develops in the upper section of the cleft between the buttocks. A pilonidal cyst is more common in individuals who have heavy hair growth in that area, and the condition is exacerbated by friction, warmth and moisture. Generally, a pilonidal cyst causes no problems unless it becomes infected—resulting in local pain, tenderness and swelling. There may be several openings from the cyst to the skin (pilonidal sinus or fistula) which discharge purulent material.

Cholecystitis is acute or chronic inflammation of the gallbladder, and is commonly associated with impaction of a gallstone in the cystic duct. The gallbladder becomes dilated and filled with bile, pus, and blood.

Cholelithiasis is the term used to describe the presence of stones or calculi in the gallbladder. Choledocholithiasis is the presence of gallstones in the common bile duct.

Major manifestations of cholecystitis are intense pain and tenderness in the right upper abdominal quadrant, nausea and vomiting. If a stone obstructs the common bile duct jaundice may be evident.

Hepatitis which is inflammation of the liver, may be viral or non-viral in origin. Viral hepatitis is classified as hepatitis A (HAV), hepatitis B (HBV), and hepatitis non A/non B (NANB).

1. *Hepatitis A* is an infectious disorder which is generally spread via the faecal-oral route, e.g. through the ingestion of contaminated food. The individual may have few symptoms, or he may experience headaches, fatigue, anorexia, pyrexia, dark urine, pale faeces, liver enlargement, jaundice, and pruritus.

2. *Hepatitis B* (serum hepatitis) is generally transmitted parenterally by contact with infected blood. The virus may also be spread via contact with body secretions such as saliva, vaginal secretions, menstrual blood, and semen. The virus may also be transmitted from an infected mother to her baby, during passage through the birth canal or via breast milk.

The incidence of hepatitis B is higher in individuals who receive blood or blood products, use or share contaminated needles, or engage in homosexual practices. An individual may be a carrier of HBV, but experience no symptoms of the disease. Manifestations of HBV are similar to those of HAV, but in a more severe form. The infection may persist for a long time, resulting in chronic liver failure and cirrhosis.

3. *Hepatitis non A/non B*, which is caused by an undentified virus or viruses, is more common in individuals who have received numerous blood transfusions. The manifestations are similar to those of hepatitis A and can be severe.

Non-viral hepatitis generally results from exposure to certain chemicals which, when ingested or inhaled, cause necrosis of hepatitic cells. Manifestations of the disorder are similar to those of viral hepatitis.

Neoplastic and obstructive disorders

Neoplasms of the digestive system may be benign or malignant. Obstruction of part of the digestive tract, e.g. the small intestine, may occur as an acute or a chronic disorder.

Polyps, which are projections of the mucosal surface of an organ, may develop in the stomach or intestine. Polyps may be benign or malignant, and the most common form is adenoma. An adenomatous polyp may begin in the benign form and later undergo malignant changes. Polyps may be asymptomatic, or they may cause diarrhoea, haemorrhage, or the manifestations of intestinal obstruction.

Familial colonic polyposis is a hereditary disorder characterized by numerous polyps, and it has a high association with colonic malignancy.

Cancer may develop in the mouth, oesophagus, stomach, intestines, rectum, liver or pancreas. Cancer of the oral cavity has been linked to heavy tobacco use and alcohol abuse. Dietary factors have been implicated in the cause of gastric cancer, along with various other causes. Dietary factors, particularly a lack of dietary fibre, are considered to be related to carcinogenic changes in the intestines and rectum. The majority of cases of liver cancer involve metastatic lesions; while cancer of the pancreas appears to be associated with diabetes, pancreatitis, smoking, and exposure to industrial chemicals.

Further information on the causes, incidence, and types of cancer, is provided in Chapter 64.

The manifestations of cancer of the digestive system vary according to the site and include dysphagia, hoarseness, anorexia, nausea, vomiting, epigastric discomfort, abdominal distension, weight loss, changes in bowel habits, bleeding from the rectum, and blood in the faeces. Pain is not usually a feature in the early stages of the disease, but the individual may experience gas pains, abdominal cramps; or discomfort associated with swallowing or defaecation. Cancer of the rectum frequently causes a sensation of incomplete evacuation and tenesmus.

Manifestations of liver cancer are related to the extent of damage to the liver cells and include weight loss, ascites, abdominal pain, liver enlargement, anaemia, and jaundice.

Pancreatic cancer causes similar symptoms to those related to cancer of the liver. Steatorrhea may occur as a consequence of pancreatic enzyme deficiency, as may the manifestations of hyperglycaemia if insulin production is impaired.

Intestinal obstruction may occur as an acute or a chronic condition. When an obstruction occurs, the passage of intestinal contents is inhibited. Part of the small or large intestine may become partially or totally obstructed.

Obstruction of the small intestine is more common and may be due to adhesions or a strangulated hernia. The small intestine may also be obstructed by foreign objects, compression of the bowel wall due to stenosis, or intussusception.

Paralytic (adynamic) ileus is a form of intestinal obstruction that may develop after abdominal surgery; or as a response to peritonitis, toxaemia, electrolyte imbalance, or certain medications. In this condition, the motility of the small intestine is decreased or absent.

Obstruction of the large intestine is related to diverticulitis, cancer, and volvulus (twisting of the colon).

Manifestations of intestinal obstruction appear when fluids, gas, and ingested substances accumulate proximal to the site of obstruction. The individual generally experiences abdominal pain, distension, and vomiting; and is usually unable to pass flatus or faeces.

If the obstruction is at the distal end of the intestine vomiting may occur late, and the vomitus has a faecal odour—caused by bacterial overgrowth in the intestinal tract.

The individual commonly exhibits the manifestations of fluid and electrolyte imbalance due to progressive dehydration and plasma loss.

Complications of intestinal obstruction include peritonitis, ischaemia and necrosis of the bowel.

Traumatic disorders

Trauma to parts of the digestive system may be related to injury or to irritation, e.g. the ingestion of a corrosive substance. Abdominal trauma may be localized, or it may involve a number of abdominal structures. When a part of the digestive system is damaged the processes of digestion, absorption, and elimination may be impaired. As a consequence, alterations in nutritional, electrolyte, and fluid status occur.

Depending on the type and extent of injury the manifestations include external bruising, abdominal distension, pain, altered bowel sounds and haemorrhage—either internal and concealed, or presenting as haematemesis and/or melaena. Complications of trauma to the digestive system include haemorrhage, shock, infection, peritonitis and obstruction.

Some disorders of the digestive system will require surgical intervention. Information on the care of an individual who requires surgery is provided in Chapter 59.

Diagnostic tests

Certain tests may be performed to assist, or confirm, the diagnosis of digestive system disorders.

Laboratory tests

Specimens which may be obtained from the patient for laboratory analysis include blood, faeces, gastric or peritoneal fluid, urine, and samples of tissue.

The blood may be tested to determine haemoglobin level, haematocrit, leucocyte count, serum electrolytes, bilirubin levels, glucose levels, or pancreatic enzyme levels.

The faeces may be tested to identify bleeding disorders, biliary obstruction, infections, and disorders of digestion or absorption. The procedure for collecting a specimen of faeces is described in Chapter 30.

Gastric fluid analysis involves examination of gastric secretions, and it may be performed by examining a specimen of vomitus or by testing a sample of the gastric contents which have been aspirated via a nasogastric tube.

The gastric acid stimulation test measures the secretion of hydrochloric acid for a predetermined time following the subcutaneous administration of a medication, e.g. pentagastrin which stimulates hydrochloric acid production.

Another test performed to measure hydrochloric acid secretion involves the administration of an oral dye, e.g. in granules mixed with water. If the gastric contents are sufficiently acid the dye is released, absorbed into the bloodstream, and excreted in the urine. Specimens of urine are collected at specified times, and laboratory testing estimates the amount of dye present.

Peritoneal fluid analysis assesses a sample of peritoneal fluid which has been obtained by abdominal paracentesis. The test may be performed when bleeding or infection is suspected. Abdominal paracentesis involves the insertion of a trocar and cannula through the abdominal wall, so that a quantity of peritoneal fluid may be aspirated.

A therapeutic paracentesis may also be performed when the individual has ascites, as drainage of the excess fluid relieves pressure in the abdominal cavity.

The urine may be tested to detect the presence of any abnormal substance, e.g. bilirubin, which may be excreted in the urine as a result of a digestive system disorder.

Biopsy. Specimens of tissue may be obtained during endoscopic examinations or surgery. The specimens are examined microscopically for changes in cellular structure, to confirm diagnosis or to determine the cause of a disease, e.g. malignancy.

Radiological examination

Plain X-rays may be taken to aid in the diagnosis of abdominal masses, bowel obstruction, trauma to abdominal organs, and ascites.

Fluoroscopy (visualization with motion) involves use of a contrast agent, e.g. barium sulphate, which can be visualized as it passes through and outlines structures in the digestive tract. Fluoroscopic examination of the digestive tract includes barium swallow, barium meal and barium enema.

For a *barium swallow* or barium meal the individual drinks the contrast medium. Its progress is observed on a fluorescent screen, and X-ray films are taken, as the substance moves through the upper digestive tract. To visualize the lower digestive tract, a barium enema is administered. The contrast medium is instilled into the colon by means of a rectal tube, then the progress of the substance is observed on a fluorescent screen and X-ray films are taken.

Cholecystography involves the ingestion of a radio-opaque substance, followed by a series of X-ray films which show the shape of the gallbladder and the presence of gallstones.

A cholangiogram is the radiographic examination of the biliary ducts and gallbladder after the intravenous infusion of a contrast medium. A T-tube cholangiogram may be performed several days following surgical removal of the gallbladder. Dye is injected into the T-tube, which was inserted at the time of surgery, so that the common bile duct may be visualized and its patency assessed.

Computerized tomography scanning (CT scan) involves the direction of a narrow X-ray beam at parts of the body, from various angles. Contrast medium is often administered intravenously to enhance visualization. A computer reconstructs the information as a three-dimensional image on a screen.

Ultrasonography (ultrasound) involves the use of sound waves to visualize body structures. A transducer is passed over the area, e.g. the abdomen, and receives echoes which are bounced off body structures. The echoes are converted into electrical impulses which may be viewed on a screen or photographed.

Endoscopy

Endoscopy is the visual examination of part of the digestive tract, using a flexible fibre-optic endoscope. The endoscope also provides a channel for the introduction of instruments for the purpose of obtaining a sample of tissue for microscopic examination. The various forms of endoscopy derive their names from the part of the body being examined:

- oesophagoscopy (the oesophagus)
- gastroscopy (the stomach)
- duodenoscopy (the duodenum)
- proctoscopy (the anus and rectum)
- sigmoidoscopy (the sigmoid colon)
- colonoscopy (the colon).

CARE OF THE INDIVIDUAL WITH A DIGESTIVE SYSTEM DISORDER

Although specific nursing actions and medical management vary depending on the disorder, the main aims of care are to:

- prevent and manage alterations in elimination
- promote comfort
- maintain skin and mucous membrane integrity
- maintain nutritional and fluid status.

Preventing and managing alterations in elimination

The two main alterations in bowel elimination, that occur in disorders of the digestive system, are diarrhoea and constipation. Information on the prevention of diarrhoea and constipation is provided in Chapter 30, together with information on the care of an individual who is experiencing altered elimination from the bowel.

Vomiting is another manifestation of certain digestive system disorders, and information on the care of an individual who is vomiting is provided in Chapter 29.

Promotion of comfort

Many disorders of the digestive system result in discomfort or pain due to gastrointestinal distension, pressure on abdominal organs, or alterations in elimination. Tolerance and reaction to pain varies with each individual, and with the severity and character of the pain being experienced. Information on promoting pain relief is provided in Chapter 36.

The nurse has a responsibility to implement care that will alleviate the individual's pain and discomfort. Nursing care includes administration of prescribed medications, e.g. analgesics, anti-emetics, antacids, anticholinergics, antibiotics, or laxatives. Any prescribed medication must be administered in accordance with nursing regulations and the institution's policies.

To help prevent or alleviate abdominal discomfort, the individual should be encouraged to avoid consuming gas-producing foods or liquids, and foods that are highly spiced or high in fat content.

Discomfort or pain may interfere with the individual's ability to meet his needs independently, therefore the nurse should assist him to meet all his physical and psychological needs. Some treatments, e.g. the creation of a stoma, cause alterations to the individual's body image and self esteem. The nurse can help to promote his psychological comfort by ensuring that he receives sufficient information and emotional support as he adjusts to any changes.

Maintenance of skin and mucous membrane integrity

The integrity of the skin or mucous membranes can be impaired in certain disorders, e.g. diarrhoea can produce excoriation of the anal area, or the skin may become excoriated from wound secretions or drainage from a stoma. The mouth may become dry if the individual is dehydrated or is unable to tolerate oral fluids. The presence of a nasogastric tube can cause irritation and breakdown of the nasal mucosa.

The individual's skin should be kept clean and dry, and protective substances such as a barrier cream may be applied to areas susceptible to excoriation. Information on the care of the skin when the individual has a stoma is provided later in this chapter. If excessive wound drainage is present, a collection bag may be applied to prevent continual contact between the skin and exudate.

Regular mouth care will help to keep the mouth moist, and will help to remove any unpleasant odours or tastes, e.g. after an episode of vomiting. A water soluble lubricant may be applied to the nostril to reduce irritation from a naso-gastric tube.

Maintenance of nutritional and fluid status

The individual's nutritional and fluid status may be impaired by disorders which affect digestive system function. Some individuals may experience periods where they are unable to consume food or fluid, due to pain, nausea or vomiting; or as part of the management of the disorder. Loss of fluids and electrolytes may occur during episodes of vomiting or diarrhoea, and through wound drainage or nasogastric suction.

If the individual is able to tolerate substances orally he should be encouraged to eat the types of foods which will meet his nutritional needs. Food that will stimulate his appetite, and not cause discomfort, should be selected. Often, small frequent amounts of food are better tolerated than large meals. An adequate intake of fluids is essential to prevent dehydration.

If the individual is experiencing nausea and/or vomiting, he should be encouraged to eat and drink small amounts slowly. Dry foods such as toast or biscuits may be more easily tolerated, and he should be encouraged to lie quietly and relax for some time after consuming any food. Antiemetic medications may be prescribed if necessary.

If the individual is unable to tolerate food or fluid orally, or if large amounts of fluids and electrolytes are lost from the body, intravenous therapy or artificial feeding may be necessary. He may require nutritional support through gastric tube feeding or total parenteral nutrition. Information on artificial feeding is provided in Chapter 29.

During the course of the disorder the individual should be continually assessed for the manifestations of dehydration and malnutrition (Table 46.1). An accurate record of his input and output, and weight, should be kept as part of the assessment.

Nursing activities

Specific nursing activities include:

- care of an individual with a nasogastric tube
- implementation of measures to assist elimination from the bowel
- observation and collection of excreta
- artificial feeding
- care of wounds and drainage tubes
- care of an individual with a stoma.

Table 46.1 Manifestations of dehydration and malnutrition

Dehydration	Malnutrition
Dry skin, loss of tissue turgor	Dry and atrophic skin and mucous membranes
Dry mouth and tongue	
Thirst	Extreme hunger or anorexia
Loss of weight	Loss of weight and subcutaneous fat
Oliguria and concentrated urine	Constipation or diarrhoea
Sunken eyes	Pale conjunctiva
Elevated temperature, lowered blood pressure	Rapid heart rate, elevated blood pressure
Irritability, confusion	Irritability, apathy, lack of energy

Gastric intubation

A tube may be inserted through the nostril, or less commonly through the mouth, into the stomach for diagnostic or therapeutic purposes to:

- collect gastric contents for analysis
- perform gastric lavage
- aspirate gastric secretions
- decompress the stomach after major surgery
- administer fluid.

Information on nasogastic tube feeding is provided in Chapter 29, while this chapter addresses the care of the individual with a nasogastric tube.

Insertion of a nasogastric tube

The insertion of a nasogastric tube (Fig. 46.1) is an invasive technique and is performed by individuals who are qualified and experienced in the technique. A suggested procedure for nasogastric tube insertion is outlined in the guidelines.

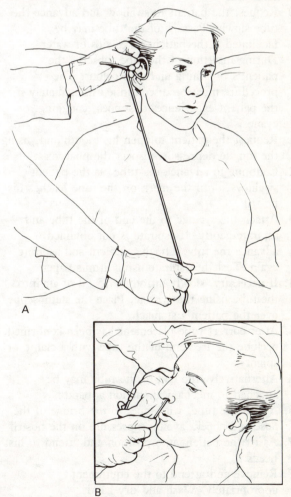

Fig. 46.1 Insertion of a nasogastric tube. (A) Estimating how far to insert the tube. (B) Inserting the tube.

Guidelines for insertion of a nasogastric tube

Nursing action	Rationale
1. Explain the procedure to the patient and provide privacy	Reduces anxiety and embarrassment
2. Unless contraindicated, assist the patient to assume a sitting position	Facilitates passage of the tube into the oesophagus
3. Place the equipment within easy reach	Facilitates performance of the procedure in an organized manner
4. Request the patient to blow his nose	Clears the nostrils of any secretions
5. Wash and dry hands. Put on disposable gloves	Prevents cross infection
6. Inspect the nostrils for any obstruction or deviated septum	Assists in selecting the most suitable nostril
7. Place the tip of the tube at the tip of the patient's nose, extend the tube to his earlobe and down to the xiphoid process. Mark this point on the tube	Determines the length of tube needed to reach the stomach
8. Lubricate the tip of the tube, without occluding the lumen	Facilitates insertion and prevents injury to the nasal passages
9. Insert the tip of the tube into the nostril, directing it downward and toward the ear on the same side	Avoids pressure on the nasal turbinates
10. Request the patient to swallow and advance the tube slowly. Passage of the tube may be facilitated if the patient takes sips of water	Assists descent of the tube into the oesophagus
During insertion of the tube, observe the patient's breathing and skin colour. The procedure must be discontinued immediately if the patient experiences dyspnoea, coughing, or cyanosis	The tube may be entering the trachea instead of the oesophagus
11. Request the patient to open his mouth and, using the tongue depressor, inspect the pharynx	Determines whether the tube is descending, or curling up in the mouth
12. Continue to advance the tube, as the patient swallows, until the mark on the tube reaches his nostril	The tip of the tube must be situated in the stomach
13. Attach the syringe to the end of the tube and aspirate gently. If aspirate is not obtained, advance the tube a further 2.5 cm and aspirate again. Test the aspirate using litmus paper	Determines correct tube placement, i.e. in the stomach and not in the oesophagus. Acid aspirate changes blue litmus paper to red
14. If necessary, slowly introduce 15 ml of air into the tube using the syringe. Place the stethoscope over the patient's stomach	A rush of air heard entering the stomach verifies correct tube placement
15. After correct tube placement has been confirmed, occlude the free end of the tube with a clamp or spigot	Prevents leakage of stomach contents
Alternatively, the end of the tube may be attached to mechanical suction apparatus	Promotes removal of gastric contents
16. Attach the tube, with tape, to the bridge of the nose and cheek, avoiding pressure on the nostril	Secures the tube in position
17. Assist the patient into position and attend to his needs.	Promotes comfort and relaxation
18. Remove and attend to the equipment appropriately. Wash and dry hands	Prevents cross infection
19. Document and report the procedure	Appropriate care can be planned and implemented

The basic equipment consists of:

— water soluble lubricant, e.g. K-Y jelly
— nasogastric tube of appropriate size
— 50 ml syringe
— tongue depressor
— receiver for aspirate
— litmus paper
— hypoallergenic tape
— clamp or spigot
— stethoscope
— scissors
— drape
— disposable gloves.

A nasogastric tube may be inserted for a short time, e.g. to obtain a specimen of gastric contents for analysis, then removed immediately. Alternatively, a nasogastric tube may remain in position for longer periods, e.g. following abdominal surgery or for the purpose of administering feedings. In some circumstances the nasogastric tube may be attached to mechanical suction apparatus, to keep the stomach empty. A wall unit suction device, which can provide intermittent or continuous suction, is commonly used.

Gastric lavage is a procedure that involves flushing the stomach and removing gastric contents, via a gastric tube inserted through the mouth or nostril. This technique may be used as an emergency procedure in the treatment of ingested poisons.

An iced saline lavage may be performed by a medical officer to help control upper gastro-intestinal haemorrhage. This procedure involves the instillation of small amounts of iced sterile normal saline into the stomach through a nasogastric tube. Approximately 50 ml of saline is instilled then withdrawn or allowed to drain out by gravity, the technique being repeated as many times as necessary. When the cool solution enters the stomach it promotes vasoconstriction, and helps to stop haemorrhage.

Care of the individual with a nasogastric tube

Care of the individual involves continued assessment of his condition, assisting him to meet his needs, and maintenance of the equipment.

● Oral and nasal hygiene should be provided to reduce any irritation, discomfort or dryness caused by the tube. The nostrils should be cleansed to remove any secretions, mouth rinses should be provided, and a protective cream may be applied to the rim of the nostril and to the lips.
● The tape securing the tube in position is replaced if it becomes loose or damp.
● Intermittent manual aspiration may be prescribed, and is achieved by attaching a syringe to the end of the tube. The plunger of the syringe is slowly withdrawn to remove any gastric contents, and the end of the tube is occluded

with a clamp or spigot following aspiration.
● If mechanical suction is used, observations are necessary to assess correct functioning of the apparatus. Any malfunction must be reported immediately.
● Aspirate is observed for amount, colour, and consistency. All aspirate or drainage is measured and the amounts are recorded on a fluid balance chart. Normal gastric secretions are either yellow—green or colourless, and have a mucoid consistency. Any abnormalities, e.g. blood, must be reported immediately.
● The individual's bowel sounds are assessed at regular intervals to check gastro-intestinal function. Absence of bowel sounds, abdominal pain or distension, or vomiting may indicate tube obstruction and must be reported immediately.
● Prior to instilling any substance, correct tube placement must be confirmed. Administration of fluid or medication through a malpositioned tube can result in the substance entering the lungs.
● Prior to instilling medications or thick fluids, the tube should be irrigated with a small amount of water. Following instillation, the tube is again irrigated with a small amount of water to clear the lumen.
● The individual should be observed for complications associated with gastric intubation, gastric suction, or gastric tube feeding:

● erosion of skin at the nostril
● inflammation of the oral cavity
● fluid and electrolyte imbalance
● diarrhoea, constipation, or vomiting
● aspiration pneumonia resulting from gastric reflux
● oesophagotracheal fistula (prolonged intubation).

Removal of a nasogastric tube requires care to prevent mucosal damage, and inhalation of fluid. Prior to its removal, the tube is irrigated with water to clear it of any gastric contents which could cause mucosal damage should leakage occur during removal. The tube is pinched, or clamped, then gently and steadily withdrawn. Following removal of the tube any tape residue is removed from the skin, and nasal and oral hygiene is provided. The individual is observed for any manifestations of gastro-intestinal dysfunction, e.g. abdominal distension or pain, nausea or vomiting.

Other nursing activities

Information on the administration of suppositories, enemata, bowel lavage; on the insertion of a rectal tube to remove flatus, and on the digital removal of impacted faeces is provided in Chapter 30. The same chapter includes information on observation and collection of a specimen of faeces. Information on artificial feeding, e.g. via a gastric tube, is provided in Chapter 29. Information on the care of wounds and drainage tubes is provided in Chapter 59.

Pre- and Post-diagnostic test care

The nurse may be required to prepare the individual prior to a diagnostic test, to provide psychological support during the procedure, and to monitor his condition following the test. By understanding how specific diagnostic procedures are performed, the nurse is able to reinforce the medical officer's explanations to the individual.

The nurse should refer to the institution's policy manual for information on preparation of the individual prior to each diagnostic test. The nurse must also know what observations, and post test care, are required. Preparation of the individual prior to a specific diagnostic test may include fluid or dietary modifications or restrictions, preparation of the bowel, e.g. administration of an enema; checking that written consent has been obtained and the administration of any prescribed medications.

Assessment of the individual following the test may include monitoring his vital signs, observing for bleeding after an invasive procedure, assessing his ability to swallow and cough before oral fluids are given, and observing him for any discomfort or pain.

Care of the individual with a stoma

Specific disorders of the digestive tract may require surgical treatment involving the creation of an artificial opening on the abdominal wall. Part of the intestine is brought through this opening to form a stoma.

A colostomy involves the creation of an artificial opening into a section of the colon, which is brought out through an opening in the abdomen.

An ileostomy involves the creation of an artificial opening into part of the ileum, usually the terminal ileum, which is brought out through an opening in the abdomen.

As a result of both surgical procedures faecal elimination occurs through the stoma, which may be created as a temporary or a permanent measure. A temporary colostomy is created to divert faecal contents, e.g. to allow healing of an incision in the distal colon or rectum. A permanent colostomy is indicated principally in colorectal cancer, after a partial or total colectomy has been performed. A temporary ileostomy is created to rest the bowel, e.g. in ulcerative colitis. A permanent ileostomy may be formed following total colectomy in the management of Crohn's disease, ulcerative colitis, or familial polyposis.

Figure 46.2 illustrates the sites where a stoma may be located. The site is selected according to which part of the bowel is affected and, if the stoma is to be permanent, with consideration of the individual's physique, his occupation, and any other factors that may influence his ability to successfully manage the care of his stoma. In many health care institutions a stomal therapist liases with the patient and surgeon to select the most appropriate site. The site of the stoma will determine the consistency of the faecal matter

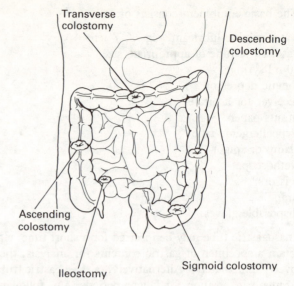

Fig. 46.2 Stoma sites.

excreted through it. The closer the stoma is to the small intestine, the more liquid the faeces well be. Faeces excreted through an ileostomy are liquid to pastelike, whereas faeces excreted through a sigmoid colostomy are semiformed to solid.

Figure 46.3 illustrates the types of colostomy or ileostomy that may be created.

Care of the individual with a stoma includes the selection and management of appliances, care of the stoma and surrounding skin, colostomy irrigation, meeting his nutritional needs, and provision of psychological support. A stomal therapist may be available to assist in the preparation of the individual and his significant others prior to the operation. She also plays a major role in providing support and education following the operation.

Ostomy appliances

Immediately following surgery, and for several days afterwards, the individual generally has a long bag (Fig. 46.4) applied over the stoma. This type of appliance is secured over the stoma by an adhesive backing, and the excess bag is folded up with the end closed off by a rubber band to prevent leakage. To empty the bag the band is removed, the bag is unfolded, and the contents are drained into an appropriate receiver. After being emptied, the bag may be flushed through with water to which a deodourizing substance, e.g. eucalyptus drops, has been added. A new long bag is applied when necessary.

Later, this appliance is replaced by a smaller bag or pouch. A variety of disposable bags and pouches are available to suit individual needs. The type of appliance which is selected should be easy for the individual to use, be com-

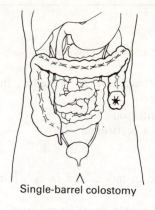

Single-barrel colostomy

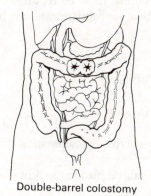

Double-barrel colostomy

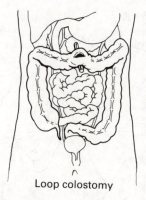

Loop colostomy

Fig. 46.3 Types of ostomy.

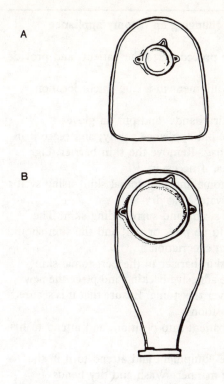

Fig. 46.4 Ostomy appliances. (A) Non-drainable stoma bag.
(B) Drainable stoma bag. Reproduced with permission from Game C,
Anderson R E, Kidd J R (eds) 1989 Medical-Surgical nursing: a core
text. Churchill Livingstone, Melbourne.)

fortable, non-irritant, leak-proof, and odour-proof. Several
styles may need to be tried before the individual finds the
one which is most appropriate.

The disposable bags or pouches are equipped with an
adhesive backing which is applied to the skin surrounding
the stoma. The adhesive backing may be applied directly
to the skin, or over a protective skin barrier, e.g. a pectin
wafer or a liquid substance, which is applied to the peristomal skin before the bag is placed over the stoma.

It is important that the opening in the bag or pouch is
centered over the stoma, and that the adhesive backing is
pressed down to provide an efficient seal. Gentle pressure
is applied to the adhesive surface from the stoma outward.

Some individuals may prefer to further secure the bag in
position with an ostomy belt. It is important that the ostomy bag or pouch is applied correctly to prevent leakage
of faeces. Leakage of faecal material causes odour and irritation of the peristomal skin, and is a source of extreme
embarrassment to the individual.

The bag or pouch is removed and replaced with a new
one as necessary, generally when it is one-third full. Correct disposal of soiled appliances involves emptying the
contents into the toilet, and placing the appliance in a plastic bag or newspaper before discarding it into the garbage
container.

A suggested procedure for changing an ostomy appliance
is outlined in the guidelines. As soon as practicable, the
individual is encouraged to care for his ostomy independently. The basic equipment for changing an appliance is:

— a bag for used appliance and soiled swabs
— a skin barrier
— clean appliance
— cotton wool swabs
— container of warm water
— scissors
— disposable gloves.

Guidelines for changing an ostomy appliance

Nursing action	Rationale
1. Explain the procedure to the patient, and provide privacy	Reduces anxiety and embarrassment
2. Place the equipment in a convenient location	Facilitates performance of the procedure in an organized manner
3. Wash and dry hands, and put on gloves	Prevents contamination
4. Remove the old appliance gently, and place it in the plastic bag. Remove the skin barrier, e.g. pectin wafer, if necessary	Avoids damage to peristomal skin
5. Wipe the stoma and peristomal skin, using swabs and warm water. Pat dry	Cleanses the skin of mucus and faecal drainage
6. Inspect the stoma and surrounding skin. The stoma should be pink or red, and the skin should be free from excoriation	Deviations from normal must be reported immediately, so that appropriate care can be planned
7. Apply the skin barrier to the peristomal skin	Protects the skin
8. Remove the adhesive backing and place the new appliance over the stoma. Ensure that it is secured firmly in position	Prevents leakage of faeces
9 Assist the patient into position, and attend to his needs	Promotes comfort
10. Remove the equipment and attend to it in the appropriate manner. Wash and dry hands	Prevents odour and cross contamination
11. Document and report the procedure	Appropriate care can be planned and implemented

Colostomy irrigation (Fig. 46.5) is a technique which, if appropriate, is performed in order to give the individual some control over elimination. Performed daily, colostomy irrigation establishes a regular pattern of faecal evacuation.

The individual is instructed in the technique while he is in hospital, so that he is able to successfully manage it independently when he leaves hospital. Colostomy irrigation involves placing an irrigation drain over the stoma, and introducing warm water into the bowel. After a period of approximately 20–30 minutes, the water and faecal material is allowed to drain out. After several weeks of daily irrigation the colostomy usually becomes regulated so that, between irrigations, the individual needs to wear only a small adhesive patch over the stoma.

A suggested procedure for colostomy irrigation is outlined in the guidelines. The basic equipment for irrigation is:

— irrigating drainage appliance
— belt to hold appliance in position
— irrigation bag containing 500–1000 ml warm water
— cone tip attached to irrigating tubing
— clamp
— stand for the container of fluid
— colostomy appliance (pouch or patch)
— disposable gloves
— water soluble lubricant.

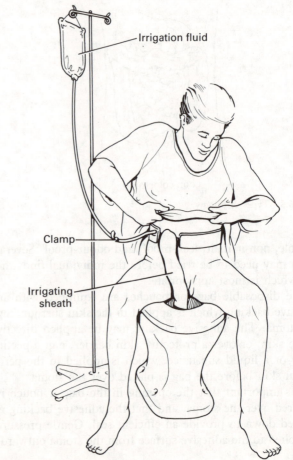

Fig. 46.5 Colostomy irrigation.

Guidelines for colostomy irrigation

Nursing action	Rationale
1. Explain the procedure to the patient	Reduces anxiety
2. Assemble the equipment where the procedure is to be performed, e.g. in the bathroom if the patient is ambulant	Maximum privacy should be provided in a convenient location. Prior assembly of equipment facilitates performance of the procedure in an organized manner
3. Wash and dry hands and put on disposable gloves	Prevents contamination
4. Fill the irrigation bag with 500–1000 ml warm water, suspend the container at patient's shoulder level, and flush a little water through the tubing. Clamp the tubing. Connect the cone to the end of the tubing	Allows water to flow by gravity Removes any air from the tubing
5. Remove any colostomy appliance and dispose of it appropriately	Prevents odours and contamination
6. Lubricate the tip of the cone	Facilitates insertion and prevents damage to the mucous membrane
7. Apply the irrigating drainage bag/sleeve over the stoma, and secure it with the belt	Appliance must fit securely over the stoma
8. Insert the cone through the opening of the irrigation bag, and insert the cone tip gently into the stoma	The cone prevents back-flow while the irrigating fluid is being instilled
9. Open the tubing clamp to allow water to slowly enter the bowel—over a period of 10–15 minutes Observe for pain	Cramping may occur if the water enters the bowel too rapidly
10. When all the water has flowed into the bowel, remove the cone and seal the distal end of the irrigating bag Encourage the ambulant patient to walk about for approximately 10–20 minutes	Ambulation stimulates elimination and return of the irrigating fluid
11. Within 20–60 minutes request the patient to sit on the toilet, and place the open distal end of the drain sleeve into the toilet	Allows fluid and faeces to drain into the toilet
12. Encourage the patient to lean forward and/or gently massage his abdomen	Stimulates the return of irrigating fluid and faeces
13. When all the fluid and faeces have drained out through the bag, remove the bag and belt Cleanse the peristomal area and put on a colostomy appliance	Avoids subsequent leakage from the stoma
14. Attend to the equipment in the appropriate manner, wash and dry hands	Prevents cross contamination
15. Document and report the procedure	Appropriate care can be planned and implemented

---

Care of the peristomal skin and stoma

Because faeces contain enzymes that are irritating to the skin, maintenance of peristomal skin integrity is essential. The skin must be kept clean and dry, and any signs of irritation or excoriation must be reported immediately. With the repeated removal of adhesive appliances, the risk of skin damage is increased.

There are various preparations available which may be applied to the peristomal skin to protect it, including adhesive wafers, lotions and pastes. The stomal therapist helps to determine which type of skin protection is most appropriate for the individual.

The stoma should be observed for normal pink or red colour, both of which indicate an adequate blood supply. Any discolouration, e.g. cyanosis, or signs of oedema, necrosis, recession or prolapse of the stoma, must be reported immediately.

When the ostomy appliance is changed, the stoma is gently wiped with damp cotton wool to remove any mucus and faecal matter.

Nutritional needs

The individual with an ileostomy or colostomy is given advice on the type of diet which will help to avoid excessive gas production, odour, diarrhoea or constipation. Dietary modifications may be necessary, and the individual will gradually learn the types of food he is able to consume without adverse effects. Adequate hydration is essential, especially for the individual with an ileostomy, as large amounts of fluid may be excreted in the drainage. An adequate oral intake is also necessary to prevent constipation, and possible blockage of the stoma.

Psychological support

The creation of a stoma generally alters body image. Changes in body structure and function are threatening to the individual, who has to learn to adjust to these alterations. The individual, and his significant others, will commonly require a great deal of psychological support and counselling to reach acceptance of this new condition.

The individual may worry about the impact of his ostomy on his relationships with other people, and he may experience anxiety that the stoma will be obvious to others. Depression and fear of rejection are common reactions to stomal surgery, and the nurse has an important role to play in helping the individual overcome any difficulties related to the stoma.

Pre-operative preparation through explanation and information giving is an essential part of providing psychological support. The individual, and his significant others, should be given the opportunity to discuss any fears or anxieties. A variety of literature is available which may be helpful in preparing the individual pre-operatively, e.g. booklets which describe and illustrate various types of stomas and appliances. Post-operatively, psychological support must be continued. The individual should be encouraged to gradually assume responsibility for the care of his stoma, and the nurse should keep in mind that adequate time is needed to recover from the surgery and to develop confidence in self care.

Discharge planning includes ensuring that the individual knows how to obtain the use appliances, and how to care for his stoma. He should be provided with education aids in the form of instruction booklets or leaflets which contain information helpful to an individual with a stoma. He whould be made aware of the need to contact the medical officer or stomal theropist immediately if any complications occur, e.g. skin irritation, stomal oedema, stomal necrosis, or stomal recession or prolapse.

Prior to his discharge from hospital, the district nursing service should be contacted so that a visiting nurse can call on the individual at home to check on his physical care and psychological adjustment. Follow up visits to his surgeon should also be arranged. The individual should also be provided with information on support groups in the area, e.g. the local Ostomy Association.

With adequate physical and psychological preparation and support, the individual will generally come to realize that a return to his usual lifestyle is possible.

SUMMARY

The functions of the digestive system are to ingest and digest foods so that nutrients can be absorbed into the bloodstream, and to eliminate wastes from the body.

Normal function may be impaired as a result of alterations in swallowing, secretory function, motility, digestion, absorption or elimination.

The major manifestations of digestive system disorders are pain, flatulence, altered eating habits, nausea and vomiting, altered bowel function, and dysphagia.

Disorders of the digestive system can be classified as those occurring from multiple causes, from inflammation or infection, as a result of neoplasms or obstruction, or as a result of injury.

Diagnostic tests used to assess digestive system function include laboratory analysis of body fluids, excretions or tissue; radiological examinations, and endoscopy.

Care of the individual with a disorder includes preventing and managing altered elimination, the promotion of comfort, maintenance of skin and mucous membrane integrity, and maintenance of nutritional and fluid status.

Nursing activities include the care of an individual who has a gastric tube, the implementation of measures to assist bowel elimination, observation and collection of excreta, and assisting with artificial feeding.

An individual with a specific disorder of the digestive tract may require the surgical creation of a stoma, through which faeces are excreted.

REFERENCES AND FURTHER READING

Brunner L S, Suddarth D S 1988 Textbook of medical-surgical nursing, 6th edn. J. B. Lippincott, Philadelphia
Chilman A, Thomas M 1987 Understanding nursing care, 3rd edn. Churchill Livingstone, Edinburgh
Game C, Anderson R, Kidd J (eds) 1989 Medical-surgical nursing: a core text. Churchill Livingstone, Melbourne, 458–544

47. The individual with a urinary system disorder

OBJECTIVES

1. State the pathophysiological influences and effects associated with disorders of the urinary system.
2. Describe the major manifestations of urinary system disorders.
3. Briefly describe the specific disorders of the urinary system which are outlined in this chapter.
4. State the diagnostic tests which may be used to assess urinary system function.
5. Assist in planning and implementing nursing care for the individual with a urinary system disorder.

INTRODUCTION

Information on the normal structure and function of the urinary system is provided in Chapter 24, and it should be referred to before studying the contents of this chapter.

The kidneys are essential in the maintenance of homeostasis as they regulate the rates of elimination of water and electrolytes from the body, and contribute to the maintenance of a constant blood pH. The kidneys also eliminate metabolic waste products and toxic substances. Therefore, any dysfunction in the formation or excretion of urine can have major adverse effects on homeostasis.

Pathological influences and effects

Alterations in normal function of the urinary system can be classified as changes in kidney structure, fluid and electrolyte balance, elimination of waste substances; and alterations in the output of urine.

Changes in kidney structure

Atrophy of the kidneys, because of destruction of the renal tissue, can occur in many chronic renal diseases. Alternatively, the kidneys can become enlarged because of a blockage of the ureters, enlargement of the prostate gland, or from invasion of the kidneys by neoplastic cells. If there is an obstruction lower down in the urinary tract, the ureters may become enlarged in diameter as they fill with urine that cannot pass the obstruction.

Fluid and electrolyte imbalance

If the kidneys are unable to control fluid volume, e.g. by concentrating the urine, the loss of a large amount of dilute urine may result in fluid imbalance.

Failure of the kidneys to excrete water affects total body function, e.g. an increase in the total circulating fluid volume impedes cardiovascular function.

Failure of the kidneys to help control the balance of electrolytes in body fluids, or to maintain normal osmolarity, poses a major threat to homeostasis. Failure to excrete potassium will disrupt the conduction system of the heart, or failure to conserve potassium may result in altered cardiac muscle contraction.

Renal disease may also result in abnormal retention or loss of sodium, calcium or phosphorous.

Elimination of wastes

Normal metabolism produces an excess of acids and, to compensate, the kidneys excrete acids and return bicarbonate to the plasma and extra cellular fluid. An acid–base imbalance (metabolic acidosis) will result if this function is impaired, i.e. if there is an increased amount of acid or a decreased amount of base in the body.

The kidneys must also continually filter and excrete nitrogenous wastes derived from protein metabolism. Renal failure can result in an accumulation of urea, uric acid, and creatinine in the blood—causing uraemia. The accumulation of uremic toxins has adverse effects on several body systems, producing, e.g. impaired neurological function.

505

Urine output

Alterations in urine output may be temporary or long term. Urine output may be decreased, e.g. in obstruction of the ureter, acute or chronic renal failure; or urine output may be increased, e.g. during the diuretic stage of acute renal failure. The passage of urine along the urinary tract may be impeded by an obstruction, e.g. a tumour or calculus.

Major manifestations of urinary system disorders

Disorders of the urinary system may produce a range of signs and symptoms which vary according to the site and severity of the disorder.

Pain

Pain is more common in acute, rather than chronic, disorders of the kidneys and urinary tract. Pain which originates from the kidneys is generally experienced as a dull ache in the lower back region which may radiate to the lower abdominal area. Pain associated with renal or ureteric colic is sudden and severe. It is felt in the lower back and may radiate to the groin area. Nausea and vomiting frequently accompany this type of pain.

Suprapubic pain may result from spasms or overdistension of the bladder, e.g. in acute retention of urine. An infection of the lower urinary tract, e.g. cystitis, commonly causes pain and burning associated with micturition. *Strangury* is the term used to describe a burning pain that can occur during or after micturition.

Changes in voiding pattern or urine output

The individual may experience increased frequency of voiding, problems controlling the passage of urine, difficulty in initiating micturition, or a sense of urgency associated with the need to void. Changes in the output of urine include voiding increased or decreased amounts, and a cessation of the secretion of urine. Information on altered patterns of micturition is provided in Chapter 30.

Changes in the urine

Abnormalities of the urine associated with urinary system disorders include changes in the normal colour, clarity, or odour of urine. The urine may be bloodstained, or it may be dark amber, cloudy, or smoky in appearance. Chronic renal disease can result in pale, almost colourless urine. A foul smelling 'fishy' odour is commonly present when there is a urinary tract infection. Information on abnormalities of urine is also provided in Chapter 30.

Other manifestations

The individual with a lower urinary tract infection commonly experiences pyrexia, malaise, nausea and vomiting, pelvic and abdominal discomfort. The individual with renal disease may experience hypertension, oedema, anorexia, nausea and vomiting, skin changes, and neurological symptoms such as headache or altered consciousness.

Specific disorders of the urinary system

Disorders of the urinary system may be classified as congenital, infectious, immunologic, degenerative, neoplastic or obstructive, traumatic, or those resulting from multiple causes.

Congenital disorders

Certain disorders may be present at birth, although the manifestations may not become evident for some time.

Vesico-ureteric reflux is a mechanical problem which may be congenital or acquired. The condition often leads to reflux nephropathy.

Vesico-ureteric reflux is an abnormal backflow of urine from the bladder to the ureter/s, which increases the hydrostatic pressure in the ureters and kidneys. Reflux into the kidney causes damage to the renal parenchyma and reflux nephropathy. In the congenital form the child is born with a short ureter, which often grows to normal size as the child develops and matures—and thus the condition resolves. Acquired vesicoureteric reflux may be caused by repeated urinary tract infections; by inadequate functioning of the detrusor muscles in the bladder, e.g. stemming from a neurogenic bladder; or from a high intra-bladder pressure due to an obstruction of the bladder outlet.

Symptoms of the disorder generally appear only in the presence of a urinary tract infection. There may be no symptoms with chronic infection, and the condition may not be diagnosed until signs of renal damage become evident.

Polycystic kidney disease is an inherited disorder which is characterized by grape-like clusters of fluid-filled cysts that enlarge the kidneys. There are two forms of this disorder; one affecting children, and the other affecting adults.

In its infantile form, the disorder manifests as bilateral masses in the kidney areas, with symptoms of respiratory distress and cardiac failure. Adult polycystic disease is frequently asymptomatic until the individual is approximately 40 years of age. Initial symptoms include hypertension, haematuria, and low back pain. Urinary tract infection is common, and progression to renal failure is gradual.

Disorders of multiple cause

Various urinary system disorders have more than one cause.

Acute renal failure is the sudden disruption of kidney function due to obstruction, reduced blood circulation, or renal damage. The condition is characterized by oliguria, electrolyte imbalance, and metabolic acidosis.

Acute renal failure generally consists of 4 phases; onset, oliguric, diuretic, and recovery. During the oliguric phase, urine output may be as little as 50–150 ml in 24 hours. At the same time, the serum creatinine and blood urea nitrogen levels rise steadily. The diuretic phase is characterized by a urine output greater than 400 ml in 24 hours. Some individuals may void large amounts of urine, e.g. over 3 litres in 24 hours. During this phase, the risk of electrolyte imbalance remains high. Recovery of renal function may proceed over a few days or may take as long as 12 months. During this phase, the serum electrolyte levels return to normal.

Chronic renal failure is the gradual loss of functional nephrons due to several causes including chronic kidney infections, polycystic kidneys, renal vascular disease, hypertensive disease, obstructive diseases such as calculi, nephrotoxic agents, and diabetic neuropathy. The condition produces major changes in all body systems.

Chronic renal failure consists of 4 phases; diminished renal reserve, renal insufficiency, renal failure, and end stage renal disease.

During the first phase renal damage occurs, but the individual may have no symptoms. With renal insufficiency the kidneys still function adequately, but urine concentration is impaired and blood urea levels are elevated. Renal failure produces uraemia, metabolic acidosis, electrolyte imbalance, and impaired urine dilution. Renal function is severely impaired in the final phase and, as a result, most other body systems are affected.

When renal function is impaired to such an extent that conservative treatment is no longer effective, dialysis therapy and/or kidney transplantation may be necessary.

A neurogenic bladder results from a variety of causes including cerebral or spinal cord disorders, and disorders of peripheral innervation. Neurogenic bladder refers to bladder dysfunction caused by impaired bladder innervation, and the condition produces a variety of effects. The individual experiences loss of perception of bladder fullness, and loss of the desire to void. As a consequence, the bladder becomes distended and overflow incontinence occurs. Because of incomplete emptying of the bladder, the individual is susceptible to urinary tract infection.

Urinary incontinence, which may result from many causes, is characterized by the inability to control the flow of urine. Information on urinary incontinence is provided in Chapter 30.

Infectious disorders

Infection may occur in any part of the urinary tract, as urine provides an ideal medium for the growth of micro-organisms. Most commonly, micro-organisms gain access to the urinary tract by ascending the urethra; although micro-organisms may also descend from the kidneys to the lower urinary tract. Hospital-acquired urinary tract infections are commonly related to the use of catheters. Repeated insertion, or prolonged use, of catheters increases the risk of infection.

Pyelonephritis, is inflammation of the renal pelvis, and may be an acute or chronic condition. Acute pyelonephritis results from bacterial invasion of the kidneys, commonly as a consequence of a lower urinary tract infection. Chronic pyelonephritis can result in the formation of renal scar tissue, which may lead to chronic renal failure. This condition most commonly occurs in individuals who experience recurrent acute pyelonephritis as a result of a urinary tract obstruction or vesico-ureteric reflux.

The individual with acute pyelonephritis experiences severe pain or a continual dull ache in the kidney region, pyrexia, nausea and vomiting, and fatigue. He may also experience rigors. Urination may be more frequent and painful, and the urine is generally cloudy, blood stained and offensive in odour.

Cystitis, which is inflammation of the urinary bladder, is usually the result of bacterial contamination. Causative organisms include *Escherichia coli*, *Proteus*, and *Pseudomonas pyocyaneus*. Because the female urethra is short and in close proximity to the rectum and vagina, cystitis is more common in females than in males. Cystitis generally results from infection in the urethra, or from sexually transmitted diseases.

The individual with cystitis experiences a burning pain during micturition, which may be accompanied by frequency, urgency, and bladder spasms. Incontinence of urine may occur. The urine is generally cloudy and offensive, and may contain blood cells. Other features of the disorder include pyrexia, pain or discomfort in the bladder area, and fatigue.

Urethritis, which is inflammation of the urethra, may result from bacterial infection or traumatic irritation. Causative organisms include *Chlamydia trachomatis* and *Neisseria gonorrhoeae*. Manifestations of urethritis include dysuria, and the presence of pus in the urine.

Immunologic disorders

This category of renal disorders is comprised of various conditions in which the kidneys are damaged, and partly destroyed, by inflammation of the glomeruli. It is generally believed that the disorders are autoimmune in origin, and that glomerular damage is the result of antigen–antibody complexes which circulate in the blood and are deposited in the glomeruli.

Acute glomerulonephritis, also called post-infectious glomerulonephritis, results from an infection that has recently occurred elsewhere in the body, e.g. the respiratory tract. The common causative organism is the *Haemolytic* *streptococcus*. The individual generally experiences signs and symptoms of glomerulonephritis within 1–3 weeks after an infection. The most common manifestations are peripheral and periorbital oedema, decreased urine output, and hypertension. The urine contains red blood cells and protein, and is smoky or dark in appearance.

Chronic glomerulonephritis is a condition where there is progressive kidney damage, with a corresponding impairment of kidney function and retention of metabolic waste products. It is characterized by hypertension, oedema, high blood urea levels; and by the presence of protein and red and white blood cells in the urine. The manifestations of chronic renal failure, e.g. nausea and vomiting, pruritus, fatigue, muscle cramps, may be early symptoms. As the disease progresses, the individual experiences severe headaches, dyspnoea, oedema, cardiac arrhythmias, and disturbances of vision. Death from uraemia may occur if the condition is not treated by means of dialysis or kidney transplantation.

Nephrotic syndrome can occur in any condition that results in glomerular damage, e.g. glomerulonephritis. The glomerular capillary membrane is damaged, thus allowing loss of fluid into the interstitial spaces. The condition is characterized by marked proteinuria, hyperlipidaemia, and oedema primarily in dependent areas of the body. Periorbital oedema may be evident, particularly in the morning. Accompanying manifestations include lethargy, anorexia, depression, pallor, and orthostatic hypotension.

Degenerative disorders

This group includes disorders includes those in which there are degenerative changes in the renal structure, e.g. in the glomeruli or tubules, or changes in the blood vessels that supply the kidney. Degeneration occurs over a long period, and the individual may not experience any symptoms until the degeneration is quite marked.

Nephrosclerosis which is necrosis of the renal arterioles, results from untreated or uncontrolled hypertension which impairs the blood supply of the kidney. Renal damage occurs as a combination of fibrosis of the blood vessels walls, and the resulting ischaemia.

Manifestation of the condition are high blood pressure, headaches, visual disturbances, and altered neurological functioning. The urine contains protein and blood. If untreated, this condition can lead to kidney and heart failure.

Analgesic nephropathy results from chronic ingestion of substances containing phenacetin. Aspirin-Acetaminophen combinations have also been found to cause similar renal tubule damage. Manifestations of the condition include low back pain, haematuria, and the symptoms of uraemia (nausea, vomiting, pruritus, muscle cramps). If end stage renal failure develops, dialysis or kidney transplantation may be indicated.

Neoplastic and obstructive disorders

Tumors which arise in the urinary system may be benign or malignant. Obstruction of the urinary tract may be caused by factors other than the presence of tumours, e.g. calculi.

Kidney tumours are generally malignant, and usually well advanced before any signs or symptoms appear. Haematuria is the most common manifestation of a renal cell carcinoma. Other features include pain as the tumour enlarges and presses on adjacent structures, nausea and vomiting, loss of weight, and metastatic symptoms such as bone pain.

Wilm's tumour is a malignant tumour of the kidneys which occurs primarily in children. With suitable treatment, the prognosis is favourable.

Bladder tumours are generally malignant, and more common than kidney tumours. The majority occur in males over the age of 50. Evidence shows that prolonged exposure to certain substances, e.g. aniline dyes, is associated with the incidence of bladder cancer. A variety of other carcinogenic substances, e.g. artificial sweeteners, are thought to be linked to bladder cancer. The prime manifestation of a bladder tumour is intermittent haematuria.

Prostatomegaly, which is enlargement of the prostate gland surrounding the male urethra, may compress the urethra and cause urinary obstruction. The cause of prostate gland hypertrophy is not fully understood, but it is thought to be related to a hormonal mechanism.

Prostatic cancer is a relatively common form of cancer and, like benign prostatic hypertrophy, it is thought to be linked to hormonal changes.

Enlargement of the prostate gland is more common in males over the age of 50 years.

The manifestations of prostatomegaly include difficulty in initiating micturition, a feeling that the bladder is not empty after voiding, and dribbling of urine following micturition. As obstruction increases urination becomes more frequent, with nocturia, urgency, and incontinence. Haematuria may be present due to rupture of dilated blood vessels at the neck of the bladder. Acute retention of urine may occur if the flow from the bladder is severely obstructed.

Hydronephrosis, which is a dilation of the renal pelvis, may result from an obstruction in the urinary tract. The build up of pressure behind the area of obstruction eventually results in renal dysfunction. Causes of hydronephrosis include prostatomegaly, urethral stricture, calculi, congenital abnormalities, and neurogenic bladder. Manifestations include dull lower back pain and tenderness, decreased urine flow, dysuria and haematuria. Infection or renal failure can occur if the problem is not corrected.

Calculi are stones which may form in the kidney and urinary tract. The majority of stones form in the kidney

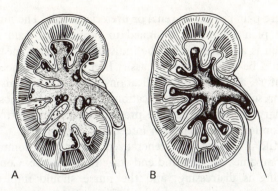

Fig. 47.1 Renal calculi. (A) Multiple small calculi. (B) A staghorn calculus.

and are passed down into the ureters or bladder. Most calculi are composed of calcium salts, or uric acid. Multiple small calculi may remain in the renal pelvis or pass down the ureter, while a staghorn calculus remains in the kidney (Fig. 47.1). Although the precise cause is unknown, predisposing factors in the formation of calculi include dehydration, metabolic factors, infection, prolonged immobility and obstruction which produces urinary stasis.

The major manifestation of calculi is pain, felt as a dull ache while the stone remains in the kidney. If a stone passes into the ureter, the individual may experience excruciating pain which is frequently accompanied by nausea and vomiting. Severe intermittent pain results as the ureter goes into spasm in an attempt to move the calculus out of the ureter by peristalsis. There may be haematuria, and small stones may be passed in the urine.

Traumatic disorders

Injuries to the kidney or urinary tract can have serious consequences. Because the kidney receives a large amount of blood from the abdominal aorta via the renal arteries, even a small laceration can cause massive haemorrhage.

Injuries to the kidney include contusion, haematoma, and laceration. The renal artery or renal vein may be ruptured. Manifestations include haematuria, back and abdominal pain, and symptoms of hypovolaemic shock if the injury is severe.

Bladder trauma may be associated with pelvic fractures, or it may occur from a blunt or penetrating injury. Manifestations of bladder injury include haematuria, dysuria, diminished output of urine, suprapubic pain and tenderness. Scrotal or perineal swelling occurs when urine escapes from the damaged bladder into those tissues.

Diagnostic tests

Certain tests may be performed to assist, or confirm, the diagnosis of urinary system disorders.

Urine tests

Urine may be obtained and tested for the presence of abnormal substances, to provide information about renal and urinary functions. Information on methods of collection and testing urine is provided in Chapter 30.

Blood tests

Blood may be obtained and tested in the laboratory to assess renal function. The tests most often performed are:

- serum creatinine measurements, which reflect the ability of the kidneys to excrete creatinine—the waste produce of energy metabolism.
- blood urea nitrogen levels, which reflect the ability of the kidneys to excrete urea nitrogen.
- uric acid levels, which may indicate renal dysfunction if elevated.
- measurement of haemoglobin and haematocrit levels, white blood cell counts, serum potassium and phosphorous levels.

Radiological investigations

Plain X-ray films may be taken to show the size, shape and position of the kidneys, or to show the presence of calculi in the urinary tract.

An intravenous pyelogram (IVP) involves the intravenous injection of a contrast medium, followed by a series of X-rays. Prior to this procedure the individual is fasted, and his bowel is cleansed, e.g. via the administration of an oral laxative, suppositories or enema.

Well-functioning kidneys excrete the contrast medium rapidly, whereas impaired kidney function delays excretion. The IVP also provides information about the size of the kidneys and ureters, and the presence of calculi in the urinary tract.

A retrograde pyelogram involves the insertion of catheters into the ureters through an instrument called a cystoscope. Contrast medium is introduced through the ureteric catheters into the pelvis of the kidneys, and x-ray films are taken.

A cysto-urethrogram involves the introduction of contrast medium into the bladder through a urethral catheter. X-ray films are taken before, during, and after micturition to show the outline of the bladder, the urethra and any backflow of urine into the ureters.

Renal angiography involves passing a special catheter into the femoral artery through a small incision in the groin. The catheter is passed into the aorta to the level of the renal arteries, then contrast medium is injected through the catheter to outline the renal arteries on x-ray film.

Computerized tomography (CT) scan of the abdomen may be performed to identify kidney size or structural alterations within the urinary system. It may be done with or without contrast medium.

A renal scan demonstrates blood flow to the kidneys, following the intravenous administration of a small quantity of radioactive isotope. Pictures are taken at various intervals following injection of the isotope.

Endoscopic examination

A cystoscopy allows visual examination of the bladder and *a urethroscopy* allows visual examination of the urethra. Both endoscopic techniques may be performed at the same time (panendoscopy). A cystoscope is inserted into the bladder via the urethra to enable visualization of the bladder wall and contents of the bladder. Via the endoscope ureteric catheters can be inserted, a biopsy obtained, and small tumours or stones may be removed.

Renal biopsy

A biopsy of kidney tissue may be necessary to enable microscopic tissue examination. Prior to insertion of the biopsy needle, the skin in the area is injected with local anaesthetic. A special biopsy needle is inserted through the skin to obtain a sample from the cortex of the kidney.

CARE OF THE INDIVIDUAL WITH A URINARY SYSTEM DISORDER

Although specific nursing actions and medical management vary depending on the disorder, the main aims of care are to:

- prevent and manage alterations in elimination
- promote comfort
- maintain skin integrity
- maintain fluid and nutritional status

Prevention and management of altered elimination of urine

Care includes assisting the patient with micturition, observation and collection of urine, maintenance of urinary continence, and care of the patient who requires internal or external urinary drainage apparatus. Information on these aspects of care is provided in Chapter 30. Information on the care of an individual who has had a urinary diversion operation performed, or who requires dialysis, is provided later in this chapter.

Promotion of comfort

An individual who has a urinary system disorder may experience discomfort or pain from a distended bladder, dysuria associated with a lower urinary tract infection, or severe pain caused by renal or ureteric calculi. The nursing care plan should be designed to provide for pain relief which is appropriate for the individual. Nursing measures should be implemented to assist him to meet his need for comfort, and analgesic medications should be administered as prescribed. Other medications such as antibiotics and urinary antiseptics may be prescribed to help control the discomfort associated with infections, e.g. cystitis.

Mild or severe generalized pruritus commonly accompanies uraemia and end stage renal disease. Constant itching is distressing, and the nurse should implement measures to relieve pruritus. Information on the relief of pruritus is provided in Chapter 41.

Maintenance of skin integrity

A number of factors contribute to the loss of skin integrity in the individual with a urinary system disorder, e.g. pruritus accompanied by scratching, loss of urinary continence, and oedema or dehydration. In addition, the individual with end-stage renal disease may have reduced mobility, altered sensation and decreased mental alertness. These factors make the individual susceptible to the development of decubitus ulcers.

The measures that should be implemented to maintain skin integrity are described in Chapters 38 and 39, and include relief of pressure, the provision of a well balanced diet and adequate fluid intake, (providing the specific renal disorder does not contra-indicate such a measure), and keeping the skin clean and free from moisture.

Information on preventing skin damage in the presence of oedema is provided in Chapter 31.

Maintenance of nutritional and fluid status

The individual with impaired renal function is at risk of altered nutritional and fluid status. He may experience anorexia, nausea and vomiting; all of which can impair nutritional status. If there are no dietary restrictions, the individual should be encouraged to eat a well balanced diet. Dietary modifications and restrictions may be indicated for the individual with impaired renal function. Commonly, salt, potassium and protein are restricted; and the individual should understand the reasons for any modification of his diet.

Excessive fluid loss may occur through the use of diuretics, in infectious processes, or through escape of fluid into the interstitial spaces (as in the nephrotic syndrome). Fluid retention occurs in some disorders, e.g. renal failure. Maintenance of fluid balance may involve either an increased or decreased fluid input. The individual is assessed for signs of fluid retention or deficit, by recording his input and output, daily weighing, and by observing for the manifestations of dehydration or fluid retention. Information on the manifestations of fluid imbalance is provided in Chapter 31.

Other nursing activities

The nurse may be required to assist in the preparation of an individual prior to specific diagnostic procedures, and to monitor his condition afterwards. Following any procedure involving the use of contrast medium the individual is observed for any adverse reactions such as numbness, tingling, or palpitations. Following a renal biopsy the individual must be monitored closely for any signs of haemorrhage, e.g. haematuria, rapid weak pulse, pallor, or low blood pressure.

Catheterization may be necessary, e.g. to obtain a specimen of urine or to treat acute urinary retention. Information on catheterization, and care of the patient who has a urinary catheter, is provided in Chapter 30.

Urinary diversion

An individual whose bladder has been removed, e.g. due to malignancy, will require urinary diversion. Various surgical techniques are available which divert the flow of urine (Fig. 47.2).

A ureterosigmoidostomy involves the implantation of the ureters into the sigmoid colon. As a result of this operation, urine is passed via the rectum.

A cutaneous ureterostomy involves bringing the ureters through the abdominal skin. The urine then drains out through the stoma/s, into an ostomy appliance.

An ileal conduit involves resection of part of the ileum. Both ureters are implanted into the proximal end of the ileal segment, and the distal end of the ileum is brought through the abdominal wall to form a stoma. The urine then drains out through the stoma into an ostomy appliance. This particular surgical technique is generally considered to be the most satisfactory if urinary diversion is required.

Care of the individual with a urinary stoma is similar to the care required by an individual who has a stoma created for the passage of faeces. Information on general stoma management is provided in Chapter 46. The main aspects of care are the selection and management of ostomy appliances, care of the stoma and surrounding skin, and provision of psychological support.

Dialysis

When renal function is impaired to such an extent that conservative treatment is no longer effective, the individual may be commenced on dialysis therapy. Dialysis combines the principles of diffusion, osmosis, and filtration. It involves the transfer of solutes across a semipermeable membrane, and the removal of waste products, excess salts

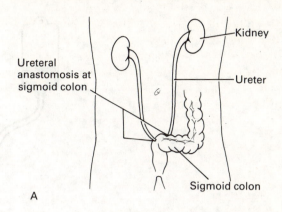

A

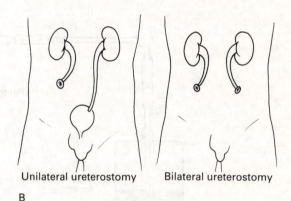

Unilateral ureterostomy   Bilateral ureterostomy

B

C

Fig. 47.2 Urinary diversion. (A) Ureterosigmoidostomy. (B) Cutaneous ureterostomy. (C) Ileal conduit.

and fluid from the blood. There are two types of dialysis:

1. Peritoneal dialysis, in which the individual's peritoneum provides the semipermeable membrane.

2. Haemodialysis, in which the semipermeable membrane is contained within a machine (artificial kidney).

The method of dialysis is determined by the individual's condition, and either method can be performed by the individual in his own home if the facilities are available. Home dialysis is the aim in order to provide the individual with greater autonomy.

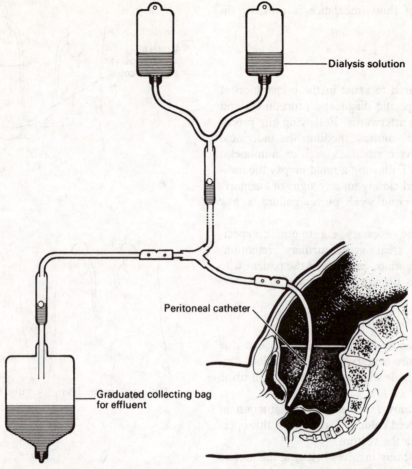

Dialysis solution

Peritoneal catheter

Graduated collecting bag
for effluent

Fig. 47.3 Peritoneal dialysis. (Reproduced with permission from Chilman A M, Thomas M (eds) 1987 Understanding nursing care. 3rd edn. Churchill Livingstone, Edinburgh.)

Peritoneal dialysis (Fig. 47.3) may be performed on an intermittent or continuous basis. A catheter is placed in the abdominal cavity, and dialysate is instilled through the catheter. *Dialysate* is an isotonic, or hypertonic, solution composed of water, electrolytes, and dextrose. Through diffusion and osmosis, waste products together with excess electrolytes and fluid are transported from the blood into the dialysate. The dialysate is drained out by gravity before fresh dialysate is instilled.

In intermittent dialysis each treatment takes approximately 9–12 hours, and is performed 3–4 times a week.

Continuous ambulatory peritoneal dialysis (CAPD) (Fig. 47.4) enables the individual to have greater mobility and independence. In this form of treatment the dialysate is run into the peritoneal cavity, through a catheter, and remains there for approximately 4 hours. The empty dialysis bag remains attached to the tubing and it can be rolled up under the individual's clothing. At the end of 4 hours the bag is unrolled, and the fluid is allowed to drain into it by gravity. After drainage, a fresh bag is connected and the procedure is repeated 3–5 times every day.

Haemodialysis is performed on an average of 3 times per week for a period of 4–6 hours. This method requires regular and convenient access to the individual's blood circulation. A variety of systems are available which provide this access including an arterio-venous shunt or the creation of an arterio-venous fistula (Fig. 47.5).

During haemodialysis, the individual's blood is passed through the artificial kidney (haemodialysis machine) and then returned to his circulation. The haemodialysis machine delivers the prescribed dialysate to the artificial kidney, which allows the removal of waste products and excess water and helps to maintain or establish correct electrolyte levels and acid-base balance.

The individual's blood is anti-coagulated during haemodialysis to prevent clotting in the tubing and machine. Heparin is used for this purpose, and it can be administered as a continuous infusion or intermittently.

Although dialysis is a life-saving treatment, it is nonetheless accompanied by risk. Table 47.1 lists the possible complications associated with either peritoneal dialysis or haemodialysis.

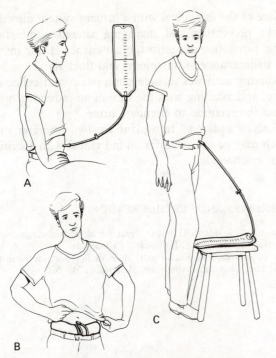

Fig. 47.4 Continuous ambulatory peritoneal dialysis (CAPD). (A) A bag of dialysate is attached to a tube in the individual's abdomen so the fluid flows into the peritoneal cavity. (B) While the dialysate remains in the peritoneal cavity, the individual can roll up the bag, place it under his clothes, and go about his normal activities. (C) The bag is unrolled and suspended below the pelvis, which allows the dialysate to drain from the peritoneal cavity.

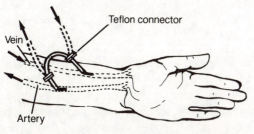

Fig. 47.5 (A) Arterio-venous shunt. (Reproduced with permission from Game C, Anderson R E, Kidd J R (eds) 1989 Medical-surgical nursing: a core text. Churchill Livingstone, Melbourne.)

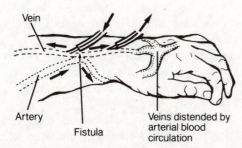

Fig. 47.5 (B) Arterio-venous fistula. (Reproduced with permission from Game, Anderson R E, Kidd J R (eds) 1989 Medical-surgical nursing: a core text. Churchill Livingstone, Melbourne.)

Table 47.1 Complications of dialysis

Peritoneal dialysis	Haemodialysis
Peritonitis	Haemorrhage, from heparinization or from accidental disconnection of the apparatus
Obstructed catheter, by a fibrin clot	
Excessive protein loss	Infection, at the insertion site or from contaminated equipment
Hyperglycaemia, if the dialysate contains high level of dextrose	
Candida or herpes zoster infections	Thrombosis at insertion site
Abdominal hernia or uterine prolapse, due to persistently raised intra-abdominal pressure	Oedema of the hand or ischaemia of the fingers, as a result of the shunt or fistula.
Perforation of abdominal structures by the catheter	Air Embolism
	Hypotension, e.g. from fluid and sodium removal
	Hypertension, e.g. from fluid overload
	Hypothermia or hyperthermia, as a result of a malfunctioning thermostat on the machine
Psychological reactions to the therapy, e.g. anger or depression	Psychological reactions to the therapy, e.g. anger or depression

Renal transplantation

As an alternative to long-term dialysis, the individual with chronic renal failure may be assessed to determine his suitability for a renal transplant. Unfortunately the waiting list for potential recipients far exceeds the availability of donor kidneys. Transplant centres establish their own criteria and guidelines regarding recipient suitability, and the procedures involved in obtaining donor kidneys.

Renal transplant is a surgical procedure in which a donor kidney, from either a living close relative or a cadaver, is transplanted into the recipient. The recipient's own kidneys may be either left or removed. The new kidney is placed in the left or right iliac fossa, outside the peritoneal cavity, and the renal vessels of the donor kidney are anastomosed to the recipient's iliac artery and vein. The donor ureter is either anastomosed to the recipient's ureter or into his bladder. The transplanted kidney may begin to produce urine within a very short time following the operation.

Close monitoring of the individual following surgery is essential to assess renal function, and to detect early signs of rejection of the new kidney. Immunosuppressive drugs are administered to prevent graft rejection, which may occur within 1–30 days or as long as several years after the transplant. To protect the individual against infection, protective isolation techniques may be implemented. Information on protective isolation is provided in Chapter 61.

A successful kidney transplant enables the individual to lead a life free from the restrictions associated with dialysis therapy. He will, however, be required to continue with immunosuppressive therapy, and to attend follow-up consultations for the evaluation of renal function and his general health status.

SUMMARY

The functions of the urinary system are the regulation of elimination of water and electrolytes, and the elimination of metabolic wastes and toxins.

Normal function may be impaired as a result of changes in kidney structure, changes in the ability of the kidneys to secrete and excrete urine, or alterations in the passage of urine through the urinary tract.

The major manifestations of urinary system disorders are pain, changes in voiding pattern or urine output, and changes in the urine.

Disorders of the urinary system can be classified as those that are congenital, resulting from multiple causes, infectious, immunologic in origin, degenerative, neoplastic or obstructive, or traumatic in origin.

Diagnostic tests used to assess urinary system function include laboratory analysis of urine, blood and tissue; radiological examination, and endoscopy.

Care of the individual with a urinary system disorder includes preventing and managing altered elimination of urine, promotion of comfort, maintenance of skin integrity, and maintenance of nutritional and fluid status.

Nursing activities include observation and collection of urine, and assisting with the care of an individual who requires intervention to eliminate urine.

Dialysis and renal transplant are two forms of therapy which may be indicated for an individual with specific end stage dysfunction.

REFERENCES AND FURTHER READING

Brunner L S, Suddarth D S 1988 Textbook of medical-surgical nursing, 6th edn. J. B. Lippincott, Philadephia
Game C, Anderson R, Kidd J (eds) 1989 Medical-surgical nursing: a core text. Churchill Livingstone, Melbourne, 548–626

48. The individual with an endocrine disorder

INTRODUCTION

Information on the normal structure and functions of the endocrine system is provided in Chapter 25, and it should be referred to before studying the contents of this chapter. The endocrine system is comprised of a number of glands, each of which secretes *hormones* directly into the blood-stream. Hormones are chemical substances that initiate or regulate the activity of an organ or a group of cells in another part of the body. Because of the complexity of the endocrine system, and its interrelation with other body systems, dysfunction of any endocrine gland can have widespread effects. Most endocrine disorders result from the over or under production of hormones.

Pathophysiological influences and effects

The pathophysiological changes which occur are generally the result of either hyperfunction or hypofunction of a specific endocrine gland.

Pituitary gland

Hyperfunction of the *anterior* pituitary gland commonly results from a tumour which causes pressure on cerebral structures with resulting neurological manifestations, or which causes excessive secretion of pituitary hormones and, consequently, increased stimulation of the target organs.

Hypofunction of the *anterior* pituitary gland can also result from a tumour in the gland, or it can be secondary to trauma of the hypothalamus. Other causes of hypofunction include infiltrative granulomotous disorders such as sarcoidosis, and infections such as tuberculosis or brucellosis.

Damage to the *posterior* lobe of the pituitary gland can result in a decreased or increased secretion of the anti-diuretic hormone (ADH). Diabetes insipidus is a condition caused by posterior lobe damage, and it results from a deficiency of ADH.

Thyroid gland

The thyroid gland can become enlarged, hyperactive or hypoactive as a result of pathophysiological changes.

An enlarged thyroid gland may be the result of a simple goiter, thyroiditis, or neoplasia. Pressure from an enlarged thyroid gland may produce dysphagia, or respiratory distress.

Hyperfunction of the thyroid gland may be caused by many factors, e.g. thyroiditis or an overproduction of thyroid-stimulating hormone (TSH). An increase in the secretion of thyroid hormones affects the basal metabolic rate, as well as the functions of other body systems. The manifestations of hyperfunction are generally related to increased metabolic processes.

Hypofunction of the thyroid gland may be congenital, e.g. cretinism is related to a deficiency of thyroxine secretion. Hypofunction may also occur later in life if the thyroid gland is removed or damaged. The manifestations of hypofunction are generally related to decreased metabolic processes.

Parathyroid glands

Hyperfunction of the parathyroid glands can result from hereditary factors, tumours, or enlargement of the glands. Secondary hyperfunction can be caused by renal disease, osteomalacia or rickets. Hyperfunction leads to an increased secretion of parathormone (PTH).

Hypofunction of the parathyroid glands can result from familial hypoparathyroidism, autoimmune disorders, or iatrogenic causes. Hypofunction leads to a deficiency in PTH secretion. Severe, or untreated, hyposecretion is manifested by hypocalcemia and tetany.

Suprarenal glands

Hyperfunction of the suprarenal glands is usually confined to the cortex of the gland, although a tumour (pheochromocytoma) of the medulla can cause oversecretion of epinephrine and norepinephrine. Manifestations of medulla hyperfunction are increased metabolism, hypertension, and hyperglycaemia.

Hyperfunction of the cortex may be caused by neoplasia or hyperplasia, or it may be iatrogenic. Other factors resulting in hyperfunction of the cortex include tumours or hyperplasia of the pituitary gland. Manifestations of hyperfunction are generally related to an excess of glucocorticoids, mineralocorticoids, and sex hormones. Three major disorders can result:

1. Cushing's syndrome
2. Primary aldosteronism
3. Virilizing changes in females, or feminizing changes in males.

Hypofunction of the cortex may be caused by primary insufficiency (Addison's disease), or secondary insufficiency arising from undersecretion of adenocortico-trophic hormone (ACTH) from the pituitary gland. Manifestations of hyposecretion are related to a decrease of glucocorticoids, mineralocorticoids, and sex hormones.

Islets of Langerhans

The islets of Langerhans in the pancreas secrete hormones, insulin, glucagon and somatostatin, that are involved in the regulation of blood glucose levels. Insulin plays the major role in the regulation of glucose metabolism.

Factors that may be involved in a deficiency of insulin include insufficient production, increased requirements by the body, a decrease in the effectiveness of available insulin and, less commonly, increased destruction of insulin by the liver. When there is a deficiency of insulin the blood glucose level rises. Manifestations of impaired function are related to disordered glucose and protein metabolism, and increased lipolysis. The resulting pathological changes can affect small and large blood vessels, leading to atherosclerosis, retinal damage, and nephropathy.

Gonads

As the ovaries and testes are involved in both the production of hormones and in the process of reproduction, the pathophysiological changes and effects associated with them are described in Chapter 49.

Thymus gland

While dysfunction of the thymus gland is uncommon, a benign tumour of the gland is thought to be associated with myasthenia gravis. Congenital thymic hypoplasia causes deficient cellular immunity, making the infant more susceptible to infections.

Pineal gland

A rare neoplasm of the pineal gland (pinealoma) may either obstruct the flow of cerebrospinal fluid causing hydrocephalus, or it may extend into the hypothalamus—causing precocius puberty.

Major manifestations of endocrine disorders

Because each endocrine gland, by the action of its hormones, affects and is affected by many other organs, the manifestations of any dysfunction are widespread and varied. As endocrine dysfunction generally results in either an under or an over secretion of hormones from the impaired endocrine gland, the manifestations of a disorder are related to the actions and effects of those hormones. In this chapter, the manifestations of endocrine gland dysfunction are described under each specific disorder.

Specific disorders of the endocrine system

Endocrine gland disorders have a variety of causes including genetic defects, neoplasia, obstruction, trauma, autoimmune reactions, infection, inflammation, and hyperplasia. Many disorders result from multiple causes and some may be iatrogenic in origin.

Disorders of the pituitary gland

Disorders of the pituitary gland can be summarized as hyperpituitarism, hypopituitarism, and diabetes insipidus.

Hyperpituitarism, or oversecretion of the pituitary hormones, produces changes throughout the body. It is a chronic, progressive disorder marked by hormonal dysfunction and skeletal overgrowth, which can appear in two forms:

1. Gigantism, which occurs in childhood, begins before epiphyseal closure.
2. Acromegaly, which occurs in adulthood, develops after epiphyseal closure.

In gigantism, there is overgrowth of all body tissues causing remarkable height increases.

In acromegaly, oversecretion of growth hormone (GH) causes atrophy of skeletal muscle and formation of new bone and cartilage. The individual develops a characteristic appearance with an enlarged lower jaw, a bulging forehead, and thickened ears and nose. The extremities become elongated and enlarged, the hands and feet increase greatly in size. Thickening of the tongue may cause the voice to sound deep and hollow.

Neoplasms of the anterior lobe of the pituitary gland are commonly the cause of hyperpituitarism, and they give rise to symptoms such as severe headaches and visual defects.

Hypopituitarism is a syndrome marked by metabolic dysfunction and growth retardation. In children, the condition may cause dwarfism and delay of puberty.

1. Fröhlich's syndrome, which is commonly caused by a tumour in the anterior pituitary gland, is characterized by dwarfism, mental retardation, lack of sexual development, and a reduction in all endocrine activity.
2. Dwarfism, which results from hyposecretion of growth hormone, is characterized by retarded growth.
3. Simmond's disease, which is due to atrophy of the anterior lobe of the pituitary gland, is a rare disorder with widespread effects. Anorexia, atrophy of sexual organs, loss of weight, hypotension, and anaemia, are clinical manifestations of the disorder.

Diabetes insipidus, which may be idiopathic in origin or develop due to a deficiency in antidiuritic hormone (ADH) or as a result of intracranial trauma, is characterized by polyuria and excessive thirst. It is a rare chronic disease in which, because of undersecretion of ADH, the kidney tubules fail to reabsorb water. This results in the passing of large volumes of dilute urine—up to as much as 30 litres in 24 hours. The individual is continuously thirsty, and drinks large amounts to compensate for the loss of fluid.

Disorders of the thyroid gland

Disorders of the thyroid gland can be summorized as hyperthyroidism, hypothyroidism, and goitre.

Hyperthyroidism is a metabolic imbalance that results from an overproduction of the thyroid hormones. It can be caused by genetic or immunologic factors, thyroid gland nodules, or chronic inflammation of the thyroid gland. There are several categories of hyperthyroidism with Graves' disease, which is an autoimmune disorder, being the most common.

The manifestations of hyperthyroidism include weight loss, raised body temperature, increased pulse and ventilation rates, hyperactivity, anxiety and irritability, moist skin, disordered menstruation, exopthalmus, and an enlarged thyroid gland. Hyperthyroidism may also be referred to as *thyrotoxicosis*.

An individual with advanced hyperthyroid disease may develop a condition known as *thyroid crisis*. Thyroid crisis may be stimulated by emotional stress, infection, trauma, or cardiovascular disease—all of which result in a sudden release of thyroid hormone into the bloodstream. In thyroid crisis, all the symptoms of hyperthyroidism are increased and heart failure is a major potential problem.

Hypothyroidism is characterized by a decreased secretion of thyroid hormones. Hypothyroidism may be congenital, or it may develop later in life.

1. *Cretinism*, the congenital form, results from absence or underdevelopment of the thyroid gland or it may occur from severe maternal iodine deficiency during pregnancy. The manifestations of cretinism are related to a marked depression of metabolic processes, and progressive mental impairment. Typically, the infant is overweight and lethargic; and has thick dry skin, coarse features, a broad flat nose, and a large protruding tongue. He exhibits hypotonic abdominal muscles, a protruding abdomen, and slow movements. Mental retardation will result if treatment is not commenced early.
2. *Myxoedema*, which is acquired hypothyroidism, develops when the thyroid gland ceases to function effectively. This may be caused by atrophy of the gland, surgical removal of the gland, irradiation therapy, autoimmune thyroiditis, or inflammatory conditions such as sarcoidosis.

The manifestations of myxoedema are widespread and include weight gain, lowered body temperature, decreased pulse and ventilation rates, slow clumsy movements, tiredness, impaired memory, dry skin, oedema of the eyelids, disordered menstruation and decreased libido. The thyroid gland may be enlarged.

When hypothyroidism is aggravated by stress, e.g. low environmental temperature, myxoedematous coma may develop—which may precipitate shock, and result in death.

Goitre is the term that refers to any thyroid enlargement, and it may be asociated with either over or under secretion of thyroid hormones. A goitre can cause local problems by exerting pressure on the trachea and, less commonly, on the oesophagus.

1. Simple goitre (nontoxic goitre) is due to an iodine deficiency which causes a compensatory enlargement of the thyroid gland in an attempt to maintain thyroid hormone production.
2. Endemic goitre occurs in regions away from the coast where there is little iodine in the soil and water. The introduction of iodised salt has reduced the incidence in most Western countries.
3. Exophthalmic goitre occurs in hyperthyroidism.

Disorders of the parathyroid glands

Disorders of the parathyroid glands can be summarized as hyperparathyroidism and hypoparathroidism.

Hyperparathyroidism may be caused by hyperplasia or neoplasm, or it can occur secondary to conditions which cause hypocalcaemia, e.g. Vitamin D deficiency or chronic renal failure. It is characterized by overactivity of one or more of the parathyroid glands, resulting in excessive secretion of parathyroid hormone (PTH). Oversecretion of PTH promotes bone decalcification and hypercalcaemia. As a result, increased renal and gastrointestinal absorption of calcium occurs.

The manifestations are widespread and include symptoms of bone decalcification such as backache, bone curvature and pathological fractures. Renal stones may develop due to high calcium output in the urine. Peptic ulceration may occur, and neuromuscular co-ordination is often impaired.

Hypoparathyroidism is characterized by underactivity of one or more of the parathyroid glands, resulting in decreased secretion of PTH. Undersecretion of PTH causes hypocalcaemia, producing neuromuscular symptoms ranging from parasthesia to tetany. Hypoparathyroidism may be caused by surgical damage to the parathyroid glands, or by autoimmune reactions.

The manifestations include anxiety, increased deep tendon reflexes and laryngeal spasm. *Tetany* is a condition in which there is hyperexcitability of nerves and muscles—due to low calcium blood levels. Tetany begins with tingling in the fingertips, the toes, and around the mouth. The tingling becomes more severe producing muscle tension and spasms, and consequent adduction of the thumbs, wrists, elbows, and toes (carpopedal spasm).

Disorders of the suprarenal glands

Various disorders may occur in the medulla *or* the cortex of the suprarenal gland. The *medulla* of a suprarenal gland can be affected by neoplastic disorders, two of which are neuroblastoma and phaeochromocytoma.

Neuroblastoma occurs primarily in children, is malignant and may metastasize to the lymph nodes, liver, lung, and bone. Manifestations depend on the size of the tumour and the site of metastasis.

Phaeochromocytoma is generally a benign tumour of the medulla, or of the sympathetic chain, which causes oversecretion of norepinephrine and epinephrine. The resultant increase in sympathetic activity manifests as episodes of hypertension, tachycardia, chest pain, pallor, sweating, headaches, anxiety, tremor, nausea and vomiting, and frequency of urination.

Disorders of the *cortex* of a suprarenal gland can be summarized as hypersecretion and hyposecretion of either glucocorticoids, or androgen steroids.

Hypersecretion of glucocorticoids produces a condition known as *Cushings syndrome*. It may be caused by various factors including hypersecretion of pituitary adrenocortico-

tropic hormone (ACTH), steroid therapy, or a tumour of the suprarenal gland/s. Manifestations of this disorder are related to hyperglycaemia, abnormal distribution of lipid, and protein wasting. Features, include obesity of the trunk with a pad of fat across the shoulders (buffalo hump), a moon face; pink–purple striae on the breasts, abdomen and legs, muscle weakness, osteoporosis, and skin fragility. Persistent hyperglycaemia may result in diabetes mellitus. Hypertension is a common feature which leads to artherosclerosis, ischaemic heart disease, and nephrosclerosis.

Hypersecretion of mineralocarticoids produces a condition known as *Conn's syndrome*, which results from a suprarenal tumour producing excessive amounts of aldosterone. Manifestations of this disorder are related to impaired reabsorption of sodium and water in the renal tubules, due to potassium depletion. Features include hypertension, muscle weakness, neuromuscular dysfunction, polyuria, polydipsia, and metabolic acidosis.

Hypersecretion of androgens can produce the conditions of adrenal virilism, and adrenogenital syndrome. Excessive secretion of androgens causes pseudohermaphroditism (a condition in which the gonads are of one sex, but one or more contradictions exist in the physical criteria of the sex) in female infants, hirsuitism and masculine body features in older females; and precocious puberty in males.

Hyposecretion of substances from the suprarenal cortex produces a condition known as *Addison's disease*. This rare condition is thought to be due to an autoimmune reaction, or caused by infective agents. Progress of the disease is slow, and symptoms do not develop until the disease is well advanced. The manifestations are related to a deficiency of all three suprarenal cortex hormones. Features of the disease include progressive weakness, weight loss, dehydration, hypotension, tachycardia, hypoglycaemia, and a brown pigmentation of the skin and mucous membranes.

Disorders of the islets of Langerhans

Diabetes mellitus is a disorder of glucose regulation, characterized by abnormal metabolism of carbohydrate, protein, and fat. A feature of the disorder is some degree of hyperglycaemia. Diabetes mellitus results from an insulin deficiency or from the production of substances antagonistic to insulin which cause it to be ineffective.

Diabetes mellitus may be caused by hereditary factors, pancreatic disorders, or by disorders of other endocrine glands, e.g. the pituitary or suprarenal glands. Diabetes mellitus is also though to be autoimmune in origin. Gestational diabetes mellitus is one form of the disorder that appears only during pregnancy, and it is characterized by impaired glucose tolerance. A woman who has had gestational diabetes runs a greater risk of developing diabetes later in life.

The two main classifications of diabetes mellitus are Type I (or insulin dependent diabetes mellitus), and Type II (non-insulin dependent diabetes mellitus).

The diagnosis of diabetes mellitus is confirmed by the presence of an elevated blood glucose level. A fasting blood glucose of 7.8 mmol/l or above, or a post-absorptive blood glucose level of 11.1 mmol/l or above is indicative of the disorder.

A deficiency of insulin causes changes in the metabolism of glucose and, as a result, these changes cause numerous physiological effects. In the liver the glycolitic enzymes are inhibited, the gluconeogenic enzymes are activated, and amino acids are used to form glucose. Consequently, additional glucose is liberated into the bloodstream. Without insulin, glucose is unable to cross the cell membranes into muscle and fat cells, and hyperglycaemia occurs. The blood glucose level eventually exceeds the renal threshold, and glucose is excreted in the urine. The most significant effect of an elevated blood glucose level is dehydration of the tissue cells because the increased osmotic pressure in the extracellular fluids causes osmotic transfer of water out of the cells. In addition, the loss of glucose via the urine causes diuresis, because of the osmotic effect of glucose in the renal tubeles.

The manifestations of diabetes mellitus vary according to whether the disorder is Type I of Type II:

1. Type I diabetes mellitus. The distinguishing features are that it can occur at any age from infancy up to approximately 40 years, there is a sudden onset of signs and symptoms—weight loss, polyuria, polydipsia, fatigue, and the presence of glucose and ketones in the urine. Hyperglycaemia and dehydration accelerate the development of metabolic acidosis and, if untreated, coma and death may result.

2. Type II diabetes mellitus. The distinguishing features are that it is more likely to occur after the age of 40, the individual is likely to be obese, and the signs and symptoms develop gradually. There may be no classic manifestations of diabetes mellitus, although some individuals do experience fatigue, polyuria, and polydipsia. It is not uncommon for Type II diabetes mellitus to be undetected until the individual presents with a condition which is commonly a complication of the disease, e.g. monilial infection, cataracts, degenerative changes in blood vessels, or peripheral neuritis.

The individual with diabetes mellitus is prone to a number of complications, especially if his blood glucose level is not controlled. Complications include:

- hypoglycaemia
- hyperglycaemia
- diabetic ketoacidosis
- retinopathy
- nephropathy
- cardiovascular and peripheral vascular disease
- neuropathy.

Diagnostic tests

Certain tests may be performed to assist, or confirm, the diagnosis of endocrine disorders. Various tests are performed to assess the function of each endocrine gland.

Pituitary function tests

Pituitary function may be assessed by estimating the level of trophic hormones, and by measuring their response to stimulation or suppression tests.

The most common tests for evaluating anterior pituitary function are the serum growth hormone test, and the insulin tolerance test. The insulin tolerance test, also called the growth hormone stimulation test, provides information about the secretion of growth hormone and adrenocorticotrophin (ACTH).

Investigations may also include an X-ray or a CT scan of the skull.

Testing posterior pituitary function includes the 'water deprivation test; which is performed when the individual's symptoms indicate diabetes insipidus. This test is based on the principle that withholding fluid for several hours stimulates secretion of ADH.

If the individual is suspected of having diabetes insipidus, his urine may be tested to determine specific gravity. A low specific gravity is suggestive of diabetes insipidus.

Thyroid function tests

A combination of tests is generally performed to evaluate thyroid function including direct tests of thyroid function, tests that measure concentration and binding of the thyroid hormones, and tests involving the use of scanning or imaging techniques.

Blood tests are performed to measure serum hormone levels, which assist in the diagnosis of hyperthyroidism and hypothyroidism.

Radioactive iodine tests, e.g. the radioactive iodine uptake test, evaluate thyroid function by measuring the amount of orally ingested ^{131}I that accumulates in the thyroid gland after 2, 6, and 24 hours.

Thyroid scanning is the visualization of the thyroid gland after administration of a radioisotope.

Thyroid ultrasonography helps to evaluate thyroid structure, and to differentiate between a cyst and a tumour on the thyroid gland.

Parathyroid function tests

Tests used to assess parathyroid function include estimation of serum calcium and serum phosphorous levels. A 24 hours urine collection may be performed to measure the total urine calcium. Hyperparathyroidism causes increased excretion of calcium in the urine, and hypoparathyroidism causes decreased excretion of calcium.

Suprarenal function tests

Both the cortex and the medulla of the suprarenal glands secrete several hormones, and tests are performed on blood and urine to measure the hormone levels.

Blood is tested to determine the serum aldosterone, serum cortisol, or serum catecholamine levels. The results aid in the diagnosis of suprarenal function, e.g. serum cortisol levels are increased in Cushing's syndrome, while decreased serum cortisol levels are seen in Addison's disease.

A 24 hour urine collection may be performed to estimate the total daily free cortisol, aldosterone, or catecholamine, levels.

CT scan or suprarenal venography may also be used to aid diagnosis of tumours.

Pancreatic endocrine function tests

The islets of Langerhans, in the pancreas, secrete three hormones which are involved in the regulation of blood glucose levels. The laboratory evaluation of endocrine function is largely concerned with the levels of glucose in blood and urine.

Urine is examined for the presence of glucose and ketones. When the serum glucose level exceeds the renal threshold, the excess *glucose* is excreted in the urine. As a result of increased lipolysis, excess *ketone* bodies accumulate and are excreted in the urine.

Blood tests are performed which estimate the body's use of glucose:

1. Glucose tolerance test. This test evaluates glucose absorption after its oral administration. An intravenous method of performing the glucose tolerance test is also available, which may be used if the results of the oral test are not conclusive.

The individual fasts overnight, then 50 g of dextrose is administered. Blood glucose levels are measured 30 minutes after administration of dextrose, then at one hourly intervals for 3 hours. Diabetes mellitus is diagnosed if the 2 hour blood glucose level exceeds 11 mmol/l.
2. Fasting serum glucose (fasting blood sugar). This test measures plasma glucose levels following a 6–8 hour period of fasting. The normal fasting blood glucose level is between 4.0 and 6.0 mmol/l. In diabetes mellitus, the absence or deficiency of insulin allows persistently high plasma glucose levels of 7.8 mmol/l or above.
3. Two-hour postprandial (after eating) serum glucose.

This test also provides information about the body's utilization and disposal of glucose. A blood glucose level of 11.1 mmol/l or above suggests diabetes mellitus.
4. Tolbutamide tolerance test. An intravenous injection of the drug tolbutamide usually stimulates the secretion of insulin. Normally, after administration of the drug, the serum glucose level will fall rapidly and return to baseline levels in $1\frac{1}{2}$–3 hours. In diabetes mellitus, the initial drop in serum glucose level is slow and there is a prolonged return to pretest levels.
5. Glycosylated haemoglobin test. This test requires only one blood test every 6–8 weeks, and its main purpose is to assess control of diabetes mellitus. Glycosylated haemoglobin is normally present but, in diabetes mellitus, it may be elevated to three times the normal level. Levels of glycosylated haemoglobin reflect the glucose level within erythrocytes rather than the serum glucose level.

CARE OF THE INDIVIDUAL WITH AN ENDOCRINE DISORDER

Because endocrine dysfunction has such widespread effects, the medical management and nursing care depends on the diagnosis of a specific disorder.

When care is being planned, the nurse must consider the effects that the disorder may have on the individual. He may experience:

• A major change in lifestyle, e.g. as a result of diabetes mellitus the individual may have to depend on life-long medication and dietary modifications.
• The prospect of facing major surgery, e.g. removal of the thyroid gland may be indicated in the presence of hyperthyroidism, goitre, or carcinoma of the gland.
• Alterations in nutritional status, e.g. weight gain often occurs in hypothyroidism, whereas weight loss is common in individuals with Type 1 diabetes mellitus. Nutritional status may also be affected if the individual is experiencing anorexia, nausea or vomiting.
• Alterations in fluid balance, e.g. excessive loss of fluid may occur in diabetes mellitus or posterior pituitary gland disorders. Loss of fluid may also occur if the individual has diarrhoea—as may be present in disorders such as hyperthyroidism and Addison's disease. Conversely, retention of fluid may occur in disorders such as Cushing's syndrome.
• Discomfort, e.g. many endocrine disorders result in problems related to body temperature regulation. An individual with hypothyroidism is very sensitive to cold, whereas an individual with hyperthyroidism commonly experiences intolerance to heat. Other factors that may cause discomfort include pruritus associated with hyperthyroidism or diabetes mellitus, and joint pain associated with acromegaly. Anxiety and nervousness associated with certain disorders, e.g. hyperthyroidism, may also cause dis-

comfort as the individual is restless and finds it difficult to relax.

● Reduced independence, e.g. extreme fatigue often accompanies endocrine disorders, and the individual may require assistance to carry out the activities of daily living. Certain disorders, e.g. Cushing's syndrome or hyperparathyroidism, may be accompanied by central nervous system involvement. Altered states of awareness or consciousness will reduce the individual's level of independence.

● Altered body image, e.g. as a result of hirsuitism associatd with suprarenal gland dysfunction, or as a result of increased skin pigmentation with Addison's disease.

The care plan designed for the individual should consider all his needs and specifically address his need for comfort, psychological support, and maintenance of nutritional and fluid status. Many individuals will benefit if they are given information about, and encouraged to contact, self-help groups such as Diabetes Associations. As diabetes mellitus is one of the more common disorders of endocrine function this chapter addresses the principles of management and care of an individual with the disorder.

Care of the individual with diabetes mellitus

Diabetes mellitus is a disorder which is thought to affect approximately 3–4% of the population of Australia. The main aims of management of an individual with diabetes mellitus are to maintain the blood glucose level within normal limits, and to implement measures that will assist the individual to live as normal a life as possible.

Diabetes mellitus is a condition that cannot be cured, but it can be controlled. Management of the condition is directed at controlling it so that the two aims stated previously can be achieved, and so that complications can be avoided.

Management of diabetes mellitus involves regulating the blood glucose level by diet, exercise, and insulin or oral hypoglycaemic agents; prevention of infection, and monitoring blood and urine glucose levels. Self management of the condition is the overall goal, and, therefore, education of the individual in all aspects of self care is an essential part of management.

Diet

The diet is an important aspect in control of both Type I and Type II diabetes mellitus. A dietitian works with the individual to develop a carefully balanced food intake which follows the principles of a recommended diet for diabetics. It is essential that the individual understands the principles, and knows how to modify or adapt his diet to meet the demands experienced during illness, injury, emotional stress, or major changes in lifestyle. Recent research has demonstrated that a diet which is high fibre, high unrefined carbohydrate, and low fat is beneficial in lowering blood glucose levels and in reducing the amount of insulin required. The aims of the diabetic diet are to:

● satisfy hunger
● provide for normal growth rate in children
● attain and maintain a desirable body weight
● maintain the level of blood glucose within the normal range to prevent hypoglycaemia and hyperglycaemia
● meet the individual's energy requirements
● prevent the development of long-term complications associated with diabetes mellitus.

Carbohydrate, particularly in a high-fibre form, should provide approximately 50–60% of the total daily intake, but the amount varies according to the individual's level of energy expenditure. Some unrefined carbohydrate should be eaten at each meal.

Refined carbohydrate foods should be limited or excluded under normal circumstances, as they cause a rapid rise in the blood glucose level.

The average daily allowance of *protein* is from 1–1.5 g per kilogram of body weight for adults, and from 2–3 g per kilogram of body weight for children.

Fats should provide approximately 15–20% of the energy in the diet, and should consist mainly of polyunsaturated fats. Polyunsaturated fats are thought to reduce blood cholesterol and triglyceride levels and, therefore, decrease the risk of vascular disease—a common complication of diabetes mellitus.

Alcohol should be limited as it is high in kilojoules, and may cause adverse reactions to some medications used in the treatment of diabetes.

Lists and charts are supplied to the individual who is instructed on their use to plan nutritious and varied meals within the prescribed limitations. The importance of regular meals and snacks is emphasized, e.g. three main meals plus a snack mid-morning, mid-afternoon, and before going to bed. The evening snack is of particular importance to prevent nocturnal hypoglycaemia. Continuing evaluation of the diet is essential, and adjustments are made if necessary. Continuing education of the individual helps him to adhere to the dietary principles.

If the individual is in hospital, the nurse must report immediately to the nurse in charge if any foods in the diet are not eaten. If the prescribed amounts of nutrients are not consumed the individual is at risk of hypoglycaemia, therefore a substitute is given.

Exercise

The amount of exercise required by the individual should be estimated, and planned to balance with his dietary intake and insulin. A well planned programme of regular exercise, which is adjusted as necessary, is beneficial in weight control, in its physiological and psychological effects, and in terms of blood glucose control.

Exercise stimulates the uptake of glucose by muscle cells, lowering blood glucose levels and increasing the absorption of injected insulin. For these reasons, exercise can increase the likelihood of hypoglycaemia. To prevent the development of hypoglycaemia following exercise, the individual needs either to increase his nutritional intake or to decrease his insulin dosage. It is essential that the individual learns to balance the level of exercise with dietary intake and insulin administration, under varying conditions.

Insulin

As insulin is essential for the normal metabolism of glucose, it is a major factor involved in the regulation of blood glucose levels. Many types of insulin are available and these may be short, intermediate, or long-acting. Information on various insulin preparations is provided in Table 48.1. Information on the technique of insulin administration is provided in Chapter 58.

As soon as possible, the individual is instructed how to inject insulin and how to care for the equipment. He is also informed about the recommended sites of the body where insulin can be subcutaneously injected. Figure 48.1 illustrates the areas which contain sufficient subcutaneous tissue and are, therefore, suitable for insulin injection.

Tissue atrophy, or hypertrophy, may occur at injection sites therefore rotation of the sites is essential. An individually designed plan for rotating sites may help the individual to select and use several areas of the body for injection.

Table 48.1 Insulin preparations

Preparation	Types	Actions
Short Acting	Regular Insulin	Onset within 30–45 minutes Duration up to 8 hours
	Neutral Insulin	Onset within 30 minutes Duration of 6–7 hours
	Insulin Zinc Suspension (Semilente)	Onset within 30–60 minutes Duration of 12–16 hours
Intermediate Acting	Biphasic Insulin	Onset within 30 minutes Duration of 18–22 hours
	Insulin Zinc Suspension (lente)	Onset within 2 hours Duration of 24 hours
	Isophane Insulin	Onset within 2 hours Duration of 20–24 hours
Long Acting	Insulin Zinc Suspension (ultralente)	Onset within 4 hours Duration of 36 hours
	Protamine Zinc Insulin	Onset within 4–8 hours Duration of 24–36 hours

Oral hypoglycaemic agents

Oral hypoglycaemic agents may be prescribed in the management of Type II diabetes mellitus which is unresponsive to diet alone, or for the individual for whom insulin is unacceptable. The oral medications used in the treatment of diabetes either act by stimulating the pancreas to release insulin, or act by delaying or impairing glucose absorption from the bowel. Oral hypoglycaemic agents include chlorpropamide, glibenclamide, gliclazide, tolazamide, and tolbutamide.

Prevention of infection

The individual with diabetes mellitus is susceptible to infection as a result of impaired body defence mechanisms. Uncontrolled diabetes may result in a number of infections, whereas if diabetes is well controlled the individual is less susceptible. The individual with diabetes mellitus is particularly at risk of developing urinary tract infections; fungal infections, e.g. Candida albicans, and infected skin lesions.

To minimize the risk of infection the individual should recognize the importance of good control of blood glucose levels, of maintaining a high standard of personal hygiene, and of avoiding unnecessary exposure to infection. The skin should be kept clean and free from excessive irritation, friction, or pressure. All injuries to or infections of the skin, however minor, should be cleaned with a mild antiseptic solution and covered by a dressing.

Skin lesions of the feet commonly occur in individuals with poor control of their diabetes. Such lesions result from, or are exacerbated by, impaired circulation and peripheral neuropathy. If a minor injury or lesion is undetected, or untreated, ulceration and infection may develop. Therefore, care of the feet and prevention of foot lesions is of prime importance. Care of the feet includes:

- Wearing well fitting socks or stockings, and shoes. Socks that are not made from natural fibres, e.g. wool or cotton, should not be worn, and care must be taken to avoid hosiery with seams that lie under the feet.
- Daily cleansing, drying, and inspection of the feet A mild soap is used and the feet should not be soaked for long periods. After washing, they should be patted dry rather than rubbed. Dry feet may be gently massaged with lanolin or oil to prevent fissures.
- Consulting a podiatrist if corns or calluses need attention.
- Trimming the toenails straight across, to avoid damage to the surrounding skin.
- Keeping the feet warm, but avoid placing the feet close to heating devices to prevent possible skin damage. If an electric blanket is used to warm the bed, it should be turned off before the individual gets into bed.

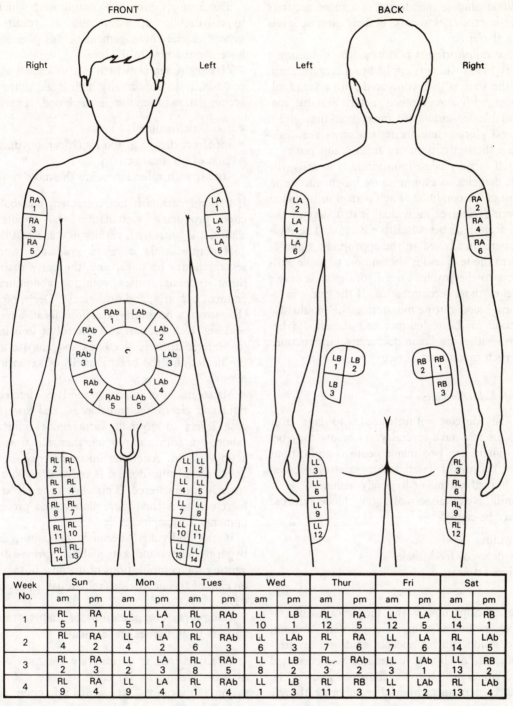

Week No.	Sun		Mon		Tues		Wed		Thur		Fri		Sat	
	am	pm	am	pm	am	pm	am	pm	am	pm	am	pm	am	pm
1	RL 5	RA 1	LL 5	LA 1	RL 10	RAb 1	LL 10	LB 1	RL 12	RA 5	LL 12	LA 5	LL 14	RB 1
2	RL 4	RA 2	LL 4	LA 2	RL 6	RAb 3	LL 6	LAb 3	RL 7	RA 6	LL 7	LA 6	RL 14	LAb 5
3	RL 2	RA 3	LL 2	LA 3	RL 8	RAb 5	LL 8	LB 2	RL 3	RAb 2	LL 3	LAb 1	LL 13	RB 2
4	RL 9	RA 4	LL 9	LA 4	RL 1	RAb 4	LL 1	LB 3	RL 11	RB 3	LL 11	LAb 2	RL 13	LAb 4

Fig. 48.1 Sites for insulin injection. (Reproduced with permission from Boore J R P, Champion R, Ferguson M C (eds) 1987 Nursing the physically ill adult. Churchill Livingstone, Edinburgh.)

- Avoiding walking barefooted, or on hot surfaces.
- Performing foot and leg exercises to increase circulation.
- Avoiding constrictive clothing, e.g. garters, and crossing the legs; both of which may reduce blood flow.
- Seeking immediate attention from the podiatrist or medical officer if there is any injury, colour change, infection, or discharge of pus or blood.

Monitoring glucose levels

Although it is less accurate than blood glucose monitoring, *urinalysis* is still used by individuals who are unable or unwilling to monitor blood glucose levels. The individual is instructed in the technique of testing his urine for glucose and ketones. Information on urinalysis is provided in

Chapter 30. Blood glucose monitoring is a more accurate method of assessing the effectiveness of diet, exercise levels and medication therapy.

Blood glucose monitoring is performed by obtaining a drop of capillary blood which is applied to a reagent strip. The colour of the strip is then compared with a standard, either visually or with a reflectance meter. Suitable machines are available for automatic finger-pricking, and a selection of blood glucose monitoring machines are available which run either on batteries or from mains power.

The aim of self blood glucose monitoring is to assist the individual with diabetes to assume more independence in the management of his condition. Each person using blood glucose monitoring receives individual instruction in the technique, e.g. from a diabetes health educator. The individual with diabetes is advised on the appropriate times at which to perform the test, and is shown how to make suitable adjustments to the insulin dose if the glucose levels are above or below those recommended. If the nurse is required to perform blood glucose monitoring she should also receive instruction in the technique, and she should become familiar with the manufacturer's instructions accompanying each monitoring device.

Complications of diabetes mellitus

Complications may develop within minutes to days, over several months, or may take several years before they become evident. There are two major acute complications which can occur because of unsatisfactory control of blood glucose levels; hypoglycaemia or hyperglycaemia.

Hypoglycaemia is an abnormally low blood glucose level, and it may be caused by:

- too much insulin
- too little, or delayed, food intake
- excess physical activity
- vomiting.

Hypoglycaemia develops *rapidly* and the early manifestations are hunger, pallor, sweating, tachycardia, yawning, nausea, blurred vision, slurred speech, confusion or irrational behaviour. If the hypoglycaemia is not corrected rapidly the individual will become comatose and, if the coma is prolonged, permanent brain damage or death may occur.

Mild symptoms can often be reversed with the ingestion of 10 g of simple carbohydrate, e.g. provided in fruit juice or honey. Insulin-dependent diabetics should ensure that they always have ready access to some form of carbohydrate that is readily absorbed, e.g. barley sugar.

If the individual is unable to ingest a carbohydrate substance, intravenous administration of glucose or glucagon will be necessary. Glucagon can also be administered subcutaneously or intramuscularly.

The *Somogyi effect* is a complication which may follow a hypoglycaemic episode, and it results in rebound *hyperglycaemia*. Management of this phenomenon involves lowering the insulin dosage.

Hyperglycaemia, which is also known as diabetic keto-acidosis, is an abnormally high blood glucose level and an accumulation of ketones in the blood. It may be caused by:

- too little insulin
- incorrect diet, e.g. too much carbohydrate
- lack of physical activity
- stress, with infection being the most common stressor.

If hyperglycaemia is not corrected, metabolic acidosis occurs, producing vasodilation and hypotension. Severe acidosis, if untreated, results in coma and death.

Hyperglycaemia develops *gradually* over a period of several hours or days, and the early manifestations are thirst, anorexia, nausea, vomiting, abdominal pain, muscle cramps, polyuria, and drowsiness. Deep, rapid ventilations (Kussmaul's breathing) develop, in an attempt to control acidosis. Dehydration and electrolyte imbalance occur due to osmotic diuresis. Ketones and glucose are excreted in the urine, and the breath smells of ketones (sweet, fruity odour).

Management of hyperglycaemia is directed at correcting fluid and electrolyte imbalances, and lowering blood glucose levels to normal. Intravenous fluids, e.g. normal saline, are administered together with intravenous short-acting insulin. After the initial decrease in blood glucose level, the insulin dosage is reduced and intravenous dextrose is administered. This allows the blood glucose levels to return to normal more slowly, and prevents the development of hypoglycaemia.

If the individual becomes comatose, as a result of hyperglycaemia and ketoacidosis, care is directed at preventing the complications of unconsciousness. Information on care of an unconscious individual is provided in Chapter 43.

Long-term complications of diabetes mellitus involve various body tissues and systems.

1. *Atherosclerosis* is a relatively common complication of diabetes mellitus, with coronary artery disease being the major complication. Myocardial infarction, cerebrovascular accident, and renal failure are the major causes of death in individuals with diabetes. Peripheral vascular disease is often widespread causing manifestations of peripheral ischaemia: cold lower extremities, intermittent claudication, diminished or absent pulses, ulcers, infection, and gangrene. If vessels in a leg become occluded, amputation of the limb may be necessary.

2. *Neuropathy*, which is inflammation and degeneration of the peripheral nerves, gives rise to disturbances of sensation such as tingling and numbness particularly in the

lower limbs. Another form of neuropathy is characterized by decreased sense of position (proprioceptive disturbances), and diminished sensation to touch, pain, and temperature. The sensory deficits increase the possibility of injury, and increase the chance of injuries being unnoticed by the individual. Peripheral motor involvement results in muscle weakness and atrophy which may lead to deformities, particularly of the feet (Charcot's arthropathy).

3. *Retinopathy* is a disorder of retinal blood vessels, characterized by haemorrhages and leakage of blood and serum into the retina. Repeated vitreous haemorrhage may result in retinal detachment or blindness.

Cataracts may also develop in the presence of diabetes mellitus.

4. *Nephropathy* may occur over a period of many years, and few signs or symptoms occur until uraemia and oedema develop. Diabetic nephropathy is more likely to develop if diabetes is poorly controlled. Renal function is gradually impaired by glomerulosclerosis, and it may progress to chronic renal failure. Prevention and treatment of any condition that may impair renal function, e.g. urinary tract infections or hypertension, reduces the development of diabetic nephropathy.

5. *Impotence* occurs in approximately 50–60% of all men with diabetes. In addition to the psychological causes of impotence, the condition is believed to be caused by damage to the nerve endings as a result of diabetic neuropathy. Diabetic neuropathy involving those nerves controlling reflex blood flow to the penis appears to result from peristently elevated blood glucose levels. Conversely, low blood glucose levels may be the most common cause of occasional impotence in diabetic males. Control of blood glucose levels, therefore, may help to prevent or alleviate the problem of impotence associated with diabetes.

The individual should be encouraged to contact the local branch of the Diabetic Association, which provides information and support. He should be advised to always carry some form of medical identification, e.g. a card, bracelet or medallion, which identifies him as a person with diabetes. Such identification helps to ensure appropriate care in emergency situations.

Education

The individual with diabetes mellitus has to learn to accept his condition and the resulting changes in life style. In order to gain confidence in managing the condition, he must acquire a considerable amount of knowledge and learn new skills.

A well-planned education programme helps to reduce the individual's anxiety about his condition, promotes greater self-reliance, and better diabetic management. Family members or significant others may also be involved in the education programme to gain knowledge and understanding. The aim of an education programme are that the individual will:

• accept his condition, and understand the importance of good diabetic control.
• acquire the technical skills needed to monitor blood glucose levels and administer medications.
• understand the importance of diet, exercise, and medications in the maintenance of blood glucose levels.
• recognize disturbances of blood glucose levels, and the development of complications.

SUMMARY

The endocrine system consists of a number of glands, each of which secretes hormones which are chemical substances that initiate or regulate the activity of an organ or group of cells in another part of the body.

Most endocrine disorders result from either over or under production of hormones, and the effects of endocrine dysfunction are varied and widespread.

Disorders of endocrine function can result from genetic defects, neoplasia, obstruction, trauma, autoimmune reactions, infection, inflammation, or hyperplasia.

Diagnostic tests used to assess the functions of an endocrine gland include estimating serum hormone levels, urine tests, scanning, and ultrasonography.

Medical management and nursing care varies according to the specific disorder. The nursing care plan is designed to help the individual meet all his needs, specifically his need for comfort, psychological support, nutrition and fluids.

Diabetes mellitus is a disorder of blood glucose regulation, and aspects of management of the disorder include diet, exercise, insulin or oral hypoglycaemic agents, prevention of infection, monitoring glucose levels, and prevention of complications.

REFERENCES AND FURTHER READING

Boore J R P, Champion R, Ferguson M C (eds) 1987 Nursing the physically ill adult. Churchill Livingstone, Edinburgh
Brunner L S, Suddarth D S 1988 Textbook of medical-surgical nursing, 6th edn. J B Lippincott, Philadelphia

49. The individual with a reproductive system disorder

OBJECTIVES

1. State the pathophysiological influences and effects associated with disorders of the female and male reproductive systems.
2. Describe the major manifestations of reproductive systems disorders.
3. Briefly describe the specific disorders of the female and male reproductive systems, which are outlined in this chapter.
4. State the diagnostic tests which may be used to assess reproductive systems function.
5. Assist in planning and implementing nursing care for the individual with a reproductive system disorder.

INTRODUCTION

Information on the normal structure and function of the female and male reproductive systems is provided in Chapter 26, and it should be referred to before studying the contents of this chapter. The biological function of both the female and male reproductive systems is propagation of the species. In addition, the reproductive organs are a means of obtaining sexual pleasure. Therefore any dysfunction of the reproductive system may affect fertility and/or sexual function.

Education

The nurse is in a key position to inform others about self examination techniques and the prevention of sexually transmitted diseases. She may also be asked for information about birth control methods.

Two techniques of self examination which, when performed regularly, can detect *early* pathological changes, are self examination of the breasts and testes. The nurse should know how to perform both examinations so that she can teach these practices to other individuals. She should in-

form others to consult with a medical officer immediately if any abnormalities are detected. Information on breast and testicular self examination, birth control methods, and prevention of sexually transmitted diseases, is provided later in this chapter.

DISORDERS OF THE FEMALE REPRODUCTIVE SYSTEM

This part of the chapter addresses various pathophysiological influences and effects on the female reproductive system, the manifestation of disorders, specific disorders, diagnostic tests and care of the female with a disorder of the reproductive system.

Pathophysiological influences and effects

Pathophysiological changes may result from structural abnormalities, hormonal imbalance, neoplasms, infection, or trauma. The major effects caused by these changes are variations in the menstrual cycle, and pelvic pain.

Changes in the menstrual cycle

The frequency of menstrual bleeding can be increased or decreased, or bleeding may occur between menstrual cycles. Increased frequency of bleeding is generally due to a reduced follicular or luteal phase of the cycle, and it is more common immediately after menarche and during menopause. Decreased frequency of bleeding is generally due to an extended proliferative phase of the cycle, which may be caused by physical factors such as ovarian disease or malnutrition, and emotional factors. Intermenstrual bleeding (metrorrhagia) may occur at the time of ovulation, or it may be caused by factors such as hormonal imbalance or neoplasms.

Variations in the amount or duration of bleeding include excessive or prolonged bleeding, and absence or suppression of menstruation. Excessive and/or prolonged bleeding (menorrhagia) may be caused by erosive lesions, endometrial hyperplasia, blood dyscrasias, or neoplasms. Absence of menstruation (amenorrhoea) is normal before puberty, during pregnancy, and after menopause. Secondary amenorrhoea generally results from anovulation due to hormonal dysfunction, e.g. decreased secretion of oestrogen.

Post menopausal bleeding may result from the administration of oestrogen (hormone replacement therapy), from an oestrogen-producing ovarian neoplasm, uterine hyperplasia or carcinoma, or atrophic vaginitis.

Pelvic pain

Pelvic pain may be caused by chronic inflammation, infection, pelvic congestion, ovulation, ovarian or uterine neoplasms, or ectopic pregnancy.

Major manifestations of female reproductive system disorders

The signs and symptoms, which vary according to the type and severity of the disorder, include pain, bleeding, vaginal discharge, pruritus, urinary problems, and breast changes.

Pain

Dysmenorrhoea (painful menstruation) is the most commonly experienced type of pain. The pain is usually perceived as intermittent, cramping lower abdominal pain which may radiate to the back, thighs, and groin. Dysmenorrhoea may be accompanied by abdominal distension, painful breasts, headaches, nausea and vomiting. The pain is thought to result from excessive amounts of prostaglandins, synthesised during the breakdown of the premenstrual endometrium, causing myometrial hyperactivity.

Dysmenorrhoea may also be secondary to endometriosis, uterine fibromas, or pelvic inflammatory disease.

Abdominal or low back pain, occuring at times other than menstruation, may be due to infection, inflammation, or neoplasms.

Intense lower abdominal pain, of sudden onset, may result from torsion of an ovarian cyst or a ruptured uterine tube the result of an ectopic pregnancy. The pain associated with a ruptured uterine tube may be referred to the shoulder if blood tracks to the diaphragm and stimulates the phrenic nerve.

Pain may also be experienced in the presence of vaginal or vulval lesions, e.g. genital herpes.

Pain associated with sexual intercourse (dyspareunia) may be due to decreased vaginal lubrication, vaginal or vulval infection, endometriosis, neoplasms, or pelvic inflammatory disease.

Pain in the breasts may be caused by congestion, inflammation, hyperplasia, or neoplasms.

Bleeding

Unusual uterine bleeding may be due to disturbances of the menstrual cycle, or due to infection, neoplasms, or systemic disease. Sometimes, the cause of dysfunctional uterine bleeding cannot be determined. Bleeding may range from 'spotting' between menstruation, to the passage of clots during menstruation, to prolonged menstrual bleeding, to bleeding after sexual intercourse. The individual may describe the bleeding as slight, irregular, or heavy.

Vaginal discharge

Although a clear or opaque white vaginal discharge occurs normally, certain disorders can cause an increase in the amount or character of vaginal discharge. Deviations from normal include an offensive odour, and a vaginal discharge which may be yellow, frothy, green, or bloodstained. Vaginal and vulval irritation and pruritus may accompany an abnormal discharge. The most common cause of abnormal vaginal discharge is infection of the vagina or cervix.

Pruritus

Pruritus vulvae is an irritative condition of the vulva. This distressing itching sensation leads to scratching, which can damage the vulval tissues. Causes include contact dermatitis, and vaginal infections that are accompanied by an irritating discharge.

Urinary problems

The most common urinary problems associated with reproductive system disorders are dysuria and stress incontinence. Causes include infection, prolapse, and pressure from a pelvic neoplasm.

Breast changes

Deviations from normal include a discharge from the nipple, pain or tenderness in the breast/s, the presence of lumps or masses, nipple inversion, and dimpling of the skin.

Specific disorders of the female reproductive system

Disorders of the female reproductive system can be classified as congenital, resulting from multiple causes, degenerative, infectious or inflammatory, neoplastic, or traumatic.

Congenital abnormalities

Abnormalities of the uterus include Müllerian aplasia,

in which the vagina ends in a blind pouch with an absent or non-functional rudimentary uterus. A bicornuate uterus results from incomplete Müllerian fusion and is characterized by a uterus that is either abnormally shaped or divided.

Vaginal atresia is complete absence of the vagina, and it is caused by fusion of the Mullerian ducts during early embryonic development.

Disorders of multiple cause

Premenstrual syndrome (premenstrual tension) is a collection of symptoms that occur approximately 4–7 days before menstruation, and which subside with the onset of menstruation. Although the precise cause is unclear, the symptoms are related to transient fluid retention. Manifestations include oedema of the legs and fingers, abdominal distension, breast tenderness, headaches, and mood changes.

Endometriosis is the presence of functioning endometrium outside the lining of the uterus. Such ectopic tissue is usually confined to areas in the pelvic cavity. The cause is unknown, but research suggests that some endometrium is expelled from the uterus into the pelvic cavity, at the time of menstruation. Manifestations depend on the location of ectopic endometrium, and include dysmenorrhoea, backache, and menstrual abnormalities.

Infertility is defined as the inability to conceive after 1 year of regular intercourse without contraception. Infertility is caused by anatomical, functional, or psychological factors. In many instances, no cause can be determined. Anatomical factors include uterine or uterine tube abnormalities. Functional factors include failure to ovulate, while psychological factors such as stress are thought to contribute to some cases of infertility.

Degenerative disorders

Uterovaginal prolapse is descent of the genital tract, which may be first, second, or third degree. First degree prolapse is the descent of the cervix to the vaginal opening. Second degree prolapse is protrusion of the cervix through the vaginal opening. Third degree prolapse (procidentia) is prolapse of the entire uterus through the vaginal opening.

Causes of prolapse include stretching of the cardinal ligaments and the pelvic floor muscles, e.g. following childbirth, and sustained increased intra-abdominal pressure. Manifestations depend on the degree of prolapse, and include backache, a 'bearing-down' sensation, cervical erosion and bleeding, and urinary problems.

A cystocele is the herniation of the posterior aspect of the bladder into the vagina; a **urethrocele** is herniation of the urethra into the vagina; and **rectocele** is herniation of the rectum into the posterior vaginal wall. All three con-ditions are caused by the same general conditions that result in uterine prolapse. Manifestations include stress incontinence of urine, urinary tract infections, and—with a rectocele—a feeling of rectal fullness and incomplete defaecation.

Menopause, although it is a natural event, may create uncomfortable symptoms for the individual. Menopause is the cessation of ovarian activity with cessation of menstruation. It may also be referred to as the climacteric. The climacteric is actually the prolonged period of declining ovarian function leading up to the cessation of menstruation.

Menopause is the natural result of declining ovarian hormone production and function, which usually occurs between the ages of 45 and 60 years. Some women have no symptoms, apart from cessation of menstruation, while others experience a variety of symptoms. These include irregular menstruation, hot flushes, night sweats, palpitations, vaginal dryness, tiredness, and mood changes. Following menopause, the lack of ovarian hormones may lead to osteoporosis, stress incontinence, and uterine prolapse.

Infectious and inflammatory disorders

Vulvovaginitis is inflammation of the vulva and vagina. Because the two structures are in close proximity, inflammation of one generally causes inflammation of the other. Causes of vaginitis—with or without vulvitis—include infection, vaginal mucosal atrophy, vulval atrophy, chemical irritants, and poor personal hygiene.

Yeast infection results from overgrowth of the *Candida albicans* fungus which is normally present in the mucous membranes and on the skin. Under certain circumstances overgrowth and infection can occur. Predisposing factors include diabetes mellitus, pregnancy, broad spectrum antibiotic therapy, and the use of oral contraceptives. Manifestations include pruritus and a thick, white, cheesy vaginal discharge.

Haemophilus vaginitis is caused by the bacteria *Haemophilus vaginalis*. This type of vaginitis is generally mild with less severe pruritus than occurs in other infections.

Trichomonas vaginalis infection is caused by a protozoan flagellate which is generally sexually transmitted. Manifestations include pruritus, vaginal tenderness, and frothy green-tinged offensive vaginal discharge.

Chlamydial vaginitis infection is caused by a microorganism of the genus *Chlamydia*, which is generally sexually transmitted. Manifestations include a thin, white, frothy vaginal discharge.

Gardnerella vaginalis is caused by the microorganism of the same name which is generally sexually transmitted. The major manifestation is profuse offensive vaginal discharge.

Herpes genitalis is caused by type 11 Herpes simplex

virus (HSV-II) which is generally sexually transmitted. Manifestations include vesicular eruptions on the genital skin and mucous membranes. The lesions are painful and are frequently associated with a burning sensation, dysuria, enlarged inguinal lymph nodes, and pyrexia. There may be some cervical or vaginal discharge. Secondary infections can recur from every few weeks to once or twice a year.

Gonorrhoea is caused by *Neisseria gonorrhoeae* which is sexually transmitted. In approximately 50%–75% of women with gonorrhoea there are no symptoms. Manifestations which may occur include dysuria, transient vaginal discharge, low abdominal discomfort, and a change in menstrual patterns. The primary site of infection is the endocervix, and the infection can spread through the reproductive tract—causing pelvic inflammatory disease (PID) and sterility. The infection may also enter the urinary tract, causing urethritis. Infants born of infected mothers can contract gonococcal ophthalmia neonatarium during passage through the birth canal. The microorganisms can also be spread to the eyes, if they are touched with contaminated hands, causing gonococcal conjunctivities. Through sexual behaviour, the organism can also be transmitted to the pharynx and rectum.

Genital warts (condylomata acuminata) is caused by the human papillomavirus which is generally sexually transmitted. Manifestations include the appearance of painless warts on the vulva, perineum, perianal area, and on the vaginal and cervical walls.

Syphilis is caused by *Treponema pallidum* which is sexually transmitted. Syphilis, if untreated, is characterized by progressive stages. As the organism incubates, there are no symptoms. The primary stage (10–90 days after incubation) involves the formation of small fluid filled lesions, called chancres. Chancres, which are usually painless, generally appear on the labia. The inguinal lymph glands enlarge, but are not painful.

The secondary stage (up to 8 weeks after the initial chancre) is characterized by a generalized rash and inguinal lymphadenopathy. In warm moist areas of the body, lesions enlarge and erode, producing highly contagious lesions called condylomata lata. Systemic symptoms such as malaise, pyrexia, and headaches generally appear.

The tertiary stage (up to 30 years after infection) is the non-infectious but destructive final stage of the disease. Manifestations involve areas other than the reproductive system, including the cardiovascular, nervous, digestive, and skeletal systems.

Chancroid is caused by Haemophilus ducreyi which is sexually transmitted. Manifestations include the appearance of soft, painful lesions on the vulva, vagina, or cervix; inguinal adenitis, headaches, and malaise.

Pelvic inflammatory disease (PID) is any acute, subacute, recurrent, or chronic infection of the uterus and uterine tubes that can extend into the pelvic cavity. PID has many causes, including infection by Neisseria gonorr-

hoea and Chlamydia trachomatis. PID can also be caused by microorganisms that are not sexually transmitted, e.g. aerobic and anerobic bacteria that are normally present in the cervix and vagina.

The manifestations of PID vary from mild to severe, with salpingitis (inflammation of a uterine tube) being the most common finding. Manifestations of PID include abdominal pain, menorrhagia and metrorrhagia, increased vaginal discharge, and slight pyrexia. The complications of PID are numerous, e.g. chronic abdominal pain, ectopic pregnancy, and infertility.

Neoplastic disorders

Benign or malignant neoplasms can develop in the ovaries, uterus, vulva, and breasts.

Benign ovarian tumours are a group of disorders which includes cysts and fibromas. Depending on type, the tumour may contain fluid or solid material. There may be no symptoms until the tumour enlarges and presses on other structures, ruptures or becomes twisted. Large, or multiple, cysts may cause pelvic discomfort or abnormal uterine bleeding secondary to disrupted ovulation. Rupture, or torsion, causes abdominal pain, distension and rigidity.

Benign uterine tumours are also called leiomyomas or fibroids. They are composed of smooth muscle cells and connective tissue, and are generally mutiple. They may be submucous, interstitial, or subserous. While the precise cause is unknown, it is thought that leiomyoma formation is hormonally influenced. Leiomyomas tend to decrease in size or disappear after menopause—when oestrogen production decreases.

Manifestations include prolonged, heavy, or painful menstruation, a feeling of heaviness in the pelvic region, frequency of micturition, and an enlarged irregular uterus.

Benign breast disease includes fibroadenomas, intraductal papillomas, cystic hyperplasia, and chronic mastitis. Fibroadenomas are mobile, round, firm, painless lumps, which occur most often in younger women. Intraductal papilloma produces a serous or serosanguinous nipple discharge, and occurs most often in women between the ages of 35 and 45 years.

Cystic hyperplasia and chronic mastitis are collectively referred to as fibrocystic disease. A painful mass decreases and increases in size in relation to the menstrual cycle. The mass is generally firm, mobile, regular in shape; and is most often present in the upper outer quadrant of the breast. Fibrocystic disease usually regresses after menopause as ovarian hormones decrease.

Uterine cancer may originate in the cervix, or in the endometrium.

1. Cervical cancer is one of the most common cancers in women, and may be one of two types: squamous cell carcinoma or adenocarcinoma. Cervical cancer begins as a

change in the epithelial covering of the cervix and, if not treated, eventually involves the epithelial layer. Invasive carcinoma extends beyond the surface, involves the body of the cervix, and may spread via the lymphatic system to surrounding structures.

Manifestations of cervical cancer do not appear in the early stages. Later manifestations are 'spotting' between menstruation, postmenopausal bleeding, bleeding after sexual intercourse, or a brown vaginal discharge.
2. Endometrial cancer is less common, and usually effects women over the age of 50 years. The major manifestation is abnormal vaginal bleeding, which may initially present as a watery blood-stained discharge.

Ovarian cancer, because it is difficult to detect in the early stages, is often not detected until metastasis has occured. Sometimes, the woman may experience an increase in abdominal girth caused by intraperitoneal accumulation of fluid (ascites).

Cancer of the vulva develops from premalignant hyperplasia, and is more common in elderly women. The major manifestations are vulval pruritus, a history of chronic vulvitis, and the presence of raised grey-white patches on the vulva.

Breast cancer is the most common cancer in women and, although it usually affects women over the age of 50 years, it can also affect much younger women. Manifestations include a unilateral increase in breast size, changes in the shape of a breast, a palpable mass, dimpling of the skin, nipple retraction or ulceration, and nipple discharge.

Pain is not a common symptom. Further information on causes, incidence, detection, prevention, and staging of cancer is provided in Chapter 64.

Traumatic disorders

A fistula, which is an abnormal passage from an internal organ to the body surface or between two internal organs, may develop in the female reproductive tract. The majority of fistulae occur following trauma to the reproductive tract or bladder; but they may also be caused by infection, malignancy, or radiotherapy. Fistulae may develop between the bladder and vagina and, less commonly, between the rectum and vagina or between the bladder and uterus. Depending on the site of the fistula, manifestations include leakage of urine or faeces into the vagina.

Haematomas and laceration of the vulva or vagina can result from a fall, intercourse injury, or from sexual assault. Manifestations include vulval bruising and swelling, and bleeding from lacerations.

Diagnostic tests

A variety of tests may be performed to assist, or confirm, the diagnosis of disorders of the female reproductive system. Certain examinations may be performed to detect pathological changes at an early stage.

Pelvic examination

Internal examination of the vagina and cervix may be performed manually or with the aid of a vaginal speculum.

Manual examination involves the medical officer inserting one or two gloved fingers into the vagina. The other hand is placed on the abdomen over the suprapubic area. The medical officer may also perform a rectovaginal examination, by inserting one finger in the vagina and another into the rectum. Manual examination enables the medical officer to palpate the uterus and ovaries for size, position, shape, tenderness, and mobility.

Instrumental examination involves the insertion of a vaginal speculum to provide visualization of the vagina and cervix, and to obtain a sample of cells and secretions. During a pelvic examination, the woman is requested to assume the dorsal or Sim's position. Refer to Figure 35.6.

Papanicolaou test

The Papanicolaou test (Pap smear) is performed to obtain a scraping of cervical cells. Micrsopic examination of the cells can determine the presence of abnormalities before the symptoms of cancer appear. The test involves the insertion of a vaginal speculum, so that the examiner can collect some cells by gently scraping the cervix with a spatula. The cells are placed on a slide, sprayed with a fixative, and microscopically examined. Papanicolaou's classification of findings is:

- Class I. Absence of abnormal cells.
- Class II. Atypical cytology, but no evidence of malignancy.
- Class III. Cytology suggestive of, but not conclusive for, malignancy.
- Class IV. Cytology strongly suggestive of malignancy.
- Class V. Cytology conclusive for malignancy.

Most experts recommend that all women should have an annual Pap. test. Some women have a greater risk of developing cervical cancer, e.g. those who became sexually active at a young age, those who have had numerous sexual partners, those who have a history of herpes virus II, and daughters of women who took diethylstibestrol (DES) during pregnancy. These women may require more frequent screening, e.g. twice a year.

Breast examination

Examination of the breasts, particularly breast self examination (BSE), is the best method of detecting early breast changes. By examining her own breasts regularly, a woman is generally able to detect any departure from normal. The earlier a breast lump, or other change, is detected, the sooner it can be investigated and treated. Although the presence of any breast lump is frightening, approximately 90% of lumps are not malignant.

Breast self examination, which should be performed after each menstrual period (or monthly after menopause) (Figs 49.1–49.5), involves:

1. Careful inspection, in front of a mirror, of each breast. The breasts are assessed for symmetry in size and shape, puckering or dimpling of the skin, retraction of the nipple, and any nipple discharge. The breasts should be inspected with the arms by the sides, with the arms raised over the head, and thrusting the breasts forward with the hands on the hips.

2. Methodical palpation, of each breast in the shower and when lying down. The breasts are palpated using a small circular movement to detect any lumps or thickening. The three patterns used in breast palpation are strips, quadrants, and circles. Whichever approach is used each entire breast, including the axillary tail, is thoroughly assessed. The woman lies down on a flat surface, with a small pillow or folded towel under the shoulder on the same side as the breast to be palpated.

Colposcopy

Colposcopy involves using a magnifying colposcope to visualize the vagina and cervix. After inserting a vaginal speculum, the colposcope is positioned to provide illumination and magnification of the tissues. A biopsy of tissue may be obtained at the same time, for microscopic examination. Prior to colposcopy, the vagina and cervix may be painted with an iodine preparation. Normal cells take up the iodine whereas abnormal cells do not. The colour of the cells may be readily observed using the colposcope.

Cervical biopsy

A specimen of cervical tissue is obtained for cytological study, using either punch biopsy or cone biopsy techniques. Punch biopsy, which may be performed in conjunction with Colposcopy, involves the removal of a small column of tissue.

Cone biopsy, performed under general anaesthetic, involves removal of a cone-shaped piece of tissue from the cervix. Possible complications following the procedure are haemorrhage and infertility—due to the removal of mucus-producing glands and the formation of scar tissue.

Laparoscopy

Laparoscopy is a surgical procedure, performed to enable visualization and exploration of the pelvic cavity and reproductive organs. Following a general or local anaesthetic, the laparoscope is inserted through a small incision near the umbilicus, and a second probe may be inserted through a suprapubic incision.

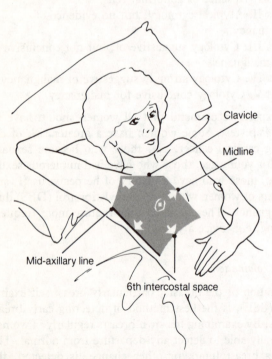

Fig. 49.1 Breast self examination: boundaries of area to be examined. (Reproduced with permission from Game C, Anderson R E, Kidd J R (eds) 1989 Medical-surgical nursing: a core text. Churchill Livingstone, Melbourne.)

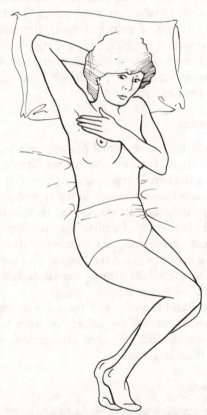

Fig. 49.2 Breast self examination: lying down position used. (Reproduced with permission from Game C, Anderson R E, Kidd J R (eds) 1989 Medical-surgical nursing: a core text. Churchill Livingstone, Melbourne.)

Diagnostic uterine curettage

Dilatation (stretching) of the cervical opening, and curettage (scraping) of the endometrium (D&C) may be performed to obtain samples of tissue for cytology. Usually, a general anaesthetic is administered, before the medical officer inserts a series of graded dilators to stretch the cervix. After dilatation, the uterine cavity is systematically scraped. A D&C may also be performed for various therapeutic purposes.

Radiography and ultrasonography

A hysterosalpingogram is a radiological examination performed to visualize the uterine cavity and uterine tubes. The procedure involves taking X-ray films as contrast medium flows through the uterus and uterine tubes.

Ultrasonography involves the generation of high-frequency sound waves that are reflected to a tranducer,

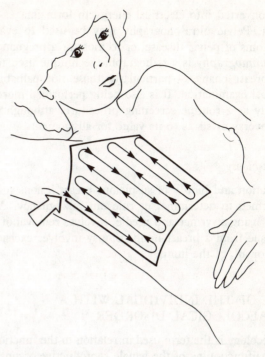

Fig. 49.4 Breast self examination: vertical strip pattern of palpation used. The large arrow indicates the starting point. (Reproduced with permission from Game C, Anderson R E, Kidd J R (eds) 1989 Medical-surgical nursing: a core text. Churchill Livingstone, Melbourne.)

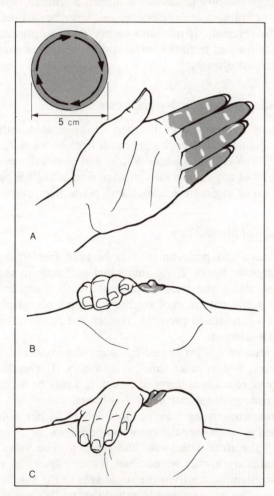

Fig. 49.3 Breast self examination.
(A) Area of fingers and circular movement used for palpation.
(B & C) Both light and firm pressure should be used in palpation.
(Reproduced with permission from Game C, Anderson R E, Kidd J R (eds) 1989 Medical-surgical nursing: a core text. Churchill Livingstone, Melbourne.)

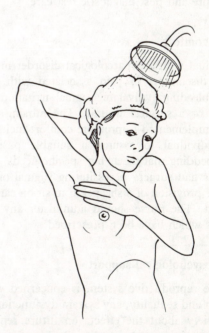

Fig. 49.5 Breast self examination. Small firm breasts can be satisfactorily examined with a soapy hand while standing in the shower with the arm raised on the side being examined. (Reproduced with permission from Game C, Anderson R E, Kidd J R (eds) 1989 Medical-surgical nursing: a core text. Churchill Livingstone, Melbourne.)

and converted into electrical energy to form images on a screen. Pelvic ultrasonography may be used to evaluate symptoms of pelvic disease, or to monitor a pregnancy.

Mammography is a radiographic technique used to detect breast changes—particularly those not palpable on physical examination. It is also being performed more frequently as a routine screening procedure, although some controversy exists as to its value for all women.

Breast biopsy

Aspiration and biopsy of suspicious breast lesions may be performed to determine, or rule out, malignancy. Aspiration, using a syringe and needle, involves removal of fluid or tissue from a breast lump. Biopsy involves excision of part, or all, of the lump.

CARE OF THE INDIVIDUAL WITH A GYNAECOLOGICAL DISORDER

Gynaecology is the term used in relation to the functioning and malfunctioning of the female reproductive organs. Although medical management and nursing care will depend on the specific disorder, the main aims of care are to:

- promote comfort
- provide psychological support
- provide perineal and vaginal care
- meet elimination needs
- provide pre and post diagnostic test care.

Promoting comfort

The individual with a gynaecological disorder may be experiencing discomfort or pain associated with heavy or prolonged bleeding, vulval or vaginal irritation, voiding difficulties, or a surgical wound. The nursing measures which are implemented to promote comfort include assisting the individual to assume a suitable position and providing bedding that meets her specific needs. If the individual has had surgery necessitating vaginal or perineal sutures, the provision of a sheepskin to sit on can enhance her comfort. The nurse should administer any analgesic medications which have been prescribed.

Providing psychological support

Because the reproductive system is concerned with both propagation and sexuality, any system dysfunction may result in anxiety about the effects on future reproductive function, femininity, and sexuality. Such anxiety can have a significant effect on the individual's body image and self concept. Some individuals will experience relief that their problem, e.g. prolonged heavy bleeding, is being rectified. In other cases individuals may experience feelings of grief

that, because of the outcome, they will no longer be able to bear children.

To assist the individual, it is essential that she is provided with adequate information. She should be informed about the physiological effects of the specific disorder, e.g. on menstruation, reproductive ability, and sexual activity. The nurse should reinforce the medical officer's explanation about any implications on the individual's lifestyle, and she should ensure that the information is understood. If gynaecological surgery is necessary, it is essential that the individual is aware of what the surgery involves, e.g. the structures which are to be repaired or removed, and the structures which will remain intact. It is important that the individual is helped to realize that loss of part of the reproductive tract, e.g. removal of the uterus, does not mean loss of femininity or sexuality.

Prior to discharge from hospital, the individual is provided with information which includes the need to continue with specific treatment, whether to expect some vaginal discharge and how to identify abnormal discharge, whether baths or showers are preferable, and when sexual activity may be resumed. It may also be necessary to provide information about fertility control and prevention of sexually transmitted diseases.

Providing perineal and vaginal care

As many gynaecological disorders are associated with vaginal discharge or bleeding, perineal hygiene measures are essential. Measures include vulval and perineal care, assessment of any vaginal loss, management of vaginal packs, insertion of vaginal medication and pelvic floor exercises.

Vulval and perineal care

The vulva and perineum should be kept free of vaginal discharge or blood. If the individual is unable to shower or bath daily, the areas are cleansed with a non-irritant solution and cotton wool swabs. The aims of vulval and perineal care are to promote comfort and healing, and to prevent infection.

Perineal care is performed following elimination of urine or faeces, and at other times as necessary. If vaginal discharge or bleeding is heavy or constant, it may be necessary to provide perineal care every 2–4 hours.

Perineal cleansing may be provided by either pouring warmed solution over the vulva and perineum, or by gently wiping the areas with swabs and solution. The vulva and perineum are always wiped from front to back, to avoid cross-contamination from the rectal area to the vagina and urethra. The areas are gently patted dry, and a clean vulval pad is applied.

Each time perineal care is provided assessment of the perineum is made. The perineum is observed for oedema, inflammation, or bruising. Assessment is also made of any vaginal discharge or bleeding, e.g. amount, character, and the presence of an offensive odour.

To promote comfort, and to assist healing, various topical treatments may be prescribed, e.g. the application of cold or heat to the perineum.

Vaginal creams or medicated pessaries may be prescribed for specific disorders, e.g. to treat infections. If the individual is able, she is instructed how to insert vaginal medications. A nurse may be required to perform the procedure if the individual is dependent. Vaginal medications are inserted using an applicator, and instructions on its use are provided with the medication. Information on vaginal medications is provided in Chapter 58.

A vaginal pack may be inserted, by the medical officer, to control bleeding, to administer medication, or to prevent vaginal adhesions. When a pack is inserted, the amount of packing used is documented.

The pack is generally left in place for 24 hours and, while it is in situ, the nurse assesses the individual for vaginal loss through the pack and for any difficulty experienced with voiding. As removal of a pack generally causes discomfort, a prescribed analgesic medication is administered prior to its removal. After removal of the pack, the amount of packing removed is documented and the individual is assessed for vaginal bleeding or discharge.

Vaginal irrigation, is the instillation of fluid into the vaginal cavity. As repeated irrigation is known to disturb the natural defence mechanism of vaginal acidity, this procedure is prescribed infrequently.

In some societies, vaginal irrigation (douching) is performed as a routine hygiene measure, as a contraceptive measure, or prior to intercourse to alter the vaginal pH—which is thought by some to influence the sex of a baby.

Vaginal irrigation involves suspending a container of solution approximately 30 cm above the pelvis. The container is fitted with tubing and a nozzle. The nozzle is inserted into the vagina, and the fluid is allowed to flow into and out from the vagina. When the irrigation is complete the individual should assume a sitting or standing position, to allow any remaining fluid to drain from the vagina.

Pelvic floor exercises

Pubococcygeal (Kegel) exercises are a regimen of isometric exercises involving a series of voluntary contractions of the pelvic floor muscles and perineum. The exercises are designed to strengthen the pelvic floor muscles, and may be necessary to promote muscle tone, e.g. following specific gynaecological surgery or after menopause. Pelvic floor exercises, if performed regularly, also help to minimize stress incontinence of urine.

The exercise regimen consists of tightening, then relaxing, the muscles surrounding the entrances of the vagina, urethra, and anus. Generally, the muscles should be tightened and held for 5 seconds followed by 15 seconds of relaxation. Alternating tightening and relaxation are repeated several times, at various intervals throughout the day.

Meeting elimination needs

Because of the close proximity of the urinary tract and rectum to the reproductive tract, disorders of the reproductive system may result in problems of elimination, e.g. stress incontinence, retention of urine, or constipation. Information of meeting elimination needs is provided in Chapter 30.

Specific bladder management may include caring for the individual with an indwelling urinary catheter, intermittent catheterization to assess residual urine, and re-establishment of a normal voiding pattern. Following most major gynaecological surgery, e.g. vaginal wall repair, the individual's bladder is continuously drained via an indwelling catheter for 3–5 days to prevent pain, dysuria, distension, and infection. After this time the surgeon may prescribe a regimen whereby the catheter is clamped for 4 hours then released. A schedule of clamping and releasing may be continued for 24–48 hours prior to removal of the catheter. This regimen assists in the re-establishment of normal bladder sensation and function.

Some individuals may experience difficulty voiding after catheter removal, because of oedema and discomfort associated with surgery. Residual urine estimations may be prescribed and made by passing a catheter immediately after the individual has voided—to determine how much urine remains in the bladder. This technique is generally discontinued when the residual urine is less than 100 ml on two consecutive occasions.

Alternatively, a *suprapubic* catheter may be used. The catheter is inserted at the time of surgery, and is not removed until the individual is voiding normally. When the individual is voiding normally, she should be instructed in the 'double-voiding' technique to empty the bladder completely. Once the individual has finished voiding she should remain sitting on the toilet for a few minutes then try to void any urine that has remained in the bladder.

Specific bowel management is directed at preventing constipation. This is generally achieved by providing an adequate fluid and fibre intake, encouraging ambulation, and by administering any prescribed medications, e.g. stool softeners or rectal suppositories.

Other nursing management of an individual with a gynaecological disorder may involve wound care and preventing post operative complications. Information on surgical nursing is provided in Chapter 59.

Providing pre and post diagnostic test care Preparation of the individual for, and care following, diagnostic tests is part of the nurses' role. The nurse must refer to the institution's policy manual for information about preparation of the individual for specific diagnostic tests. Preparation includes a general explanation of the procedure to reinforce the information provided to the individual by the medical officer. Other preparation may include dietary or fluid restriction, administration of prescribed medications, assisting the individual into a specific position, and measurement of baseline vital signs.

Postprocedural care may include assessing vital signs and vaginal loss, measuring and recording fluid input and output, administering prescribed medications, and assessing the individual for untoward signs and symptoms, e.g. abnormal vaginal discharge, abdominal pain, or difficulty with voiding.

CARE OF THE INDIVIDUAL WITH A BREAST DISORDER

This part of the chapter addresses care of the woman who requires breast surgery for malignancy. Any surgical procedure involving the breast can significantly affect body image—depending on the worth the woman places on her breasts as parts of her femininity and sexuality. Benign breast disease may be treated surgically or non-surgically, and may have only a temporary or minor affect on the individual. Malignant breast disease has a devastating impact on the individual.

Breast cancer usually develops in the epithelial breast tissue, more often in the upper outer quadrant. The epithelial cells undergo hyperplasia which may progress to carcinoma in situ and then to invasive carcinoma. Cancer of the breast can spread, via the lymphatic system and bloodstream, to various sites in the body.

Controversy exists over the treatment of breast cancer, and both localized and systemic treatments may be implemented. Treatment may include any, or a combination, of:

- surgery—lumpectomy or mastectomy
- chemotherapy
- radiotherapy
- hormone therapy.

Information on treatment of malignant disease is provided in Chapter 64.

Mastectomy, which is removal of a breast, is one of the more common surgical procedures performed in the treatment of breast cancer. A modified mastectomy involves removal of the entire breast and the axillary lymph nodes.

Prior to surgery, the individual is informed about whether breast reconstruction is a viable option. Breast reconstruction, following a mastectomy, involves the creation of a breast mound and reconstruction of a nipple and areola. It may be performed at the same time as the mastectomy, or several months later. Most surgeons prefer the latter approach, as immediate reconstruction increases the risk of complications and may have a poorer cosmetic result.

Care of the individual undergoing a mastectomy involves pre-operative preparation, emotional support, promotion of comfort, and prevention of complications.

Pre-operative preparation

In addition to pre-operative physical preparation, it is essential that the individual is provided with adequate information and emotional support. Contact with a person who specializes in breast prostheses, and with a woman who has had a mastectomy, provides a valuable opportunity for the individual to discuss the implications of surgery. The individual must be able to discuss all the possible physiological and psychosocial implications, for example:

- loss of functional breast tissue
- decreased movement and oedema of the arm on the affected side
- disfigurement
- fear of death
- difficulty in adapting to altered body image
- relationships and sexuality
- need for a support system
- available breast prostheses.

The individual's partner should, if desired by both, be included in any discussions and decision making. The nurse should provide sufficient opportunities for the individual to express her fears, and to answer any questions. She may need to re-inforce the information provided by others, e.g. the breast prostheses advisor and medical officer.

Breast prostheses are available in a range of styles. Generally a soft light-weight prosthesis is provided while the incision is healing and until all tenderness has dissipated. Commercial breast forms are available from a variety of sources, e.g. large department stores, and the individual may need to view a number of different styles before finding one that best meets her needs.

Post operative care

Physical post operative care includes providing pain relief, promoting comfort, care of the wound, prevention of complications, exercise instruction, and continued emotional support. Information on surgical nursing is provided in Chapter 59.

Exercise instruction

Postmastectomy exercises are commenced immediately after surgery to prevent shortening of muscles, contracture of joints, loss of muscle tone, and to reduce any oedema in the arm on the affected side. Range of motion (ROM) exercises (Fig. 49.6) are performed for short periods, 3 or 4 times daily. The individual is encouraged to resume self

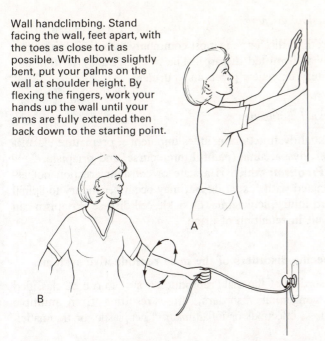

Wall handclimbing. Stand facing the wall, feet apart, with the toes as close to it as possible. With elbows slightly bent, put your palms on the wall at shoulder height. By flexing the fingers, work your hands up the wall until your arms are fully extended then back down to the starting point.

Rope turning. Hold the end of the rope on the affected side, your other hand on hip. With your arm held nearly parallel with the floor turn the rope as wide as possible. Slow at first—speed up later.

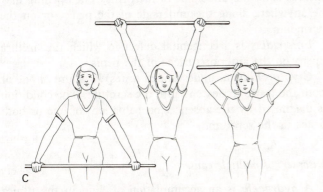

Rod or broom handle. Hold the rod with both hands about 22 cm (2 feet) apart. With arms straight, raise the rod over your head. Bend elbows lowering rod behind your head. Then do the exercise in reverse.

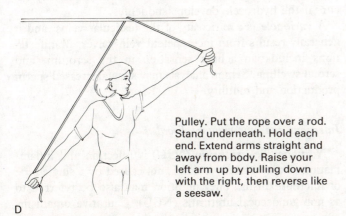

Pulley. Put the rope over a rod. Stand underneath. Hold each end. Extend arms straight and away from body. Raise your left arm up by pulling down with the right, then reverse like a seesaw.

Fig. 49.6 Post mastectomy exercises.

care activities as soon as possible to retain mobility and independence. Most health care institutions provide a leaflet that illustrates a range of postmastectomy exercises, which should be continued after the individual is discharged.

Emotional support

Continued emotional support is vital in the postoperative period. The nurse can, with other support personnel, assist the individual to adjust to her surgery and altered body image. The individual may take several days before she feels able to view the incision, and the nurse must remain sensitive to her feelings. It is important for the nurse to realize that the individual's feelings of grief are a normal response to loss of a body part. As part of dealing with her feelings of loss and anxiety, the individual may utilize a mental defence mechanism, e.g. denial or anger. Information on defence mechanisms is provided in Chapter 6.

The nurse can assist the individual who is coming to terms with the implications of a mastectomy, by ensuring that she undertands the information given to her, and by providing opportunities for her to discuss her anxieties. The individual may also appreciate the opportunity to talk with another woman who has had a mastectomy, and who is able to offer advice and answer questions from first-hand knowledge.

Prior to her discharge from hospital the individual should be given information on the need to continue with exercises, and on any follow-up treatment. She is provided with a temporary breast prosthesis and given information on where to obtain a permanent prosthesis—if one is required. She is also informed about the importance of performing regular breast self examination of the unaffected breast.

DISORDERS OF THE MALE REPRODUCTIVE SYSTEM

This part of the chapter addresses various pathophysiological influences and effects on the male reproductive system, the major manifestation of disorders, specific disorders, diagnostic tests and care of the male with a disorder of the reproductive system.

Pathophysiological influences and effects

Pathophysiological changes may result from structural abnormalities, hormonal disturbances, neoplasms, infection, or trauma. Three of the major effects caused by these changes are disturbed testosterone production, impaired sexual response, and infertility.

Disturbed testosterone production

A disease process that affects the testes generally results in either underproduction or overproduction of the hormone, testosterone. Reduced production of testosterone can result from a variety of disorders including surgical removal of the testes, viral diseases, or a pathological condition of the pituitary gland. Increased production of testosterone can be caused by primary or secondary neoplasms of the testes.

Impaired sexual response

Sexual dysfunction, which includes impotence, premature ejaculation, and dyspareunia, can result from either physiological or psychological causes. Physical factors include low testosterone levels and anatomical abnormalities, spinal cord injury and disease, and systemic disorders such as diabetes mellitus.

Impotence, which is an impairment of erectile function, may be primary or secondary. As the majority of males regard the erectile response as very important, any dysfunction usually causes extreme anxiety.

Premature ejaculation is the inability to exert voluntary control over the timing of the ejaculatory reflex. Although there may be physiological causes, psychological factors usually contribute to premature ejaculation.

Infertility

Many factors can affect the production, transport, or ejaculation of sperm.

Sperm production can be disrupted by hormonal imbalance, congenital abnormality of the testes, infections, high environmental temperatures, and by auto-immune factors.

Transport of sperm through the male reproductive tract can be impeded by adhesions,, structural weaknesses, or obstruction.

Ejaculation of sperm may be impaired by diseases that alter the autonomic response, by psychosexual factors, or by systemic diseases such as diabetes mellitus.

Major manifestations of male reproductive system disorders

The signs and symptoms, which vary according to the type and severity of the disorder, include urinary problems, urethral discharge, and sexual dysfunction.

Urinary problems

The individual may experience alterations in the pattern of urinary elimination, related to urinary tract obstruction and retention, e.g. as a result of a urethral stricture or an enlarged prostate gland. He may experience dysuria, difficulty in initiating or stopping the flow of urine, or acute or chronic retention of urine.

Urethral discharge

Urethral discharge is most commonly associated with sexually transmitted diseases. The discharge may be thin and watery or yellow-green and purulent.

Sexual dysfunction

Sexual dysfunction includes impotence, premature ejaculation, dyspareunia (painful intercourse) and priapism.

Priapism, which is a state of constant erection not associated with sexual desire, may occur secondary to spinal cord injury, leukaemia, or sickle-cell disease. Priapism can result in retention of urine.

Specific disorders of the male reproductive system

Disorders of the male reproductive system can be classified as congenital disorders, those resulting from multiple causes, infectious or inflammatory, neoplastic, or traumatic.

Congenital disorders

Hypospadias is a congenital defect in which the urinary meatus is on the underside of the penis. The opening may be anywhere along the underside of the penis, or on the perineum.

Epispadias is a congenital defect in which the urethra opens on the anterior surface of the penis.

Cryptorchidism (undescended testes) is failure of one or both the testes to descend into the scrotum. The condition is diagnosed by the absence, on palpation, of one or both testes in the scrotum.

Disorders of multiple cause

A hydrocele is an accumulation of fluid in the tunica vaginalis testis. The condition may be associated with an inguinal hernia, or it may occur following infection of or trauma to the scrotum. A hydrocele generally appears as a painless, oblong, soft mass in the scrotum. Pain only occurs if the hydrocele develops suddenly.

A variocele is a varicosity of the testicular veins, and it generally results from incompetent vein valves. Manifestations include an aching sensation in the scrotum, and scrotal swelling. Semen analysis may show decreased sperm production and motility.

Infectious and inflammatory disorders

Non-specific urethritis (NSU) is infection and inflammation of the urethra, which is not caused by a single type of microorganism. The condition may also be referred to as non-gonoccocal urethritis (NGU). Causative organisms include *Chlamydia trachomatis*, and several types of bacteria. Less commonly, NSU may be related to pre-existing urethral strictures, neoplasms, and traumatic inflammation. Manifestations include dysuria, mucopurulent urethral discharge, and occasional haematuria.

Epididymitis, which is inflammation of the epididymis, may be caused by a urinary tract infection, prostatitis, or it may result from a sexually transmitted disease, e.g. chlamydia. Manifestations include unilateral scrotal pain, inflammation and swelling.

Prostatitis, which is inflammation of the prostate gland, generally results from infection. The condition may, or may not, be sexually transmitted. Causative organisms include *Escherichia coli* and *Chlamydia trachomatis*. Manifestations include urethral discomfort, dysuria, urgency and frequency of micturition, retention of urine, suprapubic and perineal pain, and a sensation of rectal fullness. If the condition is acute, the individual will experience the manifestations of a systemic infection.

Gonorrhoea, syphilis, and herpes genitalis are three of the more common sexually transmitted diseases. Information on these disorders is provided earlier in the chapter, and listed in Table 49.1.

Neoplastic disorders

Benign prostatic hyperplasia is an enlargement of the prostate gland. The cause of this condition, which is common among males over the age of 50, is not known. It is not malignant or inflammatory, but is usually progressive and may be related to ageing or to a hormonal mechanism. Manifestations, which are related to increasing obstruction of the urethra, include urinary tract infection, acute urinary retention, hesitancy, frequency, urgency, nocturia, and declining sexual function.

Cancer of the prostate, which represents a significant health problem for males over age 50, is one of the major causes of death from cancer. Manifestations, in the early stages, are similar to those of benign prostatic hyperplasia. Metastasis is common, and metastatic symptoms include low back pain, bone pain, anaemia, and haematuria. Rectal palpation reveals a hard mass.

Cancer of the testes, generally affects males between the ages of 15 and 40. The two main types of testicular cancer are seminomas and non-seminomas. Manifestations, in the early stages, are the presence of a smooth, painless lump in the scrotum. Later metastatic symptoms include general abdominal and inguinal aching. Other metastatic symptoms include bowel or urinary obstruction and abdominal pain.

Cancer of the penis is more likely to affect non-circumcised males over the age of 50, and is thought to be related to poor personal hygiene. Pre-malignant lesions,

Table 49.1 Sexually transmitted diseases

Disease	Causative organism	Manifestations (M/F)
Gonorrhoea	*Neisseria gonorrhoeae*	Asymptomatic in many instances (F) Purulent vaginal discharge (F) Vulval pruritus (F) Dysuria (M) Purulent urethral discharge (M) Low abdominal pain (M&F) Pharyngitis (M&F) Rectal burning (M&F)
Trichomoniasis	*Trichomonas trachomatis*	Profuse thin, foamy, yellow-green offensive vaginal discharge. (F) Vulval pruritus (F) Urethritis, dysuria (M)
Chlamydia	*Chlamydia tracholatis*	Thin, white, bubbly vaginal discharge. (F) Thin, watery urethral discharge (M) Dysuria (M)
Syphilis	*Treponema pallidum*	Primary stage: • chancre (M&F) • regional lymphadenopathy (M&F) Secondary stage: • malaise, headaches, pyrexia (M&F) • inguinal lymphadenopathy (M&F) • generalized non-irritating rash (M&F) • condylomata lata (M&F) • alopecia (M&F) Latent stage: • asymptomatic (M&F) Tertiary stage: • lesions (gummae) on the skin, bone, mucous membranes, upper respiratory tract, stomach, liver (M&F) • cardiovascular manifestations (M&F) • neurological manifestations (M&F)
Herpes genitalis	*Herpes simplex* type 2 (HSV2)	Painful vesicles on the genitals (M&F) Dysuria (M&F) Inguinal lymphadenopathy (M&F) Pyrexia, malaise (M&F)
Condylomata Acuminitata (genital warts)	*Human papillomavirus*	Warts on moist surfaces: • vulva, vagina, cervix (F) • urethral meatus, scrotum, penis, anorectal area (M)

Table 49.1 (cont'd)   Sexually transmitted diseases

Disease	Causative organism	Manifestation (M/F)
Non-specific Genitourinary Infections (including NGU)	*Chlamydia trachomatis* *Haemophilus vaginalis*	Muco-purulent urethral discharge (M&F) Dysuria, haematuria (M&F) Epididymitis (M) Persistent vaginal discharge (F)
Chancroid	*Haemophilus ducreyi*	Papules on penis (M) Papules on vulva, vagina (F) Inguinal adenitis (M&F) Headaches, malaise (M&F)
Lymphogranuloma Venereum	*Chlamydia trachomatis*	Painless lesions on genitals (M&F) Inguinal lymphadenopathy (M&F) Pyrexia, headaches, malaise (M&F) Rectovaginal fistulae (F) Rectal strictures (M&F) Pararectal abscesses (M&F)
AIDS (also transmitted non-sexually)	Human immunodeficiency virus (HIV)	Vary according to classification of HIV infection Manifestations (M&F) include: • extreme and constant fatigue • recurrent pyrexia, nightsweats • rapid weight loss • lymphadenopathy • skin lesions • persistent diarrhoea • persistent or dry cough • diminished appetite • Viral, fungal, bacterial or protozoan infections. • Pneumocystis carinii pneumonia • Kaposi's sarcoma

* M = Male
F = Female

such as leukoplakia and balanitis, may progress to penile cancer. Manifestations include a small circumscribed lesion on the penis and, later, dysuria, pain, haemorrhage, and purulent discharge. Further information on cancer is provided in Chapter 64.

Traumatic disorders

Trauma to the male genitals can result from penetrating or blunt injuries, and from congestion or impairement of circulation to the area. Manifestations include laceration, haemorrhage, pain, and discolouration of the penis or scrotum.

Diagnostic tests

A variety of tests may be performed to assist, or confirm, the diagnosis of disorders of the male reproductive system.

Rectal examination

Rectal examination may be performed in order to palpate the prostate gland. The medical officer inserts a gloved finger into the anus, locates and palpates the prostate gland for size, shape, and firmness. Prostatic massage may be performed to obtain a sample of prostatic secretions for laboratory analysis.

Biopsy

Biopsy of the prostate gland or testes may be performed to detect abnormal cells, e.g. if cancer is suspected. To obtain a specimen from the prostate gland, the medical officer inserts a needle into the perineal skin and aspirates a quantity of prostatic tissue. Testicular biopsy involves incising the scrotal skin so that a specimen of tissue from the testis may be obtained. The specimens of tissue are sent for cytological examination.

Urethral culture

To identify the causative organism of urethritis or infection, the medical officer may obtain a specimen of urethral discharge. A small collecting swab is inserted 3–5 cm into the urethra, rotated gently, and withdrawn. The specimen is sent for laboratory analysis.

Semen analysis

As part of fertility testing, a specimen of semen may be obtained and the sperms examined for motility, morphology, quantity and quality. Semen is collected by requesting the individual to masturbate and ejaculate into a sterile container.

Other diagnostic tests

A series of tests may be performed to evaluate the male urinary tract, e.g. cystoscopy or intravenous pyelogram. A sample of blood may be obtained and tested to assist in the diagnosis of syphilis, prostatic or testicular cancer, or infertility.

Testicular examination

Examination of the tests, particularly self examination, (TSE) is one method of detecting early changes. By examining his own testes regularly, a man is generally able to detect any departure from normal. The earlier any change is detected, the sooner it can be investigated and treated.

Self examination of the testes, which should be done monthly, is best performed after a warm shower or bath when the scrotum is relaxed. The scrotum should first be assessed for any abnormal colour or swelling. Holding the scrotum in the palms of his hands, the individual should then examine each testis by applying the thumb and fingers in a gentle rolling action over the entire surface. He should also palpate the epididymis and the spermatic cord. A normal testis should be firm, but not hard, and should have a smooth regular surface. The testes should be similar in shape, size, and consistency. The epididymis and spermatic cord should feel slightly firm and smooth.

CARE OF THE MALE WITH A REPRODUCTIVE SYSTEM DISORDER

Although medical management and nursing care will depend on the specific disorder, the main aims of care are to:

- promote comfort
- provide psychological support
- meet urinary elimination needs.

Promoting comfort

The individual with a disorder of the reproductive system may be experiencing discomfort or pain associated with scrotal swelling, urethral inflammation, voiding difficulties, or a surgical wound. The nursing measures which are implemented to promote comfort include assisting the individual to assume a suitable position. To relieve any discomfort caused by inflammation and testicular swelling, a support to elevate the scrotum may be provided. The nurse should administer any analgesic medications which have been prescribed.

Providing psychological support

A man with a disorder of the reproductive system may experience anxiety about sexual dysfunction, infertility, and other implications of the disorder. He should be provided with adequate information about the disorder and its possible outcome. He should also be provided with opportunities to express his feelings and, if necessary, he should be referred for sex counselling.

Prior to his discharge from hospital, the individual is provided with information which includes whether some urethral discharge is to be expected, how to identify abnormal discharge, and when sexual activity may be resumed. It may also be necessary to provide information about fertility control and the prevention of sexually transmitted diseases.

Meeting urinary elimination needs

The individual who experiences altered patterns of urinary elimination will need assistance to achieve continent, pain-free, unobstructed urinary flow. Specific bladder management may include caring for the individual with an indwelling urinary catheter, or external urinary drainage appliance, and the re-establishment of a normal voiding pattern. Information on meeting urinary elimination needs is provided in Chapter 30.

FERTILITY CONTROL AND CONTRACEPTION

There are numerous methods of birth control (family planning) available, which act by preventing ovulation, preventing fertilization, or preventing successful implantation and development of a fertilized ovum. An individual who wishes to practise birth control has a responsibility to obtain information about available methods, in order to select one that is appropriate, safe, and effective.

Methods

Birth control methods may be classified as:

- hormonal contraceptives
- intrauterine devices
- mechanical barriers
- chemical barriers
- natural (ovulation)
- sterilization
- abortion.

Table 49.2 lists the types, advantages, and disadvantages of each method.

PREVENTION OF SEXUALLY TRANSMITTED DISEASES

The spread of sexually transmitted diseases (STD) can be reduced if people are aware of the preventive measures to implement. It is important that people are encouraged to discuss STD, to be informed of modes of transmission, and to recognize the manifestations of STD. Only through the dissemination of accurate information will people become aware of the preventive measures required, know that treatment is available, and the importance of seeking medical advice if they contract a sexually transmitted disease.

Transmission

Sexually transmitted diseases are acquired following sexual contact with an infected person. The microorganism that causes *syphilis* is able to pass through the placenta, thus an infected mother can transmit the organism to her unborn

Table 49.2   Methods of birth control

Method	Description	Advantages	Disadvantages/possible side effects
Oral Contraceptives	Consist of a combination of oestrogen and progestogen or progestogen only ('mini pill') Principal function is to inhibit ovulation. Other actions are changing the endometrium so that implantation is unlikely, and altering the composition of cervical mucus	Regular menstruation Reduced menstrual bleeding Reduced menstrual discomfort Continuous contraceptive coverage High level of effectiveness	Nausea weight gain fluid retention breast tenderness break through bleeding mood changes loss of libido Not suitable for women who: • smoke heavily • have a history of thrombo-embolic disease • have malignancy of the breast or reproductive system • have cardiovascular disease
'Morning-after pill'	Combination of oestrogen and progestogen in high doses. Taken as an emergency measure after unprotected intercourse	High level of effectiveness Provides birth control if mechanical barriers failed during intercourse, if unprotected intercourse occured, or if the woman forgot to take a contraceptive pill	Nausea Spotting or bleeding a few days later
Injectable and implanted hormones	Consist of long acting progestogens and oestrogens in injectable or implant form	Offer long-term contraception without frequent intervention or action	Menstrual disturbances Headaches Weight gain Not suitable for women who: • have malignancy of the breast or reproductive system • have a history of abnormal menstrual bleeding
Intrauterine devices	Device which is inserted into the uterus to prevent pregnancy	No disruption of the body's hormonal system High level of effectiveness	Increased menstrual bleeding Abdominal cramps and low back pain May be expelled from the uterus Risk of infection, and subsequent infertility. Risk of ectopic pregnancy in the event of contraceptive failure
Mechanical barrier	Condoms, diaphragms, caps. All provide a barrier between the sperm and ova	Condoms offer protection against STD Do not interfere with the menstrual cycle Used only as required High level of effectiveness Easy to use	Barrier may break or slip out of position May alter feeling and sensitivity during intercourse Possible irritation from the rubber May be considered to affect spontaneity Pregnancy may result if not used correctly
Chemical barriers	Spermicidal preparations in foam, creams, jellies and vaginal suppositories. They block the passage of sperm, and render sperm inactive	Highly effective when used in conjunction with a mechanical barrier. Help to provide vaginal lubrication. Available without prescription	Used alone, without a mechanical barrier, contraceptive failure is high. May result in irritation of mucous membranes
'Natural' methods	Birth control based on abstinence from sexual intercourse during the fertile phase of the menstrual cycle. Methods of calculating the fertile phase: 1. Rhythm/calender 2. Temperature measurement 3. Cervial mucus observation	No disruption to menstrual cycle Safe, easy, and effective if practised correctly	May be considered 'messy' to use All methods require considerable motivation and self-discipline Unreliable if menstrual cycles are irregular Infection may alter temperature pattern. Needs practice to assess cervical mucus variations

Table 49.2 (cont'd)   Methods of birth control

Method	Description	Advantages	Disadvantages/possible side effects
Sterilization	Vasectomy for the male Tubal ligation for the female Both methods are designed to prevent fertilization	Generally effective and safe Does not disrupt the normal menstrual cycle, or sexual feelings	Should be considered as an irreversible process Slight failure rate Minor discomfort after surgery
Abortion	Termination of a pregnancy before the 28th week Methods include: • endometrial aspiration • vacuum extraction • dilatation and curettage • dilatation and evacuation	Controversial	Controversial

infant. The baby may be stillborn, or suffer from a variety of physical and intellectual disabilities. The microorganisms that cause gonorrhoea, herpes genitalis and chlamydia trachomatis may be transmitted to the infant during its passage through the birth canal.

AIDS, caused by HIV, is discussed in Chapter 44. While the incidence of infection is primarily related to sexual transmission, HIV may also be transmitted non-sexually, e.g. via blood or contaminated injection equipment.

Prevention

Prevention of sexually transmitted diseases includes:

• prompt treatment of an infected individual.
• investigation and treatment of those who have had sexual contact with an infected individual.
• advising an infected individual to avoid sexual activity during the infective stage of the disease.
• avoiding sexual contact with a person known to be, or suspected of being, infected.
• using condoms during sexual activity.
• attending to genital hygiene soon after intercourse, e.g. washing with soap and water, and passing urine will rid the areas of many microorganisms.
• encouraging those who engage in sexual activity, with other than reliable sexual partners, to have periodic tests for STD—regardless of other preventive measures employed.
• implementing the recommended blood and secretion precautions as effective infection control measures (refer to Chapter 44 for guidelines).

SUMMARY

The biological function of the female and male reproductive systems is propogation of the species. In addition, the reproductive organs are a means of obtaining sexual pleasure.

The pathophysiological influences and effects of female reproductive system disorders include variations in the menstrual cycle and pelvic pain; while in the male the effects include disturbed testosterone production, impaired sexual response, and infertility.

Major manifestations of disorders of the female reproductive system include pain, bleeding, vaginal discharge, pruritus, urinary problems, and breast changes.

Major manifestations in the male include urinary problems, urethral discharge, and sexual dysfunction.

Disorders of the female or male reproductive system can be classified as congenital, infectious or inflammatory, degenerative, neoplastic, traumatic, and those resulting from multiple causes.

Tests used to assist, or confirm, the diagnosis of female reproductive system disorders include pelvic examination, breast examination; radiography and ultrasonography, biopsy and cytology.

Tests used to assist, or confirm, the diagnosis of male reproductive system disorders include rectal examination, testicular examination, biopsy, and semen analysis.

Care of the individual with a gynaecological disorder includes promoting comfort, providing psychological support, providing perineal and vaginal care, meeting elimination needs, and providing pre and post diagnostic test care.

Care of the individual who requires breast surgery includes providing pre and post operative physical care and psychological support.

Care of the individual with a disorder of the male reproductive system includes promoting comfort, providing psychological support, and meeting urinary elimination needs.

REFERENCES AND FURTHER READING

Chilman A M, Thomas M (eds) 1987 Understanding nursing care, 3rd edn. Churchill Livingstone, Edinburgh
Farrer H 1987 Gynaecological care, 2nd edn. Churchill Livingstone, Melbourne
Game C, Anderson R, Kidd J (eds) 1989 Medical-surgical nursing: a core text. Churchill Livingstone, Melbourne, 644–633, 674–690

50. The individual with a disorder of the eye or ear

INTRODUCTION

Information on the normal structure of the eye and ear is provided in Chapter 27, and it should be referred to before studying the contents of this chapter.

The eyes and ears are two of the major structures by which an individual receives information about the external environment. The eye is the means by which light, reflected from objects, travels to the retina so that an image is formed. Nerve endings in the retina transmit electrical impulses along the optic nerve to the brain for interpretation. The ear is the means by which sound waves are collected and amplified. Nerve endings in the inner ear transmit electrical impulses along the auditory pathways to the brain for interpretation. The auditory system is also responsible for maintenance of balance.

DISORDERS OF THE EYE

Pathophysiological influences and effects

Normal function of the eye can be altered by a variety of pathophysiological factors including those that are congenital, degenerative, infectious, neoplastic, or traumatic. The effects may be mild and temporary, severe, or permanent.

Congenital factors

Eye function may be altered by a variety of conditions that are genetically determined, most of which lead to progressive visual impairment, pain, or blindness. Congenital factors may cause refractive errors, motor anomalies, clouding of the lens or cornea, or optic atrophy. Other abnormalities, although not genetically determined, may be contracted by the fetus in utero, or may be contracted soon after birth. Dysfunction of the eyes and reduced vision are associated with maternal infection, prematurity, and infant oxygen intoxication or deprivation.

Degenerative factors

Degeneration of the eyes is a normal part of the ageing process, or degenerative alteration may occur secondary to disease, e.g. diabetic retinopathy. Degenerative alterations include loss of lens transparency, arteriosclerosis of vessels supplying structures of the eye, and the development of plaques on the cornea. All can affect vision with varying degrees of severity.

Infectious factors

The external eye structures may be infected by bacterial, viral, or fungal microorganisms, while infection of the margin of the eyelid causes a stye. A corneal ulcer may result from bacterial, viral, or fungal infections.

Neoplastic factors

Benign or malignant tumours may occur in the eye, eyelid, or orbit. Tumours may destroy important structures and/or interfere with normal function. Neoplasms may obstruct vision, displace the lens, cause retinal detachment, obstruct the drainage of aqueous humour, or displace the eye.

Traumatic factors

Trauma to the eye may have short or long term effects, depending on the extent and type of injury incurred. Contusions, abrasions, burns, and perforations may all lead to pain, scarring, infection, and impaired vision or blindness.

Protection and preservation of sight

The nurse is in a key position to educate people about the ways by which eyesight can be protected and preserved:

• Regular eye examinations are important, especially for individuals with a family history of eye disorders, and for people who are more vulnerable to ocular complications, e.g. those with diabetes mellitus.
• Examination of the eyes is also recommended if an individual experiences any disturbances of vision, pain, sudden appearance of floaters, photophobia, purulent discharge, trauma to the eye, or pupil irregularities.
• Prevention of eye infection includes washing the hands before touching the eyes; not sharing eye make-up, eye drops or ointment.
• Prevention of injury includes wearing eye protection when working with chemicals, or when the eyes may be exposed to dust, wood, metal, or glass fragments. Protective eye wear should also be worn during recreational or sporting activities in which sticks or balls may contact the eye, e.g. squash. Excessive exposure to strong sunlight or sun lamps should be avoided, as these may damage the eyes. A common form of cataract, which can result from frequent exposure to intense sunlight, can largely be prevented if sun hats and good quality sunglasses are worn.
• Prevention of eye fatigue includes using adequate illumination when reading or writing, resting the eyes often during prolonged use, and reducing screen glare when using a visual display unit (VDU).

Major manifestations of eye disorders

The major manifestations of disorders that affect the eye are changes in vision, pain or discomfort, excessive production of tears or dryness, and discharge.

Changes in vision

Vision changes include blurred or double vision, (diplopia) and decreased or absent vision—all of which may be unilateral or bilateral. The individual may also state that he is experiencing 'halos', which are coloured rings encircling bright lights caused by alteration in the ocular media. Small moving spots or flecks seen before the eye are commonly called 'floaters', and they may be due to the ageing process as the vitreous material degenerates. Floaters may also be caused by retinal lacerations, diabetic neuropathy, or hypertension. Photophobia (an abnormal intolerance to light) may be caused by inflammation of the cornea or the iris and ciliary body.

Pain

Pain or discomfort may range from mild aching, to irritation, to severe pain or sensations of pressure. Pain may be worse at certain times of the day, or it may be aggravated by bright light. Keeping the eyelids closed, e.g. by applying an eye pad, may relieve pain associated with infections, foreign bodies, or corneal injuries. Burning or itching is frequently caused by inflammation of the eyelids or conjunctiva from infection or irritation.

Lacrimation

The excessive production of tears may be caused by irritation of the conjunctiva or cornea, or of the iris by photophobia. Excessive tears can also result from obstruction of the lacrimal drainage system. Dryness of the eyes may be caused by a variety of conditions, e.g. hypofunction of the lacrimal glands, or it may be part of the ageing process.

Discharge

A mucopurulent drainage from the eyes usually indicates a bacterial infection, e.g. conjunctivitis. The drainage may be accompanied by inflammation and crusting of the eyelid margins.

Specific disorders of the eye

Disorders of the eye may be classified as congenital, degenerative, infectious, neoplastic, traumatic, or those resulting from multiple causes.

Congenital disorders

Strabismus is a condition of eye deviation, where the eyes appear to be crossed. Congenital strabismus is an anomaly in which there is a defect in the position and fusion ability of the two eyes. The condition is usually easily observed and, in addition to crossed eyes, the child may squint, tilt the head, or close one eye to improve vision.

Ptosis, drooping of the upper eyelid, may be unilateral or bilateral. Congenital ptosis, results from failure of the levator muscle in the upper eyelid to develop. Manifestations are usually very obvious; the lid appears smooth and flat, and the individual may tilt the head back to compensate if the lid droops over the pupil.

Retinitis pigmentosa is a hereditary disorder which involves the degeneration and clumping of the retinal pigment (primarily the rods). The disorder may be mild, or it may progress to total blindness. Manifestations, which are not generally evident before the age of 10, include night blindness, progression to tunnel vision and, ultimately, blindness.

Corneal dystrophy is the term used to encompass a group of rare hereditary disorders of the cornea. The disorders are characterized by deposits of substances on the cornea, by structural changes, and conical protrusion of the cornea. Manifestations include excessive lacrimation, photophobia, irritation of the eye, pain, cloudy cornea, and increasing visual impairment.

Degenerative disorders

A cataract is a gradually developing opacity of the lens or lens capsule. Cataracts generally develop bilaterally, with each progressing independently—with the exception of congenital and traumatic cataracts. Causes include the ageing process, inflammation, malignancy, metabolic factors, toxins, heredity, and trauma. Manifestations generally begin with painless, gradual blurring and loss of vision. Vision seems poorer in bright light, and double vision may occur. As the cataract progresses, the pupil appears milky white.

Macular degeneration is a condition which occurs because of an abnormality at the level of the retinal pigment epithelium and overlying photoreceptors. The cause is not known. Manifestations include blurred vision, distorted visual acuity, and blindness.

Infectious disorders

A hordeolum (stye) is a localized staphylococcal infection of the follicle of an eyelash, or accessary gland along the eyelid margins. Manifestations include localized inflammation, swelling, and pain.

Blepharitis is inflammation of the eyelid margins. Seborrheic blepharitis results from seborrhoea of the scalp or eyebrows, while ulcerative blepharitis is caused by a *Staphylococcus aureus* infection. Manifestations include itching, burning, redness of the eyelid margins, chronic conjunctivitis, and yellow purulent discharge crusts on the lashes.

Conjunctivitis is inflammation of the conjunctiva. The condition may be caused by exposure to toxins, allergens, chemicals; or it may be caused by bacteria, viruses, or fungi. Manifestations include hyperemia of the conjunctiva, purulent discharge, excessive lacrimation, pain, pruritus, and a scratching or burning sensation. Allergic conjunctivitis may cause considerable swelling.

Trachoma is a chronic form of keratoconjunctivitis, which causes permanent damage to the cornea and, if untreated, it can result in blindness. The condition results from infection by *Chlamydia trachomatis*, and it is associated with poor personal and community hygiene and lack of available clean water. There is a high incidence of trachoma among Australian Aboriginals. Manifestations, which may not become apparent for many years, include the signs and symptoms of a severe conjunctivitis. There is corneal inflammation and scarring, due to inward turning of the eyelids which causes the lashes to rub against the cornea. Severe corneal scarring may result in blindness.

Keratitis is inflammation of the cornea, and it may be complicated by the formation of a corneal ulcer. The condition may be caused by bacteria, viruses, fungi, exposure due to the individual's inability to close the eyelids, chemical or ultraviolet injury. Manifestations include opacity of the cornea, irritation, excessive lacrimation, blurred vision, redness, and photophobia.

Uveitis is inflammation of the uveal tract—the fibrous tunic beneath the sclera that includes the iris, the ciliary body, and the choroid of the eye. The most common form is iritis (acute anterior uveitis). Causes include infection and hypersensitivity reactions. Manifestations include pain, blurred vision, photophobia, redness, and a pupil which is small and irregular.

Orbital cellulitis is an acute infection of the orbital tissues and eyelids, which does not involve the eyeball. The condition is generally secondary to infection of nearby structures. If orbital cellulitis is not treated, the infection may spread to the sinuses or the meninges. Manifestations include unilateral eyelid oedema, inflammation of the orbital tissues and eyelids, pain, impaired eye movement, and purulent discharge from indurated areas.

Neoplastic disorders

Benign or malignant tumours may arise in the tissues surrounding the eye, but neoplasms of the eyeball are rare.

A chalazion is a small localized swelling of the eyelid, resulting from obstruction and retained secretions of the sebaceous glands. Manifestations include a painless, firm lump and, if the chalazion becomes large enough to press on the eyeball, astigmatism (asymetric focus).

A choroidal melanoma is a malignant tumour of the middle layer of the eyeball. The major symptom is visual distortion. There is generally no pain unless glaucoma develops.

Retinoblastoma is a congenital, hereditary neoplasm which develops from retinal germ cells. It is the most common malignancy of the eye in childhood. Manifestations include diminished vision, strabismus, retinal detachment, and an abnormal pupillary reflex. The tumour, which grows rapidly, may invade the brain and metastasize to distant sites.

Traumatic disorders

Abrasions are superficial scratches on the eyelid, conjunctiva, or cornea. Corneal abrasions may be caused by foreign bodies, or overwearing of contact lens. Manifestations include excess lacrimation, pain, a sensation of something in the eye, and photophobia.

Lacerations (cuts) may involve the eyelids or the eyeball. Lacerations of the eyeball may lead to intraocular infection, cataract formation, or loss of vision. Manifestations of a lacerated eyeball include severe pain and shock.

Contusions of the eyeball involves a bruising injury in which intraocular damage occurs. The injury may result in bleeding into the anterior chamber (hyphema) or into the vitreous or surrounding tissues. Contusions generally result from a severe blow to the eye, e.g. from a fist, golf or squash ball. Manifestations include impaired vision pain, bruising of the tissues surrounding the eye, and blood in the anterior chamber.

Foreign bodies may enter the conjunctiva or cornea, or they may penetrate and perforate the eyeball. Examples of foreign bodies that gain entry include eyelashes, dirt, small particles of metal, dust, and glass. Manifestations include irritation, pain, excess lacrimation, and photophobia.

Burns to the eye may result from exposure to chemicals, radiant energy, or high temperatures. The extent of damage to the eye depends on the duration of exposure and the causative agent. Manifestations include extreme pain, excess lacrimation, photophobia, inflammation or destruction of tissue, and visual impairment.

Disorders of multiple cause

Glaucoma is a condition in which the intraocular pressure is abnormally increased so that it causes atrophy of the optic nerve and loss of vision. Glaucoma occurs in various forms: primary open-angle, primary angle-closure, secondary, congenital, and absolute. The condition may be caused by overproduction of aqueous humour, or obstruction to the outflow of aqueous humour—both of which result in accumulation of fluid and a rise in intraocular pressure.

Manifestations of primary open-angle glaucoma are gradual and progressive visual impairment, where the individual is unable to perceive changes in colour, ex-

periences blurred vision and persistent aching of the eyes. Manifestations of primary angle-closed glaucoma occur suddenly. The individual experiences intense pain, loss of vision, nausea and vomiting. The affected eye appears red, and the pupil is fixed, dilated, and unresponsive.

The manifestations of secondary glaucoma are similar to those of the primary form, depending on the cause. Congenital glaucoma is a rare disorder generally associated with other anomalies, and manifests as a large diameter cornea. Absolute glaucoma is the end result of any uncontrolled glaucoma—resulting in blindness.

Retinal detachment is a condition in which the sensory portion of the retina separates from the pigment epithelium of the choroid. The condition is generally unilateral, and may be spontaneous or follow trauma. Predisposing factors include myopia, absence of the lens, and retinal degeneration. Manifestations include the appearance of a 'shadow' or 'curtain' spreading across the field of vision, floaters, blurred vision; and gradual, painless, loss of vision.

Refractive errors are a group of visual problems which includes myopia (nearsightedness), hyperopia (farsightedness), presbyopia (lack of focusing power), and astigmatism (asymmetric focus). Refractive errors may be genetically determined, or be caused by disease or injury. Manifestations include headaches, reduced visual acuity, and ocular discomfort.

Diagnostic tests

Tests used to diagnose eye disorders may be classified as subjective, objective, or special procedures. Subjective tests require oral responses from the individual, that must be interpreted by the examiner. Objective tests are those in which the examiner obtains precise measurements or directly visualizes the interior of the eye.

Subjective eye tests

A visual acuity test evaluates the individual's ability to distinguish the form and detail of an object. In the test, the individual is required to read letters on a chart from a distance of 6 m. Generally, the smaller the symbol the individual can identify, the sharper his visual acuity. Near, or reading, vision may also be tested using standardized charts.

Colour vision tests evaluate the individual's ability to recognize differences in colour. The most common colour vision tests use plates made up of patterns of dots of the primary colours, superimposed on backgrounds of randomly mixed colours. An individual with normal colour vision can identify the patterns.

Accommodation tests evaluate the ability of the eyes to adjust the curvature of the lenses. The examiner may perform this test by questioning the individual concerning his visual acuity, while placing trial lenses before his eyes.

Alternatively the test can be performed using an ophthalmoscope.

Visual field tests evaluate the functions of the retina, optic nerve, and optic pathways. The individual's peripheral and central visual fields are assessed when the examiner moves an object from outside the field into the field, on a radial line, until the individual states that he can see the object. *Tangent screen* examination detects central visual field loss. In this examination, a screen is used and test objects from 1–50 mm in size are placed on the screen. Each eye is individually tested for visualization of the objects.

Objective eye tests

Assessment of intraocular pressure is made using a tonometer. A topical anaesthetic is instilled, and the examiner places the tonometer on the apex of the cornea to determine pressure in the eye. An alternate method involves the use of an 'air-puff' tonometer that does not contact the eye. Tonometry serves as a valuable screening test for early detection of glaucoma and there are attempts to establish tonometry as a routine screening device for people over 40 in Australia.

Ophthalmoscopic examination involves the use of an instrument, the ophthalmoscope, to view the interior structures of the eye. The instrument allows magnified examination of the optic disc, retinal vessels, macula, and retina.

Slit-lamp examination allows the examiner to visualize in detail the anterior segment of the eye. Prior to the examination, dilating eyedrops (mydriatrics) may be instilled. The individual sits, with his chin on a rest and his forehead against a bar attached to a lamp.

Fluorescein staining is a technique whereby staining the eye's surface with dye provides a better view of the anterior portion of the eye. The test is generally performed when conjunctival or corneal abrasions are suspected. Surface defects absorb more dye than normal areas.

Special procedures to assess the eye

Fluorescein angiography involves rapid-sequence photographs of the fundus, following intravenous injection of a contrast medium. Flurescein angiography records the appearance of blood vessels inside the eye.

A culture, to determine the microorganism causing an ocular infection, may be obtained by passing a sterile swab over the conjunctival surface.

Computerized tomography (CT) of the orbit may be used to detect abnormalities, e.g. intraocular foreign bodies, or retinoblastoma. Contrast dye is injected and the eyeball is scanned.

Ocular ultrasonography involves the transmission of high-frequency sound waves through the eye, and measurement of their reflection from ocular structures.

Vetrasonography can identify abnormalities that are undetectable through opthalmoscopy, and may be used to locate intraocular foreign bodies.

CARE OF THE INDIVIDUAL WITH AN EYE DISORDER

While the general care of the individual with a disorder of the eye is directed towards helping him to meet his needs, the three main aspects of care are maintaining a safe environment, assisting the person to make adjustments to any visual impairment, and providing any prescribed local eye care.

Maintaining a safe environment

Any visual impairment or loss renders the individual susceptible to injury, therefore the nurse has a responsibility to protect him from environmental hazards. Some of the hazards to a person with visual impairment or vision loss are hot fluids, a high bed, articles left at floor level, unguarded heaters, and stairways.

The nurse should describe the layout of the ward to the individual and, if he is ambulant, she should encourage him to locate the various pieces of furniture so that he becomes familiar with their position in the room. The signal device must be placed within easy reach, and the individual should be encouraged to seek assistance when ambulating until he becomes oriented to the geography of the environment. Information on the provision of a safe environment and prevention of accidents is provided in Chapter 38.

Assisting the individual to adjust to visual impairment

The individual who is experiencing visual loss, which is either temporary or permanent, needs assistance to adjust to the physical and psychosocial implications. Care of the individual includes encouraging independence in the activities of living, and encouraging him to express his reactions to his visual loss.

The visually impaired person may lose the ability to observe body language and the reading and writing components of communicating. Therefore, it is important that he is helped to communicate effectively. He should be encouraged to express his frustrations at his inability to see other people or objects. Key aspects related to assisting the visually impaired individual include:

● Encouraging as much self-care as possible. The individual who is experiencing recent visual impairment may need assistance until he adjusts to his condition. An individual who has been visually impaired for some time will probably have developed considerable self reliance. The nurse should always consult the individual when she is uncertain whether assistance is required.

• Addressing him by name before reaching the bedside and before he is touched, to avoid frightening him.

• Identifying yourself, visitors or others in the room. It is more helpful to tell the individual who is there, rather than to expect him to guess from the sound of a voice. It is also useful to knock before entering, and inform him when you are about to leave the room.

• Speaking to him in the same manner as you would to a fully sighted person. The nurse must suppress the urge to speak more loudly than usual, which people often do when conversing with a visually impaired person. There is no need to exclude words such as 'look' and 'see' from normal conversation. He should be encouraged to maintain an interest in the outside environment through listening to a radio or television, and by discussing newspaper items. The individual may need to be reminded of the day, date, and time.

• Providing full descriptions of people, places, and things. It is of particular importance to thoroughly explain any procedure or treatment before it is commenced. Whenever possible, e.g. if it will not affect sterility, the individual should be allowed to feel any items to be used during a procedure.

• Leaving the furniture and his personal belongings in the same position in the room or, if anything is moved, explaining where it has been moved.

• Ensuring that any doors are either fully closed or open, as a visually impaired person can easily injure himself if a door is left ajar.

• Informing him when he is approaching stairs or steps, remembering to let him know whether they are leading up or down.

• Encouraging him to use handrails while he is ambulating or in the bathroom or toilet. When walking with the individual, the nurse should let him take her elbow and walk slightly ahead of him. This technique enables the individual to sense the direction in which he is walking. He should not be held and 'pushed' in the desired direction. The nurse should warn him of hazards, e.g. articles on the floor, as they are approached.

• Being aware of the community resources available to people with partial or total loss of vision, and of the rehabilitation programmes which help them to perform the activities of living.

Table 50.1 describes various aids which are available to assist the visually impaired.

Local eye care

Various nursing procedures involving the eye should be performed in accordance with the policies of the health care institution. The general principles which should be followed in all ophthalmic procedures include:

Table 50.1 Aids for the visually impaired

Aid	Description
Magnifiers	Hand held or standing magnifiers can be used to enlarge print, or for fine detail
Enlarged print	Large print books, magazines, and newspapers may be borrowed from the local library
Talking books	Tapes of books may be available on loan from agencies for the blind or public libraries
Telephone aids	Special dials are available for telephones in both large print and braille
Braille	The braille system of writing and printing uses tangible points or dots, which the individual feels and 'reads' with his fingers
Optical-to-tactile converters	Consist of devices which convert vision into tactile sensation, by reproducing the outline of a letter on a tactile screen
Canes	A variety of canes are available, e.g. a white or collapsible cane which helps the individual to locate obstacles in the environment. Laser canes also locate objects and can identify changes in the region as far away as 6 metres
Guide dogs	Trained dogs allow greater mobility and independence for the visually impaired person. The individual holds a U-shaped handle which is attached to a harness on the dog. Communication between the two takes place through the movements of the harness. When a guide dog is working, i.e. when it is in harness, other people should not approach or pat the dog without the handler's permission—as the dog may become distracted

• Explaining what you are going to do.

• Ensuring that the individual is sitting or lying with his head well supported.

• Ensuring that there is adequate lighting.

• Washing the hands thoroughly before and after the procedure, to prevent cross infection.

• Using gentle, unhurried movements and refraining from exerting any pressure on the eye. Avoid all sudden movements.

• Avoiding touching the cornea with the fingers or equipment, to prevent corneal damage.

• Using aseptic technique. When only one eye is infected or inflamed, the unaffected eye must receive attention first to prevent cross infection.

• Ensuring that, if an eye pad is to be applied, the eyelid is closed firmly to avoid corneal abrasion.

The application of pads and shields

A light eye pad may be applied to prevent further injury after trauma to the eye, or to avoid eye damage after administration of a local anaesthetic. A pressure pad may be applied to control postoperative oedema, or haemorrhage. If pressure is required, two or three pads may be applied. The eye may be further protected by the application of a rigid cone or shield which is placed over the eye pad. The cone or shield rests on the bony prominences of the brow, cheek, and nose, and it is secured in position with hypoallergenic tape.

Before the eye pad is applied, the individual is asked to close his eyelid firmly. The pad should be applied so that the eyelid cannot be opened. Pressure should not be applied unless it has been prescribed by the medical officer. The eye pad is secured in position using hypoallergenic tape, placing the tape diagonally from forehead to cheek.

Cleansing the eyelids

It may be necessary to cleanse the eyelids before applying a compress, before removing or inserting an artificial eye, before instilling drops or ointment, or to remove discharge from the margins of the eyelids. A technique of eyelid cleansing is outlined in the following guidelines. Equipment required:

— sterile cottonwool swabs
— sterile receiver, e.g. kidney dish
— sterile bowl of solution, e.g. sodium chloride 0.9% warmed to body temperature
— paper bag for soiled swabs.

Eye irrigation

Irrigation is a technique performed to flush secretions, chemicals, or foreign bodies from the conjunctival sac. Chemical injuries to the eye require flushing the conjunctival sac with *copious* amounts of solution. It may be necessary to cleanse the eyelids prior to irrigation, e.g. if there is excessive discharge or crusting. A technique of eye irrigation is outlined in the following guidelines. Equipment required:

— sterile undine or prepacked eye wash supplied in a disposable container
— receiver, e.g. kidney dish
— sterile cottonwool swabs
— container of solution, e.g. sodium chloride 0.9% warmed to body temperature
— paper bag for soiled swabs
— towel.

Guidelines for cleansing the eyelids

Nursing action	Rationale
1. Explain the procedure and ensure privacy	Reduces anxiety
2. Starting with the least affected eye, assist the individual into a recumbent position, with the head tilted towards that side	Minimizes the risk of accidental infection from the other eye. Facilitates performance of the procedure
3. Place the equipment in a convenient location, and ensure adequate lighting	Facilitates performance
4. Wash and dry hands thoroughly	Prevents cross infection
5. Place the kidney dish beside the individual's cheek	Provides a receiver for excess lotion, and used swabs
6. Moisten a swab with the solution and begin to cleanse the lids. Using each swab only once, swab the eyelids from the inner to the outer canthus. Use swabs to gently dry the eyelids	Reduces the risk of solution entering the lacrimal duct, or contaminating the other eye
7. Discard each swab into the receiver immediately after use	Prevents cross infection
8. If necessary, cleanse the lids of the other eye, after repositioning the head	Both eyes may need treatment
9. Assist the individual into position	Promotes comfort
10. Remove and attend to the equipment appropriately. Wash and dry hands	Promotes comfort
11. Report and document the procedure	Appropriate care can be planned and implemented

Guidelines for eye irrigation

Nursing action	Rationale
1. Explain the procedure and ensure privacy	Reduces anxiety
2. Assist the individual into a recumbent position, with the head tilted towards the affected side	Solution will flow away from the inner canthus, and will not flow across the bridge of the nose into the other eye
3. Place the towel under the head on the affected side and across the neck. Place kidney dish against his cheek, and request him to hold it in position	Prevents solution from flowing down the neck
4. Wash and dry hands thoroughly	Prevents cross infection
5. Pour irrigating solution into the undine or open the container of eye wash. Gently hold the eyelid open with one hand	The individual will instinctively try to close the eye
6. Hold the spout of the undine or the container 2.5 cm away from the eye	If the undine is held too high, fluid will flow at increased pressure causing discomfort and possible damage to the eye
7. Pour a little of the solution over his cheek first	Accustoms him to the feel of the solution
8. Direct the flow of solution towards the inner canthus	Because the head is tilted, the stream of irrigating solution will flow over the eyeball from the inner to outer canthus
9. Avoid directing the stream forcefully onto the eyeball, and avoid touching the eye's structures	Prevents discomfort and damage to the eye
10. Request the individual to move his eye in all directions while the irrigation is proceeding	Facilitates flow of solution over all parts of the conjunctival sac
11. When the irrigation has been completed, gently dry the eyelids, with a swab. Dry the individual's face. Assist him into position	Promotes comfort
12. Remove and attend to the equipment appropriately. Wash and dry hands	Prevents cross infection
13. Report and document the procedure	Appropriate care can be planned and implemented

Instillation of drops and ointment

Eye drops or ointment which may be prescribed include those that combat infection, dilate or constrict the pupil, act as a local anaesthetic, stain the cornea, reduce inflammation, or reduce intraocular pressure. Eye drops or ointment are instilled only when they have been prescribed by a medical officer, and the nurse who is instilling them must follow the nursing regulations and policies regarding administration of medications. Key aspects regarding the use of ophthalmic medications include:

• Ensuring that a registered nurse checks the name, strength, and amount of drops or ointment to be instilled. She must also check, with the nurse, the time and frequency of administration and into which eye the medication is to be instilled. The expiry date on the container must also be checked, and the medication is discarded if the expiry date has passed.
• Ensuring that a separate container of drops or ointment is supplied for each individual. Single dose packaging is

preferred, as contamination of the medication is likely to occur if the container is used repeatedly.
• Using the container correctly. To prevent cross infection eye drops are supplied in a squeeze bottle with a nozzle top through which the drops are delivered.

A technique of instilling eye drops and ointment is outlined to the following guidelines. Equipment required:

— prescribed drops or ointment
— 2 or 3 cottonwool swabs
— paper bag for used swabs
— sterile eye pad if required.

Applying heat to the eye

Heat may be applied to the eye to relieve pain, and to promote circulation of blood to the area in the treatment of conditions such as conjunctivitis or hordeolum. Heat may be applied either by hot spoon bathing or by using an electric eye heater.

Guidelines for instilling eye drops or ointment **Nursing action**	**Rationale**
1. Explain the procedure and ensure privacy	Reduces anxiety
2. Help the individual to assume a position with his head tilted well back	Facilitates correct placement of the medication
3. Wash and dry hands thoroughly	Prevents cross infection
4. Gently pull down the lower lid to form a pouch	Facilitates correct placement of medication
5. Remove the cap of the container, and hold the dropper or tube slightly away from the eye	Avoids contacting any part of the eye with the nozzle
6. If drops are being instilled, the prescribed number are dropped into the pouch of the lower lid	Medications must be inserted correctly, i.e. into the pouch of the lower lid, not directly onto the eyeball
If ointment is being instilled, the first 1.25 cm is discarded into a swab. Directing the nozzle of the tube near the lid, a ribbon of ointment is squeezed into the pouch of the lower lid	Reduces risk of introducing contaminated ointment
7. Request the individual to gently close the eyelid Wipe away any excess with a cottonwool swab Request him to blink gently several times	Facilitates distribution of the medication over the eye's surface
8. Apply an eye pad if required	A pad may be prescribed for comfort or protection
9. Attend to the individual's position	Promotes comfort
10. Remove and attend to the equipment appropriately. Wash and dry hands	Prevents cross infection
11. Report and document the procedure	Appropriate care can be planned and implemented

1. Hot spoon bathing involves the use of a wooden spoon. The concave surface of the bowl of the spoon is padded with cottonwool, which is secured firmly in position with a gauze bandage. The padded end of the spoon is placed in a jug, which is supported in a bowl, and boiling water poured into the jug. The individual is assisted to sit in an upright position, and he is instructed to lean toward the steam. He holds the handle of the spoon and, keeping his eyelids closed, brings the hot padded end of the spoon close to the affected eye. The spoon is replaced in the jug to reheat it, and the technique is repeated for approximately 15 minutes.

2. The eye heater consists of a small oval electric pad containing an element, which is positioned between the cottonwool layers of an eye pad. The pad is secured over the eye, and the electric pad is connected to a transformer. The dial on the transformer is regulated to supply the degree of heat to suit the individual. Heat is generally applied for 15 minutes at a time.

Eye prostheses

Two types of eye prosthesis are contact lenses and the artificial eye.

A contact lens is a small plastic disc that is positioned on the cornea and is held in place by surface tension. Contact lenses may be worn in place of glasses by an individual who has a refractive error, e.g. astigmatism. There are a variety of lenses available including the hard, soft, gaspermeable, and extended-wear lens. Contact lenses require care to prevent corneal damage and eye infection. Care includes:

- Cleansing with a surfactant cleaner, which is rubbed on the lens daily and rinsed off with water.
- Soaking in a chemical disinfectant when the lens is not in the eye, i.e. overnight. The disinfectant solution is changed each time the container is used. Before the lens is reinserted all traces of disinfectant must be rinsed off.
- Wetting with contact lens solution prior to insertion, to minimize any initial discomfort.
- Washing and drying the hands before inserting or removing a lens.
- Using only the recommended solutions for cleaning, soaking, and storage of the lens.
- Removing the lens before sleeping or swimming.

Table 50.2 describes the insertion and removal of a contact lens.

An artificial eye (prosthesis) may be inserted following the surgical removal of an eye. A temporary shell (conformer) is inserted into the socket until an artificial eye is available. The individual is educated how to remove, clean, and replace the temporary prosthesis. An artificial eye may be removed, the socket cleaned, and the eye replaced. Alternatively the prosthesis may remain in the socket permanently. When a prosthesis is removed from the

Table 50.2 Inserting and removing a contact lens

Insertion	Removal
1. The hands are washed and dried	1. The hands are washed and dried
2. The lens is placed on the tip of of an index finger	2. With the individual looking up, the lens is slid down off the pupil with an index finger
3. The lids are held apart with the other hand	3. The lens is gently squeezed with the thumb and index finger, and lifted off the eye
4. With the individual looking straight ahead, the lens is placed over the cornea	*Alternatively* the lens is removed using a small rubber suction extractor
5. Releasing both eyelids, the individual blinks to centre the lens over the pupil	

Table 50.3 Inserting and removing an artificial eye

Insertion	Removal
1. The hands are washed and dried	1. The hands are washed and dried
2. The socket is cleansed with warm sodium chloride 0.9% solution	2. The individual assumes a a comfortable sitting or lying position
3. The prosthesis is moistened	3. With the individual looking up, the lower lid is gently drawn down. The lower lid is depressed with an index finger to raise the edge of the prosthesis
4. With the individual looking up, the prosthesis is inserted under the upper lid	4. With the individual looking down, the prosthesis is expelled from beneath the upper lid
5. The lower lid is pulled down until the prosthesis slips in behind the lid to rest in the lower fornix	5. The prosthesis is grasped between the thumb and index finger, and lifted out
6. The individual blinks gently, and a check is made to ensure correct position of the prosthesis	

socket it is placed in clean water or sodium chloride. Table 50.3 describes the insertion and removal of an artificial eye.

DISORDERS OF THE EAR

Pathophysiological influences and effects

Normal function of the ear can be altered by a variety of pathophysiological factors including those that are congenital, degenerative, infectious, obstructive, neoplastic, or traumatic.

Congenital factors

Congenital alterations, which may either be hereditary or acquired, include structural malformations which can lead to hearing loss or deafness, disorders resulting from maternal infection during pregnancy, trauma incurred during pregnancy or delivery, and prematurity.

Degenerative factors

Degenerative changes in the bones and joints of the ossicles can result in conductive hearing loss, while narrowing of blood vessels to the inner ear can result tin tinnitus, vertigo, or hearing loss.

Gradual sensorineural hearing loss can result from a decrease in the number of hair cells and nerve fibres in the auditory system as a consequence of the ageing process.

Infectious factors

Microorganisms can cause external, middle, or inner ear infections; all of which can result in pain and varying degrees of conductive hearing loss.

Obstructive factors

Obstruction of the auditory system, which may result in conductive or sensorineural hearing loss, include impacted cerumen, foreign bodies, oedema, and neoplasms. An obstruction can impede the passage of sound waves, cause an imbalance of pressure on either side of the tympanic membrane, or it may disrupt the transmission of sound to the inner ear.

Neoplastic factors

Neoplasms, which may be benign or malignant, can affect the external, middle, or inner ear. The effects of a neoplasm include pain, discharge, vertigo, tinnitus, and hearing loss.

Traumatic factors

Trauma to the external ear includes bruising, lacerations, and frostbite. Trauma to the head can result in fractures of the temporal bone, dislocation of the ossicles, rupture of the tympanic membrane, and damage to the auditory nerve. Trauma can lead to vertigo, tinnitus, nystagmus, pain, bleeding, and hearing loss. Hearing loss can also result from sudden exposure to a loud explosive sound, or from continued exposure to loud noise.

Protection of the ear and hearing

The nurse is in a key position to educate people about the ways by which hearing can be protected and preserved:

• Regular hearing examinations are important for the early detection of hearing problems, especially for children whose ability to learn can be impaired by hearing defects. Evaluation of hearing is also important for elderly persons, because the ageing process is commonly accompanied by degenerative ear changes.

• Prevention of trauma to the ears includes teaching people never to put small or sharp objects into their ears. Excessive cleaning of the ear canal is contraindicated, as it removes the cerumen which has a protective function.

• Protection of the ears from contamination by water, when swimming or diving, is particularly important if the individual has experienced ear infections.

• Adequate treatment of infections which could involve the ear, e.g. upper respiratory tract infections.

• Protecting the ears from damage by noise. Prolonged exposure to noise levels greater than 85–90 decibels causes cochlear damage. People working in areas of high noise levels should wear protective ear plugs or muffs. Exposure to loud volume from live music, stereo equipment, and headphones should be avoided.

Major manifestations of ear disorders

The major manifestations of ear disorders are pain, discharge, tinnitus, vertigo, nystagmus and hearing loss.

Pain

Earache (otalgia) is a common manifestation of many ear disorders. Middle ear pain, associated with otitis media, is often described as deep seated and throbbing. If the external ear is infected or inflamed the individual may experience pain and tenderness. Earache may also be referred from other parts of the body via various cervical or cranial nerves, e.g. as occurs with tonsillitis.

Discharge

Discharge from the ear (otorrhoea) is generally associated with infections of the middle ear. Purulent, or haemopurulent, discharge may drain from the middle ear through a perforated tympanic membrane. Otitis externa may be accompanied by profuse discharge and irritation of the pinna.

Tinnitus

Tinnitus, which may be constant or intermittent, describes a noise in the inner ear. The noises, such as ringing, hissing, buzzing, roaring, are due to irritation of hair cells in the organ of corti. Causes include pressure from cerumen on the tympanic membrane, pharyngotympanic tube obstruction, otitis media, otosclerosis, Meniere's syndrome, and tumours.

Vertigo

Vertigo is a sensation of spinning. The individual may feel as if his head is spinning or as if the room is spinning around him. Causes of vertigo include trauma, tumours, inflammation, degeneration of the maculae in the inner ear, Meniere's syndrome, and pharyngotympanic tube obstruction.

Nystagmus

Nystagmus is involuntary, rhythmic movements of the eyes. The movements may be horizontal, vertical, rotary, or mixed. Jerking nystagmus, characterized by faster movements in one direction than in the opposite direction, may be a manifestation of certain disorders of the inner ear, although it can be caused by other factors such as neurological disorders. Nystagmus may also be induced by introducing cold or warm water into the external auditory canal.

Hearing loss

Impaired hearing, or deafness, may be conductive, sensorineural, or a combination of both types.

Conductive hearing loss results from disturbances of the sound transmission mechanism of the external or middle ear, which prevents sound waves from reaching the inner ear. Conductive hearing loss, or deafness, can result from impacted cerumen, foreign body in the ear canal, middle ear infection, ruptured tympanic membrane, otosclerosis, pharyngotympanic tube obstruction, neoplasms, or barotrauma (injury due to pressure).

Sensorineural (perceptive or nerve) hearing loss results from disturbances of the inner ear neural structures, or nerve pathways leading to the brainstem. Sensorineural hearing loss, or deafness, can result from hereditary or genetic factors, acoustic trauma, infection, neoplasms such as acoustic neuroma, advanced otosclerosis, haemorrhage or thrombosis of the cochlear vessels, and Meniere's syndrome.

Mixed-type hearing loss results from disturbances in both the conductive and nerve mechanisms.

Specific disorders of the ear

Disorders of the ear and auditory system may be classified as congenital, degenerative, infectious, neoplastic, traumatic, and those resulting from multiple causes.

Congenital disorders

Congenital disorders may be caused by a genetic defect, or may result from prenatal trauma or toxicity. Some of the disorders affect the cosmetic appearance only, while others may result in varying degrees of hearing loss. Congenital disorders include partial or total absence of the external ear (atresia), protruding ears, fused or absent ossicles, and malformation of the cochlea.

Degenerative disorders

Presbycusis is a slowly progressive, bilateral hearing loss as a result of the physiological changes of ageing. It results from a loss of hair cells in the organ or corti, and causes sensorineural hearing loss, usually of high-frequency tones. Manifestations include gradual progressive hearing loss which may be accompanied by tinnitus and dizziness, depression or irritability.

Infectious disorders

Otitis externa, which may be acute or chronic, is inflammation of the external ear canal and auricle. The most common causative organism is *Streptococcus pyogenes*, although *Proteus vulgaris*, *Staphyloccocus aureus*, *Candida albicans*, and *Aspergillus niger* may be responsible for infection. Predisposing factors include swimming in contaminated water, abrasion of the ear canal from inserting sharp or small objects to clean the ear, exposure to irritants, and constant use of earphones or ear plugs. Manifestations include otalgia which is exacerbated on chewing or opening the mouth, lymphadenopathy, pyrexia, regional cellulitis, offensive smelling discharge, pruritus, and partial hearing loss.

Otitis media, which may be acute or chronic, is inflammation of the middle ear. Causative organisms include *Haemophilus influenzae*, *Pneumococcus*, and *Beta-haemolytic streptococcus*. Predisposing factors include the wider, shorter, more horizontal pharyngotympanic tube in infants and children; anatomical abnormalities such as cleft palate, and respiratory tract infection. Manifestations include severe otalgia, pyrexia, hearing loss, dizziness, nausea and vomiting. If the tympanic membrane ruptures, there is often purulent discharge from the ear canal.

Serous otitis media, is an accumulation of serous fluid within the middle ear. The condition results from obstruction of the pharyngotympanic tube, viral infection, or allergy. Manifestations are minor, and the adult may experience a feeling of fullness or bubbling in the ear. Generally the disorder causes no pain.

Mastoiditis, which may occur following otitis media, is infection and inflammation of the air cells of the mastoid antrum. Predisposing factors include chronic otitis media, and untreated acute otitis media. Manifestations include aching and tenderness in the area of the mastoid process, swelling behind the ear, pyrexia, and purulent discharge from the ear canal.

Neoplastic disorders

A cholesteatoma is an ingrowth of epidermis from the external meatus into the middle ear. It may be congenital, primary, or secondary. Epidermis in the middle ear produces keratin, which accumulates and destroys underlying tissue. The condition may be asymptomatic, or the individual may experience conductive hearing loss in the affected ear. If secondary infection develops, there is an offensive-smelling discharge from the ear.

An acoustic neuroma is a benign tumour arising from the VIII cranial nerve, and occurring within the internal auditory canal. As the tumour grows the cochlear branch of the VIII cranial nerve becomes involved. Manifestations include tinnitus followed by an increasing high-frequency hearing loss. As the tumour increases in size, symptoms of other cranial nerve involvement occur, e.g. trigeminal pain and loss of taste in part of the tongue. Nystagmus and ataxia may occur.

Traumatic disorders

The external ear, because of its vulnerable position, may sustain abrasion of the canal, burns, or contusions of the pinna. Foreign bodies may be inserted into the canal and become lodged, or insects may fly into the ear causing great irritation.

A perforated tympanic membrane may be caused by a variety of factors such as the introduction of a sharp object to clean the canal, unskilled irrigation of the auditory canal, middle ear infection, trauma to the head, or sudden exposure to loud noise. Most traumatic perforations heal spontaneously, but a perforated tympanic membrane results in scarring and renders the individual susceptible to chronic ear infections and hearing loss. Manifestations include sudden severe pain inside the ear, loss of hearing, tinnitus, and bleeding.

Barotrauma is injury caused by changes of air pressure to the walls of the pharyngotympanic tube and mucous membrane of the middle ear. It is caused by failure of the pharyngotympanic tube to open sufficiently, resulting in unequal pressure between the middle ear and the atmospheric pressure. It may occur during 'take-off' or landing in planes or deep-sea diving. Manifestations include severe pain, decreased hearing, tinnitus, and vertigo.

Noise-induced hearing loss is a condition which develops gradually as a result of continued exposure to environmental or industrial noise at or above 85 decibels. *Acoustic trauma* is sudden hearing loss from brief exposure to a high-intensity sound at close range, e.g. gunshots. Manifestations of noise trauma include hearing loss, tinnitus, and a feeling of fullness within the ear.

Ototoxicity is a toxic reaction to medications or chemicals that can damage the auditory and/or vestibular system.

Auditory damage may be permanent, whereas vestibular damage may be reversed after the drug therapy is discontinued. A variety of substances may result in ototoxic reactions, e.g. diuretics, alcohol, lead, carbon monoxide, aspirin, and antibiotics. Manifestations include bilateral hearing loss, tinnitus, vertigo, and ataxia.

Disorders of multiple cause

Otosclerosis is a disorder whereby the spongy temporal bone becomes a dense sclerotic mass, eventually immobilizing the stapedial footplate and causing a conductive hearing loss. Although no definite cause has been identified, heredity is a significant factor. Females have a higher incidence of the disorder than males. Manifestations are a slowly progressive, bilateral conductive hearing loss, and mild tinnitus.

Meniere's syndrome is a disorder of the inner ear that results from overproduction or decreased absorption of endolymph. The resulting dilation of the membranous labyrinth can progress to herniation and rupture. Manifestations are exacerbations and remissions of three symptoms; vertigo, tinnitus, and sensorineural hearing loss. During an acute episode the individual may experience nausea and vomiting, sweating, giddiness, nystagmus, and ataxia.

Diagnostic tests

Tests used to assist in the diagnosis of ear disorders assess auditory or vestibular function.

Auditory tests

Otoscopic examination is the direct visualization of the external auditory canal and the tympanic membrane, through an otoscope (auroscope). Otoscopy is performed to detect foreign bodies or cerumen in the external canal, or to detect external and middle ear pathology.

Tuning fork tests detect hearing loss and provide information as to its type.

1. The Weber test determines whether the individual lateralizes the tone of the tuning fork to one ear.
2. The Rinne test evaluates air and bone conduction in both ears.
3. The Schwabach test compares the individual's bone conduction response with that of the examiner, who is assumed to have normal hearing.

Pure tone audiometry tests each ear separately for air conduction, via earphones, and bone conduction via a vibrator placed on the mastoid bone. The faintest point at which the individual hears the tone is called the hearing threshold level. Comparison of air and bone thresholds can suggest a conductive, sensorineural, or mixed-type hearing loss.

Speech audiometry tests the individual's ability to understand and discriminate sounds. Two-syllable words are presented through earphones, to measure how loud speech must be before it is heard.

Speech discrimination testing measures the individual's ability to distinguish phonetic elements of speech, and thus understand what is heard. The examiner presents one-syllable words through earphones.

Impedence audiometry evaluates middle ear function by measuring the flow of sound energy into the ear, and the resistance to that flow. The objective is to determine the resistance (impedence) or flexibility (compliance) of the tympanic membrane to sound.

Vestibular tests

Electronystagmography (ENG) evaluates vestibular function, by measuring the effect of the semicircular canals on the ocular muscles. Electrodes are positioned at precise points on the face and eye movements, in response to specific stimuli, are recorded on a graph.

Caloric tests compare the nystagmus produced by warm and cold stimulation in each ear. Each ear is irrigated with water to stimulate mild vertigo, and nystagmus. No response indicates that the labyrinth is nonfunctional.

Other tests used to diagnose ear disorders include cultures of secretions to detect the source of an infection, and radiological examination of the temporal bone.

CARE OF THE INDIVIDUAL WITH AN EAR DISORDER

While the general care of the individual with a disorder of the ear is directed towards helping him to meet his needs, the three main aspects of care are maintaining a safe environment, assisting the person to make adjustments to any loss of hearing, and providing any prescribed local ear care.

Maintaining a safe environment

Any hearing impairment renders the individual susceptible to accidents and injury. Those with vestibular disorders are at risk of losing balance and falling. Information on providing a safe environment is provided in Chapter 38.

Assisting the individual to adjust to hearing loss

The individual who is experiencing hearing loss, which is either temporary or permanent, needs assistance to adjust to the physical and psychosocial implications. The main way to assist the individual with impaired hearing is to maintain and improve communication. He should be encouraged to express his frustrations at his inability to hear sounds. Key aspects related to assisting the hearing impaired individual include:

• Attracting his attention before speaking to him.
• Standing directly in front of him, and in the light. This enables the individual to see facial expressions, body gestures, and to read lips. Avoid covering your mouth while speaking to him.
• Employing non-verbal cues to help convey the meaning of your conversation, e.g. facial expressions, hand gestures, pointing, writing.
• Allowing the individual time to insert or adjust any hearing aid before you speak.
• Speaking clearly and more slowly than usual. Avoid exaggerated lip movements and shouting. Shouting distorts sound, and is painful to the wearer of a hearing aid.
• Rephrasing your words if the individual has not understood. You may need to use different words to restate the message, as some words are more easily understood than others. It may be helpful to write out the message if you remain uncertain whether he has understood you.
• Encouraging the hearing impaired individual who has a speech disorder to communicate verbally. If you do not understand his communication, do not pretend to have done so. He should be encouraged to repeat himself, or to use other words and gestures to get his message across.
• Using items which are available from organizations such as the Deafness Foundation. Such organizations provide packaged kits to health care institutions, designed to assist hearing impaired individuals and the staff. The kit generally includes adhesive stickers, discs, cards, and information sheets. The adhesive stickers should be placed on all documents related to the individual's care, as they alert staff that he has special needs of which they should be aware. A disc or card is available for placing on the head of the bed, again to remind other people that the individual has a hearing impairment. The kit generally includes a small plastic card designed to allow the hearing impaired individual to easily, and discreetly, identify his disability to others. The reverse of the card provides advice on how others can assist the hearing impaired individual.
• Being aware of the community resources available to people with partial or total loss of hearing, and of the rehabilitation programmes which help them to perform the activities of living.

Table 50.4 describes various aids which are available to assist the hearing impaired person.

Hearing aid care

Hearing aids are delicate and must be protected from heat, moisture, and breakage. Key aspects related to care of aids include:

Table 50.4 Aids for the hearing impaired

Aid	Description
Hearing aid	Device which receives speech and environmental sounds through a microphone, and amplifies sound. Various styles including those worn in the ear canal, behind the ear, on the arm of spectacles, and in the form of a transmitter that is attached to the clothing (body aid) Some styles may be used with an induction coil for television, telephone, and radio
Modified telephone	Telephone fitted with volume control and induction coil
Radio and television	Used in conjunction with headphones, induction coils, infra-red and FM transmitters
Telephone typewriter	Device fitted to a telephone whereby a caller's message is typed and translated into a written message, which is either displayed on a screen or printout
Captioning devices	Added to a television set, these devices display captions or subtitles at the bottom of the screen. Not all television programmes are coded for this service
Hearing dog	Dog trained to respond to specific sounds, e.g. door bell, telephone, a baby's cry, and to alert the hearing impaired person to the source of the sound

• Ensuring that the ear mould and tubing are not blocked by wax or moisture. To clean the aid the ear mould is detached from the battery device, washed in warm soapy water, and rinsed with clear water. The ear mould must be dried thoroughly before it is reconnected.
• Keeping the aid dry and away from high temperatures, e.g. direct sunlight. It should be removed before the individual showers or washes his hair.
• Switching off the aid when it is not in use.
• Checking the battery and replacing it when necessary. Ensure that the battery is inserted correctly.
• Checking that the hearing aid is switched on when in use, and that the volume is adjusted.
• Investigating the cause of any 'whistling', which can result in embarrassment and annoyance. Causes of whistling include a poorly fitting ear mould, ear mould incorrectly positioned, cracked or broken tubing, and the volume turned up too high.
• Inserting the hearing aid correctly. The aid is turned on to be certain it is working, then the ear mould is gently inserted into the ear canal. Once the mould has been inserted, the individual adjusts the volume. The tube, if fitted, is placed over the ear and attached to the battery device.
• Notifying the audiologist, or hearing aid specialist, if the aid is malfunctioning.
Recent research has resulted in the development of a device to improve hearing—the cochlear implant. A cochlear im-

plant is an electronic device which is surgically implanted. The device picks up environmental sounds, and converts them to electrical impulses which are relayed to an implanted receiver. Direct electrical stimulation to the nerve fibres of cranial nerve VIII sometimes enables profoundly deaf individuals to hear some sounds.

Local ear care

Various nursing procedures involving the ear should be performed in accordance with the policies of the health care institution. The general principles which should be followed include:

- explaining what you are going to do.
- ensuring that the individual is sitting or lying with his head well supported.
- ensuring that there is adequate lighting.
- washing the hands thoroughly before and after the procedure, to prevent cross infection.
- warming solutions and ear drops to body temperature, as hot or cold temperatures stimulate the inner ear—causing vertigo and, sometimes, nausea and vomiting.
- placing cottonwool or gauze packing in the ear canal only if they have been prescribed, since obstruction of the canal may cause a pressure increase against the tympanic membrane.

Cleansing the ear canal

While normal hygiene practices are generally sufficient to keep the ear canal clean, extra care may be required if the individual has ear discharge. A technique of cleansing the ear canal is outlined in the following guidelines. Equipment required:

— sterile cottonwool tipped applicators
— paper bag.

Ear irrigation

The ear may be irrigated (Fig. 50.1) to cleanse the external canal, or to remove a foreign body or wax. As irrigation has the potential for causing damage, it is performed only by persons skilled in the technique. Irrigation is never performed if the tympanic membrane is ruptured, as this could cause further damage and infection.

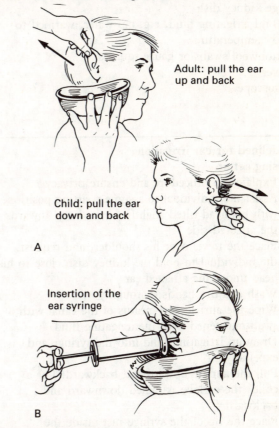

Fig. 50.1 Irrigating the ear
(A) Note that the direction of pull is different for adults and children.
(B) Insertion of the ear syringe.

Guidelines for cleansing the ear canal Nursing action	Rationale
1. Explain the procedure and ensure privacy	Reduces anxiety
2. Assist the individual into a recumbent position, with his head to one side	Facilitates performance of the procedure
3. Wash and dry hands thoroughly	Prevents cross infection
4. Pull the auricle up, back, and slightly outwards	Straightens the ear canal
5. Gently insert an applicator into the canal, rotate the applicator and withdraw it	Avoids damage to the ear. Removes secretions
Do not insert the applicator too far into the canal	Avoids damaging the tympanic membrane
6. Use a new, sterile applicator each time the canal is entered	Prevents cross infection
7. Dispose of soiled applicators appropriately. Wash and dry hands	Prevents cross infection
8. Report and document the procedure	Appropriate care can be planned and implemented

If the irrigation is performed to remove wax it may be necessary to instil a cerumenolytic agent, e.g. Cerumol aural drops for at least 30 minutes beforehand. These have the effect of softening and loosening the wax. A technique of ear irrigation is outlined in the following guidelines. Equipment required:

— aural syringe
— large kidney dish
— 500 ml irrigating fluid, e.g. tap water, warmed to body temperature
— cottonwool swabs or gauze squares
— towel
— auroscope.

Instillation of ear drops

Ear drops which may be prescribed include those that combat infection, and those that soften wax. Ear drops are instilled only when they have been prescribed by a medical officer, and the nurse must follow the nursing regulations and policies regarding administration of medications. Key aspects regarding the use of otic medications are the same as those for using ophthalmic medications, as described on page. A technique of instilling ear drops is outlined in the following guidelines. Equipment required:

— prescribed drops, warmed to body temperature
— 2 or 3 cottonwool swabs
— paper bag for used swabs.

Guidelined for ear irrigation

Nursing action	Rationale
1. Explain the procedure and ensure privacy	Reduces anxiety
2. Assist the individual to assume a sitting position, with his head tilted slightly forward and towards the affected side	Facilitates entry of the irrigating fluid into the ear canal
3. Place the towel over his shoulder, and request the individual to hold the kidney dish close to his head under the affected ear	Prevents the irrigating fluid from running down his neck
4. Wash and dry hands thoroughly	Prevents cross infection
5. Wipe the auricle and meatus of the canal with a swab moistened with the irrigating fluid	Avoids introducing debris into the ear canal
6. Draw up irrigating fluid into the syringe and expel any air	Avoids introducing air into the canal
7. Pull the auricle upward and backward. For a child, the earlobe is pulled downward and backward	Straightens the ear canal
8. Place the tip of the syringe just inside the meatus, and direct a slow, steady stream of fluid against the roof of the ear canal	Directing the stream upward prevents forcing debris further into the canal, and prevents injury to the tympanic membrane
9. Observe the individual for signs of pain or dizziness. If either occurs, stop the procedure	The individual may experience pain if too great a force is used. Dizziness may occur if the fluid is not at body temperature
10. When the syringe is empty, remove it and inspect the return flow in the kidney dish. Refill the syringe and continue the irrigation until the return flow is clear, or the obstruction has been removed	Assesses the effectiveness of the procedure
11. Remove the syringe, and inspect the ear canal with the auroscope (otoscope)	Assesses the canal for cleanliness
12. Encourage the individual to tilt his head towards the affected side	Facilitates drainage of any residual fluid and debris
13. Dry the individual's auricle and neck	Promotes comfort
14. Remove and attend to the equipment appropriately. Wash and dry hands	Prevents cross infection
15. Report and document the procedure	Appropriate care can be planned and implemented

Guidelines for instilling ear drops

Nursing action	Rationale
1. Explain the procedure and ensure privacy	Reduces anxiety
2. Assist the individual to lie on his side opposite the affected ear.	Facilitates instillation of the drops into the ear canal
3. Wash and dry hands thoroughly	Prevents cross infection
4. Gently pull the auricle up and back. For a child, the earlobe is pulled down and back	Straightens the ear canal
5. Instil the prescribed number of drops, so that they fall against the sides of the canal and not on the tympanic membrane	Avoids discomfort
6. Gently massage, or apply gentle pressure to, the projection in front of the meatus (the tragus)	Ensures that the drops flow into the canal
7 Wipe the outer ear free of excess drops	Promotes comfort
8. If prescribed, place a cottonwool swab loosely into the meatus	Prevents the medication leaking out
9. Dispose of equipment appropriately. Wash and dry hands	Prevents cross infection
10. Report and document the procedure	Appropriate care can be planned and implemented

SUMMARY

The eye is the means by which light, reflected from objects, travels to the retina so that an image is formed. Nerve endings in the retina transmit electrical impulses to the brain for interpretation.

Normal eye function can be altered by a variety of factors including those that are congenital, degenerative, infectious, neoplastic, or traumatic.

Major manifestations of eye disorders are changes in vision, pain or discomfort, excessive production of tears or dryness, and discharge.

Disorders of the eye may be classified as congenital, degenerative, infectious, neoplastic, traumatic, and those resulting from multiple causes.

Tests used to assist diagnosis of eye disorders include subjective tests such as evaluation of visual acuity, and objective tests such as assessment of intraocular pressure.

Care of the individual with a disorder of the eye is directed towards maintaining a safe environment, assisting the person to adjust to visual impairment, and providing any prescribed local eye care.

The ear is the means by which sound waves are collected and amplified. Nerve endings in the inner ear transmit electrical impulses to the brain for interpretations.

Normal function of the ear can be altered by a variety of factors including those that are congenital, degenerative, infectious, obstructive, neoplastic, or traumatic.

Major manifestations of ear disorders are pain, discharge, tinnitus, vertigo, nystagmus, and impaired hearing.

Disorders of the ear may be classified as congenital, degenerative, infectious, neoplastic, traumatic, and those resulting from multiple causes.

Tests used to assist diagnosis of ear disorders include those that evaluate auditory function such as pure tone audiometry, and those that assess vestibular function such as electronystagmography.

Care of the individual with a disorder of the ear is directed towards maintaining a safe environment, assisting the person to adjust to impaired hearing, and providing any prescribed local ear care.

REFERENCES AND FURTHER READING

Chilman A M, Thomas M (eds) 1987 Understanding nursing care, 3rd edn. Churchill Livingstone, Edinburgh
Kneisl C R, Ames S W 1986 Adult health nursing: a biopsychosocial approach. Addison-Wesley, Massachusetts

PART 5

Special aspects of nursing care

51. Admission to a health care facility

INTRODUCTION

Admission to a health care facility, e.g. a hospital, is a major event for the individual and for his significant others as they will be anxious about the admission, the illness and its implications. It is, therefore, most important that the nurse is familiar with the admission protocol in order to carry out the necessary activities in a manner which will help to reduce anxiety.

Admissions are classified as either elective or non-elective:

1. An elective admission is a planned admission, where the individual knows in advance that he will be entering a health care facility. In many instances the individual's name will have been placed on a waiting list until a bed becomes available.

2. A non-elective or emergency admission is one in which admission to a health care facility has suddenly become necessary. The individual may be acutely ill or severely injured, and the admission may be arranged by his medical officer or he may be transported directly to the emergency department of a hospital without having been seen by a medical officer.

Health care facilities adopt an admissions, and discharge, policy whereby individuals for elective admission report to the admitting department on a specified date at a specified time. Implementation of this policy promotes efficient admission procedures and subsequent care of the individual.

Prior to an elective admission the individual visits the admitting department to arrange the date and time. At this visit the individual is given a printed information leaflet which provides details about the admission. Information on the leaflet includes a list of the items the individual should bring with him, details about visiting hours, the facilities available, e.g. kiosk, telephone service, and any instructions regarding pre-admission investigations or procedures that have been prescribed.

Reactions to admission

Most individuals face admission to a health care facility with reluctance, while others may experience relief that something is being done to deal with their illness. Whether the individual is to be admitted for a brief or an extended period, any admission is associated with various potential stressors. Previous admissions can affect the individual's reactions and expectations, while an individual who is being admitted for the first time faces the unknown. Elective admission for a relatively minor condition generally causes less stress than does an emergency admission. The nurse must remember that although many anxieties about, and reactions to, admission are common to most people, each person is an individual. As such, anxieties and other reactions experienced vary from person to person.

Stress is a phenomenon in which the individual perceives environmental stimuli as taxing the physiological, psychological, or sociological systems.

Stressors, which may be classified as either physical or psychological, are factors which require a response or change.

Admission to hospital, apart from the implications of the reason for admission, is a major stressor for most people. Features of admission that produce stress, and pose a threat to self concept, self esteem, and body image, include:

- loss of independence and control over events
- disruption to relationships
- unfamiliar environment, equipment, and personnel
- possible loss of income
- possible effects on employment prospects

- the nature and implications of the illness
- painful and/or embarrassing tests or procedures
- worry to significant others
- restrictions on the activities of living
- loss of privacy and dignity
- loss of emotional or moral support
- fear of dying and death.

Reactions to stress and coping mechanisms are described in Chapter 6, and mentioned here briefly. The individual may experience:

- nervousness
- anxiety
- irritability
- emotional lability
- anger or hostility
- decreased tolerance towards other people
- forgetfulness
- confusion
- indifference
- withdrawal
- depression
- difficulty in sleeping
- physical manifestations, e.g. palpitations, headaches, loss of appetite, gastrointestinal disturbances.

The nurse should, therefore, attempt to reduce the stressors related to admission to a health care facility. She should approach the individual in a warm and empathetic manner, and provide him with information about the admission procedures and subsequent activities. The nurse should implement ways of maintaining the individual's independence, self esteem, and dignity. One of the most important ways by which this can be achieved, is to involve the individual in planning and evaluating his care.

ADMISSION

The process of admission prepares the individual for his stay in the health care facility. Admission procedures that are efficient and demonstrate appropriate concern for the individual will help to ease anxiety. Effective admission procedures are directed towards:

- verifying the individual's identity
- assessing his physical and psychological status
- promoting his comfort in an unfamiliar environment
- providing items needed for his care
- providing him with information about various practices and protocol.

Preparation of the unit

Before the individual is admitted to the unit, the nurse in charge will determine the location of his bed. Depending

on need, and availability, the individual may be admitted into a single or shared room. Before the individual arrives, the nurse should check to see that the room is in order and that all the necessary items are available. The room should contain a bed, bedside locker, overbed table, chair, and a wardrobe. The bed may need to be adapted to meet specific needs, e.g. by providing extra pillows, a bed-cradle, a sheepskin, or a fracture board under the mattress.

Although the items which are placed in the unit may vary slightly in different health care facilities, the basic items provided for each individual are:

- two bath towels
- two face washers
- an information booklet
- a thermometer in a container.

Extra items are placed in the room if required, e.g. oxygen equipment, suction apparatus, side rails for the bed, or an intravenous pole. The top of the bedclothes may be turned back or they may be folded down in order to receive an individual who arrives on a trolley.

Reception of the individual

Table 51.1 provides details of the admission assessment. Prior to his arrival in the unit, unless it is an emergency admission, the individual reports to the admitting department. Here, a member of the clerical staff obtains and records information which includes the individual's full name, age, sex, marital status, religion, address; the name, address and telephone number of his next of kin, and details about any hospital insurance. An identification band (see Fig. 38.1) is placed on his wrist. This is partly a basic safety precaution against mistaken identity and treatment. Refer to Chapter 38. Some facilities require that the individual wears two identification bands, one on the wrist and one on the ankle. The individual is advised whether he is to attend the X-ray or pathology department prior to his admission to the unit. The individual is then escorted to the unit where he is received by the nurse in charge.

The nurse who is responsible for admitting him to the unit should greet him, and any accompanying relative or friend, in a warm and friendly manner. She should address the individual by name, and introduce herself to him. The nurse escorts the individual to his room and begins the process of admission. Depending on the circumstances, his relative or friend may accompany him, or they may be offered a seat in a waiting area.

The admission procedure is basically the same in all health care facilities, but it will vary in detail in different settings, and in sequence according to circumstances.

- The individual is taken to his room, and introduced to any other person in the room. If he is sharing a room, his

Table 51.1 Admission assessment

Aspect	Normal	Deviations from normal
General physical appearance	Normal weight for age, sex, height, body build Personal hygiene and grooming satisfactory	Overweight Underweight Appears to be neglected
Skin	Normal colour for race Neither dry nor moist Normal temperature Smooth Elastic No lesions	Pallor, cyanosis, jaundice Excessively dry or moist Elevated temperature, localized warmth, or coldness Rough, or localized changes or irregularities Diminished by dehydration or oedema Rashes, bruises, scars, abrasions, ulcers, nodules
Hair	Normal texture for age, race Normal distribution Scalp clean and healthy Shiny and clean	Brittle, dry, course Areas of hair loss Dandruff, lesions, lice Dull, neglected
Nails	Transparent Smooth Convex Pink nail beds	Streaks (red or white) Ridged Concave curves Cyanosed, pale
Eyes	Sclerae and corneas clear Eyelashes turn out and away Open eyelids do not fall over pupils Pupils equal and reacting to light No discharge Tolerance to light Normal visual acuity	Pale, inflammed, jaundiced Rubbing on eyeball Ptosis (drooping) Dilated, pinpoint, unequal, non-reactive Watery or purulent discharge Photophobia (intolerance to light) Visual impairment
Ears	Normal hearing acuity Ear canal clean No discharge	Hearing impairment Inflammed, presence of excessive wax Watery or purulent discharge Itching, pain, tinnitus
Mouth	Lips pink, moist, smooth Mucosa pink, moist, glistening Gums pink, moist, smooth Teeth white, straight, smooth Tongue pinky red, moist Breath fresh	Pale, cyanosed, dry, cracked Pale, cyanosed, dry, ulcers, cracks Inflammed, swollen, bleeding, lesions Discoloured, chalky, decayed Coated, cracked Halitosis (bad breath), ketone odour

Table 51.1 (cont'd) Admission assessment

Aspect	Normal	Deviations from normal
Thorax and lungs	Normal shaped chest Normal breath sounds	Barrel-shaped Wheezing, rales, gurgles, dry or moist cough
Abdomen	Slightly convex, symmetrical	Excessively concave, asymmetrical, distended
Posture and gait	Able to sit, stand, and walk normally	Abnormal gait Postural abnormalities, e.g. kyphosis, scoliosis
Mobility	Full range of joint motion	Stiffness or instability of a joint Unusual joint movement Swelling of a joint Pain on movement
Muscle tone and strength	Normal tone and strength	Increased or decreased tone Decreased strength
Speech	Ability to speak clearly	Speech impairment, e.g. lisp or stammer
Mental and emotional status	Appropriate emotional responses	Responses inappropriate Apprehension, anxiety, depression, hostility
Level of consciousness and orientation	Alert, responsive, oriented to time, place, person	Disoriented, unresponsive to stimuli, shortened attention span
Presence of prosthesis or aids	None, although aids to sight and hearing are common	Spectacles, contact lenses, artificial eye Hearing aids Walking sticks, frames, wheelchairs, artificial limb Dentures.

privacy must be ensured. He is shown where to put his personal belongings, and the general lay-out of the room. It is important that he is shown how to use the signal device, any fitted television or radio controls, and lights.

● The individual is identification band should be checked, and compared with the card on his bed to see that they are correct.

● The individual is shown the location of the bathroom, toilet, sitting room, and telephones.

● Depending on circumstances, the individual may remain in his day clothes and be able to walk about the ward, or he may be required to change into his night clothes and get into bed.

● Although he will have been advised not to bring valuable items with him, documentation is made of any personal effects. It is not generally necessary to itemize clothing, but a list is compiled of any items of value, e.g. wristwatch, jewellery, television set, radio, and money.

Some health care facilities also require that documentation is made of any prosthesis, e.g. dentures, hearing aid, or an artificial limb. If he has a large sum of money he is advised to either send it home, or to place it in the health care facility's safe. A 'valuables' envelope is provided for the safe-keeping of money or valuable items. It is very important to inform him that the health care facility does not accept responsibility for valuable items, unless they are deposited in the safe. The nurse should refer to the facility's policy regarding the procedure to be followed when the individual's valuables are to be stored.

• The individual is shown the health care facility's booklet, which contains information about various aspects of the organization. The booklet contains details such as visiting times, meal times, how to identify the various personnel; kiosk, telephone, television, and laundry facilities available, regulations regarding smoking, and the time the individual is expected to vacate the room when he is discharged.

• As soon as practicable, assessment is made of his vital signs and weight, and the information documented. A sample of urine is obtained and urinalysis performed. Information on vital signs is provided in Chapters 32, 33, and 34, while information on urinalysis is provided in Chapter 30. The individual's height may also be measured and documented.

• Throughout the admission procedure, the nurse should discreetly observe the individual to gain information that will assist in planning his care. Assessment is made, and documented, of his:

• general physical appearance
• degree of mobility
• level of independence
• psychological status
• skin
• hearing and visual acuity
• ability to communicate
• level of consciousness and orientation
• gait and posture
• use of any prostheses or aids.

• At the time of or as soon as possible after admission, a nursing history is compiled and a nursing care plan developed. Information on these, and other aspects of the nursing process, is provided in Chapter 12.

• The individual should be provided with a flask of fluid, and offered a cup of tea or coffee—unless oral fluids are contraindicated. Anybody accompanying him may also be offered a drink, or shown where to find the kiosk. This is of particular importance if it is an emergency admission. The individual's significant others may be very distressed, and may appreciate being shown to an area where they can sit and rest for a while. The health care facility may also provide accommodation for the relatives if the individual is very ill, or a child. Information on the admission of a child is provided in Chapter 54.

• Before leaving the room the nurse should ensure that the individual, and his significant others, have been given all the information they require. The nurse should answer any questions or, if she is not able to, refer them to the nurse in charge. The nurse should also bear in mind that a person who is stressed, tends not to hear or remember all the information given to him. She should, therefore, ensure that the information is repeated whenever necessary.

DIAGNOSTIC PROCEDURES

Shortly after admission, or it any time during his stay in a health care facility, the individual may be required to have one or various diagnostic tests or examinations performed. For most people any test or examination is a cause for anxiety and apprehension. The individual may experience discomfort, pain, or embarrassment during a procedure, and he may be apprehensive about the results. The nurse is in a key position to reduce or minimize anxiety, embarrassment, and discomfort. She is generally responsible for preparing the individual prior to the test or examination, remaining with him during some procedures, ensuring that specimens are appropriately despatched, and caring for the individual after the procedure.

Prior to some procedures, particularly those that are invasive, the individual must give his informed consent. It is not the nurse's responsibility to gain the individual's consent, but she may need to *check* that it has been given prior to commencement of a procedure. Information on informed consent is provided in Chapter 10.

Examination of the individual

When he is admitted to a health care facility, each individual is given a comprehensive physical examination by a medical officer, and further examinations may be performed during his stay. The medical officer assesses the individual by using various techniques:

• *Auscultation* is the act of listening for sounds within the body to evaluate the condition of specific organs. Auscultation may be performed directly, but a stethoscope is generally used to determine the intensity, quality, and duration of the sounds.

• *Percussion* is a technique used to evaluate the size and borders of some internal organs, or to determine the presence of fluid in a body cavity. Direct percussion is performed by striking the fingers directly on a body surface. Indirect percussion is performed by striking the finger/s of one hand on the finger/s of the other hand which is placed on a body surface.

• *Palpation* is a technique whereby the examiner feels the texture, size, consistency, and location of certain parts of the body with his hands.

Preparation of the individual

Preparation of the individual prior to the examination involves:

- Providing him with a full explanation of the type of examination to be performed.
- Providing him with the opportunity to empty his bladder and/or bowel. The individual will feel more comfortable, and the examination will be performed more effectively, if the bladder and rectum are empty.
- Providing privacy by closing any doors or windows, or by drawing the screens around the bed.
- Providing a drape for warmth and privacy. The upper bedclothes should be folded to the bottom of the bed.
- Assisting him to assume the required position. Information on various positions is provided in Chapter 35. The pillows should be arranged to provide comfort and support.

The positions normally used are as follow:

- For examination of the chest and back, the individual is assisted into a sitting position. The nightgown or pajama top is undone, or removed if necessary, and a drape positioned to provide privacy.
- For examination of the abdomen, the individual is assisted into the recumbent position. The clothing is adjusted to provide exposure of the abdomen, and a drape is positioned to provide privacy.
- For a rectal examination, the individual is assisted to assume the left lateral position. A drape is positioned so that only the anal area is exposed.
- For a vaginal examination, the individual is assisted to assume either the dorsal or Sim's position according to the medical officer's instructions. Adequate draping is necessary to ensure that only the vaginal area is exposed.

Preparation of the equipment

The equipment required depends to some extent on the areas of the body to be examined, but there are certain basic requirements:

- sphygmomanometer
- stethoscope
- ophthalmoscope (to examine the eyes)
- auriscope (to examine the ears)
- tuning fork (to evaluate hearing)
- tongue depressor in a receiver, and a torch (to examine the mouth)
- patella hammer (to evaluate reflexes)
- waste container (for disposable items)
- head mirror (to reflect light into a body orifice, e.g. the throat)
- anglepoise lamp.

For a rectal examination the items required are:

- kidney dish and cover

- disposable gloves
- lubricant
- swabs
- proctoscope (may be required).

For a vaginal examination, the items required are:

- kidney dish
- disposable gloves
- lubricant
- swabs
- vaginal specula (Sim's, and bivalve)

and if a cervical smear is to be obtained

- spatula (Ayre's)
- fixing solution
- glass slides
- pencil, pathology request form.

During the examination

The nurse should remain with the individual to provide physical and emotional support. She should assist when a change of position is required, remembering to provide adequate physical support and privacy. Emotional support is partially provided by the nurse's presence, and further support may be given in the form of encouragement and explanations of what is to happen. The nurse may also be required to hand items to the medical officer, or to receive any specimen obtained.

After the examination

The individual is assisted into a position of comfort, his clothing re-adjusted, and the bedclothes are arranged to meet his needs. If a rectal or vaginal examination was performed, the individual should be provided with tissues to wipe off any excess lubricant. The equipment is removed and attended to in the appropriate manner. Any specimens are dispatched to the laboratory as soon as possible. The examination, and the individual's response to it, is reported to the nurse in charge and documented.

Diagnostic investigations

Apart from the physical examination, specific tests may be performed to assist diagnosis or to aid in evaluation of the individual's condition. Diagnostic procedures include:

- radiological examination
- ultrasonography
- blood tests
- urine tests
- histologic tests
- microbiologic tests
- endoscopy

- recording electrical activity
- CT scanning.

The nurse may be involved in preparing the individual prior to a diagnostic procedure, assisting throughout the procedure, and caring for him following the procedure. To determine the specific preparation and post-test care required for each procedure, the nurse should refer to the health care facility's policy manual.

Preparation of the individual prior to any diagnostic procedure involves both physical and psychological preparation. The nurse should:

- Explain the purpose of the test and the procedure. If the individual understands what is to happen, and why, he will be less anxious about the test. The nurse should ensure that he is informed of when, where, and by whom the test will be performed.
- Check that the individual's informed consent has been obtained. Many tests, especially those of an invasive nature, require that the individual gives his informed consent for the test to be performed.

Preparation for specific procedures

Radiography includes plain and special X-ray diagnostic studies. *Plain* X-rays are performed when dense tissue such as bone is to be examined. *Special* X-rays are performed when soft tissues are to be examined, and they involve the use of a contrast medium. Contrast medium is a radiopaque substance introduced into the body to facilitate imaging of internal structures that are difficult to visualize using plain X-rays. Contrast medium may be introduced into the body in various ways, e.g. orally, rectally, or intravenously. X-rays involving the use of contrast medium include:

- intravenous pyelogram (IVP), to outline the structures in the urinary tract
- retrograde pyelogram, to outline the structures of the kidney
- barium swallow, meal, or enema. Barium sulphate is either swallowed or introduced by means of a rectal tube, to outline the oesophagus, stomach, or intestines.
- cholecystogram, to outline the gallbladder
- intravenous cholangiogram, to outline the gallbladder and bile ducts
- bronchogram, to outline the bronchial tree
- cardiac catheterization, to outline the structures of the heart
- cerebral angiography, to outline the structure of the brain
- salpingogram, to outline the uterine (fallopian) tubes.

Some individuals are allergic to iodine and may experience a hypersensitivity reaction, therefore radiographic studies involving iodine-based contrast media require careful preparation of the individual before the test, and close monitoring of him afterward.

Prior to any radiographic examination, the individual is dressed in a plain cotton garment fastened with tapes. Any metal objects, e.g. hair clips, jewellery, or fastenings on clothing, are not worn as these will show up on the X-ray film.

Preparation for each procedure depends upon the health care facility's protocol, and upon the type of procedure to be performed. Preparation may include:

- a period of fasting
- administration of medications
- administration of rectal suppositories or enema
- shaving an area of skin
- ensuring that the bladder is empty.

Ultrasonography is a technique whereby deep body structures are represented by measuring and recording the reflection of pulsed or continuous high-frequency sound waves. Preparation involves dressing the individual in a plain cotton garment fastened with tapes. A period of fasting may be required, and it may be necessary to ensure that the bowel and/or bladder are empty. If an ultrasound is being performed during pregnancy, e.g. to determine fetal size, the individual is generally required to have a full bladder for the procedure—as this pushes the uterus out of the pelvis thus aiding visualization of uterine contents.

Blood tests involve the withdrawal of a sample of blood for laboratory analysis. Blood may be obtained from a vein, artery, or capillary; and the sample required may be whole blood, plasma, or serum. Whole blood is obtained for many haematologic studies, e.g. blood gas analysis, complete blood count, haemoglobin estimation. Plasma or serum may be obtained for biochemical, immunologic, or coagulation studies.

Venous blood, because it represents physiologic conditions throughout the body, and because it is relatively easy to obtain, is used for most laboratory studies. The quantities of blood, plasma, or serum obtained for analysis, depend on the type of test to be performed.

Preparation of the individual may include a period of fasting depending on the specific test. The individual should be sitting or lying down in case he becomes faint or dizzy.

Urine may be tested for a variety of reasons, and the test may require only a small amount or the entire urine output over a 24 hour period. Information on the collection and testing of urine is provided in Chapter 30.

Histology, the study of the microscopic structure of tissues and cells, involves the removal of a specimen of living tissue. A specimen of tissue may be obtained using an aspiration needle, a punch, or a scalpel. Depending on the size of the specimen to be obtained, and the site from where it is to be obtained, the individual may require a local or a general anaesthetic.

Preparation of the individual involves providing emotional support, as anxiety is likely to be experienced about the procedure and the test results. Physical preparation may involve:

- preparation of the skin over the site, e.g. cleansing or shaving
- a period of fasting
- administration of medications
- checking that informed consent has been obtained
- ensuring that he is supported in a comfortable position.

Microbiologic tests involve obtaining a sample of a body fluid, secretion or excretion for analysis. The sample is tested to isolate micro-organisms, and to determine their sensitivity to specific antibiotics. Microbiologic tests may be performed on urine, faeces, respiratory tract secretions, blood, wound exudate, gastric contents, genital tract secretions, secretions from the eyes or ears, and cerebrospinal fluid. Depending on the specimen to be obtained for testing, the sample may be collected in a sterile container or obtained by swabbing the area with a sterile swab-stick.

Preparation of the individual depends on each test and may include assisting him to assume a specific position, or a period of fasting.

Endoscopy is the visualization of the interior organs or cavities of the body, with an endoscope. An endoscope is an illuminated optical instrument, available in varying lengths for examining various areas of the body. Some endoscopes are flexible, while others are rigid. Areas of the body which may be examined by endoscopy include:

- gastrointestinal tract (oesophagoscopy, gastroscopy, duodenoscopy, sigmoidoscopy, proctoscopy, colonoscopy)
- respiratory tract (laryngoscopy, bronchoscopy)
- peritoneal cavity (laparoscopy)
- joints (arthroscopy)
- cervix and vagina (culdoscopy)
- urinary tract (cystoscopy).

Preparation of the individual generally involves:

- a period of fasting
- administration of medications, e.g. a sedative
- ensuring that the colon is empty before an endoscopy involving the intestines
- explanation that either a local or a general anaesthetic will be administered
- dressing the individual in a plain cotton garment with tapes
- checking that informed consent has been obtained.

Recording electrical activity involves recording the electrical current generated by specific areas of the body. The two main areas of the body to be examined are:

- the heart (electrocardiogram)
- the brain (electroencephalogram).

Electrical activity in other tissues may also be recorded, e.g.

- the muscles (electromyography)
- extraocular muscles (electronystagmography).

Preparation of the individual involves explaining to him that electrodes will be attached to specific areas of the body after the electrodes sites have been cleansed and wiped dry. If necessary, the sites may be shaved. Conductive jelly is applied to the sites, and the electrodes are positioned. Flat electrodes do not cause any discomfort whereas needle electrodes, which are less commonly used, may cause a prickling sensation. Electrodes which are placed on the limbs are secured in position with a rubber strap.

During the test the individual may be asked to remain still, or he may be requested to perform certain activities. During an *electroencephalogram*, he may initially be required to lie still with his eyes closed, then be requested to breathe deeply and rapidly for a few minutes. A strobe light may also be placed in front of him, and recordings made with his eyes opened and closed. During an *electrocardiogram* he may be required to remain still or, if a stress test is being performed, he may be required to exercise on a treadmill or bicycle. *Ambulatory electrocardiography* is the continuous recording of heart activity as the individual carries out his normal activities of living.

Computerized tomography (CT scanning) is a technique in which a scanner is used to attain a series of detailed visualizations of the tissues. CT scanning is used in diagnosing intracranial, intrathoracic, mediastinal, and intra-abdominal abnormalities. The procedure is painless, although the equipment looks formidable and may be noisy. A contrast medium may be used.

Preparation of the individual may include dressing him in a plain cotton garment with tapes, and informing him that he may experience possible side effects if a contrast medium is used. He is informed to report immediately if he experiences nausea, flushing, dizzyness, or sweating.

Post test care

Care of the individual following a diagnostic test involves implementing the appropriate care, and assessing him for side effects or complications. Depending on the specific procedure performed, care of the individual may include:

- assisting him to assume a specific position
- ensuring his physical comfort

- providing psychological support
- measuring and documenting his vital signs
- observing for any sign of bleeding, either internal or from a puncture or biopsy site
- observing for the manifestations of shock
- observing for discomfort or pain
- assessing urinary and/or gastrointestinal function
- observing for the manifestations of a hypersensitive reaction to contrast medium: urticaria, pruritus, hypotension, circulatory insufficiency, bronchospasm
- administering prescribed medications.

TRANSFER AND DISCHARGE

Transfer

Sometimes it is necessary to transfer an individual from one unit or ward at a health care facility to another, or to another facility. Transfer of an individual may be necessary for a variety of reasons, e.g. a change in his condition, demand for available beds, or if he requires to be isolated from others.

Whatever the reason, a transfer may be a distressing experience for the individual, who is likely to feel apprehensive about the need to adapt to new surroundings and personnel. Conversely, the transfer may be welcomed as an indication of an improvement in the individual's condition, e.g. being transferred from an intensive care unit to a general ward.

When an individual is to be transferred, it is essential that both he and his significant others are informed as soon as possible. A full explanation of the reasons for the transfer provides the individual with time to adjust, and provides his significant others time to make any changes necessary.

In addition to preparing the individual for the transfer, it is necessary to inform the staff in the receiving unit or facility of the individual's condition and care plan. Arrangements for transportation are made if necessary. Key aspects involved in the transfer are:

- Informing the individual of the date and time the transfer is to occur.
- Assessing whether he is able to walk, or if he requires a wheelchair or trolley.
- Arranging transportation, e.g. an ambulance, if he is being transferred to another facility.
- Notifying the receiving unit or facility of the date and time of the transfer.
- Notifying the admissions department of the transfer.
- Assisting the individual to pack all his personal possessions. The nurse should check the entire room to ensure that nothing is left behind.
- Assembling the documents that are to accompany him.

The individual's medications are either sent with him, or they may be returned to the facility's pharmacy department.

- Accompanying the individual to the receiving unit, or to the ambulance or private car.
- Introducing him to the nursing staff in the receiving unit, and remaining with him until they have received him into their care.
- Reporting to the nurse in charge and documenting that the transfer has been accomplished.

Discharge

Effective discharge from a health care facility requires careful planning and continuing assessment of the individual's needs during his stay. Ideally, discharge planning begins soon after the individual's admission. The purpose of discharge planning is to assist the individual to make a smooth transition from one setting or level of care to another, without impending the progress that has already been achieved; and to provide for other health needs that are still unmet. Discharge planning is directed towards teaching the individual, and his significant others, about his condition and its effects on his lifestyle; providing instructions for performing self-care activities, informing him of any dietary or activity restrictions, and arranging for any follow-up care that may be necessary.

The concept of continuity of care recognizes that the individual's needs change, and that the type of services necessary to support these needs also change. Health services which may be required following the individual's discharge include long-term and rehabilitation settings, nursing home or day-care centres. Services, outside the health care facility setting, include community nursing, home nursing resources, and community facilities such as 'meals on wheels'.

Discharge planning is a team approach involving the individual and his significant others, the medical officer, nurses, and other health team members, e.g. occupational therapist, physiotherapist, and dietitian. The steps involved in discharge planning are:

- assessment of the individual, and his significant others
- analysis of data to identify specific needs
- planning to meet those needs
- implementation of the plan
- evaluation of the discharge planning process and the results.

Day of discharge

When the date and time of discharge have been determined, the individual and his significant others are informed. Transport is arranged for him if necessary. Before the individual leaves the facility, the nurse should check that:

- All his personal possessions have been collected and packed, including any articles of value being held in the facility's safe.
- He is assisted to dress if necessary.
- Any dressings or bandages have been applied as necessary.
- The individual is provided with any prescribed medications, and instructions on their administration. The facility generally provides an instruction–information sheet which includes this information.
- The individual is aware of, and understands, any dietary or activity restrictions.
- The visiting nurse service has been notified, if the individual requires their services.
- The medical officer has informed the individual of any future appointments at his surgery or at a health care facility.
- The individual is confident about performing any self-care activities that were taught to him, e.g. administration of insulin, dressing a wound, or caring for a colostomy.
- The individual, and his significant others, are aware of whom to contact should there be any problems after discharge.

When the individual is ready to leave the unit or ward, he is escorted to the discharge department, and any documentation completed. He is then escorted to the exit and farewelled. In the unit, the nurse reports to the nurse in charge, and documents that the discharge has been accomplished.

Discharge against medical advice

An individual may, at any time, decide to leave a health care facility against the advice of his medical officer. If this occurs, the nurse must immediately report the incident to the nurse in charge, and the individual's medical officer is notified. If the individual cannot be dissuaded from leaving, he is asked to sign a statement to the effect that he is leaving at his own risk and that he is responsible for the consequences. If he refuses to sign, this must be documented. The document is signed by at least one witness—this may be the medical officer or the nurse in charge. The incident is fully reported in the individual's notes.

SUMMARY

Admission, elective or emergency, to a health care facility is a major event for the individual. Both he and his significant others are generally anxious about the admission and its implications.

The individual may react to admission in one or more ways, e.g. with apprehension, irritability, anger, depression, or relief.

The nurse should perform the process of admission in a warm, efficient, and empathetic manner in order to minimize any anxiety.

Prior to admission, the unit is prepared to receive the individual. Reception of the individual is directed towards verifying his identity, assessing his physical and psychological status, promoting his comfort in an unfamiliar environment, providing items needed for his care, and providing him with information.

Shortly after admission, or at any time during his stay, the individual may be required to have one or various diagnostic examinations or tests performed.

The nurse is involved in preparing the individual prior to the diagnostic procedure, and caring for him afterwards.

The individual may be transferred to another ward, unit, or health care facility. A full explanation of the reason for the transfer should be provided to the individual, and to his significant others.

Discharge planning, which commences soon after admission, is directed towards assisting the individual to make a smooth transition for one setting to another.

Discharge planning involves assessment, analysis of data, planning, implementation and evaluation.

REFERENCES AND FURTHER READING

Potter P A, Perry A G 1985 Fundamentals of nursing. C V Mosby, St Louis
Sorensen K C, Luckmann J 1986 Basic nursing, a psychophysiologic appraoch, 2nd edn. W B Saunders, Philadelphia

52. The mother and the newborn baby

INTRODUCTION

Maternity nursing involves the care of a woman during her pregnancy and labour, and the care of both the woman and her infant during and following birth. Although midwifery is a specialized profession, requiring the learner midwife to undertake a separate educational programme, the nurse may be required to assist in the provision of maternity care. It is important, therefore, that the nurse has a basic knowledge of human growth and development, the processes of normal pregnancy and labour, and an understanding of the immediate and subsequent care of the mother and the newborn infant.

PREGNANCY

Pregnancy (the gestational process) comprises the growth and development, within a woman, of a new individual from conception to birth. The average duration of pregnancy is 266 days after fertilization of the ovum, or 40 weeks from the first day of the last normal menstrual period.

Physiology of pregnancy

Pregnancy, which is a normal physiological function, produces changes in almost all the mother's body systems. Most of these changes are temporary, and most are the result of hormone actions. The mother's body is prepared, by these changes, to:

- protect the developing embryo/fetus

- provide for the demands of the fetus
- prepare to feed the baby when it is born.

Endocrine factors

The hormonal factors involved in pregnancy are listed in Table 52.1.

Physiological changes

The maternal physiological changes during pregnancy are listed in Table 52.2.

Psychological changes

During pregnancy a woman's psychological status may alter e.g. she may experience anxiety and emotional lability. The pregnant woman's psychological status depends on many factors e.g. her basic personality, whether the pregnancy was desired, the strength of her social and family support systems, and her self concept.

Confirmation of pregnancy

The manifestations of pregnancy are generally divided into three groups: possible, probable, and positive. Pregnancy is *possible* if there is:

- absence of menstruation
- morning sickness
- breast enlargement and tingling
- frequency of micturition
- increased pigmentation of the nipples
- quickening—the sensation of fetal movement felt by the mother

Pregnancy is *probable* if there is:

- a positive pregnancy test
- abdominal enlargement, and the uterus is palpable abdominally

Table 52.1 Hormonal factors in pregnancy

Gland	Hormone	Actions
Ovary	Oestrogens and progesterone—during the first few weeks of pregnancy	1. Oestrogens influence: • uterine growth • breast growth • water and sodium retention • pituitary hormone release
Placenta	Oestrogens and progesterone — when the placenta is fully developed	2. Progesterone influences: • relaxation of smooth muscle • relaxation of connective tissue • secretory changes within the breasts • development of the lactiferous ducts
	Placental lactogenic hormone	Promotes growth, stimulates development of the breasts, and plays a role in maternal fat metabolism
	Relaxin	Has a relaxant effect, especially on connective tissue
Pituitary	Thyroid stimulating hormone (TSH)	Stimulates release of thyroxine to maintain increased metabolism
	Oxytocin	Contraction of the uterus (at the end of pregnancy). Expulsion of milk (after birth)
	Prolactin	Initiates and sustains lactation (after baby is born)
Parathyroids	Parathormone	Maintains normal calcium ion concentration
Suprarenal	Increase in secretion of hormones, e.g. glucocorticoids and aldosterone	Maintain increased metabolism

Table 52.2 Physiological changes in pregnancy

Area of change	Description
Uterus	Increase in size to approximately 30 × 22 × 20 cm (at term) Increase in mass to approximately 1 kg (at term). Cervix becomes softer (in preparation for labour). Plug of mucus (the operculum) formed by, and remains in, the cervix from the eight week until labour commences. Uterus forms into two segments—the lower segment is thinner and becomes soft and dilated towards the end of pregnancy Painless, irregular contractions (Braxton-Hicks) occur throughout pregnancy
Vagina	In early pregnancy, the vagina (and cervix) changes in colour from pink to dark red/blue Acidic vaginal secretions increase in amount Increased thickness, due to venous dilation
Breasts	Increase in size and mass Nipples enlarge, and become more prominent and darker in colour Areolar becomes darker Prominent sebaceous glands (Montgomery's tubercles) appear on the areolar at approximately 12 weeks Increased sensation and tingling Colostrum (the fluid secreted during pregnancy) can be expressed at 16 weeks

Table 52.2 (cont'd) Physiological changes in pregnancy

Area of change	Description
Skin	Darker pigmentation in the nipples and areolar, on the face (chloasma) and on the abdominal midline (linea nigra) Stretch marks may appear on the abdomen, breasts, and buttocks Spider naevi (bright red lesions with minute radiating branches) may appears on the face and upper chest
Musculoskeletal system	Spinal curvature changes to compensate for the abdominal enlargement, resulting in arching of the back The symphysis pubis and sacro-iliac joints become mobile and the pelvis becomes wider—due to softening of the connective tissue in preparation for labour
Urinary tract	Relaxation of smooth muscle causes the ureters to become dilated, elongated, and kinked These changes may lead to stasis of urine and infection Frequency of micturition may occur in the early months, as the uterus occupies more of the pelvis Reduction of muscle tone in the pelvic floor, and increased pressure from the growing fetus, may result in stress incontinence towards the end of pregnancy

Table 52.2 (cont'd) Physiological changes in pregnancy

Area of change	Description
Gastrointestinal tract	Hormonal and mechanical changes, e.g. increased hormonal levels and reduced intestinal motility, may result in morning sickness, gastric acid reflux, and constipation
Cardiovascular system	Blood volume increases by 40–50% Cardiac output is increased, because of increased blood volume Haemodilution (due to increased plasma volume) results in lowered haemoglobin level Coagulability of blood is slightly increased Reduced tone in blood vessels may result in varicose veins
Respiratory tract	The rate of ventilations is increased to obtain the higher amounts of oxygen required
Basal metabolic rate (BMR)	In the second half of pregnancy, by the BMR is increased 15–25% to cope with the increased demands
Body mass	Increases by approximately 25% of the pre-pregnant weight. Weight gain is due to the growth of the uterus and breasts, the uterine contents, increase in maternal blood volume and interstitial fluid, and maternal storage of fats and protein

- Braxton-Hicks contractions (painless uterine contractions which occur throughout pregnancy)

Pregnancy is *positive* if there is:

- fetal heart sounds
- fetal movements felt by an examiner
- fetal parts felt
- ultrasonic or X-ray evidence of pregnancy.

The date when the baby is due (confinement date) may be calculated by dates, the height of the uterine fundus, or by X-ray or ultrasonic evidence.

Calculation by dates, to determine the estimated day of confinement (EDC), is made by ascertaining the first day of the last known menstrual period and adding 9 months and 7 days.

Example:
First day of the last known menstrual period 29th September; add 9 months and 7 days:
EDC = 6 July.

Calculation by assessing the fundal height (Fig. 52.1) is made by measuring the height of the uterine fundus. As the uterus enlarges steadily and predictably, the date of confinement can be determined reasonably accurately.

Calculation by ultrasound, which has largely replaced X-rays in the assessment of fetal growth, is made by using height frequency, short wavelength, and sound wave reflections to visualize the size of the fetus.

Minor discomforts associated with pregnancy

The pregnant woman may experience one or a variety of

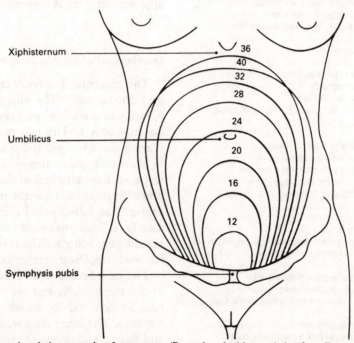

Fig. 52.1 Fundal heights of the uterus in relation to weeks of pregnancy. (Reproduced with permission from Farrer H 1990 Maternity care, 2nd edn. Churchill Livingstone, Melbourne.)

minor disorders or discomforts, many of which are the result of increased secretion of hormones or pressure from the uterus and its contents.

Table 52.3 lists the discomforts and guidelines for their management.

Development of the fetus

Conception, fertilization of the ovum, occurs in the distal third of the uterine (Fallopian) tube. The fertilized ovum (zygote) develops by simple cell division as it travels to the uterus. When it reaches the uterus, it is a sphere of cells and is referred to as a *morula*.

The morula separates into an outer (ectodermal) and an inner (endodermal) cell mass, fluid forms and fills the space between the two layers, and the structure is referred to as a *blastocyst*. The outer layer of the blastocyst becomes

Table 52.3 Minor discomforts of pregnancy

Discomfort	Management guidelines
Morning sickness	Small, frequent, dry meals Fluids in between meals Something to eat, e.g. dry biscuit, before getting out of bed in the morning Avoid fried and heavily spiced foods
Indigestion	Small frequent meals Avoid spicy foods Elevate the head of the bed
Constipation	High fibre foods Adequate fluids Exercise
Fainting	Avoid sudden postural changes Avoid constrictive clothing Avoid lying on the back during late pregnancy Avoid fatigue
Backache	Maintain correct posture Daily rest periods Wear low-heeled shoes Sleep on a firm surface, e.g. board under mattress
Varicose veins	Avoid long periods of standing Avoid constrictive clothing Elevate the legs whenever possible Wear supportive stockings Avoid sitting or standing with the legs crossed
Urinary tract infection	Adequate fluids Perineal hygiene measures, e.g. wiping from front to back after elimination
Leg muscle cramps	Avoid standing for long periods Elevate the legs whenever possible Relieve symptoms by pulling upward on toes
Haemorrhoids	Avoid constipation Relieve discomfort by applying cold compresses or ice packs

the *trophoblast* and will develop into the placenta and outer membrane, while the inner layer will develop into the embryo, cord, and inner membrane. Between these two layers, a third layer (mesoderm) will form.

Implantation, embedding in the endometrium, occurs approximately 10 days after fertilization; and normally occurs in the upper body of the uterus. Following implantation, the lining of the uterus grows over the blastocyst and pregnancy is established. From this stage onward, the lining of the uterus is termed the *decidua*.

The inner cell mass of the blastocyst differentiates into 3 distinct layers:

• The outer layer (ectoderm) will develop to become the skin, hair, nails, brain and nervous system.
• The middle layer (mesoderm) will develop to become the circulatory, musculoskeletal and urinary systems; and most of the reproductive tract.
• The inner layer (endoderm) will develop to become the intestines, internal organs, respiratory system, and the germ cells of the ovaries or testes.

As development continues, a cavity appears above the ectoderm. The lining of this *amniotic* cavity becomes the amniotic membrane which secretes fluid that makes up part of the liquor. *Liquor* is the fluid that surrounds the embryo. The amniotic cavity enlarges so that eventually the embryo is suspended by the umbilical cord in a closed sac (membranes) of amniotic fluid.

The embryo continues to develop until by the end of the second month it resembles a human, and is called a *fetus*. From this stage onward the major activities are growth and organ specialization. By the end of 40 weeks the fetus is approximately 50 cm long, and weighs between 2.7 and 4.1 kg.

Development of the placenta, membranes, liquor and cord

The placenta. The outer cells of the trophoblast develop projections (villi). The villi project into the maternal capillaries to allow the exchange of oxygen, nutrients, and waste products. The villi eventually join with an area of uterine tissue to form the placenta. The placenta continues to grow throughout the pregnancy, with one surface (maternal surface) attached to the lining of the uterus, and the other (fetal surface) has the umbilical cord arising from its centre. The fully formed placenta is disc-shaped, approximately 2.5 cm thick in the centre, and weighs approximately 500 gm. The functions of the placenta are nutritional, respiratory, excretory, and hormonal.

The membranes. The membranes are derived from part of the trophoblast, and are comprised of two membranes (the amnion and the chorion) which are attached to the placenta. The inner membrane (amnion) encloses the fetus and liquor, and covers the fetal surface of the placenta and the cord. The outer membrane (chorion) is continuous with the margin of the placenta and adheres to the wall of the uterus.

Liquor. The liquor (amniotic fluid) is the pale, straw-coloured liquid that surrounds the fetus in the amniotic sac. Derived mainly from the secretions of the cells in the amniotic membrane, liquor is 99% water plus mineral salts. The functions of liquor include protection of the fetus, and maintenance of an even intrauterine temperature.

The umbilical cord. The umbilical cord extends from the fetal umbilicus to the fetal surface of the placenta. It contains two umbilical arteries which transport deoxygenated blood from the fetus, and one umbilical vein which transports oxygenated and nutrient-rich blood from the placenta to the fetus. The vessels in the cord are embedded in a thick jelly-like substance, and the cord is covered by amniotic membrane. At forty weeks of pregnancy the cord is approximately 1.25 cm in diameter and 60 cm long.

Fetal circulation

The fetal circulation is designed (Fig. 52.2) so that the major blood flow bypasses the fetal lungs. Oxygen and nutrients move from the mother's blood into the fetal blood, and fetal wastes move in the opposite direction.

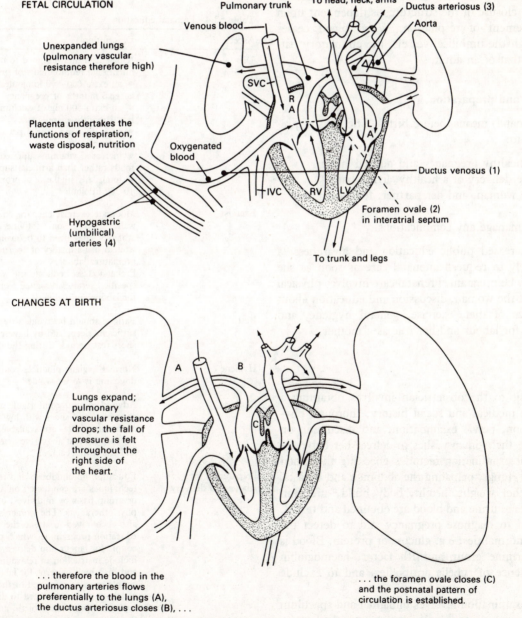

Fig. 52.2 Fetal circulation and the changes at birth. (Reproduced with permission from Farrer H 1990 Maternity care, 2nd edn. Churchill Livingstone, Melbourne.)

As blood, from the umbilical vein, flows toward the fetal heart, most of it bypasses the fetal liver through the *ductus venosus* and enters the inferior vena cava. Some of the blood entering the right atrium is shunted into the left atrium through the foramen ovale—a temporary opening in the septum between the atria. Blood that enters the right ventricle is pumped out the pulmonary trunk where it meets the ductus arteriosus—a short vessel connecting the aorta to the pulmonary artery.

Because the fetal lungs are collapsed, blood enters the systemic circulation through the ductus arteriosus. The aorta transports blood to the fetal tissues and, ultimately, back to the placenta through the umbilical arteries.

Shortly after birth the foramen ovale closes, and the ductus arteriosus collapses and is converted to a fibrous ligament. The closure of the structures is dependent upon the commencement of respiration. When blood ceases flowing through the umbilical vessels, the circulatory pattern becomes that of an adult.

Prenatal care and preparation

Prenatal (antenatal) means 'before birth'. The aims of prenatal care are to:

- promote a healthy pregnancy and normal labour
- promote the delivery of a healthy, living baby
- prepare the woman, and her partner, for labour and delivery
- detect and manage any complications.

Because of increased public education and awareness, a woman is likely to request antenatal care as soon as she thinks she may be pregnant. Prenatal care involves physical examination of the woman, discussion and education about the importance of diet, exercise, general hygiene, and preparing her for labour and her role as a mother.

Initial visit

The initial visit to the obstetrician involves obtaining a comprehensive medical and social history, thorough physical examination, pelvic examination, and discussion on selecting where the woman wishes to deliver her baby.

The physical examination includes checking the blood pressure, heart, lungs, palpating the abdomen and breasts, and assessing her weight, height, body build, and skin colour. Samples of urine and blood are obtained and tested. Urine is tested to diagnose pregnancy and to detect the presence of abnormalities, e.g. glucose or protein. Blood is tested to determine group and Rh factor, haemoglobin level, the presence of rubella antibodies, and to exclude syphilis.

The pelvic examination involves bimanual and speculum examination to assess uterine size; to observe the cervix, vagina, and perineum; and to estimate the pelvic capacity. A cervical smear and/or cervical swabs may be obtained if the woman has not had regular Pap (Papanicolou) smears or if infection is suspected.

If pregnancy is confirmed, the obstetrician will discuss with the woman possible options regarding the birth. The woman may choose to give birth in a hospital, at home, or in a birthing centre; she may also choose not to continue with the pregnancy.

Prenatal education may be provided by the obstetrician, midwives, child health nurses, or childbirth education groups. The educational aspects of prenatal care are listed in Table 52.4.

Table 52.4 Prenatal education

Aspect	Description
Diet	A balanced diet designed to meet the nutritional requirements of pregnancy: • an extra 600–800 kilojoules per day in the latter 6 months of pregnancy • an extra 500 mg of calcium per day in the last 4 months of pregnancy • an extra 3 mg of iron per day throughout pregnancy • increased vitamins supplied by suitable foods rather than artificial supplements • total daily intake of approximately 10 500 kilojoules
Exercise	Moderate exercise encouraged, e.g. a daily walk or swim. Some activities, e.g. vigorous athletics, may need to be avoided if the woman has a history of abortion or premature labour Prenatal classes educate the woman in specific exercises designed to prepare her for labour and delivery
Rest	Fatigue should be avoided by obtaining sufficient sleep, and by having numerous short rest periods during the day
Hygiene	Normal hygiene practices continued. Vaginal douching is to be avoided
Clothing	Advised to wear comfortable non-constrictive garments, and shoes with low heels Maternity girdles are available, which provide support for just above the symphysis pubis and the lower back
Preparation for labour and delivery	Education on childbirth and relaxation techniques are conducted on an individual or group basis by midwives, or physiotherapists. The woman's partner is also encouraged to attend the childbirth education programme, which prepares the couple for labour and delivery. The classes include instruction in relaxation techniques, and breathing patterns for labour. The couple are also informed of the physiology of labour and encouraged to discuss all aspects of pregnancy, birth, and care of the baby

Table 52.4 (cont'd) Prenatal education

Aspect	Description
Manifestations of complications	The woman is advised to contact her obstetrician or the hospital immediately if there is: • vaginal bleeding • abdominal or'menstrual-type' pain • severe headaches • drainage of fluid from the vagina • excessive vomiting • blurred vision • difficulty in passing urine • swelling of the hands, feet, or face
Manifestations of labour	The couple are informed of the manifestations of the onset of labour: • regular contractions • vaginal 'show' (blood-stained mucus) • drainage of amniotic fluid from the vagina (ruptured membranes)
Breasts	Maternity brassieres are designed to support the breasts as they increase in size and mass. The nipples are prepared for breast feeding by washing off any dried colostrum, and gently rolling them between the fingers each day A cream may be applied daily, e.g. anhydrous lanoline. If the nipples are flat or inverted, nipple shields may be worn under the brassiere. The shields depress the areolars and allow the nipples to extend
Sexual activity	Sexual activity may be continued throughout the pregnancy, unless there is a risk of haemorrhage, e.g. from a malpositioned placenta (placenta praevia) If the woman has a history of spontaneous abortion, she may be advised to avoid sexual intercourse during the first three months of pregnancy
Environmental hazards	Factors which are potentially harmful to the pregnancy should be avoided: • Smoking is linked to abortion, intrauterine growth retardation, and perinatal death • Alcohol, in excess, is linked to physical and mental fetal abnormalities, and fetal growth retardation • Many drugs, prescribed and unprescribed, are linked to physical and mental fetal damage • Exposure to micro-organisms, e.g. the rubella virus, in the first 3 months can result in fetal abnormalities • Immunizations generally should not be performed during pregnancy, because of possible damage to the fetus • Exposure to radiation during the early weeks of pregnancy may inhibit normal cell division • Exposure to pesticides and other chemicals may result in fetal abnormalities

Subsequent visits

The frequency with which these occur depend on the ob-stetrician and the needs of the woman, but the usual practice is to schedule the visits as follows:

* every 4 weeks until 28 weeks
* every 2 weeks until 36 weeks
* weekly until delivery.

At each visit assessment is made of:

* weight
* blood pressure
* urine (for protein, glucose, ketones)
* presence of oedema (of ankles, feet, hands)
* fundal height
* fetal position and heartbeat.

Blood tests or other investigations, e.g. ultrasonic examination, are performed as indicated.

LABOUR

Labour is the process by which the fetus, placenta, and membranes are ultimately expelled from the uterus via the vagina. Normal labour occurs spontaneously at approximately 40 weeks of pregnancy and lasts for up to 24 hours after onset. Factors which cause the spontaneous onset of normal labour include changes in hormonal levels, uterine distension, fetal pressure, and a sudden reduction of intra-uterine pressure when the membranes rupture.

Stages of labour

Labour is divided into three stages—first, second, and third. A final stage, the fourth, is the one 2 hours following the birth and delivery of the placenta. Table 52.5 lists the characteristics of each stage.

During labour, the uterus contracts rhythmically to dilate and efface the cervix, and push the fetus through the birth canal. After the baby is born, the uterus stops contracting for a brief time, then contractions recommence to expel the placenta and membranes.

Birth

The second stage of labour culminates in birth of the baby.

The woman is encouraged to adopt the position in which she feels the most comfortable for the birth. Delivery of the baby may take place with the mother lying down, standing, squatting, or kneeling. Some maternity units and birth centres are equipped with birthing chairs, in which the woman sits while giving birth.

During delivery of the baby, the obstetrician or midwife assists by gently controlling the emergence of the head to prevent perineal damage. In some instances an *episiotomy*, whereby the perineum is incised to enlarge the vaginal opening, may be necessary. Sometimes the application of

Table 52.5 Stages of labour

Stage	Characteristics
First	Contractions occur at fairly regular intervals, from approximately every 10 minutes at the onset of labour to approximately every 2 minutes at the end of the first stage The cervix is effaced (taken up) The fetal head begins to descend in the pelvis The cervix is gradually dilated The membranes rupture, and release amniotic fluid
Second	Strong contractions lasting approximately 60 seconds that become expulsive, and the woman experiences a desire to bear down The woman uses her abdominal muscles and diaphragm to assist in pushing the fetus down the birth canal The muscles of the pelvic floor are displaced by the advancing fetal head The vagina is dilated, and the perineum is thinned and flattened by the advancing head The vulva and vaginal orifice bulge, and the anus dilates as the head advances The baby is born
Third	After a brief period the placenta separates from the uterine wall Uterine contractions recommence to expel the placenta and membranes Signs of separation and descent of the placenta are: • Small rush of blood from the vagina • Cord lengthens at the vulva • The uterus is firmly contracted, and the height of the fundus drops to umbilical level
Fourth	In the 1–2 hours following delivery of the baby and expulsion of the placenta and membranes, the uterus begins the process of involution. Involution is the return of the uterus to its normal size

obstetrical forceps to the fetal head may be necessary to assist in its delivery through the birth canal.

Once the baby's head is delivered, the shoulders, then the rest of the baby's body is gently delivered. Immediately after birth, the baby is generally placed on the mother's abdomen. When the umbilical cord stops pulsating, it is clamped in two places and cut between the clamps.

Although approximately 95% of babies are born head first, a small number are born buttocks first (breech presentation). *A caesarian delivery* is the delivery of the fetus through an abdominal incision. A caesarian section may be indicated for a number of reasons, e.g. malpresentation of the fetus, maternal or fetal distress, malpositioned placenta, or failure of labour to progress.

MANAGEMENT DURING LABOUR AND BIRTH

Labour and childbirth are normal events, accompanied by a variety of emotions, e.g. excitement, fear, anxiety, and anticipation. As the management of and attitudes towards labour and birth differ widely amongst cultures, expectant women, obstetricians, and midwives, practices are developed according to needs, knowledge, and experience. This part of the chapter addresses the general aspects of care and support throughout labour and delivery.

The first stage

Care during the first stage involves monitoring the progress of labour, monitoring the condition of the woman and fetus, and promoting physical and psychological comfort.

Progress of labour is monitored by assessing the strength, frequency, and duration of contractions, by palpating the abdomen to assess the position and descent of the fetus, and by performing vaginal examinations to assess the degree of cervical dilatation and the position of the presenting part of the fetus.

The condition of the woman, and her response to labour, is monitored by checking her vital signs, by observing her urinary output and testing her urine for the presence of protein and ketones; and by observing her for the manifestations of fatigue, discomfort, or pain.

The condition of the fetus is monitored by assessing the fetal heart. As the fetal heart rate and rhythm is the main indicator of fetal condition, the fetal heart is assessed throughout labour. The heart rate should remain between 120 and 160 beats per minute, and the beats should remain strong and regular.

Assessment may be performed by listening to the heart through a stethoscope placed on the woman's abdomen, or by using a fetal monitoring device, e.g. a cardiotograph or doptone electronic machine. Fetal monitoring devices provide an audible and/or visual record of the fetal heart beat.

Another way that the condition of the fetus is assessed is by observing the passage of liquor draining from the woman's vagina. Normally the liquor remains clear and straw coloured, but green-tinged liquor indicates the presence of meconium. The passage of meconium (the dark green tarry substance that is formed in the fetal bowel) by the fetus while still in the uterus, indicates that the fetus is physically distressed due to a period of fetal oxygen deprivation.

Promoting comfort

Unless there are factors which may compromise the condition of the woman, or fetus, she is encouraged to do what ever will contribute to her comfort. She may choose to walk around, or she may prefer to sit or lie down. She may like to engage in some form of activity, e.g. read, watch television, listen to music, or knit. Some women find that frequent warm showers enhance their comfort, while other may prefer to have the midwife or partner massage the abdomen and back.

During the first stage, the woman may need to be reminded, and encouraged, to practise the relaxation and breathing techniques learnt in the prenatal classes. She is encouraged to empty her bladder at least every 2 hours, as a full bladder can inhibit uterine action.

She is also encouraged to consume frequent small amounts, e.g. 75 ml per hour, of clear fluids. Because the absorption of food is slowed down during labour, and because there is the possibility that a general anaesthetic may be necessary, solid food is generally restricted during labour. Her fluid input and output are monitored to assess for the manifestations of dehydration.

Because the process of labour requires the expenditure of large amounts of energy, the woman may become fatigued. Fatigue is minimized by encouraging rest and relaxation, and by relieving discomfort or pain.

Strong contractions may cause considerable discomfort, and the measures used to minimize and relieve discomfort will vary according to the needs of the woman. Measures to relieve discomfort aim to reduce pain and tension without causing any harmful effects to the woman or fetus. Measures include practicing relaxation techniques, assuming the most comfortable position, back and abdominal massage, using music as a distractor, and medications. Medications which may be used include sedatives, tranquilizers, and analgesics. Any medication which is administered must not cause harmful effects to the fetus, or retard the progress of labour.

Analgesic medications may be administered by inhalation, e.g. nitrous oxide and oxygen, by injection, e.g. pethidine, or by the administration of local anaesthetic solution into the extradural space surrounding the spinal cord from which the nerves supplying the uterus or cervix arise (epidural analgesia).

Throughout the first stage the nurse should provide emotional support and encouragement, and do all that she can to ensure that the labour is not a distressing experience.

The second stage

Although it may be accompanied by some anxiety, the second stage of labour is generally approached with anticipation—as it signals the imminent birth.

Progress of labour and the condition of the fetus are monitored as in the first stage but at more frequent intervals. During contractions, the midwife and/or partner should offer encouragement, and remind the woman to practise breathing and pushing techniques. To assist with the descent of the fetus, the woman takes a deep breath and 'bears down' with each contraction. Between contractions she may wish to have her lower back massaged, and she should be encouraged to rest. Small sips of fluid or ice chips should be offered to moisten her mouth, and the woman may wish to have her face wiped at frequent intervals. Labour is hard and tiring work.

Physical support may be needed to maintain the woman in a suitable position. She may wish to have her back supported by pillows—depending upon the position she adopts.

The second stage is completed when the baby is born, and it is an emotional time for everyone involved in the birth process. The baby is placed on the mother's abdomen, and both she and her partner should be allowed to look at and caress their infant. The obstetrician or midwife remains nearby so that the condition of both mother and baby can be monitored. It may be necessary to aspirate mucus from the baby's mouth to prevent inhalation.

The mother may wish to place the baby to her breast and allow it to suckle. Such close contact helps establish the attachment process between mother and baby, and sucking promotes the recommencement of uterine contractions which are necessary for expulsion of the placenta.

The third stage

During this stage the placenta and membranes are expelled. Following expulsion the woman's vulva and vagina are swabbed clean, and inspected for any lacerations. Any laceration or episiotomy is repaired. A sterile vulval pad is applied to collect the vaginal discharge.

The woman is assessed for signs of haemorrhage, and for any adverse effects of the delivery.

To assist with involution of the uterus, the uterine fundus is massaged, through the abdominal wall, to promote contraction and retraction. In some settings, oxytotic medications such as ergometrine maleate, are given to promote uterine contraction.

The placenta and membranes are assessed to see if they are normal and complete. If they are incomplete, there may be fragments retained in the uterus—preventing uterine contraction and providing a focus far infection.

POSTNATAL CARE

Following the third stage, the mother's comfort is promoted by ensuring that any wet or soiled clothing is replaced, and by offering her a drink and snack. She and her partner should be allowed to spend time together, with the baby. If the mother is exhausted she may appreciate being left to rest or sleep.

Care of the mother

The degree of care required will depend on a variety of factors, e.g. where the birth occurred, how long the mother remains in the maternity unit or birth centre, whether the birth was uncomplicated, and whether there are any post-natal discomforts or complications. Postnatal care is directed at promoting the health of both mother and baby. Aspects of care include promoting:

- adequate rest
- freedom from infection
- freedom from discomfort or pain
- establishing lactation and breast feeding
- confidence in caring for her baby.

Assessment is made of the lochia, the vaginal discharge that occurs following delivery. Lochia, which consists of blood and broken-down endometrium, is discharged for up to 3 or 4 weeks following delivery. At first it is bright red in colour, then becomes pink, and ultimately presents as a colourless or white discharge. Lochia should not have an offensive odour, nor contain any blood clots.

Perineal care involves daily showering to cleanse the area and frequent changing of vulval pads. If a tear occurred, or if an episiotomy was performed, local care may be needed to reduce discomfort and prevent infection. Local care may involve the application of cold packs to the area, or sitz baths to which salt has been added to the water. A sheepskin rug or water mattress to sit on may help to relieve perineal soreness, and analgesic medications, e.g. paracetamol, may be prescribed.

Fundal height is assessed and documented each day to monitor involution of the uterus. It may be necessary to massage the fundus to promote uterine contraction. The height of the fundus decreases by approximately 1 cm each day, until by the eleventh or twelfth day it can no longer be palpated abdominally.

The breasts and nipples are assessed each day for any red areas, oedema, cracking or bleeding. Palpation of each breast detects any areas of hardness which may indicate blocked milk ducts.

Postnatal exercises are commenced on the first day. They are designed to strengthen the abdominal muscles, and tone up the pelvic floor. An instruction sheet which illustrates the exercises to be performed is generally given to the mother.

A balanced diet, which provides adequate nutrients and fibre is provided. If the woman is breast feeding, she should consume an extra 2500–4000 kj per day above the requirements of pregnancy. This provides the extra energy required to produce milk. In addition to nutrional re-

quirements, the lactating mother requires 3 litres of fluid per day.

The lactating mother is advised to avoid consuming foods which are likely to upset the baby. The woman who wishes to breast feed should also be advised of the substances known to be excreted in the breast milk. Substances which should be avoided or taken sparingly include:

- nicotine
- alcohol
- caffeine
- laxatives
- anti-infective agents
- sedatives.

Minor postnatal discomforts

After-pains are the cramps which occur for a few days after delivery, as the uterine muscles contract during the process of involution.

Constipation may result from inadequate fibre or fluid intake, or if the mother is afraid that defaecation will cause or increase perineal discomfort.

Difficulty in voiding may be experienced initially, because of loss of bladder tone, bruising of the urethra, or perineal soreness.

Engorged breasts may occur a few days after the delivery, due to an increase in the blood supply to the breasts in preparation for lactation. The breasts become distended, hard, and uncomfortable.

Breast feeding

Breast feeding is a natural function and the optimum method of feeding the baby. While the majority of women will choose to breastfeed, there are others who, for a variety of reasons, will prefer not to. While it is important that a woman be advised of the benefits of breast feeding, it is also important that she is not made to feel guilty if she chooses to bottle feed.

Lactation

During pregnancy, development of the glandular tissue and ducts in the breasts is stimulated by the placental hormones: oestrogen, progesterone, and placental lactogenic hormone.

Colostrum is the fluid secreted by the breasts during pregnancy and the first few days after birth before lactation commences. Colostrum, a thin, yellow, serous fluid, consists of water, protein, fat, carbohydrates, and immunologically active substances.

When the placenta is expelled, following delivery of the

baby, the pituitary gland releases prolactin which activates the mammary cells to produce and release milk.

Lactation depends on the maintenance of milk production, and on the let-down 'reflex of milk ejection. Oxytocin is released from the pituitary gland in response to suckling, forcing milk out of the alveoli in the breasts. The let-down reflex, whereby milk is ejected from the breasts, is stimulated by a neurogenic reflex. The let-down reflex, which generally occurs a short time after the baby begins to suck on the nipple, can also be stimulated when the mother sees, hears, or thinks about her baby. Conversely, the reflex can be inhibited by anxiety, fear, or tension.

Breast feeding has advantages for both the mother and baby. Breast milk is free from micro-organisms, is easily digested, it contains all the essential nutrients necessary for the baby's development, and it contains immunoglobulins and other substances which protect the infant from some infections while his immune system is under-developed. Breast feeding aids involution of the uterus, and is generally emotionally satisfying for the mother. Breast feeding is also convenient and economical.

Management

The majority of women will manage to breast feed their babies without any difficulties. Initially, a woman may require some assistance to ensure that the baby's mouth is correctly positioned over the nipple. The baby's 'seeking reflex' is initiated when his cheek touches the breast, and he will turn his face to find the nipple. A few drops of breast milk can be expressed onto the nipple to encourage him to take the nipple into his mouth. The nipple should be placed into his mouth, over his tongue, and the baby's lips should be in contact with the areolar. The baby's mouth should remain wide open against the breast so that his mouth covers a substantial part of the areolar. It is important that the baby is able to breathe freely while feeding, and this is achieved by depressing the area of the breast near the baby's nose. The area should be depressed towards the nipple, so that the nipple is not pulled upwards and away from the baby's mouth.

When breast feeding, the woman should position herself so that she is comfortable and able to hold the baby securely. She should ensure that her nipples are free from any dried milk or nipple cream, before she commences the feed. The baby should also be comfortable, e.g. in a clean and dry napkin, and his arms should remain free.

During the feed, the baby should be sat up and de-winded if necessary. To detach the baby from the nipple, the mother should place a finger into the side of the baby's mouth thus letting air in the break the suction. Gentle detachment helps to prevent the development of sore nipples.

After the feed the baby is checked to ensure that he is clean and comfortable, and he should be placed in his cot without too much handling. To guard against possible regurgitation, and subsequent inhalation of milk, he should be placed on his right side, or abdomen with his head turned to the side.

The mother should ensure that her nipples are clean and dried, and she may apply a nipple cream, e.g. wool fat emollient, to protect them against soreness or cracking.

The baby is fed when he is hungry (demand feeding). Each baby is an individual, and some may require breast feeding as frequently as every 2 hours, while others will be content if they are fed every 3–4 hours. The length of time the baby feeds also varies. A baby may receive enough milk after 7 minutes on one breast, or he may require as long as 10 minutes on each breast. The baby and mother establish their own feeding routine, and the mother's milk supply adjusts according to demand.

Breast milk may be expressed, either manually or with a breast pump, if necessary. Expression may be necessary to relieve discomfort if the breasts are overfull, to help stimulate milk production, or to put breast milk into a feeding bottle, e.g. if the baby requires feeding when his mother is temporarily unavailable. Expressed breast milk can also be provided by the mother if her baby is premature or ill, and is unable to feed at the breast.

Breast feeding difficulties sometimes arise for a variety of reasons:

- maternal anxiety or frustration about breast feeding
- cracked nipples, which cause pain when the baby sucks
- inverted nipples, which are difficult for the baby to grasp
- breast engorgement, which prevents the milk from flowing readily
- overabundance of milk, which flows too quickly causing the baby to splutter and, perhaps, vomit
- failure of the let-down reflex
- inability of the baby to suck well enough at the breast.

Management of breast feeding difficulties depends on the cause, but with time, patience, and encouragement the majority can be overcome. Organizations such as The Nursing Mothers Association of Australia provide support and advice on how to prevent and deal with breast feeding difficulties.

Artificial feeding is provided for babies who are not being breast fed. Artificial feeds are generally based on cow's milk, although other preparations are available, e.g. a soy-based formula. The formula that is selected will depend on the needs of the mother and the baby. Some formulae are expensive, others may not be readily available, or the baby may require a special formula, e.g. soy-based or lactose-free.

Which ever formula is selected, the mother must know how to make it up, how to store it, and how to care for the bottles and teats. Information on artificial feeding is provided in Chapter 54.

Care of the baby

Immediately after the delivery, the midwife or obstetrician checks that the baby's airway is clear and that he is breathing normally. Initiation of ventilation is achieved in response to a high blood carbon dioxide level stimulating the respiratory centre in the medulla. In the first few breaths, air is drawn in to expand the alveoli in the lungs, thus oxygenating the blood. Because the newborn baby has a limited ability to regulate his body temperature in relation to the environment, care is taken to ensure that he does not become cold.

One minute after delivery, and again at 5 minutes, the *Apgar score* estimation is performed. The Apgar scoring system gives an estimation of the baby's condition, and is an indicator of whether special resuscitation measures are required. Table 52.6 illustrates the Apgar score chart. A total score of 10 indicates that the infant is in optimum condition; if the score is 6 or less the baby requires immediate attention. A score of 8–10 is normal, a score of 4–7 indicates the infant is moderately depressed, while a score of 0–3 indicates severe depression.

In a health care setting, e.g. hospital or birth centre, the baby is identified by placing identification bands on his wrist and ankle. An ink imprint of the baby's foot may be made as well. The identification procedure, which is performed before the baby is removed from the mother's bed is essential to prevent any mistakes in identity of the baby.

The baby is weighed and measured and the information documented. If it is the usual practice, the baby is given an intramuscular injection of Vitamin K as a preventive measure against bleeding tendencies. An initial examination of the baby is performed soon after the delivery, so that any abnormal findings can be acted upon as soon as possible. The examination assesses the baby's ventilation, colour, muscle tone, reflexes, movement, and the presence of any obvious abnormalities. Later on, a more thorough examination is performed.

Table 52.7 illustrates the characteristics of a normal newborn baby.

Subsequent care

Care of the baby following the period immediately after delivery, is directed towards keeping him adequately nourished, clean, warm, and free from infection. Careful observation is necessary to detect any problems should they occur.

In a health care setting the mother generally wishes to keep the baby in her room, although it may be necessary at times for the baby to spend some time in the nursery. When the baby remains in the room, the mother is able to care for him from the outset. This enables her to get to know her baby and gain confidence in caring for him. The midwife is available to offer guidance and encouragement in all aspects of infant care. If the baby spends time in the nursery, e.g when he requires special attention or close observation, the parents are encouraged to spend as much time with him as possible.

Hygiene and skin care. Health care settings establish their own protocol for washing or bathing newborn babies (neonates). The baby is usually washed or bathed daily. An antibacterial substance may be added to the water, or a mild pure soap may be used. It is important that the infant's skin is kept clean and dry, with special attention being paid to his scalp, skin folds, and genitals.

The buttocks and groin area are washed with plain water, or cleansed with a mild lotion, each time a wet or soiled napkin is removed. A protective cream or lotion may

Table 52.6 Apgar scoring

Factors	Scores		
	2	1	0
Heart rate	Over 100	Less than 100	Absent
Respiration	Established and almost regular	Intermittent, gasping in character	Absent
Colour	Pink all over	Centrally pink, but with blue extremities	Cyanosed or pale
Muscle tone	Good—active movements	Fair—some flexion of extremities	None—completely limp
Response to stimulation	Vigorous withdrawal	Minimal withdrawal	None

Table 52.7 The normal newborn

	Characteristics
Head	Average circumference 35 cm Anterior fontanelle—no tension or depression Posterior fontanelle—palpable May be elongated—due to moulding as the skull bones glide over each other during passage through the birth canal
Face	Nose and cheeks may have tiny white spots (milia)
Skin	Normal colour for race May be covered with lanugo (fine downy hair) May be vernix (white, greasy, protective substance) in the skin folds
Eyes	Dark blue; white sclera Blink reflex present
Thorax	Average circumference 34 cm Expands symmetrically with ventilations Breast tissue palpable in males and females
Abdomen	Prominent but not distended Moves up and down with ventilations Umbilical cord blue/white
Limbs	Symmetrical, warm, rounded Move freely Hands and feet may be slightly cyanosed
Back	Spine straight, intact, easily flexed
Genitalia	Male—large in relation to body, scrotum contains both testes, foreskin adheres to glans, urethral meatus central on tip of penis Female—prominent labia and clitoris, vaginal opening visible
Anus	Patent

be applied. Disposable or cloth napkins may be used. The mother may need some advice on how to fold and apply napkins.

The cord is observed every time a napkin is changed, until it has separated and the umbilicus has healed. The cord is kept clean and dry by using a spirit solution, and it is observed for any bleeding or signs of infection. The cord separates from the umbilicus, by a process of dry necrosis, on the sixth to eighth day. Spirit is applied to the umbilicus until it is fully healed.

If the baby's fingernails are long he may scratch his face, and the scratches may become infected. Mittens may be worn, or the baby's fingernails gently trimmed.

Elimination. After the first day, when the neonate may void only once or twice, urine is passed approximately 10–12 times per day. Any unusual colouration or odour must be reported to the medical officer.

The baby's first bowel action consists of *meconium*, the dark green tarry substance formed in the intestinal tract during intrauterine life. When the baby begins to take milk, there is a gradual transition to the normal yellow stools of the neonate. Breast fed babies pass stools that are yellow to pale brown, soft, and unformed. The stools of an artificially fed baby are yellow to pale green, firmer, and have a distinctive odour.

Nutrition. The baby is fed when he is hungry. Frequent feedings, e.g. every 2 hours, may be indicated if the baby shows signs of hypoglycaemia. In health care settings the neonate is generally weighed every second day to assess weight gain or loss. More frequent weighing is indicated if the birth weight was low, or if the baby is losing excessive weight. A loss of up to 10% of the birth weight is normal in the first 3–4 days, then the baby should begin to gain weight.

Infection control. The baby is protected from infection by normal hygiene practices, the most important aspect of which is washing the hands thoroughly before attending to the baby. Anyone with an infection is advised to limit close contact with the baby.

Temperature control. As the neonate's temperature regulating centre is not fully functional, he must be protected from extremes of environmental temperature by maintaining the room at an even, comfortable temperature, dressing the baby in suitable clothes, and wrapping him in warm, light weight rugs.

Neonatal disorders

This part of the chapter merely mentions some of the disorders which can effect the neonate. For detailed information, the nurse should refer to a current paediatric text. Disorders may be minor and temporary, major and permanent, or life-threatening. They include:

- prematurity
- low birth weight
- jaundice
- hypoxia
- atelectasis
- hyaline membrane disease
- hypoglycaemia
- persistent vomiting
- birth injuries
- congenital abnormalities.

CONCLUSION

The nurse may be required to assist in the care of a mother and her newborn baby. Therefore it is important that she has a basic knowledge and understanding of the processes of normal pregnancy, labour, birth, and the postnatal care of the mother and her baby.

REFERENCES AND FURTHER READING

Farrer H 1990 Maternity care, 2nd edn. Churchill Livingstone, Melbourne
Marieb E N 1984 Essentials of human anatomy and physiology. Addison-Wesley, California

53. The individual with a developmental disability

INTRODUCTION

Development, a life-long process that begins at conception, is influenced by both genetic and environmental factors. An individual has his own inherited genetic material which is his biological potential for development, while factors in the environment influence how that potential will be realized. It is the *interaction* between genetic and environmental factors which ultimately affects an individual's development.

The information on normal growth and development, which is provided in Chapters 2 and 3, should be reviewed before studying the contents of this chapter.

While recognizing that a developmental disability may be classified as physical, intellectual, or sociocultural, this chapter focuses on the individual with an *intellectual* disability. Intellectual disability is regarded as an cognitive (learning difficulty), rather than a medical problem. Therefore this chapter, as part of a nursing text, does not attempt to address the subject in depth. However, as nurses may work with people with an intellectual disability, e.g. in the role of residential care attendant, this chapter aims to provide the nurse with some basic information on care and provision of services.

Before addressing the area of developmental disabilities, it is necessary to define the terms, 'impairment', 'disability', and 'handicap'. In 1980, the World Health Or-ganization (WHO) adopted the following definitions:

1. Impairments: concerned with the abnormalities of body structure and appearance and with system function resulting from any cause; in principle, impairments represent disturbances at the organ level.

2. Disabilities: reflect the consequences of impairment in terms of functional performance and activity by the individual; disabilities thus represent disturbances at the level of the person.

3. Handicaps: concerned with the disadvantages experienced by the individual as a result of impairments and disabilities; handicaps thus reflect interaction with the individual's environment.

Classification of developmental disabilities

Specific developmental disabilities, which can be either congenital or acquired, may be classified as:

- Intellectual retardation, e.g. associated with Down syndrome. Intellectual disability refers to below-average general intellectual functioning, and is generally classified as profound, severe, moderate, or mild.
- Disorders of neuromuscular function, e.g. cerebral palsy, muscular dystrophy, or spina bifida.
- Learning disorders, e.g. dyslexia.
- Disorders of communication, e.g. a speech or language disorder.
- Emotional or behavioural problems, e.g. hyperactivity or autism.
- Physical disorders, e.g. visual or hearing impairments, congenital cardiac abnormalities, or limb deficiencies.

Development delay refers to a delay in the development of a child which results in functional limitations in self care and/or language, cognitive development or motor development.

Causes of developmental disabilities

A developmental disability may be either congenital or acquired. Causes of congenital disabilities include:

- chromosomal abnormalities, e.g. an extra chromosome 21 causing Down syndrome
- inherited metabolic defects, e.g. decreased phenylalanine hydroxylase causing phenylketonuria (PKU)
- maternal infections during pregnancy, e.g. rubella or toxoplasmosis
- maternal malnutrition, or chronic maternal illness such as renal or cardiac disease
- exposure to toxic agents, e.g. drugs or environmental chemicals, during intrauterine life
- exposure to high energy radiation during intrauterine life
- premature birth which may result in cerebral damage
- birth injuries, e.g. cerebral damage due to disruption of oxygen supply.

Causes of acquired disabilities include:
- trauma, e.g. brain or spinal injury
- infection, e.g. encephalitis
- exposure to hazardous substances, e.g. lead or carbon monoxide
- emotional deprivation or lack of stimulation
- inadequate nutrition, e.g. kwashiorkor caused by severe protein deficiency.

Prevention

Prevention of developmental disabilities is directed towards eliminating the causes, and includes:

- Genetic counselling for couples who at risk of producing a child with a disability, e.g. those with a family history of an inherited disorder, or those who have previously had a child with a birth defect
- Immunization against specific infectious diseases, e.g. rubella. Prenatal maternal rubella is known to be associated with fetal abnormalities such as intellectual disabilities, heart disease, cataracts, and deafnes.
- High quality prenatal care which includes advising the pregnant woman on the importance of adequate nutrition, and on the importance of avoiding exposure to harmful agents, e.g. excess alcohol, nicotine, non-prescribed drugs, and radiation.
- Good obstetric techniques which will minimize the possibility of birth injuries.
- High quality paediatric care so that a child's health status can be monitored and any impairments detected early and treated appropriately. Phenylktonuria is one disorder which, if detected early, can be treated effectively so that no brain damage occurs. Detection of this disorder involves testing a sample of the infant's blood 5–7 days after birth (Guthrie test). If the test is positive, treatment by diet is commenced immediately.

- Promoting parenting skills so that the infant's needs are met. Parents should be informed of the importance of meeting the child's emotional, as well as his physical needs. Lack of emotional security and stimulation influence a child's developmental potential.
- Early detection and treatment of any infection, e.g. encephalitis, that may result in an impairment.
- Educating people in the importance of avoiding exposure to environmental hazards which may result in intellectual disability. For example, people should be aware that ingestion of paint which contains lead can result in lead poisoning, and possible cognitive deficits.

Approaches

The reactions experienced by parents when their child is born with or develops an impairment varies according to several factors, e.g. the degree and type of impairment, how obvious the impairment is, and the response of other people. Initial feelings of shock, disbelief, anger, guilt, grief, loss, and apprehension are almost always experienced. How the situation is managed will depend to some extent on how the parents are able to deal with those feelings, and on the type and amount of support they are offered.

In the past it was quite usual to admit a person with severe impairment to an institution, for life-long custodial care. Institutional care was deemed to be the most appropriate for many reasons, e.g. an institution was viewed as being able to provide the best protection and care for an impaired individual who was unable to function 'normally' in society.

The current attitudes towards the care of an impaired person reflect the belief that such a person is entitled to the same rights and freedom as any other person in society. There is a growing realization that an individual with intellectual disability has potential for growth, development, and learning. Consequently, the emphasis is on identifying and providing the ways in which that potential can be made possible. It is now generally recognized that, regardless of whether an individual with an intellectual disability is able to remain at home or lives in alternate accommodation, the overall goal of care must be to enable him to achieve as much independence as possible.

Services

The range of services available to people with intellectual disabilities includes:

- home services, e.g. housekeeper, home help, laundry service, personal helpers, companion service, adaptations to the home, and aids to independent living.
- home-based programmes of education and care.
- volunteer groups.

- parent education, and parent support groups.
- counselling.
- adult training centres.
- neighbourhood houses.
- sheltered workshops.
- supported open employment.
- day care facilities.
- emergency or short-term relief residential care.
- consumer-based support groups.
- long-term care in hostels, small community residences, or specialized residential facilities.
- supported independent living.

The services aim to assist the intellectually impaired individual to achieve as much independence as possible by promoting family and community acceptance and involvement, providing sufficient support services, and by offering a range of accommodation options.

CARING FOR AN INDIVIDUAL WITH AN INTELLECTUAL DISABILITY

The new philosophy of care, and provision of services to intellectually impaired people, stresses the concept of 'normalization'. It emphasises the importance of helping a person with an intellectual disability, as far as possible, to live like any other person. Inherent in this concept is the belief that an intellectually impaired individual is entitled to participate in community life and to enjoy the same rights and privileges as others. The concept of normalization is applied to the provision of community services, and to the care of people with intellectual disabilities in residential facilities.

Tully (1986) states that the 'principle of normalization is generally viewed as the most important concept around which to construct appropriate and effective services for disabled people. Whilst it has been the subject of much misunderstanding and misinterpretation, it remains a central idea for identifying present deficiencies in service provision and in shaping new forms of help'.

There is much greater acceptance of the importance of family living and of participation in community life. The emphasis on residential facilities is moving away from large-scale institutional living to smaller residential homes in the community. Educational and vocational training programmes and opportunities have been increased, since the realization that intellectually impaired people benefit from an educational programme which is properly structured to meet their needs.

Thus, the provision of services for the intellectually impaired depends on recognition of their rights, promotion of community acceptance, and development of appropriate training and education programmes. Support is directed towards enabling a person with intellectual disability to achieve as much independence as possible, through intervention and support which promote independent living and vocational capacities.

The planning and implementation of appropriate educational and vocational programmes is performed on an individual basis, and takes into account any associated physical, sensory, and emotional disabilities. Some individuals with intellectual disability also have at least one additional disability, such as:

- impaired mobility
- impaired motor control of hands
- impaired speech, hearing, or vision
- seizures
- lack of bladder and/or bowel control
- emotional or behavioural problems
- impaired ability to communicate.

Assessment

Decisions about the most appropriate plan of care are made following individual assessment. Assessment is generally performed by a team which may include teachers, medical officers, social workers, nurses, psychologists, occupational therapists, speech pathologists, and physiotherapists. The purpose of assessment is to identify the specific needs of an individual so that appropriate care may be planned.

Aspects of the individual's life that require assessment include his:

- general health status
- degree of independence in the activities of daily living
- ability to participate in work and leisure activities
- ability to communicate .general educational skills, e.g. reading or writing
- ability to relate in social situations
- awareness of self and self-concept
- relationship with his family.

The team may assess the individual using a variety of methods, e.g. observation, interviewing, and testing. A checklist may be used to help identify those activities which can be performed independently by the individual, and those with which he requires assistance. Once assessment is complete, the team can plan the care to be implemented.

Planning and implementing

Using the information obtained from assessing the individual, the team can plan a programme that will meet his needs. Central to development of a programme is the concept of helping the individual to achieve as much independence as possible. Tully (1986) summarizes the stages in programming as, 'identifying skill to be developed, establishing goals, assessing present level of competence, determining the most effective teaching strategies, planning the program, implementing the program, evaluating the program.'

The plan is implemented using the appropriate teaching strategies which include instruction, demonstration, and role play. As the attention span of an intellectually impaired person may be short, each task should be simple and broken down into steps. Each specific task or skill, e.g. brushing the teeth, dressing, self-feeding, requires an individual teaching strategy. *Behaviour modification* is one method of instruction that may be utilized when an individual experiences difficulty in learning. It is a method of re-education, and is an attempt to change disordered patterns of behaviour through modification techniques. In this method of instruction, correct behaviour is rewarded (positively reinforced) and inappropriate behaviour is ignored (negatively reinforced).

Overall, behaviour management strategies build on the individual's strengths rather than focusing on his weaknesses. For example, if someone wishes to teach an individual to dress himself, each correct action performed by him would be rewarded. Reward may take the form of verbal praise or some tangible reinforcer.

For any programme to be successful, the goals and the skills to be accomplished by the individual must be clearly expressed and understood by all team members.

Evaluation

Evaluation must be performed continuously to assess whether the individual is able to perform the necessary personal and social skills, and to enable changes to be made to the programme as necessary.

Environment

Regardless of the type of accommodation in which the individual with an intellectual disability is residing, there are certain prerequisites to promote a beneficial environment:

• encouraging and teaching the individual to be as independent as possible.

• allowing the individual to exercise choice.
• recognizing the individual's right to privacy.
• establishing routines which provide a sense of security.
• providing sufficient opportunities for participation in social and leisure activities.
• providing a physical environment which is 'home-like', and which is equipped with features that facilitate independence, e.g. hand rails, ramps, access to benches and equipment.

CONCLUSION

A developmental disability may be congenital or acquired, and it may be physical, intellectual, or sociocultural.

This chapter has focused on the individual with intellectual disability, and has attempted to provide the nurse with some basic information on care and provision of services.

It is important to appreciate that intellectual impairment is regarded as an education problem and, therefore, a philosophy of care stresses the provision of suitable educational and vocational training programmes.

The current attitudes towards intellectual disability reflect the belief that such persons are entitled to the same rights and freedom as any other member of society.

The services which are provided for persons with intellectual disabilities recognize the importance of identifying and providing the ways in which the individual's potential can be made possible.

The nurse who works in the area of developmental disability, or requires further information, is advised to consult appropriate texts, such as those listed at the end of this chapter.

REFERENCES AND FURTHER READING

Clements A 1986 Infant and family health in Australia. Churchill Livingston, Melbourne
Moore T 1984 Early intervention with handicapped children-aims and methods. Workshop paper prepared for the Department of Education, Government of Victoria
Tully K 1986 Improving residential life for disabled people. Churchill Livingstone, Melbourne

54. The infant, child and adolescent

INTRODUCTION

Nursing care of infants, children, and adolescents is directed towards promoting the optimum level of health for each individual. Care involves preventing disease and injury, promoting family involvement in child care, health teaching, participating in a team approach to care, and implementing measures to meet the physical, emotional, social, and cultural needs of each individual.

It is important for the nurse to understand that both childhood and adolescence are unique phases of development, and that these phases are accompanied by special needs. In order to care for individuals from infancy to adolescence, the nurse first requires knowledge of normal growth and development. By understanding the normal the nurse is more able to recognize departures from normal and, therefore, to plan and implement appropriate nursing actions.

Growth and development

Information on growth and development is provided in Chapters 2 and 3, and it should be reviewed before studying the contents of this chapter. Growth refers to the increase in weight and size of an individual and results when cells divide and synthesize new proteins, whereas *development* relates to changes in psychological and social functioning. Growth and development affect the total person and, although separately defined, growth and development overlap and are inter-dependent. Both occur from the moment of fertilization until death. There are some of the basic principles of growth and development.

- Growth in weight (mass) and height is variable and not uniform throughout life. The maximum rate of growth occurs before birth, in the fourth month of fetal life. Growth in height ceases when maturation of the skeleton is complete. Standard growth charts are available, on which measurements of growth are periodically plotted and compared with the norm for that particular age group.
- Growth and development occur in specific directions. Development is closed related to maturation of the nervous system, and begins in the cephalocaudal direction (head to tail) i.e. head control must be achieved before walking is possible. The second direction is from the centre of the body outward (proximodistal) i.e. infants learn to control shoulder movements before they control hand movements.
- There is a sequence, order, and pattern to growth and development. There are certain developmental tasks that must be accomplished during each stage. A developmental task is a set of skills and competencies peculiar to each developmental stage, that the child must accomplish in order to deal effectively with his environment. Each stage lays the foundation for the next stage of development. The stages of development are:

- prenatal (conception to birth)
- infancy (birth to 12 months)
- early childhood (12 months to 5 years)
- later childhood (5 years to 12 years)

- adolescence (13 years to approximately 18 years)
- adulthood (18 years onward)

Development encompasses various aspects: motor, vision and hearing, speech and language, intellectual, emotional, personality, moral, and social.

Although there is an orderly pattern to the processes, the rate of growth and development varies among individuals. Growth and development are influenced by heredity, environment, physical care, mental stimulation, personal potential, and emotional security. Table 54.1 summarizes developmental progress from birth to adolescence.

Table 54.1 Developmental progress from birth to adolescence

Age	Motor, communication, manipulative, and social skills
Birth to 1 month	Primitive reflexes: can suck, grasp, and respond to sudden sounds. Crying patterns and 'cooing' noises
1–3 months	Holds head up when prone, holds head erect when held in a sitting position. Begins to vocalize. Smiles responsively. Distinguishes parents from others
3–5 months	Turns head toward sounds. Rolls from prone to supine. Makes sounds when spoken to, may squeal with pleasure. Clasps hands together and can hold a rattle. Begins to watch own hands. Smiles and vocalizes
6–9 months	Sits with support and, later, alone. Sits up from a lying position. Crawls. Babbles and vocalizes; says words like mum-mum, da-da. Picks objects up between finger and thumb. Reacts to strangers with anxiety
10–12 months	Pulls self into a standing position, may walk with support. Says single words. Obeys simple instructions. Imitates adults, e.g. will scribble with a crayon. Expresses emotion. Can hold a cup to drink
12–18 months	Walks on own, can climb stairs and onto chairs. Imitates words and has a vocabulary of 3–24 words. Turns pages, scribbles, plays with building blocks constructively. Can identify several parts of his body. Likes to play with other children
24 months	Able to run, climb, walk up and down stairs alone. Begins to put two or three words together, begins to use pronouns. Imitates adult activities, can dress himself but not do up buttons. Plays with other children
3 years	Runs confidently, jumps, can ride a tricycle. Can say his own name and sex. Listens to stories. Vocabulary of 250–800 words. Thinks ego-centrically. Plays constructively. Interacts with peers
4 years	Catches a ball, can hop on one foot. Knows many letters of the alphabet, and can count up to 10. Recites and sings. Asks lots of 'why' and 'how' questions. Vocabulary of 800–1500 words. Can use scissors. Plays co-operatively with others
5 years	Can skip and hop. Can identify colours. Increased vocabulary, enjoys jokes and riddles. Ties shoelaces, does up buttons. More independent. Strongly identifies with parent of the same sex

Table 54.1 (cont'd)   Developmental progress from birth to adolescence

Age	Motor, communication, manipulative, and social skills
6–7 years	Gradual increase in dexterity, constant activity, more aware of the hand as a tool. Vocabulary of over 2500 words, and can verbally communicate thoughts and feelings better than before. Likes to engage in quiet activities such as playing with cards, board games, paints. Less resistant and stubborn, can share and co-operate better
8–9 years	Increased smoothness and speed in fine motor control. Very active physically. Is able to count backwards, state the days of the week and months in order, describe objects in detail. Is more sociable and interacts well with a wider range of people, gets on well with adults
10–12 years	Pubescent changes may begin to appear. Body movements are more graceful and co-ordinated. Becomes more independent of adults and learns to depend on self. Enjoys reading for practical information or enjoyment. Chooses friends more selectively. Enjoys conversation. Begins to develop moral and ethical behaviour
13–18 years	Co-ordination improves until approximately 14 years of age when the individual may appear awkward. Many physical changes associated with increased production of sex hormones. Often experiences anxiety and difficulty accepting changes in appearance. Great dependence on peer groups and identifies with small select groups. Becomes independent from parents and adults. Strives for independence while still desiring dependence. Develops morals attitudes and values needed for functioning in society

Child abuse

Child abuse, or maltreatment, can be identified as any situation in which a child is non-accidently harmed physically, mentally, or emotionally. Child abuse results from psychological, sociological, cultural, and environmental factors. Studies have shown that child abuse is due to these and other factors, often in combination, and that there is no reliably identifiable single cause. Nurses may come into contact with a child who has been abused, therefore it is important that they have some knowledge and understanding about child abuse.

Many hospitals, especially those with paediatric facilities, have clearly defined protocols for the management of abused children and their families, and nurses who are working with children should make certain they understand the procedures to be followed when child abuse is suspected. Many hospitals also have multidisciplinary teams to assist in diagnosis, assessment, and treatment.

Prevention of child abuse and neglect is very important and involves:

- identifying families at risk for potential abuse
- providing supportive services, e.g. parents anonymous groups, day care facilities, foster care, volunteer co-ordinators, family aides, individual counselling

- promoting parenting skills and parental attachment
- alleviating stresses in particular families
- removing a child from an abusive, or potentially abusive, situation.

Child abuse may be classed as:

- physical abuse
- neglect
- failure to thrive
- emotional deprivation and abuse
- sexual abuse.

Signs of *physical abuse* may be readily identified, or they may be less obvious and difficult to recognize. Some of the signs which should alert medical officers, nurses, and others who work with children, include:

- delay in seeking treatment for an injury
- inadequate explanation of the cause of injuries
- multiple injuries, e.g. bruises, scratches, burns, and bite marks
- the site of injuries, e.g. localized burns on the buttocks or soles of the feet
- presentation of the parents, e.g. showing a lack of concern for the child, or inability to comfort a distressed child
- manifestations of developmental delay in a child, e.g. delay in development of language skills.

Signs of *emotional deprivation or abuse* are generally more difficult to recognize. Emotional deprivation may be evident when signs of failure to thrive are present. Failure to thrive is generally defined as an underweight, malnourished infant with a height and head circumference near to normal. Although failure to thrive may be caused by emotional deprivation, other causes are organic ones, or accidental underfeeding. Emotional abuse occurs when the child is not provided with the type of environment that is required for his optimal growth and development. The child may be subjected to continual verbal abuse, hostility and rejection.

Sexual abuse in children may present in a variety of ways:

- a history of sexual abuse from the child or a family member
- vague abdominal pains, or persistent or unexplained vaginal discharge
- sexually transmitted disease
- unexplained genital trauma
- running away from home
- sexually provocative behaviour.

PAEDIATRIC CARE

The term 'paediatric' means of/or pertaining to a child, and paediatric nursing is the area of nursing concerned with the care of infants and children. Paediatric nursing requires knowledge of normal growth and development, as well as knowledge of the needs and health problems of individuals in these age groups.

The role of a paediatric nurse can be described as that of care-giver, co-ordinator, educator, emotional support-and-resource person. The nurse who is involved in paediatric care, together with other members of the paediatric team, need to adopt a holistic attitude towards caring for the child and parent/s as a family unit. Many health care facilities recognize the need for family-centred care and adopt a philosophy to meet the needs of the family as a unit.

It is important for the nurse to recognize that children are not small adults, and that their reactions are generally quite different from the adult's reactions to illness, treatment, separation from family, and admission to hospital.

Child health services

There are a variety of child health services whose broad aims are promotion of the health of infants and children, the provision of parental support and the provision of care for the child who is ill. Many of the services are involved in preventing ill health, and are concerned with monitoring the health of children from birth. Preventive services include child health clinics and school health services.

Child health clinics play an important role in the assessment of growth and development, health education; screening for physical, metabolic, and neuro-psychiatric disorders; and in providing immunization against infectious diseases. The child health nurse aims to develop a close relationship with the mother and newborn infant as soon as possible after the birth. She provides advice on infant hygiene, nutrition, growth and development, and preventive health measures such as recommended immunization schedules (information on immunization schedules is provided in Chapter 9). She also counsels and supports parents, consults with a paediatrician on health problems, refers children and families for supportive care as appropriate, and keeps comprehensive records. These records—which include information on the child's growth and development, immunizations, and illnesses—are important tools for assessment, and for detecting situations which require early intervention and preventive action.

School health services aim to promote health by providing health education programmes, by ensuring that each child is as healthy as possible so that he may obtain the maximum benefit from educational programmes; and by assisting with the detection and management of various groups of children with impairments, disabilities, or learning difficulties. School health services perform routine medical services just prior or soon after entry into school, and selective medical examinations during school life. The school nurse plays an important role in the prevention and detection of illness and disabilities. Two of the tests which are performed on all children assess acuity of sight and hearing.

Child guidance clinics, which are staffed by educational psychologists, social workers, and psychiatrists, are available to assess 'maladjusted' children and they provide services to help such children overcome their difficulties. The services assist children who show evidence of emotional instability or psychological disturbance to attain personal, social, or educational readjustment.

Children with mental or physical impairments are provided for by health, education, and social services. Integration in ordinary schools is promoted so that all children can receive education, irrespective of the degree of their disability. In some instances this may not be possible and it may be necessary to provide education at home or in a special school. Every effort is made to ensure that a mentally or physically impaired child can develop to his fullest potential.

Disorders of infancy and childhood

Table 54.2 list the disorders which are common to infancy, childhood, and adolescence.

Needs of infants and children

The needs of children, throughout the various stages of development, are both physical and psychosocial. Physical needs include the need for food, water, oxygen, elimination, warmth, safety and protection. Psychosocial needs include the need for love and affection, security, dependence and independence, and self development. When physical or psychosocial needs are not met, the child experiences disruptions to his biological, emotional, social, and educational growth and development. When needs are not met there are a variety of effects on the child, e.g. a greater incidence of disease and accidents, failure to thrive, behavioural problems, delayed language skills; antisocial behaviour such as conflicts with the law or substance use and abuse; learning difficulties, and social inadequancy. Information on basic human needs is provided in Chapter 28, and it should be reviewed in conjunction with the contents of this chapter.

The child in hospital

When a child has a condition which requires hospitalization, the nurse should understand the effects of admission on the child and his parents. Admission to hospital may be planned or unexpected, and the nurse should realize that an emergency admission is a time of crisis for the child and his family—as there is no time to prepare them for the event. Children must *never* be threatened with hospitalization as a form of punishment, nor should they be told

Table 54.2 Common disorders of infancy, childhood and adolescence *

Disorder	Most likely to occur
Communicable diseases:	
Pertussis (whooping cough)	Under 10 years
Infectious parotitis (mumps)	Between 2 years and adulthood
Rubeola (measles)	Early childhood
Rubella (german measles)	Childhood
Varicella (chicken pox)	Early childhood
Hepatitis A	Childhood
Enteritis	Infancy, childhood
Meningitis (viral, bacterial)	Infancy, early childhood
Sexually transmitted diseases	Adolescence (or during childhood in cases of child sexual abuse)
Impetigo	Early childhood
Respiratory system disorders:	
Laryngotracheobronchitis (croup)	3 months to 3 years
Acute epiglottitis	3–4 years
Tonsillitis	Childhood to adulthood
Pneumonia	Infancy, childhood
Asthma	5–6 years and onwards
Allergic rhinitis	Childhood
Otitis media (as part of viral upper respiratory tract illnesses)	Childhood
Acute bronchiolitis	Infancy
Gastrointestinal disorders:	
Acute gastroenteritis	Infancy
Pyloric stenosis	Manifests between 2–4 weeks
Acute appendicitis	Childhood, adolescence
Umbilical hernia	Infancy to 3–4 years
Intussusception	Infancy
Helminth infestations (worms)	Childhood
Diarrhoea	Infancy, childhood
Constipation	Childhood, adolescence
Skin disorders:	
Napkin dermatitis	Infancy
Eczema	Infancy, early childhood
Seborrhoeic dermatitis	Infancy
Scabies	Childhood
Miliaria (prickly heat)	Infancy
Acne	Adolescence
Genito-urinary disorders:	
Urinary tract infection	Childhood
Enuresis (bed-wetting)	Childhood (4–8 years)
Acute glomerulonephritis	5–10 years
Menstrual problems	Pre teen and teenage years
Circulatory system disorders:	
Anaemia	Infancy, childhood, adolescence
Leukaemia	Childhood
Haemophilia	Manifests in early childhood
Atrial/septal heart defects	Congenital—manifestations appear in infancy or early childhood
Idiopathic thrombocytopenic purpura	3–7 years
Neurological conditions:	
Convulsions	6 months—6 years
Epilepsy	Generally appears between 4 and 8 years
Cerebral palsy	Infancy
Metabolic and nutritional disorders:	
Coeliac disease	Manifests within 6 months after birth
Cystic fibrosis	Manifests in infancy

Table 54.2 (cont'd) Common disorders of infancy, childhood and adolescence*

Disorder	Most likely to occur
Obesity	Childhood or adolescence
Protein-kilojoule malnutrition	Infancy
Rickets	Infancy
Musculoskeletal disorders:	
Congenital hip dysplasia	Manifests in infancy
Osteogenesis imperfecta	Manifests at birth or soon afterwards
Scoliosis	Childhood, adolescence
Traumatic disorders:	
Choking, suffocation	Infancy, early childhood
Poisoning	Early childhood
Burns	Infancy, early childhood
Foreign objects lodged in a body orifice	Early childhood
Bites, lacerations, stings, abrasions	Childhood
Fractures, dislocations	Childhood, adolescence
Sudden infant death syndrome (SIDS)	Before 2 years
Abuse (physical, sexual, emotional)	Any age—from infancy to adolescence
Behavioural or psychological disorders:	
Hyperactivity, temper tantrums, concentration problems	Childhood
Autism	Manifests in infancy or early childhood
Eating disorders; anorexia nervosa, bulimia	Late childhood, adolescence
Substance abuse	Late childhood, adolescence

*Refer to the appropriate chapters for information about specific disorders

they will be going on a holiday rather than telling them they are to be admitted to hospital.

There are a number of factors which influence the way in which a child and the child's family react when illness or an injury make it necessary for the child to be admitted to hospital. These include:

- The age of the child and his ability to comprehend the situation.
- The amount of preparation of the child by the parents prior to admission. An emotionally secure child usually adapts well if he is given a realistic explanation of hospital life, is told the reason for admission and what will happen to him and has an assurance that one or both parents will spend as much time as possible with the child. Many parents fail to prepare a child for hospitalization, and in some cases may transmit their own fears and misconceptions with the result that admission to hospital is a very frightening and traumatic experience for the child.
- The condition of the child. An acutely ill or severely injured child may not be totally aware of his situation but the parents will be distressed and apprehensive.
- The cultural background of the child. In some cultures

there is an extended and very closely knit family pattern and the child who is accustomed to the loving protection and guidance from parents, grandparents, aunts and uncles, can be quite devastated when separated from such an environment. In other situations where a child leads a lonely existence with little companionship or family support, the company of other children and the attention received in hospital may be very welcome.

- The reaction shown by the parents can markedly influence a child's reaction to illness and hospitalization. Anxiety, tension, worry or emotional outbursts on the parent's part are likely to increase the child's feeling of fear and insecurity; whereas serene, calm, confident and supportive parents can allay the child's·fears and promote a feeling of security.
- The relationship between the hospital staff and the child's parents is a very important factor, particularly in the case of an older child who will relate more readily to nurses who have established rapport with his parents.

The role of the parents during a child's illness is now acknowledged as being of the utmost importance, and most hospitals allow unrestricted visiting while many provide accommodation facilities for the parents of children who are very sick. The parent should be encouraged to participate in the care of the child with guidance and help from the nurse assigned to the particular child. When a parent is prevented from spending much time with the sick child because of home commitments or for economic reasons, the social worker may be consulted with a view to discussing and arranging help for the parent.

Preparation for admission

Children accept admission to hospital much better if they have been adequately prepared beforehand. While it is not possible to explain hospitalization to infants, children from approximately 2 years of age can be helped to adjust to this significant event by adequate preparation. Preparation is directed towards overcoming fears and anxieties such as the fear of:

- separation
- bodily injury and pain
- loss of routine and rituals
- physical restrictions
- enforced dependency and loss of independence
- strangers
- loss of body image.

Preparation for admission involves explaining what will happen in language which is appropriate for the child's level of comprehension. Many excellent publications are available, some in picture form, which may be used to reinforce explanations. Parents should encourage their child to discuss all aspects of hospitalization to help overcome any fear and anxieties. Many hospitals encourage visits to the ward prior to admission so that the child can see the area, and meet some of the personnel who will be involved in his care. Another way of preparing the child is to allow him to decide the items he wants to take to hospital, and allowing him pack his case in readiness for the trip.

In an emergency admission there is no time to prepare the child and, therefore, the event can be very traumatic for him and for his parents. Some of the child's fears and anxieties can be reduced by encouraging one or both parents to stay with him for as long as possible.

Parents also experience many fears and anxieties when their child is to be admitted to hospital. They can be helped to overcome anxiety if they are provided with information about the child's condition, and aspects of his hospitalization. They must be given opportunities to ask any questions, and to discuss their anxieties. The emphasis on parental involvement and family-centred care can do much to relieve anxiety. The parents should be informed of the facilities available if they wish to stay with their child, and they are encouraged to participate in the child's care.

Rooming-in, whereby a parent stays with the child during his period of hospitalization, reduces stress related to separation and prevents many of the disturbances which are commonly experienced by a child when such facilities are not available. Following discharge from hospital, children are generally less 'clinging' and suffer fewer emotional and behavioural disturbances than those who have been separated from their parents for any length of time. To be successful, rooming-in depends on many factors such as:

• the ability of the nursing staff to accept that parents have a right to remain with, and be actively involved in the care of, the child.
• the extent to which the parents are provided with clear information about hospital and ward policies, and their degree of involvement in the child's care.
• the ability of the parent to adapt to the hospital/ward environment.

Many children go through various phases of disturbance when they are hospitalized—particularly if they are separated from the parents. During the initial phase, that of *protest*, the child may cry or scream for his parents and refuse the attention of anyone else. It is not unusual for the child to stop protesting only when he becomes physically exhausted. During the second stage, that of *despair*, the crying generally subsides and the child may become withdrawn and apathetic. He may feel abandoned, and experience feelings of hopelessness and grief at his plight. During the third stage, that of *detachment*, the child appears to have adjusted to the separation—but in reality he is detaching himself from his parents in an attempt to escape the pain and wishing they were with him. When the parents do visit him he may react to them with disinterest and, unless the parents understand his reactions, they may become very distressed.

Nurses, need to be aware of the phases and signs of *separation anxiety* in order to intervene appropriately. Much paediatric nursing care is directed towards helping the child, and the parents, adjust to the reality of hospitalization.

Admission

Admission to hospital can be frightening for a child and distressing for his family. As most children respond to their parent's reactions, it is important that the nurse gains the parent's confidence from the time of admission. This is reassuring to the child, who is quick to sense the parent's reactions.

Prior to admission, the nurse in charge of the ward assigns a room based on the child's age and his diagnosis. Whenever possible children of the same age group with similar types of illnesses are placed in the same room. Other children in the room should be informed of the pending arrival of a new patient so that they can welcome him. The room should be prepared, and all the necessary documents and items of equipment placed nearby, so that the admitting nurse will not have to leave the child.

The admission procedure may vary slightly between hospitals, depending on hospital policy and the prevailing circumstances. Information on admission to hospital is provided in Chapter 51. Admission of a child involves assessing his vital signs, measuring his height and weight, placing an identity band on his wrist and/or ankle, obtaining a sample of urine for urinalysis, introducing him to other children in the room, and orienting the family to the available facilities, e.g. signal device, television controls, telephone, bathroom, toilet. The child and his parents should be shown the playroom and dining areas, and the parents should be provided with details about the rooming-in facilities.

During admission, the parents are encouraged to remain with the child and to assist with activities such as undressing and putting him to bed. The use of each piece of equipment should be explained, and the child may be encouraged to handle some of the items to allay his fears. Most children, and parents, will react and adapt better if they are informed in advance of the possibility of treatments involving the use of intravenous therapy equipment, drainage tubes, dressings, plasters, or oxygen apparatus.

A nursing history is obtained from the parents, and from the child if he is old enough. As much information as possible should be obtained to enable the nurse to understand the child if he is old enough. As much information as possible should be obtained to enable the nurse to understand habits and helps to establish a greater similarity between home and hospital environment. Information obtained should include:

• Family data, e.g. the child's name or nickname, date of birth and age, names of other family members, parent's occupation.

• Medical history, e.g. details of any infectious diseases suffered by the child, any known exposure to infectious diseases within recent weeks, details of immunization against infectious diseases, any known allergies, current medications, and details about any current illness or disability other than that for which the child is being admitted. It is important to ask whether the child has ever been admitted to hospital before and, if so, how he reacted to the experience.

• Activities of daily living, i.e. information about eating, sleeping, elimination, hygiene, play.

Table 54.3 lists the information which should be obtained about the child's activities of living.

General aspects of paediatric nursing

Care of children differs from the care of adults in many ways, e.g. the inability of very young children to communicate necessitates special skills of observation and

Table 54.3 Paediatric nursing history (activities of living)

Activity	Information obtained
Eating and Drinking	Food and beverage likes and dislikes Any foods he is not allowed to eat or is allergic to Usual appetite Feeding habits: cup, spoon, bottle, eats by self, needs assistance Special cultural requirements or habits If bottle fed, the formula and frequency of feeds
Sleeping	Usual time of sleep and awakening Routine before sleep: drink, bed-time story, favourite toy or blanket, night light Bed or cot Sleeps alone or with others Any problems, e.g. nightmares or sleepwalking
Elimination	Toilet trained or not Use of toilet, pot, or napkins Use of words to communicate urination and defaecation Any problems, e.g. bedwetting, constipation
Hygiene	Usual habits: bath or shower, hair and dental care Any problems, e.g. hates having his teeth cleaned Degree of assistance required Care of any prosthesis, e.g. glasses, contact lenses, orthodontic appliances, hearing aid
Play	Favourite toys and activities Attends creche, play group, pre-school, school Favourite television programmes, any restrictions Prefers to play with others, or by self Any imaginary playmate

interpretation. Each child must be treated as an individual, but there are certain aspects of care which apply to all children:

• Complete honesty is important. Simple explanations before any procedure is performed should be given in language appropriate for the child's level of development and comprehension. A child should not be told that a technique or procedure will not hurt, if in fact it is likely to do so. The nurse should be patient and be prepared to take the time necessary to help the child understand, and to allay his anxiety.

• The nurse should recognize the child's need for love and a feeling of security. Parents should be encouraged to room-in, or to spend as much time as possible with their child. If the parent/s cannot be with the child all the time, the nurse should give him extra attention and demonstrate affection for him by fondling or cuddling.

• Whenever possible the same nurse/s should care for the child during his stay in hospital. An attempt should be made to maintain a routine similar to the one the child is accustomed to at home. A similar routine makes hospital life less bewildering for a child, and promotes a feeling of security.

• Efforts should be made to minimize a hospital-type environment, e.g. by encouraging the child to wear his own clothes, to sit at a table for meals, and by allowing the child to keep as many attachments to home as possible—such as family photographs and his own toys.

• Lessen the feeling of separation from home by encouraging the child to talk about his home, family, pets, friends, and school. If the parent/s cannot be with the child all the time, it is sometimes helpful if they leave small parcels for the child to open each day. Visits by siblings, other relatives, and friends should be encouraged.

• Show respect for the dignity of the child and his right to privacy. Undue exposure, e.g. when dressing him, can cause embarrassment especially for an older child.

• Maintain the degree of independence and the behaviour patterns which were established by the parents. It can be distressing for the parents, and detrimental to the child, if a child's development is retarded as a result of a period spent in hospital.

• Allow for periods of regression during hospitalization, and recognize that regressive behaviour is a feature of illness. For example, a child who was previously toilet trained may regress to bed wetting.

• Provide opportunities for play. *Play is an activity* by which a child can practise and perfect skills, give expression to thoughts and feelings, be creative, perfect language, and be prepared for adult behaviour and roles. Play, within a hospital environment, is a valuable means of teaching and of reducing anxiety. A range of play materials should be provided which are suitable for a child's level of development, condition, and capabilities. Some paediatric facilities provide play therapists whose function is to ensure that a child is occupied, has the opportunity to play and be creative, and is provided with an outlet to release pent-up feelings.

- Provide an atmosphere and opportunities that encourage free expression of feelings by the child and parents.
- Preparation for discharge from hospital involves providing the parents, and child if he is able to understand, with information about medications or other forms of treatment or care required, arranging appointments and/or contact with the visiting nurse service, and ensuring that the parents understand that the child may experience some behavioural problems when he returns home, e.g. sleep disturbances, difficulties at school, or regressive behaviours.

Safety

The child must be protected from injury or further illness during his period of hospitalization. Children are prone to accidents because they are often unaware of potential hazards, many have no fear, and very young children in particular are defenceless in dangerous situations. The nurse has a responsibility to provide a safe environment for children in hospital:

- Cot sides must be pulled up before the nurse turns her back on the cot or moves away from it.
- Restrainers should be used only when permission has been obtained from the nurse in charge, and they must then be used with great care. Restrainers should allow mobility, should not impair breathing or circulation, and they should be fastened in such a way that would make it impossible for any ties to be wound around the child's neck. Restrainers should be removed as frequently as possible, and if an arm or leg has been restrained it should be exercised and skin care provided at frequent intervals.
- Safety gates placed across stairways should be fastened securely.
- Objects which are hazardous e.g. heaters, containers of medications or lotions, hot liquids, sharp instruments, or glassware, should be made inaccessible to children.
- A child should always be within a nurse's sight, and should be accompanied by a nurse whenever it is necessary for him to leave the ward for any reason.
- Toys should not have sharp edges or points, and they should not be very tiny or have detachable parts small enough to be inhaled or swallowed. Toys which could generate sparks, e.g. friction toys, should not be used in the vicinity of oxygen apparatus. Syringes should not be given to children to play with, as there is a risk of injury from the syringe and a risk of transmission of microorganisms.
- Clothing should be checked to see if that is safe and does not restrict the child's movements. Garments should be loose, laces tied securely, and footwear should fit properly and have non-slip soles.

- Food and drink should be at the correct temperature when given to a child, and very hot food or fluid should not be left in the vicinity of children.
- Taps should be of a type which cannot be operated by children, and the water supply to the bathrooms should be thermostatically controlled.
- Floors should have non-slip surfaces, and any spills should be wiped up immediately.
- Power points should be out of reach of children, and should be fitted with safety covers.
- Ambulatory children should be supervised at all times.
- A nurse must remain with a child when his temperature is being assessed, when he is in a bathroom, when he is on an examination table, and while a medication is being swallowed. Two nurses should attend to a child when it is likely that he will move during a procedure, e.g. administration of an injection.
- Hands must be washed and dried before and after giving care, to prevent cross infection.
- The child's identity band must be carefully checked before any care is provided or treatment performed.

Further information on safety is provided in Chapter 38.

Assessment

As nurses are with hospitalized children constantly, they have a vital role to play in assessment and accurate reporting. Changes in a child's condition can occur with alarming rapidity, and a child's reactions to illness and to treatment can be dramatic—therefore constant vigilance by the nurse is essential. Infants and young children are unable to communicate their feelings therefore they need to be closely observed for indications of pain, a change in condition, or the onset of complications. The nurse must have a sound knowledge of what is considered normal so that she is able to recognize an abnormal situation.

Table 54.4. Lists observations to be made.
Assessment of an infant or child also involves measuring the vital signs, weight, and height. Information on assessing vital signs is provided in Chapters 32, 33, and 34.

When measuring *temperature*, the route selected depends on the age and condition of the child. The axillary route is generally selected for infants and young children, whereas the oral route may be more suitable for an older child. Rectal temperature measurements are not usually performed, but if required the thermometer must be held in position throughout the procedure.

It may be easier to assess the *pulse* of an infant or young child while he is asleep, or by selecting the temporal pulse site in preference to the radial site. An infant's pulse may be assessed apically, by placing the diaphragm of a stethoscope over the apex of the heart.

Measurements of ventilations are best performed when the child is asleep or resting quietly, in order to obtain an

Table 54.4 Assessment of infants and children

	Observations
General appearance	*Facial expression*: alert, anxious, placid, pained, apathetic *Posture*: favouring a body part, e.g. knees drawn up to relax the abdominal muscles may indicate abdominal pain, or sitting up to relieve breathing difficulties; unusual gait, curvatures in posture, e.g. lateral curvature of the spine Range of joint motion *Hygiene*: cleanliness, unusual odour; condition of the hair, nails, and teeth *Nutritional status*: overweight, underweight *Behaviour*: personality, level of activity, reactions to stress, interactions with others, listless, overactive; aggressive or regressive behaviour *Development*: speech, motor skills, degree of co-ordination
Skin	Colour, texture, temperature, moisture, turgor Lesions, scratches, bruises, scaliness, evidence of infestation, scars, bite marks, inflammation, rashes, oedema
Hair	Quality, texture, distribution, elasticity, evidence of infestation
Nails	Colour, shape, texture, quality
Mouth	Condition of lips, tongue, teeth, gums. Presence of sores, coating, bad breath, ulcers, bleeding
Eyes	Pupils for size, equality, reaction to light Colour of sclera Presence of any inflammation, discharge, excessive watering, puffiness of the lids, squint, ptosis Any defects of vision
Ears	Accumulation of wax, discharge, presence of pain Any hearing defects
Chest and lungs	Shape, symmetry, movement of the chest Ventilations are assessed for rate, rhythm, depth, and quality. The character of breath sounds is noted, e.g. noisy, wheezing, grunting
Abdomen	Contour of the abdomen, e.g. distension or rigidity Condition of the skin covering the abdomen Movement, e.g. visible peristalsis Presence of hernias
Infant cries (the only way an infant can express himself)	Characteristic for each infant, but common features include: • an angry cry with fist in the mouth indicates hunger • an angry cry with excessive movement of the arms and legs indicates frustration • a shrill, spasmodic cry indicates pain • a weak, whimpering cry indicates general weakness • a fretful cry may indicate loneliness, hunger, discomfort, or boredom • a hoarse cry indicates an infection or obstruction of the respiratory tract • a shrill cry may indicate cerebral irritation

Table 54.4 (cont'd) Assessment of infants and children

	Observations
Faeces	Colour, quantity, consistency, odour, frequency A breast fed infant's stools are yellow and paste-like An artificially fed infant's stools are pale yellow to brown, firmer in consistency, and have a more offensive odour Abnormalities include: • green frothy stools • pale offensive bulky stools • watery stools • presence of blood, mucus, parasites
Urine	Colour, quantity, odour, frequency

accurate measurement. In general, particularly with infants and young children, the pulse and ventilations are measured before the temperature.

Blood pressure measurements are performed using the same techniques as those used for adults, but with equipment that is designed for paediatric use, e.g. a small cuff.

Weight (mass) is measured using a type of scale which is appropriate for the child, e.g. infants are weighed on infant scales, and older children are weighed on a chair or standing scale.

Height is measured with the older child in a standing position, while recumbent length is a more reliable form of height measurement in infants and young children.

Head circumference is generally measured in children up to 3 years of age, and in any child whose head size is questionable. The head is measured at its greatest circumference by placing a tape measure around the head— slightly above the eyebrows and around the occipital prominence at the back of the skull.

Nutritional needs of infants and children

General information on nutrition is provided in Chapter 29. Throughout all stages of development, a balanced diet is necessary to provide the nutrients required for the body's needs.

The infant

Human breast milk can supply the infant with all his nutritional needs for at least the first few months of life. In 1979, The World Health Organization stated that 'Breast feeding is an integral part of the reproductive process, the natural and ideal way of feeding the infant and a unique biological and emotional basis for child development.' Breast milk has several important qualities:

• It is ideally suited to the infant's digestive system, and effectively supplies all the nutrients needed for health and growth.

• It is free from microorganisms, and it contains immuno-globulins to provide protection against infection.
• It appears to play a role in preventing allergic illness, particularly in children of parents with allergies.
• It is delivered at the right temperature throughout a feed.
• Both mother and baby benefit psychologically from their close contact during breast feeding.
• Breast feeding allows the infant control over the amount of milk taken at each feed.

Further information on breast feeding is provided in Chapter 52.

When breast feeding is not possible substitute feeding is commenced. The choice of a specific formula depends on a number of factors such as the parents' personal preference, financial considerations, availability, and ease of preparation. Most artificial feeds are based on cow's milk, but if an infant is unable to tolerate cow's milk one of the proprietary preparations which are available must be used instead. Special formulae include those that are soy—based, or lactose free. All infant formulae are required to comply to stringent standards. It is essential that, which ever formula is selected, it supplies adequate fluid, energy, and nutrients.

Table 54.4 compares the composition of human breast milk and cow's milk.

Infant formulae preparations have clear instruction on the containers, for the reconstitution of the formula. The hands must be thoroughly washed before preparing the formula, and all items used during preparation must be sterile. Jugs, bottles, spoons, and teats may be sterilized by boiling or by using a hypochlorite solution. When using a hypochlorite solution, the manufacturer's directions must be followed precisely.

In a hospital, bottle feeds are generally made up in bulk and distributed from a central point. During preparation, stringent precautions are taken to prevent the entry of microorganisms. The risk is further decreased when pre-packed feeds in disposable bottles are provided. Prepared formula is refrigerated until it is needed. The teat should be handled by the flange only to avoid touching the part that goes into the infant's mouth. During transfer to the bedside, the teat must remain covered.

The nurse may be required to bottle feed an infant, and the important aspects of this technique include:

• Washing the hands before preparing the requirements: jug of hot water containing the prepared bottle of formula labelled with the infant's name, and a sterile covered teat.
• Ensuring that the infant is dry and comfortable. Wet or soiled napkins are changed before the feeding is commenced.
• Sitting down to feed the infant. He should be wrapped in a light blanket, and held correctly in the crook of one

Table 54.5 Composition of breast milk and cow's milk (per 100 ml)

Constituent	Breast milk	Unmodified cow's milk
Water	88 g	88 g
Protein	1 g	3.3 g
Fat	3.8 g	3.5 g
Carbohydrate (lactose)	7 g	5 g
Energy	294 kilojoules	273 kilojoules
Sodium	15 mg	50 mg
Potassium	60 mg	150 mg
Chloride	43 mg	95 mg
Calcium	35 mg	120 mg
Phosphorous	15 mg	95 mg
Iron	1 mg	0.5 mg
Zinc	4 mg	40 mg
Vitamin A	60 μg	31 μg
Vitamin C	3.8 mg	2.0 mg
Vitamin K	1.5 mg	6.0 mg
Thiamine	16 μg	40 μg
Riboflavin	31 μg	190 μg
Pyridoxine	5.9 μg	40 μg
Cobalamin	0.01 μg	0.3 μg

arm. The infant's head should be higher than the chest and he should be held close to the nurse's body. A bib is placed under his chin.
• Testing the temperature of the formula on the inner aspect of the nurse's wrist. The formula should be warmed to 37°C. The rate of flow from the teat should be approximately one drop per second.
• Holding the bottle in one hand with the palm upper-most, and with the first or second finger under the infant's chin. The teat is introduced into the infant's mouth so that it lies on top of the tongue. The bottle is kept tilted, so that the teat is always filled with formula and, therefore, the infant does not suck in air.
• 'De-winding' the infant during and at the end of the feed. The bottle is placed in the jug of hot water to keep the rest of the formula warm, while the infant is being de-winded. De-winding can be achieved by one of two techniques. The infant can be sat up, the nurse places one hand on his abdomen and, with the other hand, gently rubs or pats his back. Alternatively, the infant can be held over

the nurse's shoulder while his back is gently rubbed or patted.
- Feeding the remainder of the formula, and dewinding the infant at the end of the feed.
- Ensuring that the napkin is changed if necessary before placing the infant back in the cot. After the feed the infant is placed either on his right side, or on his abdomen with his head to one side.
- Washing the hands and recording the type and amount of formula taken by the infant. It is also important to document whether the infant passed urine or had his bowels open.
- Attending to the equipment. Non-disposable bottles and teats must be cleaned immediately and sterilized before being used again. *Bottles* are rinsed in cold water, washed in warm soapy water using a bottle brush to remove all traces of formula, and rinsed again. *Teats* are rinsed in cold water, washed in warm soapy water, turned inside out and rubbed with salt to remove the film of formula, and rinsed to remove all traces of salt and soap. Water is squirted through the hole to clean it and to ensure patency. Both bottles and teats are sterilized before re-use.

If an infant is unwilling to suck, the cause may be:

- discomfort due to wet or soiled napkin, wind, or incorrect handling by an inexperienced nurse
- blocked nose making it difficult to breathe while sucking
- painful condition of the mouth, e.g. thrush
- the formula being too warm or cold
- a teat with an opening that is too small or too large, or a teat which is too large for the infant's mouth
- exhaustion due to illness.

The nurse in charge must be notified immediately if an infant does not take all of a feed, and if he vomits during or afterwards.

The introduction of solids is generally commenced when the infant is approximately 6 months old, but this varies according to the infant's needs and development. The term *educational diet* is sometimes used to describe the gradual introduction of solids. The initial aim of introducing solids is to educate the palate to different tastes and textures, therefore eating becomes largely a learning process. Baby cereal, pureed stewed fruit and vegetables are suitable first foods. Because food allergies can be a problem during infancy, it is important that single ingredient foods are introduced one at a time. If the infant has an adverse reaction to a food, it can then be readily identified and eliminated from the diet. By 6 to 8 months of age chewing movements begin, and the infant can be introduced to coarser textured foods. When he begins to grasp objects and put them in his mouth, he is ready to be introduced to finger foods. When an infant can take fluids from a cup, at about 7–8 months of age, fruit juice may be introduced. Giving fruit juice from a bottle should be discouraged, as this may contribute to the development of dental caries.

At approximately 12 months of age, the infant should be eating a range of basic foods. The diet should consist of bread and cereals, fruit and vegetables, meat and/or other proteins foods, milk and/or milk products, and small amounts of butter or margarine. Salt, sugar, and fatty foods should be avoided.

The toddler and pre-school child

During this stage of development a child's rate of growth is slower than in infancy, and this is normally reflected by a decrease in appetite—although appetite is generally unpredictable during these years.

Children should be encouraged to eat a variety of nutritious foods, and food should be served at regular times in a calm and relaxed atmosphere. Because young children are active, between meal snacks are important. The foods offered for snacks should contribute to the nutritional needs of the child, and foods of poor nutritional value should be avoided. Small hard foods, such as nuts, are potentially dangerous for the young child as they may be inhaled. The toddler and pre-school child should be having, each day:

- 4–5 servings from the bread and cereal group
- 3–4 servings from the fruit and vegetable group
- 1–2 servings from the meat and protein group
- 600 ml of milk, or equivalent in cheese or yoghurt
- 5–10 g of butter or margarine.

The school age child

During the first 12 months of life a foundation is laid down for good dietary practices, and by the time the child is of school age eating patterns are usually firmly established. Likes and dislikes established at an early age generally continue, although the child may acquire a taste for an increasing variety of foods.

Nutritional requirements are similar to those for children of pre-school age and, although kilojoule needs are diminished in relation to body size, resources are being laid down for the increased growth needs of the adolescent period. The school age child should be encouraged to consume a balanced diet consisting of foods from each of the 5 food groups, and should be discouraged from consuming foods that have little or no nutritional value. If the child eats mainly foods that are high in kilojoules, sugar and fat, he runs the risk of childhood obesity. Iron-deficiency anaemia is another nutritional problem associated with school age children, due to inadequate amounts of iron in the diet.

Meal times

Meal times in a hospital should be pleasant unhurried occasions, and the environment should be one which enables to child to enjoy his meals:

- As far as possible meal times should be free from distractions, and adequate time should be allowed for the meal to be eaten without hurrying.
- The children should be prepared for the meal. Toilet needs should be attended to, hands and face washed, serviette or bib provided, toys put away, and the child made comfortable in bed or seated on a chair at a table.
- Painful or distressing procedures should not be performed immediately before a meal, and activities should be timed so that a child does not become too tired to eat a meal.
- Meals should be served attractively, in amounts appropriate to the age and condition of each child.
- Children should be encouraged to feed themselves, even though they may do it in a 'messy' fashion. Assistance should be given if the child is unable to manage.
- Some children may need coaxing, but a child must never be forced to eat.

Uneaten food should be removed without comment, and the nurse in charge informed. If a child's illness is causing a poor appetite, fortified milk drinks may be offered. Refusal to eat may be an attempt by the child to gain more attention, or it may be that the foods are different to the ones he is used to eating. Every attempt should be made to provide nutritious foods which the child enjoys. A lot of patience may be required to persuade a child to eat 'normal' meals if he is used to a poor standard of diet at home.

Children should be observed for any adverse reaction to food, and the nurse in charge must be informed if a child:

- vomits after a meal
- develops diarrhoea
- develops what may be an allergic reaction to a food, e.g. rash, urticaria, breathing difficulties.

Daily care

Daily care of the infant or child includes meeting the needs for hygiene, rest and sleep. The infant or child generally requires a daily bath or shower, which may be given in the morning or evening depending on the child's needs and condition. In addition, the hands and face should be washed as frequently as required, e.g. before meals, and after using the toilet or toilet utensils. The hair should be brushed, combed, and washed as necessary. Good oral care should be encouraged, and the nurse may need to assist a child to clean his teeth and rinse his mouth. Swabbing the mouth may be necessary when normal oral hygiene practices are not possible. Information on this technique is provided in Chapter 39.

Bathing an infant

Bath time should be an enjoyable occasion for the infant, and the bath should be performed as quickly and safely as possible.

Preparation for a bath includes:

- ensuring that the bathroom is warm and draught-free.
- warming the towels and clothing.
- assembling all the items required: baby bath half filled with water at 38°C, bath thermometer, two towels, facewasher, cotton wool swabs and cotton tipped applicators, mild soap or cleansing lotion, clean set of clothing and napkins; baby oil, cream, or powder; clean linen for the cot, receiver for soiled linen, hair brush, nail scissors, gown or apron.
- preparing an area, e.g. on a bench or table beside the bath, on which the infant can be placed while being undressed dried, and dressed—a towel should be placed on the bench to provide a soft and warm area on which to place the infant.

The technique of bathing involves:

- Washing the hands and putting on a gown or apron.
- Lifting the infant from the cot and placing him on the prepared area beside the bath.
- Undressing the infant, except for the napkin which is left on.
- Wrapping the infant in a towel, and washing his face with cottonwool swabs moistened with warm water. It the nostrils are clear it is not necessary to clean them. Should they require cleansing a small piece of cotton wool, or a small cottonwool tipped applicator, may be inserted gently, rotated, and withdrawn. The inside of the ears should be left alone, but the outer ear should be cleansed with moistened cottonwool. The face is gently patted dry.
- Holding the infant, wrapped in the towel so that the nurse's hand supports his neck and head and his body is tucked under her arm, he is held with his head over the bath. His hair and scalp are washed, rinsed, and patted dry.
- Placing him back on the bench, the towel is unwrapped and the napkin is removed. With well soaped hands, the infant's body is washed. Particular attention is paid to the skin folds, axillae, groin, and between the fingers and toes. The nurse rinses the soap off her hands. The child is observed for any abnormalities, e.g. skin rash.
- Lifting the infant, by sliding the left arm under his neck and shoulders to hold his left upper arm. The nurse's right arm is placed under his buttocks to hold his left thigh. The infant is gently lowered into the water, and the nurse's left arm and hand remains in position to support and control the infant's movements.
- Using the right hand, the soap is rinsed off the infant's body. He should be allowed some time to splash and kick in the water.
- Lifting the infant from the bath and placing him on the prepared bench. He is dried quickly but thoroughly, pay-

ing particular attention to skin folds and creases. Oil or cream may be applied, e.g. to the buttocks, and if powder is used it is applied sparingly.

- Dressing the infant before he becomes cold. The napkin is placed on first, then the singlet, and the gown. The hair is brushed, and if necessary the nails are trimmed.
- Returning the infant to his cot, which is made up with clean linen. A second nurse may be available to make the cot while the infant is being bathed, or the infant may be placed in an infant chair while the cot is made up. He should be placed in the cot on his side, or on the abdomen with his head to one side. Very young infants feel more secure if they are wrapped in a light blanket before the upper bedclothes are placed over them. Ensure that the sides of the cot are pulled up and fastened securely.
- Attending to the used items, and cleaning the bath before it is used again. The hands are washed and dried.
- Reporting to the nurse in charge, and documenting the procedure.

Care of the infant's buttocks is necessary to prevent excoriation. The condition of the infant's skin should be assessed each time a napkin is changed, and any signs of sore buttocks should be reported immediately. Napkin rash is a maculopapular excoriated eruption on the buttocks and/or genital area and groins. It is caused by irritation from faeces, moisture, heat, or from ammonia produced by decomposition of urine. Other possible causes of sore buttocks include using irritating soap, incorrect laundering of napkins, failure to cleanse and dry the buttocks adequately, or the frequent passage of loose acid stools.

A napkin is changed immediately it becomes wet or soiled. Warm water should be used for cleansing the buttocks, genitals, and groin, ensuring that all traces of urine or faeces are removed. Alternatively, a proprietary 'napkin change' lotion may be used to cleanse the skin. A water repellant substance may be applied after washing and drying to give protection to the skin.

The napkins provided by a hospital may be re-usable cloth types, or one of the variety of disposable types which are available.

Rest and sleep

The amount of sleep required depends on the age, activity, and physical condition of each child. As the infant grown and develops there will be a greater need for more exercise and there is a growing awareness of surroundings, which means that an infant will stay awake for longer periods. The average requirements are 10–12 hours sleep at night, plus one or more rest periods during the day. Ideally, periods of activity are followed by rest periods when the children lie in or on top of their beds.

To settle a child for sleep the nurse implements measures, e.g. a darkened room and a quiet environment, to minimize sensory stimulation. The infant or child should be made comfortable, e.g. by providing toilet facilities, washing the face and hands, brushing the teeth, straightening creased bedlinen, changing wet or soiled napkins, ensuring adequate warmth, offering a warm drink, and ensuring that the child is free from pain. If parents are not rooming-in, the child may like the nurse to read him a bed time story.

Further information on comfort, rest and sleep is provided in Chapter 35.

Paediatric procedures

Depending on the type of illness, an infant or child may be required to undergo diagnostic tests, surgical intervention, receive medication or other forms of therapy. The principles of management for a paediatric patient are similar to those for an adult, and information on these topics is provided in the relevant chapters. There are, however, special aspects to be considered when the individual is an infant or child.

To assist a child to cope with uncomfortable or painful procedures the nurse should:

- explain what will happen in terms the child can understand
- not tell the child the procedure won't cause discomfort; be honest but avoid creating undue concern
- not tell the child not to cry—as crying is a normal response to pain, fear, or stress
- not restrain the child any more than is necessary
- remain with the child and provide psychological support while the procedure is performed, e.g. allow the child to hold his favourite toy, or stroke him and talk softly to him
- involve the parent/s in the procedure if possible
- encourage the child to participate in the procedure whenever possible, e.g. he could hold a bandage or items of equipment
- provide distraction to focus his attention away from the procedure, e.g. asking him to count aloud while an injection is being administered
- hold and cuddle the child after the procedure, or encourage the parents to comfort the child.

When medications are being administered, the principles described in Chapter 58 must be followed. Factors relevant to the care of children receiving medication include:

- Explaining the purpose of the drug if the child is old enough to understand, and preparing him for an unpleasant taste of an oral medication or the discomfort of an injection.
- Essential foodstuffs should not be used as a camouflage for oral medications, as there is a risk of the child developing a dislike of that particular food as a result.

• Great patience may be needed to coax a child to take oral medications and the nurse may need to use ingenuity to devise a way of achieving this, e.g. playing a game, distracting the child's attention in some way, offering a sweet to follow the dose.

• The presence of two nurses may be required when an injection is given, so that one nurse can devote herself entirely to supporting and comforting the child.

• When oral medications are administered to an infant, they may be given from a small spoon or from a special dropper. The medication should not be forced into the infant's mouth, as this may lead to spluttering or inhalation. The infant should be allowed to suck the medication from the spoon or dropper.

• If children are unable to swallow tablets whole, the tablets may be crushed between two spoons—unless this action would alter the efficacy of the drug.

• The child should be offered a drink, e.g. fruit juice or water, immediately after swallowing an oral medication—to remove any unpleasant taste.

• Recognition and reporting of any side effects of a medication is of the utmost importance.

THE ADOLESCENT

Adolescence is a stage of development which is characterized by sudden physical changes, and social and emotional maturing. Adolescence is frequently described as a transition period between childhood and adulthood, which begins with the gradual appearance of secondary sex characteristics and ends with cessation of body growth.

Adolescence is a stage of development which is accompanied by problems of adjustment. The adolescent has to adjust to physical, psychological and emotional changes.

• Physical changes are caused by an increase in the production of sex hormones. For example, increased physical growth, increased sebaceous gland activity, and distribution of body hair. Development of the external genitalia occurs, girls develop breasts and begin to menstruate, and boys experience ejaculation of semen and nocturnal emissions.

• Psychological and emotional changes occur, whereby the parents' influence diminishes and the influences of the peer group are greatly increased. The peer group serves to support the adolescent in terms of a sense of belonging, and it provides a link between independence and autonomy. The ability to reason, assess, evaluate, and to use divergent thinking are increased during this developmental stage. Changes in emotional control and response often result in behaviour that is bewildering to others, and to the adolescent. In late adolescence the individual begins to demonstrate more mature emotions, but at times his behaviour reflects feelings of insecurity, tension, and indecision.

Further information on growth and development during adolescence is provided in Chapters 2 and 3.

The nurse who is caring for an adolescent needs to recognize that this stage of development is generally a difficult one; and that rebellion against rules and regulations, criticism of treatment and lack of co-operation by an adolescent may be due to a combination of an instinctive negative reaction against authority, and hidden anxieties and fears. Much of the behaviour observed in the adolescent is related to the struggle for independence, and the external constraints that are placed on this maturation process.

When an adolescent requires admission to hospital, the most appropriate environment is a ward or unit which has been especially designed to cater for the needs of adolescents. It is not usually appropriate for an adolescent to be nursed in a paediatric ward, nor in a ward where the patients are middle-aged or elderly. When a special ward is not available the adolescent should be placed in a room where the other occupants are approximately the same age, and the same sex.

As the adolescent is seeking independence, the nurse should try to involve him in his own care as much as possible. He should be encouraged to participate in decision making and care planning, and he should be allowed the maximum amount of independence appropriate to the situation.

The nurse should also recognize that adolescents are acutely aware of their body image and the physical changes which accompany this stage of development. The sudden growth, and maturation of the external sexual characteristics, often causes the adolescent to feel anxious and confused about his body.

A male may be concerned if he is not showing the same signs of maturation as his friends, e.g. growth of facial and body hair, growth of the penis and testes. A female may be very conscious of her increasing height, onset of menstruation, and development of the breasts. Adolescents of both sexes are often acutely aware and embarrassed by the development of pimples or acne.

Health promotion during adolescence is directed towards establishing healthy habits of daily living, education in stress-reducing techniques; and providing information on nutritional requirements, accident prevention, and avoidance of sexually transmitted diseases and unplanned pregnancies.

Disorders which are common during adolescence are listed in Table 54.2.

Accidents are the greatest cause of deaths in the adolescent age group, as their tendency for risk-taking behaviour together with feelings of indestructibility make adolescents particularly prone to accidents—especially those involving motor vehicles and sports.

During adolescence the needs which require particular

attention are:

- nutrition: related to growth spurt, and maturation of systems
- oxygen: related to increase in vital capacity of lungs
- protection and safety: related to risk-taking behaviour
- hygiene: related to increased production of sebum, and attainment of puberty
- sexuality: related to maturation of the reproductive organs, and sexual experimentation
- self esteem: related to physical appearance, peer relations, striving for independence, and establishment of identity.

CONCLUSION

To care for individuals from infancy to adolescence, the nurse first requires knowledge of normal growth and development.

Infancy, childhood, and adolescence are unique phases of development which are accompanied by special needs.

The nurse who is working with children or adolescents needs to develop certain skills in order to provide a high quality of care.

REFERENCES AND FURTHER READING

Clements A 1986 Infant and family health in Australia. Churchill Livingstone, Melbourne
Whaley L F, Wong D L 1989 Essentials of pediatric nursing, 3rd edn. C V Mosby, St Louis

55. The aged individual

OBJECTIVES

1. Discuss the changes and effects associated with physiological ageing.
2. State the stresses associated with ageing.
3. Describe the measures which can be implemented to promote independent function in the elderly.
4. State the facilities which are available to support the elderly in the community.
5. Assist in planning and implementing care of the elderly person in hospital.
6. Assist in planning and implementing care of a confused elderly person.

INTRODUCTION

The number of people over 65 years of age is increasing every day. Individuals are living longer and are healthier than ever before so that, today, the majority of people can expect to live into their seventies. It is estimated that by the end of this century there will be a considerable increase in the number of people over 80 years of age—with consequences for the whole of society.

Ageing is a *normal* process, which is accompanied by changes in body structure and function. Because of these changes the elderly have special needs, and are at greater risk of illness, chronic disease, and injuries. Information on physiological ageing is provided in Chapter 3, and summarized in Table 55.1.

Gerontology is the study of the normal process of ageing; while *geriatrics* is the branch of medical science dealing with the treatment of disease in the elderly. Information on the various *theories of ageing* is provided in Chapter 3. Research is continuing in an effort to discover more about how the body ages and new theories of ageing are continually being developed. A recent suggestion is that cell structures called mitochondria may be involved in the ageing process. Research has suggested that mitochondria appear to decrease

in number, and become more easily damaged in older people. All of the enzymes which break down nutrient substances into carbon dioxide and water, together with the enzymes which enable the transfer of released energy to stable high-energy compounds, are present within the mitochondrial structure. Therefore, it is considered that less efficient mitochondrial activity may contribute to reduced physical activity in elderly people.

It is now evident that ageing is a complicated and variable process subject to modification from environmental, chemical and physical forces, and influenced by genetic factors and disease. The effects of physical and psychological ageing may be quite varied within a group of people of the same chronological age.

It is also clear that there is no universally accepted theory of ageing, however it is important for nurses to understand that ageing is a *normal* process. It is also important that nurses, and others who work with elderly people, understand that pathological changes due to disease should not be confused with normal ageing. To help determine the difference between the natural results of ageing and the warning signals of disease, the nurse should understand that with old age:

● Not all functional changes are related to disease; many are the results of ageing and can be compensated for.
● Sensory receptors and compensatory mechanisms gradually decline so the body does not respond as vigorously to injury or disease.
● Health problems frequently occur in 'clusters'.
● There is increasing vulnerability to disease. This is because the body gradually loses its reserve capacity, its resistance to stress, and its ability to adapt.

Stresses associated with ageing

Ageing, like the other stages of development, is associated with stress. Stress can be produced by any factor that requires a response or change in the individual. Stressors can be physical, psychological, chemical, developmental, or emotional. While some stresses may be positive, others can be negative, and excessive or prolonged stress can be very detrimental. The stresses associated with ageing include:

- Fear of ageing. Many people have a fear of growing old, which is related to a fear of declining physical and/or mental function.
- Fear of isolation. Many people fear being alone or lonely when they are elderly, e.g. the threatened loss of a loved partner may create anticipatory loneliness. If a partner dies, and if there are no children living with the elderly person, he may experience much anxiety related to being on his own.
- Loss. Ageing is associated with many losses, such as the loss of income, mobility, health, strength, hearing and/or sight, or a partner and/or friends. Loss is associated with grief, as described in Chapter 65. When losses occur simultaneously, or one after another, an elderly person may experience chronic grief and may never be able to recover fully.
- Physical deterioration. Many elderly people experience depression, frustration, and anger when their bodies are no longer able to function as they once did. Physical factors such as arthritis, stiffness, loss of balance, or decreased visual acuity, may prevent an elderly person from carrying out his usual activities.
- Impaired cognitive function. An elderly person may become very anxious if he begins to experience alterations in judgment or memory. Confusion is a common reaction to stressors in old age. For example, preoccupation with losses, fears, threats to security, or a non-stimulating environment will often induce a state of confusion.

More pronounced confusional states, e.g. severe disorientation, may result from various disease processes, medication, or metabolic deficiencies.

Information on confusion, and the care of a confused elderly person is provided later in the Chapter.

- Change of environment. Adjustment to old age is made easier when the individual is surrounded by personal possessions and a familiar setting. Facing the prospect of having to move to another setting, e.g. due to illness or inability to cope, is one of the most common fears experienced by many elderly people. While some people may welcome such a change, others experience anxiety or depression when they are required to move out of their home.

How an elderly person responds to these and other stresses depends on many factors, e.g. general health status, mental state, and the amount of support available from family and friends.

Measures to promote independent function

An elderly individual can be helped to maintain independent function by teaching him how to cope with any changes in mental capabilities, sensory acuteness, appetite and elimination, and mobility. Utilization of the various community support services which are available, e.g. Meals on Wheels and Home help, often enable an elderly person to maintain independence in his or her own home.

Remaining alert

Community attitudes must change so that instead of viewing old age as a non-stimulating ad non-productive time of life associated with deteriorating physical and mental capacities, a more positive view of the value and worth of the elderly is required. A society which considers that older people are to be valued and respected for their knowledge and experience, will reduce the feelings of uselessness and rejection feared by many older people.

To remain alert and to prevent deterioration of the cognitive processes an elderly individual, like a person of any age, requires stimulation. An elderly individual should be encouraged to remain or become interested and involved in activities and social interactions. A social life is especially important for elderly individuals who are at risk of social isolation. Many older adults have relationships with family and friends, which provide on-going contact and support. Some elderly people may find support by joining senior citizen groups, where experiences and concerns can be shared, as well as participation in various social activities.

Alcohol or drug abuse can lead to cognitive impairment, resulting in confusion and slow reflexes. An elderly person should be informed of this risk, and advised to avoid substance abuse. Drugs such as sedatives and hypnotics can lower the blood pressure and interfere with neurovascular reflexes.

If an elderly person is experiencing some changes in mental capabilities, e.g. poor memory, he can be assisted to adjust to these alterations. For example, to improve memory, an elderly person could be advised to make lists. To signal that a task needs doing or a special occasion is approaching, he could mark a calendar.

Assisting the senses

An individual can be helped to adjust to the effects of ageing on his senses by suggesting ways of improving his ability to see, hear, and communicate. Evaluation of the individual's vision and hearing should be made, so that spectacles or a hearing aid can be provided if necessary.

The individual can be advised on the most appropriate form and placement of lighting so that he is able to see more easily, and so that glare is reduced. He can be recommended to eliminate unnecessary background noise, e.g. from a radio or television set, so that he can hear a person's conversation more easily. When communicating with a elderly person whose vision and/or hearing is decreased, it is important to face him and speak with a firm voice—preferably in an area which is free of background noise.

Dietary considerations

There are numerous factors that may influence the nutritional status of an elderly person:

- reduced economic status
- physical symptoms, e.g. lack of teeth on dentures, which leads to difficulty in eating
- diminished sense of taste and/or smell
- diminished gastric secretions that results in less efficient digestion
- physical disabilities, or lack of transportation, that make shopping and preparation of food difficult
- living alone decreases the interest and pleasure of preparing and eating meals.

Nutritional requirements of an elderly person are not significantly altered by ageing, except that greater amounts of vitamins C and A, iron, and calcium are required. As there is likely to be some reduction in energy demand, total kilojoule requirements usually decline. An elderly person should be advised to consume a balanced diet which provides the necessary nutrients. Information on meeting nutritional needs is provided in Chapter 29.

The nutritional intake of some elderly people may be improved if they are encouraged to eat with others, e.g. at senior citizen's centres. Meals on Wheels can provide regular nutritious meals for an elderly person who is experiencing difficulty in shopping for or preparing food.

Preventing problems of elimination

An elderly person may become constipated for a variety of reasons. Information on the causes and prevention of constipation is provided in Chapter 30. Prevention includes consuming adequate dietary fibre and fluids, and obtaining sufficient exercise.

For many people, incontinence of urine is the most distressing indignity of old age. The incidence of incontinence increases with age, but incontinence is frequently associated with a variety of reasons other than the ageing process, e.g. urinary tract infection, gynecological causes, or mechanical obstruction to urinary flow.

An elderly person who is concerned about becoming incontinent especially at night can be advised to limit fluid intake in the late evening, to keep a light on at night so as not to waste time looking for the light switch, to place a commode in the room at night if the toilet is far away, and to avoid long-acting sedative and hypnotics which may result in not awakening in response to the signal that the bladder is nearing capacity.

If an elderly person experiences incontinence of urine, a comprehensive examination by a medical officer or a continence advisor must be performed to determine the cause. Information on incontinence is provided in Chapter 30.

Maintaining mobility

Because of certain physiological changes associated with the ageing process, an elderly person may experience problems of mobility. For example, osteo-arthritis may affect the weight bearing joints and result in pain when walking. Other factors which may affect mobility include impaired vision, loss of interest in going outside the home, or insufficient exercise resulting in muscle atrophy. Immobility can have serious consequences, as described in Chapter 37, therefore it is essential that an elderly person be encouraged to remain mobile.

The elderly person should also be recommended to implement measures which reduce the risk of a fall moving about. Preventive measures which may be implemented include using available ramps rather than stairs, to avoid placing loose mats on the floor, ensuring that all floor surfaces are dry and non-slippery, wearing suitable footwear, ensuring that all areas are adequately lit, and using aids, e.g. a walking stick, if extra support is required.

If an elderly person is required to limit his mobility for a period of time, e.g. during illness, he should be encouraged to perform range of motion (ROM) exercises to prevent the development of position contractures. Information on ROM exercises is provided in Chapter 37.

Utilizing community services

Domiciliary care programmes have been developed to keep the elderly in good health in the community, and to support the elderly in the home environment—using all available medical, social, and other ancillary means. Domiciliary services are currently provided by a range of agencies.

- Home help services. Home help services are organized by local councils and by some voluntary agencies. The needs of an elderly person are assessed, and the number of hours of help required each week is estimated. The home helper assists with housework, washing, ironing, shopping, and transportation as required.
- Nursing services. Home nursing services are provided by district or visiting nurses when required and requested. Nurses assess an elderly person's needs, and plan and implement measures to meet those needs. Activities performed by district or visiting nurses include assisting the elderly person with his personal care, e.g. bathing and dressing, administering prescribed medication, performing wound dressings, and monitoring his health and wellbeing. A district or visiting nurse may also consult with the individual's medical officer and other personnel to arrange

physical adaptation of the home, e.g. the installation of rails or a bath seat in the bathroom. Further information on community nursing is provided in Chapter 62.

● Home maintenance services. A handyman service, arranged through a domiciliary service or by a service club, carries out maintenance and repairs in and around the home. This service is invaluable for elderly people who find that home maintenance activities are beyond their capabilities, or for those who are unable to afford the cost of commercial services.

● Meals on Wheels. This service provides a cooked meal once a day for, elderly people who are not able to shop for, or prepare food. A nominal fee is charged for the meals, which may be provided through local councils, hospitals, or some voluntary agencies. In addition to promoting adequate nutrition, the service provides a valuable social contact through the person who delivers the meals. In some situations this person may be the only social contact the elderly person has.

● Laundry facilities. Some hospitals provide a laundry service, e.g. for an incontinent person living at home. This service relieves a major burden from the incontinent person or his carer, who would otherwise be faced with the task of keeping up the supply of clean linen. The service supplies, collects, and launders the linen as necessary.

● Voluntary agencies. A number of voluntary agencies such as Red Cross, church organizations and others provide a range of services including transportation, supply of firewood, companionship, and the organization of social outings.

● Day Care Centres. A day care centre provides elderly people with supervision, activity, and social stimulation. Staff in attendance may include nurses, medical officer, social worker, physiotherapist, occupational therapist, and a chiropodist. The services provided by a day care centre enable many elderly people to remain in their own homes, and an individual may attend for as many hours per day or days per week as considered necessary and appropriate.

● Senior citizens clubs. Such clubs provide mental stimulation and companionship for many elderly people. Some clubs provide a cooked meal at lunchtime, and a few operate a Meals on Wheels service for people unable to attend the club. In many clubs, the programme is designed to include activities that are educational, entertaining, and recreational.

The nurse should become familiar with the various local support services which are available in the area, in order to advise elderly people of the services which may be appropriate.

Accommodation

If an elderly person is not able to live in his own home, or with friends or relatives, various types of alternative accommodation may need to be considered. The main aim of gerontic care is to provide sufficient support services which enable an elderly person to remain at home, but in certain instances relocation may be necessary.

● Senior citizen units. There are a variety of units and 'retirement villages' which have been designed and built exclusively for elderly people. The individual, or couple, live independently in a single unit within a group of units. Many have communal areas, e.g. sitting or dining areas, which can be utilized by the residents if desired. Such accommodation provides an opportunity for the elderly person to live in close proximity to other people of his age group, but still retain his independence.

● Hostel accommodation. Hostel accommodation may be suitable for elderly people who are unable to care for themselves and their homes, but are not in need of nursing care. Supervision on a twenty-four hour basis should be provided by suitably caring staff. Hostels may be attached to a geriatric hospital complex, or be part of the services provided by a number of voluntary agencies.

Accommodation usually consists of a bed-sitting room with a bathroom and toilet annexe. In some instances each resident also has a small kitchen. Most hostels have a communal dining room and sitting room.

● Nursing homes. Nursing home care may be required for elderly people who are unable to function independently because of physical or mental impairments. Nursing homes are numerous: some are administered by church or charitable organizations, while others are commercial ventures. Many of the larger nursing homes provide services such as physiotherapy, occupational therapy, and psychosocial activities and stimuli. In others, only basic custodial care is given.

● Family relief. Some hospitals provide facilities whereby an elderly person who is cared for at home by relatives can be admitted temporarily. Short-term admission of the elderly person, referred to as respite care, enables the carers some relief, e.g. to go on a holiday. Thus, family relief services play an important role in preventing the permanent admission of some elderly persons to a geriatric hospital or nursing home.

● Geriatric hospitals. Most geriatric hospitals can be broadly divided into three sections:

1. A rehabilitation unit to which individuals are admitted on a short-term basis, their rehabilitation potential assessed and an appropriate programme implemented. The aim of a rehabilitation programme is to restore an individual to his maximum level of function and independence so that he is able to return to his own home or, if that is not possible, to make it possible for him to cope with the activities of daily living under supervision in hostel or similar accommodation.

2. A minimal care section for individuals who require

some assistance with one or more of the activities of daily living, e.g. bathing, dressing, or ambulating.

3. An extensive care section for elderly individuals who require a greater degree of assistance or who are totally dependent.

Some geriatric hospitals have established sheltered workshops which offer part-time work in a closely supervised environment, where the type of work and the pace are appropriate for the individual. Such activities may be a means of re-educating certain muscles, or they may help the individual to maintain the level of activity reached in a rehabilitation unit.

Currently the problem of providing suitable accommodation for the increasing elderly population in Australia is being addressed by the government and other agencies. One of the government's long-term objectives is to ensure that nursing home places are available to those in greatest need of those services. The government also recognizes the need to provide additional hostel places for less dependent people, who might formerly have been admitted to nursing homes.

In the future, all elderly people will be classified according to the new 'outcome standards' system, whereby they are placed in categories numbered from one to five. Category 5 comprises less dependent individuals with the lowest need, and category 1 comprises more dependent persons with the highest need, e.g. those elderly people who are bedridden and dependent.

Those who are involved with the care of elderly people are concerned that there should be more efficient planning to match services to people's real needs. An elderly person must be able to live in an environment where his privacy, dignity, and freedom of choice are respected. Ideally, there should be a range of facilities and accommodation options available to cater for the needs and choices of all elderly people.

The elderly person in hospital

An elderly person may require admission to hospital because of a chronic health problem or an acute illness.

Table 55.1 lists the major physical and cognitive effects of physiological ageing, while some of the common disorders of ageing include cardiovascular problems, malignancy, musculoskeletal disorders, genito-urinary problems, gastro-intestinal disorders and cognitive disorders.

Cardiovascular problems. The ageing process results in changes in cardiac function, and loss of elasticity of blood vessel walls. Consequently the most common cardiovascular disorders associated with ageing are:

- hypertension
- postural hypotension
- angina pectoris

- cerebrovascular accident
- myocardial infarction.

Information on cardiovascular disorders is provided in Chapter 44.

Malignancy. Malignant neoplasms are second only to cardiovascular disease as a cause of death of the elderly. The most common sites of cancer include the gastrointestinal tract, lungs, breast, and genito-urinary tract. Information on malignant conditions is provided in Chapter 64.

Musculoskeletal disorders. Changes which occur as a result of the ageing process include progressive muscle atrophy, thinning of bone, arthritic changes, and changes in the intervertebral discs. Consequently, the most common disorders associated with ageing are arthritis and fractures. Information on musculoskeletal disorders is provided in Chapter 42.

Genito-urinary problems. The ageing process results in decreased kidney function, reduced bladder capacity, and some loss of bladder control may occur. In addition an elderly male may experience prostatic hypertrophy, and an elderly female may experience a degree of uterine prolapse. Consequently, the most common disorder associated with ageing is urinary incontinence. Some of the causes of incontinence of urine in elderly people are:

- retention of urine with overflow
- urinary tract infection
- gynaecological disorders
- enlarged prostate gland
- mental confusion
- bladder outlet weakness
- impaired mobility
- iatrogenic, e.g. associated with the use of drugs.

Information on genito-urinary disorders is provided in Chapters 47 and 49.

Gastro-intestinal disorders. The ageing process results in atrophy of gum tissue, reduction in the number of taste buds, reduced secretion of saliva and digestive juices, decreased intestinal motility, and reduced regenerative capacity of the liver. Consequently, the most common disorders associated with ageing include:

- constipation
- faecal impaction, with possible faecal incontinence
- diminished ability to metabolize drugs.

Information on gastro-intestinal disorders is provided in Chapter 46.

Cognitive disorders. Although the structural and physiological changes occurring in the brain during the ageing process do not necessarily alter the elderly person's functional abilities, some elderly people experience changes in behaviour and personality. Information on behavioural problems in elderly people is provided later in the Chapter.

Table 55.1   Physiological ageing

Body system	Changes	Effects
Integumentary	Loss of collagen in the dermis	Folds, lines, wrinkles appear
	Loss of subcutaneous fat	Skin fragility
	Loss of elasticity	
	Atrophy of sweat glands	Drier skin
	Number of blood vessels decreases	Increased sensitivity to cold
	Thinning and loss of hair	Cosmetic implications
	Thickening of nails	More difficult to cut
	Pigmented or non-pigmented lesions may appear	Cosmetic implications
Musculoskeletal	Progressive muscle atrophy	Weakening of muscle strength
	Tendency for muscle cells to be replaced with fibrous tissue	
	Thinning of bone (osteoporosis)	Fractures more common
	Arthritic changes	Stiff and painful joints
	Changes in intervertebral discs	Gradual loss of height and characteristic stoop
		Loss of mobility
Cardiovascular	Change in cardiac function	Heart is less able to respond effectively when under stress
	Loss of elasticity of blood vessel walls	Increased pulse and systolic blood pressure
		Decreased peripheral arterial blood supply and poor venous return
		Wound healing takes longer
Haematopoietic	Defence mechanisms decline	Slower to produce leukocytes and erythrocytes in response to antigens and blood loss
	Bone marrow and lymphatic tissue have less functional and reserve capacity	
Respiratory	Progressive decrease in the thickness of alveolar walls and in elastic recoil	Breathing less efficient
		Greater tendency to develop atelectasis/pneumonia
		Less reserve capacity and tolerance for exercise and stress
Genitourinary	Loss of nephrons leading to decreased kidney function	Reduced ability to eliminate drugs
	Bladder capacity reduced	More frequent voiding
	Bladder control may be unstable	Incontinence may develop
Gastrointestinal	Atrophy of gum and bone tissue	Loss of teeth
	Reduction of saliva	Swallowing may be more difficult
	Decreased secretion of digestive juices	More difficult to digest fried/fatty foods
	Decreased intestinal motility	Constipation
	Decreased sense of taste and smell	Diminished appetite
	Reduced weight and regenerative capacity of the liver	Decreased ability to metabolize certain drugs
Nervous	Decreased number of nerve cells in specific areas of the brain	May affect personality and/or behaviour
		Slower reaction time
	Nerve conduction slower	Diminished reflexes
		Decreased sensitivity to pain, heat/cold sensation
	Decreased kinaesthesia	Diminished sense of movement and position
Special senses	Cochlear degeneration	Gradual reduction in ability to hear high tones
	Increased size and rigidity of the lens, reduced density of lens	Decreased depth perception, night vision, visual fields adaptation, accommodation acuity
		Increased sensitivity to glare

A high percentage of elderly adults experience one or more chronic health problems. In addition, an elderly person may experience an acute illness which necessitates admission to hospital.

The elderly person who is admitted to a hospital has the *same needs* as a person from any other age group. However, because of the problems associated with the effects of ageing some needs assume a higher priority. Thus, the basic nursing care given to an elderly person does not differ from the care given to a person in any other age group but there are additional factors to be considered.

Safety

Because of the effects of degenerative changes associated with ageing, e.g. reduced mobility, loss of balance, diminished visual acuity, and slower reaction time, elderly people are more prone to accidents. Falls are one of the most common accidents experienced by elderly people. A fall can have serious consequences for the individual, e.g. a fractured bone, enforced immobility, loss of confidence, and temporary or permanent reduction in independence. Causes of falls include disorders which affect the cardio-vascular or nervous system, medications such as sedatives, and environmental hazards. Therefore the prevention of accidents is very important, and includes measures such as:

- Provision of low level beds for individuals who are able to get out of bed unaided but risk falling from a high bed.
- Provision of non-slip surfaces on floors, and the removal of loose floor mats which may slip when stepped on. Floor coverings should be kept in good repair, and any spills should be wiped up immediately.
- Ensuring that shoes fit properly and have non-slip soles. Wearing of slippers and walking in stockinged feet should be discouraged.
- Maintaining equipment, e.g. walking sticks or frames, wheelchairs, electrical appliances, in good condition.
- Providing hand grips in toilets and bathrooms, and hand rails along the walls of passages. Bathrooms and shower cubicles should be equipped with non-slip mats or strips.
- Providing chairs of a suitable style and height which will not tip or slide.
- Ensuring adequate lighting in all areas to reduce the risk of falls. Many elderly people require higher intensity of lighting to see adequately. Provision of a bed-side light promotes safety, especially if the individual needs to get out of bed during the night.
- Providing ramps to replace steps and stairs whenever possible. If stairs are being used they should be fitted with hand rails. Bright or white strips should be added to the edges of any steps as an additional safety measure.
- Ensuring that elderly people with visual or auditory loss are provided with, and use, suitable aids such as spectacles or a hearing aid.
- Ensuring that heaters and other articles which may cause burns are safe and equipped with covers or guards. An elderly person can be easily burned, as ageing causes a person's sense of touch to be less effective as a protective mechanism.
- Ensuring that adequate supervision is provided especially for elderly people who are forgetful or confused, and those whose vision or hearing is impaired.

Further information on safety, e.g. preventing transmission of infection, is provided in Chapter 38.

Physical activity

In order to maintain independence an elderly person needs to remain mobile. Physical activity is necessary to maintain circulation, muscle tone, and elimination, and to avoid the deformities that may occur with inactivity. The risk of a fall also decreases when the elderly person is able to move freely. The dangers of prolonged bedrest and inactivity are numerous, and are described in Chapter 37.

While in hospital, the individual should be encouraged to be as ambulant as possible. If it is necessary for him to remain in bed, he must participate in active range of motion exercises. If active ROM exercises are not possible, passive exercises should be performed. If necessary the elderly person should be provided with aids, e.g. a walking stick or frame, which promote safe and effective mobility.

Communication

Because of diminished sight or hearing an elderly person may experience difficulty in communicating. Following a cerebrovascular accident, an individual may experience aphasia (loss of speech). These and other factors require special measures to promote effective communication. Of prime importance is continual encouragement of the individual to communicate, so that he does not feel rejected or isolated.

Information on general communication techniques is provided in Chapter 5; information on communicating with an aphasic individual is provided in Chapter 43, and information on communicating with visually or hearing impaired people is provided in Chapter 50.

Psychological support and mental stimulation

An elderly person admitted to hospital may lose his self esteem and sense of worth because of reduced independence. One of the primary aims of geriatric care is the prevention of dependency, therefore the individual must be encouraged to remain self-sufficient and mentally active. Nurses can provide psychological support and promote mental alertness by:

- Encouraging the individual to do as much for himself as possible. Nursing care plans should allow the person to participate in decision making. He should always be consulted on matters that directly concern him and his care.
- Helping the elderly person to maintain contact with the outside world e.g. by encouraging visitors, and by ensuring that he has access to a telephone, newspapers, radio or television.
- Spending time talking with him. Many elderly people take a keen interest in current affairs and enjoy discussing them. Some older people enjoy reminiscing about past events, and can remember them vividly—even though they may be unable to remember more recent events. Nurses should welcome the opportunity to spend time with older people, as they have so much to contribute and we can all learn a great deal from them.
- Addressing the person courteously and correctly, calling him by the name he prefers. It is wrong to assume that all elderly people appreciate being called by their first name

or by a pet name such as 'Pop' or 'Gran'. Most elderly people, and their relatives, find this practice offensive.

• Avoiding insulting an individual's intelligence by treating him as a child. A nurse may find herself doing just that, particularly if an elderly person is dependent on nurses for most of his needs. Every elderly person, regardless of his circumstances, must be treated with dignity and respect.

• Showing an interest in the elderly person's activities, such as any skills learned in the physiotherapy or occupational therapy department.

• Encouraging an ambulant individual to walk in the hospital grounds when possible, or taking a non-ambulant person outside in a wheelchair.

• Encouraging social interaction with others in the ward. Nurses should remember that interaction is inhibited if people sit in rows against a wall, and is enhanced if people are facing each other or are seated in a 'circular' arrangement.

Visitors should be encouraged so that the elderly person maintains contact with family and friends. Sometimes, a visit from a loved pet does wonders for an elderly person's state of mind—particularly if that pet is his closest companion. (Many nursing homes and mental health units have introduced Pet Therapy. Many lonely or confused people will respond to an animal, and animals can provide companionship, a sense of responsibility and purpose).

• Promoting recreation programmes, whereby activities are planned which encourage individual participation and social interaction. Care must be taken not to enforce participation in activities that hold no interest for an individual. The elderly should be the people to design their own recreation programmes which meet their physical, social, and emotional needs.

It is wrong to assume that all elderly women have an aptitude for, and enjoy, craftwork, just as it is equally untrue that all elderly men prefer woodwork, leatherwork, etc. An elderly person may well prefer to read, listen to music, play chess, or engage in some other activity. It must also be remembered that many elderly people will not want to engage in any activity, and nurses must respect their choice.

• Providing opportunities whereby an elderly person can continue to pursue his religious practices. Many hospitals have visiting clergy who conduct religious services, others have Chapels which can be visited by the individual and his relatives as desired. At other times, it may be possible to arrange transportation to church or other religious meeting place.

• Providing a pleasant environment, and encouraging the elderly person to have whatever personal possessions he wishes with him. Elderly people will generally feel less anxious and less isolated when they are able to keep some familiar objects in their room.

• Encouraging preservation of self-respect by acknowledging the individual's right to privacy, his freedom to choose, and by encouraging pride in his physical appearance.

When an elderly person is admitted to hospital, the nurse should take into account the effects of the ageing process (refer to Table 55.1) when planning and implementing care. The nurse is more able to meet the elderly person's needs if she has an understanding of the physical, psychological, and social changes that accompany ageing.

The elderly person with impaired cognitive function

Cognitive impairment and behavioural changes are possibly the most distressing aspects of ageing, and can result from factors such as:

• cerebral lesions or disease
• cardiovascular problems
• infections
• loss of sight or hearing
• reactions to medication
• excessive, or prolonged, stress
• fatigue
• nutritional deficiencies
• renal insufficiency
• endocrine disorders.

The most common changes in cognitive function are memory loss, withdrawal, confusion, disorientation, and dementia.

Memory loss usually occurs progressively, and loss of short-term memory is more likely to occur than loss of long-term memory. Many factors contribute to memory loss in elderly people, e.g. stress, loss of interest, sensory deprivation, lack of social interaction, and changes in vision or hearing.

Withdrawal occurs when an elderly individual loses interest in, and withdraws from, social contacts, daily routines, and the activities of daily living. Factors such as prolonged grief following the loss of a partner, can lead to withdrawal and disinterest.

Confusion is the most common reaction to stressors in old age, and is a term used to describe a group of behaviours in which the elderly person displays memory deficits, failure to perform the activities of daily living, communication problems, and inability to make decisions. Mild confusion may simply indicate that the elderly person lacks sufficient stimulation, suffers from a sensory impairment, or does not pay sufficient attention to environmental cues such as clocks and calenders. More severe confusion often results from factors such as acute grief or a change from a familiar environment to one which is unfamiliar.

Disorientation is a condition whereby an individual is unable to state his present location, the year, month, or date, and the name of the person with whom he is interacting. While a person may be disoriented about the present, he may be able to recall past events fairly clearly.

• ***Dementia*** is a condition which is characterized by a loss of intellectual abilities such as memory, judgment, and abstract thought. Commonly, there are also changes in personality and behaviour. Characteristics of dementia include disorientation, memory loss, deterioration in a social skills, decreased inhibition, restlessness and agitation. The onset of dementia is usually gradual, the condition is most common over 65 years of age, often the cause is unknown, and it is sometimes possible for the condition to be reversed, e.g. if the cause is identified and treated.

Alzheimer's disease is one of the most common causes of dementia. Information on Alzheimer's disease is provided in Chapter 43.

Care of a confused elderly person

Confusion is a frightening and frustrating experience for an elderly person and his family. The problem may be temporary, e.g. if caused by illness or medication, or permanent. The cause of confusion should be investigated and eliminated, but if this is not possible a great deal can be done to improve the person's ability to function.

Nurses who looked after confused individuals need to be mature, calm, and patient. Frequent changes of staff can be bewildering to confused people, so as far as possible they should be given the security of nurses they know and to whom they can relate. The confused person usually requires a lot of reassurance and frequent explanations, and the nurse should be able to spend time gently and calmly talking to him.

The nurse should appreciate that many elderly people will have lucid periods when they are frightened about their bouts of confusion, and very concerned about what they might have said and done whilst confused. The nurse's attitude should be sympathetic and reassuring both to the individual and his relatives, who also find it most distressing to witness mental confusion in a loved and respected member of the family.

Following thorough assessment of the individual to determine his needs, a plan of care is developed to rehabilitate him as much as possible and to prevent further deterioration of his condition. The plan generally includes measures directed towards:

- providing reality orientation
- encouraging independent function
- encouraging socialization
- providing sensory stimulation
- promoting pride in personal appearance
- protecting from accidental injury.

Reality orientation is a form of rehabilitation used to orientate a confused or cognitively impaired individual by promoting or maintaining the individual's awareness of person, time, and place. To be effective, a reality orientation programme must be implemented on a 24 hour per day, seven days per week, basis. Implementation of such a programme stimulates the confused elderly person to maintain contact with reality, the outside world and his place in it. A reality orientation programme generally consists of measures and activities which include:

- Calling the individual by name every time you are in contact with him, after first determining by which name he prefers to be called, e.g. Mr Smith or John.
- Stating your name and showing the individual your name tag each time you are in contact with him.
- Facing the person, and speaking clearly and slowly. Reword statements if necessary.
- Maintaining a calm and relaxed atmosphere, and avoiding loud noises and hurried movements.
- Telling the person the date and time each morning, and repeating the information as often as necessary during the day.
- Reminding the person of holidays, birthdays, and other special events.
- Providing cues to reinforce verbal information, e.g. clocks, large calenders, bulletin boards listing the day's activities.
- Maintaining a normal day-night cycle, e.g. opening curtains and blinds during the day and closing them at night, and encouraging the person to dress in his own clothes during the day rather than in nightgowns or pyjamas.
- Maintaining a routine established for the individual, to encourage a sense of order and anticipation of what to expect. For example meals, bathing, television programmes, and other activities are performed to a schedule.
- Explaining what you are going to do, and why. Give short simple instructions, and avoid giving too much information at a time.
- Ask clear and simple questions, and allow enough time for a response. Give clear and simple answers to the person's questions.
- Encouraging the individual to place his personal possessions and familiar objects in his immediate environment.
- Leaving the furniture and the individual's belongings in the same place, as rearranging objects in the environment adds to his confusion.
- Encouraging the person to wear aids, e.g. spectacles or hearing aid, if necessary.
- Using touch as a means of communicating and providing sensory stimulation.
- Providing sensory stimulation by ensuring that newspapers, magazines, books, radio, and television are available. Sensory stimulation can also be provided by discussing current affairs with the individual, and by placing paintings and plants in the environment. Some elderly confused people also appreciate being able to look at, and interact with, small pets such as fish or caged birds. Larger animals such as cats or dogs provide added stimulation, as the elderly person is able to touch and stroke them.
- Encouraging the individual to participate in self-care activities, and giving immediate praise for any degree of success. He should be encouraged to participate in decision-making, e.g. choosing what to wear and when to have a bath or shower.
- Providing opportunities for social interaction, e.g. with other residents, family, or friends. In a residential care set-

ting, e.g. a nursing home, programmes should be developed whereby the individual is given the choice whether to attend arranged activities or outings.

● Ensuring that the environment is planned to minimize confusion. Measures such as distinctive colours on bathroom or toilet doors can help the confused person to identify these areas. There must also be adequate lighting in all areas to help the person become oriented to his environment.

● Avoiding reinforcement of delusions or hallucinations. If the person begins to ramble in conversation or talk unrealistically, he should be directed back to reality-oriented conversation.

● Providing purposeful things to do if the individual begins to demonstrate erratic or purposeless behaviour.

CONCLUSION

Old age is a natural stage of development which is accompanied by physical and psychosocial changes.

Physical changes associated with the ageing process involve most body systems, while the mental and psychological changes vary considerably with each individual. Many of the psychosocial changes associated with ageing occur as the result of stresses such as fear of ageing, fear of isolation, loss, physical deterioration, and change of environment.

Care of the elderly is directed towards maintaining independent function, and involves the provision of services which enable an elderly person to stay in his own home for as long as possible without deprivation. When this is not possible, suitable alternative accommodation must be available.

Alternative accommodation for elderly people includes hostels, family relief facilities, retirement villages, nursing homes, and geriatric hospitals.

An elderly person may require admission to hospital because of a chronic health problem or an acute illness. The elderly person who is admitted to hospital has the same needs as a person from any other age group, but there are additional factors to be considered, e.g. safety, maintenance of mobility, and special communication needs.

Cognitive impairment is one of the most distressing aspects of ageing, and can result from factors which include cerebral disease, infections, excessive stress, nutritional deficiencies, and reactions to medications. The most common changes in cognitive function are memory loss, withdrawal, confusion, disorientation, and dementia.

Care of a confused elderly person includes measures directed towards providing reality orientation, encouraging independent function, encouraging socialization, providing sensory stimulation, promoting pride in personal appearance, and protection against accidental injury.

REFERENCES AND FURTHER READING

Matteson M A, McConnell E S 1988 Gerontological nursing: concepts and practice. W B Saunders, Philadelphia
Shaw M W (ed) 1984 The challenge of ageing. Churchill Livingstone, Melbourne

56. The individual with a mental illness

OBJECTIVES

1. Discuss mental health and mental ill-health.
2. Assist in planning and implementing care of an individual who is anxious, depressed, aggressive, self-destructive, or hyperactive.

INTRODUCTION

Psychiatric nursing is a specialized branch of nursing for which the preparation is a specific educational programme, whose goal is the care of those with psychiatric disorders. A nurse who has not undertaken a course in psychiatric nursing may be required to assist in caring for an individual with a mental health impairment. The nurse may be required to work in a psychiatric unit or ward within a general hospital, or she may be required to assist in caring for an individual with a mental health disorder in a general medical or surgical ward. It is, therefore, important that the nurse has a basic knowledge of mental health, mental illness, and the principles of care related to an individual with a psychiatric problem.

This chapter aims to introduce the nurse to the basic concepts of mental illness and psychiatric nursing. As it is beyond the scope of this book to provide comprehensive information on psychiatric disorders and psychiatric nursing practice, the nurse who is interested in gaining such information is advised to refer to the texts listed at the end of this chapter.

Mental health

The concept of mental health is difficult to define, as mental health is much more than the absence of mental illness. There are numerous definitions of, and little consensus about, what constitutes mental health. Mental health is often referred to as a state of wellbeing whereby an individual is happy and contented, but this view does not account for the fact that mental health is a state which can change frequently and which can vary according to specific circumstances.

Mental health may be broadly defined as a relative state of mind in which an individual who is healthy is able to cope with, and adjust to, the recurrent stresses of everyday living in an acceptable way. This is far from an ideal definition as questions then arise of 'What is acceptable behaviour?', and 'Who is qualified to decide whether a behaviour is normal or not?'. People tend to evaluate the behaviour of others based on their own social, ethical, and behavioural standards. Thus, whereas one person may regard someone's behaviour as acceptable and normal, another person may view it as totally unacceptable.

It is, therefore, important for the nurse to appreciate that there is no one universally accepted definition of what constitutes 'mental health'. Whenever a nurse is assessing the mental status of an individual she should have sufficient knowledge to understand what is accepted as normal, what can legitimately be called eccentric, and what deserves the label of a psychiatric disorder. Nowadays the division between 'normal' and 'eccentric' is sometimes very difficult to discern. Nevertheless it should be noted that those nurses who have significant experience in psychology and psychiatry are capable of distinguishing the differences. Other nurses, with guidance and experience, can gradually attain some of these skills. Despite problems in defining mental health the majority of people tend to regard an individual as being mentally healthy if he:

- has a positive attitude towards himself
- develops and strives towards self-actualization
- has an accurate perception of reality
- is able to regulate his moods and emotions
- is able to withstand stress and cope with anxiety
- is able to think rationally and make decisions
- is able to accept the consequences of his own actions
- is able to obtain satisfaction from life
- is able to respond to other people, to love and be loved.

Mental ill-health

Just as it is difficult to arrive at a definition of mental health, so too is it difficult to succinctly define mental ill-health. Broadly, mental ill-health can be defined as a state in which an individual exhibits marked disturbances of emotions, thinking, and action. In the past, mental illnesses and 'madness' were attributed to a variety of factors such as the influences of the moon magic, or witchcraft; possession by the devil or evil spirits; loss of the soul, punishment by the gods, etc. Currently there are a number of explanations for 'abnormal' behaviour, which are used to determine the presence of mental ill-health.

● The medical model views abnormal behaviour as being linked to disease or illness, and those utilizing this model believe that there are physiological reasons for a variety of disorders. For example, there is evidence to suggest that some forms of severe depression are the result of abnormal neurotransmitter function, and that some genetic factor may be linked to schizophrenia. The medical model labels specific disorders according to signs and symptoms exhibited by an individual.
● The psychoanalytic model, first conceptualized by Sigmund Freud (1856–1939), attributes disrupted behaviour in the adult to tasks which needed to be accomplished at earlier developmental stages. This model assumes that behavioural disturbances result from failure to accomplish developmental tasks, remaining infantile and not separating from parents. Information on stages and theories of development is provided in Chapter 2. Freud believed that adult neuroses were caused by childhood experiences.

According to Freud, and other psychoanalysts, *unconscious* processes are largely responsible for abnormal behavioural systems. Those utilizing this model assume that no human behaviour is accidental, and that significant unconscious mental process occur frequently in normal as well as in abnormal mental functioning.

● The social interpersonal model focuses on a broader context of 'abnormal' behaviour, and on the processes by which an individual comes to be identified as abnormal. Those utilizing this model assume that mental illness is a label given to an individual by others, when that individual's behaviour does not conform to their own. It is also assumed that an individual's behaviour involves within the context of his relationships with others, and that his interpersonal experiences are the most significant factors to be considered in psychiatric care. This model also considers the importance of the social environment on an individual, and views social conditions as a major factor in causing abnormal behaviour. Furthermore, this model asserts that an individual's wellbeing depends on the amount of stress he is facing and the ways in which he copes with stress.
● The behavioural model regards the symptoms associated with psychiatric disorders as *learned* behaviours that persist because they are rewarding to the individual in some way. According to behaviourists there are two major methods of learning: operant conditioning and classical conditioning. *Operant conditioning* results in behaviour that acts upon the environment to produce or gain access to reinforcement, and operant behaviour becomes strengthened by reinforcement. *Classical conditioning* (conditional reflex) is a form of learning in which a previously neutral stimulus comes to elicit a given response through association. Information on these two methods of learning is provided in Chapter 4. Some behaviourists see the theories of classical and operant conditioning as a major factor to understanding and controlling a range of abnormal behaviour.

From the brief descriptions of these models it should be clear that a definition of mental ill-health depends largely on which conceptual framework is used. It should also be clear that there is still much to be learned and understood about people and their behaviour.

When discussing the differences between mental health and mental illness it is useful to be aware that there is a 'grey' area into which all individuals enter from time to time. Those with a psychiatric impairment occasionally dip back into sanity and reality-based living for a while and, similarly, sometimes the stresses of everyday living are so overwhelming that the most 'normal' person may experience a marked set of 'abnormal' thoughts, feelings, and actions.

It has become obvious in recent years that mental health, like physical health, is affected by biological, psychological, sociocultural, and spiritual factors. Consequently psychiatric nurses and psychiatrists are concerned with all the aspects of people's lives that distinguish them as human beings. The psychiatric nurse uses knowledge from the psychosocial and biophysical sciences, and theories of personality and behaviour, to develop a framework on which her practice is based. Psychiatric nursing may be described as an interpersonal process whereby the nurse makes purposeful use of her own personality and her knowledge of psychology and effective communication to assist an individual, or his significant others, to promote mental health, to prevent or cope with the experience of mental illness and, if necessary, to support these people through a successful rehabilitation.

Classification of mental disorders

An understanding of the diagnostic classification of mental disorders enables the nurse to understand the basis of medical diagnosis and management of an individual's problem.

For many years psychiatric disorders were divided into psychoses and neuroses but since 1982 those terms are completely out of the classification. For the sake of clarity in this chapter it is useful to define two terms which used to be used and which, sometimes, in everyday life are still used even though they no longer legitimately belong within the accepted psychiatric classification:

• *Neuroses* refers to a cluster of signs and symptoms brought on by excessive anxiety. Even though a neurotic disorder can be quite incapacitating the person who is afflicted does remain in touch with reality.
• *Psychoses* refers to those disorders which are so marked and incapacitating that the person who is afflicted is out of touch with reality, and lacks insight into his behaviour, which may be unacceptable and/or unusual.

The DSM III (Diagnostic and Statistical Manual of Mental Disorders, as described in the Third Edition) classification of clinical conditions is an internationally accepted classification. As it is an extensive classification, only the most commonly occurring disorders are listed in this chapter:

• organic mental disorders, e.g. dementia, delirium
• substance-use disorders, e.g. alcohol abuse or dependence, drug abuse or dependence
• anxiety disorders, e.g. phobias, anxiety states, neuroses
• schizophrenic disorders, e.g. paranoid or catatonic schizophrenia
• affective disorders, e.g. depression, mania
• personality disorders, e.g. antisocial personality disorder, histrionic personality disorder
• psychosexual disorders, e.g. gender identity disorders, psychosexual dysfunctions.

For detailed information on mental disorders, the nurse should refer to the texts listed at the end of the chapter.

Terminology

Terms associated with psychiatry include:
• *Affect*: emotion, feeling, tone, or mood.
• *Affective disorder*: a disorder in which the main feature is a disturbance in the feeling state of an individual; a disturbed personal coping pattern.
• *Aggression*: forceful behaviour that may be physical or verbal, as well as subtle manipulation.
• *Amnesia*: loss of memory of events for a period of time which may range from a few hours to many years.
• *Anxiety*: a feeling of apprehension, dread, or unexplained discomfort, associated with a sense of helplessness, arising from internal conflict.
• *Apathy*: lack of feeling, emotion, concern, or interest.
• *Autism*: preoccupation with the self and inner experiences; a process of introspective thinking which is often rich in fantasy.
• *Behaviour*: any human activity, either physical or mental. Some behaviour can be observed while other behaviour can only be inferred.
• *Behaviour modification*: a method of changing or controlling behaviour through the application of techniques based on the principles of classical conditioning.

• *Body image*: the conscious and unconscious attitudes an individual has towards his body, e.g. feelings about size, function, and appearance.
• *Catatonia*: a state characterized by muscular rigidity and immobility (stuporose type) and is which, at times, is interrupted by episodes of extreme agitation (excited type) and is usually associated with schizophrenia.
• *Compensation*: process by which an individual makes up for a deficiency in his self image, by strongly emphasizing some feature of himself which he regards as an asset.
• *Compulsion*: an uncontrollable persistent urge to perform an act repetitively in an attempt to relieve anxiety.
• *Confusion*: a cluster of abnormalities constituting disturbances of judgement, orientation, memory, affect, cognition.
• *Coping mechanisms*: any effort directed towards stress management. They can be unconscious (defence) mechanisms that protect the individual against anxiety, or conscious attempts to solve a problem which is creating stress. Information on defence mechanisms and stress management is provided in Chapter 6.
• *Delusion*: a fixed false belief that is resistant to modification. A delusion of grandeur is a false belief that one has great prestige, power, or money—which may be manifested in the belief that the individual is a famous person. Delusions of persecution is an individual's belief that he is in danger, being harassed, is under investigation, or is at the mercy of some powerful force. A somatic delusion is a belief that one's body is changing and responding in an unusual way.
• *Dementia*: an organic mental disorder that is characterized by a gradual onset of usually irreversible cognitive impairments.
• *Depression*: a term which can be used to denote a serious disorder of mood. Feelings of sadness dominate which are accompanied by psychosomatic features, e.g. anorexia.
• *Disorientation*: lack of awareness of the correct time, place, or person.
• *Hallucination*: a sensory experience that is not the result of an external stimulus; may be visual, auditory, tactile, or olfactory.
• *Hyperactive*: excessively or unusually active.
• *Hysteria*: a disorder in which symptoms of physical illness occur in the absence of any underlying organic pathological disorder.
• *Illusion*: misperceptions and misinterpretations of real external stimuli; may be visual or auditory or, less commonly olfactory or tactile.
• *Labile*: subject to frequent or unpredictable changes: the term is commonly used with reference to emotions.
• *Mania*: a condition which is characterized by a mood that is elevated, irritable, or expansive, accompanied by poor judgement.
• *Manic-depressive disorder*: a group of reactions whose main characteristic is mood swings ranging from profound

depression to acute mania, interspersed with periods of normality.
- *Neurotic behaviour*: a behavioural dysfunction that is characterized by anxiety, but in which there is no distortion of reality.
- *Obsession*: a persistent thought, idea, or impulse that cannot be eliminated from consciousness by logical effort.
- *Paranoia*: a serious personality distortion whereby the person is markedly suspicious and mistrusting of others, and may be convinced that they wish to harm him.
- *Phobia*: an intense fear of some situation, person, or object so that the danger is magnified out of proportion, and may result in a panic attack.
- *Psychosis*: a state in which an individual's mental capacity to recognize reality, to communicate, and to relate to others is impaired.
- *Psychotic behaviour*: dysfunctional behaviour characterized by disintegration of personality, regressive behaviour, and a panic level of anxiety.
- *Schizophrenia*: a complex condition which is characterized by withdrawal from reality, disordered thinking, regressive behaviour, poor communication, and impaired interpersonal relationships. Delusion and/or hallucinations often occur.
- *Tardive dyskinesia*: a severe side effect of antipsychotic medication which manifests as involuntary movements of the face, jaw, and tongue. It is irreversible.

Promoting mental health

Because of the lack of consensus about precise definitions of mental health and mental illness, measures which promote mental health are often difficult to identify and implement. Another reason why promotion of mental health and, thus, prevention of mental illness is a complex issue is that mental illness has causative factors which are multiple, situational, interactional, and sociocultural. Promotion of mental health is largely directed towards identifying factors which predispose to maladaptive responses, reducing the incidence of stressful life events, identifying vulnerable groups of people, and promoting constructive coping mechanisms.

Causative factors and stressors

Every person faces changes and stress during each stage of development, but various factors create major stress for some individuals. Stressors are events that are perceived by the individual as threatening, challenging, or demanding. A stressor that first has an impact on physiological functioning, e.g. a myocardial infarction, will also affect the individual's psychological and sociocultural behaviour. The nature of an individual's response depends on his appraisal of the stressor and on his appraisal of the coping resources that are available to him.

Appraisal of a stressor involves the individual's cognitive, affective, physiological, behaviour, and social responses. It is the individual's evaluation of the *significance* of an event in his life, whereby he evaluates whether a situation is damaging or potentially damaging. The way an individual interprets an event is a major factor in understanding the nature and intensity of his stress response.

The individual also evaluates his coping resources, options, or strategies by concentrating on the *availability* and *effectiveness* of possible coping methods. Coping resources include individual skills and abilities, social supports, defensive techniques, and economic assets. Therefore, how a person responds to a stressor depends on how significant it is to him, and what coping resources are available and effective.

Prolonged, or intense stress has long been acknowledged as a significant factor in mental, as well as physical, ill health. Some of the stressors which may result in ineffective coping and, consequently, which may precipitate mental illness include:

- breakdown in relationships
- chronic health problems
- multiple losses
- job dissatisfaction
- bereavement
- decreasing independence
- retirement
- change in the health of a family member
- role failures.

It is important to appreciate that, although the majority of individuals are able to withstand changes and the associated stress from time to time, if several changes occur together, or in close succession, there is a cumulative effect. Thus, the individual is more likely to experience an overwhelming stress reaction.

Vulnerable groups

It is important to realize that there are some people who are unable to adapt to, or cope with, developmental tasks and changes as adequately as others. For some individuals, at specific times in their lives, a stressor places an excessive demand on their ability to cope. Such people include those who have additional stressors placed on them, those with inadequate coping resources, and those who have had few positive experiences in life. These groups of people are particularly vulnerable or at high risk for developing maladaptive responses. *A maladaptive response* is a faulty or ineffective adaptation to stress or change, e.g. failure to make necessary changes in values or needs, or an inability to make necessary adjustments in the external world. The people or groups who are particularly vulnerable include:

- Adolescents, who face a period of enormous physical,

psychological, and social change. Some adolescents may not have sufficient resources to cope with the demands placed on them and to successfully complete the developmental tasks during this phase.

● New parents, as the stressors faced by them may include conflict over the acceptance of the pregnancy, transition from being a couple to being parents, and anxiety about the infants welfare.

● Women, because of factors such as their disadvantaged status in society, conflict arising from decisions about whether to pursue a career or become a 'home-maker', or being subjected to domestic violence or buse.

● The elderly, because of the many stresses facing them, e.g. retirement, reduced income, fear of declining physical and mental abilities, relocation, death of a partner or friends of the same age.

● Migrants, who may experience a grief reaction on leaving their homeland, friends, and family, to live in a country where they are classified as strangers. It may be difficult for some migrants to work through their grief reaction because of language barriers, financial uncertainty, and lack of support from relatives and friends. Some migrants may experience problems of adjustment, isolation and loneliness—each of which may contribute to mental illness.

● Physically disabled persons, because of factors such as isolation, lack of meaningful relationships, restrictions caused by impairments, poor self-esteem, and community attitudes towards disabled persons.

Promoting constructive coping mechanisms

Since stress is often harmful to wellbeing, learning to recognize and manage stress is very important. While information on stress and stress management is provided in Chapter 6, some important points are mentioned here. In order to recognize and deal with stress individuals need to be educated and made more aware of:

● the issues and events related to health and illness, and the importance of adhering to sound health practices, e.g. adequate nutrition, exercise, relaxation, as a way of dealing with stress

● the dimensions of potential stressors, possible outcomes, and coping responses

● how to recognize and improve their own abilities in problem—solving, tolerating stress, and interpersonal skills.

● where and how to gain access to coping resources, e.g. support groups and counselling.

Coping mechanisms are strategies which individuals develop to cope with stress and include:

● intense expression of feeling, e.g. laughter or tears
● working it off, e.g. by engaging in strenuous sports activities

● seeking support and comfort from another person
● relying on self-discipline, i.e. not seeking support from others
● seeking comfort in substances, e.g. food, nicotine, alcohol, or other chemicals
● avoidance of or withdrawal from the stressful situation
● talking about the stressful situation with another person.

The mental health team

Many people are involved in assisting an individual who is experiencing a disruption, or potential disruption, to his mental health. Psychiatric care requires an interdisciplinary team approach whereby a range of psychology, sociology, medical and nursing expertise is available whenever patient care is being discussed. The team members work together to plan, implement, and evaluate programmes that will meet the mental health needs of the individual. Ideally, members of the team include:

● *The psychiatrist*: a physician whose specialty is mental disorders, and who is responsible for diagnosis and treatment.
● *The psychiatric nurse*: a nurse with experience and expertise in clinical psychiatry.
● *The clinical psychologist*: a psychologist who has undertaken special education in the area of mental health, and whose function includes applying and interpreting psychological tests and the implementation of behaviour modification programmes.
● *The psychiatric social worker*: a social worker in the field of psychiatry whose function includes counselling and assisting individuals who are confronted by a range of social problems, e.g. accommodation placement or acquiring sickness benefits.
● *The occupational therapist*: a therapist who uses diversionary activities and creative techniques in an effort to improve interpersonal and functional skills.

Deinstitutionalization

There is a growing trend to keep people out of psychiatric hospitals, and in the community as far as possible. Deinstitutionalization is a term which refers to the current policy of the health professionals who work in psychiatry and the governments who fund psychiatric treatment. It is a policy whereby people who develop mental disorders are either treated in the community and never admitted to a treatment centre, or are discharged back into the community from a treatment centre as early as possible. Ideally, community-based psychiatric services provide appropriate networks of supports and caring interventions that are best suited to assist the person to cope in society.

To achieve this goal mental health domiciliary services, community clinics and centres have been established which provide counselling, group therapy, relaxation therapy, occupational and recreational activities. Mental health nurses are very involved in community care and play a major role in education and health promotion, as well as in the provision of continuing care and counselling for persons with a mental health problem.

Overseas experience has shown that there are some serious difficulties with deinstitutionalization, and in Australia there is a determined effort to provide programmes and support networks that adequately meet the requirements of the psychiatrically impaired. In particular, community-based programmes must be designed to meet the needs of the thousands of chronically ill people who deteriorate more and more with every episode of psychiatric illness.

Legal aspects of psychiatric care

The provision of health care for individuals suffering from mental disorders is governed by Mental Health Acts. Each Australian state has its own Act and, as these Acts are periodically revised, the nurse who is involved in psychiatric nursing has a responsibility to be aware of the current Act.

Mental Health Acts provide guidelines and directions regarding the provision of psychiatric care, e.g. criteria for determing whether a person is mentally ill, criteria for admission to hospital, and regulations and requirements regarding the periodic review of individuals suffering from mental illness. Admission to a psychiatric treatment centre may take the form of:

• Voluntary admission, whereby an individual seeks admission as a personal decision or based on the advice of family or a health professional, and is able to leave whenever he chooses.
• Involuntary admission, whereby the request for admission comes from a source other than the mentally ill person who is deemed to be incompetent. An individual may be referred for admission if he poses a danger to himself or others, requires treatment, and is too confused or disorganized to seek voluntary admission. A doctor not employed by the government psychiatric services examines the individual and, if necessary, signs the necessary recommendation documents. The admitting psychiatrist at the treatment centre then examines the individual and decides whether or not to act on the recommendation by admitting the individual.

Care of individuals with a specific problem

This part of the chapter addresses some of the more common mental states which individuals being cared for in non-psychiatric hospital settings may experience. Informa-tion is provided on caring for a person who is anxious, depressed, aggressive, displaying self-destructive behaviour, hyperactive, confused or disoriented.

The anxious individual

Anxiety is an internal feeling which is usually experienced as an unpleasant or uncomfortable emotion, and which is frequently associated with conflicts and frustrations. A certain degree of anxiety can be beneficial when it stimulates motivation and energy, however severe anxiety can be devastating and is the basis of many psychiatric disorders. Sometimes, in extreme anxiety, an individual may experience panic attacks which induce disorganised behaviour and which manifests as either immobility or hyperactivity.

Anxiety differs from fear in that fear occurs in response to a real threat or danger, whereas anxiety occurs in response to situations that are not actually dangerous. Anxiety is experienced in a wide variety of situations, and is generally the result of a threat to an individual's self-esteem or his physical integrity. Threats to self-esteem include factors such as interpersonal difficulties, change in job status, social or cultural group pressures, a change in role, or confusion over one's identity. Threats to physical integrity include factors such as decreased ability to perform the activities of living, injury or illness; or lack of basic requirements such as food, shelter, or clothing.

Anxiety, although sometimes difficult to identify, produces physiological responses, behavioural changes, and emotional reactions. Physiological responses include:

• increased heart rate
• elevated blood pressure
• hyperventilation
• difficulty in breathing
• sweating
• facial pallor
• dry mouth
• muscular tension
• fatigue and/or weakness
• headaches
• chest pains
• diarrhoea or constipation
• loss of appetite
• sleep disturbances
• disturbance of sexual function.

Behavioural and emotional changes include:

• restlessness or agitation
• tremors
• lack of co-ordination of movements and actions
• withdrawal from interpersonal interactions
• rapid speech
• chain smoking
• apprehension

- distortions of reality
- labile moods.

Emotional reactions are usually apparent in the individual's descriptions of his experience. For example he may state he feels apprehensive, irritable, angry, depressed, helpless, on edge, unable to concentrate or remember things; or he may feel detached from events and the environment. The individual may experience angry outbursts or a tendency to cry.

Care of an anxious individual is directed towards reducing intense anxiety to a more manageable level, and helping the person to use effective coping mechanisms, e.g. problem solving. In the early stages minor tranquilizers e.g. diazepam (valium) may be prescribed to suppress the sense of anxiety but, as medications do not cure the condition, long-term use is not advocated. General care involves:

- attempting to identify the cause (stressors) of the anxiety and encouraging the individual to take effective action.
- establishing and maintaining a trusting relationship.
- encouraging the person to talk about his anxiety or problems.
- discussing, with the individual, ways of resolving conflicts.
- educating the individual in measures which can be implemented to reduce stress, e.g. relaxation therapy or massage.
- encouraging the person to take an interest in events and activities.

Diversional activities can be helpful in directing his attention away from unpleasant feelings. Physical exercise, e.g. walking, may provide an emotional release and divert the individual's attention from himself.

The depressed individual

Depression may be mild, severe or profound in intensity. Severe depression gives rise to total withdrawal from people and the environment. Depression commonly occurs when an individual has experienced a loss but other causes include changes to self image, chronic illness, genetic factors and biochemical abnormalities. Most people, at various times, will experience feelings of sadness and grief but this is not the same as the depth of intensity experienced by someone who is suffering from depression. However, when an individual does not engage in the process of mourning in an attempt to deal with the sadness or grief, he may develop depression—which is a pathological grief reaction. Manifestations of depression include:

- non verbal cues (sad facial expression, slumped posture, flat and colourless voice, slow and dragging gait, lack of concern over personal appearance, and reduced activity)
- disturbed sleep patterns, e.g. insomnia or sleeping for much longer periods than usual
- self criticism
- low self esteem
- apathy, poor concentration
- agitation
- anorexia and loss of weight
- fatigue
- loss of sexual libido
- headaches, chest pains
- increased consumption of substances such as nicotine or alcohol
- delusions and/or hallucinations.

Care of a depressed individual is directed towards improving his self esteem, reducing the impact of major stressors, helping him to develop constructive coping mechanisms, and assisting him to regain interest and motivation. In some instances of severe depression, intense psychotherapy and drug therapy, e.g. antidepressants, may be necessary. General care involves:

- establishing and maintaining a trusting relationship.
- helping the individual, when the acute phase is ended, to recognize and express his emotions, e.g. through verbal and non-verbal communication which demonstrates acceptance of him and respect for his feelings.
- encouraging him to talk about his feelings.
- helping him to see that some of his goals may be unrealistic, and assisting him to set realistic goals.
- helping him to establish and maintain social contact and interpersonal relationships.
- encouraging visits by his family or significant others, in order to reduce any feeling of isolation.
- promoting his physical health and well-being, e.g. adequate sleep and nutrition.
- educating the individual in measures which can be implemented to reduce stress, e.g. relaxation techniques.
- protecting him from additional stressors as much as possible.
- assisting him to develop effective coping mechanisms, e.g. decision making and problem solving.

The aggressive or hostile individual

Anger is a feeling, experienced by most people at certain times, which generally occurs in response to fear, confusion, or frustration. Anger often occurs in response to the anxiety a person feels when he perceives a threat. The majority of people have little difficulty in handling mild anger, which is experienced as annoyance and which is usually forgotten quickly. Feelings of anger, disappointment, and frustration may be expressed verbally or non-verbally, e.g. by cursing or kicking a car when it won't start!

When a person is very frustrated, e.g. by being unable to attain an important goal, anger may become more intense. An individual who is experiencing intense anger may try to disperse the unpleasant feeling through an angry outburst or an act of aggression. Occasionally a person may be so consumed by feelings of anger that he becomes violent, and poses a threat to himself and to others nearby.

Nurses may encounter anger in the course of providing nursing care, e.g. an individual whose health is disrupted becomes frustrated, and frustration can lead to anger. Sometimes an individual expresses his anger through verbal, or physical, abuse towards a staff member. Therefore, it is important that nurses are aware of the reasons why a person may be angry, their own responses to angry feelings, and how to help an individual to express anger in a productive way.

Anger may be the result of various stressors, e.g. those that are biological, psychological, or sociocultural. Some of the factors which may cause anger or aggression in individuals who are in hospital include:

- a feeling of loss of control and/or independence
- a sense of isolation from family, and familiar environment
- a feeling of loss of identity or individuality
- feelings of fear and discomfort because of inadequate privacy
- anxiety about the possible outcomes of illness, e.g. altered body image.

Aggressive outbursts may occur when an individual is unable to find a solution to the problem which is causing fear, confusion, or frustration.

Aggressive action may be directed towards the person or object perceived as the source of the frustration, or at other persons or objects in the vicinity. *Displacement* is a defence mechanism whereby an individual discharges pent-up feelings such as anger, on a person or object other than the one that aroused the feelings.

General approaches to an angry or aggressive person include:

- Remaining calm and rational, and avoid responding to anger with anger.
- Listening to the person and helping him to identify the source of his anger if possible.
- Encouraging him to express his feelings verbally, e.g. of frustration, helplessness, or fear. When an individual is allowed to share his thoughts and feelings, and knows that he is being listened to, he is less likely to remain angry.
- Offering constructive remarks in an effort to diffuse the situation and help the individual to regain self-control.
- Refraining from becoming defensive and interpreting the individual's anger as a personal attack.
- Avoiding any tendency to ignore or make light of any expression of anger, as this may only increase his anger.
- Suggesting, if appropriate, a direct way in which the anger can be displaced, e.g. physical exercise of some kind.

- Removing the individual from the immediate environment if it appears that he is on the verge of losing control. Taking him to a quiet area, where he can talk and regain self-control, may help to reduce mounting tension.
- Informing him that there are less distressing and more acceptable ways of expressing anger. He should be provided with this information when he is calm, and not in the middle of an aggressive outburst.

Assertive behaviour is a constructive way of dealing with anger. To be assertive is to stand up for oneself while taking into account other people's interests and feelings. Information on assertiveness is provided in Chapter 6.

In a violent situation, where an angry person has lost self-control, there is the risk of injury to the individual and to others. Prevention of violence is always preferable, but not always possible. If such a situation occurs, the nurse should take measures to ensure the safety of herself and the violent person. It may be necessary, for the safety of all concerned, to remove the nurse and others who are in danger of physical harm. Personnel who are experienced in dealing with violent outbursts should assume control of the situation and implement appropriate measures.

The individual who is self-destructive

Self-destructive behaviour is that which results in physical harm and, sometimes, in the person's own death. Some indirect forms of self-destructive behaviour are eating disorders such as anorexia nervosa, alcohol or drug abuse, and failure to comply with prescribed medical therapy. Direct self-destructive behaviour includes self mutilation, and any form of suicidal or parasuicidal (attempted suicide) activity.

People may engage in self-destructive behaviour for a variety of reasons other than actually wishing to die; and self-destructive behaviour may result from any stress which is perceived by an individual as being overwhelming. An individual may engage in self-destructive behaviour in an attempt to escape from a situation that creates severe anxiety, and which has become intolerable. Factors which may result in a person committing acts of self-harm include:

- recent loss
- rejection by others
- depression
- lack of close interpersonal relationships
- feelings of aggression or hostility
- suffering from a terminal illness
- breakdown in relationships
- poor self-esteem
- mental illness.

The nurse may encounter an individual who is recovering in hospital from the effects of self-destructive behaviour, or she may come into contact with an individual who commits a self-destructive act while in hospital. The 'high-risk' time in a general hospital, when those with suicidal ideas are likely to carry out the act, is in the early morning when the night and day staff are preoccupied with handover.

The first priority in dealing with a person who exhibits self-destructive behaviour is to protect him from himself. This means that, as far as possible, the person must be prevented from self-harm. All dangerous, or potentially dangerous, objects that could be used in a act of self-harm must be removed from the individual's environment. This would include knives and other sharp implements, matches, glass; and items of clothing such as belts, scarves, or stockings that may be used by the individual to harm himself. Other general measure include:

• Observing the individual closely, e.g. for subtle indications of intent to commit an act of self harm. This may take the form of the individual giving away him personal possessions, making a will, or withdrawing from all social activities and relationships.
• Taking seriously any statement that alludes to self-harm, i.e. a threat or innuendo made by the person that he is going to harm himself.
• Helping the individual to identify the factors (stressors) that are responsible for him wanting to commit acts of self-destruction.
• Helping him to eliminate or resolve those stressors, and assisting him to develop constructive ways of coping with stress.
• Assisting the individual to increase his self-esteem, e.g. by promoting relationships with others, helping him to communicate more effectively, and by encouraging him to participate in activities he likes and does well.

The hyperactive individual

Hyperactivity can be a manifestation of an affective mental disorder, and is quite different to the normal exuberant activity engaged in by the majority of people at various times. Hyperactivity is also referred to as hypomania—a psychopathological state characterized by excitability, optimism, marked hyperactivity, talkativeness, quick anger and irritability, and a decreased need for sleep. Sometimes a person who is experiencing hypomania may also experience more extreme manic episodes, whereby all aspects of his behaviour are exaggerated and irrational. Behaviours associated with mania include:

• elation or euphoria
• inflated self-esteem
• lack of shame or guilt
• weight loss and/or dehydration
• reduced need for sleep
• lack of judgement
• flight of ideas (jumping from one idea to another without pause)
• distractibility and poor attention span
• aggression and/or irritability

• increased motor activity and speech
• delusions.

If another person attempts to restrain the individual's activities, he may be subject to irritability, rapid mood swings, and aggressive outbursts.

Care of a hyperactive person is directed towards decreasing hyperactivity, promoting self-control, establishing and maintaining the activities of daily living, and providing a safe and secure environment. General measure include:

• Establishing and maintaining a trusting relationship by being supportive but firm.
• Spending time with the individual, listening to him, and showing concern for his feelings. The nurse must be careful not to evoke his irritation, or be provoked by him or his behaviour—which at times may be hostile or obscene.
• Ensuring that the individual receives adequate nutrition, fluid, and rest.
• Reducing the amount of stimulation to which the individual is subjected.
• Preventing the person from injuring himself, either accidently or intentionally.
• Providing a structured daily programme which allows them individual opportunities to expend his energy in set activities.
• Preserving his dignity when his behaviour is a source of embarrassment to others and, when he is functioning more normally, to himself.

The confused or disoriented person

A person may become confused or disoriented for a variety of reasons. Information on the general management of a confused or disoriented person is provided in Chapter 55. While the information in that chapter relates to the elderly individual, the principles of care are the same for any age group.

CONCLUSION

Although psychiatric nursing is a specialized branch of nursing, the general nurse may be required to assist in the care of an individual who has a mental illness, e.g. if he is being cared in a general hospital.

Mental health, while difficult to define precisely, is often referred to as a state of wellbeing in which the individual is able to cope with and adjust to the recurrent stresses of everyday living in an acceptable way.

Mental ill-health may be broadly defined as a state in which an individual exhibits behavioural disturbances.

Mental ill-health can result from factors which a physiological, psychological, and sociocultural.

While no-one is immune to developing a mental disorder some groups are more vulnerable, e.g. those who have additional stressors placed on them, those with inadequate coping resources, and those who have had few positive experiences in life.

This chapter addresses some basic measures which may be implemented when caring for an individual who is anxious, depressed, aggressive, self-destructive, or hyperactive.

Further information on psychiatric nursing may be obtained by referring to the texts listed at the end of the chapter.

REFERENCES AND FURTHER READING

Beck C K, Rawlins R P, Williams S R 1988 Mental health-psychiatric nursing, 2nd edn. C V Mosby, St Louis
Stuart G W, Sundeen S J 1983 Principles and practice of psychiatric nursing, 2nd edn. C V Mosby, St Louis
Wilson H S, Kneise C R 1988 Psychiatric nursing, 3rd edn. Addison-Wesley, California

57. Emergency care

INTRODUCTION

First aid is the emergency care of a sick or injured person until medical aid is available, or until the person recovers. The nurse may encounter an emergency situation in a health care facility, in the home environment, or in a public place. Knowing what to do in an emergency situation may mean the difference between a person living or dying.

An emergency situation within a health care facility may involve a patient, a visitor, or a staff member. Under these circumstances lifesaving equipment and expert help are usually at hand, but the prompt emergency care given by the person who is first on the scene may save life.

Documentation of the incident will be required, and health care facilities provide 'incident and accident' forms for this purpose. Information to be documented includes details of the onset of the incident; the date, time, and location; the emergency care provided, and the name of any person who witnessed the incident. The nurse attending the emergency must remain with the individual and summon assistance. If the incident occurs within a ward area, the nurse in charge must be notified immediately.

This chapter addresses some emergencies and the basic care that needs to be provided. For more detailed information, the nurse is advised to consult a current first aid text. There are also a variety of courses available, conducted by organizations such as the St. John Ambulance Association in Australia, which provide valuable instruction in emergency care.

The aims of emergency care

The emergency care of a sick or injured person is directed towards:

- preserving life
- promoting recovery
- preventing a worsening of the condition
- providing basic first aid care.

The principles of emergency care

Every emergency situation must be assessed, and appropriate measures taken in the sequence which is most logical for that particular situation. A variety of factors will influence the actions taken and the order in which they are taken, e.g. the presence of life threatening circumstances, the availability of assistance, the location in which the emergency occurs, and the availability of transport. The general principles of emergency care are:

- Check whether there is danger to self, the casualty, or any bystanders. Proceed only if it is safe to do so.
- Remain calm, as calmness and efficiency will help the casualty to feel more secure.
- Assess the situation quickly, and decide the order of priorities. Perform life saving actions first.
- Remove the cause of the emergency or, if this is not practicable, remove the casualty from the cause.
- Assess the casualty. Assessment is made of his conscious state, airway, breathing, and circulation. Circulation is assessed by checking the pulse and observing for bleeding or manifestations of shock.
- Begin to manage the situation according to priorities decided on as a result of assessment.
- Provide emotional support for a conscious casualty.
- Keep the casualty lying down or in the position in which you found him, as any injury could be exacerbated if he is moved. Exceptions to this principle are when the casualty is unconscious and must be positioned to maintain a clear airway, or when resuscitation measures must be implemented.

- Seek assistance from any helpers who are available.
- Arrange for medical aid. Ask a bystander to telephone for an ambulance. Information provided to the ambulance service should include your location, the number of casualties, and the nature of the emergency.
- Maintain the casualty's normal body temperature. Use coats or knitwear if a rug is not available.
- Prevent persons from giving the casualty any food or fluids, as the ingestion of substances may cause harm or delay any surgical intervention which may be required.
- Remain with the casualty and continue to provide physical and emotional care until medical assistance arrives.
- Provide emergency personnel with information regarding your assessment of the casualty and any care provided.

Assessment of the casualty

Assessment of the casualty at the scene of the emergency involves obtaining an account of the incident, and observing for the manifestations of illness or injury.

Information about the incident, which may be obtained from the casualty or a witness, should include whether there were any contributing factors such as a dizzy spell before a fall, and the symptoms the casualty is experiencing. If the problem appears to be of a medical nature, rather than the result of an accident, the individual should be asked about his medical history, e.g. does he have a heart disorder, epilepsy, or diabetes. He should also be asked whether he usually takes any medication for the condition. The individual should be observed to see whether he is wearing a medical warning bracelet or pendant, which provides information about his medical condition.

Life threatening situations which have first priority and must be attended to before attending to other problems, involve assessing the individual for conscious state, breathing, heart beat, and severe bleeding.

Assessment of consciousness is made by observing whether the casualty responds to a verbal command, e.g. 'can you hear me?.' If he does not respond to words, observe for any response when he is touched.

If he is unconscious his airway must be checked, and cleared if necessary. If he is not breathing, expired air resuscitation must be commenced immediately.

If his carotid pulse is absent, cardiopulmonary resuscitation must be commenced immediately.

Information on resuscitation techniques is provided later in the Chapter.

Assessment of bleeding is made by observing for obvious loss of blood from an injury or orifice. Severe external bleeding must be quickly controlled to prevent shock.

The individual may be bleeding internally—into a body cavity, organ, or tissues. Manifestations of internal bleeding include a weak and rapid pulse, pale face and lips, cold and clammy skin, rapid ventilations, faintness, and restlessness or apprehension.

Following the initial assessment, for life threatening problems, the casualty is assessed for other manifestations of injury or illness:

- tenderness
- swelling
- bruising
- abrasions or minor lacerations
- deformity
- pain
- loss of movement
- abnormal sensation, e.g. tingling
- abnormal skin colour, e.g. cyanosis
- abnormality of the pupils, e.g. unequal in size
- nausea or vomiting
- difficult breathing
- disorientation.

Moving the casualty

When the casualty is to be moved, the choice of an appropriate means of transport is most important, and the factors to be considered are:

- the nature and severity of the injury or illness
- the equipment available
- the number of helpers available and their physical capabilities
- the nature of the surroundings in which the emergency occurred
- the distance to be covered.

Which ever method of transport is used, certain basic principles apply:

- The safety of the casualty and the helpers must be ensured
- The casualty should be made as comfortable as circumstances permit
- Transport of the casualty should be accomplished as speedily as possible.

To promote safety when moving a casualty the first aider should ensure that:

- The airway is clear
- Bleeding is controlled
- Supporting bandages and splints are maintained in their correct position
- The casualty is correctly positioned, and securely fastened, if a stretcher is used
- The casualty is not left unattended.

A stretcher may be improvised from any material strong enough to carry the weight of the casualty without giving way, e.g. a door, gate, ladder, or blankets attached to poles.

Ambulance personnel may use a Jordan lifting frame or scoop stretcher to move the casualty with little disturbance to the injured areas.

When a stretcher is used to transfer the casualty, care must be taken to avoid causing further injury or pain. Any straps or bandages used to secure the casualty must be placed so that they do not restrict breathing, impair circulation, or aggravate any injuries.

Casualties with minor injuries may be transported sitting in a car seat, provided that the injured parts are adequately supported.

Basic emergency management of wounds

Wounds are classified as *closed* or *open*. Examples of closed wounds include a contusion, sprain, or closed fracture; or it may be open. Open wounds are those which result in external bleeding, and they may be classified as:

- abrasions, caused by direct contact with a rough surface
- incisions, due to cutting by a sharp object
- lacerations, due to tearing by a blunt object
- bites, caused by animals or humans
- penetrating injuries, caused by a sharp pointed object.

The basic emergency management of an open wound involves:

- controlling bleeding
- cleansing the wound
- applying a clean, or sterile, dressing
- seeking medical aid.

The basic emergency management of a closed wound involves:

- resting the injured part
- elevating the injured part, if appropriate
- applying a firm bandage
- applying cold, if appropriate.

Dressings, splints, slings, and bandages

Dressings

A dressing is a covering applied to a wound to control bleeding, absorb discharge, promote comfort, and to protect the wound from further injury and infection. The dressing should have a surface that will not adhere to the wound, and it should be large enough to cover the wound. Ideally the dressing should be sterile, but in an emergency situation a dressing can be improvised from any clean, soft, non-adherent material. Items that are suitable include clean linen, towels, napkins, and handkerchiefs.

A pressure dressing may be applied to provide additional local pressure to assist in controlling bleeding. The dressing is applied over the wound, and held in position by hand pressure or a firmly applied bandage.

A ring dressing is a form of pressure dressing which may be applied around a protruding bone or foreign body, to control bleeding. The dressing is formed into a ring, placed around the wound, and secured with a bandage without applying pressure on the protruding bone or foreign object.

Splints

A splint is a device applied to a limb to provide rigid support for a fracture, to immobilize a limb when a joint injury is suspected, or it may be used in the management of snake bite. In an emergency situation a splint can be improvised from any suitable firm material, e.g. flat pieces of wood, branches, cardboard, or newspaper.

A splint should extend past the joints on either side of the injury, and padded so that pressure is not applied to bony prominences. The splint is secured with bandages, above and below the injury area, and at each end of the splint. The bandages should be applied firmly to prevent movement, but not so tight as to impair blood circulation or cause pain.

Inflatable air splints are commonly used by ambulance personnel, as a quick and effective means of immobilizing an injured limb. An air splint consists of a double-walled plastic tube, with a valve in the outer wall for inflation. The splint is fitted with a zip slide fastener to facilitate application.

Slings

A sling may be used to support, elevate, or rest an injured upper limb. It may be used to prevent the weight of the upper arm from pulling on, or moving, an injured chest or shoulder. A sling may be also used to help immobilize rib fractures. Three types of sling (Fig. 57.1) may be applied:

- collar and cuff
- arm sling
- St. John sling

A sling may be improvised by using a scarf, tie, or belt. Turning up the lower edge of a jacket being worn and pinning it to the clothing, or pinning a sleeve containing the injured arm can be effective. The principles involved in applying a sling are:

- Maintain the individual's comfort while the sling is being applied.
- Use a reef knot to secure the sling, as this type of knot is less likely to slip undone or cause pressure on the neck.
- Place the knot in the hollow above the clavicle, where it will not cause discomfort by pressing on a bone.

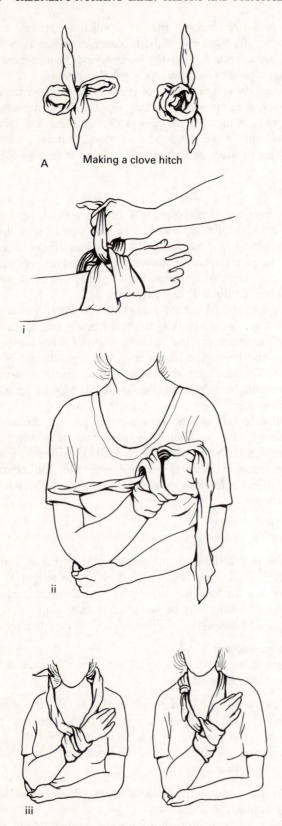

A   Making a clove hitch

i

ii

iii

Fig. 57.1   (A) Making a collar and cuff sling.

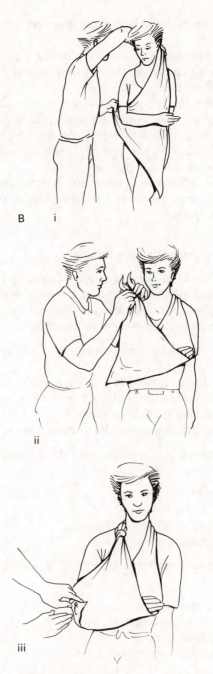

B   **i**

ii

iii

Fig. 57.1   (B) Making an arm sling.

● Place the portion of the sling lying at the back of the casualty's neck, under his collar to prevent chafing. Alternatively, a pad may be placed under that portion of the sling.

● Position the affected arm so that the wrist and hand are higher than the elbow.

Bandages

A bandage may be used to maintain pressure over a dressing to control bleeding, to retain a splint in position, to

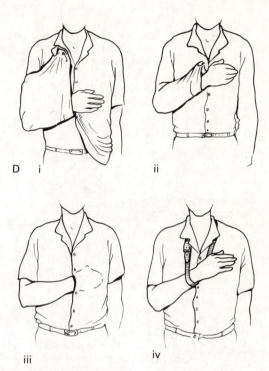

Fig. 57.1 (D) Improvised slings.

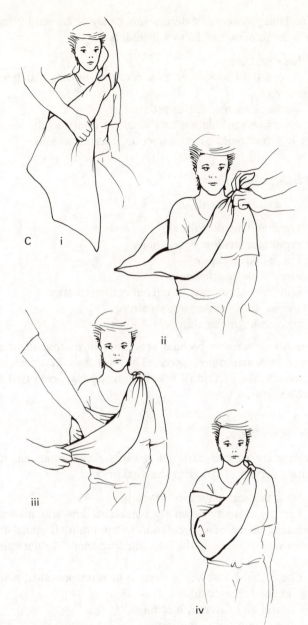

Fig. 57.1 (C) Making a St John sling.

prevent or control swelling, to restrict movement, or to apply pressure and immobilization in the management of certain bites and stings.

In many health care settings the use of bandages has diminished, as other methods have been devised to take the place of bandaging. However, there are still occasions when a bandage is required. The most commonly used bandage materials are crepe and gauze. Types of bandages include:

- roller, e.g. crepe
- triangular, e.g. slings
- tubular, e.g. gauze
- impregnated, e.g. plaster of paris.

In an emergency situation a bandage may be improvised by cutting material into strips. The general principles of bandaging are:

- Select a bandage which is the correct width, and material, for the purpose.
- Stand, or sit, opposite the individual and support the part to be bandaged.
- Position the part correctly before applying the bandage.
- Place padding, e.g. gauze, between two skin surfaces to prevent chafing.
- Hold the bandage with the head (roll) uppermost, as this ensures that the bandage unwinds smoothly and can be easily controlled.
- Unroll the bandage a few centimetres at a time, maintaining even pressure throughout.
- Apply the bandage from below upwards, so that circulation is not impaired.
- Fasten the end of the bandage, with a clip, pin, or tape, at a point where it will not cause discomfort, pressure, or friction.
- Assess the individual for manifestations indicating that the bandage is too tight and impeding circulation. Manifestations of impaired circulation are pallor, cyanosis, coldness, or swelling of the extremity. The individual may also experience pain, tingling, or numbness; or he may be unable to move the digits of the bandaged limb.

Figure 57.2 illustrates various methods of applying a bandage.

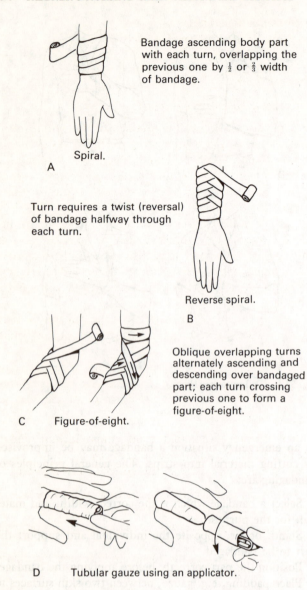

Bandage ascending body part with each turn, overlapping the previous one by ½ or ⅔ width of bandage.

Spiral.

A

Turn requires a twist (reversal) of bandage halfway through each turn.

Reverse spiral.

B

Oblique overlapping turns alternately ascending and descending over bandaged part; each turn crossing previous one to form a figure-of-eight.

C   Figure-of-eight.

D   Tubular gauze using an applicator.

Fig. 57.2 Bandaging methods.

SPECIFIC EMERGENCY SITUATIONS

Emergency situations requiring first aid management include shock, haemorrhage, seizures, unconsciousness, asphyxia, heart attack, exposure to extremes of temperature, injuries to bones and joints, poisoning, bites and stings, and injuries to the eye.

Shock

Shock is a condition in which tissue perfusion is inadequate to maintain the necessary supply of oxygen and nutrients for normal cell function, and to remove the waste products of metabolism. It may result from inadequate cardiac function, or a reduction in circulating blood volume.

Shock may develop immediately, or progressively over several hours. If severe, shock may lead to collapse of the circulatory system and death. Shock may be caused by one, or a combination of factors including:

- haemorrhage
- severe fluid loss, e.g. as a result of burns, diarrhoea, vomiting
- cardiac damage, e.g. heart attack
- excessive vasodilation as a result of injury to the spinal cord, severe pain, severe infection, certain poisons.

Manifestations of shock

The manifestations of shock include:

- rapid and weak pulse
- rapid and shallow ventilations
- low blood pressure
- anxiety and restlessness
- faintness, dizziness, or altered conscious state
- nausea and, sometimes, vomiting
- pale, cold, moist skin.

The manifestations become progressively more evident as shock becomes more severe. The skin may become cyanosed and the individual may become drowsy, confused or unconscious.

Emergency care

Emergency care is directed towards maintaining an adequate supply of blood to the vital organs:

- Seek medical assistance urgently
- Lie the casualty down with his head low and his legs elevated, to improve circulation to the brain. If spinal injuries or fractures to the legs are suspected, do not raise the legs
- Check that his airway is clear. If he is unconscious, place him in the coma position
- Control any external bleeding
- Loosen any tight clothing
- Place a blanket or coat over him to maintain body temperature, taking care not overheat him as this draws blood away from the vital organs.
- Provide emotional support.

Electric shock

Electric shock occurs when the body comes into contact with strong electrical currents which may cause cardiac arrest, respiratory arrest, and burns.

The first aider must take precautions to avoid coming into contact with electricity himself, either from live wires or from the casualty's body. Water and metals conduct electricity, therefore measures should be taken to exclude both from the rescue operation. The rescuer's hands should be protected by an insulating material, e.g. rubber, paper, wood, dry clothing.

Emergency care

Emergency care involves:

• Breaking the casualty's contact with the electrical current. Either switch off the current, or pull the cord to jerk the plug out of the socket. If either of these actions are not possible stand on a dry surface, and use an object which is a poor conductor of electricity to pull the casualty away.
• Checking the casualty's breathing and pulse
• Commencing cardiopulmonary resuscitation if necessary
• Covering any burns with a clean dry dressing
• Seeking medical aid urgently
• Providing emotional support.

Haemorrhage

Haemorrhage (bleeding) is classified according to the site and according to the type of blood vessel involved. Haemorrhage may be external and visible, or internal and concealed.

External haemorrhage is usually obvious, although the source may not be immediately evident.

Internal haemorrhage occurs into tissues, joints, organs, or cavities within the body and is not visible, although it may be revealed if blood escapes through a body orifice. Blood may reach the surface of the body in:

• haemoptysis, when blood is coughed up
• haematemesis, when blood is vomited
• a melaena stool, which is black and tarry due to digested blood
• frank blood, from the rectum/anus
• haematuria, when blood is present in the urine
• vaginal bleeding
• epistaxis (bleeding from the nostrils).

Arterial haemorrhage is bleeding from a damaged artery. The blood is bright red in colour, and the bleeding occurs in spurts which coincide with the beats of the heart.

Venous haemorrhage is bleeding from a damaged vein. The blood is dark red in colour, and the blood flows steadily.

Capillary haemorrhage is bleeding from damaged capillaries. A small amount of blood flows as a gentle ooze.

Manifestations of haemorrhage

The manifestations of haemorrhage are:

• obvious bleeding
• rapid and weak pulse
• rapid and shallow ventilations
• low blood pressure
• anxiety and restlessness
• faintness or dizziness
• pale and clammy skin
• thirst

• loss of consciousness
• escape of blood through a body orifice.

Emergency care

External haemorrhage is controlled by:

• Applying direct pressure to a bleeding wound. Pressure controls bleeding by compressing the blood vessels leading to the wound, and by retaining blood in the wound long enough for it to clot. A thick dressing is placed over the wound, and manual pressure is applied. A firm bandage is applied over the dressing to maintain pressure. If a dressing is not available, apply direct pressure with the bare hand. If bleeding is profuse, it may be necessary to grasp the sides of the wound and firmly squeeze them together
• Elevating the injured part, to decrease blood flow to that part. This action is contraindicated if a fracture is suspected
• Resting the injured part, to lessen the demand for blood by the tissues and to prevent dislodgement of the forming clot
• Placing another dressing over the first if bleeding continues, and apply manual pressure. Do not remove a dressing, as this leads to dislodgement of the clot and further bleeding

Other aspects of first aid management include seeking medical assistance and preventing shock

Epistaxis, bleeding from the nostrils, is managed by:

• sitting the casualty up with his head tilted forwards
• providing a receptacle for the blood
• applying digital pressure to the nostrils for approximately 10 minutes
• instructing the casualty to breathe through his mouth, and not to blow his nose
• loosening tight clothing around the neck, and see that there is a good supply of fresh air
• placing cold wet compresses on the neck and forehead
• seeking medical aid if the bleeding is not controlled, or if a large amount of blood was lost
• providing emotional support.

If internal haemorrhage is suspected:

• Keep the casualty at rest
• Prevent shock
• Seek medical assistance urgently
• Provide emotional support.

Seizures

Seizures are sudden attacks involving involuntary contraction of skeletal muscles, due to disturbances of cerebral function. Three forms of seizure disorders are generalized tonic-clonic (grand-mal) epilepsy, absence (petit mal), and infantile convulsions.

Petit mal attacks do not require any emergency management. Information on possible causes of seizure disorders is provided in Chapter 43.

Manifestations of tonic-clonic seizures

This type of generalized seizure generally follows a characteristic pattern:

1. An aura, the warning phase which signals an impending attack. This does not always occur, but may consist of a specific taste, smell, or other sensation experienced by the individual. He may give a characteristic 'cry' as air is forced out through the vocal cords which are in spasm.

2. The tonic stage, in which the individual loses consciousness. Muscle spasms occur, the individual becomes rigid, and the teeth are tightly clenched. The face and neck become cyanosed due to a brief period of apnoea.

3. The clonic stage, in which intermittent violent contractions of muscle cause jerky, spasmodic movements of the body. Frothing at the mouth commonly occurs, and there may be blood if the individual bites his tongue or the inside of his cheek. There may be loss of bladder and/or bowel control.

4. The comatose stage, in which the muscles relax, and the individual remains unconscious.

5. The post-epileptic stage, in which, on regaining consciousness, the individual may be confused or drowsy. In some instances the individual performs actions that are repetitive and undirected (automatism). He is unaware that he is performing these actions.

Emergency care

During a seizure the objective is to prevent the individual from injuring himself:

- Move harmful objects out of the way
- Do not attempt to put anything in the individual's mouth
- Loosen constrictive clothing, and place a folded towel or jumper under his head if the individual is lying on a hard surface
- Place the individual on his side when the convulsions begin to subside in order to maintain a clear airway
- Treat any injuries resulting from a fall to the ground, or from the seizure
- Seek medical aid if the individual is not known to have epilepsy
- Allow him to rest after the seizure
- Provide emotional support.

Manifestations of infantile convulsions

Convulsions are relatively common between the ages of approximately 10 months and 4 years. They are frequently associated with a high body temperature resulting from infection. Manifestations are:

- stiffness of the body
- twitching of the limbs
- arching of the head and back
- rolling of the eyes
- congestion of the face and neck
- cyanosis of the face and lips.

Emergency care

Emergency management of infantile convulsions involves:

- ensuring a clear airway, by holding the child with the head low and turned to one side
- loosening any tight clothing
- seeking medical assistance
- if it is a febrile convulsion, reducing body temperature by sponging the child with tepid water
- providing emotional support.

Unconsciousness

Unconsciousness may be caused by many factors, e.g. head injuries, cerebrovascular accident, drug or alcohol overdose, fainting, poisoning, or seizure disorders. The period of unconsciousness may last for a few minutes, as in fainting, or for much longer. The unconscious individual is unable to respond to external stimuli, e.g. voice and touch.

Emergency care

As the unconscious individual is unable to communicate, maintain a clear airway, or protect himself from danger, emergency care involves:

- placing him in the coma position (Refer to Figure 35.6)
- ensuring a clear and open airway
- seeking medical assistance
- checking breathing and pulse. If cardiac or respiratory arrest develop, commence cardiopulmonary resuscitation
- providing emotional support for relatives or friends who are with the individual.

Manifestations of syncope (fainting)

Fainting is a temporary loss of consciousness due to an inadequate supply of oxygen to the brain. Fainting may result from nervous shock, injury, standing still for a long time, or a sudden postural change. Manifestations are:

- giddiness
- blurred vision
- weakness
- a 'hot and cold' feeling
- yawning

- pale, cold, clammy skin
- slow and weak pulse
- loss of consciousness follows.

Emergency care

Loss of consciousness may be prevented by prompt action to restore blood supply to the brain:

- Lie the individual down, with the head and body flat and the legs raised
- Loosen tight clothing
- Ensure a good supply of fresh air
- Encourage deep breathing
- Provide emotional support
- Allow him to rest for a few minutes until he has fully recovered
- If the individual loses consciousness, place him in the coma position
- Seek medical assistance if unconsciousness persists for more than a few minutes.

Asphyxia

Asphyxia is severe hypoxia leading to unconsciousness. Lack of oxygen, if not corrected, may lead to brain cell damage, altered consciousness, absent breathing, absent pulse, and death. Asphyxia may be caused by any factor which interferes with the exchange of gases in the lungs and tissues, such as:

- drowning
- electric shock
- aspiration of vomitus
- lodgement of a foreign body in the air passages
- inhalation of toxic gas or smoke
- oedema of the lining of the air passages
- strangulation
- asthma
- chest injuries, e.g. flail chest
- cerebral injury or disease.

Manifestations of asphyxia

Manifestation of asphyxia are:

- shortness of breath
- painful, rapid, or laboured breathing
- dizzyness
- cyanosis of the face, lips, ears, nail beds
- gasping speech
- swollen veins of the head and neck
- reddening of the whites of the eyes
- confusion and restlessness
- loss of consciousness
- cessation of breathing and/or pulse.

Emergency care

Emergency care involves:

- removing the cause of asphyxia, if possible, or the individual from the cause
- clearing the airway by removing any obstructions
- placing the victim in the coma position
- commencing cardiopulmonary resuscitation, if breathing and pulse are absent
- seeking medical assistance urgently.

Resuscitation

If an individual is not breathing (respiratory arrest) expired air resuscitation (EAR) must be commenced immediately. If the heart has stopped beating and the individual is not breathing, EAR and external cardiac compression (ECC) must be commenced immediately. When the two techniques are performed simultaneously, the term cardiopulmonary resuscitation (CPR) is used.

Expired air (mouth-to-mouth) resuscitation

To perform expired air resiscitation:

- Lie the casualty on his back, and kneel beside his head
- Clear his mouth of any obstructions
- Tilt the casualty's head back, and hold his lower jaw up and forward (Fig. 57.3)
- Pinch his nostrils together
- Take a deep breath
- Open your mouth wide and place it over the casualty's slightly open mouth—making an airtight seal
- Breathe into the casualty's mouth to inflate his lungs, and observe his chest wall for movement
- Remove your mouth to allow air to be expelled from the casualty's lungs
- Observe his chest for movement, and listen or feel for exhaled air
- Give 4–5 quick breaths, then continue at a rate of twelve breaths per minute (1 every 5 seconds)

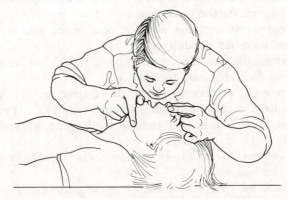

Fig. 57.3 Expired air (mouth-to-mouth) resuscitation (EAR).

• Check that the carotid pulse is present after 1 minute, then every 2 minutes
• If the chest fails to rise, check again for obstructions in the mouth, and check that the casualty's mouth is effectively sealed during inflation
• Continue with EAR until the casualty is breathing spontaneously, or until medical assistance arrives
• If breathing recommences, cease EAR and place the casualty in the coma position.

If the casualty is an infant or child, place your mouth over his nose and mouth, breathe out gently in small puffs, and inflate at the rate of twenty times per minute.

Cardiopulmonary resuscitation

When the heart stops (cardiac arrest) circulation of the blood ceases. The casualty will be unconscious and breathing will be absent. Manifestations of cardiac arrest are:

• unconsciousness
• absent pulse
• absent breathing
• pale or grey cool skin
• dilated pupils.

CPR is most effectively performed by two people, but a person acting alone can successfully perform CPR. To perform cardiopulmonary resuscitation:

• Lie the casualty on a flat firm surface
• Kneel at the side of the casualty's chest
• Locate the lower end of the sternum, and position the heel of one hand 1–2 finger widths above this point, in the midline of the sternum (Fig. 57.4)
• Place the other hand securely over the top of the first, and interlock the fingers of both hands
• Keep the fingers of the first hand off the surface of the chest, so that no pressure will be exerted directly on the ribs
• Keeping the arms straight, exert pressure through the heel of your lower hand using your body weight as the compressing force
• Perform the compressions rhythmically, with equal time for compression and relaxation
• Depress the sternum about 5 centimetres with each compression (for an adult)
• Release the pressure after each compression, but do not remove the hands from the chest wall
• Continue compressions at a rate of sixty per minute.
N.B. EAR is performed simultaneously with ECC. If one person is performing both techniques, the ratio is 2 ventilations to 15 compressions.

If two persons are involved, the ratio is 1 ventilation to 5 compressions.
• Check for the presence of a carotid pulse every 1–2 minutes

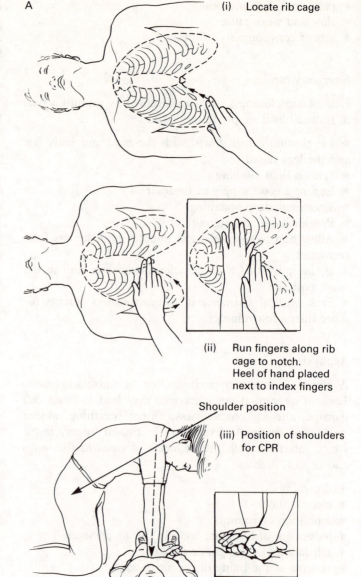

(i) Locate rib cage

(ii) Run fingers along rib cage to notch. Heel of hand placed next to index fingers

Shoulder position

(iii) Position of shoulders for CPR

Hand position

Fig. 57.4 (A) External cardiac massage. Proper hand and shoulder positions.

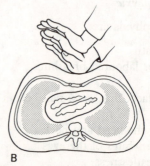

Fig. 57.4 (B) External cardiac massage. The heart lies between the sternum and the spinal column. When pressure is applied to the sternum, the heart is compressed.

• If circulation is restored, stop ECC but continue with EAR. If breathing is restored, stop EAR. Place the casualty in the coma position.

If the casualty is an infant under twelve months of age, apply compression with the tips of your index and middle fingers over the centre of the sternum. Compress to a depth of 1.5 centimetres at a rate of 100 compression per minute.

If the casualty is a child under 8 years of age, apply compression with the heel of one hand over the centre of the sternum. Compress to a depth of 2.5 centremetres at a rate of 100 compressions per minute.

Health care facilities develop their own protocol for managing a cardiac or respiratory arrest, and the nurse has a responsibility to be aware of the actions to be taken should such an event occur.

Choking

Choking occurs when food or objects pass the epiglottis to enter the larynx.

Manifestations include a fit of coughing, violent attempts at breathing, clutching the throat, and increasing cyanosis of the face, lips, and nail beds. These manifestations are followed by loss of consciousness and respiratory arrest.

Emergency care involves:

• Checking the airway and removing any visible obstruction If the obstruction is not visible and the casualty is an infant or child, place him across your lap with his head down. Give 3–4 sharp smacks between his shoulder blades, with the heel of one hand. In the case of an adult lie him face down, with his head low if possible, and strike him with 3–4 sharp blows between the shoulder blades. Alternatively, have him sitting and bend his head and shoulders forward before striking him between the shoulder blades.

N.B. the Heimlich manoeuvre is another technique to clear the obstructed airway of a *conscious* adult. It is performed by standing behind the casualty, and wrapping your arms around his waist. Make a fist with one hand, and place it thumb side against his abdomen (just above the umbilicus and below the end of the sternum). The other hand is placed over the first, and both are pressed into the casualty's abdomen with a quick upward thrust. The thrusting movement may be repeated, if necessary, in order to expel the obstruction.

• Seeking medical assistance urgently if there is any difficulty in dislodging the obstruction
• Providing emotional support
• If the casualty is unconscious, placing him in the coma position and seeking medical assistance
• If breathing stops commencing EAR immediately, and seeking medical assistance urgently.

Heart attack

A myocardial infarction (heart attack) occurs when disruption of the blood supply to the heart results in the death of part of the myocardium. Blood flow to the myocardium may be obstructed by artherosclerosis or thrombus formation (coronary occlusion). Information on cardiac disorders is provided in Chapter 44.

Manifestations of a heart attack

Manifestations, which vary, include:

• pain or discomfort in the centre of the chest. The pain may radiate to either arm, the neck or the jaw
• anxiety or apprehension
• nausea and, sometimes, vomiting
• sweating
• shortness of breath
• irregular pulse (not always)
• collapse and cardiac arrest.

Emergency care

Emergency care when a heart attack is suspected involves:

• Seeking medical assistance urgently. A delay in obtaining expert assistance is potentially critical to the individual's survival
• Making the individual as comfortable as possible while awaiting medical assistance, or while transporting him to hospital
• Placing him in the coma position if he loses consciousness
• Providing emotional support
• Commencing CPR immediately if cardiac arrest occurs.

Exposure to extremes of temperature

Injuries from extremes of temperature include burns, scalds, heat exhaustion, heat stroke, frostbite, and hypothermia.

Burns and scalds

A burn is damage to the tissues caused by excess heat, friction, chemical agents, electricity, or radiation. A scald is a burn caused by moist heat. Information on burns, e.g. classification and manifestations, is provided in Chapter 41.

Emergency care of burns is directed towards removing the casualty from the source of heat, cooling the burned area, and preventing infection and shock:

• Remove the casualty from danger
• Put out burning clothing by smothering it with a blanket, rug, an item of clothing, or by using water
• Hold the burned area under cold, gently running water

for at least 10 minutes. For chemical burns, continue to flush the areas with water for 20 minutes
• Remove any jewellery, e.g. rings or bracelets, from the burned part before swelling occurs
• Cut away clothing over the burned area, but leave any clothing that is adhered to the skin **In the event of scalding or chemical burns**, remove clothing immediately—as it may retain heat or chemicals.
• Cover the burned area with a sterile or clean non-adherent dressing
• Seek medical assistance urgently
• Provide emotional support.

Heat exhaustion and heat stroke

Heat exhaustion is due to an imbalance between heat gain and heat loss. Heat stroke may occur if the body's heat regulating mechanism fails. Individuals who are most at risk of either condition are the elderly, infants, and those who are unsuitably clad when working or exercising in hot environmental temperatures. Manifestations include:

• exhaustion
• nausea
• thirst
• faintness
• shortness of breath
• muscle cramps
• lack of co-ordination
• irritability or confusion
• flushed and dry skin.

Emergency care involves:

• moving the casualty to a cool place where there is circulating air
• removing unnecessary clothing
• sponging his body with cool water
• providing cool oral fluids
• seeking medical assistance
• providing emotional support.

Frostbite

Frostbite results from local freezing of body tissues, generally in the extremities. Severe frostbite may impair the blood supply to the limbs so badly that gangrene develops. Manifestations include:

• numbness and tingling
• insensitivity to touch
• areas may appear waxy, white, mottled blue-white
• firmness and coldness of the areas
• possible blistering.

Emergency care involves:

• moving the casualty to a warm dry place

• removing constricting garments or jewellery from the affected areas
• rewarming the areas by applying body heat
• covering blisters with a clean dry dressing
• seeking medical assistance.

N.B. Do not rub or massage the affected areas, or use artificial heat to rewarm them.

Hypothermia

Hypothermia is a condition which is caused by a loss of surface heat, followed by cooling of the deep tissues and organs. Causes include prolonged immersion in cold water, and prolonged exposure to cold environmental temperatures. Manifestations include:

• cool skin
• slow pulse
• slow and shallow breathing
• apathy or confusion
• unconsciousness.

Emergency care involves:

• moving the casualty to a warm dry place
• placing the casualty between blankets so that his body temperature can rise gradually
• giving warm sweet drinks, if he is conscious
• seeking medical assistance urgently
• placing him in the coma position if he is unconscious.

N.B. Do not speed up the warming process by applying artificial heat, e.g. electric blanket, hot water bag, or by immersion in warm water.

Injuries to bones and joints

Information on injuries to the bones or joints, including causes, types, and manifestations, is provided in Chapter 42.

Emergency care

The aim of first aid management of fractures or joint injuries is to prevent movement at the site of injury so as to prevent further damage, to minimize pain, and to prevent shock:

• Sit or lie the casualty down, and support the injured part in a position of comfort. Support the injured part in a slightly elevated position, if possible, to reduce swelling
• Immobilize the area with well padded splints, bandages, or a sling. A leg may be used as a splint for the other leg, or the torso may form a splint for an arm. Handle the injured part gently and do not use force to position it, as this could cause further injury and pain

- Cover any wounds with a sterile or clean dressing and control bleeding
- Seek medical assistance
- Provide emotional support.

If spinal or neck injuries are suspected the individual must not be moved, as movement could result in damage to the spinal cord. Spinal or neck injuries should be suspected if the casualty experiences back pain, altered sensation, loss of movement or feeling below the injury, manifestations of shock, breathing difficulties, or loss of bladder and bowel control. Emergency care involves:

- leaving the casualty where he is until expert assistance arrives
- checking that his airway is clear, and observing him for signs of respiratory failure
- placing a blanket or coat over him
- instructing him not to attempt to move
- providing emotional support
- seeking medical assistance urgently.

When he is moved, there should be at least 4 people involved. One person supports the head and neck, and the others support the torso and limbs, thus preventing any movement of the vertebrae.

Poisoning

Poisons are substances which damage cells and may destroy life when they are introduced into the body. Poisons may be solid, liquid, or gaseous and they may enter the body by:

- the mouth (swallowed)
- the lungs (inhaled)
- the skin (absorbed or injected).

Some poisons take effect immediately, while other cause delayed but rapidly progressing effects.

Manifestations of poisoning

Depending on the type of poison, and the route by which it entered the body, some or all of the following may be present:

- abdominal pain
- nausea or vomiting
- drowsiness or unconsciousness
- burning pains from the mouth to the stomach
- burns around and inside the mouth
- breathing difficulty and/or cyanosis
- headache
- blurred vision
- ringing in the ears
- odours on the breath

- contamination of the skin
- injection or bite marks.

Emergency care

Detailed information for the emergency management of specific poisons can be obtained by telephoning the nearest Poisons Information Centre (listed in the Telecom Directory) or by contacting the emergency department of the nearest hospital. General management depends on whether the casualty is conscious or not, and whether the substance was corrosive or not.

For an unconscious casualty the emergency care involves placing him in the coma position, maintaining a clear airway, and seeking medical assistance urgently. If breathing ceases commence EAR immediately, and if the pulse ceases CPR must be commenced immediately.

For a conscious casualty it is essential to determine whether the poison taken was a corrosive or petroleum based substance, or a non-corrosive substance. *A corrosive substance* is one that directly damages tissue by erosion, e.g. oven cleaner, toilet cleaner, strong disinfectants, bleach, battery acid. Petroleum based substances include petrol, kerosene, turpentine, and diesel oil.

Emergency care, where a corrosive or petroleum based substance is involved includes:

- seeking medical assistance urgently
- encouraging the casualty to drink copious quantities of water or milk, in small amounts at a time
- *not* inducing vomiting. Vomiting will increase the corrosive effect, and vomiting increases the risk of the substance being inhaled.
- providing emotional support.

Emergency care, where a non-corrosive substance is involved, and the casualty is *conscious*, includes:

- inducing vomiting. Vomiting may be induced either by stimulating the back of the casualty's throat with your finger, or by giving him Syrup of Ipecacuanha to drink—following the instructions on the bottle
- seeking medical assistance urgently
- providing emotional support
- providing the hospital, or ambulance personnel, with any poison container found in the vicinity of the casualty and any material vomited by the casualty.

Do not induce vomiting in cases of poisoning if the casualty:

- **is unconscious**
- **has swallowed a corrosive substance**
- **has swallowed a petroleum based substance**

Bites and stings

Australian snakes, spiders, and marine creatures are among

the most venomous in the world. Some of the most poisonous creatures are the:

- brown snake
- tiger snake
- taipan
- red back spider
- funnel web spider
- blue-ringed octopus
- cone shell
- stonefish
- sting ray
- box jellyfish.

Snake and spider bites

Manifestations of snake or spider bites include:

- headaches
- blurred or double vision
- puncture marks on the skin
- swelling and inflammation of the bitten area
- nausea
- faintness or giddiness
- sweating
- chest and/or abdominal pain
- breathing difficulty
- muscle weakness or spasm.

Emergency care involves:

- Keeping the casualty at rest
- Applying a pressure-immobilization bandage over the bitten area and around the limb. The bandage should be applied firmly, and it should cover as much of the limb as possible. **N.B.** A pressure-immobilization/bandage is **not** applied in the management of red back spider bite. Instead, a cold pack or compress is placed over the bitten area.
- Splinting the bitten limb. The splint should immobilize the entire limb, and be held in position with bandages
- Assessing the individual's breathing and pulse. Perform EAR or CPR if breathing or circulation ceases
- Seeking medical assistance urgently
- Providing emotional support.

Marine creatures

Manifestations of stings from marine creatures include:

- numbness of the lips and tongue
- breathing difficulties -progressing to respiratory arrest
- intense pain at the site and along the limb
- swelling at the site
- visual evidence of stinging, e.g. whip marks, or discolouration of the stung area.

Emergency care depends on the *cause* of the sting.

- Management of blue ringed octopus stings and cone fish bites is the same as for snake bite.
- Management of stonefish and sting ray stings involves removing any foreign body, bathing the area with warm water, and seeking medical assistance.
- Management of jellyfish stings involves flooding the stung area with vinegar before applying a firm compression bandage over the area.

In all instances the individual's breathing and pulse must be assessed, and EAR or CPR commenced if necessary.

Eye injuries

Eye injuries may be caused by foreign objects lodging in the eye, penetrating objects, direct blows, chemicals, smoke, or heat.

Manifestations of eye injuries

Depending on the cause of the injury, manifestations include:

- discomfort or pain in the eye
- excessive production of tears
- inflammation of the eye
- sensitivity to light
- spasm of the eyelids
- swelling of the eyelids.

Emergency care

Small foreign bodies may be washed out of the eye by the flow of tears, or they may need to be removed. **N.B.** Do **not** attempt to remove any foreign body that has lodged on the cornea or has become embedded in any part of the eye.

To remove a small foreign body, that is not lodged on the cornea or is embedded, use a wisp of cotton wool or the corner of a clean soft cloth moistened with cold water. If the object is on the lower surface of the eye, ask the individual to look up then draw the lower lid downwards and outwards. If the object is on the upper surface of the eye, ask the individual to look down and gently pull the upper lid down over the lower lid. If this fails to dislodge the foreign body, everting the upper lid over a matchstick may make removal of the object possible. Seek medical assistance if the object is not easily removed, as repeated attempts to remove it may cause further damage and pain.

Emergency care of a penetrating wound, or sharp blow to the eye, involves lying the casualty flat on his back. Apply thick pads over *both* eyes and loosely secure them with a bandage avoiding any pressure over the eye. Instruct the casualty not to move his eyes, and to remain still. Seek medical assistance urgently.

Emergency care of burns to the eye involves irrigating the eye freely and continuously with cold flowing water for approximately 20 minutes. Place an eye pad or clean dressing over both eyes, and bandage loosely. Seek medical assistance urgently.

In all instances where the eye has been injured the individual should be told not to rub the eye, as this may cause further damage.

CONCLUSION

First aid is the emergency care of a sick or injured person until medical assistance is available, or until the person recovers.

Emergency situations may be encountered in a health care facility, in the home environment, or in a public place.

This chapter has addressed some of the emergencies and the basic care that needs to be provided. For more detailed information, the nurse is advised to consult a current first aid text.

REFERENCES AND FURTHER READING

Australian first aid: the authorised manual of the St John Ambulance Association in Australia, 1983, Melbourne
Cosgriff J H, Anderson D L 1984 The practice of emergency care, 2nd edn. J B Lippincott, Philadelphia

58. The individual who requires medication

OBJECTIVES

1. Discuss the nurse's legal and professional responsibilities in drug administration.
2. State the mechanisms by which drugs are transported and metabolized in the body, and state how drugs are excreted.
3. Demonstrate understanding of the system of weights and measures used in drug prescriptions, and ability to perform calculation of dosages.
4. Assist in planning and implementing care of an individual who is receiving medication, and in monitoring the effects of medications.
5. In accordance with prescribed role and function, perform the nursing activities described in this chapter safely and accurately:
   - administration of oral medications
   - administration of injections
   - instillation of ear, eye, vaginal, and rectal medications
   - administration of medications by inhalation
   - application of transdermal medications
   - application of topical preparations.

INTRODUCTION

As she may be required to assist the registered nurse in administration of medications, and in monitoring their effects, it is essential that the enrolled nurse has sufficient knowledge to promote the safety of individuals who are receiving medications. Nurses must always work within the nursing standards established by the nurse's registering bodies, therefore they must be aware of their legal and professional responsibilities regarding drug administration. As she is responsible for her clinical actions, the enrolled nurse must be fully aware of her prescribed role and function and she must not participate in the administration of medications if this function is not part of her role. The registered and the enrolled nurse must have knowledge of pharmacology and physiology, the legal aspects of drug storage and administration, routes and techniques of drug administration, and how to monitor the effects of medications.

Pharmacology

A *drug*, or medicine, is any substance which may be administered in a variety of forms and by different routes for the purpose of preventing, diagnosing, or treating a disease or condition. *Medication*, which is another term for drug, is generally used to denote a drug which is administered with therapeutic intent. Drugs have various names:

- The chemical name provides an exact description of the drug's chemical composition.
- The generic name is given by the manufacturer who first develops the drug.
- The trade, or proprietary, name is the name under which a manufacturer markets a drug.

Pharmacology is the study of the preparation, properties, uses, and actions of drugs. Basic pharmacology includes the methods by which substances are transported in the blood, cell transport and activity, mechanisms of drug absorption, the metabolic action of the liver, and the excretory function of the kidneys.

Transportation in the body

After entering the bloodstream a drug is diluted and transported throughout the body, Movement of a drug from the blood to the tissues is influenced by several factors:

- Plasma proteins can bind many drugs, so that only the unbound portion of the drug is able to move from the blood to the tissues.
- If plasma proteins are deficient, e.g. in malnutrition or liver disease, a greater proportion of the drug is able to enter the tissues.

• If two or more drugs are administered concurrently, the drug with higher affinity will be bound and displace the other/s from the protein-binding site.

• Cardiac output and circulation affect the role and extent of distribution of a drug. Efficient cardiac output and blood circulation improve drug distribution.

• Increased vascularity and permeability, e.g. if the tissues are inflamed, leads to an increased rate of passage of drugs to the tissues.

• A drug must cross a lipid (fat layer) to diffuse into tissues and exert its action. Drugs which are highly fat-soluble pass across the fat layer and are taken up rapidly by the tissues.

• Transfer barriers, e.g. the blood-brain barrier of the central nervous system, and the placenta, are selective.

Some drug substances pass readily through these barriers, while others are not transferred.

Drug action

Drugs act by affecting, or controlling, changes in biochemical or physiological processes in the body. Drugs produce their actions in one of three ways: altering body fluids, altering cell membranes, or interacting with receptor sites.

Most drugs act at specific cell receptors. A *selective* drug acts at a receptor in a particular type of body tissue, and produces little effect on similar receptors in other organs. For example, a bronchodilator (salbutamol) has specific selectivity for receptors in bronchial smooth muscle, but produces little or no stimulation of similar receptors in cardiac muscle.

A *specific* drug forms a complex with only one type of receptor, but may produce multiple effects due to the location of those receptors in cells of different tissues or organs. For example, an anticholinergic drug (atropine sulphate) not only reduces the production of saliva, bronchial, nasal, and gastric secretions—but it also increases heart rate, stimulates ventilation, and raises intraocular pressure.

A drug may produce more than one effect:

• Desired action is the physiological response the drug is expected to cause.

• Side effects are secondary effects caused by most drugs. For example, a side effect of Acetylsalicylic acid (aspirin) is increased bleeding time.

• Toxic effects develop after prolonged administration of high doses of medication, or when a drug accumulates in the blood because of impaired metabolism or excretion.

• Allergic reactions are unpredictable responses to a drug which acts as an antigen, triggering the release of the body's antibodies. Allergic reactions may be mild and be accompanied by urticaria and pruritus, or they may be severe and be accompanied by severe wheezing and respiratory distress.

• Idiosyncratic reactions are those where the individual either over-reacts or under-reacts to a drug, or when he has a reaction which is different from normal.

• Drug interactions occur when one drug modifies the action of another drug, e.g. a drug may either increase or decrease the action of other drugs. A drug may be *synergistic*, whereby it enhances the effects of another drug, or it may be *antagonistic*—whereby it opposes the effects of another drug.

The extent of response to a drug depends on its concentration at the site of action—which depends on dosage, absorption, metabolism, and elimination. More than any other factor, the route of administration determines the onset of drug effect. Drugs which are administered directly into the bloodstream provoke a rapid response, whereas drugs which are administered orally or topically must be absorbed into the bloodstream before they can take effect.

Metabolism of drugs

After a drug arrives at its site of action, it must be metabolized into an inactive form that is more easily excreted. Transformation of the drug, into an inactive form, occurs under the influence of enzymes. The main site of drug metabolism is the liver; although the lungs, kidneys, blood, and intestines also metabolize drugs. The specialized structure of the liver oxidizes and transforms many toxic substances and harmful chemicals before they are distributed to the tissues.

The rate of drug metabolism is influenced by a variety of factors. Liver disease can result in a potentially harmful buildup of drugs within the body. The ability to metabolize drugs is reduced in very young and elderly individuals.

Drug excretion

Once a drug is metabolized, it exits the body through the kidneys, liver, bowel, lungs, and exocrine glands. The chemical composition of a drug determines the organ of excretion.

The kidneys are the main organs for drug excretion, and if an individual's renal function is impaired he is at risk of drug toxicity. Some drugs exit unchanged in the urine, while others must undergo transformation in the liver before being excreted by the kidneys.

Gaseous compounds such as general anaesthetic agents are eliminated from the lungs. Many drugs enter the hepatic circulation to be broken down by the liver and excreted into the bile. Lipid-soluble drugs are excreted by the exocrine glands.

The rate at which drugs are excreted depends on several factors, such as the type of drug and the degree of renal function. The rate of drug excretion varies from 1-2 hours to several days or weeks. Drugs which depend on renal function for excretion are eliminated more slowly in very young and elderly individuals.

Drug sources

Drugs are chemical substances which are extracted from vegetable, animal, or mineral sources; or which are prepared synthetically. Drugs of vegetable origin are the oldest and, from the earliest times, roots, leaves, seeds, and the bark of trees were used for medicinal purposes. Some drugs of vegetable origin which are in common use now are atropine, digoxin, and some antibiotics. Drugs derived from animal sources, which are less numerous, include insulin and oestrogens.

Drugs derived from mineral sources are used extensively and include sodium bicarbonate, ferrous sulphate, potassium chloride, and calcium gluconate. Synthetic drugs are made in a laboratory. Many new drugs are developed each year, following research and testing for pharmacological activity and toxicity. Although the number of synthetic drugs already available is enormous, the search for new and more effective drugs continues.

Drug forms

A drug may be presented in a variety of forms including:

- *Capsule*: gelatine container enclosing a drug in liquid, powder, or granule form.
- *Tablet*: a drug mixed with a base and compressed into a variety of shapes. Tablets are sometimes coated, and the coating delays release of the drug until the tablet reaches the intestine. Tablets are coated if the drug could cause gastric irritation, or if the drug would be destroyed by gastric juice. Another form of tablet is called 'slow release', which contains a drug that is released over a prolonged period.
- *Granules*: small rounded pellets which are usually coated.
- *Lozenge*: small tablet containing a medicinal agent in a flavoured fruit or mucilage base, that dissolves in the mouth to release the drug.
- *Mixture*: aqueous vehicle in which drugs are dissolved or suspended.
- *Suspension*: liquid in which insoluble particles of a drug are dispersed.
- *Elixir*: sweetened, flavoured alcoholic solution containing a drug.
- *Linctus*: sweetened syrup containing a drug.
- *Tincture*: alcoholic solution containing a drug.
- *Emulsion*: mixture of oil and water containing a drug.
- *Syrup*: concentrated sugar solution containing a drug.
- *Cachet*: envelope of rice paper which encloses a drug.
- *Injection*: sterile aqueous or oily solutions and suspensions containing a drug, that are administered parenterally.
- *Suppository*: solid preparation, containing a drug, which melts when inserted into the rectum.
- *Pessary*: solid preparation, containing a drug, which is administered vaginally.
- *Drops*: aqueous or oily solution containing a drug. Drops may be instilled into the eye, ear, or nose.
- *Cream*: aqueous or oily emulsion for topical application.
- *Ointment*: semi-solid greasy preparation for topical application.
- *Paste*: similar to ointment but contains a high proportion of powders. Pastes have a very stiff consistency and will adhere to lesions at body temperature.
- *Liniment*: oily or alcoholic preparation for topical application.
- *Paint*: liquid preparation for application to the skin or mucous membranes.
- *Lotion*: aqueous, alcoholic, or emulsified vehicle for topical application.
- *Powder* (dusting): medicated substance for topical application.

Routes of administration

A drug may be required to exert a local or systemic effect, and it may be administered through the alimentary tract or parenterally. Drugs administered through the alimentary tract may be given either by the oral or rectal route. Drugs administered parenterally (routes other than the alimentary tract) may be given by:

- injection: intramuscular, subcutaneous, intravenous, intradermal, intra-arterial, intrathecal, intra-articular, intra-peritoneal, intracardiac
- inhalation: into the respiratory tract
- instillation: into the eye, ear, or nose
- insertion: into the vagina or rectum
- insufflation: of a powder into a cavity
- transdermal application: to produce either local or systemic effects.

Legal aspects of drug administration

The supply, storage, and use of drugs and preparations are under the control of governments. Certain legal requirements apply to the sale, supply, dispensing and labelling of drugs and poisonous substances. These substances are listed under certain schedules which determine restrictions on their use and management. While there is no national schedule, each state has its own. For example, the schedules in Victoria are:

1. Dangerous poisons (substances in this schedule are currently under review, and are being listed in other schedules)
2. Medical poisons
3. Potent substances

4. Restricted substances
5. Hazardous substances
6. Industrial and Agricultural poisons
7. Part 1—dangerous poisons
   Part 2—special poisons
8. Drugs of addiction

The nurse must be aware of the laws governing the custody and use of drugs, follow the directives of the nurses registering body on the administration of drugs, and she must also observe the health care facility's policies designed to promote safe storage, handling, and usage of drugs. There are a number of general principles.

• All medications must be kept in a locked cupboard or medication trolley, the key of which is kept by a registered nurse at all times. Some preparations, e.g. suppositories, vaccines, insulins, require refrigeration. For storage of these drugs, a lockable refrigerator is required.

• Drugs of addiction (Schedule 8(Victoria)) are kept in a separate locked cupboard which is firmly fixed to a wall. It is customary for this cupboard to be within another locked cupboard. The key is kept by a registered nurse at all times.

• Drugs or preparations for external use are stored apart from those intended for internal use.

• A register must be maintained of all drugs of addiction and the records must contain full details of all receipt of drugs and all disposal of drugs, whether by administration to a patient, return to the pharmacy department, or by any other means.

• Drugs of addiction and restricted substances can be supplied only on a written order by a medical practrican.

• A qualified pharmacist has complete responsibility for all containers issued from the pharmacy department. No-one else is permitted to label a container, alter the wording on a label, or transfer the contents of one container to another.

• There should be a *written* order for all drugs administered to patients. Verbal orders are open to misinterpretation. A written prescription must contain the date of prescribing, the patient's full name, the name and dosage of the drug, the route of administration, the frequency of administration, and the signature of the medical officer who is writing the prescription. If the nurse has any doubt about the meaning of an order, she must contact the medical officer immediately for clarification—before the drug is administered.

• A registered nurse must check every dose of medication to be administered by a student nurse. Nursing regulations dictate that a registered nurse must accompany certain levels of student nurse, during administration of a drug.

• A nurse should administer only a medication that she has prepared personally, i.e.she should not administer any medication that has been prepared by someone else.

• The nurse who administers a drug to be taken orally must remain with the patient until the drug has been swallowed.

• Checking a drug before it is administered is essential, and is performed to ensure that the **right person** is given the **right** amount of the **right** drug by the **right** route at the **right** time. Checking a drug involves:

1. Reading the written order and noting the name of the patient; the name, dose, and route of administration of the drug, and the frequency of administration.
2. Checking, on the patient's drug sheet, the time that the last dose was given.
3. Checking the label on the drug container, noting the name and strength of the drug.
4. Checking the name on the patient's identity band, and comparing it with the name on the written order. The patient should also be asked to state his name.

If the nurse is checking a drug which is to be administered by another nurse, in addition to the safety measures already stated the checker must observe the dose being measured and witness the drug being administered.

• Health care facilities implement a protocol which conforms to the relevant state regulations whereby certain drugs (usually poisons and addictive drugs) are checked at regular intervals, e.g. every eight hours. Two nurses, one of whom should be registered, count the drugs together and document their findings. The number of drugs in the containers is compared with the number of drugs that should be there—according to the record form. Both nurses sign the form, or register, to indicate that the count is correct.

After administering any drug, the nurse records it immediately on the appropriate medication record form. Prompt recording prevents errors. Details recorded on the individual's medication sheet include the name of the drug, dosage, route, and exact time of administration. The nurse who administers the drug must sign the record sheet.

Drugs of addiction are also recorded in the drug register. The nurse who administers the drug, and the nurse who checks the drug, both sign their names in the register.

Drug groups

All drugs can be classified into groups, and the classification may be based on their origin, their pharmacological action, or their chemical structure. Table 58.1 illustrates various groups of drugs and their major actions.

Systems of delivery

Various methods are used to supply prescribed drugs to wards and units within a health care facility.

Individual patient dispensing. All prescribed drugs are dispensed in individual containers, labelled with the

Table 58.1 Common drug groups

Drug group	Major actions
Analgesics (non-narcotic and narcotic)	Alter perception of pain. Narcotic analgesics induce euphoria and drowsiness, depress respiratory and cough reflexes, increase smooth muscle tone, reduce peristalsis, stimulate the vomiting centre, and constrict the pupils
Anabolic steroids	Increase retention of nitrogen, sodium, potassium, calcium, chloride, phosphate, and water
Anaesthetics (local and general)	Local anaesthetics block nerve conduction, and produce analgesia. General anaesthetic agents are used to induce and maintain anaesthesia (unconsciousness, analgesia, and muscle relaxation)
Antacids	Neutralize gastric acidity and reduce pepsin activity
Anti-angina agents	Relax smooth muscle and reduce myocardial oxygen demand
Anti-arrhythmic agents	Prevent, alleviate, or correct cardiac arrhythmias
Antibacterial agents	Inhibit the growth of or destroy bacteria
Anticholinergics	Inhibit the transmission of parasympathetic nerve impulses. Reduce smooth muscle spasms; decrease secretion of sweat, saliva, nasal, bronchial, and gastrointestinal secretions
Anticoagulants	Prevent or delay coagulation of the blood
Anticonvulsants	Prevent or reduce the severity of epileptic or other convulsive seizures
Antidepressants (tricyclic, bicyclic, tetracyclic, monoamine oxidase inhibitor)	Prevent or relieve depression
Antidiarrhoeal agents	Reduce peristalsis and/or the amount of free water in the bowel
Anti-emetics and anti-nauseants	Prevent or alleviate nausea and vomiting
Anthelmintics	Kill or paralyse worms, or inhibit the development of eggs or larvae
Antihistamines	Reduce the physiological and pharmacological effects of histamine (a compound found in all cells)
Antihypertensive agents	Reduce high blood pressure
Anti-infective agents, e.g penicillins, cephalosporins, tetracyclines, sulphonamides, antifungal agents, antiviral agents	Destroy or interfere with the development of a living organism, e.g. bacteria
Anti-inflammatory agents	Counteract or reduce inflammation
Antineoplastic agents (cytotoxics)	Prevent the proliferation of malignant cells, by attacking them at various stages in the cell cycle
Antipruritic agents	Prevent or relieve itching
Antipsychotics (neuroleptics)	Counteract or reduce symptoms of a psychosis
Antipyretics	Lower an elevated body temperature
Antiseptics	Inhibit the growth and reproduction of microorganisms
Antisera (antitoxins, immunoglobulins, antivenoms)	Serum containing antibodies against a specific disease—administered to confer passive immunity to that disease
Antiulcerants	Assist healing of gastric and duodenal ulcers, e.g. by reducing gastric acid secretion

Table 58.1 (cont'd) Common drug groups

Drug group	Major actions
Anxiolytics (minor tranquillizers)	Sedative effect, promoting mental and skeletal muscle relaxation
Aperients	Mild laxatives that promote evacuation of the bowel
Barbiturates (sedatives, hypnotics)	Depress the central nervous system
Beta-blockers (beta-adrenergic agents)	Block the beta-adrenoceptors of the sympathetic nervous system resulting in reduced cardiac rate and output, reduced blood pressure, and bronchoconstriction
Bronchodilators	Relax the smooth muscles of bronchioles to relieve bronchospasm thereby improving ventilation
Contraceptives (oestrogens and progestogens)	Prevent conception and implantation
Corticosteroids (glucocorticoids, mineralocorticoids, adrenogenital corticoids)	Hormones, naturally associated with the suprarenal cortex, which influence or control key processes in the body, e.g. carbohydrate and protein metabolism, electrolyte and water balance, functions of the cardiovascular system, skeletal muscle, kidneys
Cough suppressants	Depress the cough centre in the medulla oblongata
Cytotoxics (antineoplastic agents)	Prevent the proliferation of malignant cells
Decongestants	Elimate or reduce congestion or swelling, e.g. of the respiratory tract
Diuretics	Promote the formation and secretion of urine
Emetics	Induce vomiting
Expectorants	Promote the expulsion of mucus and other exudates from the lungs, bronchi, and trachea
Fibrinolytic agents	Activate the endogenous fibrinolytic system to dissolve intravascular blood clots.
Haematinics	Raise haemoglobin level and red blood cell count
Hypnotics	Depress the central nervous system, and tend to induce sleep
Insulins; Insulin preparations may be: • short acting, e.g. regular, neutral, insulin zinc suspension • intermediate acting, e.g. biphasic, insulin zinc suspension, isophane • long acting, e.g. insulin zinc suspension, protamine zinc	Hormone, naturally secreted by the islets of Langerhans, which regulates the metabolism of glucose and the processes necessary for the intermediary metabolism of fats, carbohydrates, and proteins
Laxatives	Promote peristalsis and evacuation of the bowel by increasing the bulk of the faeces, by softening the stool, or by lubricating the intestinal wall
Mucolytics	Reduces the viscosity of mucus thus promoting removal of mucus secretions
Muscle relaxants	Reduce the contractility of muscle fibres
Mydriatics	Dilate the pupil by stimulating the dilator muscles of the iris
Narcotic analgesics	Alter perception of pain, induce euphoria, depress respiratory and cough reflexes
Narcotic antagonists	Reverse the toxic effects of narcotic analgesics
Neuroleptics (major tranquillizers and antipsychotics)	Induce altered state of consciousness characterized by reduced motor activity and reduced anxiety

Table 58.1 (cont'd) Common drug groups

Drug group	Major actions
Sedatives	Decrease functional activity, diminish irritability, and allay excitement
Sunscreen agents	Reduce sensitivity to ultraviolet light
Vaccines	Induce specific active artificial immunity to a specific infectious disease
Vasoconstrictors	Cause the constriction of blood vessels
Vasodilators	Cause the dilatation of blood vessels
Vitamins	Essential for normal physiologic and metabolic functioning of the body

patient's name, for administration only to that specific patient. The pharmacist dispenses the drugs, usually a five day supply, according to each patient's prescription. The dispensed drugs is stored in separate compartments, one for each patient, within a specially designed medicine trolley.

A limited range of common drugs is supplied by the pharmacy to the ward, to cover those periods when the pharmaceutical service is not available.

Unit dose presentation. In this system, all drugs are dispensed in unit packs which are designed to be opened just prior to administration. The pharmacist is responsible for ensuring that a sufficient number of doses of the correct drugs are available for each individual patient. Under this system the pharmacist dispenses a one day supply of labeled, unit-dose packages containing the prescribed drug in the dose ordered, ready for administration to the patient. This method requires that each patient's drugs are stored in a separate compartment within a medicine trolley.

With both these methods, the pharmacist visits the ward on a regular basis to obtain detailed information on the current range of prescribed drugs. He is able to monitor prescriptions, dispense the drugs, and advise patients and staff on many important aspects of the use of drugs. The pharmacist assumes responsibility for ensuring that the drugs prescribed for each patient are available in the medicine trolley.

A self-medication programme may be implemented in certain circumstances, e.g. a few days prior to an individual's discharge from a health care facility. Specially designed containers are available, e.g. a plastic box with a transparent cover, whereby the pharmacist places the prescribed drugs into various compartments within the container. In the container each day of the week is allocated four compartments—according to the time at which the drugs are to be taken. This method of supplying prescribed drugs assists the individual when he is at home to take the correct drugs at the correct time. Some styles of container are also equipped with Braille, thus enabling people with visual defects to take their drugs correctly.

When the container needs to be refilled, i.e. each week, the pharmacist or visiting nurse refers to the card which is supplied with the container. The card provides details about the drugs which have been prescribed, e.g. their name and dosage.

In a health care facility, self-medication is not commonly practised, except for those medications that patients take in emergencies, e.g. nitroglycerine taken to relieve angina pain.

Weights and measures

To promote accurate and safe administration of drugs, the nurse must understand the system of weights and measures used in prescriptions.

SI units

The international system of units (S1 units) for mass and volume are:

Mass:	1 kilogram (kg)	= 1000 grams
	1 gram (g)	= 1000 milligrams
	1 milligram (mg)	= 1000 micrograms
	1 microgram (μg)	= 1000 nanograms
Volume:	1 litre (l)	= 1000 millilitres
	1 millilitre (ml)	= 1000 microlitres

The mole and millimole (mmol)

The strength of a pharmaceutical preparation used in electrolyte replacement therapy is normally expressed in *millimoles* per tablet, or millimoles per given volume of solution.

A millimole is one thousandth of a mole, which is the molecular weight of a substance expressed in grams.

Millimoles are also used to express the concentration of substances other than electrolytes, and are used widely in laboratories, e.g. on haematology reports.

Percentages

The strength of a pharmaceutical substance may be expressed as a percentage (parts per 100 parts):

- Percentage weight in volume (% w/v). For example, 10% w/v indicates that 10 g of the active ingredient is present in 100 ml of product.
- Percentage weight in weight (% w/w). For example, 10% w/w indicates that 10 g of the active ingredient is present in 100 g of product.
- Percentage volume in volume (v/v). For example, 10% v/v indicates that 10 ml of the active ingredient is present in 100 ml of product.
- Percentage volume in weight (% v/w). For example, 10% v/w indicates that 10 ml of the active ingredient is contained in 100 g of product.

Expressing the strength of active ingredients in pharmaceutical products

Solid dose forms. In most instances, the strength of the active ingredient present in each solid form, e.g. tablet, is expressed in grams, milligrams, or micrograms.

Strengths of some solid dosage forms are expressed in units of activity. For example, a Vitamin capsule may contain 100 i.u. (international units).

Products used for electrolyte replacement are expressed in grams or milligrams, and also in millimoles. For example, a potassium chloride tablet contains 600 mg of potassium chloride or 8 mmol of K^+ and Cl^-.

Liquid oral dose forms. The amount of an active ingredient in liquid oral preparations is expressed as weight per volume (w/v). For example a liquid preparation may contain 250 mg (of the active ingredient) in 5 ml.

Liquid parenteral dose forms. Small volume injections generally bear a label expressing the strength of the product in weight per volume. Care must be taken to note the total volume contained in the ampoule. For example, the label may indicate 25 mg per 1 ml but the ampoule may contain 2 ml — therefore the amount of active ingredient in the ampoule is 50 mg.

The strength of some small volume injections may also be expressed as percentage weight per volume (% w/v).

The strength of some other injections, e.g. adrenaline, is frequently expressed as 1 in 1000. This indicates that 1 gram of active ingredient is contained in 100 ml of product — thus 1 ml of the solution contains 1 mg of adrenaline.

The strength of certain substances, e.g. insulin, is expressed in units of activity per given volume. For example 100 units per 1 ml.

Large volume parenteral products contain labels indicating the strength of the product in percentage terms. For example, a solution of sodium chloride for intravenous infusion may contain 0.9% w/v.

Calculation of dosages

Although the introduction of unit doses and prepared solutions has meant that the need for nurses to undertake calculations has decreased, there are certain situations where the nurse does need to perform basic calculations in connection with administration of drugs and other pharmaceutical products.

If drugs and other products are to be used safely and effectively, the nurse must first have a thorough understanding of the SI (Systeme International) units of mass and volume.

The calculation of dosages must be performed with total accurary, therefore the nurse must be competent in dealing with decimals, fractions, percentages, ratio, and proportion.

There are several methods of performing calculations. The nurse should refer to the health care facility's policy manual to determine which one should be used.

Formulae for calculation of drug doses include:

1. Liquid drugs

$$Amount\ of\ stock = \frac{strength\ required}{stock\ strength} \times volume\ containing\ stock\ strength$$

Example: A medical officer prescribes intramuscular morphine 10 mg. The medication in stock is available only in ampoules containing 15 mg per millilitre.

$$\frac{strength\ required\ (10\ mg)}{stock\ strength\ (15\ mg)} \times Volume\ containing\ stock\ strength\ (1\ ml)$$

$$\frac{10}{15} \times 1 = \frac{2}{3} \times 1 = \tfrac{2}{3}\ ml\ to\ be\ administered$$

2. Solid drugs

$$Amount\ of\ stock = \frac{strength\ required}{stock\ strength} \times volume\ containing\ stock\ strength$$

Example: A medical officer prescribes oral phenobarbitone 45 mg. The medication in stock is available only in tablets containing 30 mg.

$$\frac{strength\ required\ (45\ mg)}{stock\ strength\ (30\ mg)} \times volume\ containing\ stock\ strength\ (1\ tablet)$$

$$\frac{45}{30} \times 1 = 1\tfrac{1}{2}\ tablets\ to\ be\ administered$$

3. Drugs measured in units

$$Amount\ of\ stock = \frac{number\ of\ units\ required}{number\ of\ units\ in\ stock\ solution} \times volume\ containing\ stock\ strength$$

Example: A medical officer prescribes subcutaneous insulin 10 units. The insulin is available in 100 units per ml.

$$\frac{Number\ of\ units\ required\ (10)}{Number\ of\ units\ in\ stock\ solution\ (100)} \times \frac{Volume\ containing\ stock}{strength\ (1\ ml)}$$

$$\frac{10}{100} \times 1 = \frac{1}{10} \times 1 = \frac{1}{10}\ ml\ to\ be\ administered$$

4. Calculation of paediatric dosages
(a) Clarke's Body Weight Rule

$$Child's\ dose = adult\ dose \times \frac{Weight\ of\ child\ (kg)}{average\ adult\ weight\ (70\ kg)}$$

(b) Clarke's Body Surface Area Rule

$$Child's\ dose = adult\ dose \times \frac{surface\ area\ of\ child}{surface\ area\ of\ adult\ (1.7\ m^2)}$$

5. Preparation of solutions

$$Amount\ of\ stock = \frac{strength\ required}{stock\ strength} \times final\ total\ volume$$

Abbreviations

When writing prescriptions, the medical officer frequently uses abbreviations, which are derived from Latin. Many medical officers have given up using these abbreviations because they can be easily misinterpreted, and it is safer to use the English terms.

Table 58.2 illustrates some of the abbreviations which may be written on prescriptions.

Table 58.2 Abbreviations used in prescriptions

Abbreviation	Latin term	English meaning
aa	ana	of each (equal parts)
a.c.	ante cibum	before meals
aq.	aqua	water
aq. dest.	aqua distillata	distilled water
b.d. or b.i.d.	bis die or bis in die	twice a day
c	cum	with
Co.	compositus	compound
dil.	dilutus	diluted
gtt. or gutta	guttae	drops
mist.	mistura	mixture
nocte	nocte	at night
ol.	oleum	oil
o.m.	omni mane	every morning
o.n.	omni nocte	every night
p.c.	post cibum	after meals
p.r.n.	pro re nata	as required
pulv.	pulvis	powder
q.q.h.	quaque quarta hora	every four hours
q.i.d.	quator in die	four times a day
s.o.s.	si opus sit	if necessary (once only)
stat.	statim	immediately
t.d.s.	ter die sumendum	three times a day
t.i.d.	ter in die	three times a day
ung.	unguentum	ointment

ROLE OF THE NURSE IN ADMINISTRATION OF DRUGS

The nurse's role in drug administration is a complex one requiring knowledge and skill. In order to promote safe and correct drug administration, the nurse requires *knowledge* about the drugs she administers including:

- indications for use
- routes of administration
- range of dosages
- desired effects
- safe handling of hazardous substances
- storage
- legislation, and health care facility policies
- side or toxic effects
- drug interactions.

The nurse also requires certain *skills* to:

- administer drugs by various routes
- calculate in S1 units of mass and volume
- evaluate the effects of drugs
- educate individuals about drug therapy
- teach self administration
- record the drugs she administers and the individual's response to them.

Administration of drugs

To ensure that medications are administered correctly and safely, the nurse must observe the five rights of drug administration:

- the right patient
- the right medication
- the right dose
- the right route
- the right time.

Before any medication is administered the drug order sheet must be checked thoroughly and systematically to determine the name of the medication, the route, the dosage, and the time of administration which have been prescribed. The nurse compares the label of the drug container with the drug order sheet three times:

- before removing the container from the trolley or cupboard
- before removing the drug from the container
- before returning the container to the trolley or cupboard.

To identify an individual correctly, before a drug is administered, the nurse:

- checks the drug order form against his identity bracelet

- asks the individual to state his name
- addresses the individual by name.

Most *medication errors* occur when a nurse fails to follow the safety guidelines, or when she is distracted during preparation or administration of medications. To prevent drug administration errors the nurse should:

- read drug labels carefully
- be aware that many drugs have similar names
- check the expiry date on the drug label
- check the decimal point on prescriptions and drug container labels
- not administer a drug if the prescription or drug label is illegible
- be proficient in calculating dosages
- use administration equipment, e.g. a medicine glass or syringe, with distinct markings
- not administer any drug that has been prepared by another person
- have the drug checked by a registered nurse during preparation and administration
- give her full attention to the task.

Information on the procedure to be followed if a medication error does occur, is provided later in the chapter.

Administration of oral medications

Oral medications may be presented in solid or liquid form. The nurse must know whether solid medications must be swallowed whole, chewed, sucked, or whether they may be crushed for administration. Powdered medications, and some drugs in granule form, are mixed with a liquid before administration.

Effervescent powders and tablets should be taken immediately after dissolving.

Some liquids, e.g. cough syrup, produce local effects on oral mucosa therefore the individual should not take fluids immediately after swallowing such syrups.

All liquid preparations should be shaken before they are poured.

Any mixture which stains the teeth should be taken through a straw, and the individual should rinse out his mouth after each dose.

In certain circumstances oral drugs may be administered through a nasogastric tube. Tablets except those which are enteric-coated can be crushed, and capsules may be opened to mix the medications in a solution for administration through the tube. Information on care of the individual with a nasogastric tube is provided in Chapter 29.

Some medications are administered by *buccal* and *sublingual* application. These routes are indicated for drugs that tend to be destroyed by gastric juice, or those that are rapidly detoxified by the liver. Buccal tablets are placed in the space between the upper molar teeth and gums. Sub-

lingual tablets are placed under the tongue. Both forms remain in place while they dissolve.

A suggested procedure for administering oral medications is outlined in the guidelines. Equipment required:

— drug order sheet and medication record
— medicine glass
— prescribed medication
— glass of water
— drinking straw or spoon if necessary.

Administration of drugs by injection

Drugs are given by injection for a variety of reasons including:

- The drug may be one which is not absorbed when given orally
- The drug may be one which is destroyed by digestive juices
- A fast onset of action may be required
- Very precise control over dosage may be needed
- The individual may be unable to take drugs orally.

Drugs by injection may be administered subcutaneously, intramuscularly, or intravenously. Intravenous injections are generally administered by a registered nurse or medical officer. The administration of an injection is an invasive procedure that must be performed using aseptic techniques, because once a needle pierces the skin there is the risk of infection. Infection is avoided by preventing contamination of the solution, preventing needle and syringe contamination, and by preparing the skin prior to injection. A variety of syringes and needles are available, the majority of which are single use and disposable.

Syringes (Fig. 58.1) are available in a number of sizes, varying in capacity from 1–50 ml. A syringe consists of a cylindrical barrel with a tip designed to fit the hub of a needle, and a close-fitting plunger. The barrel of the syringe is calibrated, e.g. into millilitres and tenths of a millilitre or, in the case of an insulin syringe, into units.

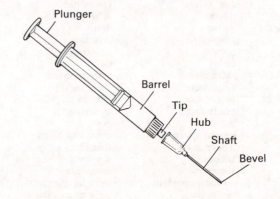

Fig. 58.1 The parts of a syringe and needle.

Guidelines for administering oral medications

Nursing action	Rationale
1. Check the drug order sheet for the individual's name, name of medication, dose, route and time of administration	Promotes correct and safe administration of the drug
2. Wash and dry hands	Prevents cross infection
3. Prepare the individual's medication by first reading the label on the container and checking it with the written drug order.	Prevents preparation errors
If the drug is in solid form:	
• calculate the correct dose	
• tip the required number of tablets or capsules into the medicine glass. Don't handle the medicines with your fingers.	Maintains cleanliness of drugs
If the drug is in liquid form:	
• calculate the correct dose	
• tip the bottle back and forth	Promotes mixing of the contents
• hold the bottle with the label against the palm of the hand	Mixture will be poured away from the label, to avoid smearing
• remove bottle cap and place it upside down	Prevents contamination of the inside of the cap
• hold the medicine glass at eye level and pour the prescribed dose (marking on the glass should be even with the fluid level at the base of the meniscus). Discard any excess	Ensures accuracy of measurement
• wipe lip of bottle with tissue or paper towel. Replace cap.	Prevents contamination of contents and prevents bottle cap from sticking
• add water to the medication if necessary (only if prescribed).	
4. Check the label of the container again	Reading the label again reduces risk of errors
5. Check the individual's identity band and ask him to state his name	Confirms the individual's identity
6. Explain the purpose of the medication and its action	Understanding improves compliance with drug therapy.
7. Assist the individual into a sitting or side-lying position when possible	Prevents aspiration during swallowing
8. Administer the medication. Offer the individual a glass of water—unless this is contraindicated	Most solid drugs are swallowed more easily with liquids
9. Remain with the individual until the medication is swallowed	The nurse assumes responsibility for ensuring that he receives the prescribed medication
10. Wash and dry hands	Prevents cross infection.
11. Record each drug administered on the medication record	Prompt documentation prevents errors
12. Report immediately if the individual refuses medication, or if he is unable to swallow a whole tablet or capsule	Appropriate care can be planned and implemented

Needles (Fig. 58.1) are available in various lengths and gauges, with different sizes of bevels. A needle has three parts: The hub which fits onto the tip of a syringe, the shaft, and the bevel or slanted tip. *Needle gauge* is determined by the lumen of the needle: as the diameter of the lumen increases, the gauge decreases. For example, a 16 gauge needle is substantially larger in diameter than a 22 gauge needle.

Selection of an appropriate syringe and needle depends mainly on the prescribed route, viscosity of the medication, amount of medication to be administered, and the individual's body size and amount of fat. Generally a 2–

3 ml syringe is adequate for subcutaneous, intramuscular, and most intravenous injections. Subcutaneous injections are generally given through a small diameter needle, e.g. 25 gauge; while intramuscular injections usually require a 21–23 gauge needle. Intravenous injections are generally administered through a 20 gauge needle.

Medications for injection are presented as liquids in glass ampoules or rubber-capped vials; or in powder form which requires reconstitution before administration. An ampoule is made of clear glass, with a constricted neck that must be snapped off to allow access to the medication. Ampoules contain volumes from 1 ml to 10 ml or more. A vial is a s ingle or multiple dose glass container with a rubber seal at the top, which is protected by a metal cap until it is ready for use. Vials contain medications in either liquid or powder form. Sterile distilled water and normal saline are commonly used to dissolve drugs in powder form—the vial label specifying the solvent to be used.

Table 58.3 illustrates preparation of medications from ampoules and vials.

Injection sites

Subcutaneous injection involves injecting medication into the loose connective tissue under the dermis. Only small volumes of medication, up to 2 ml, are administered by this route, and only medications which will not damage subcutaneous tissue are administered. Subcutaneous sites (Fig. 58.2) which are commonly used are:

- upper outer aspect (middle third) of the upper arm
- upper anterior thighs
- abdomen below the costal margins to the iliac crests.

Subcutaneous injections are administered with the needle inserted at an angle of 45° (Fig. 58.3)

Table 58.3 Preparation of medications from ampoules and vials

Ampoules	Vials
1. Tap the top of the ampoule lightly with a finger to dislodge any fluid above the neck of the ampoule	1. Remove the metal cap to expose the rubber seal
2. Place a gauze square around the neck of the ampoule to protect the fingers as the glass is broken	2. Wipe the surface of the seal with an alcohol swab, to remove any dust or grease
3. File the neck of the ampoule if necessary. Snap the neck in a direction away from the hands, to prevent shattering the glass towards the fingers or face	3. To prepare a *powdered* drug, assemble needle and syringe and draw up the amount of solvent recommended on the label of the vial in the same manner as injecting air into the vial. Refer to point 6. Gently shake or roll the vial between the hands to dissolve the powder
4. Assemble needle and syringe Remove needle cover	4. Before drawing up the solution, assemble needle and syringe, and remove needle cover. Draw back on the plunger to draw air into the syringe, equivalent to the volume of medication to be aspirated
5. Insert the needle (attached to the syringe) into the centre of the ampoule opening, being careful not to touch the needle on the rim of the ampoule—to prevent needle contamination	5. With bevel pointing up, insert the tip of the needle through the centre of the rubber seal
6. Aspirate the medication by pulling back on the syringe Keep the needle tip below the surface of the medication to prevent aspiration of air bubbles	6. Inject the air from the syringe into the vial. Hold the plunger, as it may be forced backward by air pressure within the vial
7. To expel air bubbles from the syringe, remove needle from the ampoule and hold syringe with the needle pointing up Draw back slightly on the plunger and then push the plunger up to eject the air Holding the syringe and needle upright, tap the syringe barrel to dislodge remaining air bubbles. It is important to expel air bubbles, as if air is injected it may gain entry to the bloodstream and block a blood vessel	7. Holding the syringe and plunger, invert the vial. Hold the vial in the non-dominant hand
8. Place a new needle on the syringe for administration of the medication	8. Allow air pressure to gradually fill the syringe with medication. Keep the tip of the needle below fluid level. Pull back slightly on the plunger if necessary
	9. Remove the needle from the vial by pulling back on the barrel of the syringe
	10. Tap the syringe barrel to remove any air bubbles.
	11. Place a new needle on the syringe for administration of the medication

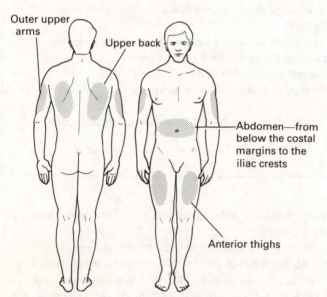

Outer upper arms

Upper back

Abdomen—from below the costal margins to the iliac crests

Anterior thighs

Fig. 58.2 Common sites for subcutaneous injections.

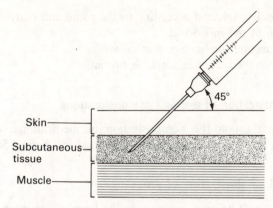

Fig. 58.3   Insertion of needles: subcutaneous injections.

Intramuscular injections involve injecting medication into deep muscle tissue. Muscle is less sensitive to irritating or viscous drugs, and up to 3 ml can be injected into muscle without causing severe discomfort. The sites chosen are areas where there is minimal risk of the needle penetrating a large blood vessel or nerve. Intramuscular sites (Fig. 58.4) which are commonly used are:

- middle third of the anterior lateral aspect of the thigh (vastus lateralis muscle)
- upper outer quadrant of the buttock (gluteal muscle) (Fig. 58.5)

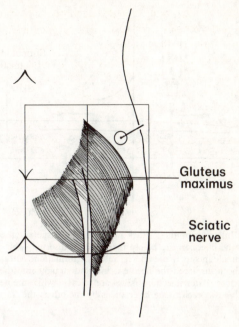

Fig. 58.5   Intramuscular injection site of the upper outer quadrant of the buttock showing the relationship to the sciatic nerve.

- upper outer aspect (middle third) of the upper arm (deltoid muscle).

Intramuscular injections are administered with the needle inserted at an angle of 90° (Fig. 58.6).

The Z-track method of injection (Fig. 58.7) is a technique used when irritating preparations such as iron-dextran complex are given intramuscularly. A new needle is attached to the syringe after preparing the drug

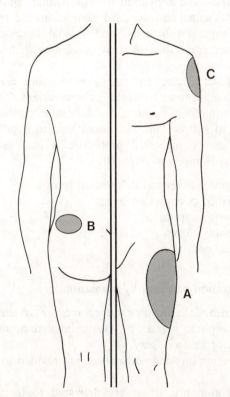

Fig. 58.4   Sites for intramuscular injections. (A) Vastus externus muscle. (B) Gluteal muscle. (C) Deltoid muscle.

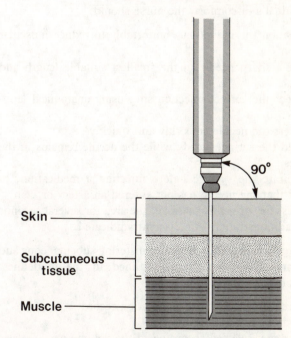

Fig. 58.6   Insertion of needles. Intramuscular injections.

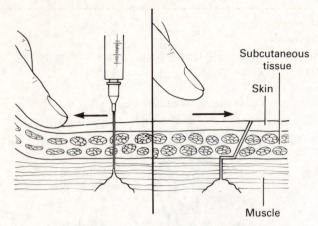

Fig. 58.7 Injection by the Z-track method. The tissue is tensed laterally at the injection site before the needle is inserted—this pulls the skin, subcutaneous tissue and fat into a Z formation. After this tissue has been displaced the needle is inserted straight into the muscular tissue. After injection tissues are released while the needle is withdrawn and as each tissue layer slides by the other, the tract is sealed.

so that no solution remains on the outside of the needle. The subcutaneous tissue is drawn to one side before inserting the needle, to promote absorption and prevent skin staining and pain. The Z-track method of injection deposits medication into the muscle without tracking residual medication through sensitive tissues.

Promoting safety and comfort

To ensure correct subcutaneous or intramuscular administration of an injectable medication and to minimize the individual's discomfort, the nurse should:

• position the individual comfortably to reduce muscular tension
• use a sharp needle in the smallest suitable length and gauge
• select the correct injection site, using anatomical landmarks
• insert the needle smoothly and quickly
• hold the syringe steady while the needle remains in the tissues
• aspirate the syringe before injecting a medication, to check that the needle has not entered an artery or vein
• press on, or gently massage, the area for several seconds after administration—unless contraindicated.

A suggested procedure for administering subcutaneous and intramuscular injections is outlined in the guidelines. Equipment required:

— drug order sheet and medication record
— kidney dish and cover
— syringe, selected according to the volume of medication to be administered

— needles, selected according to the route and body size of the individual
— antiseptic swabs, e.g. alcohol swabs
— prescribed drug in ampoule or vial.

Administration of eye and ear medications

Information on the administration of medications, e.g. drops, into the eyes and ears is provided in Chapter 50.

Rectal administration of drugs

A drug may be given rectally, in the form of suppositories or retention enemas. The rectal route may be utilized when drugs cannot be taken orally, e.g. because of vomiting or unconsciousness; or when a local action is required.

The individual may be able to insert suppositories himself, or the nurse may be required to perform the technique. Information on insertion of suppositories is provided in Chapter 30.

Instilling vaginal medications

Vaginal medications are available as creams or pessaries (suppositories). Both forms are generally administered with an inserter or applicator, which allows the medication to be placed high in the vaginal vault for maximum effect. Vaginal pessaries are presented in conical, oval, or cylindrical shapes, and are supplied in individual foil or plastic wrappers. Vaginal anti-infective medications are prescribed to treat vaginal infections, and vaginal hormone preparations are prescribed to treat conditions such as senile vaginitis.

Individuals who require vaginal medication usually prefer to self-administer to avoid embarrassment. The nurse may be required to perform the technique, or she may be required to instruct the individual how to instill vaginal medications. A suggested procedure is outlined in the guidelines. Equipment required:

— drug order sheet and medication record
— prescribed pessaries or cream
— inserter or applicator
— disposable gloves
— perineal pad.

Administration of drugs by inhalation

Drugs can be inhaled to produce a local or systemic effect via the respiratory tract by steam inhalation, nebulizer, atomizer, or aerosol spray.

Information on steam inhalations is provided in Chapter 45.

Most commonly, drugs are delivered to the lungs as sprays from pressurized aerosol dispensers, or as dry powder from an inhaler.

Guidelines for administering subcutaneous and intramuscular injections

Nursing action	Rationale
1. Explain procedure to the individual. Explain the purpose of the medication	Reduces anxiety. Understanding improves compliance with drug therapy
2. Ensure privacy	Prevents embarrassment
3. Gain the assistance of another nurse if the individual is a child, or an adult who is restless or irrational	Promotes safety during administration
4. Check the drug order sheet for the individual's name, name of medication, dose, route and time of administration	Promotes correct and safe administration of the drug
5. Wash and dry hands	Prevents cross infection
6. Calculate the dose and prepare the medication from the ampoule or vial	
7. Check the individual's identity band and ask him to state his name	Confirms the individual's identity
8. Select an appropriate injection site, and assist the individual into a comfortable position	Comfort promotes relaxation and therefore helps to reduce anxiety
9. Relocate the site, using anatomical landmarks	Insertion of medication into the correct site avoids injury to underlying structures
10. Cleanse the site with an antiseptic swab	Removes microorganisms from the skin
11. Remove the needle cap, and hold the syringe in the dominant hand. Hold the individual's skin between the thumb and forefinger and either pull it taut or pinch it up	A needle penetrates tight skin more easily than it does loose skin. Pinching the skin up may be necessary when a subcutaneous injection is given to an obese individual, or when an intramuscular injection is given to an individual with small muscle mass
12. Insert the needle quickly and firmly: at a 45° angle for subcutaneous injection, at a 90° angle for intramuscular	Quick, firm insertion minimizes anxiety and discomfort
13. Slowly pull back on the plunger. If blood appears in the syringe, the needle is withdrawn and the injection repeated at another site—using a fresh dose, syringe, and needle	Checks whether needle has penetrated a blood vessel
14. If no blood appears, inject the medication slowly	Slow injection reduces tissue trauma and pain
15. Place an antiseptic swab over the injection site and withdraw the needle	Support of tissues minimizes discomfort as the needle is withdrawn
16. Massage the area gently. Do *not* massage a subcutaneous heparin injection site	Massage improves dispersal and absorption of the drug. Massaging a heparin injection site may result in severe bruising
17. Assist the individual into position	Promotes comfort
18. Record each drug administered on the medication sheet	Prompt documentation prevents errors
19. Discard syringe and needle into an appropriately labelled rigid-walled container	Proper disposal prevents injury to personnel
20. Wash and dry hands	Prevents cross infection

Aerosol inhalers are widely used to administer bronchodilators. The drug, and its inert propellant, are maintained under pressure in a small canister. When the valve is activated, a measured quantity of propellant carrying the drug is released through the mouthpiece.

Dry powder inhalers may be used by individuals who cannot co-ordinate aerosol inhalation. When the mouth is placed on the mouthpiece, the individual inhales through the device—causing drug particles to be drawn into the respiratory tract.

Guidelines for instilling vaginal medications

Nursing action	Rationale
1. Check the drug order sheet for the individual's name, name and dose of medication, and frequency of administration. Check the individual's identity	Promotes correct and safe administration of the medication
2. Explain the procedure and the purpose of the medication	Reduces anxiety. Understanding improves compliance with drug therapy
3. Ensure privacy and assist the individual into the dorsal recumbent position	Position provides easy access to and adequate exposure of the vaginal canal
4. Wash and dry hands and don gloves	Prevents cross infection
5. Attach the applicator to the tube of cream or place the pessary in the applicator. Gently retract the labial folds	Exposes the vaginal orifice
6. Insert the applicator into the vagina in an upward and backward direction, approximately 7.5 cm Push the plunger to deposit the medication	Proper placement ensures equal distribution of medication along the walls of the vaginal cavity
7. Withdraw the applicator, wipe any residual cream from the labia, and apply a perineal pad	Promotes comfort, and perineal pad prevents staining of clothing
8. Encourage the individual to remain in the recumbent position for 10 minutes	Allows medication to melt and be absorbed into the vaginal mucosa
9. Wash applicator in warm soapy water, rinse and dry. The applicator is stored for future use by that individual only. Remove gloves. Wash and dry hands	Prevents cross infection
10. Record administration on the medication record	Prompt documentation prevents errors

A wet nebulizer adds moisture and/or medications to inspired air, using the aerosol principle. Nebulization is often used for the administration of bronchodilators or mucolytic agents. A high-pressure gas source (air or oxygen) is used to draw up the medication from a chamber. Small volume nebulizers are generally used for the administration of medications. Prior to administration of the medication, sufficient sterile 0.9% w/v sodium chloride solution must be added to the medication.

To prevent cross infection, each individual should be provided with his own nebulizer and mask for use on repeated occasions. The mask and nebulizer should be cleaned at regular intervals, and disposed of when treatment is discontinued.

A suggested procedure for using a *hand-held* oropharyngeal inhaler is outlined in the guidelines. Hand-held inhalers include the metred-dose nebulizer and the Rotohaler. Equipment required:

— drug order sheet and medication record
— prescribed drug and inhaler.

Application of transdermal medications

Certain medications can be applied to the skin to supply drugs directly into the bloodstream for prolonged systemic effect. The medications are applied via an adhesive disc or in a measured dose of ointment. Transdermal medications include nitroglycerine (to relieve angina pectoris), scopolamine (to relieve motion sickness), and oestrogen (for hormone replacement therapy). Drugs which are administered transdermally avoid first-pass metabolism by the liver. (First-pass effects mean that a large proportion of the drug is removed by the liver before it enters the bloodstream).

Adhesive discs, which are applied to the skin, are composed of an adhesive layer, a rate-limiting membrane, a drug reservoir, and a waterproof external layer. The discs are applied to a dry, hairless area of the body. The waterproof external layer enables the individual to shower or bathe without adversely affecting the drug's action. Drugs which are applied in this manner can exert their effects for as long as 24–72 hours.

Transdermal ointments are applied, in measured amounts, directly to a dry, hairless area of the body. Depending on the manufacturer's directions, the ointment may be massaged gently into the skin or placed on an application strip which is taped to the skin.

The individual is instructed in the techniques of self-administration when discs or ointments are prescribed. He

Guidelines for using hand-held oropharyngeal inhalers

Nursing action	Rationale
1. Check the drug order sheet for the individual's name, the name and dose of medication, and the frequency of administration. Check the label on the inhaler, and the individual's identity	Promotes correct and safe administration of the drug
2. Wash and dry hands	Prevents cross infection
3. Explain the procedure and the purpose of the medication	Understanding improves compliance with drug therapy
4. Assist the individual to assume an upright position	Position facilitates entry of the medication into the respiratory tract
5. Administer the medication:	
• load the inhaler with the canister of medication If a Rotohaler is being used, a *capsule* containing the drug is inserted into the device—which is twisted to break the capsule	Prepares the inhaler for administration of the medication
• remove the mouthpiece cap	
• shake the inhaler	
• instruct the individual to hold the inhaler with the mouthpiece at the bottom	
• instruct him to breathe out slowly and fully	Enables subsequent deep inhalation to be performed
• Instruct the individual to place the mouthpiece well into his mouth, close his lips firmly around it, and tilt his head back slightly	Tight seal is necessary to prevent the escape of medication into the air
• the individual inhales quickly and deeply through the mouthpiece while administering a metred dose by pressing the canister downwards	Draws the medication into the lungs
• the individual removes the inhaler, and holds his breath for as long as possible—then breathes out slowly through the mouth	Allows medication to reach the alveoli. Allows increased absorption and diffusion of the drug, and better gas exchange
• the technique is repeated, if necessary, until the prescribed dose has been inhaled	
6. Replace the cap on the mouthpiece	Prevents contamination of mouthpiece
7. Wash and dry hands	Prevents cross infection
8. Record administration on the medication sheet	Prompt documentation prevents errors

should be instructed to wash his hands after applying either form. If the nurse is required to apply transdermal medications, she should wear a disposable glove or use an applicator to apply ointment. She must wash her hands immediately after applying either discs or ointment to avoid absorbing any of the drug.

Topical applications

Topical preparations, e.g. those used in the treatment of dermatological conditions, may be presented as ointment, lotion, cream, jelly, powder, paint, paste, or spray. Drugs applied to the skin principally have *local* effects—except transdermal preparations which are designed to produce systemic effects.

Drugs may be applied to the skin by painting, spreading, or spraying medication over an area; applying moist dress-

ings, or by soaking body parts in a solution. As some locally applied medications *may* create systemic effects, gloves should be worn or an applicator used during administration. If the individual has an open wound, the nurse must use sterile techniques in applying skin preparations. The medical officer may prescribe a dressing to be placed over the medication to prevent loss of the drug or soiling of clothing.

Before applying a topical preparation, the skin should be clean. To prevent accumulation, e.g. of ointment, previous applications of the medication to the skin should be removed. When applying a prescribed topical preparation, the manufacturer's directions must be followed.

Monitoring the effects of medications

The nurse plays a vital role in monitoring the effects of

prescribed medications. Evaluation of the individual's response is essential and the nurse is required to assess, report, and record all responses to medication—including desired effects and any adverse reactions. Evaluation of the effects of medications includes assessing the individual's vital signs, urinary output, performing urinalysis, and assessing the individual for any alterations in his physical or psychological status.

To monitor the effects of any medication, the nurse must first have a good understanding of the purpose of the drug and its desired effects. Table 58.1 lists the major actions of common drugs groups, and it should provide the nurse with a guide as to the expected effects of various groups of drugs. For example, the nurse needs to be aware that an analgesic drug is administered for the purpose of alleviating pain.

Whenever medication of any sort is administered, there is always a possibility that side effects or adverse reactions may occur. Adverse reactions to a drug may be due to overdosage, idiosyncracy, toxic effects, allergy, or drug interactions. Early detection of the manifestations of an adverse reaction and immediate, factual and concise reporting of these manifestations allows prompt action to be taken. Manifestations of an adverse reaction will depend on the type of medication administered and on each individual. Table 58.4 lists possible manifestations of side effects and adverse reactions to medications.

Safe handling of hazardous substances

Cytotoxic drugs (chemotherapy) may be prescribed in the treatment of malignant disease. Cytotoxic drugs, which are toxic agents used to inhibit the growth of malignant cells, may be administered orally, intravenously, or by regional perfusion. As cytotoxic agents are harmful to normal as well as malignant cells, extreme care is required during their preparation and administration.

Although the nurse is not required to prepare or administer cytotoxic drugs, she may be assisting in the care of an individual who is receiving chemotherapy. It is essential, therefore, that the nurse is aware of and understands the guidelines. Clear guidelines, which are developed by health authorities and are available in health care facilities, set down procedures to be followed in the preparation and administration of cytotoxic agents. In addition, the guidelines specify how to deal with spillages, extravasation, and disposal of used equipment and the individual's body wastes.

Errors in administration

Errors can arise for many reasons, the main reason being failure to adhere to the principles of safe practice. Information on ways to avoid errors in administration is

Table 58.4   Side effects and adverse reactions to medications

Drugs acting on	Possible adverse reactions
Alimentary tract	constipation
	diarrhoea
	flatulence
	anorexia
	rash
	headaches
	dizziness
	nausea, vomiting
	dysphagia
	drowsiness
Cardiovascular system	headaches
	mental confusion
	visual disturbances
	bradycardia, tachycardia
	arrhythmias
	hypotension
	nausea, vomiting
	respiratory depression or arrest
	dizziness
	rash, pruritus
	depression
	flushing of the face
	sweating
	increased bleeding tendencies
Respiratory system	nausea
	drowsiness
	bronchospasm
	respiratory depression
	bradycardia, tachycardia
	hypotension
	nausea, vomiting
	muscle tremor
	headaches
	dry mouth
	palpitations
Nervous system	respiratory and cough depression
	central nervous system depression
	pallor
	sweating
	hypotension
	headaches
	drowsiness
	nausea, vomiting, diarrhoea
	muscle cramps
	confusion
	tinnitus
	rash, urticaria, pruritus
	behavioural changes
	dependence
Endocrine system	sodium and fluid retention
	potassium and calcium depletion
	hypertension
	headaches
	obesity
	hypoglycaemia
	nausea, vomiting
	tachycardia, palpitations
	arrhythmias
	sweating
	flushed face
	muscle tremors
	depression

Table 58.4 (cont'd)   Side effects and adverse reactions to medications

Drugs acting on	Possible adverse reactions
Genitourinary system	gastrointentinal disturbances headaches dizziness visual disturbances hypotension, hypertension electrolyte imbalance nausea, vomiting thirst micturition difficulties
Immune system	sedation hypotension dizziness gastrointentinal disturbances pyrexia headaches serum anaphylaxis (rare) bone marrow depression
Skin and mucous membranes	hair loss dryness of mucous membranes hypersensitivity reactions
Microorganisms (anti-infective agents)	diarrhoea allergic or hypersensitive reactions urticarial rash, pruritus bronchospasm anaphylactic shock (rare) nausea, vomiting headaches, dizziness dyspepsia ototoxicity superinfection confusion, convulsions
Malignant cells (antineoplastic agents)	anorexia nausea, vomiting diarrhoea bone marrow depression stomatitis alopecia dermatitis pyrexia impaired wound healing

provided throughout the chapter. Each health care facility has its own protocol for dealing with medication errors, and the nurse must understand and adhere to that protocol.

If the nurse makes an error, e.g. administration of the wrong drug or wrong dose, she must report it immediately to the nurse in charge. The nurse has a professional and ethical responsibility for reporting an error. Measures to counteract the effects of the error may be necessary, e.g. administration of an antidote or monitoring the drug's effects.

The nurse is also responsible for completing an incident report which describes the nature of the incident. The incident report provides an objective analysis of what happened, and is a means for the facility's safety personnel to monitor such events and to implement measures to prevent recurrence.

Continuation of medication after discharge

If an individual is being discharged from a health care facility with medications to be administered at home, the nurse must ensure that he:

- has been instructed in self-medication techniques
- understands his medication regimen
- is informed to notify his medical officer of any untoward effects from the medication
- knows how to store medications correctly and safely
- knows how to discard out of date or unwanted medications safely
- knows how to dispose of used syringes and needles safely.

A visiting nurse may be required to call on the individual at home and, with regard to medications, she can assist in monitoring his drug therapy. She is able to gain an understanding of any difficulties he may be experiencing, can offer advice on how to deal with them, and monitor his compliance with the medical officer's directions.

SUMMARY

The nurse may be required to administer medications, therefore it is essential that she has the necessary knowledge to ensure the safety of individuals who are receiving medications.

The nurse must understand how drugs are transported in the body, how they act, how they are metabolized, and how they are excreted.

Drugs are derived from vegetable, animal, or mineral sources, or they are prepared synthetically. Drugs are presented in a variety of forms, e.g. tablets, capsules, mixtures, and injectable solutions.

Drugs may be administered via the alimentary tract or parenterally.

Drugs, and other substances, are listed under certain schedules which determine restrictions on their use and management. The nurse must be aware of the laws governing the custody and use of drugs, and must follow the nurse's registering body's directions and the health care facility's policy regarding drug therapy.

All drugs can be classified into groups according to their origin, their pharmacological action, or their chemical structure.

Various systems are used to supply prescribed drugs to wards and units within a health care facility, e.g. individual patient dispensing and unit dose presentation.

To promote accurate and safe drug administration the nurse must understand the system of weights and measures used in prescriptions, and she must be competent in performing calculation of dosages.

The nurse must observe the five rights of drug administration: right patient, right medication, right dose, right route, right time.

The nurse, working within her prescribed role and function, must know how to administer drugs safely and correctly: orally, by injection, rectally, vaginally, by instillation into the eye and ear, by inhalation, and transdermally.

The nurse plays a vital role in monitoring the effects of prescribed medications, including their desired effects and any adverse reactions. She must also understand the guidelines regarding safe handling of hazardous substances, and understand the protocol for dealing with medication errors.

When an individual is discharged from a health care facility, the nurse must ensure that he understands all aspects of any prescribed drug regimen.

REFERENCES AND FURTHER READING

Havard M 1990 A nursing guide to drugs, 3rd edn. Churchill Livingstone, Melbourne

Potter P A, Perry A G 1985 Fundamentals of nursing, C V Mosby, St Louis

59. The individual who requires surgical intervention

INTRODUCTION

Surgery is a management approach whereby the surgeon intervenes in the disease process in order to remove, repair, reconstruct, or replace body tissues or organs. Surgery may be directed towards a tumour (excess of tissue), a defect (deficiency of tissue), a deformity (displacement of structures), or the removal of foreign bodies (non-living material). Surgical procedures may be classified according to their degree of urgency, their purpose, and their extent:

- An *elective* operation is one which is recommended in order to improve the individual's comfort and health, but is generally not essential for survival.
- An *essential* operation is performed to prevent a threat to the individual's life.
- An *emergency* operation must be performed with a minimum of delay, in order to remove or prevent a threat to the individual's life.
- A *diagnostic* operation is performed to determine the aetiology of the individual's disorder.
- An *exploratory* operation is performed to determine a diagnosis and/or to evaluate the extent of a lesion.

- A *curative* operation is performed to remove diseased tissue or organ/s; to build tissues and/or organs that are absent, deformed, or altered by disease or trauma; or to repair or replace tissues or organs.
- A *palliative* operation is performed to alleviate symptoms of disease, without necessarily altering the disease process.
- A *minor* operation imposes minimal trauma and/or is associated with minimal risk.
- A *major* operation imposes extensive trauma and/or is associated with serious risk.

It is important for the nurse to know the type of surgery an individual is to undergo in order to plan and implement appropriate care, and to provide appropriate psychological support. Table 59.1 lists various surgical procedures which may be performed.

Responses to surgical intervention

Surgery imposes physiological stress on all body systems, and psychological stress on the individual and his significant others.

Psychological responses

As a result of psychological stress related to surgical intervention, the individual may experience changes in mood and/or behaviour:

- anxiety
- depression
- fear
- grief
- anger
- impaired judgement
- reduced willpower
- inability to concentrate and/or remember
- intolerance of noise and other stimuli
- emotional lability
- aimless, non-productive activities.

Table 59.1 Surgical procedures

Body system	Procedure	Definition
Integumentary	Debridement	The removal of dirt, damaged tissue, and cellular debris from a wound in order to prevent infection and to promote healing
	Skin graft	A portion of skin transplanted to cover areas where skin has been lost
Musculoskeletal	Amputation	Removal of part or all of a limb
	Arthrodesis	The surgical fusion of a joint to provide stability or relief of pain
	Arthroscopy	Examination of the interior of the joint, performed by inserting an endoscope through a small incision
	Bone graft	Transplant of bone from another site—either from the individual or from a donor
	Bunionectomy	Removal of a bunion (a bony prominence and bursa) on the medial side of the first metatarsal of the big toe
	External fixation	Insertion of pins into the bone above and below a fracture. The pins are attached to an external framework to stabilize the fragments in the correct position
	Hip pinning	A type of internal fixation procedure used for repair of fractures of the proximal femur
	Hip replacement	Insertion of a prosthesis to replace a fractured or damaged femoral head
	Internal fixation	Immobilization of reduced fractures by means of rods, plates, screws, or pins
	Laminectomy	Removal of one or more laminae (vertebral bony arches)
	Menisectomy	Removal of a torn or damaged meniscus from the knee joint
	Osteotomy	A bone is cut so that it can be realigned
Nervous	Burr hole	Drilling a hole into the skull, e.g. so that an epidural haematoma may be removed
	Cranioplasty	Surgical correction of a defect in the cranium
	Craniotomy	Opening the cranium to gain access to the brain
	Ventricular shunting	Creation of an alternative pathway for removing cerebrospinal fluid from the ventricular system
Circulatory	Aneurysm repair	Resection of an aneurysm, and restoration of blood flow through replacement of the damaged section with a graft
	Angioplasty	Insertion of a balloon-tipped catheter to dilate a partially occluded artery
	Arterial bypass	Diversion of blood flow to bypass a thrombosed arterial segment, e.g. in the management of lower limb ischaemia
	Bone marrow transplantation	Replacement of diseased or deficient bone marrow, with healthy marrow from a donor
	Coronary artery bypass	Creation of a graft (from a vein or artery) to carry a new blood supply to a coronary artery
	Endarterectomy	Incision of an artery to remove an obstruction, e.g. a progressive atheroma
	Embolectomy	Removal of an occluding embolus from an artery
	Pacemaker implantation	Implantation of a temporary or permanent device (pacemaker) that supplies electrical impulses to the heart muscle
	Splenectomy	Removal of the spleen
	Valve replacement	Removal of a diseased valve and the insertion of a prosthesis
	Vein ligation and stripping	Ligation and diversion of a vein above a varicosed area, and removal of varicosed veins
Respiratory	Laryngectomy	Removal of the larynx
	Lobectomy	Removal of one lobe of a lung
	Nasal polypectomy	Removal of nasal polyps
	Pneumonectomy	Removal of a lung
	Rhinoplasty	Reconstruction of the nose
	Submucous resection of the nasal septum	Incision made in the nasal mucosa to remove cartilage or bone, to correct a deviated septum
	Thoracotomy	Opening the thorax to inspect, repair, or remove tissue
	Tonsillectomy	Removal of the palatine tonsils
	Tracheotomy	Incision into the trachea to create an opening. If the trachea is brought to the skin and sutured there, it is called a tracheostomy
Digestive	Appendicectomy	Removal of the appendix
	Bowel resection	Excision of a portion of the small or large intestine or rectum
	Choledochostomy	Incision of the common bile duct to remove calculi and to insert a T-tube
	Cholecystectomy	Removal of the gallbladder
	Colectomy	Excision of part or all of the colon
	Colostomy	Creation of an artificial anus on the abdominal surface
	Gastrectomy	Partial or total removal of the stomach
	Gastrostomy	Creation of an opening into the stomach
	Haemorrhoidectomy	Excision of haemorrhoid/s
	Herniorrhaphy	Repair of a hernia, e.g. hiatal, umbilical, inguinal
	Ileostomy	Formation of an opening of the ileum onto the abdominal surface
	Polypectomy	Removal of polyps, e.g. from the rectum or colon
	Vagotomy	Severing of the vagus nerve, to decrease gastric acid secretion

Table 59.1 (cont'd)   Surgical procedures

Body system	Procedure	Definition
Urinary	Cutaneous ureterostomy	The ureters are brought to the surface of the skin for drainage of urine
	Cystectomy	Removal of part or all of the urinary bladder
	Ileal conduit	Resection of a portion of the ileum to use as a new receptacle for the collection of urine
	Nephrectomy	Removal of a kidney
	Pyelolithotomy	Incision into the renal pelvis, e.g. to remove a calculus
	Ureterolithotomy	Incision into a ureter to remove a calculus
	Ureteroplasty	Repair or replacement of a segment of a ureter
Endocrine	Adrenalectomy	Removal of one or both suprarenal glands
	Hypophysectomy	Removal of part or all of the pituitary gland
	Parathyroidectomy	Partial or total removal of the parathyroid glands
	Thyroidectomy	Partial or total removal of the thyroid gland
Reproductive	Anterior colporrhaphy	Repair of a weakness in the anterior vaginal wall
	Breast biopsy	Removal of part or all of a breast mass for examination
	Breast reconstruction	Reconstruction of a breast following mastectomy
	Cervical cryosurgery	Application of a freezing agent to areas of the cervix
	Circumcision	Removal of the prepuce of the penis
	Cone biopsy	Removal of a cone-shaped piece of tissue from the cervix
	Dilatation and curettage	Dilatation of the cervix, and scraping of the uterine cavity
	Hydrocelectomy	Removal of a hydrocele
	Hysterectomy	Removal of the uterus—either through an abdominal or vaginal approach
	Laparoscopy	Examination of the abdominal cavity with a laparoscope, through a small incision in the abdominal wall
	Mammoplasty	Reshaping of the breast/s to lift increase or decrease their size
	Mastectomy	Removal of a breast
	Posterior colporrhaphy	Repair of a weakness in the posterior vaginal wall
	Prostatectomy	Removal of the prostate gland, either through a suprapubic or transurethral approach
	Orchidectomy	Removal of one or both testes
	Orchidopexy	Mobilization of, and bringing an undescended testis into the scrotum
	Salpingoplasty	Repair or reconstruction of uterine (fallopian) tube/s
	Tubal ligation	Ligation and, sometimes, severing of the uterine tubes
	Vasectomy	Removal of all or part of the vas deferens
	Vulvectomy	Excision of the external female genitalia
Visual system	Cataract extraction	Removal of the lens and, commonly, insertion of an intraocular lens
	Corneal transplantation	Excision of a diseased cornea, and transplantation of a donor cornea
	Enucleation	Removal of an eyeball
	Iridectomy	Removal of a small portion of the iris
	Retinal detachment surgery	Reattachment of a detached retina to its original position
	Strabismus surgery	Strengthening or weakening one or more eye muscles to correct a squint
Auditory system	Cochlear implantation	Implantation of electrodes into the middle and inner ear, to provide an 'electronic ear' that enables a deaf individual to hear some sounds
	Mastoidectomy	Incising, draining, and removing diseased mucosa and bone from the mastoid process
	Myringotomy	Incising the tympanic membrane to release fluid under pressure, and to insert ventilating tubes
	Stapedectomy	Removal of part of the stapes and the insertion of a prosthesis
	Tympanoplasty	Reconstructive procedure to repair the tympanic membrane

Table 59.2 Physiological responses to the stress of surgery

Response	Purpose
Increased peripheral vasoconstriction and blood coagulation	Prevents excessive blood and fluid loss
Increased rate and strength of heart beat, and dilation of the coronary arteries	Maintains cardiac perfusion and oxygenation
Increased reabsorption of sodium ions from the kidneys, causing retention of sodium and water	Maintains blood volume, blood pressure, and cardiac output
Decreased peristalsis in the gastrointestinal tract	Reduces metabolic activity which is non-essential in the short term emergency
Relaxation of smooth muscle that promotes dilation of the bronchioles	Improves gas exchange and tissue oxygenation
Increased breakdown of protein	Increases the availability of amino acids for repair of tissues
Proliferation of connective tissue	Promotes wound healing
Increased circulation of glucose and mobilization of stored fat	Provides required energy
Increased basal metabolic rate	Provides required energy and nutrients for the tissues

Anxiety is experienced if the individual is worried about the operation and its implications, the anaesthetic, his chances of survival, his loss of independence and/or privacy, pain, or separation from his significant others. Nursing measures that will help to reduce anxiety are described later in the chapter.

Physiological responses

The body mobilizes defences to maintain homeostasis, in response to surgical invasion. The majority of these mechanisms are generally favourable to survival and healing. If, however, the mechanisms are prolonged or uncontrolled, they may contribute to the development of complications. Table 59.2 outlines the physiological responses to the stress of surgery.

Local responses to tissue injury

Following injury, local inflammatory reactions occur in order to promote healing. The inflammatory response begins with an increase in vasodilation. The flow of blood is slowed down, and the area becomes hot and red. Capillary walls become more permeable, and an exudate of fluid and leucocytes leaves the blood stream—causing swelling and, in turn, pain due to pressure on nerve endings. The exudate provides several defence mechanisms: the fluid helps to dilute toxins, leucocytes ingest microorganisms (phagocytosis), and fibrinogen is converted to fibrin which creates a barrier to the local spread of microorganisms. Finally, fibroblasts migrate to the area and new cells are developed.

The physiology of wound healing involves a sequence of events.

1. When tissue is damaged, blood from the injured vessels fills the area. Blood platelets form a clot, and fibrin in the clot binds the wound edges together.

2. After the clot stabilizes, an inflammatory reaction begins. Wound edges swell, and leucocytes from surrounding vessels move in and ingest cellular debris.

3. As the clot diminishes in size, and as adjacent healthy tissue secretes fribroblasts, granulation tissue begins to bridge the area. Capillary blood vessels and lymphatic vessels proliferate by means of buds growing from their endothelial lining, which eventually meet, join, and establish new vessels.

4. Fibroblasts in the granulation tissue secrete collagen, a glue-like substance. Collagen fibres crisscross the area, forming scar tissue.

5. At the same time, epithelial cells at the wound edge multiply and migrate towards the wound centre. A new layer of surface cells replaces the layer that was destroyed.

6. Damaged tissue regenerates. Collagen fibres shorten, and the scar diminishes in size. Maturation takes 6–12 months to complete and, during this time, the gel-like collagen is replaced by a stronger interwoven type.

Wounds heal by first, second, or third intention:

- First intention healing occurs when the wound edges are brought together, e.g. as in a sutured surgical incision. Granulation tissue is not obvious.
- Second intention healing occurs when wound edges cannot be brought together, e.g. a gaping wound. Granulation tissue fills in the wound until re-epithelialization takes place, and a large scar results.
- Third intention healing occurs when wound closure is delayed for a few days, e.g. so that an infected or contaminated wound can be debrided. Closure of contaminated wounds is usually delayed until all layers of wound tissue appear healthy—usually within 4–10 days.

Influences on healing, and care of wounds, are described later in the chapter.

PRE-OPERATIVE CARE

The pre-operative phase begins when surgical intervention is first considered, and ends when the individual is admitted to the operating room. This phase may be of short duration if the individual is taken directly to the operating room from the emergency department, or soon after his admission to the ward. When an individual is admitted for elective surgery, the pre-operative phase may be a number of hours or days in duration. The duration depends on a number of factors such as the amount of time required to prepare the individual adequately for surgery.

An individual may be admitted for same-day surgery. In this instance he is admitted in the morning, is prepared for and undergoes surgery, is cared for following surgery, and is discharged home on the same day. The individual requires comprehensive preparation, and teaching about home recovery.

The overall aim of pre-operative preparation is to ensure that the individual is in the best physical and psychological condition possible to undergo surgery. Although certain aspects of pre-operative preparation are similar for most surgical procedures, a number of factors are specific—depending on the type of operation to be performed. Pre-operative preparation consists of:

- providing information
- teaching activities
- examining the individual—by the anaesthetist
- performing laboratory tests and diagnostic studies
- gaining the individual's informed consent
- preparing the individual psychologically and physically.

Providing information

The individual needs to be informed about pre- and post-operative procedures and care, so that he is better able to understand, predict, and feel in control of what is happening. The information given to the individual and, if necessary, to his significant others should include:

- the pre-operative procedures to be performed, and the reasons for them, e.g. restriction of food and fluids, cessation of smoking, or preparation of the operation site
- the immediate preparation, e.g. the administration of premedication and the induction of anaesthesia, and what sensations he may experience
- details of the recovery phase (in the recovery room) before returning to the ward
- postoperative situation he may expect, e.g. the presence of an intravenous infusion or wound drain, and why these are necessary
- postoperative activities, e.g. early mobilization, and why they are important
- any pain or discomfort to be anticipated, and how it will be managed
- any additional information specific to the operation to be performed.

The information must be provided in such a way that it can be understood by the individual, and it should be repeated if necessary.

Teaching activities

Pre-operative teaching can help to reduce anxiety and stress, and teaching specific activities that the individual can undertake gives him a positive role to play. In some facilities the individual is visited by an operating room nurse, who explains what will occur during induction of anaesthesia, the operation, and the period spent in the recovery room.

Pre-operative teaching of activities involves instructing the individual how to perform deep breathing and coughing techniques, leg exercises and how to move and change position. The individual is informed how important these activities are in the prevention of complications, and he is encouraged to practise them so that the techniques will be familiar when they are required post-operatively.

Deep breathing and coughing techniques, which are performed to facilitate gas exchange and expectoration of accumulated mucus, involve the individual assuming a sitting position, and taking several deep breaths followed by a short breath and cough. Alternatively, the individual may be taught to take a deep breath, hold it for 2–3 seconds, then cough several times while exhaling. The individual is informed that if coughing is painful, e.g. due to a thoracic or abdominal incision, the provision of external support (with the hands over the incision) reduces pain and therefore facilitates coughing and deep breathing.

Leg exercises, are performed to stimulate blood circulation and thus prevent venous thrombosis. The individual is instructed how to bend his knees and contract his hamstring and quadricep muscles, and how to dorsi and plantar flex his feet.

Moving and changing position helps to prevent complications, e.g. deep vein thrombosis. The nurse should inform the individual that he will be assisted to move, if he is unable to do so independently.

Physical examination

The anaesthetist and a medical officer each perform a thorough physical examination of the individual. The anaesthetist pays particular attention to the individual's cardiovascular and respiratory systems, in order to evaluate his cardiac and respiratory function. He assesses the individual for any problems which may cause difficulty during induction or maintenance of anaesthesia, e.g. an upper airway problem which may make placement of an endotracheal tube difficult.

The anaesthetist also evaluates potential sites for peripheral or central venous cannulation. After assessing the individual, the anaesthetist prescribes any pre-operative medications to be administered. He may prescribe a sedative to promote a good night's sleep before the operation, and one or more medications to be administered in the immediate pre-operative period.

Laboratory tests and diagnostic studies

Laboratory tests and diagnostic studies help to detect any risk factors or possible problems. Specific tests and studies performed depend on the individual's condition, and on the nature of the operation. They include:

- blood type and crossmatch
- arterial blood gas and pH
- blood urea nitrogen
- complete blood count
- prothrombin and/or plasma thromboplastin time
- serum electrolytes
- liver function studies
- chest X-ray
- electrocardiogram
- pulmonary function studies
- urinalysis.

Informed consent

Before an operation is performed, the individual must give his informed consent. Informed consent involves the surgeon *informing* the individual about the facts and possible risks involved, and the individual *consenting* to have the operation. Once the individual has been informed and has consented, he is required by the surgeon to sign a form documenting consent. Although the nurse is not responsible for obtaining the individual's consent, she may be required to *check* whether it has been obtained. Information on informed consent is provided in Chapter 10.

Psychological preparation

To minimize anxiety and prepare the individual psychologically for the operation, the nurse must ensure that he is provided with the relevant information as listed on page 669. People generally experience anxiety when they are facing the unknown, and anxiety is usually reduced when accurate and relevant information is supplied. The nurse must ensure that the individual, and his significant others, are given opportunities to ask questions and to express any anxieties.

It is important that the nurse recognizes that a procedure which seems minor or 'routine' to her, may not appear that way to the individual or his significant others. The prospect of any surgical intervention raises many fears about body image alteration, loss of control, pain or death. The individual may be worried about what will happen while he is unconscious, whether the surgeon will start the operation before the anaesthetic is effective, whether he will experience severe pain, how long he will have to stay in hospital, who will look after the rest of the family, how long it will be before he can return to work, and many other factors.

The family, or significant others, will also be anxious—especially in instances where the diagnosis is questionable, or the outcome of the surgery is difficult to determine. If they choose to remain in the hospital while the operation is being performed, the nurse should ensure that they know where a waiting room is located, and where they can obtain refreshments. If they prefer to remain at home, they should be given an indication of what time the surgeon will ring them, or what time and who they can ring to obtain information.

Physical preparation

Depending on the individual's condition, and the type of operation to be performed, specific measures may be implemented to minimize or eliminate any identified risks. For example, an individual with breathing problems may be required to undergo active therapy such as incentive spirometry, or elimination of pulmonary secretions by postural drainage. An individual with poor nutritional status may be admitted for some time before surgery so that nutritional deficiencies may be corrected. Or, an individual may be prescribed a special diet, e.g. one which is low in fibre content before bowel surgery. An individual with potential for infection may be prescribed prophylatic antibiotics before the operation. Other pre-operative measures may include comprehensive preparation of the gastrointestinal tract, and preparation of the skin.

Preparation of the gastrointestinal tract

Gastrointestinal activity is depressed by stress, sedation, general anaesthesia, and the inactivity associated with surgery. Depression of gastrointestinal activity predisposes the individual to retention of food and fluids and, therefore, to abdominal distension and/or vomiting. It also contributes to post-operative constipation or faecal impaction.

Before any abdominal surgery, particularly surgery of the intestines, it is necessary to ensure that the bowel is empty and cleansed—to reduce the risk of contamination and post-operative infection. Preparation of the bowel may include the administration of rectal suppositories, an enema, or bowel lavage.

A period of fasting, whereby all oral foods and fluids are withheld, aims to prevent and alleviate gastrointestinal problems. Allowing sufficient time for gastric emptying decreases the risk of regurgitation and subsequent pulmonary aspiration of gastric contents while the individual is anaesthetised. It also reduces the possibility of postoperative nausea and vomiting.

An extended period of fasting is not advocated, as it may result in fluid and electrolyte imbalances. Depending on the individual's condition, and the type of surgery, the pre-operative fasting period is generally from 6–8 hours in duration. The surgeon, and/or anaesthetist determine the length of time the individual is to fast. Minor surgical procedures, using local anaesthetics, are often performed without imposing any dietary or fluid restrictions.

When an individual is fasting, a notice reading 'Nil orally' or 'Nil by mouth' is displayed on his bed, as a reminder that he may not have anything to eat or drink. Nasogastric intubation may be prescribed if the individual is having abdominal surgery, particularly if depressed gastrointestinal function is expected or desired.

Preparation of the skin

The skin to be incised is usually cleansed before surgery, to minimize the number of microorganisms on the skin and, therefore, reduce the risk of contamination and infection of the wound. Cleansing is generally achieved if the individual showers using an antiseptic soap or solution. If he is unable to shower or bathe, the nurse may be required to cleanse the incision site with antiseptic solution.

Removal of hair from the skin, e.g. by shaving, may be performed. Current research has demonstrated that not removing hair, clipping hair, or using electric razors or depilatory cream, are associated with lower infection rates than traditional shaving. Research has also demonstrated that shaving several hours before surgery, allows time for bacterial colonization of microscopic cuts. The trend, therefore, is to remove the hair immediately before surgery— often in the operating room. Some authorities state that, unless hair near the operative site is thick enough to interfere with the surgery, it is preferable not to remove it at all.

In the operating room, when the individual is anaesthetized, the operation site is swabbed with an antiseptic, e.g. povidone-iodine, using sterile gauze squares or pads.

Administration of medications

It is important for the nurse to be aware of the medical officer's instructions regarding administration of medications. He may order that any medications the individual has been prescribed, be either administered or withheld on the day of surgery. If the individual is fasting, the medical officer may order that any prescribed medications are administered by the intramuscular route, rather than orally.

Pre-operative medications (premedications) may be prescribed for administration in the period immediately before operation. Pre-operative medications may be administered to control anxiety, reduce oral secretions, decrease gastric fluid volume, increase gastric fluid pH, or to prevent postoperative nausea and vomiting. The nurse should be familiar with common preoperative medications, their purpose, side effects and contraindications. Any medication must be administered in accordance with nursing regulations, and the agency's policy.

Preparation immediately before operation

Although preparation during the 1–2 hours prior to operation may vary slightly, depending on the individual and type of operation, preparation generally involves various standard procedures.

- Measuring and documenting his weight. Knowledge of the individual's weight (mass) enables drug dosages, based on body weight, to be calculated accurately. It is also useful for comparison as his progress is monitored postoperatively.
- Measuring and documenting his vital signs. Any deviation from normal must be reported immediately and documented, as abnormalities may result in postponement of the operation. These pre-operative measurements serve as a guide for comparison as the individual's progress is monitored postoperatively.
- Requesting the individual to pass urine, to prevent distention of the bladder during surgery. Particularly during abdominal or pelvic surgery, distension predisposes the bladder to trauma.

The *time* the individual last passes urine is documented on the pre-operation form.
- Urinalysis is generally performed and documented. Any abnormalities must be reported immediately. As the kidneys excrete most drugs from the body, any sign of kidney dysfunction is significant.
- Ensuring that the individual is not wearing any nail polish, lipstick, talcum powder, or other cosmetics that could interfere with assessment of pallor and cyanosis. Jewellery, hairpins, prosthetic devices, spectacles, contact lenses, or hearing aids should not be worn. If diathermy is used during the operation, any metal object being worn could result in the passage of electrical current to the individual and, consequently, burns.

The health care agency generally has its own policy regarding the wearing of wedding rings, e.g. a ring may be left on and secured in position with adhesive strapping.

Whether any dentures or plates are left in the individual's mouth, depends largely on the anaesthetist's instructions. Usually full upper and/or lower dentures are left in, but any partial plates or bridges that may be dislodged during endotracheal intubation are removed.
- Providing the appropriate clothing, and assisting the individual to dress if necessary. Generally, a plain cotton open-back garment with tapes is worn. A disposable paper cap to cover the individual's hair may also be worn, and some facilities also provide a style of brief that may be worn under the gown.
- Checking the individual's identification band, and the documents that are to accompany him to the operating room. The health care agency generally develops its own pre-operative forms, and the information to be entered includes:

- the individual's full name and age

- the type of operation to be performed
- latest vital signs and weight
- time the individual last voided
- results of urinalysis
- whether any dentures or partial plates have been left in or removed
- details of any specific skin preparation
- details of any known allergies
- the individual's informed consent
- details of any medications withheld or administered on that day, including the premedication
- Administering any prescribed pre-operative medications. These are administered when all the other preparations have been completed, and at the time ordered by the anaesthetist, e.g. 30–60 minutes before operation. Once the medications have been administered the individual is informed not to get out of bed, as the medication may cause drowsiness. The side rails on the bed should be raised, the signal device placed within easy reach, and the individual should be allowed to rest quietly.

Furniture in the room should be arranged so that the individual can be transfered easily onto the trolley, e.g. moving the overbed table and locker away from the bedside.

Transfer to the operating room

When the orderly arrives, the nurse should assist him to transfer the individual onto the trolley. A blanket is placed over him, and he is made as comfortable as possible. The side rails on the trolley are raised to promote safety, and the nurse accompanies the individual from the ward. She must ensure that the relevant documents are taken with the individual to the operating room. During transit the nurse should be close to, and in view of, the individual so that she can observe him and provide psychological support.

On arrival at the operating suite, the nurse hands over the documents, and the care of the individual, to a member of the operating room team.

Anaesthesia

Anaesthetics are classified as:

1. General anaesthetics—which promote unconsciousness, analgesia, amnesia, muscle relaxation, and inhibit involuntary reflex action. They may be administered intravenously, or by inhalation.

2. Local or regional anaesthetics—which block the conduction of nerve impulses to and from specific sites in the body. They may be administered through *infiltration*, where the anaesthetic is injected directly into the tissues at the operation site. An anaesthetic may also be applied *topically*, where a cream, spray, or drops, is applied to the skin or mucous membranes.

Spinal (intrathecal) anaesthesia involves the injection of a local anaesthetic into the subarachnoid space between the third and fourth lumbar vertebrae.

Epidural anaesthesia involves the injection of a local anaesthetic around major nerve roots exiting from the base of the spinal cord, outside the dura mater.

Caudal block anaesthesia involves the injection of a local anaesthetic into the caudal (sacral) portion of the spinal canal.

Peripheral nerve block anaesthesia involves the injection of a local anaesthetic into a specific site, e.g. the brachial plexus, to block a group of sensory nerve fibres.

Table 59.3 describes various types of anaesthetic agents, and routes of administration.

Table 59.3   Anaesthetic agents and adjuncts to anaesthesia

Administration	Type	Agent
Inhalation	General anaesthetic	nitrous oxide halothane enflurane methoxyflurane trichloroethylene
Intravenous	General anaesthetic	ketamine methohexitone propanidid thiopentone
Injection (infiltration)	Local anaesthetic	procaine prilocaine lignocaine etidocaine mepivacaine
Topical (surface)	Local anaesthetic	benzocaine cocaine lignocaine prilocaine amethocaine oxybuprocaine
Injection (regional nerve block)	Local anaesthetic	lignocaine procaine prilocaine etidocaine
Intrathecal injection (spinal)	Local anaesthetic	prilocaine etidocaine cinchocaine
Intravenous	Neuromuscular-blocking adjunct to anaesthesia (creates optimal conditions for endotracheal intubation, and relaxation of muscles during surgery)	flaxedil anectine pavulon tubocurarine

POSTOPERATIVE CARE

Following completion of the operation, the individual is transferred to a recovery room which is located in the operating suite. His condition is monitored closely by members of the operating team, e.g. a recovery room nurse, while he recovers from the effects of the anaesthetic. The individual is not transferred back to the ward until his motor and sensory functions begin to return, his vital signs are stable, and there are no immediate complications from the anaesthetic or surgery. While the individual is in the operating suite, the ward nurse prepares the unit for his return.

Preparation of the unit

The bed is usually stripped and remade with clean linen. The top bedclothes are folded into a pack (See Fig. 35.4) which enables them to be removed and replaced quickly. A heating pad may be placed on the bed, under the pack, to warm the bedclothes. It must be *removed* before the individual is placed back in the bed. Generally, one pillow is placed at the head of the bed, and the remaining pillows are placed in a convenient location in the room.

The furniture in the room should be arranged to provide easy access for the trolley, e.g. the bed may be positioned away from the wall, and the overbed table and locker should be positioned away from the bedside. The equipment required in the room will depend on the type of operation that was performed, but generally includes:

- oxygen and suction apparatus
- intravenous therapy pole
- postoperative assessment form
- items for assessing the vital signs
- covered emesis bowl.

Additional equipment may include:

- bedcradle
- sheepskin
- bed blocks
- fracture board (under the mattress)
- hangers/holders for drainage bottles/bags
- nasogastric tube aspiration equipment.

Immediate postoperative care

When the individual is transferred back to the ward, the nurse assists to move him gently from the trolley to the bed. He is placed in an appropriate position depending on his condition and the type of operation. The upper bedclothes are placed over him to promote maintenance of body temperature and comfort.

If an intravenous infusion is in progress, the container of solution is suspended on a pole or stand, and the infusion is assessed to determine whether it is flowing at the prescribed rate. The individual's arm, in which the intravenous cannula is inserted, is positioned so that there is nothing obstructing the tubing.

Any drainage bags or bottles, e.g. urinary or wound, are placed in a holder or hanger, and positioned to facilitate drainage by gravity.

Immediate assessment of the individual involves monitoring and documenting his:

- Vital signs. Any deviation from normal temperature, pulse, ventilations, or blood pressure is reported immediately to the nurse in charge. If necessary, oxygen is administered and oronasopharyngeal suctioning performed.
- Colour. The nurse in charge must be notified immediately if the individual appears extremely pale or cyanosed.
- Level of consciousness. Although drowsiness is normal, it should be possible to rouse the individual by verbal stimuli or touch. He may be disoriented initially, but orientation to person, place, and time gradually return. Inability to rouse the individual should be reported immediately. Restlessness should be reported as it may be due to a change in the level of consciousness; or it may be due to pain, discomfort, respiratory difficulties, or haemorrhage.
- Wound dressing. In the immediate postoperative period, assessing for haemorrhage is a major responsibility of the nurse. Both the dressing and the bed linen under the individual should be checked for signs of haemorrhage. Any increase in blood-staining on the dressing, or an increase of blood in a drainage tube/bottle, must be reported immediately to the nurse in charge.
- Drainage from a urinary catheter. If the individual has an indwelling catheter, the nurse must monitor the urinary output carefully. Any lack of, or decrease in, output must be reported. Similarly, any presence of blood in the urine must be reported.
- Presence of discomfort or pain. As the individual recovers from the effects of the anaesthetic, he may begin to feel pain. The presence of any discomfort or pain must be reported immediately, so that appropriate pain-relieving measures can be implemented.

Subsequent postoperative care

The overall aim of postoperative nursing care is the return of the individual to an optimal level of functioning and independence. Postoperative care is directed towards assisting the individual to meet his needs for oxygen and circulation of blood, comfort, nutrition and fluids, elimination, movement and exercise, hygiene, psychological support, and protection and safety.

Assessing respiratory and circulatory needs

In the initial postoperative period, the frequency with which the individual's vital signs are monitored depends on his condition. Generally, vital signs are assessed and documented every 30 minutes for the first 4 hours, then 1–2 hourly, then every 4 hours if his condition is satisfactory.

Assessment is also made of his breathing to observe for the manifestations of any respiratory tract complications. Mucus secretions may accumulate—leading to pneumonia, bronchitis, or atelectasis. During postoperative recovery, the individual is also at risk of thrombophlebitis and pulmonary embolus. Information on postoperative respiratory and circulatory complications is provided in Table 59.4.

Comfort needs

Comfort of the individual can be promoted by ensuring that a suitable position is assumed. Unless contraindicated, the individual is encouraged and assisted to assume a sitting position. This position promotes adequate lung expansion, and assists urinary or wound drainage by gravity. Pillows are arranged to provide adequate support, without restricting movement, and the placement of a sheepskin under him may further enhance his comfort. If he is unable to move independently, the nurse must assist him to change his position every 2–4 hours.

Measures are implemented to provide pain relief. Analgesic medications are prescribed and administered according to the individual's needs. With adequate pain relief the individual is able to rest, and to perform postoperative activities and exercises. Information on promoting relief of pain is provided in Chapter 36.

Nutritional and fluid needs

In the initial postoperative period, because of the effects of stress and general anaesthesia on the gastrointestinal tract, the individual may be unable to tolerate oral fluids or food. Food and fluids are generally withheld until normal gastrointestinal functioning has returned. Until this has occurred, the individual usually receives fluids and nutrients intravenously.

In some instances oral feeding is contraindicated for an extended period, or the individual may require extensive dietary therapy to rebuild tissue after the trauma of surgery. In such cases, hyperalimentation may be indicated. Information on hyperalimentation is provided in Chapter 29.

After minor or uncomplicated surgical procedures, the individual may be able to tolerate sips of fluid within a short time. If fluids are tolerated, and there are no contraindications, the individual progresses to a light then a normal diet.

Elimination needs

In order to maintain normal bowel function, the individual is encouraged to ambulate as soon as possible and to consume adequate fluids and dietary fibre, although oral fluids and food are initially, withheld until normal intestinal peristalsis returns. Return of peristalsis is indicated by abdominal peristaltic sounds and the passage of flatus. If the individual is uncomfortable, and his abdomen is distended, a rectal tube may be passed to facilitate the passage of flatus. If the individual does not have a bowel action within a few days, depending on his normal pattern of elimination and type of surgery performed, rectal suppositories may be prescribed.

Generally, early ambulation and the intake of adequate fluids stimulates micturition. Some individuals may experience difficulty in passing urine, e.g. due to pain, or the embarrassment of having to use a bedpan or urinal. If retention of urine, or inadequate emptying of the bladder, occurs it may be necessary to pass a urinary catheter.

Information on assisting the individual to meet elimination needs is provided in Chapter 30.

Movement and exercise needs

Postoperative exercises, as described earlier in the chapter, are commenced soon after the individual's return to the ward. Deep breathing and coughing, and leg exercises are performed at 2–4 hourly intervals until the individual is fully ambulant.

Mobility and activity are gradually increased as the individual's condition improves. Initially, he may experience postural hypotension and dizziness when he gets out of bed. Allowing the individual to sit on the edge of the bed and dangle his legs, then assisting him to get out of bed slowly, generally reduces these symptoms. He should be encouraged to ambulate a little more each day, and he should be informed of the benefits of ambulation. Ambulation:

- facilitates deep breathing and so prevents respiratory complications
- stimulates the circulation of blood, thus preventing vascular complications
- improves muscle tone and strength
- aids in the elimination of waste from the bladder and bowel
- reduces the risk of decubitus ulcer formation
- improves morale.

Information on movement and exercise needs is provided in Chapter 37.

Hygiene needs

Until the individual is able to meet his own hygiene needs,

the nurse assists him. Once he recovers completely from the effects of the anaesthetic, his face and hands are washed, his hair brushed, and mouth care is provided. He is assisted into his own nightwear, and any soiled or damp bed linen is changed.

Particularly in the initial postoperative period, when the individual is not taking any oral fluids, mouth care should be provided frequently to prevent dryness and soreness or cracking of the tongue and lips.

After the initial postoperative period, the individual is encouraged to resume responsibility for his own hygiene needs gradually. The nurse may be required to assist him with a shower or bath, and she should be available to supervise such activities in order to promote safety. Information on hygiene needs is provided in Chapter 39.

Psychological needs

Psychological support is provided by keeping the individual informed; allowing him to express concerns about his progress, change of body image, impact of surgery on his lifestyle; and by encouraging visits from his family and friends. His self esteem is enhanced if his independence is encouraged, e.g. by allowing him to resume responsibility for his care—without endangering his safety or recovery. Whenever possible he should be given a choice in care, and timing of activities and events. It is important that he understands the expected time-scale to full recovery, and how any problems will be managed should they arise. All procedures and activities, and the reasons for them, should be fully explained to him.

The nurse may need to help the individual, and his significant others, to develop effective coping strategies. Coping methods include:

- maintaining some control over situations and events
- obtaining additional information in order to deal with a situation more effectively
- trying out various ways of solving a problem, to see which one is most helpful
- talking over a problem with someone who has been in a similar situation
- engaging in an activity which is of interest, e.g. reading or listening to music.

Information on psychological needs is provided in Chapter 40.

Protection and safety needs

In the postoperative period, the nurse must implement measures to protect the individual from hazards in the environment. Information on protection and safety needs is provided in Chapter 38.

Wound care needs

Care of a surgical wound is directed towards promoting healing and preventing infection.

Influences on wound healing

Healing is governed not only by the condition of a wound, but also by the individual's nutritional status. Healing is further influenced by the efficiency of blood circulation to the area.

The most common causes of delayed healing of a wound are *poor circulation* and *infection*. Healing is also delayed if the individual's immune system is impaired, e.g. due to advanced age, irradiation, or immunosuppressive drugs. Excessive strain on the incision, e.g. from overactivity, can delay union of wound edges. Poor circulation reduces the supply of oxygen and nutrients to the wound site; and the presence of infection, pus, or dead tissue in a wound inhibits complete healing.

Wound healing generally takes place within 7–10 days, although the time for normal healing depends on several factors:

- the extent of tissue damage
- the amount of stress and tension placed at the incision
- the extent to which the wound edges have been approximated
- the individual's general condition.

Promotion of healing

In order to promote healing, a number of general measures may be implemented:

- Maintenance of adequate nutritional status. The individual should be provided with a diet that contains adequate kilojoules, protein, vitamins C and A, iron, and zinc.
- Promoting adequate oxygenation of the tissues. Deep breathing and coughing exercises, and early ambulation to promote full lung expansion will enhance oxygenation of the blood.
- Promoting adequate circulation of blood to the area, to transport all the substances required for healing and combating infection. Adequate blood volume can be maintained by ensuring sufficient fluid intake, and circulation can be stimulated by exercises and mobility.
- Restricting movement of the area in the early stages of healing. If strain is placed on a wound, the newly formed granulation tissue may tear. The wound area should be stabilized, rested, and supported.

Wound management

To provide the conditions necessary for healing, the wound

must be free of dead or infected tissue, protected against external agents which may delay healing, and provided with an environment which is conducive to healing.

Controversy exists about certain aspects of wound care, e.g. whether the wound should be covered, the type of dressing that should be applied, how often the dressing should be changed, and which substances should be used to cleanse the wound. Health care facilities generally develop their own protocol for wound management based on reasearch by nurses, medical officers, and infection control personnel. The nurse has a responsibility to know the protocol that has been implemented, and to be aware of current research into wound management.

Wound dressings

Wound dressing may be classified into three main types; those composed of:

- absorbent materials
- occlusive and semiocclusive materials
- special materials.

Absorbent dressings, with or without a non-adherent surface, are designed to absorb wound exudate. This type of dressing needs to be changed frequently, and it may adhere to the wound—resulting in pain and tissue damage as it is removed.

Occlusive semipermeable dressings are transparent and designed to keep the wound moist in order to promote re-epithelialization. This type of dressing may be left in position for several days, does not adhere to the wound, allows the passage of oxygen to the wound, and is impermeable to microorganisms and water. The dressing, because it is clear, also allows visual inspection of wound healing. Occlusive dressings seem to be comfortable for the individual and alleviate pain, because they protect exposed cutaneous nerve endings.

Special dressings may be required in the management of infected wounds, cavities, or ulcers. Infected wounds may be managed by the application of dextranomer beads—small spherical beads which absorb water and small molecules. Silastic foam dressings may be used in the management of open granulating wounds. Porcine skin, cadaver skin, or human amniotic membrane may be used to cover wounds where a large amount of tissue has been damaged, e.g. burns, decubitus ulcers.

A hydro-colloid dressing, composed of gelatin, pectin, and other substances, forms a hydrated gel over a wound. When the dressing is removed, the gel stays over the wound and prevents damage to the new tissue. Gauze impregnated with paraffin and, sometimes, antiseptic may be used for prophylaxis on vulnerable wounds—to reduce the risk of infection.

When wound drainage is copious and/or excoriating, a drainage bag or pouch may be placed over the wound to protect the skin. Prior to application of the pouch, an adhesive skin barrier such as a pectin wafer, is placed on the surrounding skin. The pouch is placed over the wound and secured to the barrier using gentle digital pressure. The principles of application and care relevant to a wound drainage pouch, are similar to those which apply to stomal appliances. Information on stomal appliances is provided in Chapter 46.

Several factors must be considered in the selection of dressings, e.g. allergies, the type and site of the wound, the amount of wound exudate, and the availability of various dressings.

Dressing changes, depending on the health care facility's protocol and on the type of dressing used, may be performed every few hours or daily, or a dressing may be left undisturbed until healing has occurred. Alternatively, the original dressing may be removed after 24 hours and the wound left exposed to the air.

If a dressing is to be changed, sterile equipment and aseptic techniques are used to prevent cross infection. To prevent the spread of air-born microorganisms, activities in the room should be reduced to a minimum, windows and doors should be closed, and conversation should be limited while the equipment and wound are exposed to the air.

A suggested technique for performing a dressing change is outlined in the following guidelines. Equipment required:

A sterile tray containing sterile:

— cotton wool swabs
— dressing/s
— dressing towels
— bowl/s for cleansing solution
— dressing forceps

Additional equipment:

— prescribed skin cleansing lotion
— sterile gloves
— receiver for waste
— scissors
— hypoallerginic tape or bandage.

Drainage tubes

At the time of operation, the surgeon may place a drain tube through a separate 'stab' incision near the principal wound. A drain promotes healing by providing an exit for blood, serum, and debris that may otherwise accumulate and result in postoperative swelling, pain, or infection. The type of drain inserted depends on the site and extent of the wound; and a drain may be freestanding or attached to a drainage bag, intermittent suction, or to a self-contained disposable drainage system that supplies its own suction.

1. When a freestanding drain is inserted, a sterile safety

Guidelines for swabbing and dressing a wound

Nursing action	Rationale
1. Explain the procedure	Reduces anxiety
2. Inspect the dressing	To determine dressing requirements
3. Ensure privacy and assist the individual to assume an appropriate position, ensuring that only the wound area is exposed.	Promotes comfort, and facilitates performance of the procedure
4. Ensure adequate lighting	Facilitates observation of the wound
5. Wash and dry hands throughly	Prevents cross infection
6. Assemble the required equipment, using aseptic techniques	Prevents contamination of sterile items
7. Place the equipment in a convenient location, near the bedside	Facilitates performance of the procedure
8. Wash and dry hands thoroughly, don gloves	Prevents cross infection
9. Use forceps to remove any dressing from the wound and place it in the waste receiver	Prevents cross infection
10. Position dressing towels around the wound	Creates a sterile field
11. Observe the wound for union, signs of infection, and any exudate	Evaluates condition of the wound, and stage of healing
12. Using forceps to hold the swabs, moisten a swab in the cleansing solution. Swab from a clean towards a less clean area, working from the top of the incision line to the bottom. Use each swab for only one stroke, and discard each swab into the waste receiver	Avoids transferring wound exudate and normal flora from the surrounding skin into the wound, therefore prevents wound contamination
13. Using forceps, apply a clean dressing over the wound and secure it in position. Otherwise, if ordered, the wound may be left exposed to the air	Protects the wound from infection and irritation, e.g. from clothing
14. Remove gloves and towels, and place them in an appropriate receiver	Prevents cross infection
15. Assist the individual to assume a suitable position	Promotes comfort
16. Remove and attend to the equipment appropriately. Wash and dry hands	Prevents cross infection
17. Report and document the procedure	Appropriate care can be planned and implemented

pin is usually passed through the tubing just above skin level to prevent the drain from slipping into the incision. A gauze dressing is placed between the pin and the skin. Alternatively, the drain may be secured in position by one or two sutures. An absorbent dressing may be placed over the drain to collect exudate, or a pouch or bag may be applied to the surrounding skin for drainage collection.

2. A closed-wound drain consists of tubing connected to a vacuum unit. Using aseptic technique, the container is emptied as necessary. Vacuum in the container re-established each time the container is emptied. The unit is always positioned below wound level, to promote drainage by gravity.

The drain exit site may be protected by an absorbent or an occlusive dressing.

The length of time a drain remains in position depends on several factors, e.g. the amount of drainage. Prior to its removal, a drain may be rotated and shortened, e.g. daily, to prevent the body tissues becoming adhered to it and also to promote healing.

A suggested technique for rotating and shortening a drain tube, is outlined in the following guidelines. The nurse may be required to perform this procedure if it is within her specified role and function, and if institutional policy permits. As this action may be quite painful, administration of a prescribed analgesic 30 minutes prior to the procedure is usually necessary. Equipment required:

Sterile tray containing sterile:

— cotton wool swabs
— bowl for cleansing solution
— dressing
— safety pin
— gloves
— scissors

Guidelines for shortening a drain tube

Nursing action	Rationale
Follow steps 1–12 as described in the guidelines for dressing a wound	The stab wound is cleansed to remove exudate—thus preventing contamination
13. Using the stitch-cutter, remove any suture which is securing the tube in the wound	Enables the tube to be rotated, if necessary, and shortened
14. If the tube is round, gently rotate it	Rotation of the tube frees any adherent granulation tissue
15. Withdraw the tube the prescribed length, e.g. 1.25 cm	Tube must only be shortened the prescribed length, to allow the wound to heal from within
16. Secure tube with sterile safety pin below level of planned cut	Prevents tube from slipping into the wound
17. Cut off excess tube	Prevents it pressing on the wound
18. Place and secure a clean dressing or pouch over the tube	Protects the skin from irritation from wound drainage
A gauze dressing is generally placed between the pin and the skin, and another dressing or pouch placed over the tube	
19. Remove and discard gloves and towels	Prevents cross infection
20. Assist the individual to assume a suitable position	Promotes comfort
21. Remove and attend to the equipment appropriately. Wash and dry hands	Prevents cross infection
22. Report and document the procedure	Appropriate care can be planned and implemented

Additional equipment:

— sterile stitch-cutter if necessary
— receiver for waste
— hypoallergenic tape.

The nurse should refer to the guidelines for swabbing and dressing a wound, on page 677, as the first 12 steps in the technique are identical.

Removal of a drain tube requires similar technique. Any retaining suture is removed, and the tube is withdrawn steadily and gently to minimize discomfort. If the tube is attached to a suction device, the nurse must ascertain whether suction is to be discontinued prior to removal of the tube. Generally, suction *is* discontinued, to avoid damaging the tissues as the tube is being withdrawn.

Sutures and clips

When surgery has been completed, the wound edges are approximated and held together by sutures, clips, or staples. Generally a single line of sutures or clips is sufficient for closure. In some instances, tension sutures are also required to ensure closure and to provide additional support for the wound. Suturing methods include intermittent and continuous. With intermittent (interrupted) suturing the surgeon ties each individual suture. Continuous suturing is a series of sutures with only 2 knots; one

at the beginning and one at the end of the suture line. The manner in which the suture crosses and penetrates the skin determines the method of removal. Figure 59.1 illustrates two methods of achieving skin closure.

When healing has progressed well, sutures, clips and staples are removed—usually within 7–10 days after insertion. The wound is checked for union of the edges before sutures or clips are removed. Sometimes alternate sutures or clips are removed one day, and the remainder are removed the following day. The most important principle in suture removal is never to pull the visible portion of a suture through underlying tissue, as pulling the exposed portion of the suture through tissues may lead to infection. The nurse may be required to perform this procedure if it

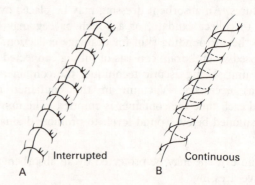

Fig. 59.1 Suturing techniques. (A) interrupted (or intermittent) suture. (B) Continuous suture.

is within her specified role and function, and if institutional policy permits.

Sutures are generally removed using a disposable sterile stitch-cutter, and staples or clips are removed using a sterile staple extractor. Figure 59.2 illustrates the technique of staple removal. A suggested technique for removing sutures or staples is outlined in the following guidelines.

Equipment required:

— sterile stitch-cutter or staple extractor
— sterile swabs and solution to cleanse the incision
— sterile gloves
— receiver for waste
— adhesive butterfly strips or paper tapes if required

Guidelines for removal of sutures and staples	
Nursing action	**Rationale**
1. Explain the procedure	Reduces anxiety
2. Ensure adequate lighting, and place the equipment in a convenient location	Facilitates performance of the procedure
3. Assist the individual into a suitable position, and ensure privacy	Promotes comfort and reduces embarrassment
4. Wash and dry hands thoroughly	Prevents cross infection
5. Remove any dressing, and swab the suture line	Removes any exudate and dried blood, thus reducing the risk of infection
6. (a) Removal of each intermittent suture involves:	
• using forceps to grasp the knot and gently raise it off the skin	
• cutting the suture as close to the skin as possible, away from the knot	Avoids risk of pulling exposed suture through the tissues
• pulling the cut suture up and out of the skin, ensuring that the exposed portion of the suture is not pulled through the tissues	Prevents infection
(b) Removal of a continuous suture involves:	
• using forceps to grasp the first knot and gently raise it off the skin	
• cutting the first suture on the side opposite the knot	
• cutting the same side of the next suture in line	
• lifting the first suture out in the direction of the knot	Minimizes discomfort and ensures that the sutures are removed in the correct direction
• repeating the process down the suture line, using forceps to hold each suture where you would grasp the knot if the suture were intermittent	
(c) To remove staples, position the extractor's lower jaws beneath the span of the first staple	
Squeeze the handles until they are completely closed, then lift the staple away from the skin. Repeat the process for each staple	The extractor reforms the shape of the staple, and pulls the prongs out of the intradermal tissue
7. Wipe the incision line gently with swabs and solution	Prevents infection, and irritation from clothing
Apply a light dressing if necessary	
If necessary, apply butterfly strips or tapes across the incision	Provides additional support, and promotes union of the wound edges if healing is not complete
8. Assist the individual to assume a suitable position	Promotes comfort
9. Remove and attend to equipment appropriately	Prevents cross infection
Wash and dry hands	
10. Report and document the procedure	Appropriate care can be planned and implemented

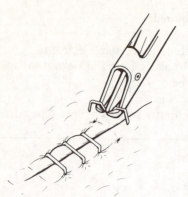

Fig. 59.2 Removing a staple.

Postoperative discomforts and potential complications

During the postoperative period the nurse must assess the individual for the manifestations of various discomforts associated with surgical intervention, and potential complications.

The nursing care plan should include any potential or actual problems; nursing measures to prevent, minimize or manage them; and the objectives or expected outcomes of the planned interventions. The nurse must know how to recognize the onset of discomforts or complications, and she must report any manifestations immediately to the nurse in charge.

Table 59.4 illustrates various postoperative discomforts and potential problems.

Preparation for discharge

Throughout the postoperative period, the individual is being prepared for discharge from the health are facility. The nursing care plan, during this time, is developed and implemented with the ultimate goal of returning the individual to an optimal level of functioning and independence. Before he is discharged the individual, and/or his significant others, should understand how to meet any specific postoperative needs. The nurse may be required to demonstrate to the individual any techniques that are to be performed at home, e.g. dressing changes.

The nurse must ensure that the individual knows how to care for his wound, whether there are any dietary or activity restrictions, whether any special exercise programme is to be followed, or prescribed medications are to be administered. The individual should be informed of the date and time he is to visit the surgeon for a postoperative check. It may be necessary to notify the domiciliary nursing service if the individual requires assistance, e.g. to care for his wound.

SUMMARY

Surgery is a form of intervention whereby the surgeon operates to remove, repair, reconstruct, or replace body tissues or organs.

Surgical procedures may be classified as elective, essential, emergency, diagnostic, exploratory, curative, palliative, major, or minor.

Surgery imposes physiological stress on all the body systems, and psychological stress on the individual and his significant others.

Following surgical intervention, local inflammatory reactions occur in order to promote healing, e.g. vasodilation, and increased capillary permeability. The healing process involves formation of a blood clot, phagocytosis by leucocytes, migration of fibroblasts, formation of granulation tissue, and migration of epithelial cells towards the centre of the wound. Healing may occur by first, second, or third intention.

Pre-operative care is directed towards ensuring that the individual is in the best physical and psychological condition possible to undergo surgery. Pre-operative care involves providing information, teaching activities, physical examination of the individual, the performance of laboratory tests and diagnostic studies, checking that informed consent has been obtained, and preparing the individual physically and psychologically.

Anaesthetic agents which are used during surgery may be classified as general or local. General anaesthetic agents administered intravenously or by inhalation promote unconsciousness, analgesia, amnesia, and muscle relaxation. Local, or regional, anaesthetic agents administered through infiltration or by topical application block the conduction of nerve impulses to and from specific sites in the body.

Postoperative care involves preparation of the individual's unit for his return to the ward, immediate assessment of his condition, and assisting the individual to meet his needs for oxygen and blood circulation, comfort, nutrition and fluids, elimination, movement and exercise, hygiene, psychological support, protection and safety.

Care of a wound is directed towards promoting healing and preventing infection. Wound management involves dressing the wound, care and removal of any drain tubes, and removing sutures or clips.

Throughout the postoperative period, the individual is prepared for discharge with the ultimate goal of returning him to an optimal level of functioning and independence.

Table 59.4 Post-operative discomforts and complications

Condition	Manifestations	Causes	Prevention	Management
Nausea and/or vomiting	Pale, cool, damp skin Sensation leading to the urge to vomit. Vomiting	Effects of anaesthetic agents. Inadequate pre-operative preparation Apprehension Sensitivity to medications	Adequate pre-operative preparation, e.g. fasting With-holding oral fluids and food until gastrointestinal function has returned	Withholding oral fluids and food. Administration of anti-emetic medications. Promotion of physical and psychological comfort
Abdominal distension	Sharp abdominal pains Swollen abdomen Inability to pass flatus	Increased production of gas in the intestines, and reduced peristalsis—causing stasis of the bowel contents	Early ambulation	Encourage ambulation. Passage of a rectal tube to release flatus
Paralytic ileus	Abdominal pain and/or distension. No passage of flatus. Nausea and vomiting	Absence of intestinal peristalsis due to the trauma of surgery	Withholding oral fluids and food until normal gastrointestinal function has returned	Insertion of nasogastric tube and aspiration of gastric contents. Withholding of all oral fluids and food Administration of fluids intravenously
Urinary retention	Suprapubic discomfort or pain Suprapubic distension. Inability to void	Pain. Micturition reflex depressed by anaesthetic agents. Anxiety or fear of pain	Early ambulation. Relief of anxiety and pain	Encourage increasing ambulation. Assistance to assume a natural voiding position. Providing sensory stimulation, e.g. the sound of running water. Ensure adequate fluid intake. *Catheterization if other measures fail*
Constipation	Abdominal discomfort and distension. 'Gas' pains. Nausea	Disruption of normal diet. Reduced mobility Reduced fluid intake Depressive effects of anaesthetic agents and/or medications	Early ambulation. Return to diet high in fibre as soon as possible. Ensure adequate fluid intake	Increase dietary fibre and fluid intake. Encourage increasing ambulation. Administration of stool-softeners or rectal suppositories if necessary
Pain	Restlessness, 'guarding' the wound. Verbal expression of pain. Pale damp skin. Rapid pulse	Tissue trauma. Anxiety	Provide adequate analgesia Promote physical and psychological comfort	Provide psychological support Promote physical comfort Administer adequate analgesic medications
Shock	Hypotension Weak, rapid pulse. Restlessness. Pale, cool damp skin. Diminished urinary output	Reduction in the volume of circulating blood. Physiological reaction to trauma	Avoid and relieve pain, fear. Prevent reduction of circulating blood volume	Restoration of blood volume to normal. Relieve pain and/or anxiety Administer oxygen. Administer prescribed medications. Maintain normal body temperature. Place the individual in recumbent position
Haemorrhage (a) reactionary	Bleeding (obvious or concealed) within the first 24 hours after surgery. Manifestations of shock	Dislodgement of clots from the cut ends of small blood vessels, or displacement of a ligature from a large blood vesel—as the blood pressure returns to normal		Arrest the bleeding. Combat shock Individual may need to return to the operating room to have the haemorrhage arrested
(b) secondary	Bleeding which occurs 7–10 days after the operation	Infection which weakens blood clots or erodes blood vessel walls	Prevent infection	Treatment of infection. Arrest the bleeding. Combat shock
Hypoxia	Tachycardia. Tachypnoea. Pallor or cyanosis Lethargy and decreased responsiveness Confusion, agitation	Ventilations depressed by anaesthetic agents or medications—resulting in poor oxygenation of the blood. Airway obstruction	Maintain a clear airway Promote adequate lung ventilation. Administer oxygen if necessary Monitor vital signs frequently	Promote adequate oxygenation and tissue perfusion

Table 59.4 (cont'd)   Post-operative discomforts and complications

Condition	Manifestations	Causes	Prevention	Management
Atelectasis	Diminished breath sounds. Increasing dyspnoea. Pyrexia	Collapse of a portion of the lung due to obstruction of part of the bronchial tree, e.g. a plug of mucus, or inhaled secretions or vomitus	Maintain a clear airway Encourage regular deep breathing and coughing exercises. Early ambulation	Promote adequate lung expansion Adminster oxygen if necessary Adminster prescribed medications
Pneumonia	Dyspnoea and cyanosis. Pyrexia. Tachycardia. Limited chest expansion on the affected side/s	Accumulation of secretions in the lung/s	Maintain a clear airway Encourage regular deep breathing and coughing exercises. Early ambulation	Promote adequate lung expansion Administer oxygen if necessary Administer prescribed medications
Pulmonary embolism	Sudden onset of dyspnoea, severe chest pain, and cyanosis Urgent desire to defaecate. Sudden circulatory collapse Sudden death	Blockage of one of the pulmonary arteries by a blood clot, air, or fat	Prevent the development of deep vein thrombosis Administration of prescribed anticoagulents Maintain normal blood volume	Administer oxygen. Administer prescribed medications Anticoagulent therapy Embolectomy may be performed
Thrombophlebitis	Calf tenderness. Pain in the leg when the foot is dorsiflexed. Oedema and inflammation of the leg Pyrexia	Venous stasis due to inadequate mobility, reduced volume of circulating blood, or damage to the veins by pressure or injury	Encourage leg and foot exercises. Early ambulation Use of anti-embolic stockings. Avoid pressure on back of legs Administration of prescribed anticoagulants Ensure adequate fluid intake	Anticoagulant therapy. Bed rest with legs elevated. Anti-embolic stockings applied. Administration of fibrinolytic substances
Wound infection	Pain, tenderness, redness, and swelling around the wound Purulent wound discharge. Pyrexia Tachycardia	Invasion of the wound by pathogenic micro-organisms	Practise aseptic techniques, using sterile equipment	Administer prescribed medications, e.g. antibiotics, analgesics. Prevent cross infection
Anxiety or depression	Behavioural manifestations such as aggression, withdrawal, apathy. Tachycardia Palpitations. Fatigue Inability to concentrate	Uncertainty about diagnosis or prognosis Loss of independence Altered body image	Provide adequate information. Promote independence. Provide opportunities for discussion of fears and anxieties	Promote physical and psychological comfort Encourage self-care
Wound dehiscence	Leakage of serosanguinous fluid from the wound Separation of the wound edges. Appearance of loops of intestine at the surface of the abdominal wound	Poor tissue healing which may be due to malnutrition, anaemia, wound infection, premature removal of sutures or clips, or stress on the unhealed incision	Prevention—management of malnutrition and anaemia Delay removal of sutures or clips until there is good union of wound edges Avoid stress on the incision	Combat shock. Cover wound with sterile dressing or towels. Provide psychological support. Prepare the individual for return to the operating room

REFERENCES AND FURTHER READING

Brunner L S, Suddarth D S 1988 Textbook of medical-surgical nursing, 6th edn. J B Lippincott, Philadelphia

Game C, Anderson R, Kidd J (eds) 1989 Medical-surgical nursing: a core text. Churchill Livingstone, Melbourne

Luckmann J, Sorensen K C 1980 Medical-surgical nursing: a psychophysiologic appraoch, 2nd edn. Saunders, Philadelphia

Potter P A, Perry A G 1985 Fundamentals of nursing. C V Mosby, St Louis

60. The individual who requires rehabilitation

INTRODUCTION

Regardless of the type of problem faced by an individual, the major goal of rehabilitation is to help the individual to achieve the highest level of independence possible.

Rehabilitation is a dynamic process in which a disabled individual is helped to achieve optimum function and independence, within the limits of the disability. The term *disability* encompasses a wide range of impairments including those that are physical, mental, emotional, or social. Disability is a general term that refers to the limiting effect of a disease or condition on an individual's ability to carry out an activity in the usual manner. An *impairment* is any anatomical, physiological, or psychological abnormality which interferes with normal structure or function.

Habilitation refers to the process in which an individual who is *born with an impairment* is helped to achieve optimal independence and function. Long-term habilitation programmes are necessary for individuals born with conditions such as spina bifida, Down syndrome, mental or physical impairment. Information on developmental disability is provided in Chapter 53.

Rehabilitation is a continuing process which, to be effective, must be a philosophy of care that is an integral part of health care delivery. Often, rehabilitation is defined as the restoration of an individual to his former capacity. In many situations complete rehabilitation is possible but, in other situations, complete recovery of function is not possible and the individual faces a permanent disability. This individual must be helped to accept, adjust to, and compensate for the existing impairment to establish an optimum level of independence.

One aspect of rehabilitation addresses chronic health problems and degenerative diseases. Although there may be no cure for such conditions, a rehabilitation programme can improve the quality of life. In this sense rehabilitation is directed towards the maintenance of optimum function and prevention of complications, or towards retaining the greatest amount of function and independence for as long as possible.

Rehabilitation begins at the onset of illness or accident, and continues until it is decided that the optimum level for a particular individual has been attained. The rehabilitation process may extend over a period ranging from a few weeks to several months or years.

Rehabilitation programmes are conducted in a variety of settings including acute hospitals, specific rehabilitation institutions, outpatient settings, the home, and in the community.

Philosophy of rehabilitation

A broad statement of basic related principles, concepts, and beliefs is termed a *philosophy*. A philosophy of rehabilitation offers a framework from which the rehabilitation process can be developed. Although rehabilitation teams devise their own philosophy, a philosophy is generally based on the premises that *rehabilitation*:

- recognizes the worth of a disabled person as a valuable human resource
- must be a major integral component of care offered by those in health services
- necessitates the active participation and co-ordination of all health team members through constant communication, to offer a comprehensive rehabilitation plan for the individual
- requires the active participation of the disabled individual to achieve optimum rehabilitation potential, i.e., the individual is viewed as a team member

- should actively involve the family or other significant people in the individual's life
- is concerned with the whole person and includes the sociocultural aspects of his life, his job or vocation, his family, his home, his place in the community, his religion, and his sexuality
- aims to achieve the highest level of independence possible for the individual.

The rehabilitation team

Effective rehabilitation involves the individual, his family or other significant people, and the whole health team. The special needs of the individual determine the fields of expertise that are represented in the team. A multidisciplinary team is required and consists of members from various disciplines, each with a vital role to play. Depending on the individual's needs some, or all, of the following team members may be involved—together with the individual's medical officer.

The nurse

Nurses spend more time with the individual than any other team member, and play a vital role in assessing, planning, implementing, and evaluating care. A nursing assessment includes an evaluation of the extent to which the individual's physical and psychosocial needs are met. Nurses develop a nursing care plan to meet those needs over a 24 hour period. In many settings nursing is the only component of the team which is represented throughout the entire 24 hours of each day, and it is frequently necessary for nurses to continue services in the absence of team members who normally provide them.

Effective nursing care during the acute phase of the illness is a major factor in preventing the development of complications which would impede the restoration of optimum functioning. For a nurse to fulfill her role as a rehabilitation team member it is necessary to:

- understand the short and long term goals of the rehabilitation programme
- appreciate the place of the nurse in the team and be aware of the need for co-ordinated effort by all team members to achieve total care
- be flexible and amenable to change
- have an understanding of the role and function of all other team members
- be able to assess accurately the individual's reactions and responses to his condition, and to the rehabilitation programme.

The physiotherapist

Physiotherapists evaluate the individual's physical capabilities and limitations, and administer therapies which are designed to correct or minimize deformity, increase strength and mobility, or alleviate discomfort or pain. Treatments include the use of specific exercises, heat, cold, and electrophysical therapy. A physiotherapist is also involved in educating members of the health team and the individual in correct methods of positioning, transferring, and mobilizing.

The occupational therapist

Occupational therapists are concerned with assisting the individual to achieve independent performance in the activities of daily living. They also assess the need for, and provide, adaptive devices e.g. aids to assist self-feeding, which help the disabled individual carry out these activities. Information on aids to daily living is provided later in the Chapter.

The speech pathologist

Speech pathologists are concerned with assessing, diagnosing, and treating communication disorders, e.g. the formation and perception of speech, ability to articulate words, and the ability to understand and initiate speech. As part of the rehabilitation process a speech pathologist may be required to assist an individual to relearn communication skills. A speech pathologist may also be involved in the management of an individual whose chewing and swallowing abilities are impaired, e.g. following a cerebrovascular accident.

The social worker

Social workers are concerned with counselling and assisting individuals and their families who are experiencing personal problems as a result of illness or injury. A social worker acts as an *advocate* by liaising with existing groups and resources, and assists the individual and the family to deal with social, domestic, financial, and emotional implications of the illness or condition.

The family or friends

The family, or significant others, are recognized as a potential support system for the individual. Members of the family are evaluated to determine their ability to help with the rehabilitation process. All families, or significant others, cannot contribute in the same way or to the same degree. In some instances the individual could return home and receive excellent care and support, while in other situations the family may be unable or unwilling to help to care for the individual. As each situation presents different problems, individual evaluation is essential.

The family, or significant others, need to understand the rehabilitative goals set for the individual and the methods selected to meet these goals. The family need to understand that their greatest contribution may be to allow the individual to do as much as possible for himself. In addition, the family can be instructed how to assist with specific therapy—thus enabling them to feel that they are playing a vital role in rehabilitation.

It is important to understand that, when illness or disability occurs, family life is interrupted and altered. The effects of illness have significant implications for the family, as well as for the individual. Plans for the rehabilitation process should, therefore, also address the needs of the family as well as those of the individual.

The dietitian

Dietitians are concerned with assessing nutritional needs and planning ways to meet those needs. As part of the rehabilitation process an individual may require specific dietary restrictions or modifications, and a dietitian works closely with the individual to plan an appropriate diet. The dietitian also plays an important role in ensuring that all those involved with the individual's care understand the importance of a specific diet to the person's recovery.

The podiatrist

Podiatrists are concerned with assessing, preventing, and treating disorders of the feet. As part of the rehabilitation process an individual may be required to relearn how to ambulate, e.g. following a cerebrovascular accident. In order to mobilize, the feet must be in good condition with no skin lesions or nail disorders, and the podiatrist plays an important role in maintaining the health and integrity of the skin and toe nails.

The prosthetist

Prosthetists are concerned with assessing an individual's need for a prosthesis, e.g. an artificial limb. Following assessment a prosthetist designs and supplies an appropriate prosthesis. Generally a temporary prosthesis is provided and trialed before a permanent one is supplied. Modifications to an existing prosthesis may be made by a prosthetist, who also checks it at regular intervals to ensure that the prosthesis is meeting the individual's needs.

Some individuals may need to be fitted with splints or braces to correct deformities or provide added support. Such mechanical devices are called *orthoses*, and include braces for the neck, arm, or leg.

The psychiatrist and psychologist

If an individual is experiencing a psychiatric or emotional problem, either a psychiatrist or psychologist is generally involved in the rehabilitation process. A psychiatrist is concerned with the causes, prevention, and treatment of mental, emotional, and behavioural disorders. A clinical psychologist is concerned with the causes, prevention, and treatment of individual or social problems—especially in regard to the interaction between the individual and the physical and social environment. A psychiatrist or clinical psychologist may be involved in the rehabilitation of an individual who is depressed as a result of the implications of his condition.

The individual

It is essential that the individual who requires rehabilitation is viewed as a *team member*. The other team members must help to motivate the individual to be actively involved in the rehabilitation process—however slow it may be. Unless he is encouraged and motivated, the individual may become discouraged and discontinue the prescribed therapy. At all stages of rehabilitation, the rest of the team must consider the individual's strengths and weaknesses, and the social and cultural influences that affect his adjustment to disability. The team must be aware of how the individual perceives his illness and disability.

Any interference with an individual's body image, e.g. paralysis resulting from a cerebrovascular accident, is devastating. The initial reaction is usually one of shock, followed by denial. As the individual gradually realizes what has happened and the implications, he may experience depression or anger, believing that life may never be the same again. While there is inevitable dependency initially, the overall aim of rehabilitation is to help the individual to achieve optimum functioning. The motivation of the individual is crucial, and it is essential that he be regarded as the most important team member, who must be encouraged to participate actively in all aspects of the rehabilitation process. The individual must be involved in planning his programme; and must learn in detail about his disability, the ways of accomplishing his goals, and the options available to him.

Conferences or team meetings are held at regular intervals where the team members discuss the progress and problems of every individual who is undertaking rehabilitation. During these meetings:

- Specific short- and long-term goals are set, with each member being aware of the other's roles in accomplishing these goals. Goals must be re-evaluated regularly, so that the team can determine whether they are realistic and/or whether they have been accomplished.
- Each team member explains to the other members the procedures and techniques that are being carried out.
- Documentation of the proceedings is made, in terms that are meaningful and valid for all persons concerned.
- The individual and/or the family may be present as both parties are encouraged to be involved in goal setting and decision making.

Process of adjustment

The process of adjustment as it relates to disability is similar to that in dying. Information on loss, grief, and dying is provided in Chapter 65. Disability involves *loss* and is accompanied by an adjustment process as the individual, and his significant others, learn to come to terms with the disability and its implications. The individual may experience loss of:

- sensation
- skin integrity
- a body part
- ability to walk
- use of an arm
- bowel and/or bladder control
- sexual function
- ability to speak, read, write, comprehend
- memory
- ability to relate to other people and the environment
- self image, sense of self-worth, self esteem, sexuality
- independence.

The recently disabled person generally experiences four stages in adjustment during the rehabilitation process:

1. Acute disorganization. The individual may express feelings of extreme anxiety, fear, and disbelief that such an event has occurred.

2. Assessment. The individual begins to assess what has happened to him. He begins to recognize and identify changes in function and ability, and may experience anger, depression, denial, and bargaining. He may hope for a spontaneous recovery or a medical miracle, and tends to resist activities designed to help him function with an impairment.

3. Mourning. The individual continues to experience anger and depression, however there is generally a new awareness of the losses involved. The individual begins to accept his most probable future, and no longer denies or ignores the disability. Eventually, he begins to participate more fully in the rehabilitation programme.

4. Re-entry. The individual resolves the depression of the mourning process, and begins to experience more positive feelings about himself and the future. He recognizes that the disability does, in fact, exist and is keen to find means to adapt his life to the disability.

It is important for nurses to understand that each individual will have his own 'time-table' for adjusting to his disability. Thus, while some people adjust in a relatively short time, others will take much longer. There is no 'normal' period of time before an individual finally accepts, and adjusts to, a disability. It must not be forgotten that the *family* also goes through a process of adjustment. The rehabilitation team plays an important role, as it supports the individual and family during the process of adjustment.

Categories of individuals requiring rehabilitation

An individual may experience a disability of acute or chronic onset, at any stage of the lifespan. Rehabilitation programmes may be developed and implemented—in hospitals, other health care settings, and in the home—for an individual who is experiencing:

- disturbance of musculoskeletal function as a result of injury, illness, or surgical intervention, e.g. fractured femur, arthritis, amputation, joint replacement.
- brain damage, e.g. following a cerebrovascular accident or head injury.
- nervous system impairment, e.g. as a result of a spinal cord injury or disease such as multiple sclerosis.
- impaired skin integrity, e.g. as a result of burns.
- removal of a body part, e.g. mastectomy, laryngectomy, or hemicolectomy with subsequent colostomy.
- cardiac impairment, e.g. following a myocardial infarction.
- impaired renal function, e.g. renal failure requiring dialysis.
- impaired bladder control, e.g. as a result of a neurogenic bladder disorder.
- respiratory impairment, e.g. as a result of obstructive disorders of the airways such as asthma or pulmonary emphysema.
- impaired vision or hearing.
- chronic pain.
- substance abuse.
- a psychiatric or emotional disorder, e.g. schizophrenia, depression, anxiety.

Assessment of rehabilitation potential

Assessment of the individual, and a realistic evaluation of his rehabilitation potential is the first step towards planning a programme. In some instances this can be a relatively simple process and, in others, it is more complicated. For example, it is comparatively easy to assess the rehabilitation potential of a healthy young adult with a fractured femur, and it is more difficult to make an assessment when the individual is elderly and has experienced a cerebrovascular accident. Assessment of each individual must take into account:

- The nature of the disability. Some conditions affect only isolated areas of the body, while others exert widespread effect. Some disorders cause progressive and diverse impairment of function.
- The overall condition of the individual and his ability to cope with a rehabilitation programme. There may be other existing conditions which could influence the choice of rehabilitation measures. For example, chronic conditions such as arthritis or emphysema may restrict the individual's ability to engage in active exercise.

• The motivation of the individual and his understanding of the situation. His motivation should stem from a realistic acceptance of his situation, and should not be the result of over optimism or a refusal to acknowledge limitations.
• The individual's home environment, and the ability of the family or significant others to be supportive.

Physical and psychological assessment of the individual is performed to evaluate his functional state, so that both short and long-term goals can be set. Assessment includes evaluating muscle function, range of joint motion, body alignment and posture, neurological function, cardiopulmonary function, and cognition.

Determining short-term and long-term goals

Short-term goals of a rehabilitation programme are those which may be achieved in a short period of time. For example, activities such as achieving a standing position, moving from a bed to a chair, feeding oneself, tieing shoelaces, or formulating a sentence, may be set as short-term goals.

Long-term goals are those which are expected to take much longer to accomplish, and depend on success in achieving the short-term goals. These may include activities such as walking, negotiation of stairs, independence in the activities of living, or returning to employment.

The value of setting goals is that both the individual and the team know what they are aiming for, and will be able to identify when they have achieved a specific goal. If *realistic* goals are to be set the entire rehabilitation team must be involved in the planning process, and must meet frequently to re-evaluate the situation.

It may be difficult for an individual to maintain a high level of motivation, as he may think that he is making little progress and that the set goals are unattainable.

He may view the rehabilitation programme as tedious, boring, exhausting, or painful. As a result, the individual may become depressed and discouraged. A nurse may help by:

• Being empathic about the situation, which involves trying to understand how the individual is feeling.
• Emphasizing what progress has been made, and expressing confidence in the individual's ability to make further progress.
• Spending as much time as possible with the individual, particularly during activities when active encouragement is required.
• Ensuring that he does not become overtired or attempt to exceed the limits prescribed.
• Encouraging the individual to concentrate on achieving one goal at a time. An over-ambitious programme may result in frustration and despair.
• Encouraging the individual to express his feelings. A relationship can be established by listening and talking to him, this creating a sense of trust so that the individual feels able to express his feelings.

Nursing aspects of rehabilitation

A rehabilitation programme is developed for each individual, and the nursing activities involved will depend on many factors such as the individual's age, degree of independence, and type of impairment. The overall purpose of rehabilitation is the restoration of an individual to normal or near-normal function, or to assist the individual to adjust to a disability, following illness or injury. The nurse, as a member of the rehabilitation team, provides support and assists the individual to meet his physical and psychological needs.

It is beyond the scope of this book to provide information about specific programmes for every category of individual who requires rehabilitation. Regardless of the specific impairment, the philosophy and aims of rehabilitation remain the same. The nurse plays a key role in assisting the individual to carry out the activities of daily living, and she must be aware that the ultimate goal is to promote independence in these activities. The achievement of *independent performance* in functional living skills is one of the most important aspects of an individual's rehabilitation. The activities of living, as identified by Roper, Logan, and Tierney (1985) are:

• maintaining a safe environment
• communicating
• breathing
• eating and drinking
• eliminating
• personal cleansing and dressing
• controlling body temperature
• mobilizing
• working and playing
• expressing sexuality
• sleeping
• dying.

Depending on the individual's disability and needs, a rehabilitation programme is planned whereby goals are set to assist him to achieve independence in the activities of living. For example, in a programme developed for an individual who has experienced a cerebrovascular accident and subsequent hemiplegia, one specific long-term goal may be that, 'The individual is able to dress himself'. In order for that goal to be achieved, short-term goals will be set, e.g. 'The individual is able to sit up in a chair'. The occupational therapist will be involved in teaching dressing and undressing techniques, and the nurse should understand the techniques the individual is using so that she can reinforce the occupational therapist's teaching.

Another important nursing function is prevention of the complications of immobility:

- decubitus ulcers
- contractures
- footdrop
- venous stasis
- pulmonary stasis
- urinary stasis
- constipation
- postural hypotension
- psychological consequences, e.g. boredom or depression.

Information on prevention of these complications in provided in Chapter 37.

Aids to daily living

There are numerous devices to help a disabled person to perform the activities of living. Such devices are invaluable as they make a degree of independence possible. Nurses should be familiar with these aids, and should be capable of teaching the individual and family the correct way to use them. Some of the aids available are:

- eating aids (as illustrated in (Fig. 29.2)
- suction devices fitted to kitchen utensils, backs of nail brushes, etc. for the benefit of a person with the use of only one hand
- boards with spikes to hold fruit or vegetables to be peeled, or bread to be buttered
- face-washers in the shape of a mitten with a pocket to hold the soap
- long-handled tongs for a person who is unable to pick items up by bending or stooping
- dressing sticks with one end covered by foam rubber to grip the sleeve or shoulder of a garment, making it easier to don and remove
- various devices to enable socks and stockings to be put on
- overlapping adhesive fastenings, e.g. Velcro, on clothing for people unable to manage other conventional types of fastening
- long handled shoe horns to make bending or stooping unnecessary
- elastic shoe laces which do not have to be untied when shoes are removed
- cuffs, which when placed over the hand, hold a pencil, toothbrush, or razor
- easy to turn tap fittings
- walking aids (as illustrated in Fig. 37.11)
- raised toilet seats
- chairs with an ejector seat which rises as the occupant leans forward
- ramps to replace stairways
- hand grips in bathroom and toilet areas

- low level fittings for occupants of wheelchairs, e.g. sinks, stoves, mirrors, light switches.

In most states of Australia there are Centres for Independent Living which provide a wide range of aids to daily living. There are a variety of community services available to assist disabled persons to remain at home, e.g. Community Health Centres, Day Hospitals and Day Centres, Drop-in Centres, Elderly Citizens Clubs, Self-help groups, Home Nursing Services, Meals-on-Wheels, and sheltered workshops. Nurses should be aware of the state-specific social welfare services and agencies, most of which are listed in the Telecom Directory.

Discharge planning

Discharge planning prepares the individual for the transition to another setting, e.g. from hospital to home. The elements of the discharge planning process should begin on the day of admission. The overall goal of discharge planning is to promote continuous health care services to meet the individual's needs. An effective discharge plan depends on the resources available to the individual who is being rehabilitated, including:

- adaptation of the home environment
- the family or significant others
- home care nursing
- social and counselling agencies
- volunteer community services
- support and special interest groups, e.g. Multiple Sclerosis Society, Diabetic Association, Cancer Society, Heart Foundation.
- medical supplies and equipment.

Nurses, together with other team members, assist in co-ordinating and developing the discharge plan, utilizing the steps of the *nursing process* to achieve the final plan.

CONCLUSION

Rehabilitation is a dynamic process in which a disabled person is helped to achieve optimum function and independence, within the limits of the disability.

A disability is any physical, mental, emotional or social impairment that limits an individual's ability to carry out an activity in the usual manner.

Effective rehabilitation involves the individual, his family or other significant people, and professional members of the health team. The nurse, as part of the rehabilitation team, plays a vital role in helping the individual to meet his physical and psychological needs as independently as possible.

REFERENCES AND FURTHER READING

Bitter J A 1977 Introduction to rehabilitation. C V Mosby, St Louis

Brunner L S, Suddarth D S 1980 Textbook of medical-surgical nursing, 4th edn. Saunders, Philadelphia, ch 4, p 179–205

Game C, Anderson R, Kidd J (eds) Medical-surgical nursing: a core text. Churchill Livingstone, Melbourne, ch 8, 63–69

Luckmann J, Sorensen K C 1980 Medical-surgical nursing: a psychophysiologic approach, 2nd edn. Saunders, Philadelphia

Roper N, Logan W W, Tierney A 1990 The elements of nursing, 3rd edn. Churchill Livingstone, Edinburgh

61. The individual who requires isolation

INTRODUCTION

In order to prevent cross infection it may be necessary to isolate an individual from others. Information on infection and cross infection, together with aspects of microbiology, is provided in Chapters 9 and 38 and it should be referred to in conjunction with this chapter.

This chapter addresses the special techniques and precautions required when an individual requires isolation from others.

Disease prevention

In order to prevent the spread of infection, the public must be informed about disease prevention and prophylactic immunization. The nurse is in a key position to educate members of the public about the ways by which communicable diseases may be prevented.

Community health depends largely on a clean water supply, sewage treatment, and proper disposal of rubbish. Personal hygiene, e.g. thorough hand washing after handling waste, after using the toilet, and before handling food is an important factor in preventing disease. Proper food handling is an important means of preventing food poisoning and the spread of infection.

Many communicable diseases can be prevented by immunization—a process by which resistance to an infectious disease is induced or augmented. Further information on immunity, and prevention of infectious diseases, is provided in Chapters 9.

Communicable diseases

Communicable (infectious) diseases are those which are caused by specific microorganisms that can be transmitted readily from person to person. Terms used in relation to communicable diseases include:

Epidemic: a large number of people in a specific geographic area, affected by the same communicable disease at one time.

Endemic: a disease is present in a community, but only a small number of people are affected at one time.

Pandemic: world-wide distribution of a communicable disease.

Nosocomial infection: acquired by an individual while in a health care facility.

Opportunistic infection: infection occurring in a host who has an immune defect.

Carrier: a person who harbours pathogenic microorganisms which may be transmitted to others. A carrier may be someone incubating a disease, or someone who is a healthy carrier of the particular microorganism without ever experiencing the manifestations of the disease.

Virulence: the power of a microorganism to produce disease.

Incubation period: the time between exposure to a pathogenic microorganism and the onset of the signs and symptoms of a disease.

Prodromal period: the period during which non-specific manifestations appear indicating the onset of an infectious disease.

Notifiable diseases: diseases which are listed in health regulations, and about which medical practitioners are obliged to notify the health authorities when cases are brought to their notice.

Quarantine: the segregation of people who have been exposed to communicable disease during the contagious period, in an attempt to prevent spread of the disease.

Isolation: the segregation of an infected person, to prevent cross infection.

Table 61.1 illustrates various communicable diseases, and the immunologic agents available to prevent those diseases.

Table 61.1 Communicable diseases

Disease	Causative organism	Incubation period	Manifestations	Available immunologic agent
Brucellosis	Brucella bacteria	From 5–21 days, up to several months	Pyrexia, muscular aches, sweating, fatigue, lympadenopathy, weight loss, depression, headaches, sleep disturbances	
Cholera	*Vibrio cholerae*	Several hours–5 days	Acute, painless, profuse, watery diarrhoea; effortless vomiting, dehydration, shock	Cholera vaccine
Diphtheria	*Corynebacterium diphtheriae*	Less than 7 days	Thick, patchy, grey-green film over the mucous membranes of the upper respiratory tract, hoarseness, rasping cough, possible airway obstruction and respiratory distress	Diphtheria toxoid. Triple antigen, which immunizes against pertussis, diphtheria, and tetanus
Gastroenteritis	Bacteria such as Shigella, Escherichia coli, Salmonella. Enteroviruses	A few to several hours	Diarrhoea, abdominal discomfort or pain, nausea, vomiting, pyrexia, malaise, dehydration	
Herpes Zoster (shingles)	Herpes virus varicella (varicella-zoster)	Not specific Reactivation of varicella virus that has lain dormant for up to several years	Pyrexia, malaise, severe deep pain, pruritus, paraesthesia or hyperaesthesia, eruption of small red skin lesions along the path of a nerve, regional lymphadenopathy	Varicella-zoster immune globulin (for passive immunization)
Influenza	Myxovirus	24–48 hours	Pyrexia, shivering, headaches, myalgia, malaise, non-productive cough, hoarseness, conjunctivitis	Influenza virus vaccine
Infectious parotitis (Mumps)	Paramyxovirus	14–25 days	Myalgia, headaches, anorexia, malaise, pyrexia, earache, parotid gland tenderness and swelling, pain when chewing or swallowing	Mumps virus vaccine
Infectious mononucleosis (glandular fever)	Epstein-Barr virus	10–50 days	Headaches, malaise, fatigue, sore throat, cervical lymphadenopathy, temperature fluctuations, stomatitis, tonsillitis	
Malaria	Genus *Plasmodium*	12–30 days	Pyrexia, shivering, headaches, myalgia, rigors	Cloroquine, Primaquine, Pyrimethamine
Meningitis (Viral or bacterial)	Enteroviruses Meningococci *Haemophilus influenzae* Pneumococci	Variable	Sudden onset of severe headaches, pyrexia, neck and back stiffness, dizzyness, photophobia, nausea and vomiting. A rash may appear. Convulsions, mental confusion, drowsiness may occur	Meningococcal polysaccharide vaccine (to prevent neisseria meningitides infections in populations at high risk)

Table 61.1 (cont'd) Communicable diseases

Disease	Causative organism	Incubation period	Manifestations	Available immunologic agent
Morbilli (measles)	Paromyxovirus (measles virus)	10–14 days	Pyrexia, nasal discharge, cough, sneezing, red and watering eyes, irritability, Koplik's spots on mucous membrane in the mouth, non-irritating red blotchy rash appearing first at the back of the ears, face and neck, then spreading to the trunk and limbs	Measles virus vaccine
Poliomyelitis	One of the poliomyelitis viruses belonging to the enteroviruses group	7–14 days	Minor manifestations only such as slight pyrexia, headaches, vague muscular aches and pains, OR paralysis may occur	Poliovirus (Salk) vaccine
Pertussis (whooping cough)	*Bordetella pertussis*	7–14 days	Sneezing, watering of the eyes, nasal discharge, a dry cough (particularly at night.) After a few days paroxysmal cough. A typical paroxysm begins with short barking coughs, difficult breathing and cyanosis. A successful inhalation then produces the characteristic high-pitched 'whoop'. The same sequence is repeated several times until the attack terminates with the expulsion of a plug of mucus, or vomiting	Triple antigen, which immunizes against pertussis, diphtheria, and tetanus
Rubella (German measles)	Rubella virus	14–21 days	Mild pyrexia, sore throat, slight cough, pink macular non-irritating rash on the face and chest — which later spreads to the neck, trunk, and limbs. Usually lymphadenopathy behind the ears and in the occipital region	Cendevax vaccine
Scarlet fever	Haemolytic streptococci	2–7 days	Pyrexia, headaches, malaise, sore throat, cervical lymphadenopathy. Tongue may be reddened with enlarged papillae (strawberry tongue). A rash consisting of red, raised spots appears on the chest, and later spreads to the trunk, neck, and limbs The face is flushed with a circumoral pallor	
Tetanus	*Clostridium tetani*	3–4 days, up to several weeks	Trismus (stiffening of the jaw muscles and inability to fully open the mouth.) Neck and back stiffness, abdominal and limb rigidity Respiratory distress Spasm of the facial muscles, producing risus sardonicus Very painful intermittent muscle spasms	Triple antigen, which immunizes against pertussis, diptheria, and tetanus. Tetanus vaccine alone Tetanus immunoglobulin — (to confer passive immunity)

Table 61.1 (cont'd)   Communicable diseases

Disease	Causative organism	Incubation period	Manifestations	Available immunologic agent
Typhoid fever	*Salmonella typhi*	12–14 days	Headaches, anorexia, constipation, increasing pyrexia. Rigors, profuse sweating, and delerium may occur. A rash may appear on the trunk Severe diarrhoea occurs about the third week of the illness	Typhoid vaccine
Toxoplasmosis	Toxoplasma gondii	Variable	If acquired during pregnancy, the infant may be premature, stillborn, or have congenital defects. Manifestations of acquired toxoplasmosis vary, and may be related to either localized or generalized infection	
Varicella (chicken pox)	Varicella-Zoster virus	10–20 days	Slight pyrexia, anorexia, malaise, headaches. A rash appears beginning with pink macules, which develop into raised papules. Vesicles develop, rupture, dry, and form crusts. The rash appears first on the face, scalp and upper trunk. As vesicles are developing, the rash becomes very itchy	
Viral hepatitis	A number of viruses, the most common of which are the Hepatitis A and B viruses	Hepatitis A: 2–6 weeks Hepatitis B: 4–24 weeks	Malaise, pyrexia, headaches, anorexia, nausea and vomiting, abdominal pain, dark urine, pale faeces. Jaundice appears in about 3–10 days, and there may be mild or severe pruritus	Immunoglobulin (to confer passive immunity) Hepatitis B vaccine

Isolation methods

While the whole concept of 'isolation' is undergoing major change and there is a trend towards implementing universal precautions, the following methods of isolation are still being practised to prevent cross infection:

1. Source isolation (barrier nursing) refers to the technique used when an individual with an infectious condition is isolated, in an attempt to prevent spread of the infection. This method, therefore, isolates the individual who is the source of infection.

2. Protective isolation (reverse barrier nursing) refers to the technique used to protect an individual against opportunistic infection when there is an immune defect or lowered resistance to infection. This method, therefore, isolates a vulnerable individual from sources of infection.

Health care facilities develop their own systems of isolation and, depending on various factors, an individual may be nursed in a private or shared room. Generally, nursing an individual in a single room is a more effective method of preventing cross infection.

There are several isolation categories, depending on the virulence of the pathogen and on the mode of transmission:

- strict isolation
- respiratory isolation
- enteric precautions
- contact isolation
- drainage/secretion precautions
- blood/body fluid precautions
- protective isolation.

Table 61.2 provides guidelines for the various isolation precautions.

The infection control officer, or team, within a health care facility plays a major role in developing specific iso-

Table 61.2 Isolation guidelines

Isolation category	Guidelines
Strict Designed to prevent transmission of highly contagious or virulent infections that may be spread by air and direct contact, e.g. chickenpox	Single room with the door closed Gowns, masks, and gloves must be worn by all persons entering the room Hands must be washed on entering and leaving the room Articles contaminated with infective material must be bagged before they are sent for decontamination and reprocessing or disposal
Respiratory Designed to prevent transmission of infectious diseases through air (droplet transmission), e.g. measles, mumps, meningitis	Single room, or individuals infected with the same organism may share a room Masks must be worn by all persons entering the room Hands must be washed on entering and leaving the room Articles contaminated with infective material must be bagged before they are sent for decontamination and reprocessing or disposal
Enteric Designed to prevent transmission of infections that are spread thrpugh contact with faeces, e.g. diarrhoea of an infectious cause, hepatitis A	Single room may be indicated Gowns and gloves must be worn by all persons entering the room Hands must be washed on entering and leaving the room Articles contaminated with faeces must be disinfected or disposed of
Contact Designed to prevent the spread of infectious diseases that are transmitted by close or direct contact, e.g. herpes simplex, impetigo	Single room, or individuals infected with the same organism may share a room Masks must be worn by persons who have close contact with the individual Gowns must be worn if soiling is likely Gloves must be worn for touching infective material Hands must be washed on entering and leaving the room Articles contaminated with infective material should bagged before they are sent for decontamination and reprocessing or disposal
Drainage/secretion Designed to prevent infections that are transmitted by contact with purulent material or drainage from an infected body site, e.g. infected wounds or infected burns	Single room not essential. Gowns must be worn if soiling is likely Gloves must be worn for touching infective material Hands must be washed on entering and leaving the room Articles contaminated with infective material must be bagged before they are sent for decontamination and reprocessing or disposal

Table 61.2 (cont'd) Isolation guidelines

Isolation category	Guidelines
Blood and body fluids Designed to prevent infections that are transmitted by contact with infective blood or body fluids, e.g. hepatitis B, HIV injection (AIDS)	Single room not generally necessary Masks and protective eye-wear, or face shields, must be worn during procedures that may result in spilling or splashing of blood or other body fluids Gloves must be worn by all persons entering the room Gowns must be worn if soiling of clothing with blood or body fluids is likely Articles contaminated with infective material must be placed in leak-proof bags before they are sent for decontamination and reprocessing or disposal Needles, syringes, and other sharp items must be placed in rigid-wall, puncture-proof containers before they are transported for disposal Care must be taken to avoid needle-stick injuries Spills of blood or other body fluids must be wiped up with wad of cottonwool soaked in a suitable solution, e.g. 1% hypochlorite solution Hands must be washed by all persons entering and leaving the room
Protective Designed to prevent transmission of infections to vulnerable individuals	Single room with door closed Gowns, masks, gloves worn by all persons entering the room Hands must be washed on entering and leaving the room Articles brought into the room must be either clean or sterile

lation precautions, and the nurse must know how and when those precautions should be implemented. An information card is generally fixed to the door of the individual's room, so that all staff and visitors are informed of the measures to be implemented.

Preparation for isolation

Before isolation precautions are implemented, the individual and his significant others require thorough explanations about the precautions and their rationale. The information provided must be comprehensive in order to prevent spread of infection through ignorance or carelessness.

The information should be provided in a sensitive manner to reduce any feelings of resentment or apprehension that the individual may experience. He may feel that he is a nuisance, is unclean, or is afflicted with some disease that makes him unacceptable to others. The individual may also be anxious that no-one will come into his room to care for or visit him.

Because isolation may lead to withdrawal or sensory deprivation, the individual is reassured that measures will be implemented to provide adequate stimulation. He should be provided with means of diversion, e.g. a television set, telephone, books and magazines, craft projects, or other forms of diversion that interest him. The nurse should also tell the individual that she will visit him at times other than those when he requires physical care. Ideally, the door should be fitted with a glass panel so that he can see people outside the room. Similarly, the room should have an outside view as a means of reducing the individual's feeling of being isolated.

The isolation unit

The individual who needs to be isolated may remain in his room, or he may be transferred to a specially designed isolation unit. The unit is set up to prevent the transmission of microorganisms to other people and areas i.e. to prevent cross infection.

Isolation techniques are based on an understanding of 'clean' and 'contaminated'. *Clean* refers to those areas or objects that are uncontaminated or free of pathogenic microorganisms. *Contaminated* refers to those areas or objects that have been in contact with infective, or potentially infective, material. If a clean area or object comes into contact with something that is contaminated, it is then considered to be contaminated.

To prevent the transmission of microorganisms, the isolation unit should contain most of the items that are necessary for the individual's use and care. Where possible disposable items are used, and the unit should contain:

— handbasin with running water
— paper towels in a dispenser
— liquid soap or antiseptic solution in a dispenser
— soiled linen receiver lined with a plastic bag
— rubbish container lined with a plastic bag
— waste basket lined with a plastic bag
— bath and/or shower
— toilet, and bedpan/urinal sanitizer
— bedpan and/or urinal, and toilet paper
— washbowl, toothmug, emesis bowl, soap dish
— telephone
— television set
— thermometer, sphygmomanometer, stethoscope
— supply of bed linen
— supply of plastic bags for waste
— paper tissues
— personal items, e.g. hairbrush, toothbrush, shaving equipment
— wall clock with a second hand.

Items to be placed immediately outside the room, e.g. in a cupboard or on a trolley, include:

— gowns
— masks
— gloves
— clean laundry and rubbish bags
— tags for marking contaminated bags.

A card is placed on the door leading into the room, which specifies which isolation techniques are being practised.

Special isolation precautions

Special precautions implemented in isolation nursing include the use of gowns and masks, double-bagging, and correct hand washing techniques.

Gowning technique

A gown is worn to prevent contamination of the clothing by pathogenic microorganisms, thus preventing cross infection. Gowns may also be worn to protect a vulnerable individual, who is being isolated for his own protection, from microorganisms that may be on the clothing of persons entering his room.

A gown may be made of paper and be disposable, or made from cotton and be re-usable. A gown should be long and large enough to cover the clothing completely, and open down the back where it is tied at the neck and waist. The inside of the gown is considered to be clean, and the outside is considered contaminated. This point is of particular importance if the gown has been worn previously and is to worn again.

To put on a gown, the hands are first washed and dried. A clean gown is picked up, and held out to allow it to unfold. The arms are slipped inside the sleeves and if it is necessary to adjust any part of the gown, this is done by handling the inside only. The neck tapes are tied, then the waist tapes are tied at the back.

To remove a gown, only the inside is handled once the waist tapes have been untied—because the outside of the gown is considered contaminated. The waist tapes are untied, the hands are washed and dried, and the neck tapes are untied. The gown is slipped off, turning it inside out as it is being removed. The gown is placed in the soiled linen container or, if it is disposable, placed in the rubbish container. The hands are washed and dried before leaving the room.

If a used gown is to remain in the room so that it can be worn again, it may be hung up so that the outside of the gown faces outward.

Face masks

Face masks are worn to prevent the spread of microorganisms from the respiratory tract. If there is a risk of splash contamination by blood or other body fluids, a more substantial face shield and/or eye goggles should be worn. Disposable masks are worn and discarded immediately after use. When a mask is used:

- it is handled only by the tapes or loops at either end
- it must cover the nose and mouth completely
- it must not be allowed to hang around the neck, as this practice results in contamination
- it must be changed as soon as it becomes damp, as moisture allows microorganisms to pass through the mask
- the hands are washed and dried after the mask is removed.

Double-bagging technique

Safe removal of contaminated articles, e.g. soiled linen, from an isolation room may require double-bagging to confine contamination and limit the spread of infection. Double-bagging is not performed routinely, but the method may be practised when the outside of a bag is visibly contaminated.

When articles need to be removed from the room, two people are required. The nurse inside the individual's room places the contaminated articles into a bag and seals the bag securely. Another person outside the door holds open a clean bag to receive the contaminated bag. Once this has been done, the person outside the room seals the clean bag securely. If the bag is not coloured distinctively, a label is placed on the outside of the bag to signify that the contents are contaminated.

Both persons wash and dry their hands after handling the bag/s.

Handwashing techniques

Effective hand washing techniques must be implemented if cross infection is to be prevented. Correct handwashing remains the most effective means of preventing cross infection. Correct handwashing technique involves:

- warm running water
- elbow-operated taps
- liquid soap or an antibacterial substance
- washing the forearms as well as the hands, and paying particular attention to the skin between the fingers, and the fingernails
- washing for at least 1 minute
- thorough rinsing after washing
- using disposable towels or a hot air blower for drying.

Clean hands with intact skin, short fingernails and no rings, minimize the risk of contamination and cross infection.

Principles of isolation techniques

Although health care facilities develop and implement their own isolation precautions, such precautions are based on the following general principles:

- Each step in the care plan is carefully devised to minimize the risk of cross infection, as one act of carelessness can result in a spread of infection. Before any nursing activity is performed, the technique to be used should be planned carefully so that the risk of cross infection is minimized. Once the nurse's hands have become contaminated, she must not handle any of her own possessions, e.g. watch, pen, scissors, or any part of her uniform. To reduce the risk of acts of carelessness, items such as a pen and scissors should be kept in the room. To avoid the need to use personal watches for measuring the individual's vital signs, the room should be equipped with a wall clock with a second hand.
- People should avoid touching their hair, nose, mouth, or eyes while caring for an individual in isolation.
- Protective clothing, e.g. gowns, masks, and gloves, are put on before entering or immediately on entering the room. Disposable clothing is preferable, or non-disposable clothing may be used once then placed in the appropriate container for decontamination and reprocessing. If a gown is to be worn more than once, it must be put on and removed as described on page 696.
- Hands should be washed on entering the room, after contact with the individual or contaminated articles, and before leaving the room. *Correct hand washing technique* is the most effective way of preventing cross infection.
- Items used during care of the individual should be disposable when possible. Re-usable items should be kept in the room and, when they are removed for decontamination and reprocessing, they are bagged, and labelled as 'infective'.
- Concurrent disinfection is practised while the individual remains in isolation.

Disinfection

Disinfection is the destruction of all pathogenic microorganisms, but not the spores.

Concurrent disinfection

Concurrent disinfection is the disinfection of an article immediately after it has been used. Disposable equipment lessens the need for disinfection and also reduces the risk of spread of infection.

Articles which are not easily disinfected, e.g. sphygmomanometer, may be kept in the individual's room throughout the period of isolation. Other items, e.g. meal tray, tooth mug and wash bowl, may also be kept in the room and used exclusively by that individual—thereby making concurrent disinfection unnecessary.

Each health care institution has its own policy in relation to disinfection techniques. Examples of practices which may be implemented are:

1. Food scraps. Food scraps may either be flushed down the toilet, or wrapped in paper and placed into a plastic bag. The bag is sealed and sent for incineration.

2. Crockery and cutlery. These should be disposable as far as possible. Non-disposable items may be disinfected by washing in hot soapy water and autoclaving.

3. Linen. Contaminated linen may be placed in a polythene bag sewn with an alginate thread which is soluble. When soda ash is added to the water in the washing machine, the thread dissolves, the bag falls apart, and the linen is liberated into the water. Before this bag is sent to the laundry, it may be placed inside another bag. The bag may be a distinctive colour, or labelled, which indicates to all personnel that special precautions are necessary when handling the bag of linen.

4. Excreta and body discharges. To minimize the risk of splash contamination occurring when a container is carried or emptied, a disinfectant solution may be placed into a bedpan, urinal, sputum receiver, or drainage bottle. The contents of the container are flushed down the toilet, as an efficient sewerage system copes with microorganisms carried by excreta. A disposable receiver for sputum should be used, and this is placed in a bag for incineration. Bedpans, urinals, emesis bowls, and drainage bottles may be disinfected in a steam pressure sterilizer.

5. Dressing materials, paper towels and tissues. These are placed in a leak-proof bag which is placed in another bag, for incineration. Disposable gloves, gowns, and masks are treated in the same manner.

Terminal disinfection

Terminal disinfection refers to the normal cleaning procedures which are performed after the transfer, discharge, or death of an individual who has been in isolation. Most Australian states require that the body of a person who had an infectious condition be placed in a special plastic bag.

The contents of the unit, and all items of equipment which have been used in the care of the individual are cleaned and disinfected. The method used should be sufficiently thorough to destroy all pathogenic microorganisms. Most health care facilities have personnel who are experienced in, and responsible for, terminal disinfection procedures.

CONCLUSION

When an individual has an infective condition it may be necessary to isolate him, to prevent the transmission of microorganisms.

As health care facilities develop their own isolation precautions and techniques, the nurse must be aware of how and when they should be implemented. The nurse must remember that even one act of carelessness could result in spread of an infection.

REFERENCES AND FURTHER READING

Benn R A V 1985 Aids to microbiology and infectious diseases. Churchill Livingstone, Edinburgh

Potter P A, Perry A G 1985 Fundamentals of nursing. C V Mosby, St Louis

Sorensen K C, Luckmann J 1986 Basic nursing, a psychophysiologic approach, 2nd edn. W B Saunders, Philadelphia

62. The individual who requires community-based care

OBJECTIVES

1. State the settings where nurses may be involved in the delivery of community-based nursing care.
2. Discuss the categories of individuals who may require home-based nursing care.
3. In accordance with specified role and function, assist in planning and implementing care of an individual and/or family in the home.

INTRODUCTION

Nursing services are provided in a variety of community settings in addition to those which are available in hospitals and other institutions. Community based nursing services are concerned with health promotion and maintenance, health education, co-ordination and continuity of care within the community.

There is an increasing emphasis on the role of community nursing in the provision of adequate health services for a variety of reasons, e.g. awareness of the importance of health promotion and disease prevention, the high cost of institutional care, and a trend towards early discharge from hospital. Areas where nursing services are provided include child health and school medical services, industry, maternal and infant welfare, family health centres, day care centres, centres for people with developmental disabilities, alcohol and drug rehabilitation centres, family planning centres, mental health centres, and people's homes. In many services nursing care is provided at a community centre, while other services provide nursing care in the home.

Community health nursing differs from hospital-based nursing in many ways, e.g. it is largely concerned with health promotion and illness prevention, it is continuing rather than episodic, and it is more family and community centred.

While community health nurses may be employed in a variety of settings, this chapter focuses on the delivery of nursing care to people in their own homes. For information on other areas of community nursing practice, the nurse is advised to refer to the texts listed at the end of the chapter.

Home nursing care is provided by a variety of organizations in each state of Australia. Nurses who are involved in the provision of home nursing care may be called community nurses, district nurses, or domiciliary nurses. Home nursing services may be provided by hospitals, local or state government agencies, church organizations, or private agencies. All domiciliary services, e.g. home nursing, hospice domiciliary care, and home help, enable people to remain at home and thus provide an alternative to hospitalization.

Individuals requiring home nursing services

Domiciliary nurses deliver continuing nursing care which may be preventive, curative, rehabilitative, or palliative, for individuals who are experiencing an acute, chronic, or terminal illness. Individuals who may require home nursing services include those who:

- Have been discharged from hospital and require continued nursing assistance, e.g. to change wound dressings, administer medications, or to care for a stoma.
- Require assistance in the performance of the activities of daily living, e.g. personal cleansing and dressing, eliminating, or mobilizing.
- Require special treatment involving the use of sophisticated equipment, e.g. dialysis, total parenteral nutrition, or ventilatory support.
- Require continued assessment of their physical or mental state and/or their ability to manage at home.
- Require care and support following the birth of a baby, e.g. assessment of the health of both mother and infant or advice on aspects of infant care.
- Require instruction in techniques which will help them to attain or maintain independence, e.g. how to administer medications by injection.
- Require counselling and emotional support, e.g. to recover from or adjust to an acute or a chronic illness, or to

699

cope with a situation such as caring for a sick or disabled relative in the home.

• Are experiencing a terminal illness. Domiciliary hospice programmes enable individuals to remain at home for as long as they wish or is possible. The visiting nurse assists in this process in various ways, e.g. implementing measures to control pain and promote comfort, administering medications, and providing support for the family.

• Require assistance to maintain their present level of functioning or to restore lost or reduced function, e.g. by performing range of motion exercises.

• Require assistance to arrange for other community support services, e.g. home help, or meals on wheels.

The individual who is receiving home nursing care, together with the family, should also be provided with information about health promotion. The domiciliary nurse, therefore, has an important educative role to play.

Goals of home nursing services

Domiciliary nursing services develop a nursing philosophy which reflects the goals of the organization. They also develop standards which serve as guidelines for evaluating nursing care. Inherent in a typical philosophy is the belief that a community has the right to expect skilled nursing care which assists ill or disabled persons to remain in the security and comfort of their own home, together with a committment to promoting the preventive, curative, rehabilitative, and palliative aspects of nursing care.

Domiciliary nursing services also recognize the importance of considering an individual's total environment which includes his family and significant others, his culture, his home, his lifestyle, and his socio-economic status. When developing standards a domiciliary nursing service considers the importance of:

• providing comprehensive nursing care to individuals and families

• assisting individuals to maintain or regain their independence

• providing support for family members or significant others who are caring for an ill or disabled person at home

• promoting understanding of the measures necessary to promote health and prevent illness

• using the nursing process to assess, plan, implement, and evaluate home nursing care.

Aspects of domiciliary care

A nurse who is involved in the delivery of nursing care to people in their own homes must appreciate the importance of:

• Recognizing the individual's right to autonomy and confidentiality, and understanding the legal implications of

nursing practice within a home nursing situation. The nurse must always remember that she is a *visitor* in a person's home and, therefore, can only implement actions at the person's invitation. It is essential that the nurse obtains an individual's informed consent before carrying out any nursing activities. A situation may also arise where an individual refuses to allow the domiciliary nurse to enter his home, or asks her to leave. If such an event was to occur the nurse must respect the individual's wishes, or she may be guilty of infringing the law of *trespass*.

• Being flexible and adaptable, e.g. to accept a variety of lifestyles and home conditions to which individuals are accustomed. A domiciliary nurse is frequently required to deliver nursing care in situations which are vastly different from those in a hospital where physical facilities and equipment are specifically designed and readily available.

• Having good assessment skills. A domiciliary nurse is required not only to assess the individual to determine his health care needs, but she may also be required to assess his social situation and his physical environment. She may need to assess the physical attributes of a home in terms of an individual's needs, usual activities, and safety. The domiciliary nurse may need to determine whether the individual would benefit from having certain changes made in the home, e.g. installation of a seat across the bath, a hand-held shower, or handrails in the toilet.

• Having knowledge of available community resources, so that she can suggest those that are appropriate, e.g. home help, meals on wheels, handyman service, day-care centre.

• Liaising with hospital, medical, and paramedical staff. For example, prior to an individual's discharge from hospital a visit from a domiciliary nurse may be requested. The nurse, in consultation with the individual and the hospital staff, discusses the discharge plan. Thus, both the individual and the domiciliary nurse are aware of the home nursing services which will be required.

• Keeping accurate and current written records of all home visits. Domiciliary nurses use the nursing process to assess, plan, implement, and evaluate an individual's care. Part of the process involves maintaining written records containing information related to nursing care and the individual's progress.

• Supervising any activities prescribed, and reinforcing instructions given, by other members of the health team, e.g. the physiotherapist or speech pathologist.

• Instructing the individual and/or family members in specific skills, e.g. changing a colostomy bag or injecting insulin.

The domiciliary nurse also plays an important role in educating the individual and/or family members in measures that promote health, and in teaching them to recognize the signs or symptoms which indicate a health problem and which should be reported to a medical officer.

It is important that a nurse who is involved in domiciliary nursing recognizes that the knowledge and skills applicable to hospital-based nursing also apply to home-based nursing care. The only difference is the *setting* in which the delivery of nursing care takes place. Therefore, a domiciliary nurse needs to be able to transfer her knowledge and skills into a community setting in order to assist an individual in the activities of living. The activities of living, as identified by Roper, Logan, and Tierney, (1985) are:

- maintaining a safe environment
- communicating
- breathing
- eating and drinking
- eliminating
- personal cleansing and dressing
- controlling body temperature
- mobilizing
- working and playing
- expressing sexuality
- sleeping
- dying.

Information on assisting the individual in each of these activities is provided in several chapters of this text.

It is also important for a nurse to understand that the notion of community health nursing, in general, is part of a thrust towards primary health care.

Primary health care is defined as:

Essential health care based on practical, scientifically sound and socially accepted methods and technology made universally accessible to individuals and families in the community through their full participation and at a cost that the community and country can afford to maintain at every stage of their development in the spirit of self-reliance and self-determination. It is the first level of contact of individuals, the family and community with the national health systems bringing health care as close as possible to where people live and work, and constitutes the first element of a continuing health care process. (WHO UNICEF 1978)

Further information on primary health care is provided in Chapter 8.

CONCLUSION

Community based nursing services are concerned with health promotion and maintenance, health education, co-ordination and continuity of care within the community.

Community health nurses work in a variety of settings, e.g. schools, industry, infant and family health centres, mental health centres, and in people's homes.

The notion of community health nursing is part of a thrust towards primary health care, which focuses on assisting people to maintain and improve their health and prevent illness.

One aspect of community nursing is domiciliary care, whereby nurses assess, plan, implement and evaluate nursing care in people's homes.

While the setting is different, the goals of domiciliary care are the same as those for hospital-based care, i.e. to assist an individual to maintain or attain independence in the activities of daily living.

REFERENCES AND FURTHER READING

Clements A 1986 Infant and family health in Australia. Churchill Livingstone, Melbourne
Green L W, Anderson C L 1986 Community health, 5th edn. Times Mirror/Mosby, St Louis
Logan B B, Dawkins C E 1986 Family-centered nursing in the community. Addison-Wesley, California
McMurray A 1990 Community health nursing: a primary health care approach. Churchill Livingstone, Melbourne
Rice V (ed) 1985 Community nursing practice. Williams and Wilkins, Adis, Balgowlah

Roper N, Logan W W, Tierney A 1990 The elements of nursing, 3rd edn. Churchill Livingstone, Edinburgh
Stanhope M, Lancaster J 1988 Community health nursing, 2nd edn. Mosby, St Louis
Vimpani G, Parry T 1989 Community child health: an Australian perspective. Churchill Livingstone, Melbourne
World Health Organization 1978 Alma ata Primary health care. World Health Organization, Geneva

63. The chemical-dependent individual

INTRODUCTION

The nurse, as a health educator and as a member of the general community, has a responsibility to be aware of the various aspects of substance abuse, misuse, and dependency. Substance abuse is one of the major problems faced by many societies, and it ranges from excessive use of products such as tobacco and alcohol—to misuse of non-prescription substances such as vitamins, aspirin, and laxatives—to the abuse of prescription drugs, and the use and abuse of illegal drugs such as heroin, cocaine, and marijuana.

In the context, of this chapter a substance refers to any chemical or drug that can be self administered. Substance abuse is a major social and health problem; and is associated with many health risks, dependence, economic effects, breakdown of relationships, criminal activities, and death. The nurse needs to be aware of the problems associated with substance abuse, e.g. the various factors which may contribute to abuse, the effects of abuse on the abuser and others, and the health problems associated with substance abuse.

Concepts of abuse and misuse

Substance abuse, or misuse is not easily defined, but it may be broadly defined as the acute or chronic use of a substance which results in impaired physical or psychosocial functioning. A substance is being *misused*, whether it is one which has been prescribed or purchased 'over the counter', if it is taken improperly or indiscriminately. A substance is being *abused* if it is taken regularly and indiscriminately in quantities that impair the individual's physiological, psychological, or social functioning.

Dependence develops with repeated use of a substance, to the extent that the individual needs the effects of that substance in order to function. Dependence may be physical and/or psychological. Physical dependence results when the individual experiences symptoms of withdrawal when the substance is discontinued. Psychological dependence results when the individual has a compulsion to continue using a substance in order to experience its effects, e.g. enhancement of self esteem and sense of wellbeing.

Tolerance to a substance develops when the body attempts to adapt to repeated exposure to specific chemical agents. With repeated use of a substance the user requires increasing amounts to produce the same effects.

Factors leading to substance abuse

Substance abuse results from a variety of factors including those that are physical, social, psychological, and cultural. An individual may begin to misuse or abuse a substance:

- as a means of relieving boredom
- to help 'solve' or avoid a problem
- as a result of peer pressure
- to seek a new experience
- to relieve stress, tension, depression, anxiety, or low self esteem
- to cope with adverse social conditions
- because of a genetic predisposition, e.g. some researchers suspect that alcoholism is caused by a genetically transmitted biochemical defect
- because substances are readily available
- as a result of media influence which portrays some substances, e.g. alcohol and nicotine, as socially acceptable.

What often begins as misuse of a substance can lead to

abuse. For example consumption of alcohol may begin with social drinking, which can lead to the consumption of larger amounts for longer periods of time and at more frequent intervals. If this pattern continues, the individual may become physically and psychologically dependent on alcohol and develop tolerance. As dependence increases, the individual may use alcohol as a means of coping with stress or of avoiding facing up to problems. After some time, he may find that he is unable to function without alcohol, and he may experience withdrawal symptoms if he stops or decreases alcohol consumption.

An individual who misuses other substances, e.g. tranquilizers, may experience the same pattern of dependence, tolerance, and withdrawal.

Effects of abuse

Substance abuse has a variety of adverse effects on the abuser and on the significant others. The effects are physical, psychological, and social. The physical effects on the abuser are illustrated in Table 63.1, and some of the effects on the abuser's significant others include:

- feelings on confusion, resentment, anger, isolation, guilt
- breakdown of relationships
- family conflicts
- economic difficulties
- impaired self concept
- physical and/or emotional abuse.

Abused substances

When the topic of substance abuse is discussed, the majority of people think only of those substances which are obtained illegally, e.g. heroin or cocaine. In fact, there are a wide variety of substances which are commonly abused. Table 63.1 illustrates the major types of abused substances and their effects.

In Australia, alcohol is considered to be the substance which is most abused. Alcohol abuse is associated with physical ill health, suicide, absenteeism, loss of income and productivity, traffic accidents, crime, and domestic violence. Therefore, while the seriousness of the abuse of substances such as heroin and cocaine cannot be overstated, it is clear that alcohol abuse seriously affects the nation's health and safety, its occupational health and safety, its productivity and social welfare structures, and the quality of family life. The National Health and Medical Research Council estimates for 1987 showed alcohol-related disease and injury cost Australian industry more than $2 500 000 a day.

Tobacco is regarded as Australia's second most commonly abused substance with smoking-related illnesses accounting for six times more working days lost than in-

Table 63.1 Substances of abuse

Substance	Administration	Effects
Alcohol	Ingested	Decreased inhibitions Euphoria Impaired co-ordination and judgment Slurred speech Nausea, vomiting Tremors, dizzyness, thirst Altered liver function, acid-base balance, and electrolyte balance Neurological damage Peripheral neuropathy Cardiac dysfunction Cirrhosis of the liver Gastritis, pancreatitis
Nicotine	Smoked (or chewed)	Stimulant Decreased appetite Craving Anxiety, restlessness Lung cancer Chronic pulmonary disease Cardiovascular disease
Caffeine	Ingested	Stimulant Tachycardia Nervousness, restlessness Extrasystoles Indigestion
Anxiolytics: barbiturates benzodiazepines	Ingested Injected	Relaxation Relief of anxiety Drowsiness Slurred speech Hypotension Confusion Depression Depressant effects enhanced by alcohol
Amphetamines	Ingested Injected	Stimulant Euphoria Impaired judgment Suppression of appetite Tachycardia Hypertension Dysrhythmias Nausea, vomiting, diarrhoea Irritability Toxic psychosis

Cannabis:
  Marijuana
  Hashish
	Smoked
	Ingested
		Loss of inhibition
		Relaxation
		Increased clarity and sensitivity
		Impaired thinking
		Apathy
		Difficulty in concentrating
		Altered libido
		Agitation, disorientation

Hallucinogens:
  LSD
  PCP
	Ingested
	Smoked
	Snorted
		Altered perception
		Hallucinations
		Illusions
		Delusions
		Dilated pupils
		Hypertension
		Ataxia
		Increased salivation
		Panic reactions
		Aggression

Table 63.1 (cont'd) Substances of abuse

Substance	Administration	Effects
Cocaine ('crack' is a form of free-based cocaine)	Snorted Smoked Injected	Euphoria Mood elevation Hyperactivity Craving Sleep disturbances Erosion of nasal mucosa Perforated nasal septum Respiratory/cardiovascular collapse Cocaine psychosis
Narcotics: Morphine Papaveretum Pethidine Codeine Heroin Opium	Ingested Injected	Pain reduction Mood changes Euphoria Drowsiness Impaired judgment Constricted pupils Slurred speech Respiratory/circulatory depression Unconsciousness
Non-narcotic analgesics, e.g: Aspirin Paracetamol	Ingested	Pain relief Tinnitus Temporary deafness Gastritis Increased bleeding time Hepatotoxicity Nephropathy
Laxatives	Ingested Inserted rectally	Defaecation Flatulence Diarrhoea Abdominal discomfort Habit forming May interfere with the absorption of fat-soluble vitamins
Inhalants, e.g: petrol paint thinner lighter fluid glue	Sniffed	Central nervous system depression Bronchial and laryngeal irritation Headaches Vertigo Ataxia Euphoria Depression Coma

dustrial disputes, and individuals with such illnesses filling more than 920 000 hospital beds each year.

Various substances, generally regarded by the majority of people to be harmless, can cause health problems if used improperly. Many 'over the counter' products such as aspirin, cold remedies, laxatives, or vitamins, have the potential for misuse, abuse, and dependence. Prescribed substances may be misused if an individual does not clearly understand the correct use and dosage. Many prescribed substances produce effects similar to those produced by illegally obtained substances, and some individual go to extraordinary lengths to obtain quantities sufficient to meet their needs.

Care of the individual

Nurses working in various settings either within the health care system or the community, are likely to come into contact with someone who is a substance abuser. Nurses need, therefore, to increase their knowledge of substance abuse to enable effective implementation of measures to assist an individual who is chemically dependent.

Whenever possible, a chemically-dependent person is admitted to a special detoxification and rehabilitation centre or unit, which is staffed by personnel who are qualified in the management of substance abuse. Such facilities are not available in all areas, therefore nurses may be involved in caring for the individual in a general hospital setting. An individual may be admitted for management of a substance abuse problem, or the problem may be detected while he is being treated for another condition.

When the care plan is developed, long and short-term goals are established. Generally, the long-term goal is to establish a pattern of abstinence from the substance. Short-term goals are directed towards implementing measures to relieve the symptoms of withdrawal, educating the individual in stress management techniques, counselling the abuser and his significant others, and promoting the use of support groups. The nursing care plan also includes measures to deal with various problems which are related to substance abuse such as sleep disturbances, nutritional deficits, altered gastrointestinal functioning, low self esteem, depression, and decreased motivation.

Acute care of an individual may involve emergency medical treatments such as the administration of narcotic antagonists, respiratory support, and treatment for withdrawal symptoms. Once the emergency situation, e.g. coma or overdose, is under control any secondary complications are attended to. Secondary complications include physical injuries related to falls, and infections. As the initial emergency situation eases, interventions continue to address physiological problems, and the individual's psychosocial needs.

Laboratory studies are generally performed to detect related health problems and complications. Specimens, e.g. of blood, urine, or gastric contents, may be collected for legal purposes. Diagnostic studies include examination of blood and urine to detect the presence of a substance, e.g. barbiturate levels or blood alcohol levels. Other diagnostic studies include chest x-ray, electrocardiogram, electroencephalogram, and complete blood count.

The management of an individual who is admitted for detoxification, i.e. to *withdraw* from an abused substance, varies according to several factors such as the philosophy of the unit, and the type and dosage of the abused substance. In detoxification units, or other centres involved in drug and alcohol abuse management, the emphasis is on individual evaluation. A detoxification programme is then designed to meet the individual's needs, and different approaches may be used depending on the substance is being abused or whether the individual is a polydrug user. Polydrug users are individuals who are using and abusing more than one substance at a time, e.g. heroin and barbiturates, or alcohol and amphetamines.

Most withdrawal (detoxification) programmes are directed towards preventing serious complications, keeping the use of other chemicals to a minimum, and providing psychological support during the process of detoxification. Withdrawal may be implemented gradually or abruptly ('cold turkey'). Gradual withdrawal aims to prevent the complications sometimes associated with sudden withdrawal of an abused substance.

Some units implement a non-medication approach, e.g. in the case of withdrawal from alcohol, where the individual is admitted and monitored closely. No alcohol or mood-altering medications are administered, and the emphasis is on providing adequate psychological support to reduce the individual's anxiety level. Alcohol detoxification generally takes approximately 72 hours.

Other units adopt a medical approach whereby specific prescribed medications are administered during the process of withdrawal. For example, during withdrawal from alcohol the individual may be prescribed diazepam. This method involves replacing alcohol with diazepam and then withdrawing the individual from this medication in a controlled way.

Units dealing with abuse of illegal substances such as heroin, may use methadone maintenance programmes. Methadone is a synthetic compound which blocks the effects of heroin. Controversy exists over the use of methadone, as one hazard of prolonged methadone maintenance is *dependence*. Those who argue against this form of treatment claim that dependence on methadone is merely substituted for dependence on heroin, and that it is a *chemical solution* which fails to encourage the abuser to find solutions to the problems that lead to substance abuse initially.

During the process of withdrawal or detoxification, the individual's vital signs are monitored every 2–4 hours, and the nurse assesses him for the manifestation of withdrawal symptoms. Symptoms of withdrawal may include tremors, sweating, nausea and vomiting, agitation, insomnia, abdominal and muscular pains, hallucinations, seizures, anxiety attacks. A properly planned withdrawal programme aims to prevent or minimize these and other symptoms.

The individual's basic needs must be met during the process of withdrawal, with particular emphasis on his need for nutrition, fluids, elimination, safety, and psychological support.

Sometimes, when a chemical-dependent individual is admitted in a drugged or intoxicated state, his behaviour may be abusive and/or manipulative. Information on the management of an individual who is abusive is provided in Chapter 56.

Management of a chemical-dependent person, once the acute phase passes, involves teaching and counselling, promoting healthy ways of dealing with stress, and encouraging participation in self-help groups. While some individuals give up substance abuse successfully, others return to their previous pattern of abuse. Nurses need to recognize that substance abuse is a long-term problem, and that prevention is generally easier to achieve than cure.

A variety of community programmes and self-help groups are available to assist the individual and his significant others. Support groups, e.g. Alcoholics Anonymous and Al-Anon, aim to assist individuals to acknowledge the problem and work toward solving it. A supportive unit, for the individual and his significant others, is especially important particularly during the first year of recovery. Substance abuse prevention programmes are being implemented in schools and community health settings, and they aim to provide accurate drug education and to assist individuals to develop self-esteem and interpersonal skills. It is important that nurses are aware of the community programmes and other available resources to which individuals in need can be referred. Some of these resources are listed in telephone directories.

CONCLUSION

Substance abuse is one of the most serious health and social problems of the time. As the problem has become more recognized, a variety of preventive programmes, support and treatment services have been established. As a health educator and as a member of the general community, the nurse has a responsibility to increase her knowledge of the problem of substance abuse.

REFERENCES AND FURTHER READING

Kneisl C R, Ames S W 1986 Adult health nursing: a biopsychosocial approach. Addison-Wesley, Massachusetts, ch 10, 231–265
Potter P A, Perry A G 1985 Fundamentals of nursing. C V Mosby, St Louis, ch 45, 1283–1303

64. The individual with cancer

INTRODUCTION

The term 'cancer' is perceived by many people to signify inevitable death, which is preceded by unpleasant treatments and pain. In the past some forms of cancer were almost always fatal, but now with early detection and effective therapy the potential for long-term cure has improved significantly.

The nurse is very likely to care for, or know, someone who has cancer, therefore in order to assist those concerned to deal with the disease it is important that she is familiar with the neoplastic process and its effects, its treatments and their side effects, its forms and their prognoses. Such knowledge is valuable in helping to plan, implement, and evaluate the care required by the individual with cancer.

Terminology

Various terms used in relation to cancer include:

- *Cancer*: any of a large group of malignant neoplastic diseases that are characterized by the presence of malignant cells. Or, a neoplasm characterized by the uncontrolled growth of cells that tend to invade surrounding tissue and metastasize to distant body sites.
- *Tumour*: a new growth of tissue characterized by progressive, uncontrolled proliferation of cells. Also called a neoplasm.
- *Benign*: not malignant, non-cancerous.
- *Malignant*: tending to become progressively worse and cause death, e.g. as in a malignant tumour.
- *Metastasis/metastases*: the process by which malignant cells are spread to distant sites in the body. A *primary* tumour is the first in order of time, place, or development. A *secondary* tumour occurs at a distant site through the process of metastasis.
- *Oncology*: the study of tumours.
- *Carcinogen*: a substance or factor that causes the development of a cancer.
- *Oncogens*: genetic material, thought to be latent in the chromosomes of some individuals, that can bring about malignant transformation.
- *Carcinomas*: malignant neoplasms arising from epithelial tissue.
- *Saracomas*: malignant neoplasms arising from fibrous, fatty, muscular, synovial, vascular, or neural tissue.
- *Leukaemias*: malignant neoplasms arising from the blood-forming organs (bone marrow, spleen).
- *Lymphomas*: neoplasms, benign or malignant, arising from lymphatic tissue.

Oncogenesis

Oncogenesis is the process by which neoplasms are produced. It is known that development of a neoplasm is related to disturbances in normal cell growth, replication, and migration. A neoplasm is a mass of cells that proliferate without normal control, to form tumours which do not have any useful function.

A neoplastic cell develops in the same way as a normal cell, i.e. the life cycle of the cell is comprised of five phases:

- resting
- synthesis of R.N.A. and protein
- synthesis of D.N.A.

- preparation for mitosis
- mitosis—during which an original cell divides to form two new cells.

Neoplastic cells are mutated cells which do not respond to the structural and chemical signals that normally regulate the replication of cells. Tumours comprised of malignant cells have certain characteristics. They:

- are invasive
- are rarely encapsulated
- usually grow rapidly
- may recur after removal
- cause death if growth is not controlled and arrested
- frequently metastasize via lymphatic channels or blood vessels to other body sites
- produce generalized symptoms such as weight loss and anaemia.

Causes of cancer

There are many factors which are known, or thought, to be related to the development of cancer. Various forms of cancer have been attributed to one or more of these factors.

Oncogenes. It is thought that, in a normal cell, the oncogenes are repressed by the products of certain regulatory genes. Therefore, for carcinogenesis to occur, these regulatory genes must be defective or repressed, e.g. by physical or chemical carcinogens. Once the regulatory genes are not functioning, carcinogenesis may take place.

Viruses. As viruses have been demonstrated to cause tumours in animals, it is considered possible that certain viruses may also influence the development of cancer in humans. The human T-cell leukaemia virus has been linked to leukaemia, and the Epstein-Barr virus to Burkitt's lymphoma. However, the evidence that viruses cause cancer is not definitive.

Genetics. Some forms of cancer arise from disturbances of the genetic material after conception. Oncogenes latent in the DNA of the parents' cells can be passed on to their children and may eventually become activated.

Immune response. Failure of the immune system to respond to tumour cells may result in cancer. Normally, the T-cell lymphocytes destroy damaged or foreign cells. Theoretically, cancer arises when certain factors inhibit the immune system, e.g. ageing cells, immunosuppressive therapy, or stress.

Environmental factors. It is thought that a high percentage of all cancers are related to environmental carcinogens such as chemicals, radiation, cigarettes, ultraviolet rays, and substances ingested in foods.

Nutrition. There is increasing evidence that dietary habits may play a role in preventing and causing cancer, e.g. a diet high in fat and protein—but low in fibre—has been linked to cancer of the colon and breast. A diet that is high in salted and pickled foods has been linked to cancer of the stomach.

Hormones. The role of hormones in carcinogenesis remains controversial, but it is thought that excessive production or use of certain hormones may produce cancer. Oestrogen has been linked to cancer of the endometrium, and synthetic oestrogen (diethylstilbestrol) to vaginal cancer in some daughters of women who received the drug during pregnancy.

Psychological factors. There is some belief that cancer may be related to psychosocial influences and stress. Although psychosocial factors are thought to play a role in cancer, the extent of this influence it remains in doubt. Some theories suggest that stress may alter or impair the immune response, thus creating a favourable environment for the development of malignant cells.

Effects of cancer

As a malignant tumour develops and grows, it produces local and systemic effects in the body. As the tumour increases in size it causes the local effects of pressure, erosion of adjacent tissue, and obstruction. The mass of cells presses on surrounding tissue causing necrosis of normal cells, and the mass may grow large enough to disrupt the flow of blood or lymph, or obstruct an organ. Haemorrhage may occur if the tumour erodes a blood vessel.

A growing tumour may produce a variety of general effects, depending on its type and location. The individual may experience anaemia, infection, loss of weight, loss of appetite, pain, anxiety or depression—as well as many other symptoms.

Pain associated with cancer may be caused by destruction of bone, inflammation, infection, necrosis, arterial ischaemia, venous engorgement, or pressure on nerves. Anxiety experienced by the individual, e.g. fear of disfigurement and death, can intensify the pain.

Weight loss results from anorexia leading to a decreased kilojoule intake, and from the increased metabolic requirements of the multiplying malignant cells.

Some of the indirect effects of malignant tumours may be life threatening, e.g. elevation of plasma calcium levels can affect the nervous system, cardiovascular system, gastrointestinal tract, and kidneys.

Prevention and early detection

The nurse is in a key position to educate the public about the prevention and early detection of cancer. Because the precise causes of many types of cancer remains unclear, it is not always possible to prevent their development; but the public should be made aware of known risk factors, the preventive measures to implement, and how to perform the techniques used to detect early evidence of tumours.

Known risk factors

The major known risk factors in the development of cancer are described in Table 64.1.

Table 64.1 Major risk factors for cancers

Site	Risk factors
Bladder	Exposure to environmental carcinogens, e.g. tobacco, nitrates, coffee, aniline dye, petroleum. Chronic bladder irritation and infection
Breast	Close relatives with a history of breast cancer Early menarche Late menopause Never given birth, or first child born when a woman is over 30 years of age Long-term oestrogen therapy for menopausal symptoms Alcohol History of fibrocystic breast disease
Colon, rectum	Familial polyposis History of polyposis or ulcerative colitis Diet high in fat and low in fibre
Liver	Exposure to environmental carcinogens, e.g. aflatoxin
Lung	Began smoking at an early age Smoking
Larynx	Heavy smoking Chronic inhalation of carcinogenic industrial and air pollutants, e.g. asbestos, radioactive dust
Mouth	Heavy tobacco use, especially when combined with alcohol use
Oesophagus, stomach	Chronic irritation, e.g. heavy smoking and excessive use of alcohol Family history of gastric cancer Dietary factors, e.g. large amounts of smoked, pickled, or salted foods
Ovaries	Family history of ovarian cancer Never given birth
Prostate gland	Not known, but may be associated with diet, hormonal status, sexuality, occupational exposure to rubber or heavy metals
Pancreas	Inhalation or absorption of carcinogens which are then excreted by the pancreas, e.g. industrial chemicals, food additives Cigarette smoking Diet high in fat and protein Chronic pancreatitis Chronic alcohol abuse
Skin	Excessive exposure to the sun Fair complexion Exposure to occupational pollutants, e.g. coal tar, creosote Sunspots (solar keratoses) Family history of melanoma
Testes	Not known, but related to factors which interfere with normal function of the testes, e.g. past history of trauma to the testes

Table 64.1 (cont'd) Major risk factors for cancers

Site	Risk factors
Uterus: • Cervix	Frequent intercourse or intercourse with many partners at an early age Herpesvirus II
• Endometrium	Abnormal uterine bleeding factors that produce Familial tendency History of uterine polyps or endometrial hyperplasia Obesity, hypertension, diabetes mellitus Excessive oestrogen stimulation
Vagina	Mother treated with diethylstilbestrol during the pregnancy
Vulva	Leukoplakia (epithelial hyperplasia) Chronic pruritis Chronic vulval granulomatous disease Obesity, hypertension, diabetes mellitus

Prevention

Prevention of cancer involves eliminating occupational and environmental carcinogens, and identifying those individuals who are most at risk. A related strategy, whereby the early manifestations of cancer are detected, is significant in reducing cancer-related deaths.

Early detection involves regular check-ups, awareness of the warning signals of cancer, and screening tests, such as breast (B.S.E.) and testicular self examination (T.S.E.). Information on B.S.E. and T.S.E., together with information on cervical smear testing, is provided in Chapter 49. Rectal and colon examinations, and testing for blood in the faeces are other screening tests which are now being performed regularly on individuals at risk of developing colorectal cancer.

Warning signals of cancer
1. **A sore that does not heal**
2. **Any unusual bleeding or discharge**
3. **Obvious change in a mole or wart**
4. **A change in bowel or bladder habits**
5. **Any thickening or lump in the breast or elsewhere**
6. **Persistent cough or hoarseness**
7. **Indigestion or difficulty in swallowing.**

Incidence of cancer

The incidence of cancer by percentage of population and site, varies throughout the world. For example, in Australia cancer is second only to heart disease as a cause of adult deaths. In Australia, cancer of the large intestine (colon and rectum) is the most common internal cancer. In the United States of America, cancer of the breast and of the lung are reported to be the most common forms. Some cancers are more common in certain groups of people, e.g. skin cancer is more common in Australian whites than in the native Aboriginal population; breast cancer is approximately six times more common in Europeans than in Japanese people. Table 64.2 illustrates the incidence of cancer in Australia, according to site.

Diagnosis of cancer

Cancer may be diagnosed by various means. A thorough medical history is obtained and a comprehensive physical examination is performed. The physical examination includes visual inspection, palpation, and percussion. Haematologic studies and tests on urine and faeces may form part of the preliminary assessment.

If there are any suspicious findings from the initial history and physical examination further investigations are undertaken which include:

- X-rays: plain and contrast
- computerized tomography
- ultrasonography
- histologic examination of tumour tissue
- endoscopy
- circulating tumour marker tests.

The individual, and his significant others, will experience many emotions while undergoing and awaiting the test results. Feelings of anxiety, dread, and apprehension are commonly experienced, because the onset of cancer is insidious and may be difficult to diagnose; the treatments may be painful, unpleasant, or disfiguring, and even early diagnosis does not necessarily guarantee a cure.

If the diagnosis of cancer is confirmed, there will most likely be a range of feelings experienced. The individual, and his significant others, may experience despair and extreme anxiety about the implications of the diagnosis. Concern may be felt about the prognosis, physical disability, pain from the disease, discomfort from the treatment, death, and many other aspects. Information on helping the individual and his significant others to adjust to the illness, is provided later in the chapter.

Classifying and staging

When cancer has been diagnosed, the neoplasm must be classified and staged, before the appropriate treatment can be offered.

Classifying the tumour means identifying it according to type and tissue of origin. Table 64.3 illustrates classifica-

Table 64.2 Leading cancer sites*
(Victorian statistics 1983)

Site	Number of cases Males	Females
Lung	1237	411
Breast	16	1476
Colon	602	677
Prostate	1032	—
Melanoma	334	417
Rectum	434	308
Bladder	488	183
Stomach	346	207
Non Hodgkin's Lymphoma	238	234
Oral Cavity	240	12
Cervix	—	231
Uterus	—	277
Ovary	—	243

*Statistics obtained from Victorian Cancer Registry 1983 Statistical Report. Anti-Cancer Council of Victoria, Melbourne, Victoria April 1987.

Table 64.3 Classification of malignant neoplasm

Origin	Type of neoplasm
Glandular epithelial tissue	Adenocarcinoma
Blood vessels	Angiosarcoma
Surface epithelial tissue	Carcinoma: squamous cell, basal cell, transitional cell Melanoma
Cartilage	Chondrosarcoma
Fibrous tissue	Fibrosarcoma
Nervous tissue (glial cells)	Glioma
Smooth (involuntary) muscle	Leiomyosarcoma
Blood-forming tissues	Leukaemia
Adipose tissue	Liposarcoma
Lymphatic vessels	Lymphangiosarcoma
Lymphatic tissue	Lymphoma, lymphosarcoma
Nervous tissue (meninges)	Meningioma
Renal embryonic tissue	Nephroblastoma
Retinal embryonic tissue	Retinoblastoma
Embryonic medulla of the suprarenal gland	Neuroblastoma
Nerve sheath	Neurofibrosarcoma
Bone	Osteosarcoma
Skeletal (voluntary) muscle	Rhabdomyosarcoma
Nervous tissue (Schwann Cells)	Schwannoma

tion of malignant tumours, according to their origin.

Staging is a system used to describe the extent of the disease. Neoplasms are staged according to tumour size, nodal involvement, and metastatic progress. Various systems may be used to stage cancer. For example the TNM classification is the internationally recognized staging system, although other systems are used for some specific cancers. The stage grouping of lung cancer, using the TNM system, is illustrated in Table 64.4.

Treatment

The major medical treatments for cancer are surgery, chemotherapy, and radiation therapy. Each treatment may be used alone, or in conjunction with one or both of the other forms. Other methods include immunotherapy, and various alternative therapies such as self-hypnosis, visual imagery, relaxation techniques, and specific dietary regimes. Controversy exists over the valve of alternative therapies, but some individuals do use them to supplement conventional therapy—and have found them helpful in enhancing their physical and psychological comfort.

Surgery

Surgery may be performed for diagnostic, curative, or palliative purposes. Curative surgery is directed towards complete removal of all malignant tissue before it metastasizes. Palliative surgery is directed towards improving the individual's comfort, rather than curing the disease, e.g. some of a tumour may be removed to relieve an obstruction or pressure on adjacent tissues.

The effectiveness of surgical intervention to cure the disease depends on many factors, e.g. the site and extent of a tumour. Generally, the earlier a tumour is detected, the greater are the chances of a surgical cure. Frequently, surgical treatment is offered in conjunction with chemotherapy and/or radiotherapy.

Information on care of an individual who requires surgical intervention, is provided in Chapter 59. The nurse

Table 64.4 Staging of lung cancer using the TNM System

Stage Ia:	T1	NO	MO
	T2	NO	MO
Stage Ib:	T1	N1	MO
Stage II:	T2	N1	MO
Stage III:	T3	NON1	MO
	Any T	N2	MO
Stage IV:	Any T	Any N	M1

Note: T refers to the primary tumour, N to regional lymph node involvement, and M to the presence (M1) or absence (M0) of metastases. The numbers added to the T and N refer to the extent of involvement.

must be aware that if an individual has had surgery for cancer, he will experience additional anxieties to those experienced in relation for other surgery purposes. He may wonder if all the cancer was removed, and whether the cancer will recur. If the individual has had extensive or 'mutilating' surgery, body image and his self esteem may be severely affected.

Chemotherapy

Chemotherapy is a form of treatment whereby specific drugs (cytotoxics) are administered to destroy cancer cells, or to inhibit their function. While there are a wide variety of specific chemotherapeutic agents available, all can be classed as one of two major types:

1. Cell-cycle specific agents which destroy proliferating (dividing) cells throughout the cycle, and phase-specific agents which destroy or arrest cells during a specific phase of the cell cycle.
2. Cell-cycle nonspecific agents that destroy both proliferating and resting cells.

Table 64.5 illustrates various cytotoxic agents used in the treatment of cancers.

Cytotoxic drugs may be administered orally, intramuscularly, intravenously, or intrathecally by regional perfusion. Combinations of high doses of cytotoxic drugs may be given intermittently—to allow normal cells to recover. Because cytotoxic agents affect both normal and malignant cells, the individual may experience one or more adverse effects which include:

- immunosuppression
- infection
- anorexia
- nausea and vomiting
- diarrhoea
- alopecia
- rash
- impaired wound healing
- stomatitis
- anaemia, neutropenia, thrombocytopenia
- bleeding
- sterility
- pulmonary, cardiac, renal, or liver toxicity

Nursing care of the individual who is receiving chemotherapy is directed towards providing him with information about the treatment, offering psychological support, promoting physical comfort, assessing him for manifestations of and minimizing the adverse effects of cytotoxic agents, and preventing infection. Guidelines for developing a nursing care plan are illustrated in Table 64.6.

Because cytotoxic agents also destroy normal cells, the nurse should be aware of health care institution's guidelines regarding safe preparation and administration of

Table 64.5 Cytotoxic (Antineoplastic) agents

Class	Agent	Route
Ankylating agents (damage DNA during all phases of cell division)	Busulphan	oral
	Chlorambucil	oral
	Carmustine	intravenous
	Cyclophosphamide	oral, intravenous
	Melphalan	oral, intravenous
	Mustine	intravenous, intramuscular, intravenous, intracavity
Antimetabolites (resemble normal human metabolites and interferes with their function, thereby inhibiting or destroying tumour cells)	Fluorouracil	intravenous, intra-arterial
	Mercaptopurine	oral
	Methotrexate	oral, intramuscular, intravenous, intrathecal
	Thioguanine	oral
Vinca alakaloids (inhibit spindle formation during mitosis, thereby arresting cell division)	Vincristine	intravenous
	Vinblastine	intravenous
	Vindesine	intravenous
Antibiotics (bind with DNA, thereby inhibiting RNA synthesis)	Actinomycin D	intravenous
	Bleomycin	intravenous, intramuscular, intra-arterial
	Doxorubicin	intravenous
	Mithramycin	intravenous
	Mitomycin	intravenous, intra-arterial
Hormones (disrupt the normal hormonal environment, making it unfavourable for the tumour cells)	Cryproterone	oral
	Drostanolone	intramuscular
	Fosfestrol	oral, intravenous
	Norethisterone acetate	oral
	Polyestradiol	intramuscular
	Tamoxifen	oral
Miscellaneous agents (some act similarly to alkylating agents, others inhibit adrenal steroid production, others act by decreasing blood levels of L-asparagine)	Cis-Platinum	intravenous
	Aminoglutethimide	oral
	Colaspase	intravenous
	Dacarbazine	intravenous
	Hydroxyurea	oral
	Procarbazine	oral

cytotoxic agents. She must be aware of the precautionary measures which are implemented to deal with accidental spillage of cytotoxic agents, and disposal of used equipment and the individual's body wastes. Further information on cytotoxic agents is provided in Chapter 58.

Radiation therapy

Radiotherapy is treatment involving forms of ionizing ra-

Table 64.6 Planning the care of an individual receiving chemotherapy

Problem (actual or potential)	Plan and implementation
Altered nutrition related to nausea, vomiting, anorexia, stomatitis	Monitor intake and output Monitor weight Encourage good oral hygiene Encourage high kilojoule intake Modify diet to enhance food and fluid intake Administer prescribed anti-emetics
Altered bowel elimination	Assess frequency and consistency of stools
• diarrhoea	Test faeces for occult blood Administer prescribed anti-diarrhoeal medications Encourage fluids, but avoid fruit juices Adjust diet to help control diarrhoea Assess for the manifestations of dehydration
• constipation	Encourage high intake of fluids and dietary fibre Encourage ambulation Administer prescribed stool softeners and laxatives
Suppressed bone marrow function, leading to infection, anaemia, bleeding	Monitor vital signs every 2–4 hours Assess for manifestations and report signs of infection, anaemia, or bleeding Implement measures to prevent cross infection Avoid invasive procedures Educate the individual in ways to avoid injury—which may result in infection or bleeding
Impaired oral mucosa	Implement preventive measures: • use of a soft toothbrush and non-abrasive toothpaste • remove ill-fitting dentures • rinse mouth after meals • avoid very hot or very cold foods or fluids Assess the mucous membranes daily for ulceration, swelling, colour change, candidiasis, and discomfort Administer prescribed antiseptic or antibiotic mouth rinses or lozenges Keep mucous membranes moist and clean Administer prescribed local anaesthetic or soothing agents if necessary
Altered urinary elimination related to dysuria, cystitis, renal calculi, oliguria	Encourage copious fluids Encourage the individual to void every 2–4 hours Observe and test urine, e.g. for blood Monitor intake and output Report immediately if output decreases below 100 ml per hour, if the urine contains abnormalities, or if the individual experiences pain or burning when passing urine
Altered sensory perception related to cytotoxicity or neurotoxicity	Assess individual for signs of impaired auditory, olfactory, tactile, or visual acuity Report immediately if there are signs of sensory impairment

Table 64.6 (cont'd) Planning the care of an individual receiving chemotherapy

Problem (actual or potential)	Plan and implementation
Impaired gas exchange related to pneumonia, atelectasis, pulmonary fibrosis	Assess for manifestations of respiratory distress Observe for cough, production of sputum, haemoptysis Encourage position changes, and deep breathing and coughing techniques
Injury to tissues related to the effects of cytotoxic agents, e.g. phlebitis or tissue sclerosis from intravenous medications	Assess intravenous sites every 2–4 hours, and report signs of inflammation or extravasion
Personality changes related to fatigue, altered body image, pain, anxiety, depression	Offer psychological support Provide information about the treatment and dispel misconceptions Promote physical comfort Promote open and honest communication Assess for and report manifestations of anxiety or depression
Impaired skin integrity, e.g. rash, urticaria, erythema, skin fragility, alopecia	Encourage high standard of personal hygiene Inform the individual that hair loss is temporary Avoid damage to, and irritation of, the skin Observe for rashes and other skin reactions Administer prescribed medications to promote comfort

diation, which is delivered to destroy malignant cells. Radiation which may be delivered from an internal or external source, may be used as first-line management, in conjunction with other forms of therapy, or for palliative symptom control. In human tissue, ionizing radiation produces physical and chemical changes in cells by interfering with cellular reproduction.

Sources of radiation can be external from an X-ray machine, or internal from a solid source which is implanted into a body cavity or tissues. Internal radiation may also be delivered systemically by intravenous injection or oral ingestion of radioisotopes.

When the source of radiation is external, the area to be irradiated is determined precisely and marked. Adjacent body structures are protected by the placement of special cones and lead shieds, which are positioned in the path of the beam to absorb unwanted radiation. An individual who receives external radiotherapy is not radioactive, and does not pose any risk to those who are caring for him.

Internal radiotherapy involves the implantation of radioactive material into a body cavity or directly into the tumour. An individual who is receiving internal radiotherapy is considered radioactive, and personnel who are caring for him must implement measures which protect themselves against exposure to radiation.

Requirements for controlling radiation exposure

Adequate isolation of the individual
Separate toilet for use by the individual, who is instructed to flush it twice after each use
Warning signs clearly displayed, e.g. the international radiation symbol (Fig. 64.1)
Attending personnel to wear a film badge, which detects and monitors the amount of radiation to which they have been exposed
Careful planning of care to enable adequate nursing without exposing personnel to excessive radiation
Procedures to be carried out as quickly as possible, and as far from the radioactive source as practicable
Precautions to prevent the transfer of radioactive materials from body secretions, fluids, and excreta to others:

- Disposable items used whenever possible
- All used items disposed of into appropriate containers labelled with the international radiation symbol

Gloves to be worn to handle contaminated or potentially contaminated materials.
Lead apron to be worn if of reproductive age, to prevent damage to ova or sperm
Personnel not to attend the individual if they know or suspect they are pregnant
KNOW what to do in cases of spills or leaks of radioactive material
CHECK for dislodgement of the implant, e.g. into the bed clothes. If an implant does fall out, it is handled only with long forceps and placed in a lead container.
The radiotherapist must be notified immediately
NEVER touch the radioactive source, including those in sealed containers, with bare hands.

For specific information on guidelines for time and distance exposure, methods of collecting and isolating body secretions, the nurse should consult the health care facility's policy manual and the radiotherapy department. As the individual may experience anxiety about spending so much time on his own during internal radiotherapy, it is important to minimize his anxiety by explaining the need to avoid radiation exposure to personnel. His significant

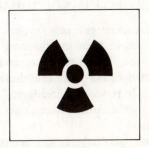

Fig. 64.1 The international radiation symbol.

others must also be informed of the reasons for precautionary measures.

Because radiation therapy destroys or damages both normal and malignant cells, the individual may experience one or more adverse effects which include:

- local skin reactions: erythema, dry desquamation with flaking, or moist desquamation with shedding of surface epithelium
- dysphagia
- fatigue
- nausea and vomiting
- bone marrow depression
- pneumonitis and pericarditis
- tissue necrosis and fistula formation may occur with long-term treatment.

Nursing care of the individual who is receiving radiotherapy is directed towards providing him with information about the treatment, offering psychological support, promoting physical comfort, assessing him for manifestations of and minimizing the adverse effects of radiotherapy, and preventing infection.

Guidelines for developing a nursing care plan are similar to those in Table 64.6. In addition to implementing measures to prevent or minimize the adverse reactions stated in Table 64.6, the individual who is receiving external radiotherapy requires care to maintain skin integrity. Integrity of the skin can be impaired by the local effects of radiation on the skin. Care involves instructing the individual in the principles of good skin care:

- Avoid vigorous rubbing with towels, wet shaving, pressure, constrictive or abrasive clothing; avoid application of any soap, perfumed talc or lotion; avoid exposure to direct sunlight.
- Keep the skin area dry—do not wash the treated area
- Avoid washing off the markings (used to define the area to be irradiated)
- Check skin area for increased erythema, dryness, burning, discomfort, or peeling. The radiotherapist is notified if any of these occur
- Institute prescribed measures used to relieve adverse skin reactions.

GENERAL CARE OF THE INDIVIDUAL

The diagnosis of cancer generally evokes emotional responses more profound than the diagnosis of any other illness. It is important for all people to understand that a diagnosis of cancer does not mean that death from the disease is inevitable. It is worth considering the significant slogan developed by the Anti-Cancer Council, 'Cancer is a word not a sentence'.

Many individuals who have cancer are treated successfully and achieve a total cure, going on to lead a normal life. For many malignancies, the individual can be offered realistic hope for long-term survival or remission. In instances where the cancer is incurable, the individual, and his significant others, requires a great deal of supportive care. Information on assisting people to deal with loss, grief, terminal illness, dying and death, is provided in Chapter 65. For the nurse to provide appropriate physical care and psychological support when a diagnosis of cancer is made, she must have a good understanding of the disease and its implications.

The care required by the individual, and his significant others, depends on many factors, e.g. whether he is in a health care facility or at home, the prognosis, the treatment, the amount of discomfort or pain he is experiencing, and his overall physical and psychological status. Care is directed towards promoting physical comfort, minimizing any adverse effects of treatment, offering psychological support, helping the individual and his significant others to develop effective coping skills, and assisting the individual to achieve optimal function and independence.

After assessing the individual and determining his needs, a care plan is developed. Factors to be considered as the plan is developed include the physical and psychological impact and implications of the disease, and the physical and psychological implications of treatment.

Promoting physical comfort

Physical comfort is promoted when the individual's needs are met. Of particular relevance for an individual with cancer are meeting the needs for pain control, nutrition, elimination, skin care, and freedom from offensive odours. The priority of needs may change, depending on the individual.

Pain control

Of all the aspects of cancer and its treatment, the factor that generally causes the most anxiety is the fear of pain, e.g. how much pain will be experienced, and whether it will be controlled. Pain associated with cancer is often the result of a tumour compressing, obstructing, or infiltrating surrounding tissue. Pain produces anxiety, and anxiety intensifies pain. Control of cancer pain *is* possible, and the goals of an effective pain control programme are to eliminate the pain or reduce it to a tolerable level, and to increase the individual's ability to cope with any residual pain.

If the pain is short-lived and self-limiting (such as pain experienced following successful surgical intervention), administration of prescribed analgesic medications and nursing measures to promote comfort are generally effective. In instances where the pain is chronic and/or unrelenting, other pain-relieving measures are necessary.

Each individual must be treated as such, as success in

managing cancer pain depends more on this than on any set formula or predetermined routine. Two forms of treatment can decrease cancer pain: one attacks the neoplasm itself, and the other disrupts the nerves transmitting the pain.

Treatments which attack the neoplasm include surgery, chemotherapy, and radiotherapy. These treatments remove the tumour, or part of it, which is causing compression or obstruction; or shrink or destroy the malignant cells. Treatments which disrupt the transmission of pain impulses include analgesic medications, transcutaneous electrical nerve stimulation (TENS), nerve blocks, and acupuncture. Other nonpharmacological approaches to pain management include relaxation techniques, visual imagery, biofeedback, and hypnosis.

Whatever treatment is prescribed for the individual, a pain control programme is developed which involves several factors:

● Breaking the pain cycle. *Pain produces anxiety, and anxiety intensifies pain*. Measures to relieve pain, e.g. analgesic medications, should be given in sufficient dosages at intervals which adequately control the pain. This way, the individual's pain cycle is disrupted so that he does not anxiously anticipate the return of pain—or actually experience pain before receiving medication
● Not withholding medication through fear of over medication or dependence. The correct dose is the amount that will free the individual from pain, or make his pain bearable. Cancer pain defies the stereotyped notions of what is a correct dose of analgesic medication. Many individuals with cancer stay alert while receiving amounts of medication, e.g. morphine, that far exceed what is considered the 'usual and safe' amounts. For example, an individual may be prescribed from 8–20 mg of morphine at four hourly intervals following surgery to remove the gallbladder. An individual with *chronic cancer pain* may require as much as 120 mg of morphine every two hours to control pain adequately. Doses as high as 600 mg have sometimes been required for pain control in terminal stages of cancer. The individual with chronic or severe cancer pain is addicted to freedom from pain—not to the psychotropic effects of the drug.
● Encouraging the individual, whenever possible, to be responsible for administering his own medications. This way, he feels that he can alleviate his own discomfort and that he has control over his pain relief.

If an individual is experiencing intractable pain, which is not controlled by conventional methods, continuous intravenous administration of a narcotic analgesic may be necessary. Continuous infusion provides better and more uniform pain control. Another method of controlling intractable pain is continuous intraspinal infusion of a narcotic analgesic, e.g. morphine. Further information on pain, and pain control, is provided in Chapter 36.

Nutrition

The individual may experience alterations in nutrition as a result of a dry or ulcerated mouth, difficulty in swallowing, decreased sense of taste or smell, anorexia, nausea and vomiting, diarrhoea, or from intestinal mucosal alterations following radiotherapy.

The individual, in consultation with a dietitian, plans a diet that will meet his nutritional requirements and include the types of foods he prefers. He is encouraged to consume foods that will supply adequate kilojoules, protein, vitamins, and dietary fibre. Frequent evaluation is necessary, and dietary modifications are made as required.

All meals and snacks should be presented attractively in an attempt to stimulate his appetite. If he prefers home-cooked foods to those available in a health care facility, every effort is made to see that these are provided. A variety of commercial food supplements are available, and these may provide an agreeable alternative if he is unable to tolerate solid foods. If he does not feel like eating at mealtimes, every effort should be made to provide him with foods he desires at times that suit him.

Anti-emetic medications may be prescribed to alleviate nausea and vomiting, thus enabling him to eat and drink more comfortably.

If the individual is unable to consume sufficient food or fluid, it may be necessary to supply nutrients and fluids via parenteral or enteral tube feeding.

Information on meeting nutritional and fluid needs is provided in Chapters 29 and 31.

Elimination

The individual may experience alterations in bowel and/or bladder elimination as a result of immobility, decreased food and fluid intake, or as a result of the effects of treatment. Nursing measures are implemented to prevent or alleviate diarrhoea, constipation, retention of urine, and urinary tract infection. Information on meeting elimination needs is provided in Chapter 30.

Skin care

The individual's skin may require extra care if he is immobile, emaciated, incontinent, or is receiving radiotherapy. Information on preventing skin discomfort during radiotherapy is provided earlier in this chapter. Care is directed towards maintaining skin integrity, and the measures which are implemented to achieve this goal include:

● keeping the skin clean and free from moisture
● protecting the skin from the excoriating effects of excreta, and wound or stomal drainage
● applying moisture-repellant creams or lotions
● assisting the individual to change his position every two to four hours

- using pressure-relieving devices, e.g. sheepskin
- avoiding prolonged pressure on bony prominences
- moving him gently and correctly to avoid skin trauma
- maintaining or improving his nutritional status
- assessing his skin every 2–4 hours for the manifestations of impaired circulation or skin breakdown.

Further information on skin care is provided in Chapters 37 and 39.

Control of offensive odours

Offensive odours may result from malignant lesions, exudate, drainage, or if the individual is incontinent. The individual will experience great anxiety if he is aware that he or his environment is causing an offensive odour. Further distress will be experienced if the individual is aware that the odour is apparent to other people. The most effective means of controlling an offensive odour is to remove the source:

- any wet or soiled clothing is changed and removed from the room immediately
- wet or soiled dressings are replaced as often as necessary. Special dressings impregnated with a substance which absorbs odours may be used
- appliances, e.g. drainage bags or colostomy bags, are checked frequently and changed as necessary
- good skin, mouth, and perineal care is provided.

The room is kept well ventilated and commercial deodorant substances may be used if necessary. Fresh flowers in the room can help to provide a pleasant perfume.

Providing psychological support

The diagnosis of cancer can be a catastrophic event for the individual and his significant others. The disease and its implications threaten the individual's sense of control over his own life, and his significant others may be greatly affected as they try to come to terms with the diagnosis.

Those concerned are likely to experience a variety of emotions including denial, anxiety, hope, depression, and despair. The feelings experienced are related to factors such as the fear of death, fear of pain, altered body image, altered role, financial concerns, effects of cancer treatments, and fear of the unknown.

The nurse can offer psychological support by demonstrating genuine concern for the individual, by providing good physical care and privacy, and by promoting an atmosphere in which open communication can take place. Communication between the individual, his significant others, and health care personnel is more likely to be effective if:

- the individual and his significant others are addressed by name

- touch is used in communication
- information is supplied and questions are answered
- the individual, and his significant others, are listened to
- his significant others are physically comfortable, e.g. provided with chairs and privacy
- health care personnel demonstrate concern and caring.

The nurse may be involved in helping the individual and his significant others to develop effective coping skills. How a person copes, or what he does about a problem, depends on many factors including:

- how he has dealt with past problems
- his perceptions of the present problem
- whether his general attitude is basically optimistic or pessimistic
- how flexible he is
- his relationships with other people
- his age, and stage of development.

A coping behaviour is ineffective when it causes more distress or pain than the disease or treatment warrants, when it stops the individual from seeking treatment or interferes with his treatment programme, or when it causes the individual to give up everyday functions and his usual sources of gratification.

People cope or behave in a certain way that has been effective for them in the past, or because it is the only way they have of coping with stress. Coping methods, which are as variable as are individuals, include:

- crying and getting depressed
- worrying
- ignoring the problem
- daydreaming or fantasizing
- taking out tensions on someone else
- drinking alcoholic beverages, taking drugs, smoking, overeating
- looking at the situation objectively
- seeking advice
- trying to maintain control over the situation
- accepting the situation as it is
- trying out different ways to solve the problem.

Some of the ways by which people can be helped to cope effectively include:

- Providing the information needed. The individual, and his significant others, should be helped to attain and maintain control by giving them information, e.g. the purpose of any treatments, and how to minimize any adverse effects. Specific questions should be answered, but the individuals should not be bombarded with non-essential information. Information may need to be repeated if it becomes evident that it has not been remembered or understood.
- Encouraging the expression of feelings and concerns. The individual, and his significant others, should be made

aware that the nurse will be available if they want to discuss their feelings. If the nurse does not feel competent to do this, she should seek support and guidance from more experienced nursing colleagues. The nurse must be able to discuss her own feelings and concerns about cancer and its implications, with someone who can provide understanding and support. Some health care facilities provide a counsellor for this purpose.

The individual with cancer may need assistance to identify problems or to break down seemingly unsolvable problems into solvable ones.

The individual and his significant others should be given time and privacy to share their feelings and concerns.

• Encouraging the individual to maintain his sense of control as long as possible. He should be able to make decisions regarding planning, implementation, and evaluation of his own care.

• Understanding that, at times, the best form of psychological support is provided by being available when the individual wants company. An individual can gain great comfort by having someone just sitting quietly with him. Words may not be necessary, and the nurse can demonstrate kindness and caring by a smile, a hand on the shoulder, or a hug. If the individual and his significant others feel comfortable in the nurse's presence, they are more likely to feel free to express their true feelings and concerns. By trying to understand how the person is feeling and being sensitive to his needs, the nurse is more able to offer appropriate psychological support.

The individual and his significant others may gain comfort and support from self-help groups. Many communities provide support groups such as a Cancer Support Service, ostomy or laryngectomy Associations. The nurse should be aware of the support groups which are available and the services they offer, so that relevant this information is supplied to those in need.

The process of *rehabilitation* begins as soon as a diagnosis of cancer is made. All care given to the individual is aimed at achieving the highest level of function and independence possible. Physical rehabilitation includes aspects such as nutritional support, occupational and physiotherapy, enterostomal therapy, and reconstructive surgery. The overall aim of rehabilitation is to improve the quality of life, by assisting the individual to retain the greatest amount of function and independence for as long as possible. If the disease progresses, rehabilitation can offer alternative ways of carrying out the activities of daily living with the help of support personnel and adaptive devices.

SUMMARY

To assist in the care of those involved when a diagnosis of cancer is made, the nurse must be familiar with the neoplastic process and its implications.

Oncogenesis is the process by which neoplasms are produced, and malignant cells develop in the same way as do normal cells. Malignant tumours have certain characteristics, e.g. they are invasive, usually grow rapidly, and frequently metastasize to other body sites.

Factors contributing to the development of cancer are oncogenic, viral, genetic immunologic environmental nutritional hormonal and psychological.

As a malignant tumour develops, it produces local and systemic effects in the individual's body.

Prevention of cancer is directed towards eliminating known carcinogens, early detection, and developing public awareness of the known risk factors and warning signals.

The incidence of cancer varies throughout the world, both by percentage of population affected and by cancer sites.

Cancer may be diagnosed through various means, including thorough physical examination and special investigative procedures. When cancer is diagnosed the neoplasm is classified and staged, so that appropriate treatment can be offered.

Treatment for cancer includes surgery, chemotherapy, and radiotherapy.

General nursing care of the individual with a diagnosis of cancer, is directed towards promoting physical comfort, offering psychological support, and rehabilitation.

REFERENCES AND FURTHER READING

Boore J R P, Champion R, Ferguson M C 1987 Nursing the physically ill adult. Churchill Livingstone, Edinburgh

Game C, Anderson R, Kidd J (eds) 1989 Medical-surgical nursing: a core text. Churchill Livingstone, Melbourne, ch 13, 123–130

Kneise C R, Ames S W 1986 Adult health nursing: a biopsychosocial approach. Addison-Wesley, Massachusetts, ch 12, 317–360

Snyder C C 1986 Oncology nursing. Little, Brown and Company, Boston

65. Loss, grief and death

OBJECTIVES

1. Describe the various stages of grieving.
2. Assist in planning and implementing care of a grieving individual.
3. Assist in planning and implementing the specific care required by an individual who is dying.
4. Perform last offices.

INTRODUCTION

Loss, grief, and dying are part of life; and every person at various times, will experience each of the three phenomena.

To assist individuals and their significant others, the nurse requires knowledge and understanding of many aspects of loss, grief, dying, death, and bereavement. Only by understanding these phenomena, and by coming to terms with her own feelings about them, can a nurse adequately assist others who are experiencing loss and grief.

Loss

Loss can be actual or perceived, temporary or permanent, and it occurs when someone or something can no longer be seen, heard, known, felt, or experienced. It is important for nurses to appreciate that loss and grief apply to events other than bereavement and dying. Loss may be of:

- a familiar environment
- a part of the self, e.g. a body part or function, or self esteem
- independence
- relationships
- financial security
- social status
- a loved person
- one's own life.

Loss of an aspect of the self can be devastating, severely affecting an individual's body image and self esteem. Loss of a body part, or loss of a physiological function, commonly results in the individual experiencing much grief over his loss. He may also experience temporary or permanent changes in body image and self esteem, as a person's self esteem is influenced by how he views his physical characteristics and abilities.

An individual who is admitted to a health care facility is separated from a familiar environment and is, therefore, experiencing a loss. If the admission is for a short time only, the effects of this loss are not likely to be great. However, if an individual is deprived of a known environment for an extended period, the effects of that loss can be severe.

Some individuals experience several losses at the one time. For example, a terminally ill person may experience loss of independence, body image, social status, financial security, plans for the future, and relationships. The same types of loss may be experienced by an aged individual who is admitted to a long-term care facility.

Reactions to loss

Reactions to loss are influenced by a variety of factors including:

- stage of growth and development
- cultural and spiritual beliefs
- socioeconomic status
- relationships with significant others.

Reactions to loss are influenced by the type of loss experienced, e.g. loss of a loved person through death usually results in deep grief. It is important to remember that individuals respond to loss in different ways, depending on its significance.

Grief is a natural response to loss. Grieving, or mourning, are normal reactions which help an individual to recover slowly from a significant loss. An individual who is faced with a serious loss, begins to grieve before the loss actually occurs. The process of grieving for a dying person before death (anticipatory grief) is a process of 'letting go'.

Acute grief is a reaction that begins at the time of a loss, e.g. loss of a person through sudden death, or loss of a limb as the result of an accident.

It is important for the nurse to realize that all individuals do not grieve in exactly the same way. However, certain patterns of grieving have been observed and documented, and the concept of stages of grieving can be useful in helping the nurse to recognize and deal with grieving persons.

Stages of grieving

The various stages of grief are the normal processes which most people experience as they face up to their loss. By recognizing the stages through which a grieving person passes, people are better able to respond appropriately to that person. It is important to recognize that every person does not necessarily experience all the stages, nor does a person necessarily experience them in any precise order. It is sometimes impossible to differentiate clearly between each of the stages as a person never moves neatly from one stage to another. Generally, a person moves back and forth between the stages of grief until final resolution occurs.

The nurse should understand that the stages of grief are not experienced only by a dying individual, but that they are also experienced by an individual who is facing other serious losses. It is important to recognize that the individual's significant others commonly experience similar feelings and reactions.

Dr Elisabeth Kubler-Ross (1970) a psychiatrist and renowned authority on the process of dying, analyzes the grieving process as five stages:

- denial and isolation
- anger
- bargaining
- depression
- acceptance.

Other researchers have proposed somewhat different stages. G.L. Engle (1964) describes the grieving process as occurring in three stages:

- shock and disbelief
- developing awareness
- reorganization and restitution.

Bowlby (1961) and Parks (1964) have described mourning as a three-phase process following acute grief:

- protest
- despair
- detachment.

Table 65.1 illustrates the various stages of grief, and the behaviours which are common to those stages.

Assisting the grieving person

Periods of grieving and mourning vary widely, and it should be remembered that while some people will return to normal life functioning within a few months, many people require longer to resolve their grief. Total absence of grief is not a healthy sign, and unresolved grief can lead to delayed or distorted reactions.

The grieving person may experience a wide range of feelings; shock, anger, sadness, guilt, depression, despair, relief, hope, acceptance. Expressions of these feelings may include; crying, wailing, withdrawal from people; lack of energy, interest, motivation; hostile behaviour, and physical symptoms such as inability to sleep, eat or concentrate, chest pain, headaches, or gastrointestinal disturbances.

The person must be allowed and encouraged to work through his grief, and to help him the nurse requires a caring, understanding, empathic approach, and an ability and willingness to listen. The grieving person really needs someone who is prepared to take a risk and get involved—

Table 65.1 Stages of grieving

Stage	Behaviours
1. Initial response: • shock and disbelief • denial • protest	This stage is accompanied by thoughts such as, 'This can't be happening—its not true'. The individual emotionally denies the loss which has occurred, or is about to occur. He commonly withdraws from social interactions, and may seek the opinion of several medical officers—hoping that the initial diagnosis was incorrect. This phase may be accompanied by physiological responses such as tachycardia, sweating, nausea, faintness.
2. Middle stage: • anger, bargaining, depression • developing awareness • despair	The individual begins to realize that the loss is real and may experience thoughts such as, 'Why me, why is this happening, why now'. He may experience anger, frustration, guilt, depression, as he begins to realize that nothing can be done to alter the situation. 'Bargaining' occurs when the individual tries to postpone reality by making a 'deal', e.g. with God.
3. Final stage: • acceptance • restitution and recovery • detachment	The individual realizes the inevitability of the situation, and accepts the loss. He is neither depressed nor angry about his fate, and is able to talk about his loss. If death is the cause of loss, the dying individual may gradually withdraw himself from people and objects.

someone who is not afraid of intensity of feeling but who will encourage the expression of it as part of healing. In caring for a grieving person the nurse needs to acknowledge the loss, facilitate the expression of thoughts and feelings, and support the person as he moves through the stages of grieving.

Facilitating the expression of feelings

Listening to an individual express feelings is possibly the most important thing a nurse can do. An individual may need to begin to resolve grief before being able to discuss his feelings, or he may be embarrassed about showing his emotions. If a person chooses not to share feelings, the nurse should make it clear that she will be available if needed.

A grieving individual may react to loss by expressing anger. The nurse should realize that expressions of anger are not really directed towards her personally—but that they are the individual's way of responding to a situation. The nurse should not engage in avoidance, but encourage the individual to express his anger. If the nurse can accept the individual's right to be angry, the person will be more able to express anger and so begin to resolve grief. The individual's significant others may be hurt and bewildered by the expression of anger, and in such a case the nurse may be able to help them by explaining that anger is one way of dealing with a stressful situation.

The nurse should always show a willingness to be with the grieving individual when he needs her. When she is with him, she should communicate her concern and understanding, and use effective listening techniques. The individual is more likely to express his feelings if he knows that the nurse is prepared and willing to listen.

Platitudes offer no support or assistance in times of grief, and they should be avoided. Almost everyone, at times, uses platitudes such as 'Don't worry', or 'I know how you feel', because they do not know what else to say. Words are not necessarily the most important aspect of effective communication, and the individual may obtain comfort if a nurse sits with him and indicates her willingness to *listen* attentively and not make judgements. Sometimes placing an arm around his shoulders or simply holding his hand enables a grieving person to express feelings. Just staying with the person and allowing him to feel and say what he needs to is often the most empathic form of communication.

At times the nurse may feel personally unable to facilitate effective communication. Caring for a grieving person can be difficult. The nurse should seek advice from more experienced nursing colleagues, who are proficient in dealing with grief. Some health care facilities provide 'grief counsellors', who assist people who are experiencing grief and the nurses who are caring for them.

Nurses and others who are uncomfortable in interacting with a grieving person often avoid discussion with him by:

- changing the subject
- silence and turning away from him
- making light of the matter
- philosophizing
- referring, e.g. 'You'll have to ask the doctor'.
- denying
- moralizing.

There are no easy answers and this chapter does not attempt to provide them for questions on how to deal with dying and death. Instead the nurse is advised to attend seminars and discussion groups, and to refer to recommended texts such as those listed at the end of the chapter.

Although the death of any person is a stressful event, the death of a child is usually accompanied by overwhelming grief. Many parents find support and comfort from self-help groups that are composed of others who have experienced a similar situation.

Death and dying

The nurse, in the course of her profession, will have contact with people who are dying and with their significant others. As the dying individual and his significant others look to the nurse for emotional support it is important that the nurse has examined her own feelings about, and attitudes towards, death. It is important that nurses develop their own philosophy on the subject of death and the process of dying.

Attitudes towards death

Values, attitudes, beliefs, and customs are the cultural aspects of an individual's life-style that influence his reaction to death and his expressions of grief. A personal philosophy about the meaning of death also influences an individual's reactions. Religion plays an important part in the lives of many people, particularly when they are facing death, while other people have no religious belief in a supreme being or an afterlife.

The nurse needs to understand and accept that there are a diversity of feelings and attitudes towards death and dying. A knowledge base of various religions and cultures will help the nurse to relate to an individual's spiritual needs. While some people view death as a natural event which holds no fears, many others experience great anxiety about dying and death. Common fears associated with dying and death include:

- fear of pain and isolation while dying
- fear of nonexistence
- fear of what happens after death
- fear of an afterlife which may not be pleasant.

A nurse needs to understand the stages through which a dying person may pass before reaching the stage of accepting impending death, and the behaviour patterns characteristic of each stage. (Refer to Table 65.1).

An individual who is facing severe loss, e.g. his own death, may ask the nurse difficult questions such as, 'Am I going to die?' Many nurses are uncomfortable with such questions and do not know how to answer them. The type of response to such a question depends on many factors:

- Has the medical officer told the individual and/or his significant others of the prognosis?
- What is the individual's stage of growth and development?
- Have the significant others requested that the individual's prognosis be withheld from him?
- Have the nurses caring for grieving persons being prepared adequately to deal with such questions?

There are no easy or standard answers.

There are several steps a nurse may take to achieve a greater depth of understanding of death and dying, e.g.

- read recommended literature particularly in relation to an individual dying in a health care setting
- discuss aspects of death and dying with experienced nursing colleagues and bereavement counsellors.

Discussing death and dying is still considered by many people to be morbid or in poor taste. However, it is only by discussing these topics that a person can come to understand and accept that death is a natural and inevitable event.

CARING FOR A DYING INDIVIDUAL

Where to die

Whenever possible, a dying individual should be cared for in the environment of his choice. His significant others must also be allowed to participate in choosing the most appropriate setting. Some people choose to remain at home, while others may feel that a hospital or hospice is better able to meet their specific needs.

Many people express the wish to die at home, and some health care services provide personnel and equipment to enable fulfillment of this wish. When an individual prefers to die at home, the nurse may be involved in assisting his significant others in providing care. She may also be required to provide counselling, and teaching services, e.g. teaching a person how to administer medications by injection. A home care programme may be provided by a palliative care service.

Palliative (hospice) care is an approach or philosophy regarding the care of terminally ill people. The term 'hospice' refers to a philosophy of palliative care, and palliative care is the type of care which is appropriate for an individual whose illness cannot be cured. The hospice movement evolved primarily from the work of Dame Cicely Saunders, who founded St. Christopher's Hospice of London in 1967.

The philosophy of hospice/palliative care recognizes that dying is a normal process, and focuses care on the relief of symptoms associated with dying—without either postponing or hastening death. The hospice movement also recognizes that the individual's significant others have a need to be involved in the care, and provides support for them as well as for the terminally ill individual. The palliative care concept involves a multi-disciplinary team approach, counselling and support, an active approach to prevent and control symptoms, involvement of volunteers in various capacities, and bereavement follow-up.

Palliative/hospice care may be provided within a 'hospice' institution, or it can be hospital based, e.g. in a palliative care unit. The trend is towards providing *community-based* palliative care or hospice programmes.

Nursing a dying individual

Care of the dying is one of the most challenging tasks nurses face. It is demanding and stressful, but it can also be very rewarding. Although a nurse cannot control the inevitability of death, there is much she can do to make the final stages of life as comfortable as possible for the individual and for his significant others.

It is important for the nurse to recognize that a dying person is also a living person who has the same needs as anyone else. As a result of the dying process, some of those needs assume a greater priority than others. The overall goal of care is the promotion of physical and emotional comfort. During the dying process the individual should be helped to retain his independence, and when this is no longer possible care should be provided in a manner which preserves self-esteem and dignity.

Promoting physical comfort

The dying process is often accompanied by discomforts and problems including breathing difficulties; and alterations in nutrition, hydration, elimination, mobility, and sensory perception. In addition, the dying person may experience acute or chronic pain.

The nursing care plan is developed after assessing the individual's needs and, while each individual may have different needs, there are some common problems and appropriate nursing interventions.

Impaired mobility. When ambulation is no longer possible, maintenance of proper body alignment is an essential comfort measure. The individual should be positioned comfortably, with bedding and pressure-relieving devices placed to enhance comfort. He should be repositioned gently and correctly every 2–4 hours to promote maximum comfort and to prevent contractures and decubitus ulcers.

Breathing difficulties. The individual may experience shortness of breath, and he may be unable to cough or expectorate to clear his airways. When possible, he should be nursed in a sitting position to facilitate breathing. When this is not possible, he should be positioned on his side to prevent aspiration of secretions. Oxygen therapy and oronasopharyngeal suctioning may be required to make breathing easier.

Inadequate nutrition and hydration. The individual may be unable to swallow and/or tolerate oral foods or fluids, or he may need assistance with eating and drinking. If he is able to eat and drink, he should be provided with foods and beverages of his choice at the times he feels like eating. Mouth care, and offering alcoholic beverages are sometimes useful measures to stimulate the appetite. Nausea and/or vomiting may be relieved by administering anti-emetic medications, and by providing chips of ice to suck or soda water to sip.

If gag or swallowing reflexes are decreased, semisolid, soft or liquid foods should be offered. If the individual cannot swallow, nasogastric feeding or intravenous therapy may be implemented to prevent or relieve thirst.

Problems of elimination. Common problems experienced include constipation, impacted faeces, retention of urine, and incontinence. The measures which should be implemented to prevent or alleviate these problems are described in Chapter 30 and include:

• laxatives to prevent constipation
• rectal suppositories to relieve constipation
• catheterization to relieve retention of urine
• external urinary drainage devices to prevent discomfort and skin breakdown from urinary incontinence
• maintenance of clean, dry bedding and an odour-free environment.

Dry mouth. Mouth care is extremely important, particularly if the individual is unable to swallow. To prevent the mouth from becoming dry and coated, it should be swabbed gently every 2–4 hours. A light film of cream should be applied to the lips to prevent or relieve discomfort.

Eye problems. Dryness and corneal irritation can occur as a result of loss of the blinking reflex. Measures to prevent or alleviate discomfort include cleansing the eyelids to remove crusts, instillation of artificial tears, and instillation of eye ointment.

Skin breakdown. If the individual is emaciated and lacks sufficient adipose tissue to 'pad' the bony prominences, or if he is unable to move, the risk of developing decubitus ulcers is increased. To prevent breakdown, the skin should be kept clean and dried and a cream or lotion applied to counteract any dryness. Pressure-relieving devices such as sheepskins should be placed under him, and his position should be changed every 2–4 hours.

Pain. Adequate analgesic medications should be prescribed and administered to alleviate or minimize pain. Information on pain relief is provided in Chapter 36.

Altered sensory perceptions. The individual may experience decreasing visual or tactile acuity. To minimize any anxiety associated with diminished sensory perception, the room should be kept bright and the individual's personal possessions should be placed where he can see or touch them. Visitors should sit close by him and, if his vision is poor, they should tell him who is there. Although the sense of touch may be diminished, the individual is generally able to feel the *pressure* of touch, therefore it is important to maintain physical contact.

Hearing is usually *not* diminished, therefore it is important to continue to speak to him in a normal manner. Even if the individual appears to be unaware of his surroundings, all personnel should assume that he is still able to hear. Some individuals gain comfort from hearing their favourite pieces of music.

If the individual is unable to speak the nurse should attempt to anticipate his needs, and people should continue to speak to him even though he cannot reply.

Confusion and restlessness. These states can be caused by physical discomforts such as pain or retention of urine, or they may be due to medication, e.g. analgesics, hypnotics, and antiemetics. The cause is first determined, then appropriate care is implemented. If no cause can be found, or if the individual remains restless and confused, a phenothiazine tranquilizer may be prescribed.

Promoting psychological comfort

The nurse can help to promote the individual's psychological comfort by:

• spending as much time as possible with him to prevent loneliness and fear of isolation
• explaining all care and treatments
• allowing him to express feelings
• listening to him
• answering his questions honestly
• providing comfort by touch, when appropriate
• respecting his wishes about extraordinary means of supporting/prolonging life
• responding to any request for a visit from a member of the clergy
• respecting his need for privacy when his significant others are present.

The nurse is often involved in assisting the dying individual's significant others. Generally, they will want to be with the dying person and will want to do what they can for him. The nurse can assist by:

• helping them to learn to interact with the dying person—if they are experiencing difficulties

- allowing them to help with simple care measures such as feeding or bathing
- providing them with privacy when they prefer to be alone with the dying person
- ensuring that they are informed of areas within a health care facility where they can rest or obtain meals and refreshments.
- allowing them to express their feelings and fears
- providing comfort by touch, when appropriate
- informing them of the individual's condition, and of his impending death
- enabling them to be with the individual at the moment of death if this is what they wish.

Promoting spiritual support

The spiritual needs of dying individuals can be defined as a search for meaning or a sense of forgiveness, hope, and love. Not all dying people experience all of these needs, or feel them with equal intensity. The nurse should be sensitive to the spiritual needs of each individual, and implement actions which may help him to meet those needs. Some people meet spiritual needs through the rituals and sacraments of organized religion. Other sources of spiritual support include reading, music, art, meditation, and imagery.

Pastoral care is a specialty within the ministry of religion which includes clinical experience, and crosses denominational and cultural barriers. Ideally, a hospital chaplain working in pastoral care and visiting clergy work together to provide spiritual care for individuals in need.

Signs of impending death

As a person approaches death, physiological changes occur which indicate impending death:

- Loss of muscle tone, which results in relaxation of the facial muscles, difficulty in swallowing, decreased peristalsis, diminished body movement, and possible incontinence of urine and faeces.
- Slowing of the circulation, which results in mottling and cyanosis of the extremities and cold skin.
- Changes in the vital signs: decreased blood pressure, weaker pulse, and changes in breathing. The ventilations may become rapid, slow, shallow, or irregular. Cheyne-Stokes breathing may occur.
- Changes in sensory perception: blurred vision, and impaired sense of taste and smell.

Signs of *imminent death* include dilated and fixed pupils, loss of reflexes, faster and weaker pulse, noisy breathing due to an accumulation of secretions in the throat, and inability to move.

It is important to remember that hearing is usually the last of the senses to fail.

Death and certification of death

Death is precipitated by failure of one or more of the three major body systems: the central nervous system, the cardiovascular system, or the respiratory system. Death may be anticipated, as in the case of a terminal illness, or it may be unexpected, e.g. as the result of a road accident. When death occurs, the time is noted and a medical officer is notified immediately. The death must be confirmed by a medical officer who issues a death certificate.

Brain death

Death may be broadly defined as 'the final cessation of body functions', but with the advent of modern technology and transplant procedures a more precise definition of death has become necessary. Determination of death must be made in accordance with accepted medical standards. There are established standards for determining brain death which is defined as 'irreversible cessation of total brain function, determined by clinical examination'. Clinical examinations are generally performed by two independent medical officers at two specified times, e.g. 24 hours apart. Certain conditions must be present before the examinations are performed, e.g. the individual's body temperature must be within normal limits, and sufficient time must have elapsed for any drugs to be excreted from the body. In most instances, before brain death can be diagnosed, the individual must meet specific conditions:

- total unreceptiveness and unresponsiveness to his environment
- absence of spontaneous movement, including breathing
- absence of reflexes
- 'flat' electroencephalogram (EEG).

These, or similar, criteria are designed to help demonstarate beyong any doubt that an individual has no cerebral activity.

Rigor mortis

Rigor mortis occurs approximately 2–4 hours after death. The condition, which is due to lack of adenosine triphosphate (ATP) required for muscle relaxation, is characterized by rigidity of the muscles. The body begins to cool at a rate of approximately 1°C per hour, and discolouration of the skin due to pooling of blood becomes apparent in dependent areas such as the back and buttocks.

Care of the bereaved

Once death has occurred, the significant others may experience shock and disbelief even if the individual's death was anticipated. Reactions to the death will vary from numbness and immobility, to outbursts of weeping or wailing. The nurse should not discourage bereaved persons from expressing their grief. If the nurse is also affected by the death and feels like crying with the bereaved, she should do so. People who have lost someone dear to them are often touched to see that the nurse who cared for that person is also grieving.

If the significant others were not present at the moment of death, they are asked if they would like to view the body. Although it is a painful and sometimes frightening experience, research has demonstrated that the bereaved are more able to accept that death has occurred if they view the body.

When a baby is stillborn or dies soon after birth, the parents should be given the opportunity to spend as much time as they want with their baby. Photographs may be taken of the baby, and the parents may gain great comfort from having some material evidence to show that their baby was real.

To make the experience more beneficial, the significant others should be informed of certain facts before they view the body. It is necessary to explain what to expect, e.g. the skin will be pale and mottled and may feel cool to touch. The bereaved should be accompanied into the room and, depending on their wishes, the nurse either remains with them or leaves them in privacy to say goodbye.

When the body has been seen, the bereaved should be shown to an area where they can sit down, and they are given the opportunity to discuss their response to the experience. Following a death the bereaved are required to carry out various functions, such as collecting the individual's belongings, informing friends and relatives, and arranging a funeral or memorial service. The nurse should inform the bereaved of the availability of support persons and groups in the community.

Care of the body

In a health care facility when death has been confirmed by a medical officer, the body is straightened and all pillows are removed except one flat one which is left under the head. The limbs are straightened and the arms should be placed at the sides of the body. All equipment, e.g. oxygen apparatus, is disconnected and removed from the bedside. The eyes are closed, and damp swabs may be required on the eyelids to keep them closed. If dentures were removed they should be replaced, and it may be necessary to place a rolled towel under the jaw to prevent it from sagging. The relatives should be consulted before any jewellery is removed from the body. Whether any jewellery, e.g. a wedding ring, was removed or left in position is documented. If a ring is left on, it should be taped in position to prevent dislodgement and subsequent loss. Blankets and quilt are removed, and the body is covered by a sheet which is drawn up over the face.

The locker and wardrobe are emptied and a list is usually compiled of the individual's possessions, which are then given to the relatives who sign to acknowledge receipt of the articles. Any items which were deposited in the safe are collected, given to the relatives, and a receipt obtained.

Last offices are performed as soon as possible after the death. This term describes the preparation of the body for removal to the mortuary. If an individual dies unexpectedly, or under suspicious circumstances, last offices may be postponed and an autopsy performed. An *autopsy* is a postmortem examination which may be performed to determine the cause of death. Special procedures must be followed in preparing the body for removal from the ward prior to autopsy. Generally any tubes, e.g. drainage or intravenous, are left in position, although this policy varies.

Each health care facility has its own protocol regarding last offices, and the nurse should refer to the policy manual for directions. The equipment required may be kept in each ward, or distributed from a central point, and it may be known by one of several names: mortuary bundle, mortuary box, or mortuary pack.

Some groups have precise teachings regarding dying and death. Death is viewed in many ways, and cultural attitudes towards death can be broadly classified as accepting, denying, or defying. Table 65.2 lists some of the rituals and beliefs associated with death and dying. Before commencing last offices the nurse must determine whether there are any special cultural or religious beliefs or practices to be performed by members of that particular group. For example, Judaism generally requires that the body be washed and prepared by members of that religion.

The bed is screened and the procedure is carried out in a quiet, respectful manner. If there are other individuals in the vicinity, the nurses should be guarded in their comments and avoid any conversation which could be distressing to others.

Table 65.2 Rituals and behaviours related to dying and death

Group	Rituals and behaviours
Roman Catholic	Sacrament of the sick Baptism for infants
Judaism	Body washed by members of the group Body not left unattended No embalming, or flowers at the funeral Mourning extends in stages over 1 year
Buddhism	Last rite chanting at the bedside
Islam	Body turned towards Mecca Body washed and prepared by family
Anglican	Last rites optional
Mormon	Baptism essential
Hindu	Body washed by family
Eastern Orthodox	Administration of holy communion is mandatory

In some facilities the body is washed and cottonwool inserted into the body orifices, but this practice is not usual. Tubes, e.g. wound drainage or intravenous, are usually removed, and waterproof strapping applied to seal any wounds. The hair is combed and arranged in the individual's usual style. A facial shave may need to be performed on a male. The body is dressed in a mortuary shroud, unless the relatives have requested that the individual's own garments be used. A tag which bears the full name of the deceased, age, sex, religion, and time and date of death, is attached to the shroud or garment. Another tag carrying the same information is attached to part of the body, e.g. the ankle. The body is then wrapped in a mortuary sheet or placed in a special plastic bag, and transferred to the mortuary on a special trolley. If the individual had an infective condition, special precautions are taken to prevent cross-infection. The nurse should refer to the facility's policy manual for information on the prescribed protocol.

In the mortuary the body is placed in a special cooling unit to slow decomposition. Many mortuaries are equipped with a viewing room, so that people may view the body if they wish. A nurse may be required to accompany a person to this area, and she should be sensitive to the fears and feelings that the person may be experiencing.

Ethical issues

There are, particularly with the advent of modern technology, certain ethical considerations and dilemmas in caring for dying individuals. This chapter does not attempt to discuss these issues, instead the reader is advised to refer to current information which is available on:

- living wills, and Right-to-Die acts
- the individual's right to know his prognosis
- resuscitation versus no-resuscitation
- euthanasia
- organ donation.

CONCLUSION

Loss, grief, and death are phenomena which will be experienced by every person. To assist individuals for whom she is caring, the nurse requires knowledge and understanding of the many aspects associated with loss, grief, dying, and death. Only by understanding and coming to terms with her own feelings about these phenomena, can a nurse respond appropriately to people who are experiencing them.

REFERENCES AND FURTHER READING

Bowlby J 1973 attachment and loss, vol II, Basic Books, New York
Engle G L 1964 grief and grieving. American Journal of Nursing 64: 93
Kübler-Ross E 1969 On death and dying. Macmillan, New York
Potter P A, Perry A G 1985 Fundamentals of nursing. C V Mosby, St Louis, ch 46, 1305–1322
Roper N, Logan W W, Tierney A 1990 The elements of nursing, 3rd edn. Churchill Livingstone, Edinburgh

Prefixes and suffixes

Complex nursing and medical terms, which are often derived from Latin or Greek, are easier to understand if they are broken down into their separate parts. Many terms consist of two or three parts: the prefix (at the beginning), the root (in the centre), and the suffix (at the end).

Prefix	Meaning
A- or Ab-	Away from, lack of, without
Abdomino-	Pertaining to the abdomen
Ad-	To; toward
Adeno-	Pertaining to a gland
Adipo-	Pertaining to fat
Alb-	White
Alg-	Pertaining to pain
Ambi-	On both sides
Angio-	Pertaining to a blood vessel
Ante-	Before in time or in place
Anti-	Against
Arterio-	Pertaining to an artery
Arth-	Pertaining to a joint
Aur-	Pertaining to the ear
Auto-	Pertaining to self
Bi- or Bin-	Two; twice; both
Bio-	Pertaining to life
Brachi-	Pertaining to the arm
Brady-	Slow
Bronch-	Pertaining to the bronchus
Bucc-	Pertaining to the inside of the cheek
Calor-	Pertaining to heat
Capit-	Pertaining to the head
Carcin-	Pertaining to cancer
Card-	Pertaining to the heart
Cat- or Cata-	Down; under; against
Caud-	Pertaining to a tail
Centre- or Centro-	Centre
Cepral-	Pertaining to the head
Cerebr-	Pertaining to the cerebrum
Cheil-	Pertaining to the lip

Prefix	Meaning
Chemo-	Pertaining to a chemical or to chemistry
Chole-	Pertaining to bile
Chondr-	Pertaining to cartilage
Chromo-	Pertaining to colour
Chron-	Pertaining to time
Circum-	Around
Cleido-	Pertaining to the clavicle
Co-	Together; with
Colo-	Pertaining to the colon
Colp-	Pertaining to the vagina
Contra-	Against
Cost-	Pertaining to a rib
Cranio-	Pertaining to the cranium or skull
Cryo-	Pertaining to cold
Crypt-	Hidden
Cut-	Pertaining to the skin
Cys- or cyst-	Pertaining to the bladder
Cyt- or cyto-	Cell, or Cytoplasm
Derma- or Dermo-	Pertaining to the skin
Di-	Two; twice, apart, away from
Diplo-	Double
Dis-	Separation or reversal
Dorsi- or Dorso-	Pertaining to the back
Dys-	Painful; disordered
Ecto-	Outside
Electro-	Pertaining to electricity
Em- or En-	In; on
Endo- or End-	Within; inward
Enter- or Entero-	Pertaining to the intestines
Epi-	On; upon
Ergo-	Pertaining to work

Prefix	Meaning
Erythro-	Red
Eu-	Well; good
Ex-	Without; away from; outside
Exo-	Outside; outward
Extra-	Beyond; in addition to; outside
Ferri- or Ferro-	Pertaining to iron
Fibro-	Pertaining to fibre
Fiss-	Pertaining to a split or cleft
Gastr- or Gastro-	Pertaining to the stomach
Ger- or Gero-	Pertaining to old age
Gloss- or Glosso-	Pertaining to the tongue
Gluco- or Glyco-	Pertaining to glucose
Gyn- or Gyne-	Pertaining to the female sex
Haem-	Pertaining to blood
Hemi-	Half
Hepat- or Hepato-	Pertaining to the liver
Hetero-	Pertaining to other, different
Hist- or Hipto-	Pertaining to tissue
Homeo-	Sameness; similarity
Homo-	The same
Hydi- or Hydro-	Pertaining to water
Hyper-	Excessive; above; beyond
Hypo-	Deficient; under; beneath
Hyster, Hystero-	Pertaining to the uterus
Iatro-	Pertaining to a physician or to treatment
Idio-	Pertaining to self, personal
Ileo-	Pertaining to the ileum
Infra-	Beneath
Inter-	Between
Intra-	Within
Iso-	Equal
Kine-	Of or pertaining to movement
Lact-, Lacto-	Of or pertaining to milk
Laparo-	Pertaining to the loin or flank or the abdominal wall
Laryng-	Pertaining to the larynx
Latero-	Pertaining to the side
Leuko-	White
Lip-, Lipo-	Fat
Lith-, Litho-	Pertaining to a stone or to a calculus
Macro-	Large; or abnormal size
Mal-	Abnormal
Mast-, Masto-	Pertaining to the breast
Mega-, Megalo-, Mego-	Great or huge
Ment-	Mind

Prefix	Meaning
Meta-	Change or exchange; after or next
Micro-	Small
Mono-	One
Multi-	Many
My-, Myo-	Pertaining to muscle
Myel-, Myelo-	Pertaining to marrow
Nas-, Naso-	Pertaining to the nose
Necro-	Pertaining to death or a corpse
Neo-	New
Neph-, Nephro-	Pertaining to the kidneys
Neur-, Neuro-	Pertaining to nerves
Odont-	Pertaining to the teeth
Olig-, Oligo-	Few; little
Oo-	Pertaining to an egg or ovum
Orchi-	Pertaining to the testes
Oro-	Pertaining to the mouth
Ortho-	Straight; normal; correct
Oso-, Osteo	Pertaining to bone
Ot-, Oto-	Pertaining to the ear
Pachy-	Thick
Pan-	All
Para-	Similar; beside
Peri-	Around
Phleb-, Phlebo-	Pertaining to a vein
Phon-, Phono-	Pertaining to sound
Phot-, Photo-	Pertaining to light
Pneuma-, Pneumo-	Pertaining to the lungs or to air
Pod-	Pertaining to the foot
Poly-	Many or much
Post-	After or behind
Pre-	Before
Prim-	First
Pro-	First, or in front of
Proct-	Pertaining to the rectum
Pseud-	False
Psych-	Pertaining to the mind
Pulmo-, Pulmon-	Pertaining to the lungs
Pyel-, Pyelo-	Pertaining to the pelvis of the kidney
Py-, Pyo-	Pertaining to pus
Quadri	Four
Ren-	Pertaining to the kidneys
Retro-	Backward; behind
Rub-	Red
Sacro-	Pertaining to the sacrum
Semi-	One half
Sens-	Perception or feeling
Seps-	Pertaining to decay

Prefix	Meaning
Soma-, Somato-	Pertaining to the body
Splen-	Pertaining to the spleen
Steno-	Contracted or narrow
Stereo-	Solid; three-dimensional
Sterno-	Pertaining to the sternum
Sub-	Under; near
Super-	Above; excess
Supra-	Above or over
Sym-, Syn-	Union or association
Tachy-	Swift or rapid
Tact-	Pertaining to touch
Tetra-	Four
Therm-, Thermo-	Pertaining to heat
Thrombo-	Pertaining to a clot
Tono-	Pertaining to tone or tension

Prefix	Meaning
Tors-	Twisted
Toxico-, toxo-	Pertaining to poison
Tracheo-	Pertaining to the trachea
Trans-	Across; through
Tri-	Three
Tricho-	Pertaining to the hair
Ultra-	Beyond
Uni-	One
Ur-, Uro-	Pertaining to urine, urinary tract, or urination
Vas-, Vaso-	Pertaining to a vessel, e.g. blood vessel
Veno-	Pertaining to a vein
Vesico-	Pertaining to the urinary bladder
Vita-	Pertaining to life

Suffix	Meaning
-aceous	Pertaining to something specified
-aemia	Pertaining to a blood condition
-algesic	Pertaining to sensitivity to pain
-algia	Pain
-an, -ian	Belonging to; characteristic of
-asis	An action, process, or result of
-asthenia	Lack of strength; weakness; debility
-biosis	Life
-blast	Embryonic state of development
-cele	Tumour or swelling
-cide	Killing
-clonia	Condition involving spasms
-coccus	Round-shaped organism
-cyte	Cell
-demic	Relating to disease in a specified region
-ectomy	Surgical removal of
-flect	To bend
-genetic	Pertaining to generation; producing
-gram	A drawing
-graph	Product of drawing or writing
-iasis	A disease produced by something specified
-iatric	Relating to medical treatment
-iform	In the form of
-ism	Condition of; practice of; theory of
-itis	Inflammation of
-lalia	Disorder of speech
-lexia	Reading
-lith	A calculus
-logy	A science; science of
-lysis	A breaking down
-lytic	Pertaining to decomposition
-malacia	Softening of tissue
-mania	Specified state of mental disorder

Suffix	Meaning
-megaly	Enlargement of a specified body part
-morphosis	A development or change
-oma	A tumour
-osis	A specified action, process, or result
-ostomy	Surgical creation of an opening
-otomy	Cutting into; a surgical incision into
-pathy	Disease
-penia	Lack of; decreased number of
-pexis or -pexy	A fixation of something specified
-phagia	Eating; swallowing
-phasia	Speech disorder
-phobia	Abnormal fear of something specified
-plasm	Cell or tissue substance
-plasty	Plastic surgery on a specified part
-plegia	Paralysis
-pnoea	Breath or breathing
-poiesis	Production of
-rrhagia	A fluid discharge of excessive quantity
-rrhaphy	A suturing in place
-rrhythmia	A condition of the heart beat
-rrhoea	Fluid discharge
-scope	An instrument for observation
-scopy	Observation
-stasis	Stoppage or inhibition
-strophy	A twisting or turning
-taxia	A condition of impaired intellectual or physical control
-thermia	A state of body temperature
-trophy	A condition of nutrition or growth
-uria	The presence of a substance in the urine
-venous	Pertaining to veins

SI units

Système International (SI) is the international system of units which is widely used in medicine, and is the current version of the metric system. The SI system has seven basic units, and *derived* units are obtained by appropriate combinations of basic units.

Quality	Name of unit	Symbol for SI unit
Length	kilometre	km
	metre	m
	centimetre	cm
	millimetre	mm
	micrometre	μm
Surface area	square metre	m^2
	square centimetre	cm^2
Mass	kilogram	kg
	gram	g
	milligram	mg
	microgram	μg
Thermodynamic temperature	kelvin	K
Temperature	degree celsius	°C
Energy	kilojoule	kJ
	joule	J
Amount of substance	mole	mol
Substance concentration	millimole	mmol
Time	day	d
	hour	h
	minute	min
	second	s
Electrical current	ampere	A
Luminous intensity	candela	cd
Volume and Capacity	litre	l
	millilitre	ml
Power	watt	w
Pressure	pascal	Pa
	kilopascal	kPa
Frequency	hertz	Hz

The following *prefixes* are used to form decimal multiples and submultiples of SI units.

Factor by which unit is multiplied	Name (prefix)	Symbol
10^{12}	tera	T
10^{9}	giga	G
10^{6}	mega	M
10^{3}	kilo	k
10^{2}	hecto	h
10^{1}	deca	da
10^{-1}	deci	d
10^{-2}	centi	c
10^{-3}	milli	m
10^{-6}	micro	n
10^{-9}	nano	n
10^{-12}	pico	p
10^{-15}	femto	f
10^{-18}	atto	a

Normal blood values

Haematologic values	Normal range	
	Conventional	SI units
Erythrocyte count	4.2–5.9 million/mm³	$4.2-5.9 \times 10^{12}$/l
Reticulocyte count	0.5–1.5% red cells	0.005–0.015
Mean corpuscular volume (MCV)	80–94 n m³	80–94 fl
Mean corpuscular haemoglobin (MCH)	27–32 pg	1.7–2.0 fmol
Leucocyte count	4300–10 800/mm³	$4.3-10.8 \times 10^9$/l
Thrombocyte count	150 000–350 000/mm³	$150-350 \times 10^9$/l
Clotting factors:		
Factor I (fibrinogen)	0.15–0.35 g/100 ml	4.0–10.0 μmol/l
Factor II (prothrombin)	60–140%	0.60–1.40 μmol/l
Factor III (thromboplastin)		
Factor IV (calcium)		
Factor V (proaccelerin, labile factor)	60–140%	0.60–1.40 μmol/l
Factor VI (not named)		
Factor VIII (SPCA)	70–130%	0.70–1.30 μmol/l
Factor VIII (antihaemophilic)	50–200%	0.50–2.0 μmol/l
Factor IX (PTC)	60–140%	0.60–1.40 μmol/l
Factor X (Stuart)	70–130%	0.70–1.30 μmol/l
Factor XI (PTA)	60–140%	0.60–1.40 μmol/l
Factor XII (Hageman)	60–140%	0.60–1.40 μmol/l
Factor XIII (Fibrin stabilizing)		
Bleeding time (Template method)	2–8 minutes	2–8 min
Prothrombin time	9.5–11.8 seconds	9.5–11.8 s
Partial thromboplastin time	25–36 seconds	25–36 s
Haematocrit—female	37–48%	0.37–0.48
—male	45–52%	0.45–0.52
Haemoglobin—female	12–16 g/100 ml	7.4–9.9 mmol/l
—male	13–18 g/100 ml	8.1–11.2 mmol/l
Haemoglobin F (fetal)	Less than 2%	<0.02
Erythrocyte sedimentation rate		
— female	1–20 mm/h	1–20 mm/h
— male	1–13 mm/h	1–13 mm/h

Blood plasma serum values

Blood plasma serum values	Normal range	
	Conventional	SI Units
Oxygen saturation (arterial)	94–100%	0.94–1.00
pH	7.35–7.45	7.35–7.45
pO_2	90–100 mmHg	90–100 mmHg*
pCO_2	35–45 mmHg	35–45 mmHg*
Carbon dioxide content	24–30 mEq/l	24–30 mmol/l
Serum calcium	8.5–10.5 mg/100 ml	2.1–2.6 mmol/l
Serum chloride	100–106 mEq/l	100–106 mmol/l
Serum magnesium	1.5–2.0 mEq/l	0.8–1.3 mmol/l
Serum potassium	3.5–5.0 mEq/l	3.5–5.0 mmol/l
Serum sodium	135–145 mEq/l	135–145 mmol/l
Creatinine	0.6–1.5 mg/100 ml	60–30μmol/l
Glucose (fasting)	70–110 mg/100ml	3.9–5.6 mmol/l
Cholesterol	120–220 mg/100 ml	3.10–5.69 mmol/l
Triglycerides	40–150 mg/100 ml	0.4–1.5 g/l
Protein (total)	6.0–8.4 g/100ml	60–84 g/l
Urea nitrogen	8–25 mg/100 ml	2.9–8.9 mmol/l
Serum glutamic-oxaloacetic transaminase (SGOT)	10–40 U/ml	0.08–0.32 nmol
Adrenocorticotropic hormone (ACTH)	15–70 pg/ml	3.3–15.4 pmol/l
Human growth hormone (HGH)	Below 5 ng/ml	<233 pmol/l
Luteinizing hormone (ICSH):		
• males	6–18 mU/ml	6–18 μ/l
• females—pre or post-ovulatory	5–22 mU/ml	5–22 μ/l
—mid-cycle peak	30–250 mU/ml	30–250 μ/l
—post menopausal	50–100 mU/ml	50–100 μ/l
Prolactin	2–15 ng/ml	0.08–6.0 nmol/l
Thyroid-stimulating hormone (TSH)	0.5–3.5 u U/ml	0.5–3.445 mU/l
Serum thyroxine (T_4)	4–12 ug/100 ml	52–154 nmol/l
T_3 Resin uptake	25–35%	0.25–0.35
Serum insulin (fasting)	6–26 uU/ml	43–187 pmol/l
Parathyroid hormone	<10ud equiv/ml	<10 ml equiv/l
Serum oestrogens:		
• premenopausal females, at stages of menstrual cycle, 1–10 days	24–68 pg/ml	
11–20 days	50–186 pg/ml	
21–30 days	73–149 pg/ml	
Plasma progesterone:		
•premenopausal females at stages of menstrual cycle		
— follicular phase	< 2 ng/ml	< 6 nmol/l
— luteal phase	2–20 ng/l	6–64 nmol/l
Testosterone (adult male)	300–1100 ng/100 ml	10.4–38.1 nmol/l
Serum bilirubin (direct)	0.4 mg/100 ml	<6.8 μmol/l

*Still used in SI system

Index